# Northfield's Surgery of the Central Nervous System

EDITED BY

## J. D. MILLER

MD, PhD, FRCS(Ed & Glas),
FACS, FRCP (Ed)

*Professor of Surgical Neurology*
*University of Edinburgh*

WITH

D. W. CHADWICK    G. F. G. FINDLAY
P. M. FOY    J. S. GARFIELD
P. R. D. HUMPHREY    R. V. JEFFREYS
B. R. KENDALL    J. B. MILES
M. D. M. SHAW

SECOND EDITION

BLACKWELL SCIENTIFIC PUBLICATIONS

EDINBURGH OXFORD LONDON

BOSTON PALO ALTO MELBOURNE

© 1987 by
Blackwell Scientific Publications
Editorial offices:
Osney Mead, Oxford, OX2 OEL
8 John Street, London, WC1N 2ES
23 Ainslie Place, Edinburgh, EH3 6AJ
52 Beacon Street, Boston Massachusetts 02108, USA
667 Lytton Avenue, Palo Alto, California 94301, USA
107 Barry Street, Carlton, Victoria 3053, Australia

First published 1973
Second edition 1987

Printed and bound in the United Kingdom by
Butler & Tanner Ltd, Frome, Somerset

DISTRIBUTORS

USA
  Year Book Medical Publishers
  35 East Wacker Drive
  Chicago, Illinois 60601

Canada
  The C. V. Mosby Company
  5240 Finch Avenue East,
  Scarborough, Ontario

Australia
  Blackwell Scientific Publications (Australia) Pty Ltd
  107 Barry Street
  Carlton, Victoria 3053

British Library
Cataloguing in Publication Data

Northfield, Douglas William Claridge
  Northfield's surgery of the central
  nervous system.—2nd ed.
  1. Nervous system—Surgery
  I. Title   II. Miller, J.D.   III. The
  surgery of the central nervous system
  617'.48   RD593

ISBN 0-632-01601-9

# Contents

# CONTENTS

# Contributors

D. W. CHADWICK DM, MRCP. Consultant Neurologist, Mersey Regional Department of Medical and Surgical Neurology, Walton Hospital, Liverpool.

G. F. G. FINDLAY BSc, MBChB, FRCS. Consultant Neurosurgeon, Mersey Regional Department of Medical and Surgical Neurology; Clinical Lecturer, University of Liverpool.

P. M. FOY MBChB, FRCS. Consultant Neurosurgeon, Mersey Regional Department of Medical and Surgical Neurology.

J. S. GARFIELD MA, MChir, FRCP, FRCS. Consultant Neurosurgeon, Wessex Neurological Centre, Southampton General Hospital; Clinical Teacher in Neurosurgery, University of Southampton.

P. R. D. HUMPHREY MA, DM, MRCP. Consultant Neurologist, Mersey Regional Department of Medical and Surgical Neurology and Wrexham Hospitals.

R. V. JEFFREYS MChir, FRCS(Ed). Consultant Neurosurgeon, Mersey Regional Health Authority and Clwyd District Health Authority; Director of Neurosurgical Studies, University of Liverpool.

B. R. KENDALL FRCP, FRCR. Consultant Neuroradiologist, Lysholm Radiological Department, The National Hospital, Queen Square, London.

J. B. MILES MBChB, FRCS. Consultant Neurosurgeon, Mersey Regional Department of Medical and Surgical Neurology; Clinical Lecturer, Associated Unit of Neurological Sciences, University of Liverpool.

J. D. MILLER MD, PhD, FRCS(Ed & Glas), FACS, FRCP(Ed). Forbes Professor of Surgical Neurology and Chairman, Department of Clinical Neurosciences, University of Edinburgh; Consultant Neurosurgeon, Western General Hospital and Royal Infirmary of Edinburgh.

M. D. M. SHAW MA, FRCS. Consultant Neurosurgeon, Mersey Regional Department of Medical and Surgical Neurology; Clinical Lecturer, Associated Unit of Neurological Sciences, University of Liverpool.

# Preface

When Douglas Northfield started his training in neurological surgery, he found no book that covered the subject. He acquired his knowledge from his mentor's teaching and from personal experience which, while excellent methods, were slow and limited in content. Since then there have been many advances in the subject and a vast increase in the literature. Northfield's aim in writing the First Edition of this book was to make available to the trainee neurosurgeon a practical textbook that would form a basis for his craft. That remains the intention of this edition.

The task of revising and producing a Second Edition after so long an interval was a daunting prospect, as in many respects, the original edition was a personal statement by Douglas Northfield of his neurosurgical philosophy, reflecting his thoughtful painstaking approach with scrupulous attention to detail and his exhaustive familiarity with the classical neurosurgical literature. There were compelling reasons for pursuing the project, no matter how difficult. In conveying his own approach to neurosurgery, Douglas Northfield exemplified the teachings of a school of neurosurgery, stemming from his close association with Cairns and Pennybacker, and drawing from the teachings of Jefferson and Dott, that has come to be seen elsewhere in the world as the British school of neurosurgery. The essence of that school was meticulous attention to clinical detail, both in obtaining the history and in conducting and recording the neurological examination and operative findings, then continuing and developing the relationship between surgeon and patient by careful follow-up, often including the programme of rehabilitation. The original exponents of this school are no longer with us, and their immediate pupils are now approaching retirement, but the philosophy continues in neurosurgical units throughout the world.

There have been a number of major changes in the neurosurgical scene since the First Edition appeared, and these have been incorporated in this Edition. The radiologists and engineers who have developed the new techniques of imaging the brain and spinal column have not only enhanced the definition of normal and abnormal craniospinal structures in a way that was undreamed of 20 years ago, but also they have been able to do so almost noninvasively, in other words without the need to puncture major arteries or the dural and arachnoid membranes that envelop the central nervous system. Advances in microelectronics and computing have enhanced and extended the use of clinical neurophysiological studies to the operating theatre and intensive care unit. Neurosurgical intensive care has become a recognizable entity in its own right, particularly in the care of the severely head-injured patient and with special emphasis on monitoring of the intracranial pressure. Administration of powerful glucocorticoid drugs has entirely transformed the management of patients with brain tumours and other focal brain lesions of a chronic nature, inducing dramatic reversal of impending coma and the signs of raised intracranial pressure and brain herniation and making all forms of operative management, from burr hole biopsy to complete surgical extirpation, very much safer. Neuropathology and neuroanaesthesia have both witnessed parallel and equally significant advances, and in neurology, now beginning to benefit from the contributions of molecular biology to clinical medicine, there have been major reclassifications of cerebrovascular disease and epilepsy and exciting advances in drug therapy. Neurosurgical approaches to the management of intractable pain, epilepsy and movement disorders have changed over the past 15 years. The adoption of microsurgical techniques in virtually every neurosurgical centre in the world has extended the range of surgically treatable craniospinal lesions.

There is in this book a bias towards clinical neurosurgery, a deliberate emphasis on neurology and physiology. There is a risk that these absorbingly interesting subjects may be subordinated to the ingenious and highly successful procedures now available for local diagnosis. Sound judgement in choosing the best treatment depends upon a high level of clinical acumen, for the best treatment is that which is best for the patient, not necessarily what is 'best' for the tumour or aneurysm. Furthermore, careful attention to the clinical manifestations and the course of the illness will reveal problems suitable for research or enquiry; an important part of training is to seize upon such a problem, however humble, and devote to it constructive thought.

This book provides information on most aspects of surgery of the central nervous system with the exception of surgical techniques. To include these techniques would have made the book unwieldly, and in any case the trainee learns his craft by assisting at operations. At this stage in his education, apprenticeship is the best method of acquiring surgical skill. Illustrations of techniques often appear to make procedures seem easy which can be dangerous for the inexperienced surgeon.

The text is deliberately extensively referenced. Guidance in the choice of reading is an important part of postgraduate tuition. Northfield's original selection of references has been reviewed, and where appropriate, new and replacement papers have been added.

I hope that, despite the inclusion of so much new material, necessary because of the very many neurosurgical and neuroscience developments of the past decade, sufficient of the clinical essence of the original edition of Northfield's *Surgery of the Central Nervous System* remains as a lasting testimony to the neurosurgical teachings of those British pioneers who gave so much to the world of surgical neurology.

J. Douglas Miller
Edinburgh
1986

# Chapter 1
# Introduction:
# A syllabus of surgical neurology

J. D. MILLER

The specialty of neurological surgery, or to use Wilfred Trotter's term, surgical neurology, has not long celebrated its golden anniversary, but during its short life a breathtaking series of technical and biomedical diagnostic and therapeutic advances have quite transformed the working life of the neurosurgeon and improved the prospects for the neurosurgical patient in a way that could hardly have been guessed at even 25 years ago.

For the neurosurgical trainee and the trained neurosurgeon alike it is hard even to keep abreast of those major advances in the neurosciences and in medical technology that soon impinge on clinical practice. The volume of neuroscience-based literature is now enormous and the trainee embarking upon a neurosurgical career may wonder where to begin. This text is strictly a clinical handbook intended to serve as a guide to the neurosurgeon in training, providing background to the clinical experience that is being gained from patients and their neurosurgical problems, and encouraging comparisons between personal experience (an invaluable, but slow learning process) and the greater experience of others as recounted in the neurosurgical literature. As a learning experience, the value of regular attendance at brain cutting, biopsy and autopsy sessions cannot be overemphasized, ensuring that the pathological findings from each patient have been personally reviewed with, and not simply left to, the neuropathologist. Witnessing and assisting in medical and neurological consultations, neuroradiological procedures, ophthalmology and otology consultations and preparation of clinical cases for presentation and review at clinical meetings, both small and large, are all essential parts of the training of the critical neurosurgeon.

Since the 1960s there has been an explosive growth in the neurosciences, in which neurosurgeons have been privileged to play an important role. Clinical knowledge must be based and built on understanding of the basic neurosciences and at least the principles of the major technical advances that have so changed and become part of daily clinical practice. There is a need, therefore, for the assembly of a personal syllabus of surgical neurology, so that the accumulating clinical experience can be built upon a sound understanding of the structure and function of the nervous system affected by the disorder being studied. The detailed contents of such a syllabus are far beyond the scope of this book. In any case, the person who expects to find all the necessary information within a single volume or series of volumes has already failed to grasp the fundamental point that for many of the questions in the neurosciences there are not yet final answers, but only a preponderance of evidence for a particular hypothesis, and full understanding can come only from considering more than one line of evidence. Furthermore, the very act of developing a personal neurosurgical syllabus is a learning process itself, as is consulting multiple sources on a particular topic. In addition, the enquiring neurosurgeon will soon find particular interests that demand additional research before a satisfying level of knowledge is attained. Common to these needs and the need for a revision syllabus in preparation for specialist examinations, however, are a number of topic headings that can be used as a check list.

## Neuroanatomy

Clearly, topographical and surface anatomy is fundamental knowledge for any surgeon. The neurosurgical need for this knowledge is dictated by the different surgical techniques that have been developed as a result of the advent of the microsurgical approach to so many neurosurgical operations on the brain and spinal cord. This has brought a new perspective to the surface anatomy of the brain and spinal cord, demanding understanding of the fine arachnoid compartments that surround the major arteries at the base of the brain so that dissection to reach an aneurysm arising from one of these vessels can be cleanly, precisely and delicately accomplished. The more aggressive surgical approaches to tumours lying within the substance of the brain demand that the surgeon appreciate the disposition of the white matter tracts within the cerebral hemisphere. The development of the transphenoidal, transoral and translabyrinthine microsurgical approaches to tumours in the sella turcica, clivus and cerebellopontine angle respectively means that the neurosurgeon must include the fine structure of the skull base in the anatomical syllabus. The practice of stereotactic surgery, now guided by computer-assisted tomography, has meant that there are no longer any areas of the brain 'forbidden' to the neurosurgeon, but the close packing of the crucial elements in many of the parts of the brain explored by the stereotactic surgeon means that anatomical knowledge of these structures must be both detailed and precise, with information on the range of variation to be expected in normal and diseased subjects.

To provide the necessary perspective on neuroanatomy required by the neurosurgeon it is important, many would say essential, to go to the laboratory and examine and dissect human brain specimens under an operating or dissecting microscope, comparing this with the naked eye appearances of the brain surface, the vessels at the base and within the Sylvian fissures, the choroidal fissure and the ventricles. The major white matter tracts should be dissected and the surgeon should be familiar with the anatomical structures revealed on the standard coronal, saggital and transaxial sections used by the neuropathologist, in computer-assisted tomography and in magnetic resonance imaging.

Included with neuroanatomy is the embryology of the nervous system, knowledge of which is fundamental to the understanding and management of spinal dysraphic states, craniofacial anomalies and certain disorders of the cerebral vasculature and the cerebrospinal fluid system.

**Topic list for neuroanatomy**

*Topographical relationships and structure of:*

  skull vault and base
  covering membranes
  cerebrum
  cerebellum
  brain stem
  cranial nerves
  vertebral column
  spinal cord
  cauda equina
  cerebrovascular system
  spinal vascular system
  somatic sensorimotor system
  extrapyramidal system
  limbic system
  visual system
  auditory system
  hypothalamopituitary axis

*Embryology of:*

  cranial, facial and spinal skeleton
  ventricular system and subarachnoid space
  cerebral arteries and veins
  sensorimotor systems
  brain stem structures

## Physiology, neurochemistry and pharmacology

Some neurosurgical patients are critically ill in the systemic sense. Examples are patients with multiple injuries that include head injury, deeply comatose patients who suffer systemic complications of the damaged brain such as gastrointestinal haemorrhage or neurogenic pulmonary oedema, infected patients who develop septic shock or patients with complex endocrine disorders. The neurosurgeon will not spend very long in clinical practice before encountering these problems and realizing that the modern intensive management of the critically ill patient in an intensive care unit demands sound knowledge of the general physiological principles governing control of respiration, oxygenation and acid base balance, cardiovascular sufficiency, fluid and electrolyte balance and nutrition.

Knowledge of cerebrovascular physiology, brain energy metabolism and the factors that determine the intracranial pressure and produce cerebral ischaemia, brain shifts and distortion and cerebral oedema is so central to understanding the majority of neurosurgical problems that these topics are discussed in some detail in this book.

Definition of central neurotransmitter, noradrenergic, dopaminergic, serotonergic and other peptidergic pathways using immunofluorescent staining techniques has widened enormously our understanding of the way that data may be processed in the nervous system and visceral processes controlled.

Recognition of the importance of the arachidonic acid cascade with production of eicosanoids, free radical compounds and other agents that can damage cell membranes has been applied to the understanding of mechanisms of production of brain damage, and in turn treatment regimens have been developed from this knowledge.

Discovery of sites within the brain specifically structured to bind with the exogenous drug morphine sulphate, followed by the discovery of endogenous peptides in the brain with morphine-like activity, have added an entire dimension to our understanding of the mechanisms of pain and of the measures required to control it in patients. The discovery that peptide molecules found originally in the gut, such as cholecystokinin, are also found in the brain in even greater quantities, has immense significance for our understanding of brain function since several of these neuropeptides satisfy many of the criteria of neurotransmitters.

Amino acid sequencing and recombinant DNA technology have led to the identification, delineation and synthesis of a number of hormone releasing factors active in the hypothalamus and the hypothalamopituitary axis. The precise molecular genetic defects responsible for a large number of specific, though mostly rare, neurological disorders have now been identified, so that the age of molecular clinical neurobiology can truly be said to have arrived.

Clinical neurophysiology has taken on a new importance in neurosurgery with the developments in electronics and computing that now make it possible to obtain artefact-free recordings of the electroencephalogram and evoked potentials in the electrically hostile environments of the intensive care unit or operating theatre. Condensed formats of the EEG make it possible to record the EEG continuously for long periods of time, and the surgeon can now expect to obtain visual, auditory and somatosensory evoked potentials in the operating theatre, yielding valuable information about the integrity of the appropriate pathways through the nervous system.

There are, however, numerous potential pitfalls in the recording of electrical activity in the nervous system, and the neurosurgeon must be aware of the limitations as well as the indications for neuroelectrical testing, the effects of drugs, changes in the physical environment. Understanding of the basics of these complex and demanding studies will enhance enormously the value of the interchange that can take place between the neurosurgeon and the clinical neurophysiologist.

**Topic list for physiology**

*General metabolism*

fluid and electrolyte balance
acid base balance
consequences of shock
disorders of pulmonary function
principles of general and local anaesthesia
use of relaxants and artificial ventilation
nutrition in the comatose patient

*Cerebral haemodynamics and metabolism*

energy metabolism in the brain
control of cerebral blood flow
cerebral ischaemia and hypoxia
cerebrospinal fluid and hydrocephalus
intracranial pressure
blood–brain barrier and cerebral oedema
drugs used in neurosurgery
eicosanoids and neuropeptides

*Neurophysiology*

properties of receptors
classification and properties of peripheral
    nerve fibres
contraction of smooth and striated muscle
neuromuscular junction and relaxants
functions of neurotransmitters and
    neuropeptides
excitatory and inhibitory postsynaptic
    potentials
autonomic nervous system
reticular activating system
sleep, arousal and coma
spinal pathways
brain stem nuclei and cranial nerve function
cerebellar function
control of posture and vestibular function
regulation of tone
motor and premotor cortex
pyramidal pathways
extrapyramidal pathways
reflex arcs
cortical sensory and association area

somatic sensation
pain perception and pathways
olfaction
vision and eye movement
audition, language and comprehension
memory and the temporal lobes
neuroendocrine hypothalamo-pituitary
    functions
emotion and the limbic system

# Neuropathology

The practice of neurosurgery must go hand in hand with that of neuropathology. It is not only the revelations of the brain biopsy or the autopsy that shed so much light on neurosurgery, but it is through the neuropathologist that most neurosurgeons are likely to encounter for the first time the applications of the newer techniques in neuroscience research, such as ultrastructural and immunohistochemical methods using specific markers derived from monoclonal antibodies and recombinant DNA technology.

**Topic list for neuropathology**

cytopathology of neurons and glia
tumours of the central and peripheral nervous
    systems
congenital malformations of the nervous system
cerebral and spinal vascular disorders
brain and spinal cord trauma
brain shifts and herniation
degenerative diseases
demyelinating diseases
bone disease in the skull and vertebral column
brain abscess, subdural empyema and epidural
    abscess
meningitis and encephalitis of bacterial and
    viral origin
toxic and deficiency disorders of the brain and
    spinal cord
immunopathological disorders
techniques of biopsy and tissue preparation

## Bacteriology, virology and parasitology

Infective disorders of the nervous system are of paramount importance because they are often preventable and almost always treatable yet they continue to exact a fearful toll in terms of both mortality and morbidity. Meningitis following head injury is still frequently fatal. Dangerous opportunist infections can arise in the neurosurgical intensive care unit and antibiotics must be used with economy, understanding and care. The neurosurgeon's knowledge of virology must now include the agents responsible for slow virus infections, hepatitis and the acquired immune deficiency syndrome. With the widespread use of long distance air travel, even tropical parasitic infections and infestations are being encountered in the temperate countries, so that an understanding of the patterns of neurological disorders seen in other countries in the world is as important for the neurosurgeon who practices in a single country as for the neurosurgical traveller.

## Medical physics

It is now quite impossible for the neurosurgeon to complete a day's work without being confronted by the products of modern technology. A working knowledge of the electronics involved in recording arterial and intracranial pressure and brain electrical activity, the optics of the operating microscope, surgical lasers, radioisotopes used in brain scanning, the principles of computerized tomography and nuclear magnetic resonance imaging, will all greatly enhance understanding of the ways in which these techniques can help in the diagnosis and treatment of neurosurgical disorders and of their inherent limitations.

## The neurological examination

Despite the wide range of advances in methods available for diagnosis of nervous system disorders, the clinical mainstay of the neurosurgeon will continue to be the neurological examination carried out at the bedside or in the clinic, and repeated to demonstrate improvement or deterioration and the rate of that change in status. With the least possible delay, the neurosurgeon in training must develop and practise a comprehensive, thorough, yet fairly rapid technique for evaluating the function of the nervous system. This can be perfected only by carrying out a very large number of such examinations at a relatively early stage in training; no amount of observation obtained at a later stage can quite substitute for this experience. The smooth and orderly progress of a competent neurological examination instils confidence in the patient and minimizes the risk of making inappropriate diagnostic and therapeutic decisions, while the stuttering, erratic performance of an inexpert and inadequate examination declares incompetence to patient and observer alike.

While the detailed history of events is an integral and crucial part of the clinical evaluation of very many patients with neurological disorders, one of the major clinical strengths of the neurosurgeon should be the examination of the comatose patient, who by definition is unable to cooperate in the examination process. The underlying principle of this examination is graded stimulus and measured response, from which the functional integrity of the neuroanatomical pathway under test is inferred.

The Glasgow Coma Scale, described in more detail in Chapter 23, is a formalized means of assessing arousal, as tested by eye opening, and responsiveness, as tested by the motor and verbal reactions to graded stimuli (verbal command, then pain if that first stimulus is unsuccessful). The aim is to establish the highest level of function of which the nervous system is capable at that time, whether it is being adversely affected by a general disorder, such as hypoxia, sepsis or global ischaemia, or by a more localized lesion, such as tumour or an infarct. In practice, even localized brain lesions often have additional general effects, such as raised intracranial pressure, and it is of paramount importance to be able to make a rapid and reliable assessment of the level of response and the degree of clinical urgency, no matter the nature of the brain or spinal cord lesion.

Assessment of the level of consciousness in the comatose patient must always be accompanied by measurement of several brain stem reflexes: the pupillary response to light, the eye movement reflexes (oculocephalic and oculovestibular), the corneal reflex, and the lower level reflexes, cough, gag, and the oculocardiac reflex (slowing of the heart in response to pressure on the closed eye).

In conducting the neurological examination in cases of focal lesions in the nervous system, an orderly approach should be used toward the localization in the brain or spinal cord. This is of importance in selecting the appropriate investigation, although it must be admitted that the advent of computerized tomography, in which the entire brain is scanned, makes this a less crucial matter than previously; for example, the erroneous choice of air encephalography as the first investigation in a patient with a large frontal brain tumour could have fatal consequences. The first priority is to establish the level of the lesion in rostrocaudal terms (supratentorial, infratentorial, spinal cord or cauda equina). The laterality of the lesion must next be established. It should be noted that dysphasia, homonymous visual field defects and focal epilepsy all indicate supratentorial lesions, and that the neurological signs arising from supratentorial lesions are always contralateral to the lesion. Infratentorial (cerebellar or cranial nerve) lesions always produce ipsilateral signs of dysfunction. An attempt should be made to deduce the cause of the neurological dysfunction: vascular, neoplastic, traumatic, infective, congenital or degenerative. The location and extent of the lesion may suggest an arterial territory of distribution. Finally, the neurosurgeon must try to assess the rate of progress of the disorder, so as to determine the urgency of definitive investigation and therapy. Appreciation of the pace of neurological deterioration is pivotal to the clinical skills of the neurosurgeon.

In reviewing the results of his or her own work, and especially in comparing it with the results of others, the neurosurgeon must understand the basic principles of analysis of data, and assessment of outcome, so that a critical appraisal can be made of reports in the literature. Of particular importance is the classification and description of patients so that like can be compared with like; this in turn depends upon knowledge of the influence of particular variables upon outcome, for example age or level of consciousness. Many newer operative and nonoperative neurosurgical treatments are costly and may involve added risk to the patient, so that any reported data must be evaluated with due care and an understanding of fundamental epidemiological and biostatistical principles.

## Some suggestions for further reading

ADAMS J.H., CORSELLIS J.A.N. & DUCHEN L.W. (1984) *Greenfield's Neuropathology* 4th edition. Edward Arnold, London.
BAIN W.H. & TAYLOR K.M. (1983) *Handbook of Intensive Care.* John Wright & Sons, Bristol.
BRODAL A. (1981) *Neurological Anatomy in Relation to Clinical Medicine* 3rd edition. Oxford University Press.
CROCKARD A., HAYWARD R. & HOFF J.T. (1985) *Neurosurgery: The Scientific Basis of Clinical Practice.* Blackwell Scientific Publications, Oxford.
GORE S.M. & ALTMAN D.G. (1982) *Statistics in Practice.* BMA Publications, London.
HEIMER L. (1983) *The Human Brain and Spinal Cord.* Springer-Verlag, Berlin.
HUBEL D.H. *et al.* (1979) The Brain. *Scientific American,* **241,** 44–232.
JOHNSON R.T. (1982) *Viral Infections of the Nervous System.* Raven Press, New York.
LOU H.C. (1982) *Developmental Neurology.* Raven Press, New York.
PLUM F. & POSNER J.B. (1980) *The Diagnosis of Stupor and Coma* 3rd edition. F.A. Davis, Philadelphia.
ROSE G. & BARKER D.J.P. (1986) *Epidemiology for the Unitiated* 2nd edition. BMA Publications, London.
RUSSELL D.S. & RUBINSTEIN L.J. (1977) *Pathology of Tumours of the Nervous System* 4th edition. Edward Arnold, London.
SIEGEL G.J., ALBERS R.W., AGRANOFF B.W. & KATZMAN R. (1981) *Basic Neurochemistry* 3rd edition. Little, Brown & Co., Boston.
WELLER R.D. (1984) *Colour atlas of Neuropathology.* Harvey Miller, Oxford University Press.
WOOD J.H. (1980) *Neurobiology of Cerebrospinal Fluid.* Plenum Press, New York.

# Chapter 2
# Normal and increased intracranial pressure

J. D. MILLER

## Introduction

Intracranial pressure is the term applied to the pressure of the cerebrospinal fluid (CSF) within the cranium but it is most frequently measured by introducing a hollow needle into the subarachnoid space in the lower lumbar region. In a relaxed person with normal intracranial conditions lying in the lateral position, so that the midline of the head is in the same horizontal plane as that of the lumbar region, the pressure measured from the subarachnoid space will be the same as that recorded from a catheter inserted into the cranial subarachnoid space or the lateral ventricle. The pressure measurement can be expressed in $mmH_2O$ (more strictly mm of CSF), in mmHg or in SI units as kilopascals (kPa). To convert the units, 10 mmHg is equivalent to $136 mmH_2O$ and 1 kPa is equal to 7.5 mmHg. In the presence of any abnormality within the cranium or spinal canal which interferes with the free passage of fluid from one part of the craniospinal axis to another, the pressure in the lumbar CSF may not be a true indication of the intracranial pressure (ICP). When some form of obstructing lesion is present the true ICP is measured from the rostral part of the craniospinal axis, usually the lateral ventricle or supratentorial cerebral subarachnoid space.

A moderate range of pressures can be recorded from recumbent healthy persons; in the adult the range 0–15 mmHg (0–2 kPa) can be regarded as normal (Lundberg 1960). In babies and infants however the upper level of normal ICP is lower at 5 mmHg (Welch 1980).

The recording of ICP shows two forms of pressure fluctuation. There is a rise with each cardiac systole and a slower change in pressure, falling

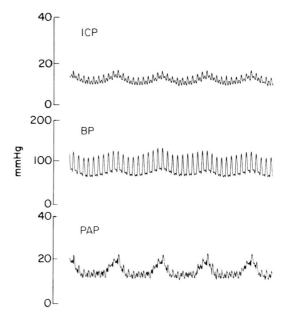

**Fig. 2.1.** Chart recording of intracranial pressure (ICP) arterial blood pressure (BP) and pulmonary artery pressure (PAP) showing the normal arterial pulse and slower respiratory oscillations in all three pressure recordings.

with each inspiration and rising with expiration (Bradley 1970, O'Connell 1943, 1970). The cardiac fluctuation is due to the distention of the intracranial arterial tree which follows systole, the respiratory fluctuation is due to changes in venous distention secondary to pressure changes within the thoracic cage (Fig. 2.1). Coughing, straining, compression of neck veins can also cause sudden and considerable rises in pressure. These simple observations emphasize that ICP is not a static state, but one that is influenced by several factors. A clear understanding of these is essential before considering the causes of pathologically raised ICP, its effects and how it may be relieved. Success in neurosurgery depends upon this knowledge; the high mortality which characterized early endeavours of surgeons to operate on brain tumours was largely the result of ignorance of this basic knowledge.

For several decades after the pioneering studies of Cushing and his predecessors on raised intracranial pressure (Cushing 1902, 1903), there was reluctance to believe that raised ICP was common in severely head injured patients and others with critical neurosurgical conditions. This was because the recorded CSF pressure from the lumbar subarachnoid space was low in many such cases (Browder & Meyers 1936). Despite the studies of Smyth and Henderson (1938), showing differences between the CSF pressure in the lumbar theca and lateral ventricle in patients with brain tumour, it was only with the systematic clinical studies of intraventricular pressure of Guillaume and Janny (1951) and Lundberg (1960), coupled with the detailed experimental study of Langfitt et al. (1964, Weinstein et al. 1968) that the development of craniospinal pressure gradients was clarified. This resulted in acceptance of the view that raised supratentorial ICP was extremely common and that in many such cases a gradient developed across the tentorial hiatus so that lumbar subarachnoid CSF pressure remained much lower, even normal in some cases.

The brain, the CSF and the blood are encased by the cranium except at the foramen magnum where there is communication with the spinal canal and its contents. In addition the tentorium and falx cerebri impose a semi rigid internal compartment formation and there is additional minor communication via the various outlet foramina from the skull for the passage of nerves and blood vessels. CSF can be displaced through the foramen magnum into the spinal theca; the spinal dural sheath can accept a quantity of CSF as it does not fit the spinal canal closely, being surrounded by a layer of loose areolar fatty tissue and the plexus of epidural veins which communicate freely with extra spinal veins. Blood from these can be expelled into the extra spinal venous system to accommodate thecal disten-

tion. In states of raised ICP there may also be an increase in passage of blood through venous emissaries. This has been ascribed to obstruction to venous outflow from the brain by Noell and Schneider (1948) and is sometimes a striking feature in infantile hydrocephalus when distended scalp veins are clearly visible, subsiding immediately upon satisfactory reduction of ICP consequent upon a CSF shunting procedure. The conception of the cranium acting as a near rigid container of virtually incompressible substances in the form of brain, blood and CSF is known as the Monro–Kellie doctrine. As stated in its original form, by Alexander Monro in Edinburgh in 1783, and corroborated by the pathologist, George Kellie in 1825, the doctrine failed to take account of the presence of CSF within the craniospinal axis. It was left to Sir George Burrows (1846) to add this factor, an essential part of the doctrine as it is understood today. Detailed explanations of the concept of interchangable fluid volumes in the process of accommodating intracranial mass lesions and expansions of one compartment at the expense of the other have been provided by Flexner et al. (1932) and by Langfitt (1969).

Intracranial pressure is therefore, a function of at least two factors: the CSF, which is constantly being secreted and, after circulating through a tortuous pathway, absorbed at an equal rate; and the intracranial circulation of blood. CSF circulation is slow, 0.35–0.50 ml/min (Davson 1967, Welch 1975) or 500–700 ml/24 hours, while cerebral blood flow is copious, 50 ml/100 g brain/min, equivalent to 700 ml/min or 1000 L/day. This blood is delivered to the intracranial cavity at a pressure of 100 mmHg. Resistance to flow is provided mainly by arterioles so that the pressure head falls from 100 mmHg to 30 mmHg at the entrance to the capillary bed, emerging at a pressure of around 12 mmHg and falling slowly thereafter, in the cerebral venous system. Any obstruction to venous outflow will entail an increase in the volume of intracranial blood and a rise in ICP. Under most conditions there is a close link between the level of ICP and the cerebral venous pressure; as ICP is increased the cerebral venous pressure increases in parallel so as to remain 2–5 mm higher. Were this not the case and ICP exceeded the cerebral venous pressure, the venous system would collapse (Miller *et al.* 1972, Johnston & Rowan 1974). Because of this relationship, the cerebral perfusion pressure, which should strictly speaking be derived from the difference between arterial and venous pressure within the cranium, can be satisfactorily estimated from the difference between arterial and intracranial pressure. Using the difference between arterial and jugular venous pressure as an estimate of cerebral perfusion pressure is invalid because this venous pressure is unaffected by ICP, needing only to remain above atmospheric pressure to remain patent, and the intervening rigid, dural venous sinuses separate the jugular system from the true thin-walled cerebral veins. As will be seen, the cerebral perfusion pressure is only one of several factors which govern the regulation of blood flow to the brain in response to changes in its function and to physiological and pathological stresses and challenges.

## Increased intracranial pressure

The genesis and effects of increases in ICP have been studied in two ways: first, by experiments in animals in which the ICP has been artificially increased by injection of artificial CSF into the subarachnoid space, by distention of a small balloon placed within the cranial cavity, by creation of focal cerebral oedema, contusion or other forms of lesion; secondly, by observing in man, at the bedside, changes in ICP, in blood pressure, and in other variables and associating these with alterations in the level of consciousness and presence of abnormal neurological signs. The experimental approach provides the opportunity to study under controlled conditions the full range of changes from normal ICP to severe intracranial hypertension leading to death. It has the disadvantage however, of generating the increased pressure from an outside source, so that these models study mainly the consequences

of raised ICP rather than its genesis. In the CSF infusion model, fluid is infused continuously at a series of predetermined rates. When a limited quantity of saline is injected into the subarachnoid space, the ICP is only transiently elevated because CSF will soon be absorbed and the pressure returns to normal. If the infusion is very rapid, for example 0.3 ml/sec in the cat, 2 ml/sec in man, then the rise in pressure is a measure of the elastic properties of the brain and other contents of the craniospinal axis and the return of pressure to normal is a function of both the CSF outflow resistance and of the elastic properties of the brain as the tissue yields to stress (Miller 1975). Marmarou *et al.* (1975) have calculated a pressure volume index from the rise in ICP generated by a bolus injection of saline into the CSF space. This index is expressed in terms of the extrapolated volume of CSF that would have been required to produce a ten fold increase in CSF pressure. This extrapolation is possible because the relationship between added CSF volume and CSF pressure is logarithmic and therefore predictable. The normal range in adult man is 25–30 ml. Marmarou has also developed an equation for calculation of CSF outflow resistance from the rate of decay of the CSF pressure after a bolus injection of saline into the CSF space. While this estimate of CSF outflow resistance (2–12 mmHg/ml/min) is subject to some error under normal conditions, there is experimental evidence that under conditions of raised intracranial pressure, such as may be encountered clinically, it is possible to estimate the CSF outflow resistance accurately (Sullivan *et al.* 1979, Takizawa *et al.* 1985).

When saline is injected more slowly in a continuous mode, the ICP rises to a plateau level at which the increased level of CSF absorption keeps pace with the infusion rate of CSF and a new equilibrium is set. This has been used as the basis for a CSF infusion test by Katzman and Hussey (1970), and refined by Børgeson *et al.* (1978) to obtain measurements in humans of conductance to CSF outflow.

The intermittent expansion of an intracranial balloon causes only a transient rise in ICP at

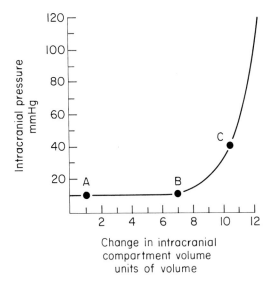

Fig. 2.2. Three stages in brain compression. At A compression has just started, intracranial pressure (ICP) does not increase because of spatial compensation. At point B, ICP is still normal but spatial compensation has become exhausted, and a smaller increase in volume to point C is accompanied by a marked rise in ICP.

first; when sufficient CSF has been absorbed to accommodate the volume of the balloon the ICP returns to normal. Expansion of the balloon to a critical volume does, however, eventually cause persistent intracranial hypertension which thereafter increases logarithmically with increasing balloon volume (Fig. 2.2). The ICP finally rises to the level of the arterial pressure, which itself begins to increase, accompanied by bradycardia or other disturbances of heart rhythm in accordance with the vasopressor response described by Cushing (1902, 1903). The concept of stages of spatial compensation, followed by intracranial hypertension, then progressive decompensation, has been recognized for over 100 years. Cushing was directed to his researches on intracranial hypertension by Kocher (1901) who, along with Von Bergmann (1880) and Duret (1878) clearly appreciated the significance of expanding intracranial mass lesions.

Key experimental observations were made by Wolff and Forbes (1928), by Wolff and Blumgart (1929) and by Fog (1933). The pial vessels of

the brain were observed through glass windows inserted in the skull during elevation of intracranial pressure; dilation of small pial arteries was observed, accompanied by some slowing of the flow of blood in the veins followed by improved and pulsatile venous flow. Noell and Schneider (1948) found that a rapid elevation of ICP diminished blood flow in the sagittal sinus but this returned to normal and even increased temporarily when the experimental elevation of ICP was terminated. Wright (1938) observed localized constriction of cerebral veins in the subarachnoid space close to the sagittal sinus during experimental intracranial hypertension. Artificial elevation of ICP to the level of systemic arterial pressure extinguishes cerebral circulation which will restart only if arterial pressure rises sufficiently beyond the ICP to restore cerebral perfusion pressure. If this response fails, as it appears to do after several vasopressor waves, cerebral perfusion will cease and brain death occurs. Angiography in patients in extremis from raised ICP has confirmed this failure of the cerebral circulation (Fig. 2.3). The opaque medium fills the carotid artery as far as its entry into the subarachnoid space at the

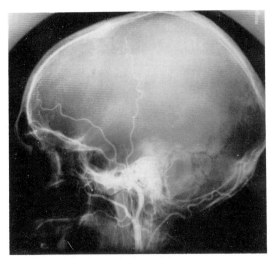

Fig. 2.3. Lateral view of carotid angiogram in a patient with severely increased intracranial pressure due to a temporal haematoma. Note that the internal carotid artery fills only to the base of the skull, while the external carotid branches fill normally.

anterior clinoid process and then abruptly terminates or continues for a short distance as a thin streak (Heiskanen 1964). This radiographic appearance, known as 'false occlusion' of the carotid and/or vertebral artery, is sometimes not absolute, and if serial films are taken over an extended period a thin trail of contrast is seen to slowly fill the cerebral circulation, but at a rate too slow to provide nutritionally significant cerebral blood flow.

Actual measurements of cerebral blood flow (CBF) during intracranial hypertension have been carried out by many investigators. Kety *et al.* (1948) showed that CBF was maintained at a normal level in patients with brain tumours until ICP exceeded 30 mmHg, after which CBF was reduced. In experimental studies when ICP is raised by CSF infusion, CBF remains constant until intracranial pressure is elevated to the point where the difference between ICP and arterial pressure, the cerebral perfusion pressure, falls to 40 mmHg (Häggendal *et al.* 1970, Miller *et al.* 1972, Johnston *et al.* 1974, Symon *et al.* 1973). The initial preservation of normal cerebral blood flow has been linked to the early observations in pial window studies of dilation of small arteries in the brain surface as ICP rises, and ascribed to a process of autoregulation similar to that by which CBF is preserved during falling arterial pressure. This is dealt with in more detail below, but at this stage it should be noted that if autoregulation is impaired because of cerebral ischaemic or traumatic insults, then CBF will not be preserved when ICP increases.

It is worthwhile at this stage to describe in more detail the experiments carried out by Cushing in Berne at the turn of the century after he had completed his early surgical training and prior to devoting himself to a career in neurosurgery. In dogs under general anaesthesia, the surface of the cortex was exposed by a trephine opening in the cranium so that the pial vessels could be observed through a glass window. The ICP was increased by injection of normal saline into the subarachnoid space and by other methods. When ICP nearly approximated the blood pressure, the latter rose and the heart rate

slowed; periodic respiration then developed, the blood pressure fell while the heart rate increased and the animal then died. This classical, so-called, 'Cushing reaction' may be observed in patients with rapidly rising intracranial pressure which results from traumatic extradural haemorrhage. By using the recently developed method of measuring blood pressure by a sphygmomanometer, Cushing was able to make this clinical observation in 1903. He ascribed the rise in blood pressure to a direct response of the medullary vasomotor centres to asphyxia. Cushing noted that it was abolished by bilateral thoracic sympathectomy and by instillation of local anaesthetic into the cisterna magna, but was unaffected by section of the brain stem rostral to the pons or by division of the carotid sinus and aortic nerves. Wright (1938) found that the bradycardia did not occur if vagus nerves were blocked. Hoff and Reis (1970) found that the centres in the medulla that are associated with this vasopressor response are pressure sensitive areas in the lower part of the floor of the fourth ventricle and on the anterolateral surface of the medulla. They showed also that simultaneous with the increase in arterial pressure there is a considerable increase in the neuronal firing rate in the sympathetic outflow nerves (Hoff & Mitchell 1972).

Langfitt (1969) made extensive studies of the changes in arterial pressure, intracranial pressure and cerebral blood flow during these agonal phases of experimental brain compression. He noted that where ICP had been high for a prolonged period, sudden lowering of this pressure by abrupt deflation of the intracranial balloon could be followed after a short interval by rapid return of intracranial hypertension, associated now with cerebral vasodilation and a tremendous increase in cerebral blood volume which could lead in turn to diffuse haemorrhages and oedema of the brain. Langfitt described this phase, during which intracranial pressure was close to the level of arterial pressure and varied passively with any change in arterial pressure, as 'vasomotor paralysis', so as to denote the loss at this stage of all contractility of the cerebral arterioles manifest both by loss of autoregulation and loss of the vascular response to carbon dioxide or oxygen (Langfitt *et al.* 1965). This type of model has also been used to study brain oedema, which develops later in the abruptly decompressed hemisphere.

**Venous drainage in raised intracranial pressure**

When ICP becomes elevated cerebral venous blood volume and pressure both increase (Bedford 1935). This is the capacitance portion of the cerebral vascular bed and the increase in venous capacity is achieved by a change in their cross sectional shape. At normal pressures, veins in the subarachnoid space are oval in cross section; very little increase in intravenous pressure expands the vein to a circular cross section. Further increases in venous capacity are then dependent upon increase in vascular radius. Escape of blood from the skull is facilitated by enlargement of emissary veins. While it is doubtful whether local venous compression by tumours plays a significant part in the genesis of increased ICP, abrupt occlusion of a major venous sinus, such as may occur with a depressed skull fracture, is almost always associated with a considerable increase in intracranial pressure and consequent increase in venous pressure. It is the latter that makes the surgical correction of these injuries so difficult and hazardous. Postural adjustments can help in reducing intracranial and cerebral venous pressure; avoidance of sharp neck flexion or angulation will ensure that the jugular veins remain patent and a moderate degree of head up tilt is helpful. When the patient is in the upright position under normal conditions the cerebral venous pressure will be below zero, as is the ICP. Under these circumstances, if an emissary vein is opened, during exposure of the posterior fossa for example, a considerable quantity of air may be entrained in the open venous channel with severe resulting air embolism. When intracranial pressure is increased and venous pressure is, therefore, increased as well, this danger may be diminished but it should always be kept in mind.

In recent years there has been an increasing reluctance by neurosurgeons to use the sitting position for neurosurgical procedures, precisely because of this risk.

**Diagnosis of increased intracranial pressure**

Accuracy in diagnosis requires that the symptoms and signs of intracranial hypertension be distinguished from those due to the localization of the lesion and by its pathological nature. This separation is usually possible, particularly when the onset is abrupt and the fulminating evolution of the picture may aid diagnosis. The neurosurgeon must be trained to recognize immediately the severity of raised ICP which demands immediate treatment in order to preserve life. The urgency of the condition may not allow the time otherwise necessary for determining precisely the nature of the lesion; appropriate interim measures, operative or otherwise, may successfully relieve a dangerous degree of intracranial hypertension, save the patient's life and permit orderly investigation of the underlying cause.

*Headache* is the commonest symptom of intracranial hypertension. It is however, an extremely common symptom, associated with many other causes both organic and nonorganic. Nevertheless, the headache of rising intracranial pressure has characteristic distinguishing features (Northfield 1938). The headache occurs often in the morning, directly the patient awakes or when rising from bed, or it may awaken him at an early hour. At first it subsides within an hour or so, becoming persistent only at a late stage. It is usually frontal or temporal and bilateral, occasionally it may be unilateral, affecting always the same side. This is however, an unreliable indicator of the side of the lesion. With increasing severity the headache involves the whole head and renders the scalp sensitive to touch. It frequently occurs in paroxysms of unbearable intensity and may be described by the patient as 'bursting'. Sometimes the headache is occipital and may even be described as a neck pain rather than headache. The neck may become stiff and flexion precipitates or aggravates the pain. Tumours in the posterior cranial fossa associated with tonsillar herniation are particularly likely to cause this form of headache with neck pain and stiffness. To mistake this for meningitis and recommend lumber puncture is to court disaster. On the other hand, a purely frontal location of headache by no means excludes a posterior fossa lesion. The character of the headache is often throbbing, aggravated by sudden changes in posture, particularly by stooping and straining. The severity gradually increases as ICP mounts and the recognition of progression is an important point in distinguishing this from headache due to other causes. When ICP is high the headache may last throughout the day but even then it may fluctuate in intensity. A headache which has been present to the same degree, day in and day out for months is most unlikely to be due to intracranial hypertension. When the headache is paroxysmal and extremely severe, as in the later stages of intracranial hypertension, there may be lack of attention or alertness, clouding of consciousness with mental confusion and the patient may show transient signs of neurological dysfunction.

*Vomiting* occurs only in the later stages and is more commonly observed in children than in adults. It is more likely to occur with lesions which cause a rapid rise in ICP such as a haematoma or abscess and in tumours of the posterior cranial fossa, particularly those arising within the fourth ventricle. In these latter cases, it is likely that the vomiting is due as much to direct irritation of the vomiting centre in the medulla as to a rise in ICP. The vomiting associated with intracranial hypertension is often sudden, violent and without preliminary nausea. For these reasons it has been described as 'projectile' and its timing may not necessarily be coincidental with headache.

*Vision* may be affected in a variety of ways. Mistiness of vision, transient at first and later continuous, progressing to an impairment of acuity is usually associated with papilloedema.

Severe headache may be accompanied by transient total amblyopia or by hemianopia. These amblyopic attacks, which may occur when rising from the sitting or lying position, must be regarded as a serious warning that if intracranial hypertension is not soon relieved, complete blindness with optic atrophy may result. Visual hallucinations are rarely due to raised intracranial pressure. They have a localizing significance; if they consist of formed images they suggest a lesion in the temporal lobes, if they consist only of flashes of light or other unformed visual sensations they suggest occipital lobe lesions. Blurring of vision may be due to diplopia in which the images are not sufficiently separated to be perceived by the patient as two images. The patient may, however, volunteer the information that the blurring is abolished by covering one eye. When the diplopia is slight a weakness of one of the ocular muscles may not be immediately apparent on clinical examination and may require detailed ophthalmological analysis to determine its presence. Abducens paresis is the most common cause of diplopia in raised intracranial pressure; it is usually unilateral but may be bilateral. The side of the paresis is not an indication of the side of the lesion responsible for raised ICP and is, therefore, often spoken of as a false localizing sign of intracranial hypertension. The lateral rectus muscle is rarely completely paralysed from this cause. Diplopia may also be due to weakness of those muscles supplied by the oculomotor nerve brought about by herniation of the temporal lobe, as will be discussed below. Divergent squint and skew deviation of the eyes, as part of disturbances of conjugate eye movement, can also give rise to diplopia.

*Disturbance of consciousness* occurs in the late stages of raised intracranial pressure. Observations and accurate, sequential, recordings of the level of consciousness are of the greatest importance in assessing the urgency of this condition. The patient is at first apathetic, disinterested and seemingly lacks awareness of the surroundings, appearing drowsy with a sluggish response to stimuli. As drowsiness deepens, coma supervenes and there is no longer a purposeful response to verbal, and then even to painful, stimuli. When recording these changes in a particular patient, terms such as stupor or semicoma should be avoided in favour or simple statements of the behaviour of the patient in response to standard stimuli. This is formalized in the Glasgow Coma Scale which records the responses of the patient in terms of eye opening, the motor response and the verbal response. This is described at greater length in Chapter 23, on Head Injury (*see* Fig. 23.9). Coma is defined as the state in which there is no eye opening even to painful stimuli, failure to obey simple commands and failure to utter recognizable words. Grading the patient sequentially at frequent intervals reveals the physiological responsiveness quite clearly; the course of events from hour to hour can be quite accurately traced and appropriate action taken. These observations are made and recorded by nursing staff and any deterioration should be immediately reported. Progressive impairment of consciousness is evidence of a dangerous degree of intracranial hypertension and the speed with which consciousness is lost bears some relation to the rate at which causative lesion is developing. In a patient with a slowly growing brain tumour with a history of several months or years duration, drowsiness may be present for several days before deepening to coma. On the other hand, in the case of traumatic extradural haemorrhage, an alert patient complaining of severe headache may pass into deep coma within a matter of hours. Loss of consciousness depends upon two factors, diminution in the cerebral blood flow below a critical level and interruption of brain stem function. Preservation of consciousness is dependent upon the integrity of the brain stem, particularly upon the ascending reticular activating system, and its connections with the cerebral hemispheres. The relative share of the two factors, impairment of cerebral blood flow and brain stem interruption, varies with the nature of the causative lesion, its location and its speed of evolution. In slowly evolving lesions such as benign supratentorial or infratentorial tumours, severe dislocation of the brain stem can take place, as

demonstrated by computerized tomography (CT), without consciousness being disturbed. In chronic subdural haematoma, where the rate of evolution is faster, the patient may be in coma with a similar degree of brain stem displacement yet at operation the intracranial pressure is frequently not raised. In cerebellar tumours an extremely high intracranial pressure (more than 50 mmHg) may be recorded yet the patient can remain alert (Lundberg 1960, Miller *et al.* 1972). The degree of accommodation to conditions which imperil cerebral blood flow and jeopardize integrity of the brain stem depends, therefore, upon the rate of development. It is, perhaps, understanding of the dynamic developing nature of these symptom complexes, their significance (and their urgent management) that is at the core of the clinical skills of the neurosurgeon.

Disturbance of consciousness may not always be progressive, for there may be periods of confusion alternating with lucidity before the onset of coma. At times this becomes a delirium accompanied by physical restlessness to a degree requiring restraint. This state is often not recognized as symptomatic of raised ICP; this is a dangerous pitfall in cases of head injury where the delirious state may be mistakenly treated by narcotic drugs with serious consequences, extending even to a fatal outcome resulting from respiratory depression and hypoxia.

*Papilloedema* is most commonly caused by raised intracranial pressure. Using injection of wax into the subdural space, Bordley and Cushing (1909) were able to produce papilloedema experimentally. Paton and Holmes (1911) suggested that the oedema of the optic nerve head is the result of venous stasis brought about by the elevated pressure of CSF in the arachnoid sheath of the optic nerve and for many years this explanation was generally accepted. The central retinal vein traverses this sheath as it emerges from the optic nerve to empty into the orbit and pterygoid venous plexus, and elevated CSF pressure acting at this strategic point will raise pressure within the retinal vein. Hayreh (1964) studied papilloedema in monkeys produced by gradual distention of an intracranial balloon and showed convincingly the link between papil-loedema and raised ICP, transmitted by the extension of the subarachnoid space along the sheath of the optic nerve. If the sheath of one optic nerve was opened within the orbit that optic disc did not develop swelling. If the sheath was opened after papilloedema had become established, the swelling rapidly subsided.

It is now considered more likely that the phenomenon of papilloedema represents a block to axoplasmic transport in the optic nerve with the swelling at the head representing an accumulation of axoplasm (Wittschafter *et al.* 1975). The experimental results of Hayreh are still compatible with this view, but it is probable that a combination of both increased retinal venous pressure and axoplasmic transport block is responsible for the appearances seen at fundoscopy in papilloedema.

While the presence of papilloedema is generally a reliable indication of the presence of raised ICP, absence of papilloedema is no guarantee that ICP is not elevated. It is absent in about one third of cases of acute brain abscess and in some cases the eyes are affected to a dissimilar degree without lateralizing significance. Selhorst *et al.* (1985) found papilloedema in only 4% of a large series of head injured patients, in whom there was certain evidence of raised ICP in 50% of cases. In this instance the onset of raised ICP may be too acute to permit the development of papilloedema; in other cases where papilloedema is absent, yet ICP elevated, the causes may relate to anatomical variations in the extent to which the subarachnoid space extends along the optic nerve. A well recognized syndrome occurs when a slowly growing tumour presses upon one optic nerve, causing optic nerve atrophy, and papilloedema develops in the other eye. This is known as the Foster Kennedy syndrome and is seen most often in the presence of meningiomas growing from the medial part of the sphenoid wing. The preretinal or subhyaloid haemorrhages, which may accompany subarachnoid haemorrhage and are due to suffusion of blood along the optic nerve, should not be confused with papilloedema.

In certain conditions, such as benign intracranial hypertension, it is most important to establish whether papilloedema is truly present or not or whether unusual appearances of the optic disc may be due to congenital or other causes. In such cases fluorescein angiography is extremely useful in distinguishing true papilloedema from other changes (Johnston & Paterson 1974).

Papilloedema is encountered in many conditions and at times its cause may be difficult to determine. Some of the less common causes are included in the following list:

1   low grade pyogenic meningitis and tuberculous meningitis
2   cortical thrombophlebitis and dural sinus thrombosis (Kalbag & Woolf 1967)
3   benign intracranial hypertension (Foley 1955)
4   malignant arterial hypertension
5   chronic pulmonary disease with hypercapnia (Freedman 1963, Stevens *et al.* 1963)
6   pulmonary hypertension due to raised venous pressure
7   endocrine disorders (Jefferson 1956, Greer 1963)
8   tetracycline (Fields 1961)
9   vitamin A deficiency or excess (Bass & Fisch 1961, Morrice *et al.* 1960)
10   polycythaemia and anaemia (Pears & Pickering 1960, Shaw & Simpson 1961, Capriles 1963)
11   Guillain-Barré syndrome (Drew & Magee 1951, Morley & Reynolds 1966) and certain neuropathies (Brain 1963)
12   lead encephalopathy (Popoff *et al.* 1963)
13   spinal tumours (Rohr & Hoffmann 1959)
14   optic nerve tumours (Meadows 1959)
15   retrobulbar neuritis and other optic nerve intrinsic disease (Greaves 1959).

Mild papilloedema may be indistinguishable in appearance from the papillitis of optic myelitis but the effects on vision usually allow a correct diagnosis. True papillitis is characterized by rapid and early failure of vision with development of a central scotoma while the peripheral field is unaffected. In papilloedema, by contrast, deterioration of visual acuity is late and develops slowly in conjunction with constriction of the periphery of the visual field and enlargement of the blind spot.

## The cerebrospinal fluid

The cerebrospinal fluid (CSF) contains nothing that can be identified as uniquely characteristic, and from this fact stem many of the difficulties encountered in studying its formation, flow and absorption. That its origin is mainly in the ventricles of the brain rests securely upon the common experience of morbid anatomy. If obstruction occurs within the third ventricle, the aqueduct of Sylvius, the fourth ventricle or by occlusion of the foramina of Luschka and Magendie, then the ventricles, thus isolated from the subarachnoid space, dilate. If one foramen of Monro becomes obstructed, that lateral ventricle dilates. It is important to hold fast to these simple facts of repeated and acknowledged observation amid the confusion of the many experimental observations which were made in subsequent decades. Dandy (1919) contended that the choroid plexus was responsible for the formation of the CSF by observing formation of fluid from the exposed choroid plexus after CSF had been removed from the lateral ventricle. Massermann (1934) removed small quantities of fluid from the lateral ventricle and determined the time taken for the pressure to return to the original level and used this to compute a CSF formation rate in the human of 0.2 ml/100 ml/minute. Dandy and Blackfan (1914) used injections of the dye phenolsulphonphthalein into the cisterna magna and followed its excretion via the kidneys to calculate CSF formation rate. Their classical experiments were reviewed in detail by Davson (1967) who recalculated their results and obtained a figure of 0.3 ml/100 ml/minute. The introduction of radioisotopes into medical research was soon applied by a number of investigators to estimates of the formation and flow of CSF. Davson reviewed these studies and esti-

mated that the rate of CSF secretion in man was 0.3 ml/100 ml/minute. If the total quantity of CSF in the normal adult is between 120 and 140 ml then these estimates suggest a secretion rate of approximately 0.5 ml/minute.

More recent reviews of the subject by Cserr (1974) and Pollay (1975) indicate that the overwhelming evidence is now that CSF formation is predominantly (70% at least) derived from the secretion of the choroid plexus within the ventricular system. Sodium–potassium activated ATPase is involved in the active secretory process responsible for producing CSF, and drugs that interfere with the activity of this ATPase will also affect the rate of CSF production. While CSF production rate is influenced by changes in the cerebral metabolic rate for glucose and oxygen, it remains on the whole a remarkably stable factor unaffected by moderate changes in cerebral perfusion pressure or blood flow. Under conditions of severely increased intracranial pressure, however, sufficient to cause significant cerebral ischaemia, CSF production rate falls (Weiss & Wertman 1978).

In seeking the mechanism whereby CSF is absorbed, the facts of common observation should be borne in mind. CSF is continually being formed and if there were no outlet into the subarachnoid space this would cause hydrocephalus. When lesions, such as basal meningitis or a tumour obstructing the cisterna ambiens within the tentorial opening, prevent CSF from spreading from the outflow foramina of the fourth ventricle over the cerebral hemispheres, hydrocephalus also occurs. Hydrocephalus results, in addition, if the subarachnoid spaces are obstructed by particulate matter which induces an intense leptomeningeal reaction and obstruction. The facts of morbid anatomy therefore, indicate that for absorption to occur, the CSF from the ventricular system must gain the subarachnoid space over the cerebral hemispheres. This might be in order to provide a vascularized surface of an adequate number of arachnoid villi. Interest has long been attracted to the arachnoid villi and their overgrown homologues, the Pacchionian granulations. These provide histological evidence of a close relationship between the CSF space and the blood stream. With the advent of sequential scanning of the radioactive emission from isotopes injected into the CSF space proof has been obtained of the direction of flow of the bulk of the CSF (McComb 1983). In the normal subject, scanning shows that the isotope emerges from the ventricular system into the cisterna magna, passes through the basal systems up over the cerebral hemispheres with concentration in the Sylvian fissures towards the vertex. The isotope is regularly last seen as a concentration on both sides in the parasagittal region. Although isotope scanning has not directly established the Pacchionian granulations in CSF absorption, it has provided powerful evidence that this region of the subarachnoid CSF space provides the main drainage system.

Like the choroid plexus, the arachnoid villi are anatomically unique. They project through the walls of dural venous sinuses and are particularly profuse in the superior sagittal sinus. Villi and granulations have a fundamentally similar structure, the granulations being villi that are large enough to be visible to the naked eye. Infants possess only villi. A mesh of fibres, continuous with the pia-arachnoid, forms the stalk and core of the granulation. Covering its summit, and extending to a variable degree into the stroma of the granulation, is a collection or cap of epithelial cells which has a papilliferous or villus surface abutting against the blood within the sinus (Le Gros Clark 1921). Various experiments have been devised to determine the function of the granulations. The older experiments of Key and Retzius (1875) and Weed (1914) are open to the objection that the experimental conditions were artificial and the substances used to follow the absorptive process may have damaged cell membranes. The injection of fine particulate matter (kaolin) into the subarachnoid space did not shed light on the problem because this aroused the phagocytic activity of mesothelial cells, led to a sterile meningitis and is most widely used now as a model for producing experimental hydrocephalus.

The advent of electron microscopic studies of arachnoid villi shed new light on the possible absorptive mechanism for CSF. Tripathi and Tripathi (1974) demonstrated vesicles within arachnoid villi that were joined to form tortuous channels through which fine particulate material could pass. Butler et al. (1983) suggested that as ICP increased these potential channels through arachnoid villi could open up thus explaining the increasing rate of CSF absorption in parallel with increased ICP. Levine et al. (1982) conducted studies in primates in which the arachnoid villi were perfusion fixed at different and progressively greater levels of ICP and demonstrated that this was indeed the case: the greater the level of ICP the more the arachnoid villus channels opened. McComb (1983) provides a useful review of this topic. Upton and Weller (1985) examined human arachnoid granulations by scanning electron microscopy and emphasized the role of villi and granulation as CSF filters as well as conduits for bulk flow of CSF.

The pressure of blood within patent cerebral veins must always be greater than the CSF pressure, for otherwise their thin walls would collapse and blood flow would be extinguished. Noell and Schneider (1948) measured intracranial venous pressure. They blocked the superior sagittal sinus in front and behind and inserted a cannula into the intervening portion of the sinus whose pressure was deemed to be the same as the veins entering it. Raising the CSF pressure by increments they recorded corresponding rises in venous pressure. Johnston and Rowan (1974) directly cannulated veins in the subarachnoid space of primates and similarly recorded progressively increasing venous pressure as ICP was experimentally elevated by CSF infusion. Flexner and Weed (1933), Bedford (1942) and Shulman (1965) all found, however, that the pressure at the posterior portion of the superior sagittal sinus and within the torcular was persistently lower than the CSF pressure. This is possible because the shape and structure of the dural venous sinuses is such that they possess sufficient rigidity to resist the intracranial pressure. This means that there is a pressure gradient along the length of the superior sagittal sinus. There is therefore a pressure gradient for CSF to enter the dural sinus blood stream via the arachnoid villi, and to be at a pressure slightly above that within the venous system at that point. For the same reasons it seems likely that there will be no absorption of CSF into cortical cerebral veins. Using excised portions of dura mater containing intact arachnoid villi, Welch and Friedman (1960) showed that one way flow of fluid could be observed across the villi with any pressure gradient over 20 mm of water (1.5 mmHg). While the results of such *in vitro* experiments must be interpreted with caution, and there may be species differences, detailed neuroanatomical observations of the structure of the arachnoid villus perfusion fixed at different levels of CSF pressure indicate that there is indeed a physical substrate for such observations (Levine *et al.* 1982).

### The cerebrospinal fluid in diagnosis

Normal intraventricular or lumbar CSF pressure does not preclude an expanding intracranial lesion, particularly when this has been present for a prolonged period, as in the case of a large frontal meningoma. Not uncommonly, the pressure within a chronic subdural haematoma is normal and in cases of hydrocephalus the intraventricular pressure may not be raised even though the patient shows well marked signs of brain damage associated with ventricular dilation. Although, the resting pressure may not be increased, a subsequent challenge of an increase in intracranial volume may produce a marked, prolonged, and pathological increase in ICP. This may happen spontaneously due to the cerebral vasodilation that occurs during periods of rapid eye movement sleep, or in association with an episode of airway obstruction or it may be produced by certain anaesthetic agents, notably the volatile agents such as halothane or trichlorethylene (Miller 1975). In these circumstances the additional cerebral blood volume produced by the episode of cerebral vasodilation may increase ICP rapidly from normal levels to levels of 50 mmHg or more. In a certain number of patients these elevations occur spontaneously and rhythmically, producing characteristic plateau waves of increased ICP in which the pressure remains elevated for between 5 and 20 minutes subsiding spontaneously to normal levels (Lundberg 1960). It is because of these episodic increases in CSF pressure that it is recommended that if the neurosurgeon wishes to exclude raised ICP, a period of continuous pressure recording should be undertaken; and since two thirds of episodes of elevated ICP occur at night, the period of continuous recording should include at least one overnight record (Marshall *et al.* 1978). The state of reduced intracranial compliance may be detected by deliberately challenging the craniospinal system by the bolus in which small changes in intracranial volume induce large changes in pressure injection of small volumes (1 or 2 ml) of saline into the ventricular system. An excessive rise in CSF pressure (>2 mmHg/ml) signifies reduced compliance (Miller & Leech 1975).

Headache after a lumbar puncture in a patient not harbouring an intracranial space occupying lesion is usually due to intracranial hypotension (Pickering 1948, Wolff 1963). The pain is eased by raising the foot of the bed and by increasing the intake of water. It rarely follows the use of a fine lumbar puncture needle and if the patient is kept recumbent for 24 hours afterwards. The low CSF pressure is due to loss of fluid through the puncture hole in the arachnoid (Brown & Jones 1962). The continued leakage of CSF through the puncture hole may be aggravating factor in the delayed development of a neurological deficit in patients with spinal tumours who have a complete block of the subarachnoid space. Headache is much less common following cisternal puncture, presumably because in the erect position the pressure of the cerebrospinal fluid in the cistern is practically zero.

When should diagnostic lumbar puncture be permissible? In patients with no evidence of raised intracranial pressure there is little risk. In patients with increased intracranial pressure and particularly when papilloedema is present, lumbar puncture should be avoided unless the information it may supply is absolutely essential for diagnosis or treatment. This would be true only of cases of meningitis so that specific treatment can be started immediately. The advent of CT has meant that it is usually possible to screen the patient first to confirm the absence of a space occupying lesion before conducting a lumbar puncture, and in some cases of spontaneous subarachnoid haemorrhage the CT itself may be sufficiently diagnostic to avoid lumbar puncture altogether. Another solution is to carry out ventricular puncture first. It should be noted however, that when an analysis of CSF is necessary a sample of ventricular fluid cannot replace a sample of lumbar CSF. Many of the diagnostic abnormalities appear only in the lumbar fluid. The normal ventricular fluid has a lower content of cells and protein than the lumbar fluid; thus the normal protein level in lumbar fluid is 200–400 mg/L but in ventricular fluid it may be as low as 100 mg/L. The abnormalities that occur in the spinal fluid secondary to disease of the central nervous system are liberally documented in standard reference books, but some of those accompanying conditions frequently encountered by neurosurgeons will be considered here.

*Glioma* In most cases the fluid is normal. If the tumour is adjacent to the wall of the ventricle there may be a slight increase in the cell count and protein level and sampling from each lateral ventricle may reveal some discrepancy. If the cell count is increased (up to 100 cells/mm³) and some cells necrotic, and if the protein is markedly raised with xanthrochromic CSF, the tumour is more likely to be glioblastoma. Intraventricular and subarachnoid spread of tumour is associated with considerable increases in protein to 2 g or more per litre. Medulloblastoma may be associated with a marked increase in the cell count with a combination of malignant cells and polymorphonuclear leucocytes raising a possible diagnosis of meningitis. When the CSF cell count

is increased and tumour suspected then cytological examination is often helpful in making a diagnosis of neoplasia (Spriggs 1954).

*Meningioma* The CSF protein is frequently increased, at times considerably, up to 2 g/L, while the cell count remains normal.

*Acoustic neurinoma* The CSF protein is nearly always, but not invariably, increased; levels of up to 3–4 g/L have been recorded. In a series of 50 large acoustic neurinomas, McMenemey and Cumings (1959) found only 1 case in which the CSF protein was less than 500 mg/L.

*Pituitary adenoma and craniopharyngioma* The CSF is unaffected in the majority of cases.

*Intraventricular lesions* In choroid plexus papilloma, cells and protein may both be increased and the fluid xanthochromic. Hydrocephalus has been attributed both to increased CSF production and obstruction due to cellular fragments in the CSF. In colloid cyst of the third ventricle there is no abnormality in the constituents of the CSF, and hydrocephalus is due to obstruction at the foramina of Monro.

*Haemangioblastoma* There may be an elevation of protein with no change in cell count. If there has been any bleeding, slight xanthrochromia and an increase in cell count may be found.

*Subdural haematoma* The CSF may be xanthrochromic, or more frequently entirely normal.

*Brain Abscess* While a moderate increase in CSF protein and a small increase in the number of cells is not uncommon, the striking fact in many cases of brain abscess is the absolute normality of the CSF.

*Blood in the CSF* This may be traumatic in origin, from head injury, or due to the rupture of an aneurysm, arteriovenous malformation, or to the other causes as discussed in Chapters 11 and 12. It may however, also be caused by the trauma of the lumbar puncture. When there is doubt the CSF specimens should immediately be centrifuged. The supernatant fluid will be yellow, xanthrochromic, if the bleeding took place more than a few hours previously.

*Intraspinal tumour*   The spinal fluid is affected in two ways. First by transudation of protein from a tumour lying within the arachnoid sheath or presenting on the surface of the spinal cord and secondly, as a result of the partial or complete loculation of CSF caudal to a tumour that blocks the subarachnoid space. The main changes increasing the CSF protein level are caused by the second mechanism and are considered in detail in Chapter 21.

In many ways the CSF can be viewed as an extension of the extracellular fluid of the brain. In addition to the routine measurements of the content of glucose, protein and cells in the CSF, numerous studies have been made of the clinical significance of variations in the content of a variety of substances within the CSF. Alterations in CSF pH, $CO_2$ and bicarbonate levels, in CSF lactate and potassium concentrations have all been used as an index of the severity of traumatic or hypoxic brain insults (Taylor & Crockard 1972). Changes in CSF levels of cyclic AMP (Fleischer *et al.* 1977) and brain specific creatine kinase (Maas 1977, Nordby & Urdal 1982) have also been used in this way. In general, while there is a significant difference between mean levels of these constituents in groups of normal and abnormal subjects, the scatter of data reduces the value of such measurements in individual patients (Bakay & Ward 1983).

## The cerebral circulation

The brain accounts for only 2% of total body weight yet its blood flow represents 15% of the resting cardiac output and it uses 20% of the total amount of oxygen consumed by the human body at rest. Cerebral blood flow is therefore copious and continuous; the effects of sudden cessation of flow are both dramatic and disas-

trous. Within 15 seconds of total arrest of the cerebral circulation, consciousness is lost, brain electrical activity ceases, and if flow is not restored within 5 minutes, structural changes begin to appear in cerebral neurons that are progressive, and eventually irreversible leading to ischaemic cell change, an appearance characterized on microscopy by shrunken, distorted, darkly staining neurons. Because of its encasement by the bony vault of the skull, the circulation of the brain has always been a difficult subject for study and early observations in the human subject depended upon the opportunities afforded by wounds of the head or, by the latter end of the 19th century, elective intracranial surgery. Thus, Horsley observed pallor of the cerebral cortex when the ipsilateral common carotid artery was occluded (Spencer & Horsley 1881, 1889), and Cushing (1901) used inspection windows in the skull for his experimental observations of the behaviour of cortical vessels when intracranial pressure was raised. These pial window studies were extended and refined by Forbes (1928), Wolff and Lennox (1936) and Fog (1933, 1937, 1939) and continue today with sophisticated apparatus which can automatically measure in absolute terms (micrometers) any change in the diameter of any chosen cortical vessel, venous or arterial (Kontos *et al.* 1978, Wahl & Kuschinsky 1979).

A major advance in understanding of the physiology of the cerebral circulation came, however, in 1945 with the development by Kety and Schmidt of the inert gas clearance method of measuring total cerebral blood flow in man. By an ingenious adaptation of the Fick principle, which states that the consumption of a substance by an organ is the product of its blood flow and the arterovenous difference for that substance, Kety and Schmidt used the metabolically inert and freely diffusible tracer, nitrous oxide, assumed that at saturation the brain concentration of tracer equalled the cerebral venous concentration, and obtained a value for cerebral blood flow measured in mls/minute/unit weight of brain from the differences and total amount of nitrous oxide in samples of arterial and jugular venous blood taken at intervals during continuous inhalation of the tracer over a short time (10 minutes). By this method they arrived at a value of 50 ml/100 g brain/min at rest in normal, conscious man. The validity of this figure for total cerebral blood flow/unit weight of brain has been validated using several different methods of flow measurement over succeeding years. Once the quantitative measurement of blood flow had been accomplished, it was possible to derive figures for the cerebrovascular resistance (CVR) from:

$$CVR \, (mmHg/ml/100\,g/min) = \frac{cerebral \; perfusion \; pressure \; (mmHg)}{cerebral \; blood \; flow \; (ml/100\,g/min)}$$

By simultaneously measuring the cerebral arteriovenous difference of other substances such as oxygen or glucose it was also possible to calculate a cerebral metabolic rate (the rate of consumption or production of the substance) from the following equation:

$$CMRO_2 \, (ml \; O_2/100\,g/min) = \\ A - VO_2 \; difference \, (ml/100\,ml) \times \\ CBF \, (ml/100\,g/min)$$

It was possible also to study the response of cerebral blood flow to changes in physiological conditions. It was thus established that cerebral blood flow in man remained constant over a wide range of arterial pressures, becoming reduced only when arterial pressure fell below 60 mmHg (Lassen 1959, Harper 1966). CBF was found to be exquisitely sensitive to changes in arterial $PCO_2$, rising by 2 or 3 ml/100 g/min for every torr increase in $PCO_2$ in a range of arterial $PCO_2$ values between 20 and 80 torr (3–10.5 kPa) (Kety & Schmidt 1948, Reivich 1964, Harper & Glass 1965). Small elevations in intracranial pressure were found not to influence cerebral blood flow, but when ICP exceeded 30 mmHg there was usually a decrease in CBF (Kety et al. 1948).

As a result of studying epilepsy, Penfield (1933) observed changes in surface vessels in the brain during seizures and Schmidt and Hendrix (1937) noted a focal increase in cerebral blood flow accompanying an increase in activity of a part of the brain in experimental animals, a finding confirmed in man by Walter and Crow (1964). The Kety–Schmidt technique is not appropriate for measuring focal changes in cerebral blood flow because it assumes uniform flow throughout the brain (the sample of jugular venous blood is assumed to be representative of venous outflow from both hemispheres). With the availability of radioisotopes of the gases Krypton and Xenon, which also functioned as inert, freely diffusible tracers, but the radioactive emanations of which could be detected outside the intact skull by focused collimated detectors, the technique of measurement of regional cerebral blood flow was developed simultaneously by Harper et al. (1961) in Glasgow and by Ingvar and Lassen (1961) in Scandinavia, though the latter were the first to report its use in man. Although at first the regions of the brain from which blood flow was measured were large, so that only sizeable abnormalities could be detected, much useful information emerged from these studies conducted in the decade between 1960 and 1970. Investigations carried out in patients with stroke, brain tumours and head injuries indicated that autoregulation of blood flow to changes in arterial pressure and the response of cerebral vessels to changes in arterial $PCO_2$ could be impaired on a focal basis, leaving the remaining, normal brain intact (Palvölgyi 1969, Paulson 1970, Fieschi et al. 1974). In the focally abnormal areas blood flow might be reduced but could also be increased. This abnormal hyperaemia was associated with early filling veins on angiography, and at operation with the appearance of 'red veins', suggesting that the increase in blood flow was non-nutritional, since there was no corresponding increase in the uptake of oxygen from the blood. Lassen (1966) coined the term 'luxury perfusion' to describe this state and proposed that it was due to a local decrease in the pH of extracellular fluid consequent upon a preceding period of anaerobic glycolysis in neurons, resulting in outpouring of lactate. This observation led to development of the concept of intracerebral *steal*. In this condition, when blood flow to the rest of the (normal) brain was increased by administration of carbon dioxide, there was no corresponding increase in flow in the focally abnormal area because the vessels in that area were already dilated and unresponsive to $CO_2$. Under these conditions it was possible for blood flow to be reduced in the focally abnormal area, consequent on diversion of blood to the rest of the brain. The practical consequence of this observation was that the practice of administering small amounts of carbon dioxide to patients with acute strokes so as to stimulate an increase in cerebral blood flow was quickly abandoned when it was recognized that not only were these patients not improved but there was now a pathophysiological explanation for the deterioration that occurred in some cases. A further development in this thinking was the concept of *inverse steal*; this consisted of an increase in flow in the focally abnormal area resulting from induction of vasoconstriction elsewhere in the brain by hyperventilation and reduction in arterial $PCO_2$. This led to the advocacy of therapeutic hyperventilation in patients with head injury and stroke.

These measurements of regional cerebral blood flow proved to be an excellent tool for studying the effects of occlusion of the carotid artery, either temporarily, as during carotid endarterectomy, or permanently as for proximal carotid ligation in the case of certain aneurysms arising from the internal carotid artery. Measurements of the change in regional cerebral blood flow in the appropriate hemisphere after temporary occlusion of the ipsilateral carotid artery proved to be a more accurate predictor of inadequate cerebral perfusion than did recording of angiographic cross-filling, carotid artery back pressure, EEG changes, or jugular venous oxygen content during temporary carotid occlusion. Leech *et al.* (1974) showed that provided cerebral blood flow was reduced by no more than 25% from control values during temporary occlusion then permanent carotid ligation could be accomplished without subsequent neurological deficit. If blood flow was reduced by between 25% and 35% then ligation could be tolerated,

provided that carotid artery back pressure did not fall below 60 mmHg.

To this point, measurements of regional cerebral blood flow had to be made by direct injection of 133 Xenon in saline into the carotic artery. Obrist *et al.* (1975) developed a noninvasive technique whereby 133 Xenon in gaseous form could be inhaled. By using a computer programme to adjust or deconvolute the curve of radioactivity recorded from the head as the tracer arrived in, and was cleared from, the brain according to the activity recorded in expired air, this provided an estimate of the washout curve of radioactivity from the brain that would have been present had the isotope been directly introduced into the cerebral arterial circulation. Clearly this less invasive method found wider application, since it no longer had to be combined with carotid angiography. The decade between 1975 and 1985 has witnessed the development of a number of new techniques for measuring regional cerebral blood flow in both experimental laboratory subjects and in man, some of which will be described briefly in Chapter 4. With autoradiographic techniques it is now possible to measure microregional cerebral blood flow and glucose metabolism in exquisite detail in laboratory animals and there is now ample confirmation of the original findings of Schmidt and Hendrix recorded under such difficult conditions many years ago.

It is now quite clear that the cerebral circulation functions in two ways. Firstly, to match blood flow precisely to local neuronal demand; thus, visual stimulation will produce marked increases in blood flow in the superior colliculi and the occipital cortex. The second function of control mechanisms for cerebral blood flow is to protect the brain against potentially harmful stresses such as hypotension or hypoxaemia.

While this is a field that is still subject to an almost exponential increase in knowledge it is possible to state fairly briefly the principal findings concerning the major aspects of the control of the cerebral circulation.

## Arterial blood pressure

In all mammalian species, including man, cerebral blood blow remains constant for rather a wide range around the normal resting level of blood pressure (Fig. 2.4). In man, cerebral blood flow is constant until arterial pressure reduces below 60 mmHg. If the cause of arterial hypotension is haemorrhage, blood flow begins to decrease at this point; in drug-induced arterial hypotension (as is practiced during some forms of neurosurgical anaesthesia), or if haemorrhagic hypotension has been accompanied by a surgical or drug-induced sympathectomy, then arterial pressure can be reduced to 40 mmHg before blood flow begins to fall (Fitch *et al.* 1975). Thereafter, there is a rapid reduction in CBF till this ceases effectively below arterial pressures of 20 mmHg mean. When arterial pressure is increased, blood flow also remains constant until a mean arterial pressure of around 150 mmHg, beyond which there is an increase in blood flow, often referred to as the 'breakthrough' of autoregulation (Strandgaard *et al.* 1974). Maintenance of constant blood flow despite a change in perfusion pressure implies a corresponding change in cerebrovascular resistance. The substrate for such a change, verified by pial window studies of cerebral cortical vessels during controlled changes in arterial and intracranial pressure, is an appropriate alteration in the calibre of cerebral arteries and arterioles. Thus, as pressure rises, the vessels constrict and when pressure falls the resistance vessels dilate. The larger vessels, 100–200 microns in diameter, are the first to dilate as arterial pressure falls; the smaller vessels, 70–90 microns diameter, dilate at lower levels of arterial pressure (Kontos *et al* 1978).

In chronically hypertensive patients these threshold levels for decreased and increased blood flow appear to be reset; thus, in the hypertensive patient blood pressure can rise to higher levels before any increase in flow is observed; conversely, but of more practical importance, the level of arterial hypotension that can be tolerated before CBF falls is much less. Thus in the hypertensive patient, reduction of mean arterial pressure below 90 mmHg may be accompanied by a fall in CBF.

When CBF is reduced to 40% of control levels, that is from 50 down to 20 ml/100 g/min, neurological dysfunction occurs, with EEG changes, consisting of slow waves followed by disappearance of neuroelectrical activity. As CBF continues to fall, a cascade of cellular events follows, including potassium efflux and calcium influx, leading eventually to neuronal cell death (Astrup 1982).

The normal autoregulatory response may be impaired by physiological or pathological mechanisms. If arterial $PCO_2$ is increased with consequent vasodilation, and arterial pressure is then reduced, CBF falls in a pressure passive relationship and no indication of autoregulation (Harper 1966). This protective response is also impaired following ischaemic or hypoxic insults to the brain, brain compression, concussional brain injury, subarachnoid haemorrhage, and focally in relation to ischaemic stroke, brain tumours, abscesses and areas of encephalitis (Lewelt *et al.* 1980).

## Carbon dioxide tension

Cerebral blood flow doubles when arterial $PCO_2$ is raised from 40 mmHg to 80 mmHg (approxi-

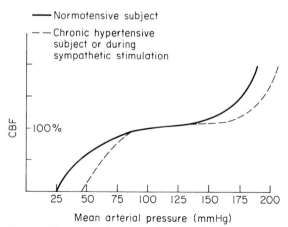

**Fig. 2.4.** Diagram to show normal autoregulatory relationship of cerebral blood flow to changes in arterial pressure.

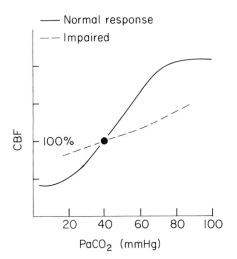

**Fig. 2.5.** Diagram to show response of cerebral blood flow to changes in arterial carbon dioxide tension.

Evenvoldsen & Jensen 1978, Obrist *et al.* 1979, Lewelt *et al.* 1982).

## Arterial oxygen tension

With progressive reduction of arterial $PO_2$ there is little effect on cerebral blood flow and metabolism until the point is reached where desaturation of blood begins to occur (Fig. 2.6). This usually begins below an arterial $PO_2$ of 55 mmHg (7 kPa) but the precise level will depend upon the configuration of the oxyhaemoglobin dissociation curve and the extent to which it is altered by changes in the pH and temperature of the blood in accordance with the Bohr effect. The oxygen content of arterial blood is normally around 20 ml/dL and of cerebral venous blood 14 ml/dL so that the cerebral arteriovenous oxygen content difference is 6 ml/dL; multiplying this by the normal cerebral blood flow of 50 ml/100 g/minute yields a normal cerebral oxygen consumption rate of 3 ml oxygen/100 g brain/minute. As arterial oxygen content falls, the cerebral venous oxygen content can be reduced so as to maintain a constant difference. With further hypoxaemia however, cerebral vasodilation begins to occur, cerebral blood flow

mately 5–10 kPa). CBF halves when arterial $PCO_2$ is lowered from 40–20 mmHg (Fig. 2.5). This reduction in cerebral blood flow with hypocapnia has been held as harmful by some; it is associated with slowing of the EEG and an increase of lactate in the CSF, findings similar to those induced by mild hypoxaemia. On the other hand it has never been demonstrated that the cerebral vasoconstriction and relative cerebral ischaemia induced by hyperventilation can produce structural brain damage; this mechanism is in widespread therapeutic use for control of raised intracranial pressure because of the reduction in cerebral blood volume that results from the hypocapnic vasoconstriction.

The cerebrovascular response to carbon dioxide is a basic and powerful one, tending to override other competing influences for the cerebrovascular resistence vessels. Thus, when arterial blood pressure is low and cerebral blood flow beginning to be reduced, the superimposition of hypo- or hypercapnia can still alter CBF. In clinical practice, complete loss of the cerebral circulatory response to a change in arterial $PCO_2$ is a very late manifestation of brain damage in head injury, subarachnoid haemorrhage or other brain insult, amounting almost to a premortem state. (Overgaard & Tweed 1974,

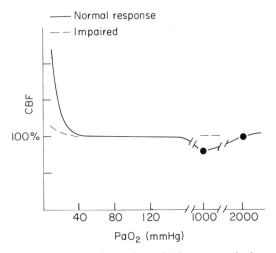

**Fig. 2.6.** Diagram to show relationship between cerebral blood flow and arterial oxygen tension.

increases to compensate for the decrease in arteriovenous difference, and cerebral oxygen delivery and consumption remain constant (McDowall 1966). By the time the arterial $PO_2$ has fallen to 30 mmHg (4 kPa) cerebral blood flow may have tripled. After severe brain insults, focal or general, when the cerebrovascular response to $CO_2$ has been abolished, there is no longer a vasodilator response to hypoxaemia.

With progressive increases in arterial $PO_2$ above the normal level there is a degree of cerebral vasoconstriction, reaching a maximum of 25% reduction in cerebral blood flow at arterial $PO_2$ levels of 900–1200 mmHg. As these are above atmospheric pressure (760 mmHg) such levels can be achieved only in a hyperbaric chamber, breathing 100% oxygen. This hyperoxic cerebral vasoconstriction is immediately reversed by administration of carbon dioxide, indicating once again the fundamental and powerful nature of this particular stimulus to the cerebral circulation (Miller & Ledingham 1971). If arterial $PO_2$ is increased further to 2000 mmHg or more (achieved by breathing 100% oxygen at 3 or more atmospheres absolute ambient pressure) the previous vasoconstriction disappears and progressive vasodilation occurs, accompanied by metabolic indications of cerebral oxygen toxicity (Miller 1973).

## Intracranial pressure

The relationship between the intracranial pressure and cerebral blood flow is twofold. Elevated intracranial pressure will eventually act as a limiting factor, reducing CBF finally to zero. On the other hand, increases or decreases in cerebral blood flow can have a corresponding effect on the level of intracranial pressure, a fact which is of considerable importance in the intensive therapy of neurosurgical patients.

In experimental models of intracranial hypertension, where the pressure has been raised by CSF infusion, or by the inflation of intracranial balloon, CBF remains constant despite considerable increases in intracranial pressure until

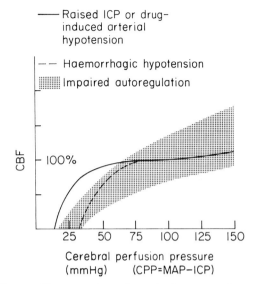

Fig. 2.7. Diagram to show relationship between cerebral blood flow (CBF) cerebral perfusion pressure (CPP), when this is defined to the difference between mean arterial pressure (MAP) and intracranial pressure (ICP). The shaded area indicates the range of flow levels that may occur in states of impaired autoregulation, i.e. CBF may be above or below normal.

the difference between intracranial pressure and arterial pressure reaches 40 mmHg (Miller *et al.* 1972, 1973). This pressure difference may be achieved at widely varied levels of ICP, depending upon the level and response of the arterial blood pressure (Fig. 2.7). It is not uncommon for arterial pressure to rise considerably as part of the vasopressor response during the late stages of intracranial hypertension. When the perfusion pressure is less than 40 mmHg the reduction in CBF is progressive until blood flow ceases at the point at which intracranial and arterial pressure are equal. This corresponds to the point at which pseudo-obstruction of the cerebral vessels occurs during attempted angiography in patients with raised intracranial pressure. Once that point has been reached, however, subsequent reduction of intracranial pressure and reestablishment of the cerebral perfusion pressure may fail to result in adequate reperfusion of the brain. While this mechanism has been most closely studied in experimental animals, this also represents the mode of death in approximately half of fatal head injuries (Miller *et al.* 1977). In addition, opportunistic monitoring of ICP in patients following subarachnoid haemorrhage who have subsequently suffered a recurrent haemorrhage indicates that in most cases intracranial pressure immediately following the subarachnoid haemorrhage rises to the level of arterial blood pressure, and loss of consciousness in these cases is probably due to temporary cessation of cerebral blood flow (Steiner *et al.* 1975).

In the earlier stages of intracranial hypertension, maintenance of normal CBF depends upon retention of intact autoregulation; if this has previously been abolished, so that blood flow is pressure passive to changes in arterial pressure, then it will be immediately reduced by any increase in ICP.

When CBF is increased, as for instance during hypercapnia or hypoxaemia, the vasodilation leads to an increase in cerebral blood volume, but not in the arterial part of the circulation; blood flow in vessels is proportional to the fourth power of the radius so that relatively small changes in arterial radius can result in large changes in flow. The increase in volume is due to distention of the venous, or capacitance, part of the vascular bed. The extent to which ICP will increase is a function, not only of the increase in venous pressure transmitted through the capillary bed and the total increase in blood volume, but also of the pressure-volume status of the craniospinal axis (Miller 1975). When compliance has been reduced by, for example, the existence of a large space-occupying lesion such as a tumour, then even a small increase in blood volume may be responsible for a very large and potentially fatal rise in ICP. In addition, because the largest part of the cerebral vascular network lies above the tentorium, any general vasodilating influence will have most effect in the supratentorial compartment, and should there be a tendency for pressure gradients to develop across the tentorial hiatus, an episode of intracranial hypertension induced by vasodilation will increase this pressure gradient and favour further brain herniation (Fitch & McDowall 1971). This topic will be considered in more detail.

## Drugs and neurogenic influences

For many years it was believed that the cerebral circulation was independent from the effects of the autonomic nervous system, indeed the term *autoregulation* is an indication of this belief. The peripheral sympathetic system appears to have little effect on cerebral blood flow but much recent research on the cerebral circulation has related to discoveries about the central innervation of cerebral blood vessels and the modulating effects on cerebral blood flow made by the central noradrenergic, dopaminergic and serotonergic systems (Heistad & Marcus 1978, Purves 1978). The effects of neurotransmitter agents have also been studied in detail, and it is now better appreciated that much depends upon whether the agent in the blood stream crosses the blood–brain barrier to be delivered to the vessel wall in the extracellular fluid. Some effects of neurotransmitter on cerebral blood flow are secondary to their effects on brain metabolism (McCulloch & Edvinsson 1984). Another area of intense interest is the vascular actions of eicosanoids in the central nervous system, substances which include the primary prostaglandins (PGE and PGF); cyclic endoperoxides ($PGG_2$, $PGH_2$), prostacyclin, the thromboxanes and leukotrienes. The net effect of these agents on the cerebral circulation may well be determined by the balance between agents that have opposing effects on cerebral blood vessels (Moncada & Vane 1978). Thromboxane $A_2$ is a powerful arterial vasoconstrictor and promotes platelet aggregation. Prostacyclin, in contrast, dilates cerebral vessels and inhibits platelet aggregation. $PGE_1$ is a vasodilator while $PGF_2a$ is a vasoconstrictor. Leukotrienes inhibit prostacyclin synthesis, inhibit platelet aggregation but promote capillary permeability.

Drugs that effect eicosanoid synthesis also have effects on the cerebral circulation, but since several systems may be simultaneously influenced the effects are complex and difficult to interpret. Detailed discussion of these topics is beyond the scope of this book and the reader is referred to recent reviews on this subject

(Walker & Pickard 1985, Leslie & Watkins 1985).

The practising neurosurgeon should be aware of the effects on the cerebral circulation of drugs that are used in neurosurgical practice. Volatile anaesthetic agents such as halothane cause cerebral vasodilation (McDowall 1967). While this may be helpful in ensuring a well perfused brain, the neurosurgeon should be aware that administration of such a vasodilating agent to a patient who has a large brain tumour may result in large, and possibly dangerous, increases in ICP (Jennett *et al.* 1969, Miller 1975). The calcium channel blocking drugs that recently have been introduced have similar effects and should be used with great care in the same circumstances. In contrast, barbiturates and neuroleptanalgesic agents cause a reduction in cerebral blood flow and in brain metabolism. This has been the basis of their application in cases of intracranial hypertension in an endeavour to reduce the ICP. Unfortunately, most of these drugs also act to reduce arterial blood pressure and the arterial hypotension may be proportionally greater than the reduction in ICP, resulting in a net fall in cerebral perfusion pressure (Miller 1985). The effects of mannitol on the cerebral circulation are complex and remain controversial. Mannitol appears to cause a small increase in cerebral blood flow under certain circumstances, and no change in others (Bruce *et al.* 1973). Muizelaar and his colleagues have recently suggested that mannitol causes cerebral vasoconstriction when autoregulation is intact, and have claimed that this is the basis of the reduction in ICP produced by mannitol; when autoregulation is impaired, the small increase in blood pressure and large increase in cardiac output caused by mannitol infusion produce a secondary passive increase in cerebral blood flow and ICP is not reduced (Muizelaar *et al.* 1983, 1984). Other effects of mannitol on ICP are referred to below.

## Brain oedema

The simplest definition of brain oedema is an increase in volume of brain as a result of an increase in brain water content (Fishman 1975). Because this definition depended upon absolute measurements of brain water content *in vitro* it was for many years a definition of interest mainly to pathologists and experimental neurochemists. The water content of the normal brain is 80% of the wet weight in the grey matter, and 68% of the wet weight for white matter. Typical water content values in oedematous brain are 82% in grey matter and 77% in white matter (Pappius & Gulati 1963). Thus in most instances, the increased water content is accommodated mainly in the white matter. This is confirmed by inspection of the oedematous brain *post mortem*. Expansion of the white matter is the most striking finding in nearly all cases. More recently, it has, for the first time, become possible to identify brain oedema *in vivo* by CT or by magnetic resonance imaging of the brain (*see* Chapter 3). These techniques offer the possibility to study the dynamics of formation, resolution and treatment of brain oedema in neurosurgical patients (Penn 1980). Nevertheless, most of the current information on the genesis and propagation of the various forms of brain oedema is still derived from experimental studies.

Of more immediate concern is the persisting confusion that exists regarding the differences between brain swelling and brain oedema, compounded by the fact that many neurosurgeons use the latter term, not in its strict sense as described above, but in the sense of raised intracranial pressure or even clinical deterioration in which some form of brain swelling or expansion or oedema is suspected as a cause. This semantic confusion has a rather long history extending back to the German literature of the 19th Century in which conditions of *Hirnödem* and *Hirnschwellung* were described and separately defined. *Hirnödem* was defined as a state in which the brain at autopsy was soft and swollen, and from the cut surface of which water dripped out; this then was the early definition of brain oedema. *Hirnschwellung* was the term for a state in which the brain was swollen but firm and did not drip water. It was proposed that in this state of brain swelling there was an excess of intracellular water whereas in the case of brain oedema the water was extracellular. In modern terminology both of these states, if truly associated with an increase in brain water content, would be described as brain oedema, in the first case extracellular, and in the second intracellular. Nowadays, the term brain swelling should be restricted to a state in which the increase in brain volume is due to vascular dilation or congestion and it might be better titled 'congestive brain swelling'.

### Causes of brain oedema

Because all forms of brain oedema are associated with an increase in tissue water content, the factor common to all types has to be some increase in the net outflow of water from the vascular bed into brain tissue (Miller 1979). For some years research in this area was made difficult by the mistaken belief that the extracellular space in the brain was negligible and that accumulation of water in brain tissue must therefore be mainly intracellular. This misconception arose at the time of introduction of electron microscopy and was probably related to artifacts produced during the complex fixation and preparation processes that were required for transmission electron microscopy. It is now accepted that in the brain an extracellular space of approximately 20% is present and there is therefore ample space for extravasated water to accumulate between, rather than within, brain cells. Because of the different cellular and structural architecture of grey and white matter, however, it is easier for water to accumulate in white matter where the fibre tracts can be relatively easily separated, in contrast to grey matter, in which there is a much more dense packing of cells and a feltwork of small blood vessels, where it is less easy for water to accumulate in large quantities. This can be envisaged as differences in tissue compliance and accounts for the different increases in water content seen in extracellular brain oedema in grey and white matter. The factors which regulate retention of outflow of water in the capillary bed of the brain are complex and are outwith the scope of this text. They are however, reviewed in detail by Rapoport (1976). As a starting point, however, it is worthwhile to consider the Starling model (1896) in which passage of water across the capillary bed is governed by the relationship:

capillary hydrostatic pressure + tissue colloid osmotic pressure = tissue hydrostatic pressure + plasma colloid osmotic pressure.

From this model it can be deduced that the most important factors disturbing this equilibrium in favour of water passing into the brain will be

**Table 2.1.** Causes of raised intracranial pressure.

| Types of brain oedema | Caused by | Associated with |
|---|---|---|
| Vasogenic | Vessel damage | Tumour, abscess, contusion |
| Cytotoxic | Cell membrane pump failure | a) Hypoxaemia, ischaemia |
|  |  | b) Toxins |
| Hydrostatic | High vascular transmural pressure | Loss of autoregulation; post brain decompression |
| Hypo-osmolar | Low plasma osmotic pressure | Hyponatraemia: dilutional or due to SIADH |
| Interstitial | High CSF pressure | Obstructive hydrocephalus |
| *Other causes of raised ICP* | | |
| Mass lesion | Tumour, abscess, haematoma | Primary intra or extracerebral, secondary (metastatic) |
| CSF accumulation | Hydrocephalus | Developmental; post infection or haemorrhage; obstructive |
| Brain swelling | Increased blood volume | Arterial dilation and hypertension; venous congestion |

increased intravascular hydrostatic pressure, damage to vascular endothelium, causing both water and colloid molecules to pass into the extracellular space, and reduction of plasma colloid osmotic pressure, such as might be induced by severe haemodilution.

When intracellular water accumulation does occur, there will again be a difference between grey and white matter, since most cell bodies lie in the former, with the exception of the special case of the myelin sheath splitting oedemas referred to below.

The first major step in defining different types of oedema was made by Klatzo (1967) who differentiated between vasogenic oedema and cytotoxic oedema. Langfitt and his colleagues (Schutta *et al.* 1968) expanded the definition of oedema to include hydrostatic oedema; Fishman (1975) added in his review of brain oedema the concept of interstitial oedema. Miller (1979) listed and compared six forms of brain oedema. These varying types of brain oedema have different causes and have different therapeutic implications. It is therefore, important for the neurosurgeon to differentiate between them (Table 2.1).

### Vasogenic brain oedema

Klatzo defined this form of brain oedema as arising from damage to the blood brain barrier, following which oedema fluid, consisting of water, sodium and protein, entered the extracellular space. The process begins mostly in grey matter, since this is where most blood vessels lie, but, because of the architecture of the white matter, water accumulates here where the tissue compliance is greater. This form of oedema was produced experimentally by Klatzo and his colleagues by application of intense cold to the cerebral cortex. This produced a small area of ischaemia and necrosis surrounded by a zone of increased vascular permeability from which the oedema fluid diffused widely in finger-like extensions in the white matter. Staining with Evans Blue, to label the protein molecules, showed the spread

of the 'oedema front' from the lesion through the white matter over time. Accumulation of tissue water from such a lesion was maximal between 24 and 72 hours from the time of making the lesion, decreasing and resolving thereafter. The rate of accumulation of tissue water was accelerated by any factor which caused an increase in intravascular pressure or vasodilation, such as elevation of arterial pressure, inhalation of carbon dioxide or pyrexia. Conversely, vasoconstriction and arterial hypotension impede the rate of formation of oedema, but in the latter case at the expense of producing brain tissue ischaemia.

Reulen *et al.* (1978) studied the process of resolution of vasogenic oedema. They were able to trace the passage of labelled extravasated protein molecules across the white matter and ependyma and into the lateral ventricles, where it was postulated that oedema fluid was cleared in the CSF. They discovered that elevated intracranial pressure slowed down the rate of resolution of the oedema, whereas reducing intracranial pressure to normal increased the rate of resolution.

More recently double labelling studies have indicated that the outward spread of oedema into the tissue is more complex than indicated by simply following the rate of spread of labelled protein. It appears that substances of different molecular size and electrical charge migrate at different rates and to a different extent through the white matter extracellular space. Moreover, labelled protein may be taken up by astrocytes and blood vessels during the passage of the 'oedema front' towards the lateral ventricle, and a small proportion of labelled protein even emerges in the lymphatic drainage of the head and neck.

In the clinical context, vasogenic oedema is the form most important to the neurosurgeon. It is this type of oedema that forms around brain tumours, abscesses, brain contusions and in the periphery of cerebral infarcts at the interface with normal brain. It is also this form of oedema that is most effectively treated by steroids.

## Cytotoxic oedema

As originally proposed by Klatzo, this form of oedema is associated with either energy failure in the brain cell or its poisoning by an external toxin. More recently it has been recognized that these probably constitute separate subgroups of cytotoxic oedema. In the first, the energy failure in the cell leads to a breakdown of the pump mechanisms with an efflux of potassium from cells into extracellular space, an influx of sodium, chloride and water with consequent swelling of the cells, particularly astrocytes. Calcium influx sets in motion a chain of destructive processes leading to lipid peroxidation, release of free radicals and further membrane damage. This form of brain oedema is thought to occur in ischaemic cerebral infarcts or in the case of hypoxic brain damage.

The other, toxic, form of cytotoxic brain oedema is induced by the agents triethyltin or hexachlorophene. In both cases, the main defect appears to be in myelin sheaths, the layers of which unravel with accumulation of water between the separated myelin layers. Electron microscopic studies indicate that it is the intracellular part of the myelin sheath that is affected. Because it is within myelin, the water accumulation is largely confined to white matter in the brain. This form of brain oedema is of most interest to the experimental worker.

## Hydrostatic oedema

Schutta et al. (1968) described a form of oedema that was produced by major increases in intravascular pressure in the cranium that were transmitted to the capillary bed because of the absence of the compensatory increase in cerebrovascular resistance in the precapillary segment that would normally protect the capillary bed from the full head of pressure. This failure of the cerebrovascular resistance vessels to constrict may result from direct trauma, excessive arterial hypertension, hypercapnia or hypoxaemia. In this form of oedema, the vascular endo-thelium is not considered to be specifically damaged and the fluid which pours into the extracellular space is not protein rich. Thus it is proposed that the Starling equilibrium is mainly upset because of the increase in intravascular hydrostatic pressure. It is usually a diffuse phenomenon, unlike vasogenic oedema which is focal and clearly related to the causal lesion.

Another model for the production of this form of oedema was proposed by Evans and his associates in Chicago (Ishii et al. 1959). They used an intracranial balloon to induce experimental brain compression almost to the point of tentorial herniation for a period of 24 hours or more. After this, the balloon was abruptly deflated and considerable swelling of the previously compressed brain ensued. Water content measurements of the swollen brain showed this to be due to an extracellular fluid collection of protein poor fluid. There are clearly clinical parallels to this model and every neurosurgeon is familiar with the problem of the patient in whom urgent decompression relieves only temporarily the increased intracranial pressure associated with a large intracranial haematoma, the ICP again rising inexorably over the succeeding hours. In its earlier stages this phenomenon may be to a greater extent an example of congestive brain swelling where the increase in brain bulk is due to distended vessels, but after 24 or 48 hours it can quite clearly be shown on CT that the swollen hemisphere is reduced in radiodensity and is oedematous, progressing to infarction.

## Interstitial oedema

Since the advent of CT it has been recognized that in certain patients with hydrocephalus, notably those cases in which the CSF pressure is high because of an obstructive process, there is a zone of increased radiolucency around the lateral ventricles. It has been suggested that this represents passage of water from the CSF across the ependyma into the periventricular white matter consequent upon the increase in CSF pressure. Not all authorities agree however, on the consistency of this explanation of the findings on CT.

## Hypo-osmotic oedema

It was shown some years ago that experimental reduction of plasma osmolality, usually produced by infusion of distilled water into the peritoneal cavity, could produce elevated ICP and an increase in brain water content (Stern & Coxon 1964, Meinig *et al.* 1973). There is almost certainly a clinical parallel of this model, in which patients with head injury or other forms of brain damage, being managed in an intensive care unit develop hyponatraemia. This may arise as a result of the syndrome of inappropriate secretion of antidiuretic hormone or because of over replacement of electrolyte-rich fluid losses by 5% dextrose solutions intravenously. This is a very real danger in clinical practice. When serum sodium concentration falls below 120 mEq/L, raised intracranial pressure is likely, and if such patients die, diffuse brain oedema is a frequent finding at autopsy.

## The effects of brain oedema

There is no direct evidence that the presence of an increased water content in brain tissue *per se* causes a decrease in cerebral neuroelectrical function. The ill effects of brain oedema are mediated by three mechanisms which are to some extent interlinked. The first of these is elevation of intracranial pressure which results when the volume of extravasated water exceeds the limits of spatial compensation. Eventually the rise in intracranial pressure can reach the point where it becomes a limiting factor for cerebral blood flow so that brain ischaemia results. In the second mechanism it is possible that the accumulation of water in the tissue produces and increase in cerebrovascular resistance because of distortion or compression of the vascular bed and this in turn also results in a decrease in regional cerebral blood flow. In the third mechanism, dys-

function is produced because of the distortion and shift of the brain which results from the mass effect of the area of oedema, particularly when this is of the perifocal vasogenic type. This aspect is discussed in more detail below.

Since cerebral ischaemia may itself be a cause of one type of brain oedema it is not difficult to see how a vicious circle can develop, in which oedema and brain ischaemia become progressive. In this context it is worthwhile to allude to the concept of 'thresholds' in the genesis of ischaemic brain damage. If cerebral blood flow is progressively reduced there is preservation of neuroelectrical function until blood flow falls to less than 40% of control. At this point EEG activity disappears and evoked potential responses are profoundly changed. If flow is immediately restored, neuroelectrical activity returns and there is no structural brain damage. If, however, the reduction in blood flow continues to 30% of control, another threshold is crossed, at which point there is an increase in extracellular potassium concentration, when intracellular stores of potassium are released because the membrane pumps begin to fail. At the same time the level of extracellular calcium falls as these ions migrate into the cells. At this point, brain oedema of the ischaemic, cytotoxic type begins to develop and once this threshold has been crossed the subsequent reperfusion of the brain with restoration of blood flow will serve only to increase the rate of oedema formation (Astrup 1982, Bell *et al.* 1985).

## *In vivo* diagnosis of brain oedema

Increases in brain tissue water content appear on CT as decreases in radiodensity. The pattern of a tumour or brain abscess or contusion surrounded by a halo of decreased radiodensity is now one familiar to neurosurgeons. Often, the finger like extension of oedema fluid in the white matter of the centrum semiovale can be clearly discerned. There are, however, other causes of decreased radiodensity, including brain ischaemia and, as will be clarified in Chapter 3, caution

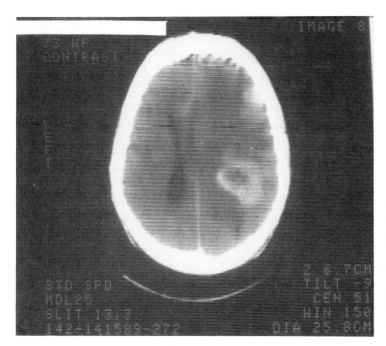

**Fig. 2.8.** Computerized tomographic scan of patient with a right posterior cerebral metastasis from a bronchial carcinoma. There is pronounced surrounding hypodensity, indicative of perifocal oedema. Note the mass effect with effacement of the right lateral ventricle and dilation and shift of the left ventricle from right to left.

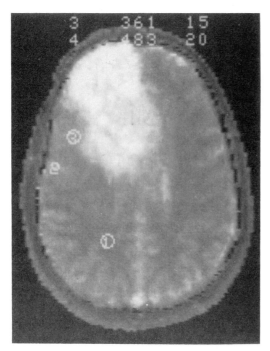

**Fig. 2.9.** Magnetic resonance ($T_1$-weighted) image from a patient with a deep frontal brain tumour (malignant glioma). Note the area of oedema anterior to the tumour, extending to the frontal pole (by courtesy of Professor J.J.K. Best).

needs to be exercised in making the diagnosis of brain oedema on CT (Fig. 2.8).

Because magnetic resonance imaging is largely directed towards the excitation of protons it should be an ideal method for detecting and quantifying changes in brain tissue water content (Fig. 2.9), McDonald *et al.* (1985) have recently compared directly measured brain tissue water content obtained from excised lobectomy species with the $T_1$ relaxation times in corresponding areas of brain subjected to magnetic resonance imaging within 24 hours of surgery. A close correlation was obtained between water content and $T_1$ values in both grey and white matter, confirming the value of this technique and raising the possibility of its use to study the effects *in vivo* of treatments for brain oedema. The treatment of brain oedema will be considered along with the general management of raised intracranial pressure later in this chapter.

# Brain displacements and internal herniation

It is matter of clinical experience that increased ICP is much more serious and poses a greater threat to life if due to a space-occupying lesion than if none is present. An example is in a patient with acute meningitis who may or may not be harbouring a brain abscess. If no abscess is present there is no obstruction to the free flow of CSF through its pathways, pressures in the CSF are of a similar order in different parts of the craniospinal axis and the level of ICP can be lowered by releasing some fluid by lumbar puncture. By contrast, a localized expanding lesion causes displacements of the brain which obstruct the flow of CSF thereby directly aggravating the degree of intracranial hypertension. Relief cannot be obtained by releasing lumbar cerebrospinal fluid because pressures can no longer be equalized; indeed, cisternal or lumbar puncture carried out under these conditions are both potentially highly dangerous. According to the rapidity of expansion of the mass lesion, ischaemia of the adjacent brain may be caused by compression. Dislocation of brain by the mass may lead to interference with its blood supply not immediately explained by the local lesions. This section examines the secondary effects of an expanding intracranial lesion which render it such a dangerous cause for intracranial hypertension. The topic has also been reviewed by Miller and Adams (1984).

With slowly growing tumours, months or years may elapse before symptoms of raised ICP develop. The volume of the tumour is accommodated at first by loss of the subarachnoid CSF space and by indentation and possibly shrinkage of the brain tissue in contact with the tumour. This is a common occurrence in meningioma, for the tumour often forms a deep cavity for itself in the brain (Fig. 2.10). In gliomas the tumour often replaces part of the brain tissue. A rapidly growing malignant glioma may attain a large size, causing severe neurological deficit yet cause little intracranial hypertension because it replaces brain to a degree nearly coextensive

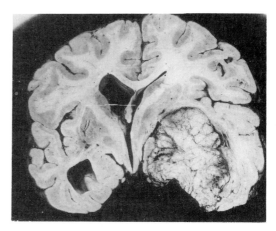

**Fig. 2.10.** Large meningioma arising from floor of middle cranial fossa, deeply embedded in brain and causing atrophy, compression and displacement, but little swelling of the brain tissue.

with its size. However, the brain surrounding a tumour often becomes swollen, recognized by expansion of gyri overlying the tumour and narrowing of the sulci. When the cut surface of the brain is inspected *post mortem*, the swollen part bulges slightly, appears more watery than the rest of the brain and is softer to the touch. This condition is due to peritumoural brain oedema, the nature and aetiology of which have just been considered. The incidence and extent of brain oedema vary considerably but seen to bear some relationship to the rapidity of growth of the tumour and to its nature. The importance in the present context is that the peritumoural oedema is effectively space-occupying and therefore magnifies the mass effect of the tumour itself (Fig. 2.11). When this process is severe, the affected hemisphere is much larger than its fellow and the brain is usually found to fill the dura mater so tightly that little or no CSF is found over the convexity or in subarachnoid CSF cisterns. In this way circulation of the CSF is obstructed and in its turn this further elevates ICP. A delay in return to normal ICP which is particularly common after the removal of large meningiomas is probably due to persistent obstruction of the subarachnoid CSF cisterns. These have been very clearly described by Spatz and Stroescu (1934). Of particular importance is blockage of the peri-

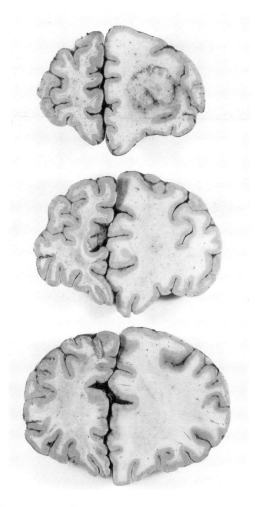

**Fig. 2.11.** A small metastatic carcinoma accompanied by a prounounced degree of oedema.

1   loss of surface subarachnoid space;
2   compression of the ipsilateral ventricle;
3   displacement of midline structures to the opposite side;
4   displacement of the medial part of the temporal lobe through the tentorial hiatus;
5   caudal displacement of the brain stem.

Infratentorial masses cause:

6   compression and displacement of the aqueduct and fourth ventricle;
7   rostral displacement of the superior vermis;
8   caudal displacement of tonsils through the foramen magnum.

These items will be considered in some detail:

1   At autopsy even before the dura is opened the brain can be seen pressed hard against the dural surface. The gyri are flattened against the dura and the surface subarachnoid space is virtually absent.
2   The whole, or only part, of the lateral ventricle may be compressed according to the location of the mass relative to the lobes of the hemisphere, to its depth or superficiality and the degree of surrounding oedema. Generally speaking the further the mass lies from the wall of the ventricle the more diffuse is its effect, as in a chronic subdural haematoma; the nearer the mass is to the ventricle the more restricted is the abnormality so that it may become a rounded mass which encroaches directly on the ventricle. In some cases, as in an abscess with considerable surrounding oedema, the lateral ventricle is reduced to a mere slit. The ventricle is also displaced towards or even across the midline.
3   The medial surface of the hemisphere bulges under the falx. This process is called subfalcine or cingulate herniation. It is more marked with lesions at the anterior part of the hemisphere where the falx is narrow. The pericallosal or callosomarginal arteries may be compressed by the hernia. The third ventricle is compressed from side to side and with the brain stem is displaced towards the opposite side. The displacement of the compressed brain stem can be seen in coronal section on ventriculography, CT

mesencephalic cistern, the cisterna ambiens. Obliteration of this cistern around the midbrain can be identified on CT and is a strong indicator of the presence of raised intracranial pressure (Teasdale *et al.* 1984).

In rapidly growing tumours, serious symptoms demanding attention occur earlier. The increase in the size of the mass and any peritumoural swelling of oedema not only displaces and expands adjacent brain tissue but, in time, causes displacement and compression of more distant structures. Supratentorial masses (Fig. 2.12) cause:

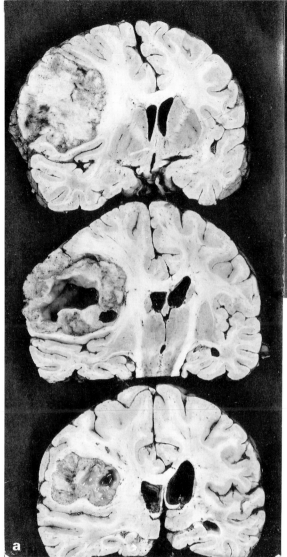

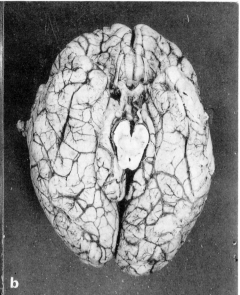

**Fig. 2.12.** Necrotic right frontal metastatic tumour. (a) displacement of midline structures, compression of third ventricle, dilation of opposite lateral ventricle. (b) bilateral herniation of uncus and hippocampus through tentorial hiatus, resulting in characteristic grooving and side-to-side compression of midbrain.

or magnetic resonance scanning; the form of the displacement is an indication of the location of the mass. When the mass is situated in the temporal lobes, the third ventricle remains a vertical slit displaced across the midline to the opposite side. When the mass lesion is situated nearer the vertex the upper part of the third ventricle is tilted to the opposite side. The accompanying compression of the brain stem is usually sufficient to render it obviously flattened and asymmetri-

cal. When this lateral shift is severe, the contralateral crus cerebri is pressed against the sharp edge of the tentorium on the opposite side. This may cause necrosis at the margin of the crus (Fig. 2.13). This is often termed Kernohan's notch following the description by Kernohan and Woltman (1929); they provided excellent histological illustrations of this lesion which may penetrate the cerebral peduncle to considerable depth.

4   The inferior surface of the temporal lobe is

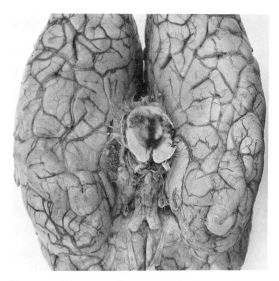

**Fig. 2.13.** Abscess in right temporal lobe: haemorrhagic necrosis of margin of left crus due to compression against tentorial edge (Kernohan's notch).

supported by the tentorium, except for its medial margin, consisting of the uncus and the hippo-campal gyrus, which overlap the free edge of the tentorium to a variable extent. The extent of this overlap is to some extent determined by the size of the tentorial hiatus, variations of which have been studied by Corsellis (1957). Spatial accommodation for a supratentorial mass is to a certain extent gained by displacement of brain through the tentorial opening. If the opening is small only the brain stem is displaced downwards, but if it is of average or larger size, the overlapping margin of the temporal lobe is also displaced downwards over the sharp tentorial edge. The amount of prolapsed brain is related to the extent to which the medial edge of the temporal lobe in company with midline structures is displaced to the opposite side. The tentorium is not flat. It lies obliquely, with its free edge higher in the cranial cavity than its peripheral attachment. The effect in conjunction with the downward thrust on the brain stem and temporal lobe is to impress a deep groove in the uncus and the hippocampal gyrus which is readily identifiable *post mortem*. Necrosis and swelling of the prolapsed brain may lead to its incarceration in the hiatus, wedged between

the free margin of the tentorium and the side of the brain stem. Because of this, the herniation and the damage to the hippocampus and uncus may persist even after the causative mass has been removed; the tentorial hernia can continue to compress the brain stem, with serious results. Lateral displacement of the brain stem is therefore due partly to the general shift of midline structures and partly to temporal lobe herniation.

Temporal lobe herniation is understandably severe and occurs early in expanding lesions within the temporal lobe, but it develops as a result of any expanding lesion above the tentorium. In some cases the great size of the tumour, even at a distance from the tentorial opening, causes massive displacement of intervening brain tissue. In others, severe oedema acts similarly. An extradural or subdural haematoma over the convexity is strategically placed to exert a downward thrust on the hemisphere towards the tentorial opening. Hydrocephalic distention of the lateral ventricles causes a downward thrust on the brain stem and also may be accompanied by bilateral hippocampal herniation.

When the mass lesion is located anteriorly as in a frontal lobe tumour, posteriorly as in an occipital lobe tumour, or bilaterally as in the case of bilateral subdural haematomas, the posterior part of the hippocampal gyri are more involved and produce a herniation through the posterior part of the tentorial hiatus compressing the dorsal aspect of the midbrain including the tectal plate. This is responsible for a different form of clinical presentation, described below.

5  Caudal displacement of the brain stem is of considerable pathophysiological importance. This was pointed out by Scheinker (1945) and in experiments with implanted intracranial balloons by Thompson and Malina (1959) and by Weinstein *et al.* (1968). This downward shift of the brain stem results from a general drift of brain through the tentorial hiatus from a region of high pressure to the infratentorial compartment which has a lower pressure. The brain stem is affected both by intrinsic stresses and

by ischaemia. Johnson and Yates (1956) and Hassler (1967) have shown that the downward displacement of the brain stem produces stretching and narrowing of the mid-line perforating vessels arising from the basilar artery. This may lead to ischaemic necrosis in the brain stem, or to haemorrhage.

6 Compression, deformity and displacement of the aqueduct and the fourth ventricle occur with masses in the posterior cranial fossa. In former times these changes could be clearly demonstrated by ventriculography but are now best demonstrated by magnetic resonance imaging, not as well by CT. The flow of CSF is often obstructed and the rostral portion of the ventricular system, the third and lateral ventricles, dilate.

7 Tumours which occupy a rostral position within the cerebellum may cause upward herniation of the superior vermis or the upper surface of the lateral lobe of the cerebellum through the tentorial hiatus. A more diffuse lesion such as a posterior fossa extradural or subdural haematoma displaces the entire cerebellum upwards and forwards. The shape and obliquity of the tentorium resembles the section of a funnel so that the hernia is wedged against the midbrain, compressing it and displacing it upwards and forwards. The pons and medulla are compressed anteriorly against the clivus.

8 The most common shift of cerebellar structures consequent upon an expanding mass in the posterior fossa is, however, in a caudal direction, through the foramen magnum. This is almost constantly evident in cerebellar lesions. The tonsils are displaced either symmetrically, or one side more than the other, over the dorsolateral aspect of the spinal cord. In severe cases the cerebellar tonsils may be displaced beyond the level of the posterior arch of the second cervical vertebra, the axis (Fig. 2.14).

The first recorded description of tonsillar herniation is possibly that of Spencer and Horsley (1891) but the significance of this form of brain displacement does not appear to have been appreciated until Cushing (1917) noted its presence in some cases of acoustic nerve tumour.

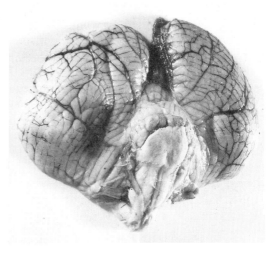

**Fig. 2.14.** Tonsillar herniation in a case of intrinsic cerebellar tumour.

Pathologists have been aware that in the most severe cases the prolapsed tonsils may be necrosed and actually separate from the brain entirely.

### Mesencephalic haemorrhages

At post-mortem examination in cases of severe tentorial herniation, haemorrhages are frequently found in the midbrain and pons. These may be petechial, linear or irregular, extending axially for several centimetres, even into the internal capsule. The haemorrhages usually occupy the tegmental portion of the brain stem near the midline and parallel to it. In some cases haemorrhages are absent but softening and necrosis are present, indicative of ischaemic damage. It is now generally agreed that these haemorrhages are of arterial origin, though Moore and Stern (1938) and Scheinker (1945) thought previously that they were venous in origin.

The close association of midbrain haemorrhage with tentorial herniation makes it likely that mechanical deformation or dislocation of the brain stem is the major factor in their causation. It is exceptional for them to occur if the tumour is infratentorial. Displacement of the brain caudally necessarily carries with it the perforating branches of the basilar artery while the artery itself is linked through the elements of the circle of Willis with the carotid arteries which are anchored to the skull base. Transtentorial axial displacement of the brain stem therefore leads to stretching and even rupture of the central perforating branches of the basilar artery. This has been elegantly demonstrated by the post-mortem injection studies of Hassler (1967). Furthermore, Johnson and Yates (1956) pointed out that when the brain stem is compressed from side to side its anteroposterior diameter is thereby increased; since the central perforating branches of the basilar artery traverse the anteroposterior diameter, these are elongated and therefore narrowed, contributing further to ischaemia in their territories of distribution.

Klintworth (1966) commented on the frequency of brain stem haemorrhage following surgical decompression of lesions that had led to extensive tentorial herniation. He offered the opinion that the subsequent reperfusion of the affected brain stem vessels following decompression might lead to bleeding in areas of previous infarction and thereby be responsible for the haemorrhages.

### Cortical infarction

Haemorrhagic infarction of the calcarine cortex and subcortical white matter is a further recognized complication of tentorial herniation. It may coexist with brain stem haemorrhages or occur with a macroscopically normal brain stem. The lesion is usually unilateral on the side of a temporal lobe hernia and lies within the territory of the posterior cerebral artery. The lesion was at one time considered to result from venous infarction but is now generally believed to result from distortion of the posterior cerebral artery due to advancing uncal and hippocampal gyrus herniation, leading to such a low rate of perfusion through that vessel that ischaemic infarction ensues.

Cortical infarction can also be found in the territory of distribution of the pericallosal or callosomarginal arteries and is ascribed to a similar mechanism during subfalcine herniation. Infarction also occurs in the posterior hypothalamus and pituitary gland (Wolman 1953), and is thought to be due to mechanical distortion of the blood vessels in the pituitary stalk.

Cortical infarction elsewhere in the brain has to be ascribed to a different mechanism. At some point in the evolution of an intracranial mass lesion, ICP begins to increase in the supratentorial compartment and and will eventually reach a level at which the perfusion pressure falls below the autoregulatory threshold and widespread brain ischaemia results. The fall in perfusion pressure may be delayed for a time because of the development of paroxysmal elevations of arterial pressure, the Cushing response, triggered off by either mechanical distortion of the lower brain stem or focal ischaemia. When ischaemic brain damage does occur, due to raised ICP in the supratentorial compartment, it is not entirely uniform in distribution. There is some predilection for the arterial boundary zones between the anterior and middle and the middle and posterior cerebral arteries; infarction also occurs in the basal ganglia, and there is the selective vulnerability of certain cell layers in the cerebral cortex and in parts of Ammon's horn (Adams & Graham 1976, Graham et al. 1978). Eventually the Cushing response begins to fail and arterial hypotension due to medullary failure ensues. At this point cerebral ischaemia becomes generalized and severe and brain death usually ensues.

The importance of internal brain herniations is therefore, two-fold. These mechanical responses of the viscoelastic properties of brain tissue produce actual movements of tissue with obstruction of the normal pathways of CSF absorption in the subarachnoid space generally, and particularly around the midbrain. Consequently, they play a large part in elevating intracranial pressure. The shifts of brain tissue also give rise to clinical disturbances which by reason of their intensity or extent can overshadow or even obliterate those signs produced by the causative lesion. This is particularly the case from frontal lobe or anterior temporal lobe lesions.

As early as 1898, Hill wrote of 'pressure discontinuity' between the cerebral and cerebellar chambers and between the cranial and vertebral cavities effected by plugging of the isthmus tentorii cerebelli and the foreman magna by the translocation of the brain mass. Spencer and Horsley described tonsillar herniation and Cushing called this foraminal impaction. The definitive clinical descriptions of herniation are those of Meyer (1920), Vincent *et al.* (1936) and Jefferson (1938). Sunderland (1958) has provided meticulous reproductions of anatomical dissections to show the relationships of structures at the level of the tentorial opening and a monograph by Finney and Walker (1962) emphasized the clinical importance of the syndrome of tentorial herniation, found in the vast majority of fatalities from cerebral hemisphere glioma, and provided a comprehensive account of the syndrome and the early descriptions of it.

Smyth and Henderson (1938) performed simultaneous ventricular and lumbar puncture in patients with raised ICP due to brain tumours and confirmed in a small number of cases that the supratentorial pressure was significantly greater than the spinal pressure. In all of these cases in which a pressure gradient was demonstrated, tentorial herniation was confirmed *post mortem*. In cases in which the ventricular and spinal pressures were equal, no tentorial herniation was found. These important findings were confirmed much later by Kaufmann and Clark (1970). They demonstrated, in a series of cases terminating fatally, that if the intraventricular pressure was more than 10 mmHg greater than spinal CSF pressure subsequent post-mortem confirmed tentorial herniation. In patients with a smaller or absent pressure differential tentorial herniation was not present. Langfitt *et al.* (1964) carried out an extensive series of experiments in primates and conclusively demonstrated the genesis of transtentorial pressure gradients during the course of inflation of a supratentorial intracranial balloon.

Fitch and MacDowall (1971) made important contributions to understanding the dynamics of transtentorial herniation and development of pressure gradients. They inflated a supratentoral balloon to the point where tentorial herniation was imminent but had not yet fully occurred. Maintaining the balloon volume constant they then administered the anaesthetic agent halothane to the subjects and observed that this drug, which produces cerebral vasodilation, caused a considerable increase in ICP above the tentorium but not below; simultaneously ipsilateral pupillary dilation, indicative of transtentorial herniation, developed. These findings have also been confirmed using carbon dioxide inhalation to produce cerebral vasodilation. Fitch and McDowall (1977) also studied the development of the systemic vasopressor response with this model.

Thompson and Malina (1959) studied the respiratory and cardiovascular responses to elevation of ICP and found the threshold for production of such responses lower when pressure was raised primarily in the supratentorial compartment than when it was evenly raised by fluid injected into the lumbar theca. The threshold to a given supratentorial increase of pressure could be lowered by decompressing the posterior cranial fossa, thereby preventing any rise in pressure below the tentorium. These investigators concluded that the trigger to the cardiorespiratory responses were the physical effects of distortion of the brain stem on its nervous activity rather than brain stem ischaemia, a finding supported by Hoff and Reis (1970). Jennett and Stern (1960) carried out experiments to investigate the cause of the pupillary dilation that occurs during tentorial herniation, studying closely the means by which the oculomotor nerve was distorted during the process of tentorial herniation. The location of this nerve between the posterior cerebral and superior cerebellar arteries makes it particularly vulnerable to uncal herniation through the tentorial hiatus.

More recent studies by Sullivan *et al.* (1978) and Takizawa *et al.* (1986) on the genesis of transtentorial pressure gradients have shown that, with progressive inflation of an intracranial balloon, ICP rises in both compartments at an equal rate until a pressure of approximately 20 mmHg is obtained. Thereafter, the rate of increase in ICP differs in both compartments. ICP still continues to rise in the infratentorial compartment, but at a slower rate, so that as supratentorial pressure rises there is a progressive underestimate of its level by measurements taken from below the tentorium. By carrying out bolus injections of fluid into the CSF spaces above and below the tentorium during balloon inflation, Takizawa *et al.* were able to demonstrate that with each bolus a small volume of fluid can pass across the tentorial hiatus, but that it appears that fluid can pass more easily in an upward direction than in a downward direction. The reasons for this are not yet clear but may be simply mechanical, related to the funnel-like shape of the tentorial hiatus.

### Neurogenic pulmonary oedema

The association between raised ICP and disturbances of the rate and rhythm of respiration are well known. Plum and Posner (1980) suggest that different disturbances of respiratory rate and rhythm have a localizing significance for dysfunction at a particular location in the depths of the hemispheres or in the brain stem. North and Jennett (1974) disputed this claim but noted the increasing frequency of respiratory disorders with structural lesions that involve the brain stem as compared with lesions confined to the cerebral hemispheres.

Neurogenic pulmonary oedema is much less common, although much more dramatic. In a patient, usually young, who is severely ill with brain damage that involves brain stem structures, the abrupt onset of pulmonary oedema is signalled by a profuse outpouring of frothy pink fluid from the airways, tachypnoea, cyanosis, tachycardia and arterial hypotension. The condition is frequently fatal even if the intracranial hypertension is relieved. Although the term 'neurogenic' has been applied to this condition,

its cause is not yet clear. Autonomic discharges from the brain stem have been suggested as a cause by Ducker *et al.* (1968), while Millen and Glauser (1983) have shown that in an experimental model of concussive head injury prodromal stages of pulmonary oedema formation exist even with fairly low intensity injuries. It is likely that the dramatic syndrome described represents only the extreme end of a spectrum of pulmonary dysfunction which frequently occurs related to brain damage. In its mildest form this would be detected only by the measurement of an abnormal oxygen tension gradient between the alveolar and arterial gases (Cooper & Boswell 1983, Frost 1979).

### Clinical signs of brain herniation

Herniations of the brain not only aggravate intracranial hypertension but give rise to recognizable clinical syndromes, recognition of which is of the greatest importance in assessing the urgency of the conditions. In some patients, the neurological disturbance characteristic of the site and nature of the original causative lesion may be similar to the effects of herniation and the latter will only constitute an aggravation of these signs. In other patients however, the primary lesion may produce little or no neurological deficit and the manifestations of the herniation syndrome may be erroneously attributed to a primary lesion. Herniation can produce signs which appear incompatible with the suspected localization of the tumour, so called false localizing signs. These may be such as to lead to a diagnosis of a lesion on the wrong side of the brain, for example ipsilateral hemiparesis in a case of subdural haematoma. It is important therefore, to consider the symptoms and signs of brain herniation at this point rather than in the section and diagnosis of tumours because these signs are common to all varieties of expanding intracranial lesions whether these be tumours, abscesses or haematomas and they clearly represent a special and crucial part of the clinical picture associated with raised intracranial pressure.

## Clinical signs of temporal lobe herniation

Herniation of the uncus and of the hippocampal gyrus over the sharp free edge of the tentorium causes progressive enlargement of the ipsilateral pupil which loses its reaction to light, whether stimulated directly or consensually. Ptosis develops in the same eye, and if the patient has not lost consciousness, examination of the movements of the eye reveals weakness of the superior and medial rectus muscles appropriate to the third nerve palsy. Post-mortem observations confirm that the oculomotor paralysis can be caused in various ways. Pressure of the herniating uncus downwards onto the nerve which lies immediately ventral is perhaps the commonest cause and has been demonstrated experimentally by Reid and Cone (1939). In some cases, grooving of the ventral surface of the nerve is seen to have been produced by counter pressure against the petroclinoid ligament (Cairns 1939) or against the lateral margin of the clivus (Fischer-Brugge 1951) or the nerve may be grooved on its upper surface by the posterior cerebral artery which is dragged downwards by the transtentorial caudal shift of brain stem (Sunderland & Bradley 1953). Sunderland and Hughes (1946) pointed out that the pupilloconstrictor fibres in the oculomotor nerve are concentrated in its upper part as it passes from midbrain to the cavernous sinus. Pupillary dilation is likely to be due to damage to the superior part of the nerve at an early stage and this, therefore, favours the mechanism of damage by the posterior cerebral artery as the most important contributor to the syndrome.

Displacement of the temporal lobe medially causes pressure on the lower part of the internal capsule, and the medial margin of the hippocampus will compress the crus cerebri. Either or both give rise to a contralateral weakness which may rapidly progress to a spastic hemiplegia with exaggerated tendon reflexes and extensor plantar responses. In the later stages the limbs adopt the abnormal flexion or extensor postures sometimes termed decorticate and decerebrate respectively. The decorticate or abnormally flexed posture indicates that the internal capsule is mainly affected, the decerebrate or extensor posture that the herniation is mainly affecting the midbrain. Unilateral extensor rigidity may be accompanied by deviation of the head and eyes upwards and to the opposite side due to transtentorial displacement and pressure in the pretectal region (Denny-Brown 1962). Spasm of the neck muscles and the hamstrings is often present in the early stages of temporal lobe herniation. This is a valuable sign and should not be mistakenly ascribed to meningism.

As herniation increases in severity, the signs become bilateral. Both pupils are dilated and nonreactive, all four limbs spastic and paralysed in a symmetrical state of extensor rigidity. The spinal muscles take part in the extensor rigidity so that the head is extended and the back arched in the position of opisthotonus, a posture peculiar to man. All tendon reflexes are exaggerated, although the rigidity may be so severe as to make them impossible to elicit. Both plantar responses are extensor. Painful stimulation only evokes more severe rigidity. At this late stage the lateralizing signs previously present have now been lost so that there are no longer means of deciding on which side of the brain the compressive process has started except from history or earlier observations.

By the time that transtentorial herniation has caused unilateral pupillary dilation the level of consciousness has usually fallen and when hemiplegia develops the patient is deeply unconscious, making only reflex movements to painful stimuli. During this period of deterioration, the body temperature commonly rises, episodes of general flushing and sweating occur; the pulse rate slows, blood pressure usually increases the respirations deepen and may become periodic in rhythm. Without appropriate treatment, the patient may go on to develop pulmonary oedema, the heart rate quickens and the blood pressure falls and death occurs from respiratory arrest. In individual patients the sequence of bradycardia followed by tachycardia, and arterial hypertension followed by hypotension may not occur;

the clinical lesson is that although bradycardia and rising blood pressure are typical, they are not essential for a diagnosis of increased ICP with transtentorial herniation.

Preceding and during the evolution of extensor rigidity there may be remarkable episodic fluctuations in the clinical state, occurring several times within an hour. They may arise spontaneously or be evoked by a stimulus such as passive limb movement. The conscious patient experiences headache of the violent paroxysmal variety described earlier, may vomit and becomes drowsy, inattentive, or confused and restless; within a few seconds or minutes bilateral decerebrate rigidity and opisthotonus can develop, together with the vegetative disturbances described above; thereafter the patient's condition may return to the previous state. In patients already exhibiting the extensor state there may be a temporary increase of rigidity and other signs. These episodes have long been recognized under various descriptions such as cerebellar seizures (Stewart and Holmes 1904) or tonic fits (Kinnier Wilson 1920), but are now recognized as manifestations of tentorial herniation.

Continuous recording of intraventricular pressure coupled with close observation of the clinical state of a large number of patients with brain tumours and other supratentorial lesions by Lundberg (1960) shed much light on the aetiology and associations of these clinical states.

Lundberg distinguished three patterns of spontaneous fluctuation of ICP. 'A' waves or plateau waves occurred at intervals of 30 minutes or more and consisted of a steep spontaneous rise of pressure from normal or near normal values to a plateau at between 50 and 100 mmHg remaining at that level for 5 to 20 minutes, or sometimes even longer followed by a spontaneous decrease to normal levels (Fig. 2.15). During the periods of intracranial hypertension, patients would show worsening of the extensor state if this was present and/or signs of vegetative dysfunction such as headache, facial flushing, but often remarkably little in the way of cardiovascular changes. Further studies by Risberg *et al.* (1969) have shown that these plateau waves coincide with periods of increased cerebral blood volume and it is now considered that the plateau wave results from a combination of cerebrovascular dilation and increased blood volume occurring at a time of reduced craniospinal compliance, when the pressure volume curve is steeply configured. Rosner and Becker (1983) have proposed that the most common trigger to vasodilation is a critical reduction in cerebral perfusion pressure produced either by a fall in arterial pressure or a small preliminary rise in ICP.

'B' waves as described by Lundberg consisted of peaked waves of intracranial pressure with a periodicity of once every 0.5–2 minutes (Fig. 2.16). In some patients these waves coincide

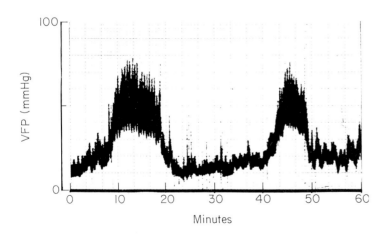

**Fig. 2.15.** Chart recording of ventricular fluid pressure (VFP) showing Lundberg A waves.

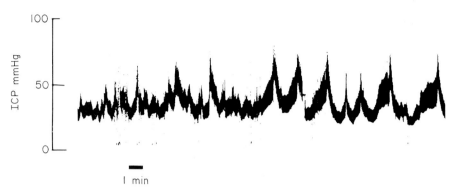

**Fig. 2.16.** Chart recording of intracranial pressure (ICP) showing typical Lundberg B waves.

with periodic respiration and are thought to represent phasic changes in arterial $PCO_2$ levels and therefore, changes in cerebral blood volume related to the degree of vasoconstriction or vasodilation that is present. In other patients however, 'B' waves can be demonstrated during periods of artificial ventilation, when arterial $PCO_2$ levels remain constant. The waves are however, considered to represent alterations in cerebral blood volume. Finally, 'C' waves occur at a higher frequency than 'A' or 'B' waves and are related to phasic changes in arterial blood pressure.

Because of the association between plateau waves, cerebral vasodilation and episodes of severe headache, it has been suggested that the headaches associated with raised intracranial pressure originate from cerebral arteries and perhaps veins (Northfield 1938, 1968).

The speed at which events develop varies considerably. If the lesion is an extradural haematoma, the patient may be in deep coma, with periodic respiration and bilateral extensor rigidity within three hours of the accident. If the lesion is a tumour, the same picture may take several days to evolve. However, oedema around the tumour, expansion in the size of the tumour by cyst formation or spontaneous haemorrhage and swelling of herniating brain increase the rate of clinical progress unpredictably. For this reason, the clinical signs of tentorial herniation always indicate a clinical situation of grave urgency.

Some variations occur, related to the site of the primary brain compression. Massive frontal lobe lesions may give rise to bilateral ptosis, defective upward conjugate movements of the eyes and fixed dilated pupils before consciousness is lost. Johnson (1957) has pointed out that brain displacement in an anteroposterior direction drives the undersurfaces of the occipital lobes downwards through the posterior part of the tentorial hiatus onto the dorsum of the midbrain in the region of the superior colliculi. Similar herniation occurs in chronic subdural haematoma and in hydrocephalus; in the latter the pressure on the midbrain may be due to a distended suprapineal CSF pouch. In infants with severe hydrocephalus, the eyeballs are often deviated downwards, due probably to similar mechanisms; this is the so-called 'sunset sign'. Improvement in the range of eye movement follows reduction of ICP and the hydrocephalus by appropriate CSF shunting procedures.

### Clinical signs of cerebellar herniation

Tonsillar herniation gives rise to painful neck stiffness, aggravated by movement. Passive flexion of the neck may give rise to sensations like electric shocks travelling down the trunk, the sign of L'Hermitte. The neck stiffness may be mistaken for meningism and young patients with cerebellar tumours may mistakenly be subjected to lumbar puncture with disastrous consequences. Occasionally, direct pressure of the cerebellar tonsils upon the posterior columns of the upper cervical cord causes impairment of postural sensibility and counter pressure against the rim of the foramen magnum may interfere with conduction in the pyramidal and spinothalamic pathways. The clinical evidence for this is extensor plantar responses and diminution of sensation below the collar level. These signs may disappear after posterior fossa decompression.

Dysarthria, vomiting, drowsiness, ataxia and slowing of respiration are probably effects of the direct thrust of the mass lesion exerted on the pons and medulla. Jefferson and Johnson (1950) drew attention to loss of consciousness in expanding lesions in the posterior fossa describing this as 'a trance like state resembling normal sleep'.

Upward herniation of the cerebellar vermis through the tentorial opening should be suspected if there are attacks of extensor rigidity, so called 'cerebellar fits'. It is important to obtain a clear description of such phenomena for their confusion with an epileptic convulsion may lead to the erroneous diagnosis of a supratentorial lesion. Upward herniation through the tentorial hiatus may be precipitated by abrupt and overzealous ventricular drainage in cases of obstructive hydrocephalus due to posterior fossa mass lesions.

Sudden death is liable to occur when cerebellar herniation is marked, usually as a result of sudden respiratory arrest, or less frequently because of vomiting and aspiration. It may occur in a patient who, until moments before, was conscious, speaking and obeying commands.

Brain herniation is a final outcome of rising intracranial pressure, in the sense that if it is not relieved rapidly it causes the death of the patient. Early recognition of herniation syndromes and appropriate treatment are matters of the gravest urgency. Treatment undertaken after the brain stem has already sustained ischaemic damage is unlikely to sustain life, or, perhaps worse, the patient may never regain consciousness but survive, decerebrate, in a persistent vegetative state (Jennett & Plum 1972).

The clinical picture of herniation gradually evolves from that of mounting intracranial pressure; the early signs are slight and may easily escape notice. Severe and rapidly worsening headache, vomiting, a fall in the level of consciousness and slowing of the pulse rate should lead one to suspect incipient herniation. Inequality of the pupils, skew deviation of the eyes, neck stiffness, a positive Kernig sign, deepening or irregularity of respiration with the use of accessory muscles are among the early changes. Minimal increases in limb tone, less restlessness on one side compared with the other, a suggestion of pronator movements of the limbs, squirming or athetoid distortion of otherwise normal movements may be noticed by the careful observer before any disturbance of reflexes or more obvious postural abnormality appears. Flinging or ballistic types of movement of the arms not infrequently occur before the development of rigidity. These subtle signs, often regarded as simple restlessness, correspond to disturbance of the pretectal region as described by Denny-Brown (1962).

**False localizing signs**

Collier set down in 1904 the important diagnostic principle that 'local signs appearing late in the course of intracranial tumours where general signs alone have pre-existed are often of false portent'. The late appearance of abnormal neurological signs may be due to a rapid change within a tumour such as a haemorrhage but these late signs may be incongruous with the presumptive localization. If so they are commonly due to pressure on remote structures by an internal brain hernia. Oculomotor nerve palsy has already been described. Abducens palsy had been ascribed to tension of this thin long nerve by caudal shift of the pons but Cushing (1910) demonstrated that the nerve was grooved by the internal auditory artery against which it was compressed. Trigeminal pain and sensory loss may be caused by a plug of brain herniating through a deficiency in the dural covering of the Gasserian ganglion, or herniation of cerebellar tissue into Meckel's cave. Occasionally, a peripheral type of facial palsy is seen in a patient whose tumour is remote from the facial nerve. Herniation of tumour or brain into the internal auditory meatus is the likely explanation. Ipsilateral hemiparesis arises from grooving of the contralateral cerebral peduncle or crus by the tentorium as has been mentioned earlier. If there is no other evidence of lateralization the lesion may be diagnosed in the wrong hemisphere. This false localizing sign (associated with the pathological change of Kernohan's notch) usually occurs in slowly developing lesions such as meningioma or chronic subdural haematoma. Gradual displacement of the brain stem provides sufficient time for blood vessels to accommodate in the presence of these chronic lesions, and pressure on the contralateral cerebral peduncle occurs before ischaemia of the brain stem. The sign is also seen in slowly growing tumours situated laterally in the posterior cranial fossa such as large acoustic nerve tumours. Transient or permanent hemianopia as a false localizing sign can be very confusing because it is readily accepted as evidence of an occipital mass lesion. It results, however, from ischaemia of the calcarine cortex as a result of impairment of circulation through the posterior cerebral artery. This clinical sign is, however, extremely rare because so few patients in whom tentorial herniation is of this degree of severity are conscious or survive; the finding is much more common in fatal cases proceeding to autopsy. Gassel (1961) provides an interesting analysis of the false localizing signs in a large series of patients with frontal meningiomas.

At the beginning of this chapter, emphasis was placed on the need to distinguish the symptoms and signs of raised intracranial pressure from those of the causative lesion. To this may be added the need to further distinguish the symptoms and signs of brain herniation and shift. Finally, there must be accurate assessment of the speed of evolution of these three symptomatic components. The importance of this lies, not only in the capacity to refine the differential diagnosis,

but as a guide to the urgency with which investigative and management measures must be carried out.

## Monitoring of intracranial pressure

Although short duration measurements of CSF pressure from the lumbar subarachnoid space and from the lateral ventricles have been obtainable for over a hundred years the possibility of making long term continuous measurements and registration of CSF pressure was not possible until the development of the electronic pressure transducer after the Second World War. Guillaume and Janny made their first observations on continuous monitoring of intraventricular pressure in neurosurgical patients in 1951. Unfortunately, their observations went largely unheeded until they were referred to by Lundberg (1960) in his classic dissertation *Continuous Recording and Control of Ventricular Fluid Pressure in Neurosurgical Practice*. In this work, which should be read by every neurosurgeon, Lundberg describes in full detail prolonged continuous measurements of CSF pressure made from a catheter placed in the frontal horn of the lateral ventricle of more than a hundred patients suffering from a wide variety of neurosurgical disorders. The relationships between the various forms of elevated ICP, including the waves already described, and the clinical status of the patient, the heart rate, the blood pressure and other physiological variables are all presented with the greatest lucidity. In addition, Lundberg was able to show that this procedure carried a minimal risk of complications by infection or haemorrhage. Despite that, neurosurgeons were rather slow to adopt this form of continuous monitoring of brain state in severely ill patients. A further ten years were to elapse before the technique of continuous monitoring of ICP came into general neurosurgical use, aided by the widespread development of intensive care units in which surgical, and then neurosurgical, patients were nursed. Langfitt, more than anyone, was responsible for drawing the attention of the world of

neurosurgery to the valuable contribution made
by Lundberg.

For full information on the experimental and
clinical applications of intracranial pressure
monitoring the reader is referred to the six volumes of *Proceedings of International Intracranial
Pressure Symposia*. Only a brief account will be
given here of the indications, methods, risks, data
analysis and findings of intracranial pressure
monitoring in neurosurgical patients. In general
terms, comatose patients being nursed in an
intensive care unit, are potential candidates for
ICP monitoring. If the patient is to be paralysed
and artificially ventilated then there are strong
indications for continuous measurement of both
arterial and intracranial pressure (so that the
calculated perfusion pressure can also be measured). In terms of disease conditions, the most
common current indications for ICP monitoring
are severe head injury, followed by hydrocephalus, by subarachnoid haemorrhage associated with depression of the conscious level, followed by smaller numbers of patients suffering
from post hypoxic encephalopathy, encephalitis
and meningitis, metabolic disorders, and a number with brain tumours, both supra- and infratentorial, awaiting surgical treatment (Miller
1978).

The standard against which all methods of ICP
measurement have to be compared remains the
intraventricular catheter attached by a fluid filled
line to an external transducer. This provides a
fathful record of the pressure, and recalibration
and zero resetting can be easily carried out; the
disadvantages lie in the necessity of puncturing
the brain and in locating the lateral ventricle
which may be narrowed in cases of head injury
or brain swelling due to infective or metabolic
causes. Alternative means of intracranial pressure measurement are to insert a screw in the
skull after opening the dura and connect this via
a fluid-filled line to an external transducer, thus
measuring ICP from the supratentorial subdural
space or simply to insert a fluid-filled catheter
directly into the space. If ICP rises above
30 mmHg there is an increasing tendency for
the true ICP to be underestimated by subdural

measurements (Mendelow *et al.* 1983). Minia-
ture pressure transducers are now available
which can be inserted into the extradural or
subdural space and the most modern of these
have facilities for resetting the atmospheric zero
level *in situ*. The risks of ICP monitoring have
recently been reviewed by Mayhall *et al.* (1984).

The signal from the pressure transducer can
be displayed on a bed head monitor, either in
analogue or in digital form, but there remains a
considerable advantage in recording the pressure
fluctuations on a continuous feed paper chart
recorder. The pattern of elevation of ICP over
time may be just as important as the absolute
level at any moment, which may in any case
fluctuate considerably from minute to minute.
With increasing application of microchip computer technology to bedside monitoring systems
it is also possible to process ICP and arterial
pressure data so as to produce a condensed record over time, to store it in memory, and to
perform simple calculations such as computation
of pulse pressure and perfusion pressure and the
ratio between these two variables. When a continuous record of ICP is required in a patient
this should always include at least one period
of pressure recording overnight. This is because
more than two thirds of pathological elevations
of ICP occur at night, related to episodes of cerebral vasodilation occuring during sleep (Hulme
and Cooper 1968, Marshall *et al.* 1978). It may
be as important to exclude high intracranial pressure as it is to confirm it, for if ICP is normal the
patient can be spared needless therapy.

Normal intracranial pressure, under the usual
conditions of bedside monitoring in the neurosurgical intensive care unit, lies between zero
and two kPa (0–15 mmHg). The neurosurgeon
should be aware of the simple factors which may
either spuriously increase the pressure or may
result in an inaccurately low pressure. Common
causes of elevation of ICP include incorrect placement of an external transducer, which should be
on a level with the upper level of the cranial
subarachnoid space. If the patient's head has
been elevated and the transducer not raised by
a corresponding amount, then an erroneous

record of intracranial pressure will be obtained, increased by the hydrostatic pressure difference between the level of the patient's head and the level of the transducer. Other causes for elevated ICP are obstruction of neck veins due to flexion of the neck or turning the head too far to one side or the other. The patient who is coughing or straining against a ventilator because muscle relaxants have worn off will also exhibit high ICP, as will the patient who has an elevation of body temperature. The patient's airway should also be checked for obstruction due to bronchial secretions or gastric aspirate.

An unexpectedly low ICP is generally due to a fault in the measuring system, usually a leak of fluid from a poorly fitting joint. Another common cause of under reading of the true ICP is blockage of the recording system either by collapse of the ventricles around the ventricular catheter or by herniation of brain tissue into the end of a sub-dural screw or catheter. Finally, it must be remembered that a sudden fall in arterial pressure will also cause a reduction in ICP.

## Management of raised intracranial pressure

When applying treatment, the neurosurgeon must be clear what is being treated. Is it raised ICP, brain oedema or brain shift and herniation? This is of extreme importance because a treatment that significantly reduces ICP may have no beneficial effect whatsoever on brain shift, indeed it may even make it worse. In the modern neuro-surgical and intensive care unit, with the patient paralysed and artificially ventilated, there is a very real risk that treatment for raised ICP may be pursued to the detriment of certain patients with intracranial mass lesions, such as haema-tomas, in whom the real need is to evacuate the mass lesion and thus remove the cause of both the intracranial hypertension and the brain shift. In the common situation where the neuro-surgeon is working in partnership with the anaesthetist this possibility must be borne in mind at all times and by all concerned. In intro-

Table 2.2. Treatment for raised intracranial pressure.

| General measures | clear airway, ensure free respiration |
| | ensure adequate circulation |
| | correct neck flexion or rotation |
| | head up tilt |
| | reduce elevated body temperature |
| | correct hyponatraemia |
| Induced cerebral vasoconstriction | hyperventilation |
| | hyperbaric oxygen |
| | hypothermia |
| Osmotherapy | mannitol |
| | glycerol |
| | urea |
| Anaesthetic agents | thiopentone |
| | pentobarbitone |
| | gamma hydroxybutyrate |
| | althesin* |
| | etomidate* |
| Other agents | frusemide |
| | acetazolamide |
| | lignocaine |
| | dimethyl sulphoxide |

*Not available for use in UK.

ducing this section, therefore, it must be empha-sized that wherever possible, the best treatment for raised intracranial pressure, brain oedema and brain shift herniation is the removal of the causative lesion, whether this be a haematoma, an abscess or a tumour. That said, it is possible to outline a strategy for management of these major neurosurgical problems (Table 2.2).

### Symptomatic treatment

Headache is often eased by rest in bed with the head and shoulders elevated and by simple anal-gesics such as acetyl salicylic acid, paracetamol or codeine phosphate. More severe headaches may call for stronger analgesic agents, but head-ache of this severity suggests high ICP and meas-ures directed at reducing the intracranial pres-sure should be instituted forthwith. Morphine or other analgesic drugs with respiratory depress-ant properties should not be given. They may ease the pain but the depressed respiration induces retention of carbon dioxide, promotes cerebral vasodilation and thereby increases the ICP. This renders the patient more drowsy, makes diagnosis more difficult and, when the raised ICP is unevenly distributed in the intracranial compartments, may promote transtentorial herniation.

Vomiting is often relieved by rest, by limiting the amounts taken by mouth although if this is severe, nasogastric suction may be required. Cyclizine or other antimetic drugs may have some effect but should not be given in doses sufficient to make the patient drowsy.

Although the exact level of increased ICP at which brain function is disturbed varies depending upon the cause of the intracranial hypertension, it is of practical value to nominate a level of ICP above which management measures should be instituted in the intensive care unit. The most frequently used level is 25 mmHg mean. When ICP exceeds this level for more than two minutes the nursing staff should immediately check for the obvious causes of intracranial hypertension outlined above and if these are not present, or their correction fails to reduce ICP, medical staff should be notified and the first in an orderly series of treatment measures instituted.

### Hyperventilation

The principle of hyperventilation is that it reduces arterial $PCO_2$, induces cerebral vasoconstriction which in turn reduces the pressure and blood volume in the capillary bed and venous capacitance part of the circulation. This, in turn, causes a reduction in CSF pressure. In practice, lowering of arterial $PCO_2$ from 5 to 3 kPa (37–22 mmHg) causes approximately 30% reduction in ICP. There is also a reduction in cerebral blood flow, and if hyperventilation is pronounced, there may be some physiological changes suggestive of brain hypoxia such as appearance of slow waves on the electroencephalogram. There is however, no evidence that hyperventilation can produce such profound cerebral ischaemia as to cause structural brain damage, but further hyperventilation will fail to produce further cerebral vasoconstriction. Extreme hyperventilation by intermittent positive pressure ventilation can in certain cases cause arterial hypotension due to interference with the venous return to the heart because of the high levels of intrathoracic pressure that are generated. For this reason it is imperative to monitor the arterial pressure in all patients in whom ICP is being measured and, when applying treatment for raised ICP, to ensure that this treatment does not result in arterial hypotension. It cannot be emphasized sufficiently that if intracranial hypertension is bad for the patient then arterial hypotension is even worse.

### The role of dehydration

For many years it was considered desirable to induce a mild degree of dehydration in patients with raised intracranial pressure. This was produced by magnesium sulphate enemas and a decrease in the intravenous fluid intake. This approach is no longer advised. It carries a substantial danger of producing a latent hypovolaemia in neurosurgical patients which may be revealed only when these patients are given barbiturates or other short acting anaesthetic agents, either for a surgical procedure, such as an orthopaedic intervention some days after a head injury, or as part of a regimen to control intracranial hypertension (see below). In the dehydrated hypovolaemic patient, administration of even a small dose of barbiturate may cause profound reduction in arterial pressure.

### Osmotherapy

More effective and more rapid relief of intracranial hypertension can be obtained by intravenous injection of hypertonic solutions which raise the osmotic pressure of plasma, withdraw water from tissues and promote diuresis. The blood–brain barrier renders the penetration of osmotic agents into the brain slower than into the general extracellular space. The brain concentration, therefore, equilibrates with that in the plasma much more slowly and the consequence of the delay is a relatively greater withdrawal of water from the brain. The effectiveness of hypertonic solutions was at first thought to depend entirely upon this selective action. More recent information however, implicates other mechanisms in the lowering of intracranial pressure induced by intravenous osmotherapy.

The first hypertonic substance to be used intravenously was a 15% solution of sodium chloride in experiments conducted by Weed and McKibben (1919) and Foley (1921). The effect of this agent was short lived however, and followed by reversal of effect as the salt was excreted and the plasma concentration fell below that in the brain. Subsequently, hypertonic solutions of dextrose and sucrose were used, but again the effects were only transient.

The effect of intravenous urea in lowering CSF pressure was first noted by Fremont-Smith and Forbes (1927) and experimentally by Smythe *et al* (1950). Javid (1958) first applied intravenous urea in clinical neurosurgery, followed shortly by Stubbs and Pennybacker (1960). A solution of 30% urea in 10% invert sugar was used in a dose of 1–1.5 g urea/Kg body weight. A rapid and substantial fall in ICP could be observed, maximal 20–30 minutes after infusion had started, with the effect persisting for 2–3 hours (Reed & Woodbury 1962). The disadvantages of this agent were the diminution of effect with repeated doses, thought to be due to leakage of the relatively small urea molecule through areas of blood brain barrier damage so that the osmotic gradient between blood and brain tissue was progressively reduced, and the grave tendency of this agent to cause extensive tissue damage if extravasation of the solution into the tissues occurred at the site of intravenous infusion.

Intravenous 20% mannitol solution was introduced into neurosurgical practice by Wise and Chater (1961). It is inert and nontoxic, its penetration is mainly confined to the general extracellular space and rate of excretion is fairly rapid.

The hypertonic solutions can be heat sterilized, are stable and inexpensive. The usual dose is 0.5–1.0 g/kg body weight, the exact dose depending upon the effect of the previous dose on ICP. As with urea, the effect on ICP is maximal 20–30 minutes after infusion and persists for 3 or 4 hours as a rule. If repeated doses are required, however, the baseline serum osmolality gradually increases. When this exceeds 330 mOsm/L, mannitol therapy should cease. Any further dose is unlikely to be effective against intracranial hypertension and very likely to induce renal failure.

Diuretic agents, such as frusemide, have been advocated either alone as a gentle means of reducing ICP or in conjunction with mannitol to hasten its excretion and to reduce the baseline serum osmolality prior to the next dose.

Several theories have been advanced concerning the mechanisms by which the mannitol reduces ICP:

1   The simplest explanation is that the mannitol induces a blood:brain osmotic gradient, resulting in withdrawal of brain tissue water into the blood stream and its subsequent excretion. This theory has been modified to take account of the impairment of blood–brain barrier integrity that occurs in and around brain tumours, contusions, abscesses and other focal lesions. It was therefore proposed that mannitol did, in effect, withdraw water from the rest of the normal brain but did little to reduce oedema in these affected areas. This was proposed on the basis of experimental data by Pappius and Dayes (1963) but doubt about this has recently been expressed by Bell *et al.* (1986) who have studied the effects of intravenous mannitol solution on brain water content in patients with peritumoural oedema by nuclear magnetic resonance imaging. In these studies mannitol was found to reduce the water content of brain in and around the tumour but to have no significant effect on brain water content in the remaining normal brain tissue.

2   Takagi *et al.* (1983) proposed that intravenous mannitol solution caused withdrawal of water across the ependyma of the ventricular

system into the blood stream and thereby reduced ICP in a manner analogous to that produced by ventricular drainage.

3  Muizelaar *et al.* (1983, 1984) have proposed that the effect of intravenous mannitol is to cause cerebral vasoconstriction and that the resultant change in cerebral blood volume is responsible for the reduction in ICP. This effect is present only when autoregulation is preserved in the bulk of cerebral circulation, and these authors propose that the initial effect of mannitol is to induce an increase in cerebral blood flow which is then countered by a compensatory vaso-constriction. When autoregulation is widely impaired mannitol will not reduce ICP. This finding was reported in earlier studies by Bruce *et al.* (1973) who found in very severely head injured patients, in whom autoregulation had been lost, that intravenous mannitol caused an increase in cerebral blood flow and no reduction in ICP.

It is likely that mannitol can lower intracranial pressure in patients with intracranial hyper-tension by more than one mechanism, but despite uncertainty about its means of effect this agent remains extremely valuable in clinical neurosurgical practice. One drawback that is fre-quently referred to is the 'rebound' phenomenon. This has received considerable attention in the literature but has been based mainly on exper-imental studies (Davson 1967). The phenom-enon consists of a rise in ICP to greater than the pretreatment level after the effect of the osmotic agent has worn off. While this has been ascribed to the progressive leak of the osmotic agent across the defective blood brain barrier and a reversal of the osmotic gradient, it is more likely that the so-called 'rebound' phenomenon merely represents a return to a progressive elevation of intracranial pressure, the cause of which has not been treated, but the manifestation of which has been only temporarily alleviated by the treat-ment.

Some clinical cautions in the use of osmo-therapy should be mentioned. A large dose of intravenous mannitol is often given to patients suspected of harbouring an intracranial hae-matoma before their transfer to the neuro-surgical unit in another hospital. Upon arrival at the neurosurgical unit, the patient's condition may have improved to such an extent that the proper sense of urgency in diagnosing and treat-ing the original cause of the deterioration may be lost, only to witness the patient's subsequent and much more serious deterioration within a short time. In patients who are harbouring an intracranial haematoma, the fear has been expressed that because of the increase in cardiac output, administration of osmotic agents may in fact worsen intracranial bleeding and increase the size of an intracranial haematoma as the bulk of the remaining brain diminishes. This is largely a theoretical concern and it is better to have the osmotherapy than no treatment at all during the hopefully short interval of time between instituting diagnostic measures and beginning the urgent evacuation of the haema-toma. When mannitol is being given as a once or twice only administration, pending the identi-fication and evacuation of a haematoma, a large dose (1 g/kg body weight) should be used. When mannitol is being given in repeated doses in intensive care unit, the correct dose is the small-est one which will produce sufficient reduction in ICP. It may under these circumstances be worthwhile to look at the effect of a dose of 0.25 g/kg.

**Cerebrospinal fluid drainage**

In patients in whom ICP is being monitored by an intraventricular catheter, a further mechanism is available for the reduction of ICP; that is by controlled drainage of CSF. It is worthwhile therefore, to devote a short section to the means of locating the lateral ventricle and catheterizing it safely. The burr hole is made in the non-dominant frontal region as a rule, unless the mass lesion is on that side, in which case the burr hole will be made over the opposite lateral ventricle. The incision is located just in front of the coronal suture, in line with the inner margin of the iris of the ipsilateral eye. The burr hole is made, the dura opened and coagulated under direct vision, an avascular part of the brain is chosen for the site of puncture with a ventricular catheter with stilet. This is passed towards the estimated position of the frontal horn. The tip of the catheter is directed downwards as if aiming for the pituitary fossa, using the plane of the inner canthus of the eye on the same side as a guide to the medial direction of the cannula. If this is unsuccessful a second pass can be made directed towards the bridge of the nose, and if this is also unsuccessful a third and final pass can be made to the plane in line with the inner canthus of the opposite eye. (This is a more medial burr hole location and direction of cannulation than that usually employed, but takes account of the fact that in many patients with raised ICP the ventricles are narrowed towards the midline). The tip of the catheter should be felt to 'pop' through the ependyma at a depth of 5–6 cm from the surface in adult patients. When the ventricle is entered it is important not to let more than a drop or two of CSF escape and, therefore, to have ready the entire fluid filled line and three-way tap for joining to the ventricular catheter.

In patients with very small ventricles, in whom difficulty in cannulation is anticipated, it may be preferable to join the catheter in advance to the pressure measuring system and to use the appearance of a pulsatile wave form as the indication that the lateral ventricle has been entered.

When the ventricular catheter has been correctly located and securely anchored to the skin, and the full connection to the pressure measuring device and recording system established, CSF drainage can be set up. It is extremely important that this should be carefully controlled and always set against a positive pressure, usually 10–20 cm above the head. This is essential because lower pressure drainage may cause a siphoning effect with collapse of the ventricle and loss of capacity either to record ICP or to drain further fluid. When the lateral ventricles are enlarged and prolonged CSF drainage is anticipated, as in certain cases of obstructive hydrocephalus, the drainage system can be converted to a closed, internalized ventriculoperitoneal shunt system. When prolonged continuous drainage is not required, but a need for further periods of CSF drainage or ICP measurement is foreseen, a Rickam or Ommaya CSF reservoir may be implanted in the frontal burr hole, attached to a ventricular cannula. CSF drainage and/or ICP monitoring can easily be established by percutaneous needle puncture of the reservoir.

## Corticosteroids in reduction of intracranial pressure

The introduction in the post-war years of effective preparations of ACTH and of cortisone permitted the development of pituitary ablation for the amelioration of certain types of advanced carcinoma and it was found that their use in the surgery of pituitary adenomas and craniopharyngiomas allowed a more radical extirpation; it was also noted that the post-operative recovery of these patients was smoother than heretofore. In the knowledge of the 'anti-inflammatory' effects of steroid agents in other diseases it was considered that this improvement in the postoperative course might be due to the prevention of brain oedema, secondary to the neurosurgical procedure. This led to the use of cortisone and newer corticosteroid agents in patients with intrinsic tumours and other conditions as reported by Lippert *et al.* (1960), and by Galicich and French (1961). With the introduction of the powerful glucocorticoid agents dexamethasone, betamethasone and methylprednisolone, steroid therapy soon found a substantial place in the therapeutic armamentarium of the neurosurgeon, increasing the safety of many surgical procedures to a degree that would have been undreamt of 10 or 20 years earlier. As an example, in patients who presented to the neurosurgeon drowsy with focal neurological deficit due to a large intrinsic brain tumour the procedure of needle biopsy of the brain to obtain tissue for diagnosis was often followed by fatal brain swelling; in such cases it was essential to keep the patient on the operating table until the pathologist could make a secure diagnosis of malignant glioma. With two or three days of pre-treatment with corticosteroids this procedure can now be carried out without upset to the patient, and the younger neurosurgeon of today can have no idea of the apprehension which such apparently simple procedures produced in his older colleagues.

In an excellent review of the clinical use of corticosteroids in neurosurgery, Maxwell et al. (1972) succinctly surveyed the possible uses of these agents in neurosurgery and defined the indications in a way that has not been bettered since; all subsequent trials of steroid therapy have so far been shown to comply with their predictions. In their review, it was emphasized that the conditions most amenable to steroid therapy were those which were focal and chronic in the brain, while those in which steroid therapy was least effective were acute and diffuse. Thus steroid therapy is effective in patients with brain tumours and peritumoural oedema, in brain abscess with surrounding oedema, and of possible but unproven value in the case of focal brain contusion with surrounding oedema. Steroid therapy is ineffective in brain swelling following cardiac arrest and resuscitation, in post hypoxic brain damage, in acute stroke and in acute diffuse traumatic brain damage.

The mechanisms of effect of steroids remain unresolved. At the subcellular level, cortico-steroids may act by reducing the increased cell membrane permeability which has been brought about by lipid peroxidation in the fatty acid chains of the phospholipid part of the cell membrane. Experimental evidence that steroids reduce the water content of brain white matter affected by (cold-induced) vasogenic oedema has not been confirmed in clinical studies using CAT and MRI (Penn 1980, Bell et al. 1986). The neurological condition of the patient is improved long before there is any substantial effect on ICP. The baseline intracranial pressure is not reduced until after 2 or 3 days of therapy, whereas patients are clinically improved within 12–24 hours. Headache and drowsiness clear, focal

neurological deficits such as dysphasia or limb paresis resolve, in some cases completely. Waves of increased intracranial pressure do tend to disappear at an earlier stage, usually after 24 hours of therapy (Kullberg & West 1965, Brock et al. 1976). Studies by Miller and his colleagues (Miller & Leech 1975, Miller et al. 1976) have shown that steroid therapy in patients with brain tumour changes the viscoelastic properties of the swollen tight brain, within 24 hours of therapy making it more compliant, even though baseline intracranial pressure is not reduced for another 24 or 48 hours. Other investigators have suggested that corticosteroids also contribute to reduction in ICP by reducing the rate of CSF formation (Weiss & Nulsen 1970) but this has been disputed by others (Martins et al. 1974).

The dose of dexamethasone used most frequently in clinical neurosurgery is 10 mg as a loading dose followed by 4 mg 6 hourly. This is an effective dose in the conditions cited above; where it is ineffective, as in some cases of recurrent brain tumour, some have suggested that even higher doses, up to 80 mg/day may be effective. This has not been conclusively demonstrated.

## Barbiturates and other anaesthetic agents

Shapiro et al. (1974) advocated the use of short acting barbiturates as a means of lowering raised intracranial pressure. The principle upon which this was based is that barbiturates, like hypo-thermia, reduce brain metabolism; this, in turn, reduces cerebral blood flow and the resultant fall in cerebral blood volume reduces the intracranial pressure. For several years this was used only by anaesthetists in the context of neurosurgical operations in which acute brain swelling occurred during neurosurgical operations. Marshall and Shapiro subsequently reported the results of administering barbiturate therapy to head injured and other comatose patients in the intensive care unit and reported that this form of treatment was successful in reducing intra-cranial pressure in a group of patients in whom all other methods had failed (Marshall *et al.* 1978, 1979, Rockoff *et al.* 1979). These reports were seized upon with great enthusiasm in many parts of the world and quickly became accepted into routine neurosurgical intensive care practice. As was pointed out by Miller (1979), however, there had to that point been no evidence for the effectiveness of barbiturate therapy obtained under the conditions of a randomized controlled trial. Two randomized controlled trials of the use of barbiturates in severely head injured patients have now shown no superior effectiveness over conventional therapy in reducing the incidence or severity of intracranial hypertension in such patients (Schwartz *et al.* 1984, Ward *et al.* 1985).

When barbiturates are administered to patients there is frequently a reduction in arterial pressure; under these circumstances this will immediately be reflected in a fall in ICP. If arterial pressure is not monitored the neurosurgeon may gain the impression of considerable benefit resulting from administration of this agent, whereas in fact the perfusion pressure may actually be less (Miller 1985). This is not to deny, however, that under carefully controlled conditions in patients who are well hydrated and normovolaemic, the administration of intravenous infusions of thiopentone will frequently result in satisfactory, though temporary, reduction in ICP (Rea & Rockswold 1983). The initial infusion rate is 12.5 mg/kg body weight/hour, reducing to 5 mg/kg body weight/hour.

An additional benefit has been claimed for barbiturates; this is a protective effect on the ischaemic brain; by reducing cerebral metabolism and, therefore, energy demand, the brain is put into a 'state of hibernation' in which the processes of tissue restitution can proceed. Unfortunately, most of the evidence for a beneficial protective effect of barbiturates is based on experimental studies and, usually, studies in which the barbiturates have been administered before, or simultaneous with, the insult. These experimental conditions do not of course simulate the clinical situation in which the advent of therapy is often delayed for hours after the insult.

In the search for other agents which can similarly reduce ICP and protect the brain without reducing arterial pressure and cerebral perfusion pressure many agents have been tried including etomidate and gammahydroxybutyrate (Strong 1984, Dearden & McDowall 1985, Leggate *et al.* 1986). At this stage it is premature to state whether or not such agents will be of any greater effectiveness than thiopentone.

## Surgical decompression for intracranial hypertension

When raised intracranial pressure has primarily been caused by an intracranial space occupying lesion such as a tumour, haematoma or abscess, the most effective means of dealing with the problem is surgical extirpation of the mass. This should not only reduce the ICP but also correct the brain shift and distortion produced by the mass. Safe performance of the operative procedure may, however, require prior therapy with mannitol or steroids. If intracranial hypertension has been prolonged and severe, even successful surgical decompression may be followed by recurrent intracranial hypertension, due initially to intracranial vasodilation, then to postcompression brain oedema. Thus operative treatment may still require to be followed by other forms of therapy.

In the early days of neurosurgery cases of benign intracranial hypertension and certain cases of brain tumour were treated by surgical decompression. The principle of the procedure was in increasing the capacity of the cranium by removal of bone and a plastic procedure to split and cover the dura mater. This was usually done in the subtemporal area where the bulging brain could be further covered by the protection of the temporalis muscle. It is a measure of the effectiveness of the methods available today for reducing intracranial pressure that such surgical procedures are now seldom carried out. Furthermore, there are sound reasons for believing that when the brain is extremely tight and swollen, to open the dura and remove bone so as to allow brain to bulge into the defect is not likely to prove an effective treatment. The herniating brain impinges on the margins of the bone defect, cortical venous drainage is interrupted, and further brain swelling tends to ensue. CT scanning in such cases, performed several days after the surgical decompression, frequently shows that the protruding brain has infarcted (Cooper & Hagler 1979). In some cases life may be saved but only at the expense of causing massive cerebral hemispheric damage. Notwithstanding, there undoubtedly exist cases where conservative measures have failed to control intracranial pressure and where judicious performance of a surgical decompression has resulted in satisfactory control of intracranial hypertension without causing a disabling amount of further brain damage. Where lesions are located at the frontal or temporal poles then lobectomy can be carried out, on one side only, without increasing neurological deficit. Bilateral brain damage or resection produces severe neuropsychological deficits.

The other form of surgical decompression, employed when external CSF drainage has been satisfactory, is to install a ventricular peritoneal shunt.

## Conclusions

A basic understanding of the processes regulating normal intracranial pressure and cerebral blood flow and responsible for intracranial hypertension, brain oedema, brain shift and herniation and ischaemic brain damage is fundamental to the practice of neurosurgery. The timely application of diagnostic and therapeutic measures depends upon such knowledge. At all times it must be appreciated that it is the whole patient and the whole problem that must be managed. The neurosurgeon must not fall into the trap of treating a given level of intracranial pressure while ignoring the fact that it might have a surgically remediable cause, treatment of which may not only reduce the ICP but also reduce brain shift and herniation and remove the source

of the brain oedema which is contributing to these problems. In addition, the neurosurgeon must recognize that reduction of intracranial pressure is helpful only when arterial pressure and arterial oxygenation are preserved. The goal of treatment should be to restore adequate perfusion and oxygenation of the brain and to reduce any shift and distortion of its structure. Lastly, the rapidity with which deterioration can occur cannot be overemphasized. It is better by far to anticipate trouble or to apply simple treatment at the early stages than to have to apply Draconian measures in a last attempt to save a dying brain.

## References

ADAMS J.H. & GRAHAM D.I. (1976) Neuropath. appl. Neurobiol., 2, 323.
ASTRUP J. (1982) J. Neurosurg., 56, 482.
BAKAY R.A.E. & WARD A.A. (1983) J. Neurosurg., 58, 27.
BASS M.H. & FISCH G.R. (1961) Neurology, 11, 1091.
BEDFORD T.H.B. (1935) Brain, 58, 427.
BEDFORD T.H.B. (1942) J. Physiol., 101, 362.
BELL B.A., SYMON L. & BRANSTON N.M. (1985) J. Neurosurg., 62, 31.
BELL B.A., MACDONALD H.L., KEAN D.M., SMITH M.A., BARNETT G.H., MILLER J.D. & BEST J.J.K. (1986) J. Neurol. Neurosurg. Psychiat., 49, 467.
BORDLEY J. & CUSHING H. (1909) J. Amer. med. Ass., 52, 253.
BRADLEY K.C. (1970) J. Neurol. Neurosurg. Psychiat., 33, 97.
BAIN W.R. (1963) Lancet, 1, 179.
BØRGESEN S.E., GZERRIS F. & SØRENSEN S.C. (1978) Acta Neurol. Scand., 57, 85.
BROCK M., WIEGAND H, ZILLIG C., ZYWIETZ C., MOCK P. & DIETZ H. (1976) In Dynamics of Brain Edema (Ed. H.M. Pappius & W. Feindel) pp 330–6. Springer-Verlag, Berlin, Heidelberg.
BROWDER J. & MEYERS R. (1936) Amer. J. Surg., 31, 403.
BROWN B.A. & JONES O.W. (1962) J. Neurosurg., 19, 349.
BRUCE D.A., LANGFITT T.W., MILLER J.D., SHUTZ H., VAPALAHTI M.P., STANEK A. & GOLDBERG H.I. (1973) J. Neurosurg., 38, 131.
BURROWS G. (1846) Disorders of the Cerebral Circulation. London.
BUTLER A.B., MANN J.D., MAFFEO C.J. & JOHNSON R.N. (1983) In Neurobiology of Cerebospinal Fluid (Ed. J. Wood) pp 707–26. Plenum Press, New York.
CAIRNS H. (1939) Brit. J. Surg., 275.
CAPRILES L. (1963) Arch. Neurol., 9, 147.
COLLIER J. (1904) Brain, 27, 490.
COOPER K.R. & BOSWELL P.A. (1983) Chest, 84, 29.
COOPER P.R. & HAGLER H. (1979) Neurosurgery, 4, 296.
CORSELLIS J.A.N. (1957) J. Neurol. Neurosurg. Psychiat., 21, 279.
CSERR H.F. (1974) Physiol. Rev., 51, 273.
CUSHING H. (1901) Bull. Johns. Hopk. Hosp., 12, 290.

CUSHING H. (1902) *Amer. J. med. Sci.*, **124**, 375.
CUSHING H. (1903) *Amer. J. med. Sci.*, **125**, 1017.
CUSHING H. (1910) *Brain*, **33**, 204.
CUSHING H. (1917) *Tumours of the Nervus Acusticus*. W.B. Saunders Co., Philadelphia.
DANDY W.E. (1919) *Ann. Surg.*, **70**, 129.
DANDY W.E. & BLACKFAN K.D. (1914) *Amer. J. Dis. Child.*, **8**, 406.
DAVSON H. (1967) *The Physiology of the Cerebrospinal Fluid*. Churchill, London.
DEARDEN N.M. & MCDOWALL D.G. (1985) *Brit. J. Anaesth.*, **57**, 361.
DENNY-BROWN D. (1962) *Proc. roy. Soc. Med.*, **55**, 527.
DREW A.L. & MAGEE I.C.R. (1951) *Arch. Neurol. Psychiat.*, ,66 744.
DUCKER T.B. & SIMMONS R.L. (1968) *J. Neurosurg.*, **28**, 112.
DUCKER T.B., SIMMONS R.L. & ANDERSON R.W. (1968) *J. Neurosurg.*, **29**, 475.
DURET H. (1878) *Etudes Experimentales et Cliniques sur les Traumatismes Cerebrau*. Paris.
ENEVOLDSEN E.M. & JENSEN F.T. (1978) *J. Neurosurg.*, **48**, 689.
FIELDS J.P. (1961) *J. Pediat.*, **58**, 74.
FIESCHI C., BATTASTINI N. & BEDUSCHI A. (1974) *J. Neurol. Neurosurg. Psychiat.*, **37**, 1378.
FINNEY L.A. & WALKER E.A. (1962) *Transtentorial Herniation*. Thomas, Springfield, Illinois.
FISCHER-BRUGGE E. (1951) *Acta. Neurochir.*, **2**, 36.
FISHMAN R.A. (1975) *New Engl. J. Med.*, **23**, 706.
FITCH W & MCDOWALL D.G. (1971) *Brit. J. Anaesth.*, **43**, 904.
FITCH W. & MCDOWALL D.G. (1977) *J. Neurol. Neurosurg. Psychiat.*, **40**, 833.
FITCH W., MACKENZIE E.T. & HARPER A.M. (1975) *Circ. Res.*, **37**, 550.
FLEISCHER A.S., RUDMAN D.R., FRESH C.B. & TINDALL G.T. (1977) *J. Neurosurg.*, **47**, 517.
FLEXNER L.B. & WEED L.H. (1933) *Amer. J. Physiol.*, **104**, 681.
FLEXNER L.B., CLARK J.H. & WEED L.H. (1932) *Amer. J. Physiol.*, **101**, 292.
FOG M. (1933) *Acta Psychiat. Neurol. Scand.*, **8**, 191.
FOG M. (1937) *Arch. Neurol. Psychiat.*, **37**, 351.
FOG M. (1939) *Arch. Neurol. Psychiat.*, **41**, 260.
FOLEY F.E.B. (1921) *Surg. Gynec. Obstet.*, **33**, 126.
FOLEY J. (1955) *Brain*, **78**, 1.
FORBES H.S. (1928) *Arch. Neurol. Psychiat.*, **19**, 751.
FREEDMAN (1963) *Brit. J. Ophth.*, **47**, 290.
FREMONT-SMITH F. & FORBES H.S. (1927) *Arch. Neurol. Psychiat.*, **18**, 550.
FROST E.A.M. (1979) *J. Neurosurg.*, **50**, 699.
GALICICH J.H. & FRENCH L.A. (1961) *Amer. Practit.*, **12**, 169.
GASSEL M.M. (1961) *Arch. Neurol.*, **4**, 70.
GRAHAM D.I., ADAMS J.H. & DOYLE D. (1978) *J. Neurol. Sci.*, **39**, 213.
GREAVES P. (1959) *Trans. Ophth. Soc. UK*, **79**, 109.
GREER M. (1963) *Neurology.*, **13**, 439.
GUILLAUME J. & JANNY P. (1951) *Rev. Neurol.*, **84**, 131.
HÄGGENDAL E., LÖFGREN J., NILSSON N.J. & ZWETNOW N.N. (1970) *Acta. Physiol. Scand.*, **79**, 262.
HARPER A.M. (1966) *J. Neurol. Neurosurg. Psychiat.*, **29**, 398.
HARPER A.M. & GLASS H.I. (1965) *J. Neurol. Neurosurg. Psychiat.*, **28**, 449.
HARPER A.M., GLASS H.I. & GLOVER M.M. (1961) *Scott. Med. J.*, **6**, 12.
HASSLER O. (1967) *Neurology*, **17**, 368.

HAYREH S.S. (1964) *Brit. J. Ophth.*, **48**, 52.
HEISKANEN O. (1964) *Acta. Neurol. Scand.*, **40**, (Suppl 7) 1.
HEISTAD D.D. & MARCUS M.L. (1978) *Circ. Res.*, **42**, 295.
HILL L. (1898) *The Physiology and Pathology of the Cerebral Circulation*. Churchill, London.
HOFF J.T. & MITCHELL R.A. (1972) In *Intracranial Pressure* (Ed. M. Brock) pp 205–9. Springer-Verlag, Berlin and Heidelberg.
HOFF J.T. & REIS D.J. (1970) *Arch. Neurol.*, **22**, 228.
HULME A. & COOPER R. (1968) In *Progress in Brain Research*, vol. 30, *Cerebral Circulation* (Ed. W. Luijendijk) p 77, Elsevier, Amsterdam.
INGVAR D.H. & LASSEN N.A. (1961) *Lancet*, **2**, 806.
ISHII S., HAYNER R., KELLY W.A. & EVANS J.P. (1959) *J. Neurosurg.*, **16**, 152.
JAVID M. (1958) *Surg. Clin. N. America.*, **38**, 907.
JEFFERSON A. (1956) *J. Neurol. Neurosurg. Psychiat.*, **19**, 21.
JEFFERSON G. (1938) *Arch. Neurol. Psychiat.*, **40**, 857.
JEFFERSON G. & JOHNSON R.T. (1950) *Folia Psychiat. neerl.*, **53**, 36.
JENNETT B. & PLUM F. (1972) *Lancet*, **1**, 734.
JENNETT W.B., BARKER J., FITCH, W. & MCDOWALL D.G. (1969) *Lancet*, **1**, 61.
JENNETT W.B. & STERN W.E. (1960) *J. Neurosurg.*, **17**, 598.
JOHNSON R.T. (1957) In *Modern Trends in Neurology*, 2nd Series (Ed. D. Williams) pp 274. Butterworth, London.
JOHNSON R.T. & YATES P.O. (1956) *Acta. Radiol.*, **46**, 250.
JOHNSTON I.H. & PATERSON A. (1974) *Brain.*, **97**, 301.
JOHNSTON I.H. & ROWAN J.O. (1974) *J. Neurol. Neurosurg. Psychiat.*, **37**, 392.
JOHNSTON I.H., ROWAN J.O., HARPER A.M. & JENNETT W.B. (1974) *J. Neurol. Neurosurg. Psychiat.*, **37**, 585.
KALBAG R.M. & WOOLF N.L. (1967) *Cerebral venous thrombosis*. Oxford University Press.
KATZMAN R. & HUSSEY F. (1970) *Neurology*, **20**, 543.
KAUFMANN G.E. & CLARK K. (1970) *J. Neurosurg.*, **33**, 145.
KELLIE G. (1824) *Trans. med. chir. Soc. Edin.*, **1**, 84.
KERNOHAN J.W. & WOLTMAN H.W. (1929) *Arch. Neurol. Psychiat.*, **21**, 274.
KETY S.S. & SCHMIDT C.F. (1945) *Amer. J. Physiol.*, **143**, 53.
KETY S.S. & SCHMIDT C.F. (1948) *J. clin. Invest.*, **27**, 484.
KETY S.S., SHENKIN H.A. & SCHMIDT C.F. (1948) *J. clin. Invest.*, **27**, 493–9.
KEY A. & RETZIUS G. (1875) *Anatomie des Nervensystems und des Bindegewebes*. Norstedt und Sönnen, Stockholm.
KINNIER WILSON S.A. (1920) *Brain*, **43**, 220.
KLATZO I. (1967) *J. Neuropath. Exp. Neurol.*, **26**, 1.
KLINTWORTH G.K. (1966) *J. Neurol. Neurosurg. Psychiat.*, **29**, 423.
KOCHER T. (1901) In *Nothnagel's spezielle Pathologie und Therapie*, Vol. 9, pt. 2, p 81.
KONTOS H.A., WEI E.P., NAVARI R.M., LEVASSEUR J.E., ROSENBLUM I. & PATTERSON J.L. JR (1978) *Amer. J. Physiol.*, **234**, 371.
KULLBERG G. & WEST K.A. (1965) *Acta. Neurol. Scand.*, **41** (Suppl. 13), 445.
LANGFITT T.W. (1969) *Clin. Neurosurg.*, **16**, 436.
LANGFITT T.W., WEINSTEIN J.D., KASSELL N.F. & GAGLIARDI L.J. (1964a) *J. Neurosurg.*, **21**, 998.
LANGFITT T.W., WEINSTEIN J.D., KASSELL N.F. & SIMEONE F.A. (1964b) *J. Neurosurg.*, **21**, 989–97.
LANGFITT T.W., WEINSTEIN J.D. & KASSELL N.F. (1965) *Neurology*, **15**, 622–41.
LASSEN N.A. (1959) *Physiol. Rev.*, **39**, 183.

LASSEN N.A. (1966) *Lancet*, **2**, 1113.

LEECH P.J., MILLER J.D., FITCH W. & BARKER J. (1974) *J. Neurol. Neurosurg. Psychiat.*, **37**, 854.

LEGGATE J.R.S., DEARDEN N.M. & MILLER J.D. (1986) In *Intracranial Pressure VI*. (Eds. J.D. Miller, G.M. Teasdale, J.O. Rowan, S. Galbraith, A.D. Mendelow). pp 754–7. Springer-Verlag, Heidelberg, Berlin.

LE GROS CLARK W.E. (1921) *J. Anat.*, **55**, 40.

LESLIE J.B. & WATKINS D. (1985) *J. Neurosurg.*, **63**, 659.

LEVINE J.E., POVLISHOCK J.T. & BECKER D.P. (1982) *Brain Research*, **241**, 31.

LEWELT W., JENKINS L.W. & MILLER J.D. (1980) *J. Neurosurg.*, **53**, 500.

LEWELT W., JENKINS L.W. & MILLER J.D. (1982) *J. Neurosurg.*, **56**, 332.

LIPPERT R.G., SVIEN H.J., GRINDLAY J.H., GOLDSTEIN N.P. & GASTINEAU C.F. (1960) *J. Neurosurg.*, **17**, 583.

LUNDBERG N. (1960) *Acta Psychiat. Neurol. Scand.*, **36**, (Suppl. 149) 1.

McCOMB J.G. (1983) *J. Neurosurg.*, **59**, 369.

McCULLOCH J. & EDVINSSON L. (1984) *J. Cereb. Blood Flow Metabol.*, **4**, 129–39.

MacDONALD H.L., BELL B.A., SMITH M.A., KEAN D.M., TOCHER J.L., MILLER J.D., BEST J.J.K. (1985) *Brit. J. Radiol.*, **58**, 817.

McDOWALL D.G. (1966) In *Oxygen Measurements in Blood and Tissues*. (Eds. J.P. Payne and D.W. Hill) pp 205–214. Churchill, London.

McDOWALL D.G. (1967) *Brit. J. Anath.*, **39**, 186.

McMENEMY W.H. & CUMINGS J.N. (1959) *J. clin. Path.*, **12**, 400.

MAAS A.I.R. (1977) *J. Neurol. Neurosurg. Psychiat.*, **40**, 666.

MARMAROU A., SHULMAN K. & LAMORGESE J. (1975) *J. Neurosurg.*, **43**, 523.

MARSHALL L.F., SHAPIRO H.M. & RAUSCHER A. (1978a) *Crit. Care Med.*, **6**, 1.

MARSHALL L.F., SMITH R.W. & SHAPIRO H.M. (1978b) *Neurosurgery*, **2**, 100.

MARSHALL L.F., SMITH R.W. & SHAPIRO H.M. (1979) *J. Neurosurg.*, **50**, 26.

MARTINS A.N., RAMIREZ A., SOLOMON L.S. & WISE G.M. (1974) *J. Neurosurg.*, **41**, 550–4.

MASSERMAN J.H. (1934) *Arch. Neurol. Psychiat.*, **32**, 523.

MAXWELL R.E., LONG D.M. & FRENCH L.A. (1972) In *Steroids and Brain Edema*. (Eds. H.J. Reulen and K. Schurmann) pp 219–232. Springer-Verlag, Heidelberg, Berlin.

MAYHALL C.G., ARCHER N.H., LAMB A.Y., SPADORA A.G., BAGGETT J.W., WARD J.D. & NARAYAN R.K. (1984) *New Engl. J. Med.*, **310**, 553.

MEADOWS S.P. (1959) *Trans. Ophth. Soc. UK.*, **79**, 121.

MEINIG G., REULEN H.J. & MAGAWLY C. (1973) *Acta Neurochirurgica*, **29**, 1.

MENDELOW A.D., ROWAN J.O., MURRAY L. & KERR A.E. (1983) *J. Neurosurg.*, **58**, 45.

MEYER A. (1920) *Arch. Neurol. Psychiat.*, **4**, 387.

MILLEN J.E. & GLAUSER F.L. (1983) *J. Appl. Physiol.*, **54**, 666.

MILLER J.D. (1973) *Europ. Neurol.*, **10**, 1.

MILLER J.D. (1975) *Clin. Neurosurg.*, **22**, 76.

MILLER J.D. (1978) *Brit. J. hosp. Med.*, **19**, 497.

MILLER J.D. (1979a) *Ann. Neurol.*, **6**, 189.

MILLER J.D. (1979b) *Brit. J. hosp. Med.*, **20**, 152.

MILLER J.D. (1985) *Brit. J. Anaesth.*, **57**, 120.

MILLER J.D. & ADAMS J.H. (1984) In *Greenfield's Neuro-*

*pathology*. 4th Edition. (Eds. J.H. Adams, J.A.N. Corsellis & L.W. Duchen) pp 53–84. Arnold, London.

MILLER J.D. & LEDINGHAM I.M. (1971) *Arch. Neurol.*, **24**, 210.

MILLER J.D. & LEECH P.J. (1975) *J. Neurosurg.*, **42**, 274.

MILLER J.D., BECKER D.P., WARD J.D., SULLIVAN H.G., ADAMS W.E. & ROSNER M.J. (1977a) *J. Neurosurg.*, **47**, 503.

MILLER J.D., STANEK A.E. & LANGFITT T.W. (1972) *Progr. Brain Res.*, **35**, 411.

MILLER J.D., STANEK A.E., LANGFITT T.W. (1973) *J. Neurosurg.*, **39**, 186.

MILLER J.D., SAKALAS R., WARD J.D., ADAMS W.E., VRIES J.K. & BECKER D.P. (1977b) *Neurosurgery*, **1**, 114.

MONCADA S. & VANE J.R. (1978) *Pharmacol. Rev.*, **30**, 293.

MONRO A. (1983) *Observations on the Structure and Function of the Nervous System*. Creech and Johnston, Edinburgh.

MOORE M.T. & STERN K. (1938) *Brain*, **61**, 70.

MORLEY J.B. & REYNOLDS E.H. (1966) *Brain*, **89**, 205.

MORRICE G., HAVERNER W.H. & KAPELANSKY F. (1960) *J. Amer. med. Ass.*, **173**, 1802.

MUIZELAAR J.P., WEI E.P., KONTOS H.A. & BECKER D.P. (1983) *J. Neurosurg.*, **59**, 822.

MUIZELAAR J.P., LUTZ H.A., BECKER D.P. (1984) *J. Neurosurg.*, **61**, 700.

NOELL W. & SCHNEIDER M. (1948) *Arch. Psychiat. Nervenheilk.*, **118**, 180.

NORDBY H.K. & URDAL P. (1982) *Acta Neurochir.*, **65**, 93.

NORTH J.B. & JENNETT S. (1974) *Arch. Neurol.*, **31**, 338.

NORTHFIELD D.W.C. (1938) *Brain*, **61**, 133.

NORTHFIELD D.W.C. (1968) In *Handbook of Clinical Neurology*. (Eds. P.J. Vinken and G.W. Bruyn) Vol 5, p 172. North Holland, Amsterdam.

O'CONNELL J.E.A. (1943) *Brain*, **66**, 204.

O'CONNELL J.E.A. (1970) *Proc. roy. Soc. Med.*, **63**, 507.

OBRIST W.D., THOMSON H.K., WANG H.S. & WILKINSON W.E. (1975) *Stroke*, **6**, 245.

OBRIST W.D., GENNARELLI T.A., SEGAWA H., DOLINSKAS C.A. & LANGFITT T.W. (1979) *J. Neurosurg.*, **51**, 292.

OVERGAARD J. & TWEED W.A. (1974) *J. Neurosurg.*, **41**, 531.

PALVÖLGYI R. (1969) *J. Neurosurg.*, **31**, 149.

PAPPIUS H.M. & DAYES L.A. (1965) *Arch. Neurol.*, **13**, 395.

PAPPIUS H.M. & GULATI D.R. (1963) *Acta. Neuropath.*, **2**, 451.

PATON L. & HOMES G. (1911) *Brain*, **33**, 389.

PAULSON O.B. (1970) *Neurology*, **20**, 63.

PEARS M.A. & PICKERING G.W. (1960) *Quart. J. Med.*, **29**, 153.

PENFIELD W. (1933) *Ann. Intern. Med.*, **7**, 303.

PENN R.D. (1980) *Neurosurgery*, **6**, 249.

PICKERING G.W. (1948) *Brain.*, **71**, 274.

PLUM F., & POSNER J.B. (1980) *The Diagnosis of Stupor and Coma*. 3rd Edition. Davis, Philadelphia.

POLLAY M. (1975) *J. Neurosurg.*, **42**, 665.

POPOFF N., WEINBERG S. & FEIGIN K. (1963) *Neurology*, **13**, 101.

PURVES M.J. (1978) *Ann. Neurol.*, **3**, 377.

RAPOPORT S. (1976) *Blood Brain Barrier in Physiology and Medicine*. pp 316. Raven Press, New York.

REA G.L. & ROCKSWOLD G.L. (1983) *Neurosurgery*, **12**, 401.

REED D.J. & WOODBURY D.M. (1962) *J. Physiol.*, **164**, 252.

REID W.L. & CONE W.V. (1939) *J. Amer. med. Ass.*, **112**, 2030.

REIVICH M. (1964) *Am. J. Physiol.*, **206**, 25.

REULEN H.J., TSUYUMU M., TACK A., FENSKE A.R. & PRIOLEAU G.R. (1978) *J. Neurosurg.*, **48**, 754.

RISBERG J., LUNDBERG N. & INGVAR D.H. (1969) *J. Neurosurg.*, **31**, 303.

ROCKOFF M.A., MARSHALL L.F. & SHAPIRO H.M. (1979) Ann. Neurol., **6**, 194.

ROHR V.H. & HOFFMANN W. (1959) Nervenarzt, **30**, 391.

ROSNER M.J. & BECKER D.P. (1983) In Intracranial Pressure V. (Eds. S. Ishii, H. Nagai & M. Brock) pp 301–306. Springer-Verlag, Heidelberg, New York, Tokyo.

SCHEINKER I.M. (1945) Arch. Neurol. Psychiat., **53**, 289.

SCHMIDT C.F. & HENDRIX J.P. (1937) Ass. Res. nerv. Dis. Proc., **18**, 229.

SCHUTTA H.S., KASSELL N.F. & LANGFITT T.W. (1968) Brain, **91**, 281.

SCHWARTZ M.L., TATOR C.H., ROWED D.W., REID S.R., MEGURA K. & ANDREWS D.F. (1984) Canad. J. neurol. Sci., **11**, 434.

SELHORST J.E., GUDEMAN S.K., BUTTERWORTH J.F., HARBISON J.W., MILLER J.D. & BECKER D.P. (1985) Neurosurgery, **16**, 357.

SHAPIRO H.M., WYTE S.R. & LOESER J. (1974) J. Neurosurg., **40**, 90.

SHAW D.B. & SIMPSON T. (1961) Quart. J. Med., **30**, 135.

SHULMAN K. (1965) J. Surg. Res., **5**, 56.

SMYTH G.E. & HENDERSON W.R. (1938) J. Neurol. Psychiat., **1**, 226.

SMYTHE L., SMYTHE I. & SETTLAGE P. (1950) J. Neuropath., **9**, 438.

SPATZ H. & STROESCU G.J. (1934) Der Nervenartzt, **7**, 481.

SPENCER W. & HORSLEY V. (1891) Phil. Trans. roy. Soc. Lond., **182**, 201.

SPENCER W. & HORSLEY V. (1889) Brit. med. J., **1**, 457.

SPRIGGS A.I. (1954) J. clin. Path., **7**, 122.

STARLING E.H. (1896) J. Physiol., **19**, 312.

STEINER L., LÖFGREN J. & ZWETNOW N.N. (1975) Acta. Neurol. Scand., **52**, 241.

STERN W.E. & COXON R.V. (1964) Amer. J. Physiol., **206**, 1.

STEVENS P.M., AUSTIN K.F. & KNOWLES J.H. (1963) J. Amer. Med. Ass., **183**, 161.

STEWART T.G. & HOLMES G. (1904) Brain, **27**, 522.

STRANDGAARD S., McKENZIE E.T., SENGUPTA D., ROWAN J.O., LASSEN N.A. & HARPER A.M. (1974) Circ. Res., **34**, 435.

STRONG A.J. (1984) Lancet, **1**, 1304.

STUBBS J. & PENNYBACKER J. (1960) Brit. med. J., **1**, 1094.

SULLIVAN H.G., MILLER J.D., GRIFFITH R.L. & BECKER D.P. (1978) Amer. J. Physiol., **234**, 167.

SULLIVAN H.G., MILLER J.D., GRIFFITH R.L., CARTER W. & RUCKER S. (1979) Ann. Neurol., **5**, 228.

SUNDERLAND S. (1958) Brit. J. Surg., **45**, 422.

SUNDERLAND S. & BRADLEY K.C. (1953) J. Neurol. Neurosurg. Psychiat., **16**, 35.

SUNDERLAND S. & HUGHES E.S.R. (1946) Brain, **69**, 301.

SYMON L., PASZTOR E., DORSCH N.W.C. & BRANSTON N.M. (1973) Stroke, **4**, 632.

TAKAGI H., SAITO T., KITAHARA T., MORRII S., OHWADA T. &

YADA K. (1983) In Intracranial Pressure V. (Eds. S. Ishii, H. Nagai & M. Brock) p 729. Springer Verlag, Heidelberg, New York, Tokyo.

TAKIZAWA H., GABRA-SANDERS T. & MILLER J.D. (1985) Neurosurgery, **17**, 63.

TAKIZAWA H., GABRA-SANDERS T. & MILLER J.D. (1986) Neurosurgery, **19**, 1.

TAYLOR A.R. & CROCKARD H.A. (1972) Clin. Neurosurg., **19**, 121.

TEASDALE E., CARDOSO E., GALBRAITH S. & TEASDALE G. (1984) J. Neurol. Neurosurg. Psychiat., **47**, 600.

THOMPSON R.K. & MALINA S. (1959) J. Neurosurg., **16**, 664.

TRIPATHI B.S. & TRIPATHI R.C. (1974) J. Physiol. (Lond), **239**, 195.

UPTON M.L. & WELLER R.O. (1985) J. Neurosurg., **63**, 867.

VINCENT C., DAVID M. & THIEBAUT F. (1936) Rev. Neurol., **65**, 536.

VON BERGMANN E. (1880) In Deutsche Chirurgie (Eds. T. Billroth & G.A. Luecke) **30**, 226, Enke, Stuttgart.

WAHL M. & KUSCHINSKY W. (1979) Pflügers Arch., **382,**, 203.

WALKER V. & PICKARD J.D. (1985) In Advances and Technical Standards in Neurosurgery, **12**, 5–64. Springer Verlag, Wien, New York.

WALTER W.G. & CROW H.J. (1964) EEG Clin. Neurophysiol., **16**, 68.

WARD J.D., BECKER D.P., MILLER J.D., CHOI S.C., MARMAROU A., WOOD C., NEWLON P. & KEENAN R. (1985) J. Neurosurg., **62**, 383.

WEED J.H. (1914) J. med. Res., **31**, 21.

WEED L.H. & McKIBBEN P.S. (1919) Amer. J. Physiol., **48**, 512.

WEINSTEIN J.D., LANGFITT T.W., BRUNO L., ZAREN H.A. & JACKSON J.L.F. (1968)) J. Neurosurg., **28**, 513.

WEISS M.H. & NULSEN F.E. (1970) J. Neurosurg., **32**, 452.

WEISS M.H. & WERTMAN N. (1978) Arch. Neurol., **35**, 527.

WELCH K. (1975) Advances in Neurology, pp 247–332. Raven Press, New York.

WELCH K. (1980) J. Neurosurg., **52**, 693.

WELCH K. & FRIEDMAN V. (1960) Brain, **83**, 454.

WISE B.L. & CHATER N. (1961) Arch. Neurol., **4**, 200.

WITTSCHAFTER J.D., RIZZO F.J. & SMILEY B.C. (1975) Surv. Ophthalm., **20**, 157.

WOLFF H.G. (1963) Headache and Other Head Pain. Oxford University Press.

WOLFF H.G. & BLUMGART H.L. (1929) Arch. Neurol. Psychiat., **21**, 795.

WOLFF H.G. & FORBES H.S. (1928) Arch. Neurol. Psychiat., **20**, 1035.

WOLFF H.G. & LENNOX W.G. (1930) Arch. Neurol. Psychiat., **23**, 1097.

WOLMAN L. (1953) Brain., **76**, 364.

WRIGHT R.D. (1938) Aust. N.Z.J. Surg., **7**, 215.

# Chapter 3
# Special investigations—neuroradiology

## B. R. KENDALL

## Introduction

Radiology is a crucial part of the investigation of all lesions of the nervous system but particularly those of potential neurosurgical significance. Precision and safety have been enhanced greatly in recent years by the application of computerized tomographic, magnetic resonance and digital subtraction techniques and the development of non-ionic contrast media.

Cushing had the foresight to introduce radiography into his unit in the Johns Hopkins Hospital in 1896 (Fulton 1946); 30 years later Sosman (1927) was able to report that by inspection of skull radiographs the position of a mass could be predicted in 50% of cases and its nature in 33%. This information was valuable when angiography of appropriate vessels was the most effective method to elucidate lateralized or posterior fossa masses, whereas encephalography or ventriculography were indicated for deeply placed or poorly localized lesions. This no longer applies when computerized tomography (CT) and/or nuclear magnetic resonance (NMR) are available. Plain skull X-rays (SXR) are usually noncontributory to the early diagnosis of important intracranial pathology (Hillemacher 1982) and the indications for SXR as a primary study in modern departments are very limited.

## The skull: X-rays and CT

Current indications for SXR include:

1   Differential diagnosis between meningioma and other tumours when doubt remains on CT or NMR.

2   Clinical or CT evidence of craniofacial anomaly or involvement of the vault or base of the skull by dysplasia or craniostenosis.

3   More detailed examination of abnormal bone noted on CT if the aetiology is not evident; in practice, this rarely allows a more precise diagnosis.

4   Assessment for skull involvement by certain types of scalp lesion, including neoplasm, inflammation, angioma or superficial soft tissue swelling of undetermined origin.

5   Severe head trauma, especially to show depressed fractures. Study for cervical spine injury is often indicated also. A history of mild head injury in asymptomatic patients or associated only with superficial bruising, headache or dizziness does not merit skull radiographs (DeLacey et al. 1980).

If neither CT nor NMR is available, plain film examination, which can often be restricted to a single lateral exposure without compromising diagnosis (Tress 1983), is performed in many more situations. Patients are not infrequently referred to the neurosurgeon with X-rays already made; facility with interpretation of skull X-rays is therefore advantageous and many of the skull abnormalities discussed in this section can also be observed on CT images displayed at appropriate window settings.

For correct interpretation of SXRs a basic understanding of the conventional radiographic projections is necessary (Du Boulay 1980).

The common projections include:

*Lateral*   The patient lies supine with one side of the head against a vertically supported film and the sagittal plane of the head parallel with the

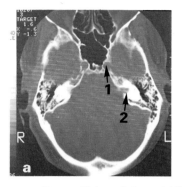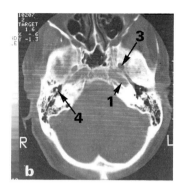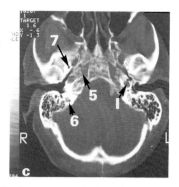

**Fig. 3.1.** High resolution axial CT scan. Window settings to show bone. (a, b, c). Contiguous 5 mm thick sections. Carotid canal (1), internal auditory meatus (2), foramen ovale (3), middle ear with ossicles (4), foramen lacerum (5), cochlear aqueduct (6), foramen spinosum (7).

film. The horizontal central ray should pass through the sella turcica.

*Anteroposterior (AP)* The head rests with the occiput on the film, the face directed towards the X-ray tube, which is tilted slightly towards the feet with the central ray in the sagittal plane. This view reveals details of the occipital and petrous bones. Tilting the tube further towards the feet (30°) projects the foramen magnum between the medial ends of the petrous bones (Towne's view).

*Postero-anterior (PA)* The forehead is against the film, giving clear definition of the frontal bones and orbits. If the central ray is inclined more obliquely, the petrous bones are projected within the orbits.

*Submentovertical* The neck is extended so that the vertex rests upon the film; the central ray passes through the base of the skull, caudal to the chin. The boundaries of the middle cranial fossa, the basisphenoid and basi-occiput, the sphenoidal air sinuses and the basal foramina are shown. All these structures are shown to good advantage on high resolution axial CT sections (Fig. 3.1).

*Optic foramen (see* Fig. 3.18c) The long axes of the foramina diverge and they are often obscured in the standard PA by the lateral mass of the

ethmoid. Separate projections along the orbit will show the optic foramen, superior orbital fissure and the floor of the anterior fossa outlined by the orbital rim; they are also demonstrated to good advantage incidentally on CT studies of the orbit and optic nerves (*see* Fig. 3.11).

The skull may reveal evidence of intracranial disease in a variety of ways. In most cases the significant bone changes are visible on high resolution CT using appropriate windowing, though they are then often of little importance if the causative abnormalities are demonstrated. Raised intracranial pressure, regardless of aetiology and the situation of a lesion, may cause specific changes. Localized skull thinning, thickening, bulging or increased vascularity may be due to a nearby tumour. The skull may also be affected in generalized diseases of bone and it may exhibit congenital malformations.

Abnormal calcareous deposits within the cranial cavity may signify certain tumours, vascular abnormalities, inflammatory or metabolic diseases. The displacement from their normal situation of the pineal body or the choroid plexus is indirect evidence of a mass.

In order to minimize the risk of overlooking abnormality, inspection of images should be carried out methodically. In the case of the skull, particular parts are examined for alteration in shape, size, situation and texture. The more important structures to inspect seriatim are the vault, its tables and vessel markings and suture lines; the sella turcica and sphenoid; the petrous bones, the basal foramina and upper cervical vertebrae. The area within the vault is searched for pathological calcification and for any deviation from the normal situation of calcification in the pineal body and the choroid plexuses.

## Increased intracranial pressure

In infants, separation of the sutures may occur within hours of elevation of intracranial pressure and the head may enlarge. Head enlargement also occurs in older children with prolonged elevation of intracranial pressure. It is often accompanied by elongation of the digitations of the sutures. In older children and adults, the radiographic signs are essentially the result of bone resorption; pressure must have been elevated for at least four weeks if radiographic signs are present. In children from about two to nine years, general thinning and/or increased convolutional marking may occur (Fig. 3.2); convolutional markings are normal in regions where the growing brain is closely applied to the vault but do not extend up to the vertex. Increased markings are not seen in the infant, probably because there is normally at that age a greater quantity of cerebrospinal fluid over the convexity which damps the pulsations from the cortex and, in addition, the bones can easily separate. In the adult, pathological convolutional markings suggest long-standing increased intracranial pressure. It is generally accompanied by sellar erosion, but may be the dominant feature in raised intracranial pressure associated with craniostenosis.

Erosion and eventually loss of the cortical lining of the floor and dorsum sellae is the commonest radiographic evidence of raised intracranial pressure in the adult skull (Fig. 3.3). In advanced cases, the sella turcica may be enlarged (Du Boulay and El Gammal 1966) (Fig. 3.4). In lesions causing chronic obstructive hydrocephalus, especially in young patients, enlargement of the sella may mimic that due to a supra-

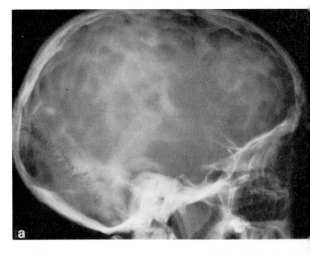

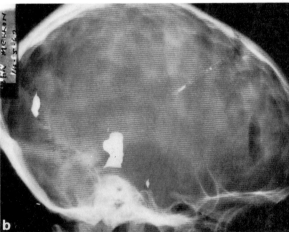

Fig. 3.2. Obstruction of the aqueduct, aged 14 years, probably due to benign stenosis. (a) Increased convolutional markings, truncated dorsum sellae. (b) Myodil/air ventriculogram. Myodil in the posterior end of the third ventricle fills the trumpet-shaped mouth of the aqueduct; the great size of the lateral ventricles is evident from the air in the tips of the anterior horns and the Myodil in an occipital horn.

or intrasellar tumour. These changes in the sella turcica are usually due to the downward distension of the floor of the third ventricle, which approaches the mouth of the sella and straddles the stunted dorsum.

Raised intracranial pressure may cause excavations elsewhere in the skull base, usually most marked in the middle fossae. Small herniations of brain are forced through weak points in the

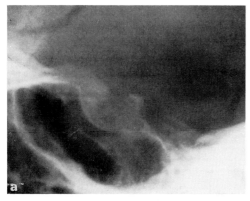 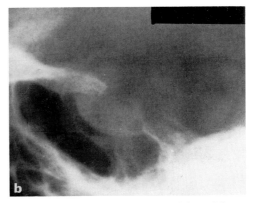

**Fig. 3.3.** Raised intracranial pressure. (a) There is loss of the cortex over most of the dorsum and floor of the sella turcica. (b) Six months later. The cortex of the whole sella and of the tuberculum has been absorbed.

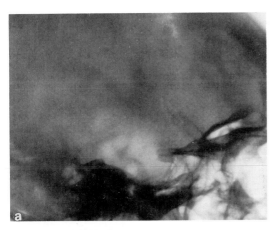

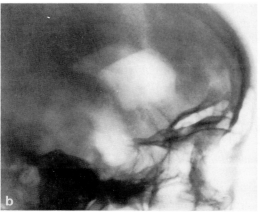

**Fig. 3.4.** A case of meningioma in the posterior cranial fossa. (a) The sella turcica is deep and the dorsum sellae absorbed. (b) Air ventriculogram, lateral brow-up, with head hyperextended. The dilated third ventricle fills the sella.

dura mater and excavate the bone. The sphenoidal ridge, seen ordinarily as a well defined curvilinear shadow, may be demineralized. Congenital hypoplasia of the sphenoid, which occurs in neurofibromatosis, is unilateral and has typical distinguishing features on SXR and CT (Fig. 3.5).

In addition to the general changes induced in the skull by increased pressure, especially in children, localized moulding can occur over a superficial cyst or a tumour, usually a glioma, situated in or immediately under the cortex (Fig. 3.6).

## Abnormal vessel markings

There are three main groups of diploic venous channels: frontal, parietal and occipital. They are recognized by their uneven calibre and irregular course; they join and divide like the channels of a river delta. Their development varies so much that it is unreliable to regard prominent diploic vessel markings as pathological. Enlargement of emissary veins occurs with raised intracranial pressure; they become particularly evident in the region of the torcular Herophili.

Abnormal grooving of the inner table by enlarged meningeal arteries and veins occurs in the vicinity of a meningioma or dural arterio venous malformation (Fig. 3.7). These channels

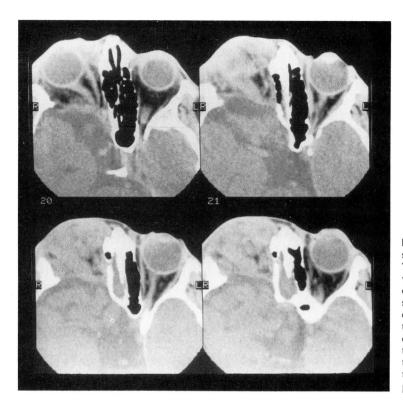

Fig. 3.5. Neurofibromatosis. CT scan, middle fossa and orbits. There is hypoplasia of the right wing and right side of the body of the sphenoid bone. The right side of the middle fossa is expanded and encroaches on the wide but shallow orbit, causing proptosis. There is thickening of the soft tissues in the upper part of the orbit and the right side of the face by a plexiform neurinoma.

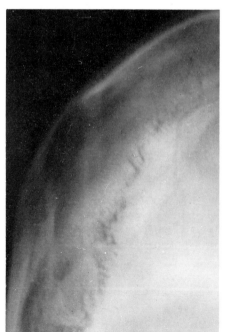

Fig. 3.6. Thinning and bulging of the vault over a subjacent glioma.

may correspond with the normal situation of the branches of the middle meningeal arteries, or they may develop elsewhere in the vault. They can be distinguished from diploic channels by their even calibre and from fractures by their smooth sinuous course; when they branch they do so with an angular junction. A large middle meningeal artery may cause enlargement of the foramen spinosum. Not to be confused with pathological enlargement of meningeal vessels is the occasional deep, wide groove of a spheno-parietal sinus, which passes smoothly upwards and backwards in the position of the anterior branch of the middle meningeal artery; it may be present on each side, does not branch, and reaches the vertex at or behind the coronal suture. In association with the pathological enlargement of meningeal vessels the bone in one area may have a fine, but irregular, spotted appearance where the excessive vascular channels often converge. This is the site of tumour attachment: at operation the inner surface of

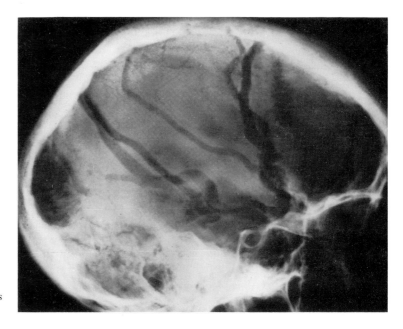

**Fig. 3.7.** Dural angiomatous malformation. Lateral skull radiograph. There is gross enlargement of meningeal vascular grooves on both sides of the vault.

the bone is roughened and penetrated by small vessels from the abnormally adherent and vascular dura mater. Computerized tomography shows the tumour itself, and angiography will show the excessive vascularity derived from the meningeal circulation.

## Local destruction of bone

A typical example of erosion of bone by adjacent pressure is that of the sella turcica produced by an intrasellar mass (Fig. 3.8). The enlargement of the sella may occur due to 'modelling' brought about by resorption and laying down of bone;

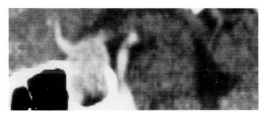

**Fig. 3.8.** Pituitary adenoma. Enhanced CT, reformatted in sagittal plane, showing sella enlarged by the mass of the adenoma, which extends through the chiasmatic cistern into contact with the optic chiasm and anterior recesses of the third ventricle.

with slowly growing tumours the sellar cortex has a crisp outline. With more rapidly progressing lesions resorption generally predominates; this is characterized by an indefinite edge without there necessarily being any enlargement of the pituitary fossa. Pituitary microadenomas may cause focal thinning and/or expansion, but similar appearances of the sella have been shown at post-mortem studies with normal pituitary glands and with nontumorous cysts, and are not a reliable indication of a tumour or its site in the gland (Muhr et al. 1981). Larger masses cause more diffuse erosion (Fig. 3.9). In advanced cases the dorsum sellae and posterior clinoid processes may disappear or the posterior clinoid processes may persist, apparently unsupported, and could be mistaken for pathological calcification. The sphenoidal air sinus may be encroached upon. The anterior clinoid processes may be sharpened or displaced upwards due to the moulding effect of the tumour on the interclinoid ligaments. A tumour extending laterally through the region of the cavernous sinus may cause erosion of the posterior wall of the orbit and/or enlargement of the superior orbital fissure. Enlargement of the sella turcica may be asymmetrical: this is very evident on CT

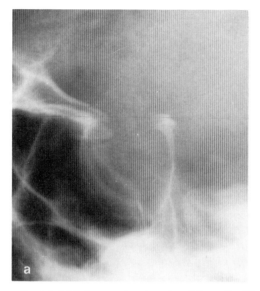 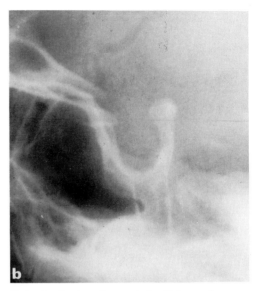

**Fig. 3.9.** (a) Enlargement and erosion of the walls of the sella turcica due to a chromophobe pituitary adenoma.
(b) Reossification of sella 5 years after surgery.

images but may be shown more subtly as an excessive tilt on AP and multiple contours on lateral X-rays. Asymmetrical erosion occurs also with parasellar tumours and aneurysms.

Enlargement of the sella may occur in association with intrasellar extension of the chiasmatic cistern. This may be a consequence of previous surgical or radiotherapy treatment, or spontaneous infarction causing regression of a pituitary tumour. More commonly, it occurs in the presence of a deficient pituitary diaphragm in otherwise normal patients, or in association with raised intracranial pressure (Foley & Posner 1975). In nontumourous cases the sella is usually symmetrical and may be disproportionately deep. It may, however, be asymmetrical and indistinguishable from an intrasellar tumour. High resolution CT (Fig. 3.10) or NMR is generally diagnostic; CSF within the sella outlines the infundibulum, descending to pituitary tissue lying against the sellar floor (Haughton *et al.* 1980).

Gliomas of the optic chiasm and of the third ventricle characteristically erode the chiasmatic sulcus, causing forward extension of the sella relative to the anterior clinoid processes.

Tumours involving the optic nerve may cause enlargement and rounding of the optic canal which is normally about 4.5 mm × 6.0 mm. Meningiomas of the sheath of the optic nerve also may expand the optic canal and/or cause sclerosis of its margins. These tumours are diagnosed at an earlier stage by CT or NMR, in which the bone changes are evident but of secondary importance (Fig. 3.11).

The sellar region may also be eroded due to invasion of the sphenoid bone by a chordoma or a malignant growth (Fig. 3.12), or to osteitis secondary to infection of the sphenoid air sinus.

Resorption is the predominent bone change in under 10% of meningiomas and is much less typical than local productive change. It is important to distinguish the normal corticated excavations of the inner table produced by venous lakes and Pacchionian granulations. These are most common adjacent to the superior sagittal sinus groove but may occur elsewhere in the vault.

Excavation of the porus acusticus (Fig. 3.13) suggests acoustic neurinoma, but it also occurs with other masses in the auditory canal, including meningioma, facial neuroma and exophytic

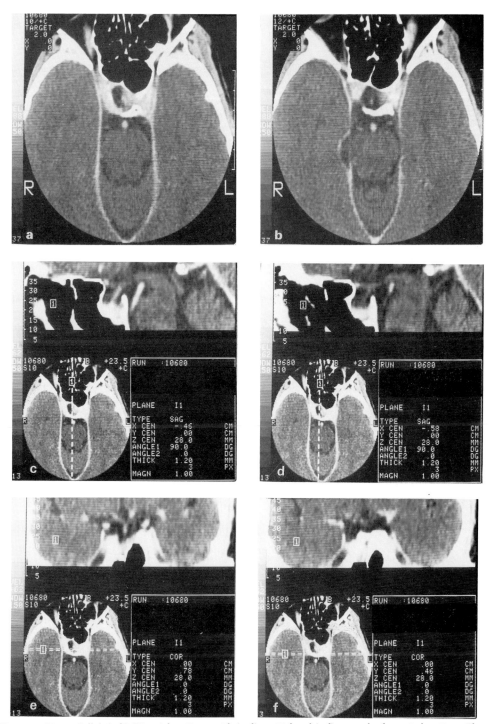

**Fig. 3.10.** 'Empty Sella'. (a, b) CT, axial sections, with (c, d) sagittal and (e, f) coronal reformatted sections. The sella is asymmetrical. The chiasmatic cistern extends deeply into the right side of the sella, outlining the pituitary stalk.

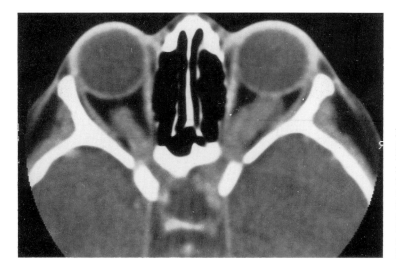

**Fig. 3.11.** Bilateral optic nerve gliomas. The orbital and intracranial segments of the right optic nerve are thickened; the optic foramen is expanded and the adjacent part of the tuberculum eroded. The orbital segment of the left optic nerve is enlarged. The intracranial segment and the left optic foramen are normal.

brain stem astrocytoma. Clean cut erosion of the tip of the petrous bone is typical of trigeminal schwannoma, though a meningioma of the cerebellopontine angle also may invade any part of the petrous bone. Enlargement of the jugular and of the anterior condyloid foramina occurs with tumours of the nerves traversing them, though these are rare (Chapter 8). Ill-defined erosion and enlargement of the jugular foramen is usually due to a glomus jugulare tumour (Fig. 3.14).

Occasionally foraminal erosion is due to a metastasis (Fig. 3.15).

An epidermoid arising within the bone produces a characteristic appearance; an oval or round area of translucency, with a scalloped

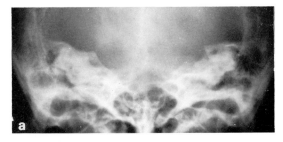

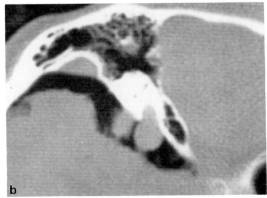

**Fig. 3.12.** Carcinoma of the nasopharynx. CT scan made with bone window. The tumour has eroded through skull base, forming a mass within sphenoid sinuses and destroying the posterior part of the body of the sphenoid, including the sella.

**Fig. 3.13.** Acoustic schwannoma. (a) SXR, Towne's projection, showing enlargement of internal auditory meatus. (b) Air meatogram (another patient) showing tumour extending out into cerebellopontine angle.

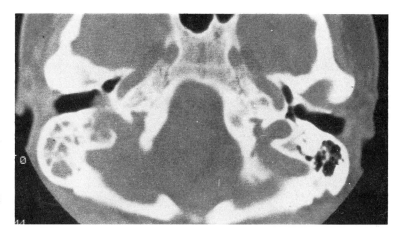

**Fig. 3.14.** Glomus jugulare tumour. CT scan, axial sections. There is erosion of the lateral border of the vascular compartment of the right jugular foramen. The right mastoid air cells are opaque and a soft tissue mass extends into the middle ear cavity.

margin clearly defined by a rim of new bone. Tangential views or CT show the tables to be 'expanded' or separated from one another (Fig. 3.16). Cavernous haemangioma (Fig. 3.17) causes a circular area of osteolysis, sometimes with a trabeculated texture, and a tangential film with low penetration may reveal superficial new bone formation with no peripheral rim of bone. Osteolytic lesions of the skull, usually round in shape, though not necessarily so, with no surrounding reactive sclerosis, are caused by a great variety of conditions and in many the skull lesion is a local manifestation of general disease. In histiocytosis X the skull lesions may be multiple, and other bones may be affected. Multiple areas with ill defined margins may be due to

carcinomatous metastases or to multiple myelomata; typically there is no excessive vascular marking and no expansion of the tables. Solitary myeloma also give rise to a somewhat irregular region of localized bone destruction with a poorly defined margin, and sometimes with reactive new bone and prominent meningeal vessels. Primary sarcoma of the skull is uncommon; the bone destruction is diffuse, its margin ill-defined and a tangential view with soft rays may show radiating spicules of new bone within the tumour.

In acute osteomyelitis of the skull no radiological change can be detected for at least two weeks, then irregular osteolysis occurs as the infection spreads unevenly through the diploe. Dense islands may remain and ultimately constitute sequestra, often comprising the outer table only and visible on tangential projections.

### Increased bone formation

*Localized*

Excessive bone formation may cause increased density (sclerosis), and/or increase in size (hyperostosis). These changes may be due to a primary tumour of bone (osteoma), a reaction of the bone to a contiguous tumour or inflammatory focus, or may be the result of systemic disease. Osteoma of the skull occurs as a smooth sessile mass aris-

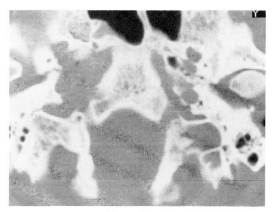

**Fig. 3.15.** Metastasis left hypoglossal canal. CT shows erosion of margins of the canal, with loss of cortex. Note normal asymmetry of jugular foramina.

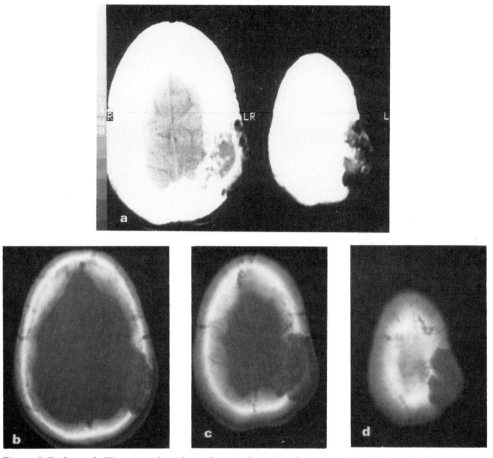

**Fig. 3.16.** Epidermoid. CT scan, made with windows to show (a) soft tissue and (b, c, d) bone. The lesion arises within the diploe, expanding and destroying the bone. There is a thin, dense line of new bone formation corticating the edge of the region of destruction. There is no evidence of any extension of the lesion beyond the expanded bone and the underlying brain substance is normal.

ing anywhere from the outer table; fairly frequent, small, dense, pedunculated, pea-like excrescences seen within the frontal sinuses are osteomas or ossifying fibromas. Occasionally they obstruct the nasal duct or, arising from the ethmoid bone, reach such a size as to involve ethmoidal and frontal sinuses and expand into the orbit. Orbito-ethmoidal osteomas can erode the skull base and give rise to serious intracranial complications.

Meningioma frequently causes new bone formation adjacent to its dural attachment, which may form a projection into the base of the tumour. Sometimes, with parasagittal men-

ingiomas in particular, the thickening affects the outer table as well as the inner, so that there is an external boss of bone over the tumour (Fig. 3.18a). Meningiomas arising from the wings of the sphenoid (Fig. 3.18b & c) and from the tuberculum sellae usually cause diagnostic thickening; involvement of the orbit may cause proptosis. These massive and dense reactions to meningioma are usually accompanied by some adjacent soft tissue tumour shown on CT, though this may be very thin with meningioma *en plaque*. Occasionally metastatic carcinoma of the prostate (Fig. 3.19) or breast, or a lymphoma, causes similar changes. In these cases the

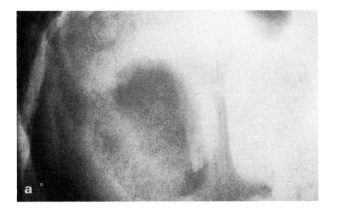

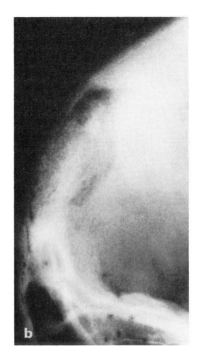

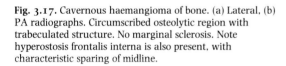

**Fig. 3.17.** Cavernous haemangioma of bone. (a) Lateral, (b) PA radiographs. Circumscribed osteolytic region with trabeculated structure. No marginal sclerosis. Note hyperostosis frontalis interna is also present, with characteristic sparing of midline.

primary neoplasm or other metastases are usually evident and there is generally no adjacent soft tissues mass on CT. Hyperostosis frontalis interna or Morgagni's syndrome gives a typical appearance of nodular thickening of the inner table of the frontal bone, usually on both sides but sparing the midline (*see* Fig. 3.17), and when advanced it has the appearance of cobblestones. The condition is most frequently seen in postmenopausal women; its cause is obscure and there are no related symptoms.

Dense, structureless, rather irregularly shaped masses of bone, single or multiple, arising from the base of the skull, sometimes also from the facial bones and jaws, are likely to indicate fibrous dysplasia. In some cases the abnormal bone is less dense due to a local accumulation of fibrous connective tissue with little ossification. The condition may simulate a meningeal hyperostosis of the sphenoidal wing causing proptosis, but it has usually been evident from childhood and has no adjacent soft tissue mass of CT. The disease may involve the long bones and skull and

be associated with cutaneous pigmentation and sexual precocity (Leeds & Seaman 1962).

*Diffuse*

Diffuse increase on the density of bone is characteristic of osteopetrosis (marble bones or Albers-Schonberg disease), and it becomes evident soon after birth. In osteitis deformans (Paget disease) the skull becomes thickened, particularly the outer table which may show a patchy increase in density (Fig. 3.20). In the early stages of the disease the affected bone may be rarefied, and when well delineated is termed osteoporosis circumscripta; the bone is soft, so that the weight of the skull causes basilar invagination, the basi-occiput being impressed into the cranial cavity.

Acromegaly is a clinical diagnosis. Uniform thickening of the skull is usually evident, with large air sinuses and mastoids and enlargement of the mandible.

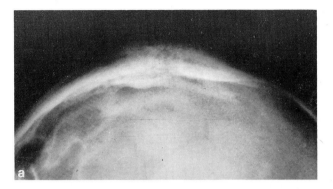

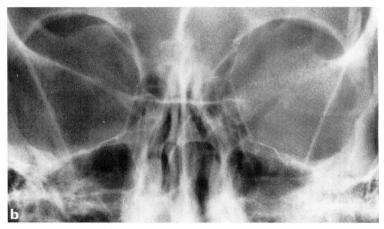

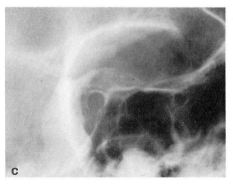

Fig. 3.18. (a) Meningiomatous hyperostosis of vault. (b) Meningiomatous hyperostosis of lesser wing of sphenoid. (c) View for optic foramen. Meningiomatous hyperostosis of anterior clinoid and upper strut of lesser wing of sphenoid.

*Other changes*

Abnormalities of the shape of the skull may be congenital or acquired. Monstrous conditions of the skull, such as anencephaly and cyclops, are clinically evident. Circular defects on the bone, usually near the sagittal plane, are asssociated with protrusion of cranial contents in meningocele or encephalocele. Anteriorly there may be a defect in the cribriform plate of the ethmoid or in the frontal bone, with protrusion into the nasopharynx, nasal cavity and/or at the bridge of the nose. Hamartomatous masses of brain tissue, termed nasal gliomas, may simulate

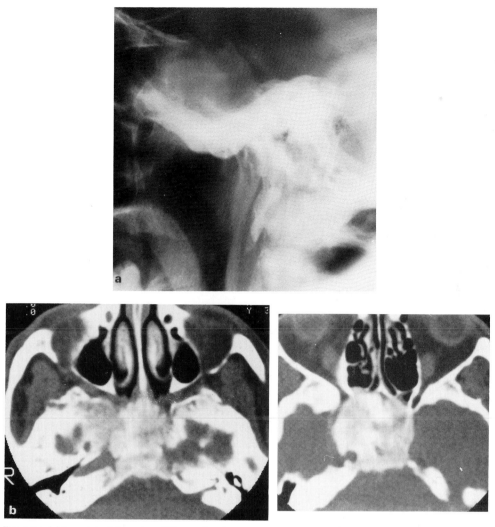

**Fig. 3.19.** (a) Invasion of the sphenoid by a sclerotic metastatic carcinoma of prostate. (b) CT scan. The extent of the bone sclerosis and expansion involving the body and greater wings of sphenoid is well shown.

these herniations. Posterior herniations occur through the occipital bone and sometimes an upper cervical spina bifida also.

The contents of the sac, the presence of any other malformation of the brain and of hydrocephalus are elucidated by ultrasound, NMR or CT.

Normally there exists in each parietal bone, near the midline and slightly anterior to its posterior border, a minute foramen which transmits an artery and a vein, the latter communicating with the sagittal sinus; occasionally these 'parietal foramina' are large.

In 'lacunar skull' there are areas of thinning, larger than convolutional impressions, separated by trabeculae or buttresses of thicker bone. The condition is often associated with other congenital abnormalities (Chapter 16). Close to the midline small defects of bone may occur, through which part of the sagittal sinus, or an abnormal

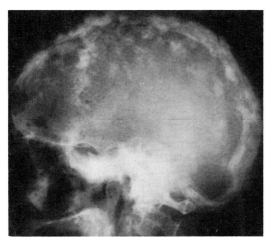

**Fig. 3.20.** Paget disease, with basilar impression.

dural sinus communicating with it, may bulge, causing the defect to pulsate; the condition is termed 'sinus pericranii'.

Premature closure of the sutures, cranio stenosis or synostosis cranii prevent the capacity of the skull from keeping pace with the growing brain. If the sutures are unequally affected plagiocephaly results and the head is asymmetrical and often of bizarre shape (Chapter 16).

### Platybasia, basilar invagination or impression

The basal angle, between the sagittal axis of the floor of the anterior cranial fossa and of the posterior cranial fossa, is usually 115–140°. It is demonstrated by a line drawn on the X-ray from the frontonasal suture to the centre of the pituitary fossa, and from there to the anterior lip of the foramen magnum. Flattening of this angle (platybasia) has no clinical consequences. Displacement upwards into the cranial cavity of the basi-occiput and its condyles may occur as a congenital anomaly, or due to invagination in conditions causing softening of bone (Fig. 3.20). Elevation of the odontoid may be caused by erosion of the supporting bony structures, most commonly by rheumatoid arthritis, occasionally by neoplasms; this may give rise to neurological disturbance (Chapter 16).

### Intracranial calcification

Calcification occurs normally in certain situations, it also occurs in pathological processes and is visible at much lower concentrations than on SXR with CT, which also has the major advantage of showing associated abnormality of attenuation or mass effect. The pineal body calcifies as age advances; calcification is uncommon in children but is visible on SXR in about 50–70% of adults (Du Boulay 1980). The calcified gland varies in size, density and texture but is usually about 0.5 cm in diameter and normally lies within 2 mm of the midline. In the lateral view the pineal is a short distance above and behind the petrous bones. Calcification in the habenular commisure has similar localizing value. It may form a characteristic C shape on the lateral and a circle on the sagittal radiograph.

Pineal calcification more than 1.0 cm diameter should be elucidated by CT as the calcification could be in a tumour. Any swelling within or overlying a cerebral hemisphere frequently causes lateral displacement of the pineal body; displacement in the sagittal plane may also be recognized (Epstein & Davidoff 1953).

Calcification in the choroid plexuses is less frequent than in the pineal body, being visible on X-rays in up to 13% of individuals. It typically occurs in the glomus in the vestibule of the lateral ventricle, but may affect any part of the plexus;

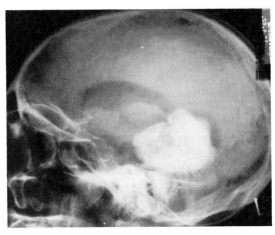

**Fig. 3.21.** Calcified papilloma of choroid plexus.

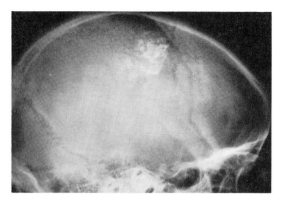

Fig. 3.22. Calcification in oligodendroglioma.

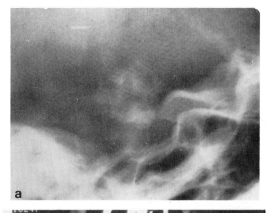

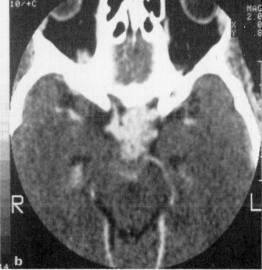

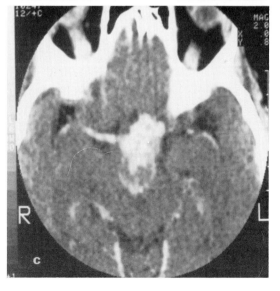

it may be unilateral or bilateral and is usually asymmetrical. The calcification consists of a collection of small spots, often forming a rounded, sometimes irregular aggregate or ring, commonly measuring up to 1.5 cm in diameter but occasionally larger. A large, densely calcified, unilateral mass is likely to be pathological and in a meningioma or papilloma (Fig. 3.21). In coronal projections the choroid glomus calcification is normally seen about halfway between the midline and the lateral wall of the cranium; in the lateral view the glomus calcification lies about a centimetre below and behind the pineal. On CT the relationship to the choroid and ventricle will be demonstrated directly.

Ossification often occurs in the dura mater, particularly in the elderly. In the falx it often shows clearly in the sagittal views as dense, limpet shaped opacities, with the flat base in the midline. Calcification in the walls of the superior sagittal sinus may form a V-shaped shadow adjacent to the groove. Linear calcification may join the anterior and posterior clinoid processes, pass backwards and downwards from the posterior clinoid process in the petroclinoid ligaments, or line the free edge of the tentorium.

Fig. 3.23 (*right*). Calcification in craniopharyngioma. (a) Lateral skull radiograph. The sella is flattened, the dorsum truncated. (b, c) Enhanced CT scan. Partly calcified suprasellar mass. The posterior part is of lower density, with ring enhancement; it was cystic.

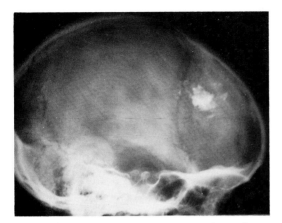

**Fig. 3.24.** Calcification within meningioma. The overlying vault is thinned, the vascular markings are excessive.

Neoplastic calcification is most common in gliomas in which it occurs in a variety of patterns: the commonest is irregular grouping of small and large deposits, as streaks with curvilinear outlines which may be present throughout in only part of the tumour. These patterns may occur in any form of slowly growing glioma, but smooth, wavy, homogeneous bands are relatively common in oligodendrogliomas (Fig. 3.22). Tuberose sclerosis may cause typical scattered, small, calcified nodules in the subependymal regions and parenchyma; the bones of the skull may be sclerosed.

The tumour which most frequently calcifies is the craniopharyngioma. The incidence is as high as 70% overall about 30% in adults, 80–90% in children (Du Boulay 1980) and it may be visible in infants. Calcification varies from a single fleck, a curvilinear band in a cyst wall, or a speckled collection in solid tumours. The situation is of importance in diagnosis; commonly it is in the mouth of the sella turcica or immediately above it (Fig. 3.23a), less frequently within the sella. In the sagittal projection it is usually close to the midline; its precise position and relation to the tumour will be evident on CT (Fig. 3.23b & c). Calcification in the wall of an aneurysm or the capsule of a pituitary adenoma, in a glioma or teratoma and, rarely, in a meningioma, may simulate the calcification of a craniopharyngioma. The sella turcica is seldom normal if a craniopharyngioma is present; the fossa may be enlarged or flattened, or have a stunted dorsum sellae.

Calcification is less frequently visible in other tumours. In meningiomas, distinct from the hyperostosis at its base (Fig. 3.24), in papilloma of the choroid plexus, in chordoma and bracketing the margins of a lipoma of the corpus callosum.

In vascular malformations calcification may be dense or so slight that it is seen merely as faint flecks. A characteristic appearance of wavy double lines following the sinuous course of those sulci in the axis of the X-rays occurs when cal-

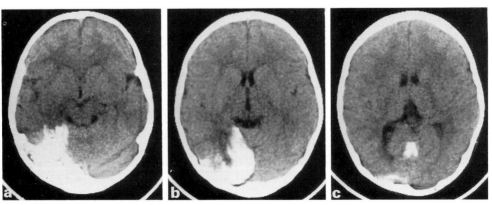

**Fig. 3.25.** Sturge–Weber syndrome. (a, b, c) CT scan. There is calcification, which was not visible on skull radiographs, superficially in the right occipital lobe. The overlying posterior part of the hemicranium is relatively small due to local cerebral atrophy.

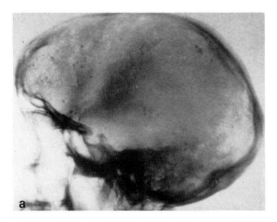

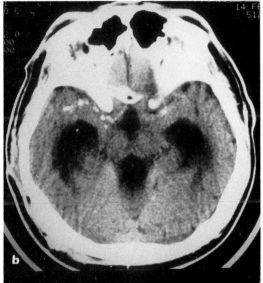

**Fig. 3.26.** Calcified cysticerci. (a) Lateral skull radiograph. Multiple calcified scolices are shown. (b) CT scan, sections through level of Sylvian fissure and posterior fossa. Multiple calcified cysticerci are present in the Sylvian fissure, mainly on the left side. The basal cisterns are almost obliterated by fibrous reaction which is causing marked four-ventricular hydrocephalus.

cium is laid down in the cortical grey matter. This pattern is particularly well seen in the Sturge–Weber syndrome in which the occipital lobes are usually first and most severely affected; calcification is not usually visible on X-rays before the age of 2 years (Alexander & Norman 1960) but is revealed much earlier by CT (Fig. 3.25). The abnormal brain is usually atrophic and the ipsilateral hemicranium is then diminished in volume and may be thickened.

Atheromatous plaques in the internal carotid artery may cast a typical curvilinear, tubular density across the sella turcica in the lateral and a circular density in the parasellar region on sagittal projections. The calcified wall of an intracranial saccular aneurysm is seen as an arc, rarely as a complete circle. The membrane enclosing a chronic subdural haematoma occasionally calcifies.

Calcification may occur in tissues devitalized by inflammatory or ischaemic lesions. It may be seen in cysticerci (Fig. 3.26) as a series of seed-like opacities, smaller than those occurring much more frequently in the muscles. High density in healed abscesses is produced by calcification or by radio-opaque media (Thorotrast, barium sulphate) which used to be injected to control treatment by aspiration. Treated tuberculous meningitis may be followed by calcification in the fibrous meningeal reaction around the brain stem in cisterna ambiens and the cisterna chiasmaticus (Lorber 1958) (Fig. 3.27); the diagnosis is confirmed by the past history. Congenital toxoplasmosis may give rise to scattered curvilinear and nodular flecks anywhere in the cerebral

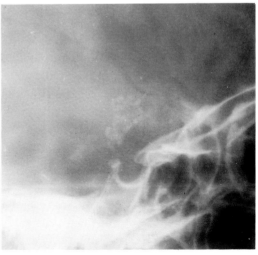

**Fig. 3.27.** Suprasellar calcification following recovery from tuberculous meningitis may simulate that within a craniopharyngioma, but the sella is normal.

hemispheres. Cytomegalovirus infection tends to cause curvilinear calcification around the lateral ventricles, which may be dilated from atrophy or hydrocephalus.

Hypoparathyroidism, pseudohypoparathyroidism and other rare disorders of metabolism and unknown aetiology may lead to calcification in the basal ganglia and, less frequently, in the dentate nuclei and deep hemospheric white matter.

### Intracranial translucence

This is usually due to the entrance of air. It occurs in fractures involving the paranasal sinuses, roof of the nose or mastoid. The aerocele may be a minute bubble in a basal cistern or a large collection within the substance of the brain. Air may also enter the cranium as a result of erosion by a tumour, commonly an orbito-ethmoidal osteoma, or it may be contained within a mucocoele of a frontal or sphenoidal air sinus. An abscess may contain gas due to bacterial activity.

A lipoma is demonstrable by less marked radiolucency. The site of predilection is the corpus callosum as a sausage shaped mass which may be bracketed by curvilinear calcification.

## The ventricles and subarachnoid spaces

### Ventriculography and encephalography

Ventriculography was devised by Dandy (1918); a small hole was bored in the skull and a cannula passed into the lateral ventricle, through which air was introduced. In the following year he showed that air introduced by lumbar puncture would ascend into the ventricules and intracranial subarachnoid spaces. This elaboration, air encephalography (AEG), proved as valuable as ventriculography in appropriate cases.

When CT or NMR are available, encephalography and ventriculography are rarely indicated. Limited pneumoencephalography is used with CT for diagnosis of small, mainly or entirely

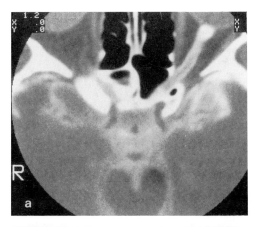

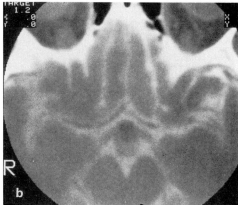

**Fig. 3.28.** Computed cisternogram. (a) Through optic canals, (b) above canals, through orbital roofs. The chiasmatic cistern with optic chiasm and proximal parts of optic tracts (b) and optic nerves and pituitary stalk (a) are well shown. The supraclinoid segments of the internal carotid arteries are in the lateral parts of the cistern (a) and the anterior cerebral and middle cerebral branches enter the Sylvian fissures (b). The left optic nerve sheath is fully opacified and the optic canals are traversed (a).

intracanicular acoustic neurinomas (*see* Fig. 3.13) (Bassi *et al.* 1985); NMR is likely to replace this procedure as soon as it is freely available. More frequently, intrathecal nonionic contrast media are used in conjunction with CT to increase the density of narrow subarachnoid spaces in which the depth of CSF is insufficient to offset partial volume; it reveals the cranial nerves and cisternal anatomy (Fig. 3.28) (Manelfe & Bonafe 1980) and can, for example, be particularly valuable in defining brain stem tumours and cerebellar ectopia. Also, because

CT provides higher resolution than gamma detectors, nonionic contrast media is more useful than radioactive isotopes for study of CSF dynamics. Since the introduction of simple methods of pressure monitoring, dynamic studies are uncommonly used in distinguishing atrophy from communicating hydrocephalus (Hindmarsh & Greitz 1977), but opacification of arachnoid cysts will differentiate these from other low density, superficial, nonenhancing masses. Conventional ventriculography is very occasionally used for elucidation of the anatomy of an intraventricular obstruction, but even in these rare instances intraventricular nonionic media are generally preferable.

*Ventriculography: technique*

Except in children and individuals who are very nervous or unable to cooperate, the procedure is with advantage carried out under local anaesthetic, so that the patient can help in the various manipulations which are necessary in order to bring the air or contrast medium into the appropriate parts of the ventricular system, and with the radiographic positioning. A burr hole is made in the right frontal region, on the coronal suture, about 2–3 cm to the right of the midline. The frontal horn is cannulated and a measurement of the CSF pressure is made with a manometer. The depth to which the cannula enters the brain before fluid escapes is a rough guide to the size of the ventricle. In the normal adult the roof of the ventricle lies approximately 5 cm from the surface of the cortex.

Precautions against an excessive fall of pressure should be observed. Informative radiographs depend on a sufficient quantity of air or positive contrast medium; when the ventricles are small much of the fluid needs replacing in order to obtain good pictures. When the ventricles are greatly enlarged, a large bubble occupying one third the length of the ventricle can be conveniently manoeuvred from one part of the system to another (*see* Fig. 3.4). Extensive replacement with air causes a severe reaction,

and may lead to subdural haemorrhage as a result of the cortex falling away from the vault. Thus, from the practical point of view, when carrying out the fluid replacement it is wise to collect and measure. The quantity and the ease with which it flows will give a rough indication of the size of the ventricles. If after 25 ml of fluid has escaped the flow practically ceases, it is clear that the ventricles are not much enlarged, if at all, and more fluid should be coaxed out by turning the head, by slight jugular compression and by injecting slightly more air. If 50 ml escapes, and the flow is still copious, the ventricles are large.

In positive contrast ventriculolgraphy, nonionic contrast medium is injected with the head markedly flexed or turned to one side, so that it flows into the frontal horn and remains there until the necessary manipulations are made. Introduction through a catheter in the frontal horn with fluoroscopic control is the preferable method. The head is gradually extended sufficiently to cause the contrast medium to flow through the foramen of Monro into the third ventricle. Films are exposed as necessary to document the procedure (*see* Fig. 3.2).

*Dangers of ventriculography and encephalography*

1 Rapid aggravation of the raised intracranial pressure due to vasodilatation or increased secretion of cerebrospinal fluid.
2 Shift of a mass.
3 Increase in temporal lobe or tonsillar herniation.
4 Hypothalamic crisis in hydrocephalus, probably due to congestion and oedema of the walls of the third centricle.
5 Haemorrhage into the ventricle as a result of striking the choroid plexus; into the brain during the passage of the cannula; into a tumour if the cannula traverses it; as a result of lowering the intracranial pressure, by rupture of a cortical vein, if the brain collapses in marked hydrocephalus causing an acute subdural haemorrhage.

Many of these dangers can be mimimized if ventriculography is immediately followed by craniotomy in the event of a lesion being demonstrated. The dangers are also lessened by avoiding large replacements, by avoiding an excessive lowering of the intracranial pressure and by releasing the pressure immediately after the films have been taken. Nevertheless, air ventriculography remains potentially dangerous in patients with large tumours or high pressure, and is only used when alternative diagnostic methods are not available. Positive contrast ventriculography with an ionic contrast medium has been shown to cause moderate intracranial hypertension. Positive contrast ventriculography with non-ionic media causes little disturbance of intracranial pressure and dangerous sequelae are uncommon.

In air encephalography (*see* Fig. 3.62), performed in modern radiology departments in patients with raised intracranial pressure, the dangers were similar to those of ventriculography, for example aggravation of pressure and internal herniation. They may be averted by taking prompt action, for example tapping the ventricle to allow the trapped air to escape, giving mannitol, immediate craniotomy. The films exposed after the first injection of air will reveal abnormality suggestive of herniation; the use of small quantities of air lessens the risks (Falk 1953). In normal and in atrophic lesions the dangers are negligible, though haemorrhage from an unsuspected vascular malformation has been encountered. Headache, vomiting and neck stiffness are unpleasant sequelae which vary considerably in degree but sometimes persist for several days. The patient requires rest in bed, sedation, analgesics and anti-emetics; raising the foot of the bed usually relieves headache. For a detailed study of pneumography the reader should consult Robertson (1957) or Norlen and Wickbom (1958).

### The normal ventricular and cisternal anatomy

The anatomical features noted in this section apply to the CSF spaces as revealed by any type of imaging, including pneumography, and as sectional images on CT and NMR. In a pneumogram it is usually necessary to build up the outline of the ventricular system from radiographs made in various positions of the head (Fig. 3.29).

In coronal and axial images the thin, clear, central vertical line of the septum lucidum separates the lateral ventricles. Anteriorly each of these comprises three areas formed by the curve of the floor of the body of the lateral ventricle as it approaches the foramen of Monro, with the thinning frontal horns as they diverge from the midline anteriorly, and the cella media posteriorly leading to the vestibule (atrium), which extends downwards, laterally and then medially into the temporal horn. The anterior end of the temporal horn lies behind the orbit, approximately midway between the midline and lateral plane of the skull, as a crescent-shaped shadow with a clear and convex lateral border and a concave inner margin, indented by the pes hippocampi. The third ventricle forms a narrow oval

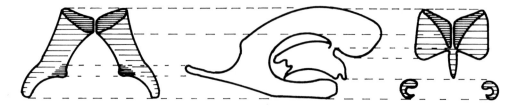

**Fig. 3.29.** Tracing of the lateral view of the lateral and third ventricles based on the cast by Retzius (Ranson & Clark 1947). If air fills approximately one half of their capacity, the AP, brow-up, ventriculogram takes the form shown on right, the PA, brow-down, that on the left. The zones of differing density depend upon the depth of the column of air traversed by the X-ray. The frontal horns are faint because they become thin anteriorly owing to the development of the forceps minor which displaces the medial walls laterally.

shadow, strictly in the midline, below and in the same axis as the septum lucidum.

In sagittal projections, the frontal horn lying anterior to the foramen of Monro has a bulbous shape, thinning anteriorly as it spreads out over the head of the caudate nucleus which bulges into the ventral part of its lateral wall, and the two horns are separated by the forceps minor; further back they are separated only by thin septum lucidum. The body or cella media, extending back from the foramen of Monro as far as the vestibule (trigone or atrium), is normally narrow with smooth contours, the roof and the floor both convex superiorly. The vestibule is bulky, and from it pass the posterior and the temporal horns. The floor of the body sweeps smoothly round the posterior body of the thalamus (covered by the fornix) to form the roof of the temporal horn. Lying on the floor of the cella media is the choroid plexus; it extends round the posterior border of the thalamus to lie in the roof of the temporal horn. It is bulkier in the vestibule, where it forms the slightly lobulated glomus. If a brain cannula strikes it and causes haemorrhage, enlargement with clot may simulate an intraventricular tumour. The temporal (descending) horn is narrow and usually terminates at a point just posterior to the coronal plane of the dorsum sellae. The posterior horn extends backwards from the vestibule; it varies in length, diameter and shape on one side compared with the other.

The third ventricle is a thin chamber, consequently its precise boundaries are often difficult to determine in the lateral view in the normal, though dilatation makes them much clearer. Anteriorly it passes downwards and forwards from the plane of the foramen of Monro, pointing towards the sella turcica; its extremity is notched by the optic chiasm so as to form supraoptic and infundibular recesses. Posteriorly the third ventricle extends backwards and slightly upwards, its roof running parallel to and separated from the floor of the body of the lateral ventricle by a narrow interval. The floor makes a smooth convex curve from the infundibular recess upwards, backwards and downwards, to

join the aqueduct of Sylvius. The anterior boundary, from the supraoptic recess to the foramen of Monro, is formed by the lamina terminalis. The posterior extremity of the third ventricle has a blunt-ended, irregular shape: inferiorly it is continuous with the aqueduct; above this is an expansion into the base of the pineal body and above this a further bulge. These are the pineal and suprapineal recesses. The former is small, and the latter varies in size but in some cases of hydrocephalus may be enlarged to form a pouch several centimetres in length. The massa intermedia forms a relatively clear area in about the middle of the third ventricle shadow; it varies considerably in size and if large may be mistaken for a tumour.

The aqueduct of Sylvius is a narrow channel, 16 mm in length, providing a linear shadow of even calibre, taking a gentle curve backwards and ventrally to open up into the fourth ventricle. In the norm it may be difficult to detect, particularly in the sagittal views, but when dilated it is shown readily; its demonstration is of great importance in the diagnosis of masses in the posterior cranial fossa. If a line is drawn from the upper extremity of the dorsum sellae through the midpoint of the aqueduct to the vault (Sahlstedt 1935), the aqueduct normally lies at the junction of the anterior and the middle one third of the line.

The fourth ventricle forms a triangular or tent-like shadow on the sagittal image, its broad base lying practically vertical forms the floor of the ventricle, comprising pons and medulla. The superior and inferior leaves of the roof may show as straight or slightly curved lines; on occasion they may be deeply indented by the superior and inferior vermis, which may be mistaken for tumour. The middle of the fourth ventricle lies on the midpoint of a line joining the tuberculum sellae and the internal occipital protuberance (Twining 1939). The contrast-filled fourth ventricle in the conventional semi-axial projection appears rhomboid or butterfly-shaped. Immediately rostral to it may be seen the posterior part of the third ventricle: a denser, central, round area formed by the emerging aqueduct end-on, joined to the upper end of the fourth ventricle by the thin streak of the vertical part of the aqueduct.

The lower extremity of the fourth ventricle normally terminates just above the foramen magnum. At its lower end the fourth ventricle communicates with the cisterna magna through the foramen of Magendie and at its lateral recesses through the foramina of Luschka into the basal or pontine cistern; patency of these foramina can be proved by outlining with or the passage of contrast media.

The cisterna magna, lying behind the lower medulla and upper cervical cord, appears oval or crescentic, with the lower poles of the cerebellar tonsils separated by the vallecula dipping into it. The cistern varies markedly in size; it may expand the occipital bone and even transgress the tentorium and may be asymmetrical. A megacistern does not displace the fourth ventricle, as may be expected from a similarly placed arachnoid cyst. The cisternae medullaris pontis and interpeduncularis are in continuity, adjacent to the clivus, in front of the brain stem.

In continuity above, and surmounting the dorsum sellae and sella turcica, is the cisterna chiasmaticus. On axial section the cistern usually appears hexagonal with the posterior margins of the frontal lobes anteriorly, separated from the medial borders of the temporal lobes, which form the lateral borders of the cistern, by the Sylvian fissures. The posterior border is formed by the cerebral peduncles or if the section is sufficiently oblique it passes through the pons and the cistern then appears pentagonal. The obliquely lying optic nerves, chiasm and pituitary stalk can usually be identified; the vessels of the circle of Willis outline their perimeter and are usually visible on enhanced CT scans.

Continuing laterally from the pontine are the cerebellopontine angle cisterns, leading into the internal auditory meati and containing the 7th and 8th cranial nerves and frequently a loop of the anterior inferior cerebellar or the internal auditory artery. All these structures are evident on high resolution computerized cisternography and NMR. The cerebellar flocculi form nodules low in the cistern and the lobulus simplex encroaches on its upper part (Stevens & Kendall 1985). These structures should not be mistaken for acoustic neurinomas or tumours of the 5th cranial nerve, which traverses the superomedial aspect of the cistern between the pons and the cavernous sinus.

The wings of the cisterna ambiens, which surround the pulvinars of the thalami, cross the same transverse plane as the upper end of the aqueduct, passing in a forward and downward direction. The ambient cistern outlines the midbrain and leads into the quadrigeminal cistern, which profiles the colliculi and blends posteriorly with the superior cerebellar cistern lying above the superior vermis.

The Sylvian and interhemispheric fissures and the cortical sulci, which were inconsistently shown on pneumography, are of localizing value on CT and NMR, especially in the supraventricular regions which constitute about 25% of the brain substance. The central white matter is continuous with that forming each gyral core and is surmounted by the rim of cortical grey matter.

Many attempts have been made to fix a norm for the size of the ventricles as seen radiologically (Bruijn 1959). Last and Tompsett (1935) have made measurements of casts of presumed normal lateral ventricles which are about 20% smaller than corresponding measurements on ventriculograms. They noted considerable variation; thus in the specimen with the biggest brain volume, from a subject aged 68 years, the volume of the ventricles was 13.3 cm$^3$; in the smallest brain, in a subject of 29, the ventricular volume was 25.5 cm$^3$. There is also considerable variation in the width of normal cortical sulci, which may reach 4 mm in width before being recognizable as definitely abnormal. Physiological changes have been observed in the size of the CSF spaces, amounting to as much as 15% in linear measurements in the same individual within a short time, and are presumed to be related to variations in the volume of intracranial and intraspinal blood vessels. There is a tendency to an increase in the volume of the ventricular system and cortical sulci after the age of 60 years, related to involutional changes which may be considerable without intellectual deterioration or neurological abnormalities. These factors necessarily mean that there is overlap between the upper range of normal size and the early pathological, especially as regards linear measurements. Volume measurements are more reliable but are impractical as a routine without special computer programmes, which are not generally available. In practice, the ratio between the maximum width of the frontal horns and the maximal internal biparietal diameter of the skull (Evan's ratio; Evan 1942) is commonly used as an index of ventricular size, taking 30% as the upper limit of normality. Alternative measurements which have been recommended include the bifrontal diameter ratio (Hahn & Rim 1976), the ventricular index (Hirashima *et al.* 1983) and the ventriculobrain ratio (Synek & Reuben 1976). Other absolute measurements have been calculated from pneumographic studies and can be applied to CT and NMR with appropriate magnification corrections.

## Ultrasound

Since ultrasound (US) is reflected from bone, use of the method is generally limited to cases with a sonic gap. It is particularly valuable in new born, especially premature babies, (London *et al.* 1980) for detection of intracranial haemorrhage or hydrocephalus (Fig. 3.30) and is also useful in older infants prior to closure of the anterior fontanelle, and in postcraniectomy patients for the diagnosis of hydrocephalus, subdural effusion, arachnoid, Dandy Walker and intracerebral cysts; large aneurysms and angiomas will also be evident (Babcock & Han 1981).

Ultrasound through the intact skull is less accurate than computerized tomography in detection of midline shift and hydrocephalus, but may be useful when other facilities are not freely available. Intraoperative US may be used for accurate siting of tumours for biopsy, location of cysts and of the lateral ventricle prior to catheter insertion, and for controlling the removal of abnormal tissue (Rogers *et al.* 1984).

## Radioisotope scanning

Pertechnetate uptake following intravenous administration is increased in most lesions, with an enlarged blood pool or defective blood brain barrier. These include most malignant gliomas, meningeal tumours, neurinomas, inflammatory lesions, subacute haematomas and recent infarcts. However, the gamma camera has relatively low resolution so that uptake under 1 cm in diameter, unless it is very intense, is not com-

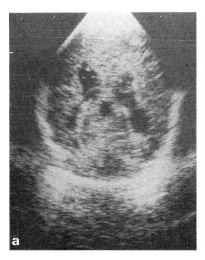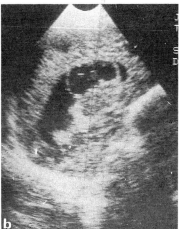

**Fig. 3.30.** Premature baby. Ultrasound study, (a) axial, (b) lateral. Intraventricular haemorrhage. Dilatation of lateral and third ventricles. Adhesions in lateral ventricles.

monly detected, especially if it lies deeply; also, normal brain and the effects on the lesion upon it, including oedema and shift, are not revealed. CT and NMR appearances are much more specific and sensitive in the diagnosis of all mass lesions, but can also detect conditions in which the blood brain barrier is intact, including low grade gliomas, nontumorous cysts, atrophies and malformations.

Only when CT is not available are isotopes used routinely in neurosurgical diagnosis. They can be usefully applied in screening for metastases from a known primary neoplasm, in detection of CSF leaks and flow patterns, for blood flow using iodoamphetamines and for showing increase of osteoblastic activity in bone metastases and premature suture closure using bone seeking isotopes. Indium labelled leukocytes may also be useful in confirming pyogenic abscess and the distinction from ring enhancement in tumour, though occasional false negatives and positives have been reported with this technique (Rehncrona *et al.* 1985).

## Computerized tomography

In CT, scintillation detectors are used to accurately measure and computers to localize X-ray absorption characteristics at all points within a planar section of any part of the body. These are expressed on an arbitrary scale of Hounsfield Units (HU) on which the reading of water is zero, dense bone 1000 HU, and air − 1000 HU. CT is sufficiently sensitive to discriminate 0.5% changes in absorption (5 HU) and has a spatial resolving capability of 0.5–1.0 mm.

X-ray absorption is determined fundamentally by:

1  The density of electrons within a tissue, which can be considered for practical purposes to be proportional to specific gravity, and in the diagnostic range to be independent of the energy of the X-rays used to produce the CT.

2  The concentration of heavy atoms, the effect of which is considerably influenced by the X-ray

energy used. Calcium (Ca) is the only element present in sufficient concentration to influence plain CT; each 1 mg Ca/ml increases absorption by 2.0 HU at 130 kV and by 2.5 HU at 100 kV. Iodide contrast medium, given by both intravenous and subarachnoid injections for enhanced scans, increases absorption by 25 HU/mg/ml at 120 kV. The contrast medium is retained within the blood–brain barrier so that the slight enhancement of normal brain substance reflects its blood volume. The capillaries of other tissues are permeable; the normal enhancement of muscle, dura and choroid plexuses is mainly due to extravasation.

Plain CT, supplemented if necessary by enhancement with intravenous contrast medium, is currently the most accurate, more or less readily available radiological study, and since it is only minimally invasive it is the imaging method of choice for detection and localization of intracranial abnormalities. In many cases it is also the most accurate study for prediction of the nature of a pathological process.

In practice, CT studies are viewed as images in which the digital values are expressed on a grey scale of about 15 shades extending between black and white which can be placed electronically to cover the densities relevant to each particular diagnostic problem.

Normal intracranial anatomy (Huckman *et al.* 1977, Gado *et al.* 1979) is well shown by differential contrast of CSF (0–6 HU), white matter (20–30 HU) and grey matter (35–45 HU) enclosed by the dura (Naidich *et al.* 1977a, 1977b) and dense bone of the skull. Fat (− 20–100 HU) muscle (c.20 HU) and air (− 1000 HU) define the anatomy of the orbit, face and pharynx.

Morphological abnormalities (Fig. 3.31), malformations, (Kendall & Kingsley 1978), atrophy (focal, regional or generalised), hydrocephalus and displacements are all recognized from modifications of the anatomy.

Pathology may be visualized directly when it causes alteration in tissue density outside the normal range of abnormal enhancement with contrast media.

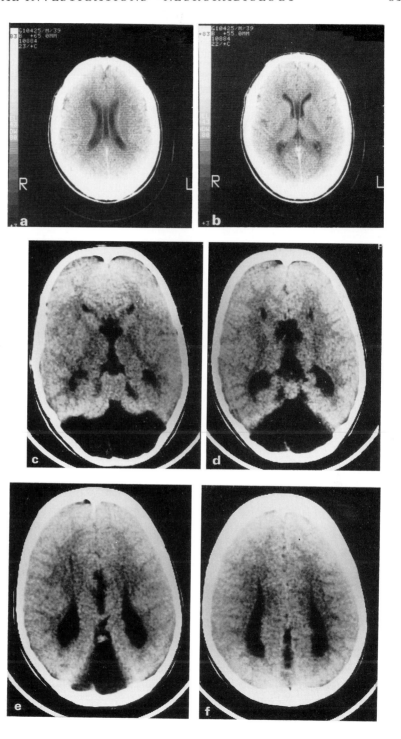

**Fig. 3.31.** Morphological variants and malformations. (a, b) A cavum septi pellucidi cum vergae separates the anterior horns and bodies of the lateral ventricles. The cisterna velum interpositum is shown between it and the third ventricle. (c, d, e, f) Agenesis of corpus callosum plus Dandy Walker syndrome. CT contiguous sections. The lateral ventricles are abnormally separated, with the third ventricle extending superiorly between them. The interhemispheric fissure reaches to the third ventricle through the region normally filled by the corpus callosum. There is absence of the vermis and hypoplasia of the cerebellar hemispheres.

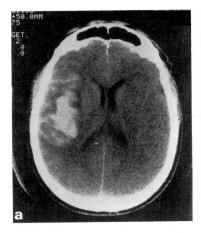 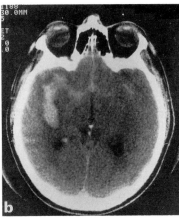

**Fig. 3.32.** Subarachnoid haemorrhage. CT, at level of (a) lateral ventricle and (b) third ventricle and suprasellar cistern. There is high density due to clotted blood in the right Sylvian fissure. There is a little low density around the fissure and the haematoma is causing sufficient mass effect to compress the right lateral ventricle. Subarachnoid haemorrhage is also present in the suprasellar cisterns and left Sylvian fissure.

Densities greater than normal grey matter may be due to:

1  recent blood clot;
2  calcification;
3  high protein content;
4  density packed cell structure.

Recent blood clot rarely exceeds 80 HU but causes the highest noncalcified tissue density (Fig. 3.32). Higher values indicate calcification unless foreign materials have been introduced.

Calcification with 80 HU density is visible on a plain skull X-ray; both higher and lower concentrations may occur normally in the pineal gland, choroid plexuses and in dural plaques and may contribute to CT density of neoplasms and granulomas, or may follow trauma, haemorrhage or metabolic disturbances.

Dense calcification is evident in 15% of meningiomas, over 70% of oligodendrogliomas (Fig. 3.33), 30% low grade astrocytomas and 10% of malignant astrocytomas. Calcification is also common in ependymomas and not infrequent in primitive neuroectodermal tumours (Fig. 3.34) and angiomatous malformations (Fig. 3.35). It is almost invariable in childhood craniopharyngiomas (see Fig. 3.23) but uncommon in other suprasellar tumours.

Compact cell structure (Fig. 3.34), often with a vascular stroma, accounts for the density of many medulloblastomas, lymphomas and fibrous meningiomas.

Protein concentration causes the high density in typical colloid cysts (Fig. 3.36) and also accounts for the relatively high readings in some nonhaemorrhagic tumour cysts.

Density readings between those of white matter and cerebrospinal fluid generally indicate increased water content in the affected tissues (Fig. 3.33). The water may be within relatively wide extracellular spaces or in microcysts which are commonly present in low-grade gliomas. Also, degeneration in the interstitial tissues of tumours especially mucoid changes commonly present in oligodendrogliomas and hydrotrophic mucinous or lipid degeneration within the cells of meningiomas, cause low density. Cavity formation within tumours also usually results in density regions within this range.

Density lower than that of cerebrospinal fluid but higher than air is usually due to long chain fatty acids; these predominate in lipomas (Fig. 3.37) and vary in concentration within dermoids and epidermoids.

Abnormal enhancement after intravenous contrast medium may indicate increased blood volume within large (Fig. 3.38, 3.39) or abnormally numerous vessels (Fig. 3.35) or extravasation from neocapillaries (Fig. 3.43), tumour vessels (Fig. 3.34, 3.40) or brain vessels injured by trauma, inflammation, infarction or demyelination, or a combination of these features. Thus enhancement is nonspecific but its distribution and form contribute to the reflection of

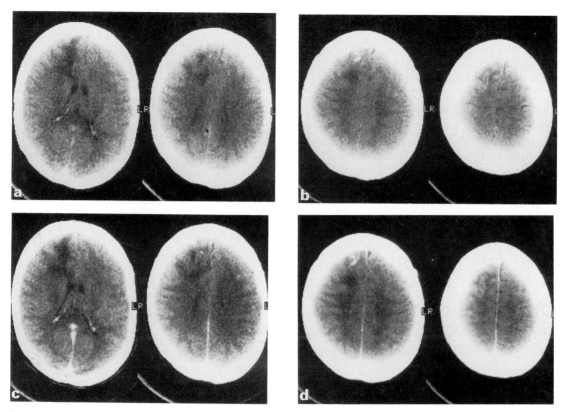

**Fig. 3.33.** Oligodendroglioma. CT scan, contiguous sections, (a, b) plain. (c, d) enhanced. The tumour causes a low density, nonenhancing region containing curvilinear calcification in the right frontal lobe. It has virtually no mass effect.

morphology which may be sufficiently characterisic to suggest a particular diagnosis.

Oedema fluid extravasating into brain substance, from a region of increased capillary permeability of any aetiology, extends through the extracellular spaces and eventually permeates into the ventricles or subarachnoid space, or is absorbed into the veins draining brain substance, or into astrocytes by pinocytosis. The extracellular spaces in the white matter, and especially those in the centrum semi-ovale and deep hemispheric white matter, are larger and more distensible than those in other parts of the brain and relatively larger amounts of oedema fluid tend to accumulate within them. This causes low density on CT with the characteristic distribution (Stevens *et al.* 1983) recognizable as vasogenic oedema (Fig. 3.41). Though not specific for any particular pathology, it is frequent around

inflammatory and malignant neoplastic processes and tends to be relatively less prominent around benign neoplasms with the exception of some meningiomas. Vasogenic oedema generally lessens with steroid therapy or after removal or resolution of the causative lesion. However, the extracellular spaces can become irreversibly dilated or rupture, forming microcysts and resulting in permanent low density on CT.

Tumour spread does not follow the pattern of vasogenic oedema but indiscriminately affects both white and grey matter; this feature may be useful in recognizing the low grade of gliomas, usually grade I astrocytomas, which present on CT as low density nonenhancing lesions.

Intracellular oedema, which typically accompanies ischaemia and infarction (Fig. 3.38), involves both grey and white matter and remains circumscribed in the damaged brain;

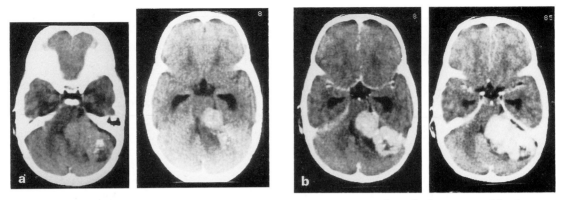

**Fig. 3.34.** Primitive neuroectodermal tumour. CT scan, (a) plain, (b) contrast-enhanced. There is a mixed density mass in the left cerebellar hemisphere, compressing the fourth ventricle and displacing it to the right and causing hydrocephalus, as evidenced by dilated temporal horns. Most of the tumour is composed of compact masses of cells; it is of high density and enhances considerably. There is calcification and a low density, nonenhancing cystic component in the lateral part of the tumour.

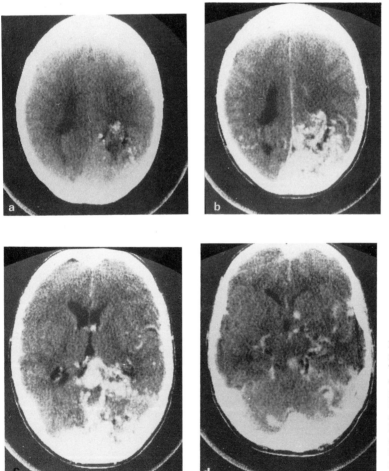

**Fig. 3.35.** Angiomatous malformation. (a) Plain scan. There is a high density, partly calcified lesion in the left posterior parietal and occipital lobes. (b) Enhanced scan at same level as (a), and (c, d) at lower levels. There is extensive enhancement of the vessels of the AVM and of the enlarged feeding arteries and draining veins.

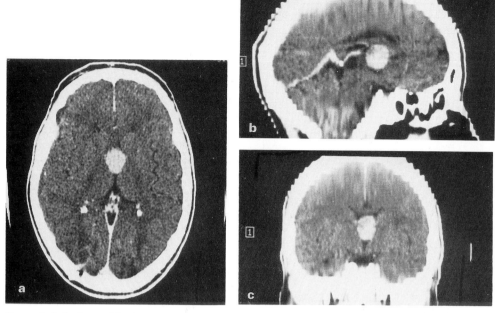

**Fig. 3.36.** Colloid cyst of the third ventricle. Enhanced CT scan, (a) axial, and reformatted sagittal (b), and coronal (c) sections. The cyst forms a high density, nonenhancing ovoid mass in the anterior third of the third ventricle, encroaching on the foramina of Monro. Lateral ventricular hydrocephalus has been controlled by a ventriculoperitoneal shunt.

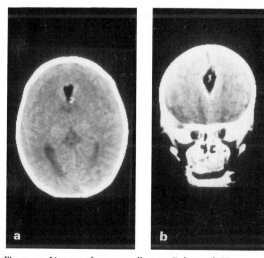

**Fig. 3.37.** Lipoma of corpus callosum. Enhanced CT scan, (a) axial, (b) coronal section. The lipoma is lower in density than the cerebrospinal fluid in the ventricles and quadrigeminal cisterns. There is slightly increased density in its periphery due to calcification. The central high density on the coronal section is the enhanced anterior cerebral artery, which, as is usually the case, passes through the lipoma.

surrounding vasogenic oedema can modify the CT appearances.

Focal cystic fluid collections may be initiated by haemorrhage, necrosis, exudation from inflammatory lesions or tumours, or loculation of cerebrospinal fluid. They form nonenhancing regions with density dependent on the nature of their contents.

Unclotted blood is of slightly higher density than brain; contraction of clot causes the typical high density of acute haematomas (Fig. 3.39) which is slowly lost over days or weeks as liquefaction and absorption occur (Weisberg *et al.* 1984). Intracerebral haemorrhage damages the adjacent brain and this is generally evident on CT as a well defined rim of low density around the retracted clot. Surrounding vasogenic oedema is not usually marked but within days of the ictus it may contribute to mass effect. Enhancement may commence after five to ten days in the immediate surrounds of the haematoma in tissue indistinguishable from brain

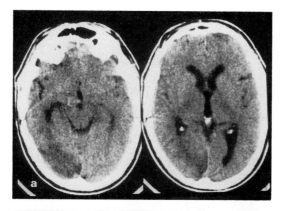

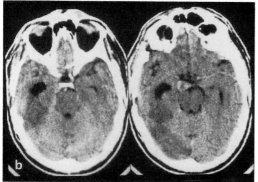

**Fig. 3.38.** Aneurysm, plus infarct. CT scan, (a) plain, (b) enhanced. The aneurysm arose from the distal basilar artery and was partly thrombosed. It causes the mixed, slightly increased density mass in the right side of the chiasmatic and right crural cisterns; there is enhancement of the patient medial part of the lumen of the aneurysm.

The infarct causes low density in the white and grey matter of the right occipital lobe, extending into the temporal lobe. Local atrophy causes dilatation of the temporal horn.

haemorrhage, where angiography is indicated, an enhanced scan is not required.

Infarction of brain may progress to scarring and atrophy, but large infarcts may liquify and produce cavities with low density fluid contents. Infarction leading to necrosis is common in malignant tumours and produces cavities which are sometimes multiple, with irregular, thick enhancing walls and surrounding oedema (Fig. 3.42). The fluid is usually of density higher than CSF and lower than brain but a haemorrhagic component may raise the density above that of brain.

In inflammatory processes, abscess formation (Fig. 3.43) or caseation produces cavitation. Pus is indistinguishable from other, moderately low density fluid; the inflamed wall is usually dense relative to the cavity and surrounding brain and forms a thin, smooth, enhancing ring with considerable adjacent vasogenic oedema. Although the CT appearances are not specific the diagnosis is generally evident in the clinical context. Tuberculomas (Fig. 3.47) are usually isodense, but may have central, low density or regions of higher density from calcification. They are often multiple and may enhance evenly or as a ring.

Some tumour cells secrete fluid which may form cystic spaces within or adjacent to the neoplasm. The cysts have thin, smooth walls with tumour forming a local thickening or nodule projecting from the wall. They are frequent with haemangioblastomas (Fig. 3.44) and low grade astrocytomas and occasionally occur with meningiomas and malignant neoplasms. Ring enhancement, while reflecting differences in tissue composition, is not infrequent in solid tumours (Fig. 3.45); sometimes the ring will fill in on several serial scans made up to 60 minutes after contrast medium has been injected. Cavities can only be identified conclusively when gravitational layering of contents of different specific gravity and attenuation are evident (Fig. 3.46). This is usually due to precipitation of high density debris from the walls of necrotic neoplasms or, occasionally, to bleeding. Fat may be released into dermoids or teratomas and form an ascendant layer: rupture allows fat globules to enter the

substance on the plain CT and it may persist throughout the period of clot resorption. Haemorrhage into a tumour does not usually destroy all the neoplastic tissue and the latter may remain as an enhancing ring around the haematoma or an irregular nodule adjacent to it, visible from the time of the ictus. Angiomatous malformations and aneurysms may also be evident from the presence of early enhancement. Haematomas of aneurysmal origin usually extend close to the basal vessels and high density of blood in the subarachnoid spaces is usual. In this situation and in isolated subarachnoid

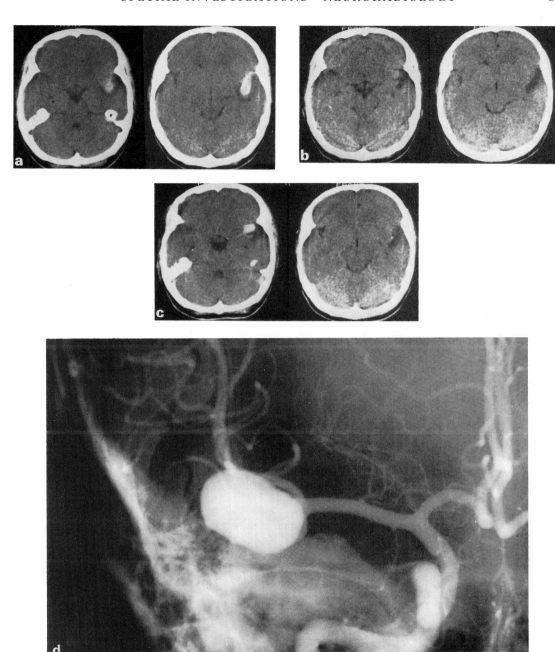

**Fig. 3.39.** Haematoma with aneurysm. CT scan, (a) plain. There is a high density mass (80 HU) due to recent haematoma anteriorly in the left temporal lobe encroaching on the Sylvian fissure. There is a surrounding, well demarcated, low density region due to damage in adjacent brain.

CT scan 10 days later, (b) plain, (c) contrast-enhanced. The haematoma is now only slightly denser than brain. There is a clearly defined enhancing aneurysm at a left middle cerebral bifurcation.

Left carotid angiogram, AP projection (d). A large unilocular aneurysm protects laterally from the second cortical bifurcation of the left middle cerebral artery.

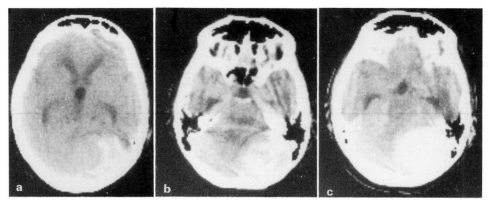

**Fig. 3.40.** Meningioma. CT scan, (a, b) plain, (c) after intravenous contrast medium. There is a partially calcified mass, of slightly higher than brain density, lying adjacent to the left cerebellar convexity. It enhances densely and homogeneously after contrast medium and has a well defined edge. The fourth ventricle is not visible due to compression by the mass, and there is hydrocephalus of the lateral and third ventricles.

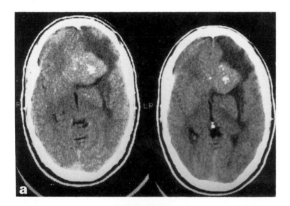

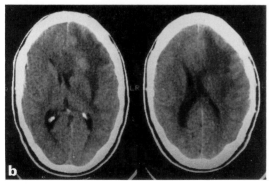

**Fig. 3.41.** Vasogenic oedema. (a)–(b) CT contiguous sections. There is a well defined, partly calcified, subfrontal meningioma, extending more to the left side. There is extensive vasogenic oedema in the left hemisphere.

cerebrospinal fluid and they may layer in the ventricles or become fixed in the subarachnoid space. Intravenous contrast medium also may form a dependent layer in necrotic cavities, usually within malignant neoplasms, and in subdural effusions.

The combination of single or, in the case of metastases, haemangioblastomas or tuberculomas (Fig. 3.47), multiple masses with cystic, haemorrhagic, necrotic or calcified regions and surrounding vasogenic oedema frequently results in complex mixed attenuation patterns and regional variations in enhancement, reflecting various pathologies.

It should be noted that, although the enhancing edge of a glioma generally reflects the macroscopic limit of the neoplasm, tumour cells are commonly present in both oedematous and apparently normal brain beyond the macroscopic edge of a malignant tumour on both brain sectioning and on CT; occasionally CT may fail to reveal a symptomatic tumour at a time when NMR is abnormal or when it is manifest on a futher CT study made after a few weeks (Wulff et al. 1982). Metabolic methods using positron emission tomography are probably the most accurate for plotting the extent of gliomas

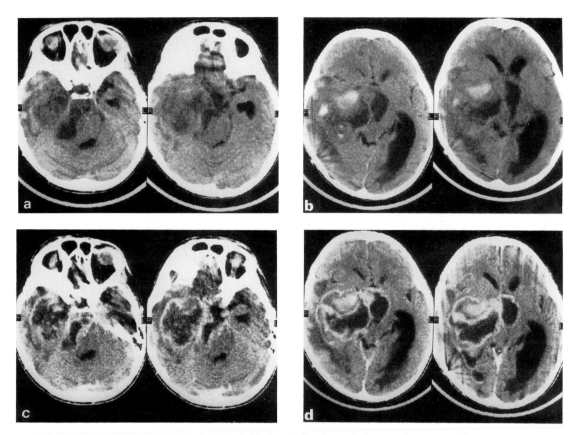

**Fig. 3.42.** Malignant astrocytoma. CT scan, (a, b) plain (c, d) enhanced. There is a large, mixed density mass in the right temporal lobe, extending through the suprasellar cisterns and into the right cerebellopontine and pontine cisterns. Most of the mass is low in density and shows irregular ring enhancement. There are higher density components, probably containing calcification, which show diffuse enhancement. The tumour extends around the walls of the posterior part of the right temporal lobe and occipital horns and third ventricle. There is hydrocephalus of the contralateral ventricle.

(Di Chiro *et al.* 1982). However, these are restricted to a few research centres, and CT currently provides all the essential information necessary to proceed to surgery or stereotactic biopsy in virtually all cases.

## Magnetic resonance imaging (NMR)
(Pykett *et al.* 1982)

Atomic nuclei with an odd number of nucleons, for example $^1H$, $^{31}P$, $^{23}Na$, tend to align in a strong magnetic field and to precess, at a speed unique for each particular nucleus, around the axis of the field. A pulse of radio waves at the same frequency as the rate of the precession applied to the nuclei in the field, will deflect them from the axis of the field to an extent determined by the amplitude and duration of the pulse. On cessation of the pulse the nuclei emit the absorbed energy as a minute radio frequency signal during the time when they are realigning with the field. The strength of this signal and its decay in a complex exponential fashion with time is influenced by five factors:

1   The strength of the magnetic field.
2   The concentration of the energized nucleons.

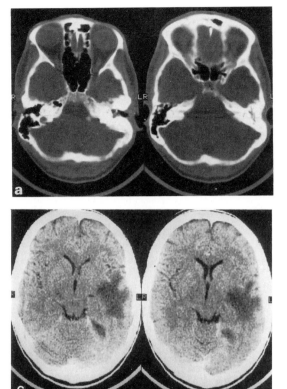

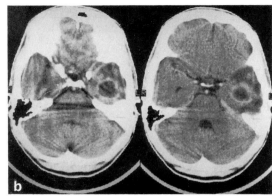

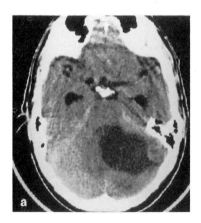

Fig. 3.43. Abscess. (a) plain CT, with bone windows. The left middle ear and mastoid are opaque. (b & c) Contiguous enhanced sections through middle fossa. In the right temporal lobe there is thin walled ring enhancement in the abscess capsule, with central low density due to pus within the abscess and surrounding vasogenic oedema. There is also a low density region with marginal enhancement just above the tentorium due to an empyema.

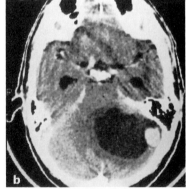

Fig. 3.44. Haemangioblastoma. CT scan, (a) plain, (b) enhanced. The tumour cyst is a well defined, non-enhancing region; the nodule is of about brain density and enhances markedly. The mass displaces the fourth ventricle to the right and compresses it, causing hydrocephalus, as is evident from the dilated temporal horns.

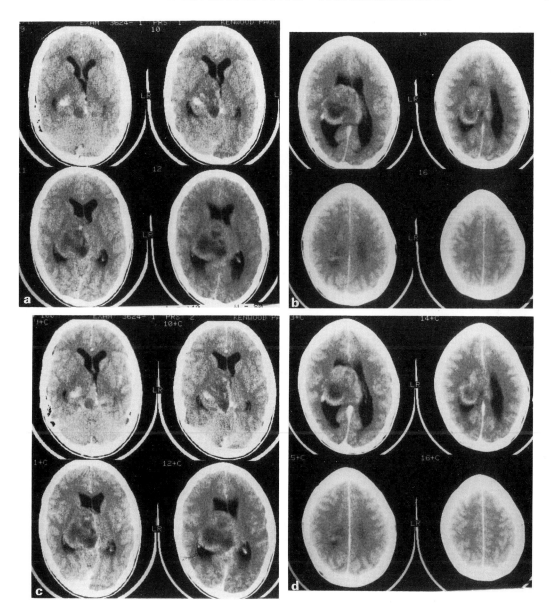

**Fig. 3.45.** Astrocytoma, Grade 2. CT scan, (a, b) contiguous plain sections, (c, d) similar levels after contrast medium. There is a mixed density mass, with regions of calcification, expanding the right thalamus, encroaching on the right lateral ventricle and displacing the third ventricle to the left and partly obstructing it, causing moderate hydrocephalus. There is patchy and irregular ring enhancement, sparing the low density parts of the tumour, which proved at surgery to be solid. There is no evidence of oedema in the surrounding brain.

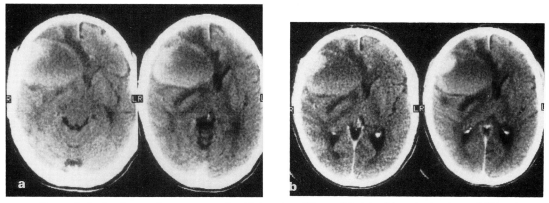

**Fig. 3.46.** Cystic adenocarcinoma metastasis with layering. CT scan, (a) plain, (b) contrast-enhanced. There is a well defined mass in the right frontal lobe, displacing the midline structures to the left and occluding the ipsilateral sulci. It is of mixed density, with an enhancing solid component adjacent to the convexity, and a medial component showing thin-walled ring enhancement. There is layering in the medial part indicating a cavity containing fluid, which was haemorrhagic at surgery. Vasogenic oedema causes low density in the white matter adjacent to the mass.

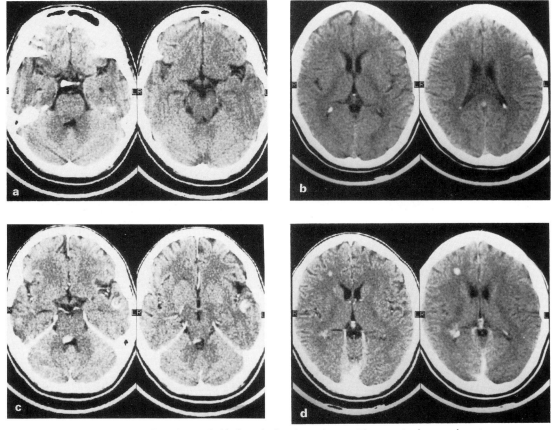

**Fig. 3.47.** Multiple masses. (1) Tuberculomas. (a, b) plain, (c, d) enhanced scans. There are isodense, enhancing small masses, with only minimal adjacent oedema, in both temporal lobes, the right frontal lobe and right side of the pons. (2) Metastases (bronchal carcinoma).

The low proton density in air and cortical bone accounts for the low energy signal from them on proton NMR images.

3 The interaction of the nucleons with surrounding molecules reflected in the time ($T_1$) taken for realignment with the field or return to thermal equilibrium. $T_1$ is referred to as the spin lattice relaxation time. Examples of the influence of $T_1$ in proton NMR include: $T_1$ is short in triglyceride fat and long in muscle, contributing to the high signal from the former and low from the latter; the relatively high water content of grey matter prolongs its $T_1$; white matter gives

relatively more signal with short pulse repetition times and the intensity from grey matter increases and exceeds it as the interval is prolonged (Fig. 3.48). The very long $T_1$ of normal CSF is particularly valuable, not only in clearly delineating the margins of the subarachnoid space (Fig. 3.49), but also in the diagnosis of cystic processes such as syringomyelia and hydromyelia (Fig. 3.90) and distinction from cavities containing proteinaceous fluid, which occur in association with neoplasms and following haemorrhage and necrosis. Increase in protein shortens $T_1$; NMR is sufficiently sensitive

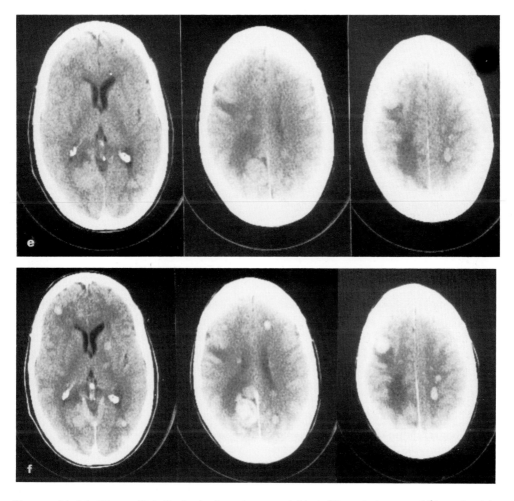

**Fig. 3.47.** (e) plain CT scan, (f) similar levels after enhancement. Most of the metastases are visible on the plain scan, being slightly denser than normal brain, with either slight or moderate adjacent oedema. All the visible metastases enhance considerably and one or two are only evident after enhancement.

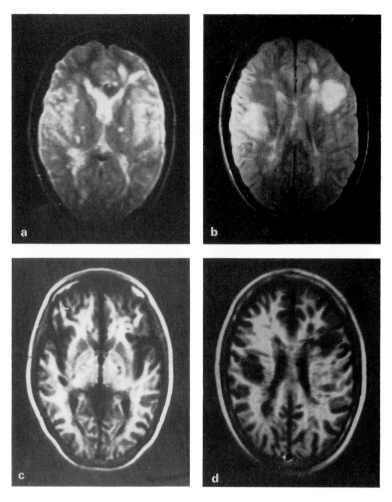

**Fig. 3.48.** Multiple sclerosis. MRI, (a, b) long spin echo, (c, d) inversion recovery. Note high signal from the CSF and higher signal from grey than white matter on the long spin echo series; the opposite is true of the inversion recovery series. Multiple small and large plaques involve the white matter and periventricular regions. Their signal intensity is high on the SE and low on the IR, associated with increase in $T_1$ and $T_2$. Note that the large lesions have virtually no mass effect or vasogenic oedema around them.

to reflect minor differences in protein content of normal intra- and extraventricular CSF (Brant-Zawadzki *et al.* 1985).

4 The interaction between the energized nucleons, reflected in the time ($T_2$) for loss of coherent resonance, caused by slight non-uniformity of the magnetic field. $T_2$, referred to as spin–spin relaxation time, is generally much shorter than $T_1$, and marked decay in the signal intensity from a tissue over very short periods generally indicates a short $T_2$. For example, in proton NMR $T_2$ is long in CSF relative to brain, hence the intensity of signal from the CSF decreases more slowly than that from brain and the CSF appears relatively brighter as the time

between excitation and reading the signal is prolonged. On early readings the relatively higher signal from nervous tissue causes positive contrast between it and the CSF, which is lost with more prolonged delay.

5 The rate of flow of nucleons in vessels passing through the field. Rapidly flowing protons give a reduced or absent signal with conventional NMR imaging techniques; slow or absent flow in vessels will increase the signal from them. Large aneurysms (Fig. 3.50) and the arterial and venous components of an angiomatous malformation can be clearly defined and thrombosis in large vessels can be recognized. Programmes to quantify blood flow have been developed.

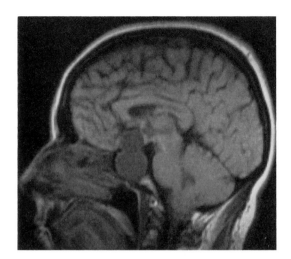

**Fig. 3.49.** Short spin echo, sagittal, midline sections. In this sequence the low signal intensity of cerebrospinal fluid outlines the surface anatomy of the subarachnoid space. A large pituitary tumour is shown expanding the sella, displacing the third ventricle superiorly and posteriorly and splaying the anterior recesses. The cerebellar tonsils are slightly depressed. Note the high signal from fat in the subcutaneous and suboccipital regions.

NMR signals can be converted to an image by applying a magnetic gradient across the field and using a double Fourier transformation technique which allows the intensity of the signal to be localized by phase and frequency encoding.

Tissue characteristics (active nucleon density, $T_1$, $T_2$) can be estimated by varying the time between radio frequency pulses and measuring the signal at various intervals after pulsing using spin echo techniques.

Hydrogen is present in high concentration in most tissues and is the most suitable nucleus for imaging; the commercial NMR machines currently available produce proton images.

NMR produces anatomical sectional information resembling, in many ways, that produced by CT and with a similar spatial resolution, but it has certain advantages over CT including:

1 It does not use ionizing radiation and, as far as is known, at field strengths used currently for imaging it lacks biological hazard. Magnetic materials, (certain aneurysm clips) or devices susceptible to radio waves (for example, cardiac pace makers) may, however, be influenced by it.

2 Many pathological processes have similar X-ray absorption characteristics and some are not distinguished from adjacent brain substance by CT. Each of the several parameters which influence signal intensity on NMR can be the dominant factor producing contrast in a particular image. By varying pulse sequences, series of images can be made which have already been shown to resolve many CT isodense lesions, including plaques of demyelination, (Fig. 3.48) ischaemic myelopathy and low-grade gliomas, in some of which CT has been absolutely normal (Brant-Zawadzki *et al.* 1984a). In general, the pathological processes revealed by CT are shown to be more extensive on NMR; internal structure tends to be shown more clearly, especially by inversion recovery modes. The detection of transcallosal or brainstem spread of glioma or of multiple lesions, which may influence the decision for or against surgical treatment, is often possible with NMR before it is evident on CT.

3 NMR images can be produced with similar resolution in any plane (Figs. 3.49, 3.50). For practical purposes CT images in certain planes, for example, the sagittal, can only be obtained by computer reconstruction of multiple thin section images produced in mechanically accessible planes, usually the axial. This process is inevitably accompanied by some loss of resolution and is prone to distortion by patient movement. NMR images in vertical planes are of particular value in assessing mass lesions of the suprasellar, parasagittal and juxtaconvexity regions, brainstem and spinal cord. The relationship of tumours to the Sylvian fissure is also best demonstrated in coronal sections. Also, a clearer indication of the volume of a lesion is possible by display in three planes.

4 NMR is free of the bone-induced artefacts which may limit CT diagnosis, especially in the posterior fossa. The lack of signal from cortical bone makes NMR particularly appropriate for study of the intrapetrous structures, including small acoustic neuromas (Young *et al.* 1983).

5 The topographic relationships of lesions to

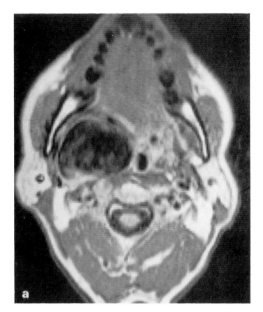 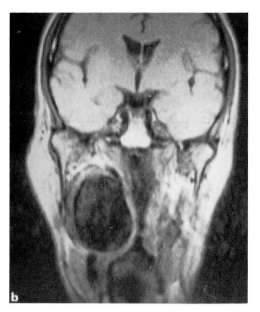

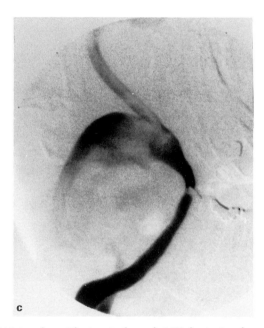

**Fig. 3.50.** Aneurysm right internal carotid artery in the neck. MRI short spin echo sequences, (a) axial, (b) coronal. The flowing blood in the normal vessels and in the aneurysm has low signal intensity. Note high signal from the subcutaneous fat and fatty marrow. Low signal from the CSF shows the normal anatomy of the frontal horns and third ventricle and of the suprasellar cistern and supratentorial subarachnoid space in the coronal section.

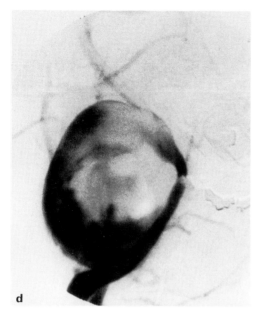
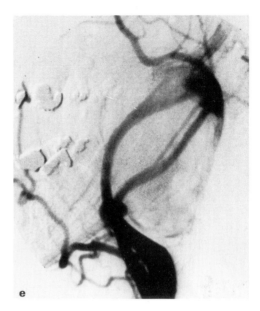

**Fig. 3.50.** Aneurysm. Digital subtraction right carotid angiogram, (c, d) AP, (e) lateral. The aneurysm displaces the internal carotid artery anteriorly and medially and the external carotid laterally. The contrast medium jets from the neck of the aneurysm into the blood pooled in its lumen.

major blood vessels is possible using flow sensitive sequences.

6 Blood flow has already been measured by NMR. $^{23}$Na images and *in vivo* localized $^{31}$P spectra have been produced so that the potential of the method for measuring physiological parameters is exciting; for example, decrease in adenosine triphosphate levels may prove a useful index of ischaemic changes in the brain studied *in vivo*, and shift of inorganic phosphate peaks may be used to measure pH.

Paramagnetic ions influence the magnetic environment of protons in a way that reduces the relaxation times and potentially enhances contrast on the NMR image. The iron in methaemoglobin is paramagnetic and accounts for the reduced $T_1$ which allows the recognition of sub acute or chronic haematomas, both at the time when they are of high density on CT and also during the isodense and into the diminishing density phase. Some paramagnetic ions, such as gadolinium, can be administered in biocompatible compounds which are retained by the

normal but penetrate the abnormal blood–brain barrier, and thus give similar information to enhancement on CT (Fig. 3.51; Carr *et al.* 1984). Increase in signal : noise ratio reveals more structure in complex lesions and may reveal more diagnostic features; distinction between oedema and the underlying tumour or inflammatory mass is generally accentuated. It must be acknowledged, however, that, as yet, the main information from NMR imaging has been the anatomical distribution of disease processes. Tissue specific characterization of individual pathological lesions is much less common; thus oedema of all types, infarction and regions lacking myelin, whether physiological in infancy or due to dysmyelinating or demyelinating processes, including post-infection encephalitis and plaques of MS, have prolonged $T_1$ and $T_2$ relaxation times; subacute and chronic haematoma (Fig. 3.52) and triglyceride fat, as, for example, in lipoma (Fig. 3.53), dermoid or atheromatous plaques, have short $T_1$ and prolonged $T_2$ relaxation times. $T_1$ and $T_2$ values alone are insufficient for precise tumour characterization,

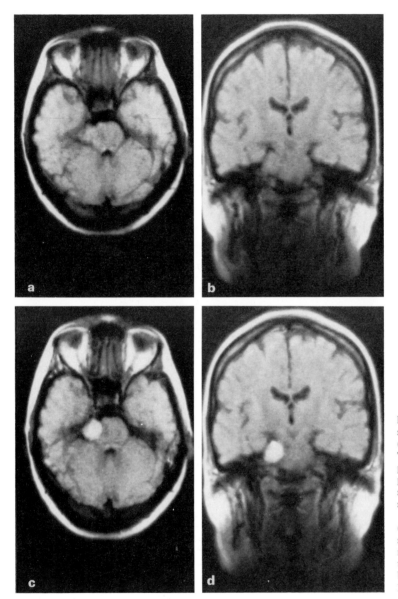

**Fig. 3.51.** Meningioma. NMR spin echo, TR 544 ms, TE 44 ms, (a) axial, (b) coronal sections. There is a mass at the right petrous apex displacing the pons. The signal from it is similar to that from brain substance.

After Gadolinium-DTPA, (c, d) similar sections. The signal intensity of the tumour is markedly increased reflecting the absence of a blood–brain barrier (Courtesy of Dr Graeme Bydder).

though they supplement the morphology of the lesion in influencing diagnosis. (Mills *et al.* 1984).

A further limitation of proton NMR is that hydrogen poor tissues such as cortical bone and calcified lesions produce little signal, so that the exquisite bone detail possible on CT is not available.

Absence of signal with all programmes allows recognition of calcification and/or ossification but any contribution to diagnosis of the patterns of calcification is lost.

The quality of NMR images is dependent upon the homogeneity of the magnetic field and a significant factor influencing the speed of acquisition of the images and minimum thickness of section with acceptable signal : noise level is field

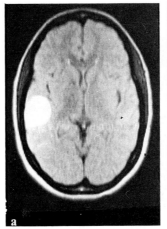 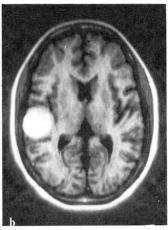

**Fig. 3.52.** Haematoma right temporal lobe. Inversion recovery, TR 3600, TI 500, subacute haematoma gives a high signal.

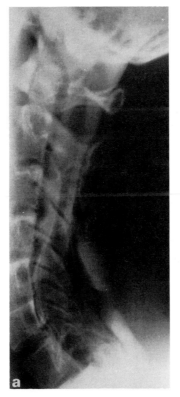 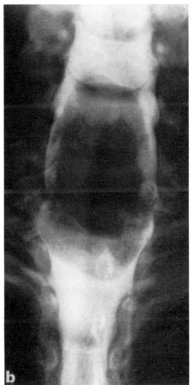

**Fig. 3.53.** Lipoma of spinal cord. Iohexol myelogram, (a) lateral, (b) AP projection. There has been a laminectomy of the 3rd to 7th cervical vertebrae. The spinal cord is expanded between C4 and T1 levels and is atrophic above C4 level.

Computed myelogram. (c) The expansion of the spinal cord is shown to be due to a mass of fat density which extrudes from the posterior surface. The spinal cord is expanded at the level of the lipoma. (d) The atrophic cord above the lipoma is confirmed.

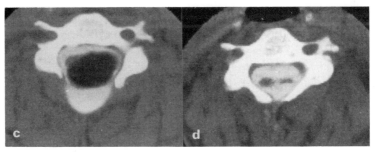

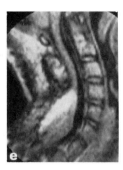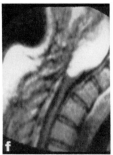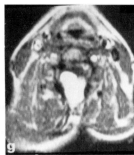

**Fig. 3.53.** Lipoma of spinal cord. MRI, spin echo (TR500, TE40), sagittal (e) at and above and (f) at and below the level of the lipoma, (g) axial section. The lipoma gives a high signal associated with a short $T_1$, similar to that of the fat in the subcutaneous and intermuscular planes. The extension of the lipoma from the spinal cord through the posterior subarachnoid space and laminar defect into the retrospinal tissues is evident.

strength. Overall, the most satisfactory images are produced by the relatively expensive machines incorporating superconducting magnets.

Such factors suggest that, though NMR will become the primary method for detection of CNS pathology (Brant-Zawadzki *et al.* 1984), CT, which presently occupies this position, will retain it for several years to come. CT will remain the optimum method for examining bone structure and will always be a powerful supplement and alternative to NMR.

## Angiography

Introduced by Moniz (1927), cerebral angiography was accepted relatively slowly as a diagnostic procedure. This was due to difficulty in perfecting a safe technique and in developing an innocuous contrast medium.

In due course, organic compounds of iodine were fabricated culminating in the nonionic contrast media, and several virtually nontoxic, satisfactory preparations which cause only minimal discomfort are now available.

Percutaneous puncture of the carotid was described by Lindgren in 1947 and the method was applied to vertebral angiography in 1949 (Sugar *et al.* 1949, Lindgren 1950). In order to avoid puncturing major arteries in the neck and to facilitate examination of the vasculature of the whole brain, selective injection is now made through a catheter which has been introduced into a systemic artery, usually the femoral, and manipulated under fluoroscopic control so that its tip is within the relevant cervical vessel. Direct puncture is reserved as a complementary method for cases in which catheterization is contraindicated or has proved difficult.

Currently three angiographic methods are used and each has particular applications:

1 High resolution technique, generally with selective arterial catheterization using magnification and screen film combination. Vessels as small as 200 $\mu$m can be resolved; smaller vessels form a capillary blush. This method is optimal for detailed study of aneurysms and vascular morphology.

2 Arterial catheterization with digital recording has the advantage over conventional angiography of requiring only one third the concentration of contrast medium, which gives rise to less discomfort and can be delivered through a relatively fine catheter, lower overall contrast dosage, of particular importance in small children, and film economy. Radiographic contrast can be electronically enhanced to show densities which would be invisible on conventional angiograms, but spatial resolution is reduced to about 0.5 mm. The method is entirely adequate in practice for diagnosis of virtually all angiographic abnormalities (Brant-Zawadzki *et al.* 1982), and it is especially useful for control of interventional procedures.

3 Intravenous digital angiography avoids arterial catheterization. The patient is required to remain completely still for up to 30 seconds

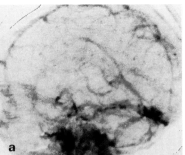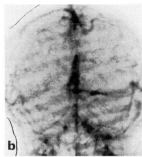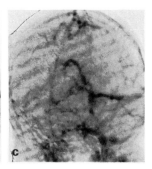

**Fig. 3.54.** Superior sagittal sinus occlusion. Digital subtraction angiogram. Injection into right atrium (a) lateral, (b) AP, (c) oblique projections. The posterior third of the superior sagittal sinus is occluded. The right transverse sinus is poorly opacified and could possibly be partly obstructed.

during the imaging and relatively large amounts of contrast medium are injected, which may be contraindicated in patients with cardiac or renal disease. Overlap of vessels is often problematical, but the method is of special value as screening for large arterial occlusive disease of severity sufficient to be considered for surgery (Foley *et al.* 1984) and for venous sinus abnormalities (Fig. 3.54) (Carmody *et al.* 1982). It is adequate for follow-up studies for operated aneurysms and arteriovenous malformation (AVM). Differential diagnosis of AVMs or large aneurysms from tumour is established, but presurgical planning may require detailed intra-arterial studies.

The complications which follow angiography include deterioration of the level of consciousness in patients suffering from high intracranial pressure, and focal deficits, usually transient but occasionally permanent and rarely fatal. Field *et al.* (1962) carried out a survey of the published accounts of complications attributable to direct puncture cerebral angiography. The mortality ranged from 0.3% to 3.3% and complications from nil to 22.5%; the diversity depends partly upon the criteria chosen to define a complication. In their personal series of 2000 patients the mortality was 0.4% and complications occurred in 2.1%, the commonest being hemiparesis. Occasionally haematoma formation in the neck may embarrass respiration, and cause hypercarbia and cerebral anoxia. Aneurysms may arise at the site of puncture (Liverud 1958). The report on the 'Cooperative Study of Intracranial

Aneurysms and Subarachnoid Haemorrhage' contains a more detailed study of the complications arising in this particular group of cases; the incidence was 7.6% and the mortality rate 0.82% (Perret & Nishioka 1966). These figures greatly exceed those encountered in modern neuroradiological practice; more representative is a recent large series of catheter cerebral angiograms (Mani *et al.* 1978) in which permanent neurological defect occurred in only 0.02% and the mortality was 0.04%.

### Indications for angiography

1   The detection of abnormalities of the blood vessels in the investigation of the cause of spontaneous intracranial haemorrhage and selected ischaemic lesions. These include aneurysm, vascular hamartoma and stenosis or occlusion of arteries and veins.

2   Demonstration of the vascular pattern of a lesion detected by CT or NMR to further determine its pathological nature in selected cases.

3   When CT and NMR are not available, the detection and localization of space-occupying lesions, including tumour, abscess and haematoma. When CT or NMR is available, angiography may be considered necessary in selected cases in difficult locations to show the relationship of blood vessels to the tumour prior to surgery.

**The normal angiogram**

The anatomical features conveniently described
as shown by angiography also apply to the vessels as revealed in less detail by CT and NMR.

*Internal carotid circulation*

In the lateral projection (Fig. 3.55), the internal
carotid artery takes a sinuous course through
the cavernous sinus, forming the U or S loop
convex forwards termed the 'carotid siphon';
occasionally a double loop is seen. The limbs of
the loop are stacked approximately parallel with
the sagittal plane. The highest limb of the siphon,
passing backwards to emerge from under the
optic nerve on its lateral border, turns upwards
and forwards to terminate by dividing into its
anterior and middle cerebral branches. The position of the termination of the carotid artery
varies but it is usually several millimetres above
the level of the anterior clinoid process. Within
the cavernous sinus, inferior hypophyseal and
meningeal branches arise. In the normal angiogram they are barely visible, but in some cases
of pituitary tumour or a neoplasm or AVM
involving the tentorium or the dura mater covering the clivus, these meningeal branches enlarge
considerably (Wallace *et al.* 1967).

Beyond its cavernous course three small branches of the internal carotid artery are usually
seen. The ophthalmic artery, arising from the
anterior border of the highest loop of the siphon,
passes forwards to enter the orbit; it may be
enlarged to serve as a major collateral, when the
internal carotid artery is obstructed below this
level, and in some cases of tumour within the
orbit. The posterior communicating artery leaves
the posterior border of the carotid artery, where
it turns upwards from the superior limb of the
siphon; it is often visible only for a few millimetres
to the point where it fuses with the posterior
cerebral artery, but it gives origin to the anterior

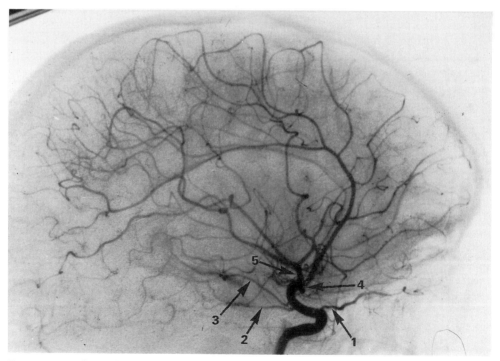

**Fig. 3.55.** Normal carotid angiogram, lateral projection, arterial phase. (1) ophthalmic, (2) posterior
communicating, (3) anterior choroidal, (4) anterior cerebral, (5) middle cerebral artery.

thalamoperforating arteries which contribute to the blood supply of the hypothalamus and medial thalamus. In about 20% of cases a primitive anatomical pattern persists in which the posterior cerebral artery takes origin from the internal carotid artery and forms a prominent feature in the arteriogram.

A few millimetres above the posterior communicating artery, the anterior choroidal artery arises from the posterior surface of the vertical portion of the internal carotid artery, it passes diagonally upwards, backwards and laterally to enter the choroidal fissure supplying the adjacent parts of the temporal lobe, the medial third of the cerebral peduncle, the optic tract, globus pallidus, genu and posterior limb of the internal capsule and the choroid plexus of the temporal horn. It may be enlarged in choroid plexus meningioma, papilloma (see Fig. 3.64) and angiomatous malformation.

The middle cerebral artery passes in a horizontal plane laterally to reach the Sylvian fissure, where it divides into branches on the insula. There is an axis of general direction of the Sylvian group which is of significance in angiographic localization. Jimenez and Goree (1967) describe a line drawn through the base of the incisor teeth and the anterior border of the siphon which, when extended upwards and backwards, forms a good guide to the normal Sylvian axis. The stem of the middle cerebral artery follows the lower border of the insula, which is crossed by those branches which are distributed to the frontal and parietal convexity. These make an acute bend at the sulcus demarcating the superior margin of the insula in order to emerge from the lateral fissure over the opercula. These bends or loops can be identified in the lateral angiogram and, together with the parent trunk, outline the insula in the pattern of a triangle. Tumours of the adjacent brain cause displacement and deformity of this vascular triangle (Serrats et al. 1968). The branches of the middle cerebral artery are liable to variations, described in detail by Ring (1962); the posterior temporal, the angular and the posterior parietal arteries are the most constant of these branches.

The anterior cerebral artery leaves the carotid artery by passing medially upwards and forwards to reach the under surface of the genu of the corpus callosum and the midline, where it is joined to its fellow of the opposite side by the anterior communicating artery which lies on a plane about 15 mm above the planum sphenoidale. This portion of its course is approximately horizontal with variable anterior inclination, the degree of which determines the way in which it may be displaced by suprasellar masses extending from the base; if the vessel runs on a plane in front of the sella it may not be elevated by even very large superior extensions of pituitary masses. The artery then passes forwards, gives off orbitofrontal and the fairly constant frontopolar branch, and then divides into the pericallosal and callosomarginal arteries. These are easily recognized as, at first, they run a fairly parallel course, making a broad sweeping curve convex forwards as they pass round the front of the genu and then backwards, the pericallosal artery hugging the corpus callosum and reflecting the position of its superior surface; it may be regarded as the direct continuation of the anterior cerebral artery and occasionally can be traced curving around the splenium.

In the anteroposterior film (Fig. 3.56) the loops of the carotid siphon are represented by a more or less vertical shadow of varying degree of width and density. The denser, rounded areas correspond to the limbs of the loops and may be mistaken for aneurysms. The terminal portion of the artery ascends from the siphon with a slight inclination outwards and the anterior cerebral and the middle cerebral arteries leave it almost at right angles, passing, respectively, medially and laterally.

The middle cerebral artery can be traced laterally to the cortical branches which form a convoluted pattern on the insula with an axis directed vertically; the terminal branches can be traced upwards and outwards towards the calvarium, the fine branches hugging the inner table as they ascend towards the vertex.

The ophthalmic artery may be seen leaving the upper part of the siphon, passing laterally

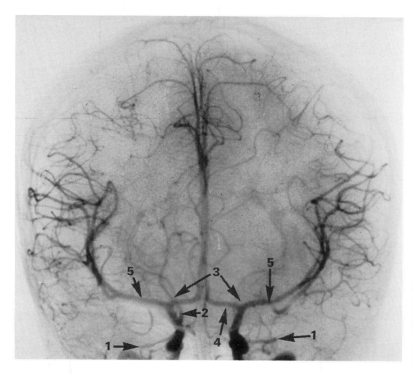

**Fig. 3.56.** Normal carotid angiogram, AP projection, arterial phase. (1) ophthalmic, (2) posterior communicating, (3) anterior choroidal, (4) anterior cerebral, (5) middle cerebral.

roughly parallel and inferior to the stem of the middle cerebral artery.

The anterior cerebral artery passes approximately horizontally to the midline to join its fellow; the vessels on either side may be relatively small (15%) or hypoplastic (5%). It ascends in the midline and the main branches form a leash of vessels ascending to the vertex, approximately bisecting the skull, giving off lesser branches laterally to the medial surface of the cortex. The frontopolar branch passes diagonally upwards and laterally.

The fine lenticulostriate central or basal arteries of the brain (Lazorthes 1961) are shown as a leash ascending first convex medially and then laterally in an S-shaped course from the horizontal portions of the anterior and middle cerebral arteries to supply the basal ganglia and internal capsule.

Films taken about 2–5 seconds later show a general opacification of brain substance, termed the cerebrogram or capillary phase. The contrast medium is in the vessels, under 100 $\mu$m in diam-

eter, too small to be individually identified on conventional magnification angiography. The greater vascularity of the deep grey matter and the cerebral cortex and the unopacified ventricles are generally evident and distortion by mass lesions can be recognized.

From the region of the Sylvian fissure the veins radiate in two main groups, passing towards the convexity to empty ultimately into the lateral sinus. Two veins are usually prominent, that of Trolard, which links the Sylvian vein or veins with the sagittal, and that of Labbé, which links the Sylvian veins with the lateral sinus.

By about 5 seconds after injection there is much more extensive filling of the veins and the medium is outlining the great dural sinuses. In the lateral film, the superior sagittal sinus can often be traced as a ribbon-like shadow hugging the bone at the vertex and gradually widening as it passes posteriorly. Below it, but shorter and narrower, may be seen the inferior sagittal sinus which merges with the straight sinus; anteriorly it normally describes a gentle curve, but it is

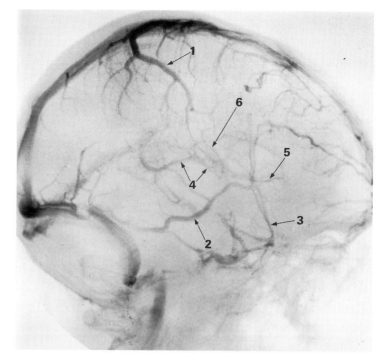

**Fig. 3.57.** Internal carotid angiogram, normal veins, lateral projection. Superior anastomotic vein (Trolard) (1) draining to superior sagittal sinus; inferior anastomotic vein (Labbé) (2) draining to transverse sinus; superficial middle cerebral veins (3) draining towards cavernous sinus; internal cerebral vein (4) draining the ventricular veins and commencing at the confluence of the septal (5) and thalamostriate veins (6) near the foramen of Monro.

straight posteriorly and resembles the shape of the blade of a scythe.

The deep venous drainage of the hemisphere (Fig. 3.57) usually, but not invariably, fills later than the superficial veins and appears in this phase. In approximately the centre of the field, two thin, short veins, that of the septum pellucidum coursing backwards and the thalamostriate forwards, meet at an angle and generally form the origin of the internal cerebral vein. This takes a sinuous course backwards and receives the basal vein of Rosenthal from the medial border of the temporal lobe. At this point the vein is a large vessel; it takes a bold curve upwards to enter the straight sinus at its junction with the inferior sagittal sinus. The point at which the vein of the septum lucidum and the thalamostriate vein fuse, termed the 'venous angle' by Krayenbühl and Richter (1952), is characteristically at or near the foramen of Monro and is important in angiographic localization of deep tumours. In the AP projections of the phlebograms, the surface of the cerebral hemisphere is well defined and subependymal veins indicate the position and size of the lateral ventricles.

*External carotid circulation* (Fig. 3.58)

The ascending pharyngeal artery extends to the skull base between the internal carotid artery and the pharynx, supplying branches to the carotid body, pharyngeal wall and middle ear and to tumours arising from them. It also supplies lower cranial nerves and meningeal branches which anastomose with branches from the cavernous segment of the internal carotid artery and the vertebral artery.

The facial artery passes superiorly towards the inner canthus; it anastomoses with the ophthalmic artery and may be an important collateral when the internal carotid artery is occluded. Venous drainage from the distribution of the facial artery passes through the superior ophthalmic vein and the vein can be well visualized by external carotid angiography.

The occipital artery supplies the descending

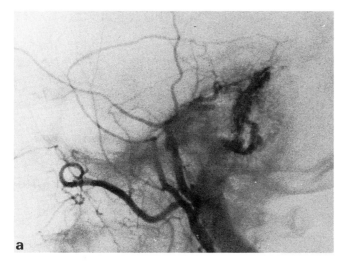

**Fig. 3.58.** External carotid angiogram, dural angiomatous malformation (AVM), (a, b) lateral and AP projections. External carotid injection filling superficial temporal and maxillary arteries. The dural AVM is around the wall of the sigmoid sinus and there is early filling of the sinus and jugular vein from it. The AVM is supplied by the posterior division of the middle meningeal artery, which normally supplies the dura of the cerebellar convexity, and by the posterior branch of the superior division, which normally supplies the low cerebral convexity dura.

(c) Occipital artery injection. Multiple branches from the artery pass both in the meninges and superficially to penetrate the bone near the sinus and supply the AVM. Early filling of the sinus and jugular vein is again evident.

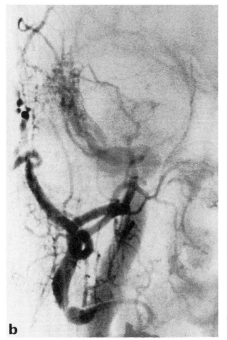

b

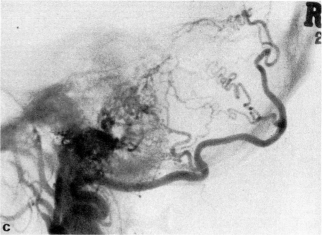

c

segment of the facial nerve and meningeal branches to the posterior fossa; muscular branches which anastomose with those of the vertebral artery are a potential route for stray emboli introduced during therapeutic occlusion procedures.

The superficial temporal artery supplies most of the scalp and part of the face, anastomosing with the ophthalmic artery.

The maxillary artery provides the major supply to the intracranial dura mater through the middle meningeal artery and to a lesser extent the accessory meningeal artery and artery of the foramen rotundum. It also gives some supply to the 3rd–7th cranial nerves. Its distal branches share the blood supply of the nasal mucosa with the ethmoid branches of the ophthalmic artery;

the former vessels are accessible to embolization in cases of intractable epistaxis. Though not very common the anomaly of origin of the ophthalmic artery from the maxillary artery should be specifically sought prior to any embolization procedure.

*Vertebral circulation* (Fig. 3.59)

In the lateral projection, the intracranial portion of the vertebral artery and the basilar artery follow a smooth course, lying close to the basi-occiput and sphenoid, ending behind and within 1.5 cm of the dorsum sellae. The largest branch of the vertebral artery is the posterior inferior cerebellar (PICA), usually arising from the vertebral artery just after it enters the skull. It takes a wavy course dorsally around the foramen magnum, a loop of the artery sometimes entering the foramen, and then ascends behind the medulla to divide into vermis and tonsillohemispheric branches. The former runs close to the lobes of the inferior vermis; the latter outlines the cerebellar tonsil and inferior surface of the hemisphere. The contralateral PICA commonly fills as a result of the reflex of contrast medium into its parent vertebral artery.

The basilar artery supplies perforating and paired circumferential arteries to the pons, which are usually visible on subtraction films, and larger paired anterior inferior cerebellar arteries (AICA), the size and distribution of which vary inversely with that of the corresponding PICA. The AICA forms a tight loop adjacent to the flocculus and porus acusticus, easily identified in the cerebellopontine angle on angiography. It then supplies brainstem and cerebellar branches. The superior cerebellar arteries leave the basilar artery shortly before it terminates, and pass backwards and slightly upwards, separated from the posterior cerebral arteries by the third nerves and tentorium. They supply branches to the midbrain, superolateral branches to the cerebellar hemisphere and superior vermis branches. The posterior cerebral arteries are of large calibre and normally arise as terminal bifur-

cation of the basilar artery. Their general direction is backwards and upwards, to irrigate the occipital, posterior temporal and parietal lobes. The first few centimetres of their course, from which arise the tiny but important posterior thalamoperforating branches supplying the hypothalamus and medial part of the thalamus, are gently curved convex downwards. At the posterior end of this portion they break up into larger branches, of which the posterior choroidal arteries continue the gentle curve upwards and then forwards; they enter the choroidal fissure to reach the choroid plexus.

Detailed assessment of diplacements is facilitated by obtaining angiograms in both semi-axial and anteroposterior projections with the chin elevated, using subtraction techniques. The vertebral artery is seen pursuing its winding course through the foramen transversarium and around the lateral mass of the atlas vertebra, to pass medially and join its fellow to ascend vertically as the basilar artery. The posterior inferior cerebellar arteries run a course on each side of the medulla, before the vermis branches run together close to the midline in the paravermian sulcus. The basilar bifurcation into posterior cerebral arteries may take the form of a Y or T junction. The posterior cerebral arteries pass upwards and backwards, first diverging and then converging around the midbrain in a goblet shape; this corresponds to the part on the lateral projection where the arteries make a gentle curve convex inferiorly. In this portion of their course their position relative to the midline is approximately symmetrical. Thereafter they become sinuous and break up into cortical branches.

*Congenital variations*

The anterior communicating artery is normally a single short trunk 1–3 mm in length and about half the calibre of the anterior cerebral arteries, but it may be replaced by several small or large vessels forming a complex of channels, a persistence of the fetal network of vessels; rarely it may be absent (Busse 1921).

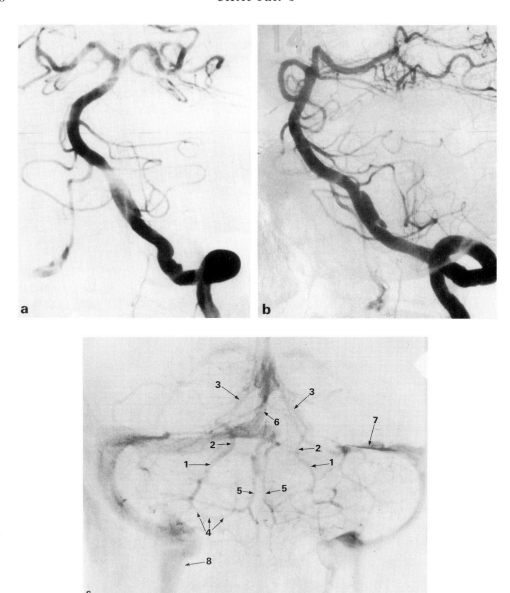

**Fig. 3.59.** Left vertebral angiogram, with normal reflux down right vertebral artery, (a) AP, (b) lateral projection (slightly oblique).

The right vertebral artery is congenitally small and the left one large. This is a common anatomical variation and not of significance in normal circumstances. The left PICA arises normally. The right one arises with the AICA from the basilar artery. The basilar artery bifurcates at a slightly proximal level and the SCAs and PCAs arise from common trunks. Note there is fibromuscular hyperplasia of the left vertebral artery just below the skull base and there is an associated short dissecting aneurysm of the intracranial segment of the vessel.

(c) Normal veins, AP projection. Brachial veins (1); lateral mesencephalic veins (2); posterior mesencephalic veins (3); vein of lateral recess of fourth ventricle (4); inferior vermian veins (5); superior sagittal sinus (6); transverse sinus (7); internal jugular vein (8).

The anterior cerebral artery may be absent on one side or may be a vestigial thread-like vessel; the other is then large and bifurcates at the midline to supply both hemispheres. Occasionally the vessels reunite under the genu of the corpus callosum before finally separating. The important finding is that carotid injection on one side fills both anterior cerebral arteries and injection on the other side fills neither. Variation of filling in the same patient may occur due to fluctuations of pressure in the injected artery. A 'cross-circulation' test may be made in order to determine whether the anterior part of the circle of Willis is functionally patent and will permit an adequate flow of blood, which may be important prior to treatment of aneurysms. During the injection into one carotid artery, the contralateral vessel is compressed by an assistant. If there is good communication, there is opac-

ification of the contralateral anterior cerebral circulation and usually, also, of the contralateral middle cerebral distribution, though this may alternatively or partly be supplied through the posterior communicating artery.

The posterior cerebral artery is well filled by common carotid injection in about 20% of cases and by internal injection in almost 40%. In such cases the posterior communicating artery is of large calibre. In other cases the artery is hypoplastic and the circle of Willis in such circumstances is ineffective in conducting blood from the vertebral artery to the carotid tree, important if the carotid artery were occluded. The posterior cerebral artery may arise from the carotid artery, just below the origin of the middle cerebral artery, as a large direct branch, a persistence of the primitive arrangement. Communication with the basilar artery may be

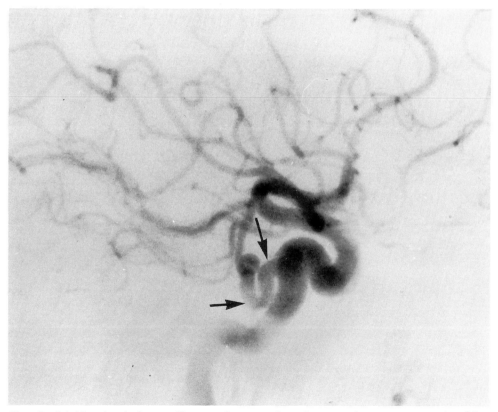

**Fig. 3.60.** Primitive trigeminal artery. The anomalous artery (arrow) connects the precavernous region of the internal carotid artery to the basilar artery inferior to the superior cerebellar arteries.

thread-like or even absent on one or on both sides and the circulation of the whole cerebral hemisphere is dependent upon the carotid flow. The vertebrobasilar network of vessels is described in great detail by Huber *et al.* (1982). The recognition of variations in the circle of Willis is important if the treatment of a cerebral aneurysm by carotid ligature is contemplated.

*Carotid–basilar and carotid–vertebral anastomoses*
These are important because they are often associated with hypoplasia of the vertebrobasilar system below the anastomosis, they may cause an unexpected distribution of an ischaemic lesion, and there is an increase in the incidence of berry aneurysm in affected patients.

A persistent primitive trigeminal artery may be seen in about 0.2% of angiograms joining the intracavernous portion of the internal carotid artery, through a curved course posteriorly and medially with the basilar artery near its termination (Fig. 3.60). It may accompany the trigeminal nerve into Meckel's cave, pass medially to the ganglion and then enter the cavernous sinus to join the carotid artery, or may enter the sinus through a separate and more medial dural

opening (Sunderland 1948, Harrison & Luttrell 1953); in other cases the anastomosis has pierced the dorsum sellae. Occasionally the primitive trigeminal artery supplies only one of the cerebellar arteries. Other persistent primitive connections between the cervical internal carotid and the basilar artery pass through the anterior condylar canal (hypoglossal artery), or between the cervical internal or external carotid and intracranial vertebral artery, passing through the foramen magnum (pro-atlantal intersegmental artery). These are less common.

**The abnormal angiogram**

*Displacement and compression of vessels* (Figs 3.61, 3.62, 3.63)

According to the size and the situation of a mass, a major group of arteries may be displaced or there may be only separation of lesser branches. Tumours lying near or on the surface of the cortex cause greater displacement than deep ones and the displacement is greater with slowly growing tumours than with rapidly invasive

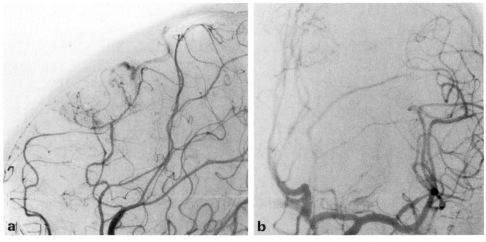

**Fig. 3.61.** Left medial frontal malignant glioma. Left carotid angiogram, (a) lateral, (b) AP projection. There is abnormal circulation in the medial frontal region supplied by branches of the callosomarginal artery and with early drainage to the superior sagittal sinus. The mass causes local deviation and splaying of the branches of the callosomarginal artery around it and rounded shift of the anterior cerebral artery to the right side. The anterior meningeal (falx) artery is prominent and probably gives a small supply to the mass which was adherent to meninges in the parasagittal region.

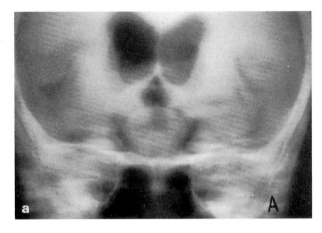

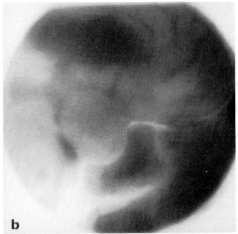

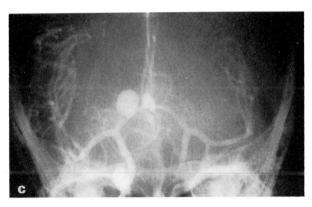

**Fig. 3.62.** Pituitary tumour and aneurysms.
Air encephalogram, (a) AP and (b) lateral
midline tomogram. A smooth well defined mass extends
from the enlarged pituitary fossa, through the
chiasmatic cistern which is increased in depth by the
wedge effect of the tumour, to elevate the chiasmatic
recess of the third ventricle and separate it from the
infundibular recess. There is mild dilatation of the
lateral ventricles. The symmetrical Sylvian fissures are
well outlined and the sulci on the medial surface of the
hemispheres are filled.

Right carotid angiogram, with compression of the
left carotid artery, (c) AP projection. The first parts of
both anterior cerebral arteries are elevated by the
tumour. There are aneurysms arising from the right
anterior cerebral and anterior communicating arteries.

ones. Incongruity between relatively slight displacement and outspoken neurological deficit favours a malignant growth. Oedema around a tumour increases the degree of displacement; if the oedema is eccentric, the centre of the deformity will not accurately indicate the site of the tumour. Herniation of brain produces dislocation of the anterior cerebral arteries to the opposite side (subfalcine herniation) and of the posterior cerebral artery downwards (tentorial herniation) (Chapter 2).

There may be delay in the circulation through the arteries in the neighbourhood of a mass. Mass effect may be evident as an area of lack of filling, beyond which there may be crowding together of vessels. Arteries in the immediate vicinity of the mass may be narrowed. Apart from the displacement and approximation of

arteries, they may be so stretched around the tumour that their normal wavy course is lost; a vessel immediately over the summit of the tumour may appear as a straight line. The position of any mass can be logically deduced from these general principles.

*Pathological circulation*

The nature of the tumour can frequently be diagnosed if it has a sufficiently rich blood supply to be revealed by angiography. Pathological vessels may fill unusually early or they may retain contrast medium after the normal phlebogram. The nature of the tumour may be deduced from the architecture of the tumour vessels, their shape, size, evenness or irregularity of calibre, the

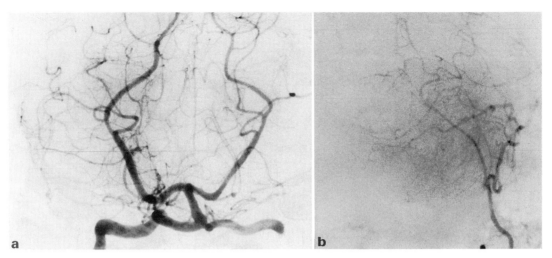

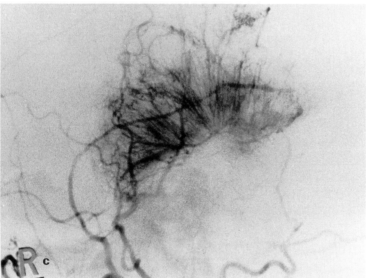

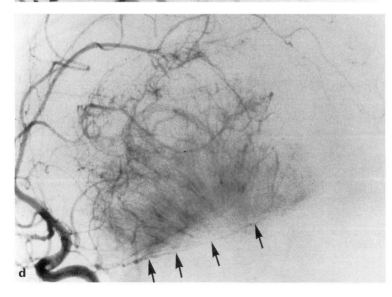

**Fig. 3.63.** Meningioma (same patient as Fig. 3.40). Vertebral angiogram, (a) the left posterior inferior and superior cerebellar arteries lateral to the brainstem are deviated medially and the vermis branches are displaced to the right. There is no abnormal circulation. Left occipital angiogram, (b) there is a rich meningioma blush supplied by the meningeal branches of the artery.

Meningioma arising from floor of middle cranial fossa and tentorium. External carotid angiogram, lateral projection (c), there is a rich blood supply from the inferior division of the middle meningeal artery. The vessels radiate into the tumour from its attachment.

Internal carotid angiogram, lateral projection (d), there is a rich circulation from the tentorial artery (arrows). The Sylvian branches of the middle cerebral artery are elevated and the temporal cortical branches descend over the tumour.

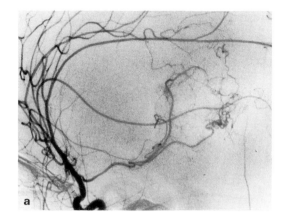

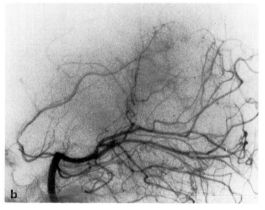

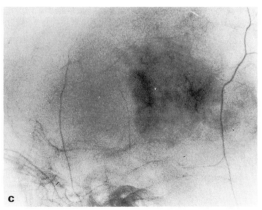

**Fig. 3.64.** Choroid plexus papilloma. Left carotid angiogram, arterial phase, lateral projection (a), left vertebral angiogram, arterial phase, lateral projection (b), vertebral angiogram, venous phase (c). The anterior and posterolateral choroidal arteries are enlarged and give rise to multiple branches which supply a large tumour in the left trigone. Pathological circulation is evident in the arterial phases and an irregular blush is present within the tumour in the capillary phase.

margin of the area and the character of major arteries and veins which feed and drain the tumour.

Meningiomas often opacify diffusely, causing a well circumscribed, evenly distributed density (Fig. 3.63). The edge is clear cut and separate vessels may not be defined. This 'blush', caused by capillary circulation in the tumour, is often not apparent until the early phlebogram phase; a later film may show encircling veins accentuating the edge of the tumour. Individual tumour vessels are frequently visible in meningiomas, especially on magnification angiography. The vessels tend to taper like those of normal tissue and may form a radiating pattern from the site of tumour attachment. Less commonly meningiomas, especially of the angioblastic type, contain early filling, irregular vessels and may show arteriovenous shunting. Meningiomas arising in the ventricular system occur most often in the lateral ventricular trigones. They are supplied by choroidal arteries and drain to subependymal veins. A similar angiographic appearance occurs with choroid plexus papillomas (Fig. 3.64); these usually affect children and are more frequently associated with generalized hydrocephalus.

Enlarged meningeal arteries, most frequently derived from external carotid branches, less often from the infraclinoid segment of the internal carotid or the vertebral arteries and entering the tumour at its of origin from the meninges, are significant in the diagnosis of meningioma. Meningeal supply is, however, by no means pathognomonic of meningioma; it may occur in any vascular mass which is adherent to or invading the meninges (Fig. 3.61).

Haemangioblastomas give rise to diverse appearances in the angiograms. There is most frequently a persistent 'blush' with or without a surrounding network of large vessels. There may be a large avascular area displacing normal vessels, caused by the cyst which often accompanies this type of tumour; in such cases, subtraction films may be necessary to identify a tiny opacified mural nodule. The combination of a large cyst and vascular tumour in the adult cerebellum is most suggestive of this diagnosis (Fig. 3.65).

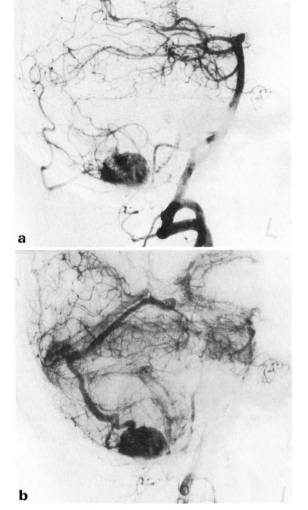

a

b

**Fig. 3.65.** Haemangioblastoma. Vertebral angiogram, lateral projection, (a) arterial, (b) late arterial–capillary phase. There is early and dense opacification of a vascular haemangioblastoma nodule in the left tonsil, with early venous drainage through the vermian veins to the straight sinus.

Multiple vascular cerebellar nodules may be the presenting feature of von Hippel–Lindau disease and should be considered in the differential diagnosis of posterior fossa metastases.

Other benign tumours may show an increased circulation composed of normally tapering vessels or a capillary blush. These include neurinomas, about 20% of which are hypervasc 268

sometimes with arteriovenous shunting in their capsules; a minority of pituitary adenomas, mainly supplied by branches of the cavernous segments of the carotid arteries; paraganglionomas supplied in the neck by branches of the external carotid (Fig. 3.66) and with intracranial extensions fed by meningeal vessels derived from both external and internal carotid and vertebral artery branches. Chordomas are usually poorly vascularized, but they may obtain rich circulation from meningeal vessels.

Over one third of cases of malignant astrocytomas show characteristic pathological vessels. The vascularity varies in degree and extent and has no discrete border. Individual vessels are increased in number and highly irregular in shape, direction and calibre; there may be bizarre enlargements in the course of a relatively small vessel (Bramwell 1887). Several patches of pathological vessels may be distributed irregularly within the tumour area. Both arteries and veins take part in this caricature of a circulation and in places they may form arteriovenous fistulae. These effect a rapid flow of blood, consequently the tumour circulation appears in the arterial or early in the capillary phase when one or more large veins draining to superficial or subependymal veins or both may be apparent (Fig. 3.61).

Another third of malignant astrocytomas have patchy, sparse circulation and the rest of malignant astrocytomas are avascular.

Other forms of glioma reveal pathological vessels much less frequently and usually the area is small compared with the size of the tumour as indicated by vessel displacement; the network of pathological vessels, often in the central part of the tumour, is present in about 20% of grade II–III gliomas and some capillary blush in only 10% of grade I–II gliomas.

Overall, about 40% of carcinoma metastases are vascular on angiograms; the vessels tend to be somewhat irregular, like those of glioblastomas. The circulation often delimits the whole tumour, giving it a discrete appearance, sometimes resembling a meningioma (Fig. 3.67); when the metastasis has undergone

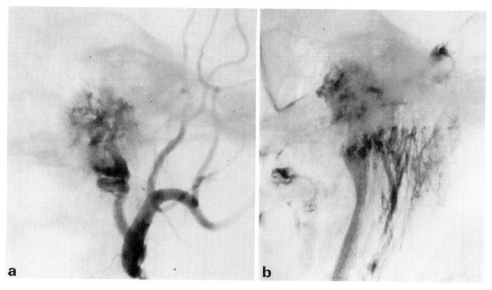

**Fig. 3.66.** Paraganglioma (glomus jugulare tumour). (a) Maxillary angiogram. The highly vascular tumour is supplied by a hypertrophied anterior tympanic branch. (b) Ascending pharyngeal angiogram. The tumour is supplied by the inferior tympanic branch. There is early filling of the internal jugular vein and retrograde filling of the petrosal sinuses, which drain the tumour.

central necrosis it may opacify as a thick-walled ring.

Aneurysms (Fig. 3.68) arising from the intracranial arteries are filled from carotid or from vertebral injections according to their disposition. The indications for angiography are dealt with in Chapter 13. An aneurysm may give rise to symptoms of increasing pressure upon neighbouring nervous structures without rupture and consequently may be revealed in a patient suspected of having a tumour (Fig. 3.69). The sac may be globular, pear-shaped, or multilobular. Additional oblique projections may be necessary to demonstrate precisely the neck of the aneurysm and its site of origin. Contrast filling occurs during the arterial phase but may be retained in the sac through the venous phase. Rapid serial angiography shows that the sac may fill more slowly than the arteries, with a swirling movement of the medium as it first sweeps around the periphery, then gradually fills in the centre. A large aneurysm frequently contains mural clot, so that its opacified lumen is smaller than the volume of aneurysm and may not be

globular, but may have sinuous inflections of parts of its outline. Angiograms made within a week of a subarachnoid haemorrhage show smooth, tubular or tapered narrowing of arteries in 60% of cases due to vascular spasm. This is frequently localized to the region of the haemorrhage but it may be widespread.

Vascular malformations are readily identified; only exceptionally are they likely to be mistaken for any other lesion. They occur anywhere in the brain, though most commonly in the cerebrum and more frequently in the territory of the middle cerebral artery. They vary in size, from those so small as to be inconspicuous among the normal arteries, to large lesions which may cause difficulty in demonstration of normal vessels because the steep arteriovenous pressure gradient in the lesion diverts most of the contrast medium through it and away from the surrounding brain circulation. Those arteries which feed the malformation tend to enlarge, as happens with arteriovenous fistulae elsewhere in the body (Fig. 3.70). Small malformations may have only one supplying artery which can be identified

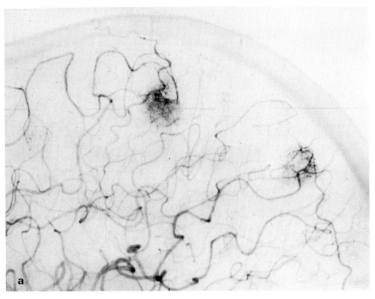

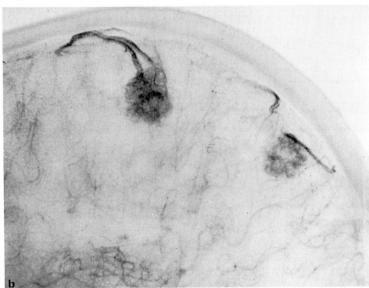

**Fig. 3.67.** Typical metastases. Carotid angiogram, lateral projection, (a) arterial, (b) capillary phase. There are two small, discrete regions of abnormal circulation consisting of irregular vessels with early filling superficial veins. They are in the frontoparietal and parietal regions, and there is stretching of the vessels adjacent to them suggesting local swelling.

on angiograms, but in large and deeply situated AVM's several major vessels may be involved and from both sides of the brain. Meningeal vessels contribute to the blood supply in about 25% of all cases. In about half of these, and much more frequently in the posterior fossa, the arterial supply is entirely dural and is best and sometimes only shown by external carotid angiography.

Dural AVM's may drain directly into an adjacent dural sinus, but not infrequently thrombosis occurs and results in venous drainage being away from the sinus through cortical veins.

In the arterial phase the angioma appears as an irregular, closely knit tangle of vessels of even calibre, though of varying sizes, and in the same film one or more broad sinuous veins are usually

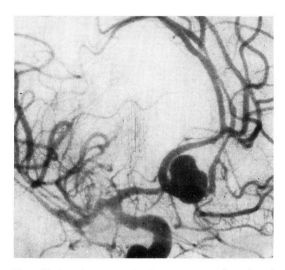

Fig. 3.68. Anterior communicating aneurysm; subarachnoid haemorrhage. Right carotid angiogram, right anterior oblique projection. The second parts of both anterior cerebral arteries fill from the right carotid. The first part of the left anterior cerebral artery was hypoplastic. There is a bilocular aneurysm projecting superiorly from the anterior communicating artery between the second parts of the anterior cerebral arteries. The aneurysm and adjacent haematoma separate these vessels, which are irregular in calibre due to spasm.

beginning to fill (Fig. 3.70). Enlarged draining veins may cover an area much greater than the malformation itself, and they may flow in multiple directions over the cortex and to the deep cerebral veins. In judging whether the angioma can be treated, the size and situation of the knot of vessels seen during the arterial phase is important rather than the extent of the venous drainage. Not infrequently saccular aneurysms are shown on supplying arteries and there is aneurysmal dilation of the veins. Small angiomas, inadequately filled, may rarely resemble the pathological circulation of a glioblastoma or a meningioma. The irregularity in calibre, in shape, in distribution, and in extent of the glioblastoma vessels which are usually separated by tumour tissue, contrasts with the more compact, more regular and even vascularity of the angioma.

Many angiomatous malformations can, with due precautions to avoid injuring normal tissues,

be embolized using particles of lyophilized dura or synthetic materials such as polyvinyl alcohol (ivalon) or rapidly setting acrylic compounds. Such emboli must reach the abnormal vessels and not occlude more proximally feeding arteries, which would merely induce collateral flow into the AVM.

A direct fistula between a major artery and venous sinus or vein is usually caused by trauma in young people, though it may occur as a congenital anomaly or, especially in the elderly, it may be due to rupture of a vessel affected by atheroma or an aneurysm.

The most frequently encountered fistula between the internal carotid artery and the cavernous sinus (Fig. 3.71) causes rapid filling of the sinus and of the outflow channels from it including the ophthalmic veins. Large fistulas are associated with poor filling of the intracranial vessels from the artery supplying the fistula. Rapid opacification of the sinus may hide the actual site of the shunt, and it may be better demonstrated by retrograde flow through the posterior communicating artery by vertebral angiography. Low vertebrovertebral fistula has become more common with the use of the central venous line, due to inadvertant trauma to the vertebral artery during attempts at puncture of the internal jugular vein. Congenital large vessel fistulas are usually in the suboccipital region and either vertebrovertebral or between the external carotid branches and vertebral or jugular veins. Maxillomaxillary and large spinal arteriovenous fistulas also occur.

All these lesions are amenable to occlusion using various embolization techniques.

## Mass effect

When a mass differs in density, enhancement characteristics or signal intensity from adjacent tissues on CT and NMR studies, swelling is of secondary importance in localization, though its degree and extent have diagnostic implications and may influence management. When mass

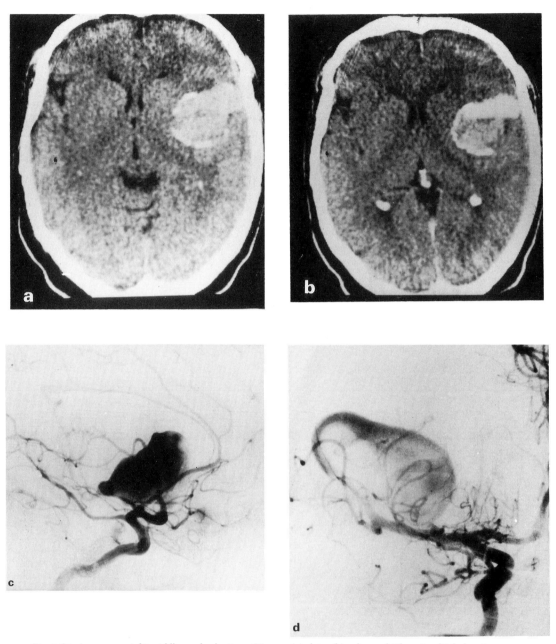

**Fig. 3.69.** Aneurysm, right middle cerebral artery. CT scan, (a) plain, (b) enhanced. There is a high density mass with peripheral curvilinear calcification in the lateral posterior frontal region. The anterior half of the mass shows dense homogeneous enhancement. Right carotid angiogram, (c) lateral, (d) AP projection. The aneurysm arises from a cortical branch of the middle cerebral artery. Only the enhancing anterior part of the aneurysm is opacified, the posterior part was filled with clot.

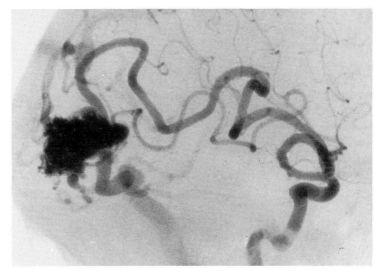

**Fig. 3.70.** Cerebral angiomatous malformation. Carotid angiogram, lateral projection. The angular branch of the middle cerebral artery is enlarged and is the main supplying vessel to a temporo-occipital angiomatous malformation (AVM). There is a small supply from the posterior temporal artery. There is early filling of superficial veins draining the AVM towards the sigmoid and superior sagittal sinuses.

effect is the main radiological abnormality, localization is generally less precise and depends on appreciation of displacements of those anatomical landmarks which can be recognized by particular imaging methods; it is facilitated in unilateral lesions by comparison with the nornal side. The visibility of normal CSF on CT and NMR allows recognition of displacement or compression of the subdivisions of the ventricles and major fissures and sulci away from the centre of a swelling, without the trauma of adding air or opaque contrast medium which was formerly necessary on conventional X-ray studies. Superficial arteries and veins provide an interrupted outline of the subarachnoid surfaces and subependymal veins adequately delineate the ventricles; angiography is rarely indicated for localization in modern departments.

Masses lying deep within brain substance generally produce smooth and widespread compression or displacement of the adjacent ventricle or subarachnoid space; conversely, tumours situated close to a surface tend to cause more localized and well defined displacements. Small superficial and extrinsic swellings may be accommodated in adjacent CSF spaces without displacing brain (*see* Fig. 3.13); eventually all masses cause compression and/or destruction combined with displacement of brain substance.

*Intrinsic masses* These cause centrifugal displacements which are modified by restraining forces from the skull and dural septa. They cause focal compression and deviation of the part of the ventricular system adjacent to the mass away from the tumour, together with displacement of the grey matter towards the vault and narrowing or occlusion of the overlying sulci (*see* Fig. 3.46). Knowledge of normal anatomy allows logical deduction of the displacements of CSF spaces, and the vessels associated with them, which will be produced by masses in any location (Fig. 3.73).

*Intraventricular masses* (Kendall *et al.* 1983). These are partly outlined in the ventricular cerebrospinal fluid. Their site of origin may be evident, but encroachment against or secondary adhesion to the wall of the ventricle may obscure it. The ventricle is expanded around larger masses and eventually obstructed by them. Classical intraventricular tumours include:

1 Colloid cysts (Fig. 3.72). These form smooth or lobulated masses arising just behind the foramen of Monro; they expand within and tend to occlude the anterior third of the third ventricle or, less frequently, the foramina themselves. On CT they are usually hyperdense and nonen-

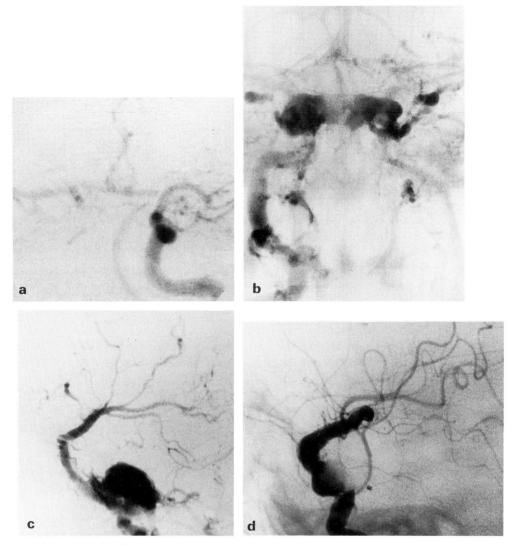

**Fig. 3.71.** Caroticocavernous fistula. 81-year-old lady with bilateral ophthalmoplegia and blind right eye. Left carotid angiogram (a). There is good spontaneous cross flow filling of right carotid distribution through the anterior communicating artery. Right carotid angiogram, (b) AP, (c) lateral projection, later phase. A fistula between the right carotid artery and cavernous sinus causes early dense opacification of both cavernous sinuses. Drainage is through ophthalmic veins and petrosal sinuses and there is retrograde filling of cerebral cortical veins.

Right carotid angiogram, (d) lateral projection, after balloon occlusion of fistula. The balloon, with its tip containing a metal pellet, lies within the cavernous sinus and fistula. The carotid flow is restored and intracranial vessels are outlined.

hancing. Low density and isodense colloid cysts occur, but glioma and cysticercosis should be considered as alternative diagnoses if there are any atypical features. Reformatted coronal and sagittal sections distinguish large third ventricular tumours from suprasellar craniopharyngiomas and terminal basilar aneurysms.

2   Choroid plexus tumours. On CT (Fig. 3.74). dense, sometimes partly calcified, well marginated, enhancing masses in the lateral ventricular

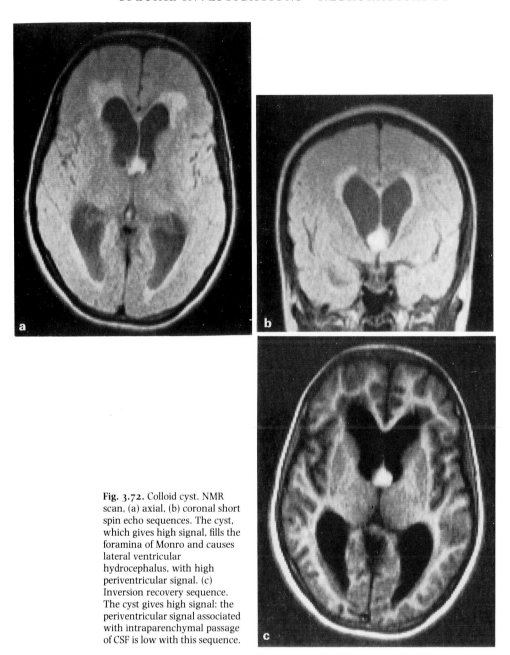

**Fig. 3.72.** Colloid cyst. NMR scan, (a) axial, (b) coronal short spin echo sequences. The cyst, which gives high signal, fills the foramina of Monro and causes lateral ventricular hydrocephalus, with high periventricular signal. (c) Inversion recovery sequence. The cyst gives high signal: the periventricular signal associated with intraparenchymal passage of CSF is low with this sequence.

choroid of children are likely to be papillomas or carcinomas; in adults they are usually meningiomas. In the third and fourth ventricles, papillomas are more common than meningiomas.

3 Gliomas invading the ventricular system usually destroy the wall and the intra-axial component tends to compress and displace the ventricle and to produce vasogenic oedema. However, even benign intraventricular tumours may attenuate or penetrate the wall and cause

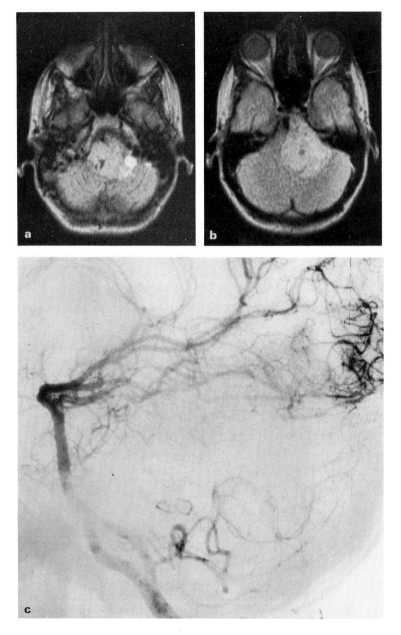

**Fig. 3.73.** Brainstem glioma. MRI scan, (a, b) short spin echo axial sections. There is increased signal from the tumour, which occupies most of the brainstem and extends from it into the left cerebellopontine angle and left side of the pontine and chiasmatic cisterns. The very high signal seen in (a) is due to a recent bleed causing a clot within the tumour.

oedema in the white matter, and, conversely, ependymomas especially may be almost entirely intraventricular.

Astrocytomas tend to cause irregular thickening of the wall, most easily recognized when the septum pellucidum or fornices are involved. Seeding metastatic spread of glioma, especially microglioma, pinealoma and medulloblastoma, may form a high density enhancing lining of the ventricles or a multinodular pattern of superficial enhancement.

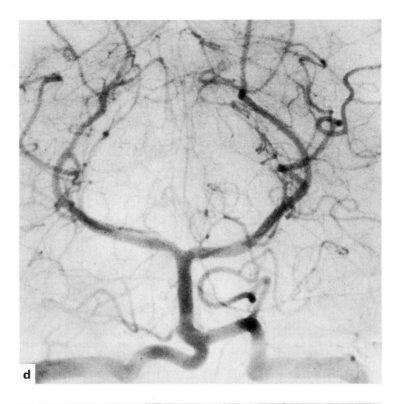

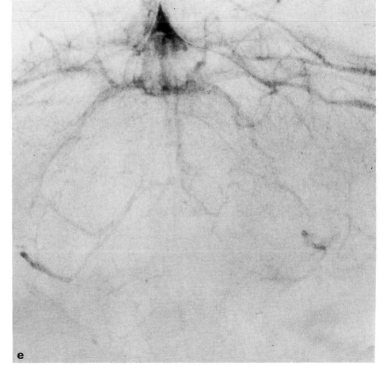

**Fig. 3.73.** Vertebral angiogram, (c) lateral, (d) AP arterial phase. The cerebellar and posterior cerebral arteries around the brainstem are stretched apart and the branches posterior to the brainstem are displaced posteriorly, indicated a mass expanding the brainstem. The basilar artery is displaced posteriorly and one posterior communicating artery is elevated by the exophytic component. (e) AP venous phase. All the veins outlining the brainstem are stretched apart by the mass expanding it. The left crural vein and veins in the left cerebellopontine angle are distorted by the exophytic component.

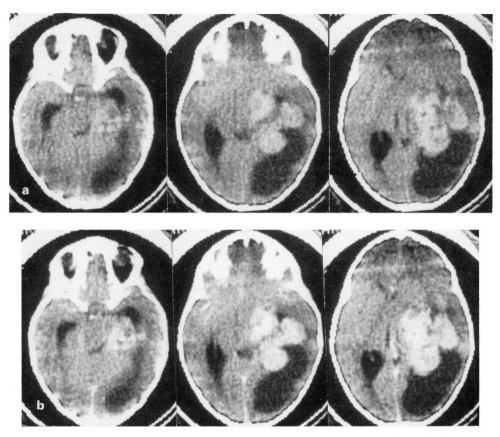

**Fig. 3.74.** Choroid plexus papilloma. CT scan, (a) plain, (b) enhanced, at similar levels. There is a high density lobulated mass, which enhances considerably, within the trigone of the right lateral ventricle, extending into the temporal horn and choroidal fissure. There is obstructive hydrocephalus of the posterior part of the right lateral ventricle and mild hydrocephalus of the left lateral ventricle, possibly caused by compression of the third ventricle.

Epidermoids tend to be slightly higher than CSF density and dermoids to be of lower density due to the presence of fat; calcification may occur in either type of tumour. Enhancement is limited to the capsules. Teratomas also may contain fat and calcium; sometimes differentiated osseous or dental structures are evident and enhancing soft tissues are usual. Arachnoid and ependymal cysts both occur as focal expansions of the ventricle with obstruction. They are confirmed by iohexol CT studies; they show as filling defects of CSF density which may opacify on delayed studies.

The arterial supply to true intraventricular tumours is entirely from the choroidal arteries, which enter through, and may define, the site of attachment; they drain to subependymal and choroidal veins. Conversely, intracerebral tumours are supplied and drained by parenchymal vessels, usually connecting to superficial in addition to choroidal arteries and subependymal veins.

*Extra-axial masses* These blend with the dural partitions or bone of the skull and extend through the adjacent subarachnoid space, acting in wedge-like fashion to widen the space and displace the brain (Fig. 3.75). Similar appearances could be caused by a tumour fungating from the brain substance, but more general

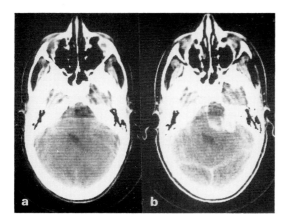

**Fig. 3.75.** Acoustic neurinoma. CT scan, axial sections, (a) plain, (b) enhanced. There is a mass in the left cerebellopontine angle which is displacing the pons and fourth ventricle posteriorly and to the right side. The mass has a lateral isodense, enhancing component, and a medial low density, ring-enhancing component which was necrotic.

expansion of the brain substance involved by the intrinsic tumour is usual.

The margins of an extra-axial mass tend to be sharply demarcated from the brain surface; displaced cortex and white matter may be visualized by CT or NMR. Large cortical vessels and, in the case of extradural lesions, venous sinuses, also, are displaced centrally by the tumour. These displaced vessels are the basis of angiographic diagnosis (*see* Fig. 3.63); they are also frequently shown on enhanced CT and NMR. Any intrinsic or extrinsic mass may cause pressure, with focal thinning and/or expansion of the overlying bone. Some extra-axial masses invaginate brain substance and attenuate or penetrate the surface from a narrow base; especially when associated with vasogenic oedema, these tumours may simulate intrinsic masses. Angiographic demonstration of a dominant meningeal blood supply may distinguish an extrinsic mass.

Giant aneurysm (Fig. 3.69) is an important differential diagnosis of basal tumour. A patent aneurysm may be recognized on CT as a well demarcated mass of similar density to the blood and showing dense enhancement occurring simultaneously with the normal blood vessels; often there is peripheral calcification. A thrombosed aneurysm is of greater density and there may

be tumour-like enhancement. Both NMR and intravenous digital angiography will show flowing blood in a patent aneurysm but intra-arterial studies may be necessary for the more subtle distinction between a largely thrombosed aneurysm and a tumour.

Progressive mass effect eventually causes herniation of brain substance away from the originally involved compartment. With unilateral supratentorial masses, medial hemispheric structures are displaced under the anterior two-thirds of the falx cerebri. The progressively increasing depth of the falx posteriorly causes characteristic deformity of the roof of the anterior horn and body and protects the posterior part of the ventricular system. The sharp free edge of the falx may compress cortical branches of the anterior cerebral artery sufficiently to cause ischaemic low density in their peripheral distribution.

The contents and margins of the tentorial hiatus are well shown by CT and NMR. Unilateral descending herniation of the uncus or hippocampus causes asymmetrical encroachment on the suprasellar and/or quadrigeminal cisterns compressing and rotating the midbrain and causing inferomedial deviation of the basal vein and posterior communicating and/or posterior cerebral arteries. Eventually the cisterns are obliterated and the hiatus occluded. Distortion of the brain stem causes haemorrhages, which are usually small but may be large enough to be visualized on CT and NMR. Posterior cerebral artery compression may infarct the occipital and posterior temporal lobes and occlusion of the posterior part of the third ventricle causes hydrocephalus of the uncompressed contralateral ventricle, which sometimes affects only the temporal horn. In the early stages, contralateral hydrocephalus tends to limit midline shift but increases descending herniation.

Bilateral supratentorial brain swelling, which occurs not infrequently with head injury, bilateral subdural effusions and central tumours, tends to depress the third ventricle and brainstem, with or without the paramedial parts of both temporal lobes, and to occlude the basal cisterns.

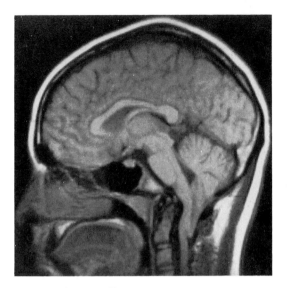

**Fig. 3.76.** Chiari I malformation. MRI, sagittal image. The inferior vermis of the cerebellum is elongated and extends into the spinal canal as low as the inferior border of the 2nd cervical vertebra. The medulla, also, is depressed. It is compressed posteriorly, opposite the adontoid, and shows the typical kink posteriorly at cervicomedullary level.

Depression of the gyrus rectus into the anterior part of the chiasmatic cistern is the only easily recognized radiological feature of the downward herniation over the sphenoidal ridge which may occur with frontal masses.

Upward herniation of cerebellum may displace the brainstem anteriorly and even invaginate the posterior margin of the third ventricle. Occlusion of superior cerebellar branches may increase the displacement by causing cerebellar ischaemia with swelling.

Displacement of the inferior poles of the cerebellar tonsils and medial parts of the biventral lobules through the foramen magnum is easily recognized in images made in the vertical planes. Tonsillar herniation occurs more frequently with posterior fossa masses than as a secondary feature of transtentorial herniation; the tonsillar depression tends to displace the spinal cord anteriorly. Tonsils expanded by tumour invasion may simulate herniation, but they usually differ in physical characteristics from normal brain tissue. Extrusion into the cisterna magna of tumours from the medulla or spinal cord and

masses arising within the fourth ventricle tend to displace the tonsils superiorly and can generally be distinguished from tonsillar herniation. In cerebellar ectopia the tonsils are elongated and the clinical presentation differs from the conditions causing herniation. In the more severe Chiari malformation the brainstem, also, is elongated into the spinal canal and syringohydromyelia is frequent; this is best investigated by NMR (Fig. 3.76) or computerized cisternography.

## Hydrocephalus and atrophy of the brain

Hydrocephalus is due to obstruction, previous or persisting, between the ventricular system, or any part of it which contains choroid plexus, and the major site of absorption of cerebrospinal fluid in the Pacchionian granulations; rarely it is due to increased fluid production by a choroid plexus papilloma or carcinoma. Mass lesions causing hydrocephalus can usually be demonstrated by CT and NMR. Hydrocephalus may also be due to congenital or acquired stenosing lesions, or to adhesions or granulation tissue in the sub arachnoid spaces (Fig. 3.77), or blocking of Pacchionian granulations by blood, cell debris, neoplastic cells, proteinaceous fluid or cholesterol. Though the site of the block may be surmised when there is obvious dilatation of CSF spaces proximal and not distal to a particular point, exact localization may require opacification of subarachnoid or ventricular CSF.

Atrophy or loss of brain substance follows damage by trauma, infection, infarction, radiotherapy or conditions of unknown aetiology, including multiple sclerosis and other demyelinating diseases and the presenile dementias, hereditary ataxias and Huntington disease. In some instances the clinical presentation may resemble a tumour; also, when the underlying condition has ceased to operate, a quantitative estimate of the degree of damage may be of limited value in assessing prognosis; the operative treatment of epilepsy depends upon the identification of a responsible focal abnor-

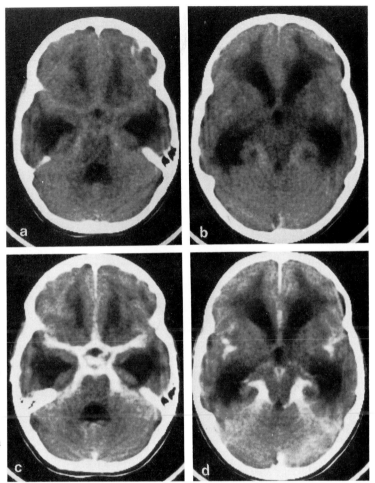

**Fig. 3.77.** Tuberculous meningitis with hydrocephalus. CT Scan, (a, b) plain, (c, d) similar levels enhanced. There is granulation tissue with density slightly greater than brain and markedly enhancing in the basal cisterns and Sylvian fissures. There is four-ventricular hydrocephalus and periventricular lucency.

mality of brain tissue and radiological studies may reveal localized scarring or widespread brain damage. CT and/or NMR, by demonstrating both brain substance and CSF spaces, allow the best estimate of the extent and distribution of damage.

Focal enlargement of CSF spaces is facilitated by comparison with more normal regions and generalized or progressive dilatation by comparison with previous studies. Generalized cerebral atrophy causes enlargement of the whole ventricular system, together with the fissures and sulci. In some diseases atrophy is more selective; widening of cerebral sulci may be an isolated abnormality in alcoholism and in some forms

of syphilis and the cerebellar sulci in cerebellar cortical degeneration. In so-called central atrophy, when the ventricular system is predominantly involved, the distinction from hydrocephalus on CT, NMR or pneumography may be difficult unless signs indicating or suggesting increased ventricular pressure are present. These include:

1 Passage of CSF into the periventricular white matter. The periventricular extracellular spaces are distended most prominently around the frontal horns and evident as a low density halo on CT (Fig. 3.77) and as an increased signal due to prolongation of $T_2$ on NMR in appropriate spin

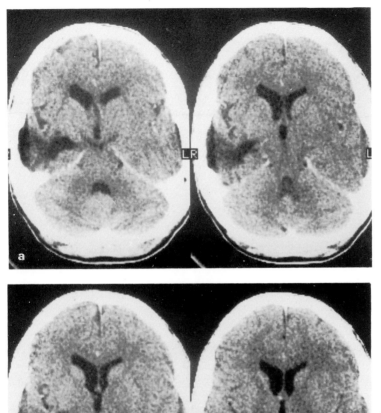

**Fig. 3.78.** Post-traumatic atrophy. CT scan, (a, b) contiguous sections. The right lateral ventricle is dilated, particularly the temporal horn, and there is widening of the right Sylvian fissure. There is low density in the right posterior temporal white matter consistent with postcontusion encephalomalacia.

echo sequences (*see* Fig. 3.72). It is most frequent with moderate acute ventricular dilatation rather than mild acute or chronic severe hydrocephalus.

2  Symmetrical lateral ventricular dilatation. There is elevation of the more lateral parts of the roofs of the lateral ventricles, causing reduction of the angle between the roofs of the ventricles and also relative prominence of the temporal horns (*see* Fig. 3.44; Sjaastad & Nordvik 1973). Isolated dilatation of the temporal horns may suggest early hydrocephalus; this may be a valuable feature in conditions such as acute trauma and subarachnoid haemorrhage, in which relative increase in ventricular size could reflect resolution of brain swelling or onset of hydrocephalus.

3  Dilatation of the third ventricle, with ballooning of the anterior medullary velum and the third ventricular recesses and with extension of the infundibular recess towards or into the sella turcica (*see* Fig. 3.4).

4  Dilatation of the fourth ventricle, with convexity of the superior medullary velum.

5 Enlarged basal cisterns, and in some cases Sylvian fissures also, with small or normal upper convexity cortical sulci. Small arachnoid cysts may simulate CSF pools over the cerebral cortex which may occur with focal atrophy; erosion of bone may result in local thinning or expansion over the cyst.

6 Changes in ventricular size may occur quickly with hydrocephalus. Even the most rapidly changing atrophic processes, which usually relate to encephalitic illnesses, takes weeks rather than days to show progression.

Brain atrophy due to previous trauma may be generalized, with dilatation of the ventricles and subarachnoid spaces, or may be focally more severe, especially with penetrating injuries, and sometimes underlying a depressed fracture. In closed head injury, focal atrophy subsequent to contusion and/or haematoma most frequently involves the inferior parts of the frontal lobes and the temporal poles and CT may reveal low density in the white matter reflecting encephalomalacia (Fig. 3.78). Hydrocephalus after head injury may be acute and transient or chronic; it is usually communicating, due to subarachnoid haemorrhage, but occasionally obstructive.

Major vascular occlusions cause atrophy in the distribution of the affected artery. When they occur in early childhood, and especially in the perinatal period, infantile hemiplegia may follow with hemiatrophy in which the affected hemisphere is small and the hemicranium is small, with vault thickening, with widening of the cerebral sulci and/or enlargement of the lateral ventricle. Large angiomatous malformations and the Sturge–Weber syndrome may be associated with focal or hemiatrophy (see Fig. 3.25). Some encephalitic illnesses also may cause predominantly, but not entirely, unilateral atrophy.

The term 'porencephaly' was introduced by Heschl (1859) to describe a congenital defect of brain extending from the surface to the ventricle, commonly in the region of the Sylvian fissures. If the destructive process occurs early in development, there may be interference with the migration of neuroblasts and abnormal gyri may

border the defect; destruction in a well formed cerebral mantle occurs with insults later in embryonic life. Cavities, which develop in late embryonic or postnatal life following a variety of insults, commonly vascular, but excluding cystic degeneration in tumours, are more correctly referred to as cystic encephalomalacia, or simply as cavitation; such cavities may be enclosed within brain substance or communicate with the ventricular system or subarachnoid space.

When there is considerable discrepancy between the size of the two lateral ventricles as a result of loss of brain substance, or when a diverticulum is present, the septum lucidum and third ventricle are often displaced towards the side of the dilatation.

## Radiographs of the spine

Anteroposterior and lateral X-rays of the spine are obtained when the clinical presentation suggests the possibility of spinal pathology which could be amenable to surgery. Supplementary oblique views display further details of the cervical and lumbar neural arches, apophyseal joints and the structures bordering the intervertebral foramina; they may be useful when there are clinical features of involvement of cervical nerve roots and for elucidation of some fractures, subluxations or dislocations.

The size and shape of the spinal canal, which determines the total amount of space available for the spinal cord and meninges, varies markedly between individuals. Charts showing the normal range at each vertebral level are available (Burrows 1963, Hinck et al. 1966). The smallest dimension in the cervical region is the sagittal diameter; if the distance from the conjoined laminae to the posterior border of a vertebral body is under 12 mm, cervical spondylosis is likely to cause cord compression (Fig. 3.79). The available space varies with posture, especially if there is instability, and this may be elucidated by lateral radiographs in full flexion and extension.

The thoracic spinal canal is round. The

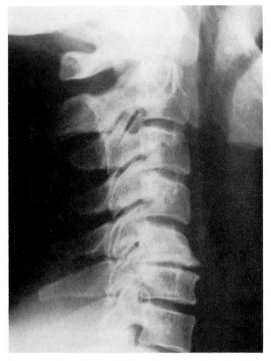

**Fig. 3.79.** Cervical spondylosis with myelopathy. Cervical spine, lateral projection. The sagittal diameter of the spinal canal, corrected for magnification, between the most anterior convexity of the conjoined laminae of the 5th cervical vertebra and the nearest point of the posterior surface of the body, is 13 mm. The C5–6 disc space is narrowed, with marginal osteophytes which encroach on the canal and further reduce the sagittal diameter to 9.5 mm.

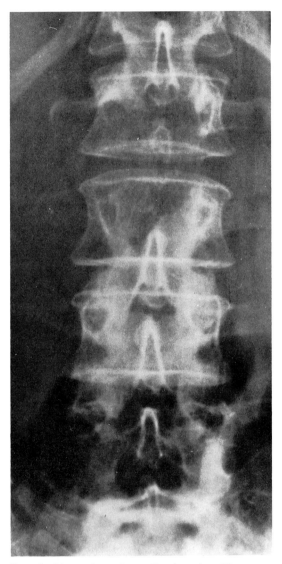

**Fig. 3.80.** Metastatic carcinoma. Lumbar spine, AP projection. There is destruction of (1) the right pedicle, laminae and inferior articular process of L1, (2) the superior articular process and right lamina of L2, (3) the right transverse process of L3, (4) much of the body of L4. The intervertebral discs are preserved.

triangular lumbar canal is narrowest in the sagittal plane, and in congenitally small canals the 'lateral recesses' are usually most severely compromised. The available space in the lumbar canal is best assessed using CT, and, indeed, once a pathological process has been detected and localized in any region, CT may be considered for further elucidation.

Malignant neoplasms within a bone cause irregular destruction and/or new bone formation; any paravertebral soft tissue mass tends to be confined by periosteum and intervertebral discs are usually preserved (Fig. 3.80).

Both pyogenic and granulomatous inflammation tends to involve intervertebral discs or, less commonly, the apophyseal joints, destroying the contiguous bone (Fig. 3.81) and forming adjac-

ent soft tissue swellings which tend to spread along soft tissue planes.

Rheumatoid arthritis of the cervical spine usually produces its most severe effects at atlanto-axial level. Anterior subluxation of the atlas is present when the distance between the odontoid

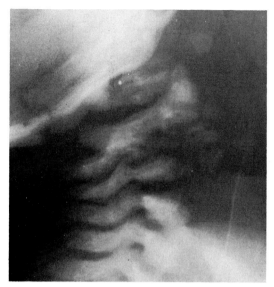

**Fig. 3.81.** Osteomyelitis. Cervical spine of infant, lateral projection. The body of C3 and the lower border of C2 are destroyed. There are fragments of residual dense bone in a soft tissue swelling in the prevertebral region.

and anterior arch of atlas exceeds 3 mm in an adult and 5 mm in a child in any position of the spine (Fig. 3.82).

Slowly growing intraspinal tumours or cystic processes erode the adjacent bone by pressure, with a tendency to recortication. This causes focal enlargement of the spinal canal at the level of the mass, with flattening of the pedicles and concavity of the posterior surfaces of the vertebral bodies (Fig. 3.83). A difference in canal diameter of more than 2 mm at adjacent levels should be viewed with suspicion. Schwannomas may arise from nerves within and cause enlargement of intervertebral foramina; schwannomas may also be dumb-bell, both intraspinal and foraminal, or arise peripherally, causing a paravertebral mass.

Enlargement of the spinal canal without erosion or flattening of the medial borders of the pedicles suggests diastematomyelia; a tendency towards intervertebral fusion is commonly present and a bony spicule extending into the spinal canal is confirmatory (Fig. 3.84).

Radiographs taken for abnormal spinal curvatures may reveal developmental vertebral anomalies or destructive lesions: curvature with-

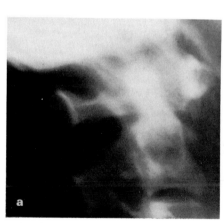

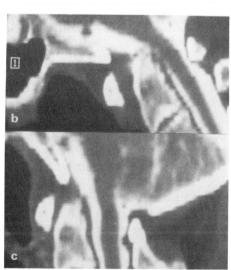

**Fig. 3.82.** Rheumatoid arthritis. Lateral tomograms C1–2 (a). There is erosion of the odontoid process. The atlas is subluxated anteriorly on the axis.

Computerized myelogram (b, c). Reformatted sagittal sections cervicocranial junction, neck in flexion (b) and extension (c). The atlas subluxates anteriorly on flexion and the spinal cord is compressed against the odontoid. Note that some deformity of the spinal cord persists when the compression is relieved in extension.

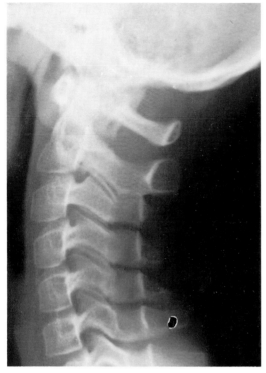

**Fig. 3.83.** Intramedullary tumour. Cervical spine, lateral projection. The sagittal diameter at C3–C7 levels is increased, most markedly in the midcervical region. The depth of the bodies is reduced and the normal anterior convexity of the conjoined laminae is flattened. The tumour was a low-grade ependymoma. Slow progression allows bone remodelling and the cortical bone is intact.

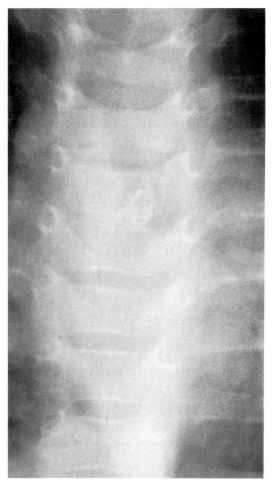

**Fig. 3.84.** Diastematomyelia. Dorsal spine, AP radiography. There is increase in the interpedicular distance in the mid-dorsal region with preservation of the normal medial convexity of the pedicles. A spur of corticated bone divides the canal at the widest point.

out additional abnormality may be associated with a spinal tumour or syringomyelia.

Overt dysraphism is evident clinically; radiographs confirm the extent of spina bifida. It is usually associated with a Chiari II malformation and hydrocephalus due to fourth ventricular outlet block; hydromyelia is frequent. The whole condition is best elucidated by NMR, if available, or by myelography plus computed myelography. Occult dysraphism also is associated with spina bifida, abnormalities of fusion of vertebral bodies and arches, narrowing of disc spaces and varying stages of duplication, the commonest being diastematomyelia which is present in over 30% of the Chiari II malformations (Emery & Lendon 1973). Up to 9 months of age, realtime ultrasound can show the position of the lower end of

the spinal cord and the presence of any associated congenital cyst or hamartomatous intraspinal lesion, and is useful in routine screening of infants with overt or suspected occult dysphraphism (Scheible *et al.* 1983).

Congenital and developmental dysplasias of the craniocervical junction are frequent in association with hindbrain maldevelopment, especially with Arnold–Chiari malformation and developmental syringohydromyelia. These dysplasias include atlanto-occipital assimilation and failure of segmentation, basilar impression and atlanto-axial subluxation (Burrows 1981).

## Radioisotope studies

An increase in osteoblastic activity can be detected by bone-seeking isotopes. Though non-specific, a pathological process may be confirmed before any abnormality can be shown on radiographs or CT in inflammations and neoplasms. Radioisotopes are particularly useful in demonstrating multiple bone metastases from a known primary malignancy (Patten & Woolfenden 1977).

## Computerized tomography of the spine

Density discrimination between structures contained within the relatively small spinal canal, surrounded by the intermittent dense bone of the spinal column, is an exacting test for CT. Indeed, the spinal cord can be shown consistently only when the surrounding subarachnoid space is at least 2 mm wide.

Adequate scans can be obtained using machines with:

1  Rapid scan times to limit movement artefacts.
2  Scout film-cursor line facility and tilting gantry to allow selection of the optimum scanning plane; for most conditions this is perpendicular to the long axis of the spinal canal or along the plane of an intervertebral disc.
3  Variable section width, between approx 1.5 mm for high spatial resolution with minimal partial volume effect, sometimes essential for visualization of cervical disc protrusion and for good resolution reformations from the axial data, and 1.0 cm for the high contrast discrimination necessary if plain scan diagnosis of spinal cord-lesions, such as syringohydromyelia, is to be successful.
4  Software capability for reasonably rapid image reformatting in any desired plane.

## Application of spinal CT without intrathecal contrast injection

1  Spinal trauma (Brant Zawadzki *et al.* 1981). Fractures of neural arches and vertical fractures of vertebral bodies (Fig. 3.85) are well shown with CT. Horizontal fractures are often shown on conventional X-rays but require reformatting of axial data for good visualization by CT. Foreign bodies, herniated intervertebral discs, displaced bone and haematoma can be visualized, together with the degree of encroachment on the spinal canal. Loss of soft tissue planes due to contusion or swelling may prevent distinction between cord swelling and extrinsic soft tissue compression by plain CT; iohexol myelography or computerized myelography will elucidate if required.
2  SXR evidence of bone destruction and/or sclerosis, or a soft tissue mass. CT shows any contiguous soft tissue swelling to better advantage than radiographs and is a valuable complementary study (Fig. 3.86). Intraspinal extension of a paravertebral mass may be shown (Fig. 3.87).
3  Spinal canal stenosis. The shape and outline of the spinal canal are shown ideally by high resolution CT (Fig. 3.88). It should be noted that the exiting nerve root traverses the largest part of the intervertebral foramen adjacent to the pedicle, behind the vertebral body and in front of the pars interarticularis above the plane of the intervertebral disc and facet joints. The facet joint and superior articular facet form the posterior border of the lateral recess with the intervertebral disc and vertebral body below it forming the anterior border. The nature of a stenosis such as congenitally short pedicles, facet joint osteoarthritis and spondylolisthesis is evident and the degree of stenosis can be measured (Ciric *et al.* 1980).
4  Prolapsed intervertebral discs. On CT these are denser than spinal theca, which contains CSF, and of similar density to other disc substance; unless totally extruded and sequestrated, they are in continuity with normally situated disc substance. Occasionally, and more frequently in the thoracic region, they are partly

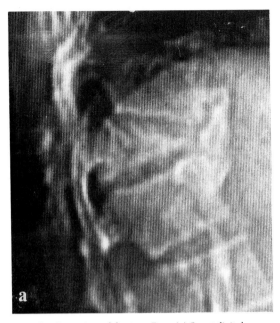

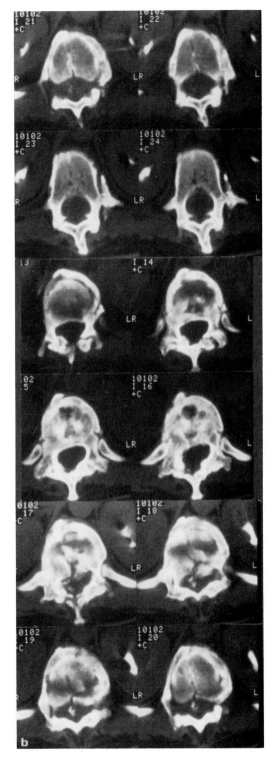

**Fig. 3.85.** Comminuted fracture D11. (a) Scout digital radiograph. The vertebra is wedged and its posterior border is displaced into the spinal canal. (b) Sections D10–12. The comminuted fracture of D11 body extends into the spinal canal and posteriorly displaced fragments narrow the sagittal diameter of the canal. The neural arch is also fractured. Separated bone fragments in the left half of the canal extend to the midline and must directly involve cord substance.

calcified. Disc substance does not enhance after intravenous contrast medium; this may be useful in distinguishing recurrent disc prolapse from enhancing postoperative fibrotic tissue. Generalized bulging of a degenerate disc can be distinguished from focal protrusion or prolapse (Williams *et al.* 1982a). The disc is contrasted against or locally effaces the epidural fat; displacement or compression of the dural sac, nerve root sheaths, or the nerve roots beyond the sheaths, may be shown; thus lateral discs which are not impinging on the theca or root sleeves can be revealed (Williams *et al.* 1982b). CT scanning is accurate in the detection of lumbar disc prolapse (Fig. 3.89), but it must be performed at the correct clinical levels from the level of the pedicle above to that below if all extruded fragments are to be detected. A weakness of CT, relative to myelography and NMR, is failure to exclude tumours of the cauda equina and conus

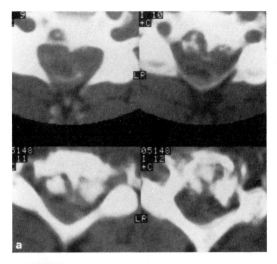

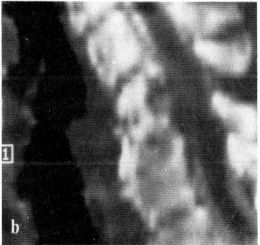

Fig. 3.86. Osteomyelitis. Computerized myelogram, (a) axial, (b) reformatted sagittal sections. There is irregular destruction of the bodies of two vertebrae and the intervening disc, with posterior angulation. There is a large extradural mass of inflammatory tissue and displaced bone lying anteriorly in the spinal canal, compromising the theca and spinal cord.

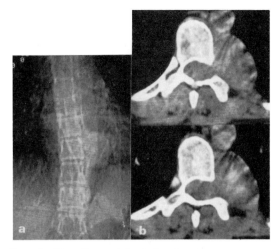

Fig. 3.87. Neurofibroma left 9th dorsal nerve root. CT scan, (a) scout film (digital radiograph). There is a left sided paravertebral mass at D9 level. (b) axial sections. A dumb-bell neurofibroma causes a mass of density slightly higher than the other contents of the spinal canal. It expands the spinal canal, enlarges the D9–10 intervertebral foramen and forms a paravertebral mass.

region and these possibilities should be considered in negative studies.

5   Dysraphism (Naidich *et al.* 1983). Bony malformations are clearly revealed and diastematomyelia, aberrant laminae and spina bifida are best assessed by CT. Lipoma, both subcutaneous and deep, including any extension into the spinal canal and infiltration of the neural placode, and meningocoees are shown. Details of intrathecal structures including the position of the conus medullaris, any tethering of the cord and site of origin of nerve roots, generally require intrathecal iohexol to elucidate.

6   Lesions with markedly abnormal attenuations are shown. High attenuation lesions include some meningiomas (Fig. 3.90), calcified discs (Fig. 3.91) and large, recent haematomas. Low attenuation lesions include lipomas and some dermoids. Cerebrospinal fluid attenuation within the cord substance occurs in syringo-hydromyelia and most post-traumatic cysts. Some tumour cysts are of low density, but most intramedullary tumours are of approximately the same density as the normal spinal cord and may not be recognized without intrathecal contrast medium. Abnormal enhancement is occasionally shown in angiomas, haemangioblastomas and meningiomas, but it is rare in gliomas. NMR has proved particularly valuable in the diagnosis of intramedullary masses in which the contribution of CT has been limited.

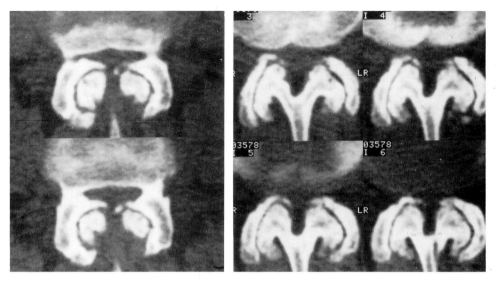

**Fig. 3.88.** Lumbar spinal canal stenosis. CT scan sections, descending from just above the level of the pedicle down to subadjacent intervertebral disc. Developmentally short pedicles and medially placed apophyseal joints, with superadded osteoarthritis causing marked narrowing of lateral thirds of spinal canal.

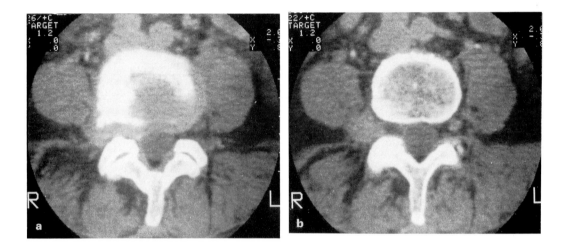

**Fig. 3.89.** Prolapsed intervertebral disc. CT scan, (a) at level of disc, (b) above disc at level of intervertebral foramen. There is protrusion of disc substance into the right lateral aspect of the spinal canal and intervertebral foramen. The disc substance is in contact with the exiting nerve root.

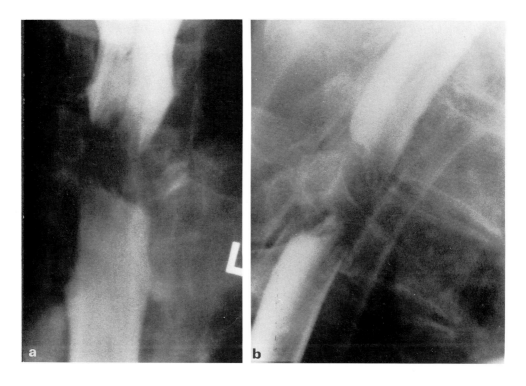

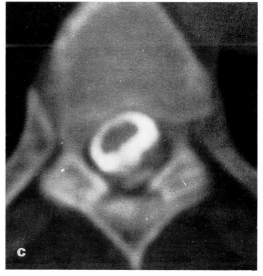

**Fig. 3.90.** Meningioma. Iohexol myelogram, (a) AP, (b) lateral projection. There is an extramedullary mass in the left side of the spinal canal in the upper dorsal region posterolateral to the spinal cord. It was partly intradural and partly extradural. The mass contains calcification and slightly flattens the adjacent pedicle.

Computerized myelogram, (c) the deformity of the spinal theca and flattening of the spinal cord by the partly calcified mass are better demonstrated.

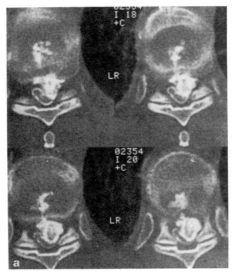 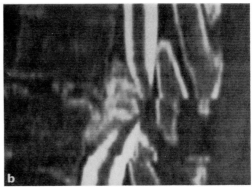

**Fig. 3.91.** Prolapsed thoracic disc. CT, (a) axial sections, (b) reformatted sagittal section. The nucleus pulposus is partly calcified and much of the calcified disc substance is in the extradural space, anterior of the theca, mainly on the left side. The spinal cord is markedly compressed posteriorly and to the left side.

## NMR of the spine

Images with high signal to noise ratio, best obtained using surface coils and high resolution, using at least a $256^2$ matrix with thin (3 mm) contiguous sections, which are probably best achieved by using a high field strength magnet (*circa* 1.5 Tesla) and gating to compensate for respiratory movement in the thoracic region, are all advantageous. Longitudinal images display the spine and thecal contents to best advantage; on axial images, scout film indication of the level at which they are attained is important. NMR interpretation is rendered difficult by severe scoliosis.

The prolonged $T_1$ and $T_2$ values of CSF can be used to advantage; the intensity of the signal generated from the fluid varies markedly, depending upon the imaging parameters used. With short echo delays and repetition times on spin echo sequences, the signal, from the CSF is low and it appears dark, outlining the spinal cord and medulla, the cerebellum, including the tonsils (*see* Fig. 3.76), and the nerve roots. Contrast between cerebrospinal fluid and epidural structures (Fig. 3.92) may be better with this type of sequence or with higher signal CSF obtained by more prolonged echo delays and repetition times depending on the signal intensity of the adjacent structures. Subarachnoid blood vessels are best revealed against CSF imaged with high intensity. Lesions containing CSF, including syringomyelia (Fig. 3.93) and hydromyelia and arachnoid cysts, generally show similar intensities to the free CSF, though an increase in protein can reduce the $T_1$ and $T_2$ values. Highly proteinaceous fluid in tumour cysts is distinguishable from cerebrospinal fluid, and solid intramedullary tumours (Fig. 3.94) can generally be distinguished from both cysts and normal spinal cord.

The cortex of the vertebrae, in common with that of other bones, gives virtually no signal, whereas the fatty and vascular medulla produces a high signal and reveals the anatomy of the spine. With the exception of angiomas of bone and the effects of radiotherapy, which results in replacement of the marrow by fat, pathologies destroying bone generally reduce the signal from the marrow. Increased signal is present from lipomas (*see* Fig. 3.53) and in the fatty components of dermoids and teratomas, and NMR is

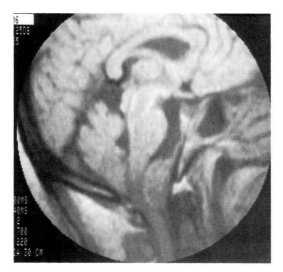

Fig. 3.92. Meningioma. NMR, sagittal section (spin echo TR500, TE40). The tumour is of similar signal intensity to brain. It is outlined by low intensity CSF. The medulla and upper cervical spinal cord are displaced posteriorly and compressed.

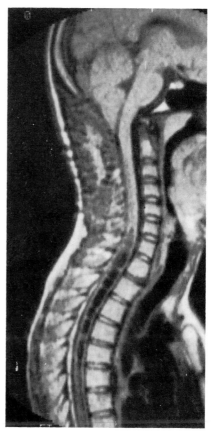

Fig. 3.93. Syringomyelia. NMR, sagittal section spin echo sequence (TR500, TE40). The linear lobulated low signal region, with similar intensity to that of CSF in the subarachnoid space, within the expanded lower cervical and whole of the thoracic segments of the spinal cord, is typical of a syrinx. There is cerebellar ectopia.

helpful in the detailed evaluation of dysraphic abnormalities with which these tumours are frequently associated.

The water content of the nucleus pulposus is about 85% at birth and, though it drops progressively with age, the normal nucleus has a higher $T_1$ and $T_2$ value than the much less hydrated annulus. Disc herniation and the degree of canal narrowing caused by it are well shown (Fig. 3.95), though this becomes more difficult as the water content decreases with age and in disc degeneration.

Flow sensitive sequences will show large vessels associated with angiomatous malformations and some tumours, and the short $T_1$ and T2 of subacute and chronic haematoma allows recognition in any location.

## Myelography

Air (Dandy 1919), oily (Strain *et al.* 1942) and ionic contrast media (Arnell & Lindstrom 1931) were previously used as myelographic contrast media, but each had particular disadvantages.

Air provided poor contrast and caused acute discomfort; oily media caused arachnoiditis, and withdrawal from the subarachnoid space prolonged the study and often caused discomfort; ionic media caused arachnoiditis and were sufficiently neurotoxic, in general to limit their application to lumbar radiculography. Even so, painful spasms of the back and lower limb muscles were occasionally precipitated and, less frequently, epilepsy. These media have been replaced by nonionic contrast agents which can be used safely in all regions of the subarachnoid space. They opacify the CSF itself avoiding the surface tension effects of the gaseous and oily

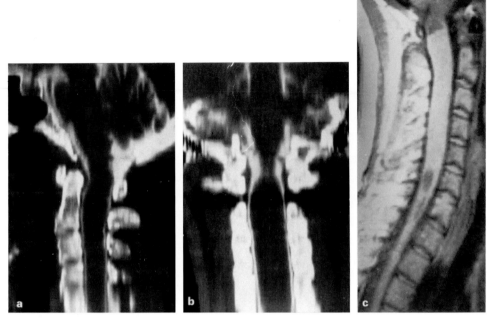

**Fig. 3.94.** Intramedullary tumour (ependymoma). Computerized myelogram, reformatted (a) sagittal, (b) coronal sections. The cervical spinal cord and lower medulla oblongata are diffusely swollen, MRI, (c) sagittal section, spin echo sequence (TR1200, TE180). There is higher signal from the solid tumour which expands the whole cervical spinal cord. There are small cysts near its upper and lower extremities, which give lower signal than the tumour and brain substance but higher signal than the CSF.

media. Thus the outline of the subarachnoid space is accurately defined and even the fine peripheral extensions of the nerve root sheaths are penetrated.

These media, in the concentrations in clinical use, do not cause arachnoiditis, even in the presence of subarachnoid blood (Haughton & Ho 1982). The most recent of the nonionic media, iohexol (Omnipaque), is not epileptogenic and transient discomforts such as headache, nausea, vomiting and backache, which are of particular importance in influencing patient cooperation for computerized myelography, are not severe. A relatively large volume containing up to 4 g iodine can be given, which facilitates examination of long segments of the spine. At diagnostic concentrations the opaque medium is heavier than cerebrospinal fluid and can be transferred by gravitational posturing to exam-

ine any region of the subarachnoid space, though mixing with cerebrospinal fluid occurs and may reduce density below that necessary for conventional myelography, particularly if the examination is prolonged.

Satisfactory apparatus for myelography should include:

1 a tilting table, preferably capable of 60° head and 90° foot down tilt;
2 a supporting system capable of taking the patient's weight during either direction of tilt;
3 a spot filming device;
4 a facility for easy lateral filming and, preferably, fluoroscopy also.

Myelography is not a painful procedure and requires patient cooperation. Explanation and reassurance prior to the study is almost always sufficient to ensure success but mild pre-

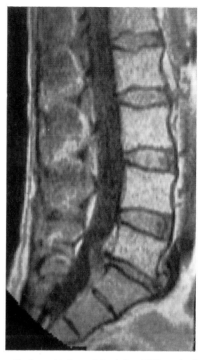

**Fig. 3.95.** Prolapsed intervertebral disc. MRI, sagittal section, short spin echo. The herniated L5–S1 disc substance is contrasted against the low signal from the cerebrospinal fluid in the lumbar theca.

medication may be given in very apprehensive individuals. General anaesthesia is used in young children and requires endotracheal intubation and muscular relaxation to ensure the airway and avoid coughing. Dehydration, which delays excretion of the contrast medium and increases the incidence of side effects, should be avoided and fluids should be pressed after the study to facilitate rapid absorption from the subarachnoid space and renal excretion. Anticonvulsant cover is unnecessary if iohexol is used.

The site of injection of the contrast medium should be selected so as to avoid the region of the suspected pathology, using lumbar puncture unless contraindicated. Cervical puncture as a primary procedure should be specifically avoided if a high or possibly obstructing cervical lesion is anticipated. It is particularly indicated:

1 to show the upper border of an obstructing lesion demonstrated by lumbar injection;

2 when the lumbar subarachnoid space is anticipated to be very narrow or possibly occluded by a pathological process;
3 when lumbar puncture has failed; or
4 when there is infection in the lumbar region.

The contrast medium is injected through a 22–24 gauge needle on the fluoroscopy table, under screen control, with the patient optimally positioned to demonstrate the pathology. This is usually prone for lumbar and cervical lesions, and lateral with the table head lowered but head raised to trap the contrast medium for the dorsal region, followed by filming in the supine position. Supine filming is necessary, also, to adequately show the foramen magnum region.

Following water soluble myelography, the contrast medium should be directed towards the sacral sac; by keeping the trunk as erect as the lesion permits, absorption from the lower theca is encouraged and this reduces minor side effects. Bed rest does not reduce the incidence and severity of side effects and is not necessary (Macpherson & Teasdale 1985). Headache, nausea, vomiting and exacerbation of radicular, lumbar or cervical pain are the most common side effects and are treated symptomatically. Rare complications of myelography include intraspinal bleeding, especially in patients with disturbances of blood clotting, and infection causing meningitis or discitis, which is avoided if sterile precautions are observed.

Extra-arachnoid contrast medium is usually easily recognized during injection and the needle should be satisfactorily repositioned; apart from generally producing a nondiagnostic study it is not of significance. When extradural it tends to flow along nerve roots and muscle planes away from the spinal canal. When subdural (Fig. 3.96) it tends to remain predominantly anteriorly or posteriorly, but it may flow throughout part or the whole of the subdural space and, if this is not recognized, it could be misinterpreted as a swollen cord or as an unusual obstructing lesion. Intramedullary injection is a rare complication of cervical puncture (Johansen et al. 1983), which is usually tolerated in small volumes and

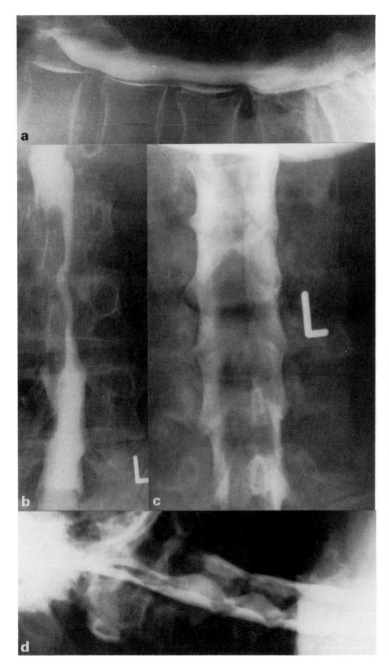

**Fig. 3.96.** Subdural injection of contrast medium. Lumbar region, prone (a) lateral, (b) AP. Contrast medium in the subarachnoid space layers anteriorly in the cerebrospinal fluid. Most of the contrast medium is subdural; it lies pocketed posteriorly, displacing the arachnoid and with a convex border towards it. On the AP the pocket is an irregular bizarre shape.

Cervical region, prone, (c) on the AP projection the subdural contrast medium has an irregular outline, but a central lower density simulates the spinal cord and the nerve roots are visible. (d) The lateral projection shows that the contrast medium is not layering in the fluid in the subarachnoid space, but forming an irregular peripheral layer in the non-fluid-containing subdural space.

should be recognized early as the contrast medium forms a lanciform density within the cord in two planes.

The spinal cord descends from the medulla oblongata, commencing at about the level of the foramen magnum, and terminates at the conus medullaris which normally lies between the lower borders of D12 and L2 vertebrae. The cord is approximately cylindrical, with slight enlargements in the lower cervical and dorsolumbar

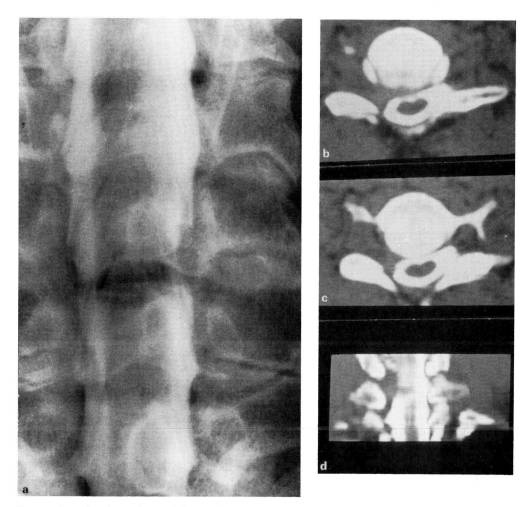

Fig. 3.97. Lateral prolapse of cervical disc. Myelogram, (a) there is occlusion of the right C7 nerve root sheath. There is also incomplete peripheral filling of the left C7 nerve root sheath. Computerized myelogram, (c, d) contiguous axial sections, (d) coronal reformatted section. C7 root sheath compression is confirmed. The epidural fat in the medial part of the foramen is obliterated. A herniated disc fragment was removed.

regions corresponding to the cervical and lumbosacral innervations, and lies symmetrically in the subarachnoid space.

The nerve roots pass laterally from the anterolateral and posterolateral margins of the cord at each segmental level, with progressively increasing obliquity of descent from cervical to sacral levels. Each root carries a sheath of arachnoid extending towards the point where it penetrates the dura to gain the appropriate intervertebral foramen. The normal sheath has a rose thorn configuration; deformity or occlusion of the sheath is an important sign of compression by an extradural mass (Fig. 3.97). Small dilatations, sometimes referred to as perineural cysts, may occur on the root sheaths. They are common in the cervical and lumbosacral regions, may fill relatively slowly with contrast medium and are not of clinical significance (Larsen et al. 1980).

The anterior spinal artery may be visible as a linear structure approximating to the line of the anterior median sulcus of the spinal cord; the

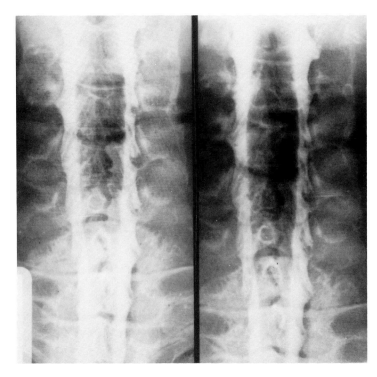

**Fig. 3.98.** Spinal angiomatous malformation. Iohexol myelogram, AP radiographs. There are large, tortuous vessels superimposed on the cervical and upper dorsal segments of the spinal cord.

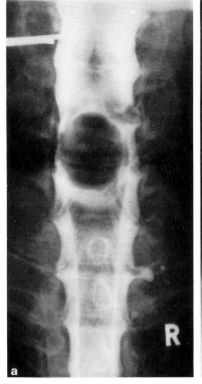
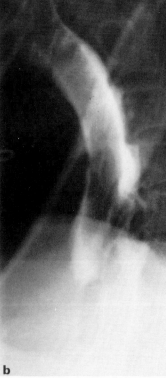

**Fig. 3.99.** Meningioma. Iohexol myelogram, (a) AP, (b) lateral projection. There is an intradural, extramedullary mass lying anterior to the spinal cord at C5 level, displacing the cord posteriorly and compressing it. The tumour forms a lobulated filling defect within the subarachnoid space which is widened around it.

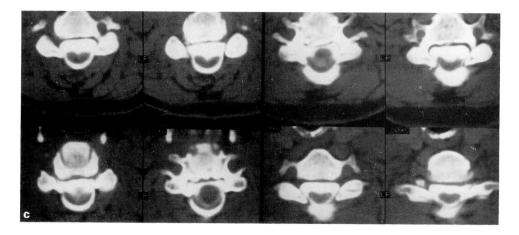

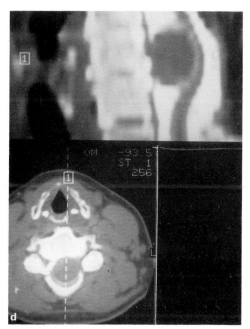

Fig. 3.99. Meningioma. Computerized myelogram (c) axial, (d) reformatted sagittal sections. There is marked compression, displacement and deformity of the cord by the anteriorly placed tumour.

major anterior radiculomedullary arteries may also be shown passing superiorly to join the anterior spinal artery at acute angles, forming hairpin loops.

Veins of the coronal plexus may cause a tortuous curvilinear pattern on the posterior surface of the spinal cord, best seen on supine films. An arteriovenous malformation, or fistula, draining into the coronal spinal venous plexuses generally causes more prominent dilatation of these veins which produce vermiform filling defects (Fig. 3.98). The coronal veins may also become somewhat similarly distended when the epidural veins are partly obstructed, but the causative lesion will also be shown encroaching on the subarachnoid space.

Enlargement of the cord shadow in one plane may be due to either flattening (Fig. 3.99) or swelling, distinguished simply by a further projection taken at right angles or by an axial CT

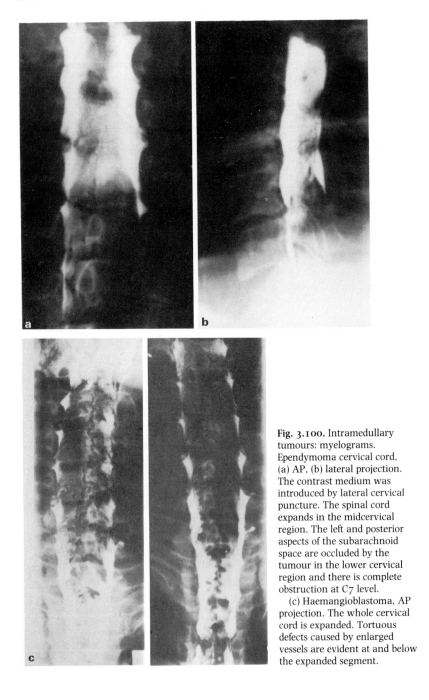

**Fig. 3.100.** Intramedullary tumours: myelograms. Ependymoma cervical cord, (a) AP, (b) lateral projection. The contrast medium was introduced by lateral cervical puncture. The spinal cord expands in the midcervical region. The left and posterior aspects of the subarachnoid space are occluded by the tumour in the lower cervical region and there is complete obstruction at C7 level.

(c) Haemangioblastoma, AP projection. The whole cervical cord is expanded. Tortuous defects caused by enlarged vessels are evident at and below the expanded segment.

section. Cystic cord swellings of any aetiology may be distinguished from solid masses if variation in size with posture occurs (Stevens *et al.* 1985), a phenomenon most frequent with syr-

ingomyelia. Congenital type syringomyelia is usually associated with cerebellar ectopia and less frequently with other lesions compromising the cisterna magna; such conditions should be sought on supine views or with computed myelography whenever a smoothly expanded cord is shown at myelography (Fig. 3.103).

Syringomyelia and cystic myelopathy following traumatic inflammatory or cord softening of other aetiology occurs, also, in spinal cords of normal or small diameter; in appropriate clinical circumstances it should be sought using NMR or computed myelography. Though extensive smooth expansion may occur with cord tumours, they tend to cause more focal and sometimes irregular expansion (Fig. 3.100a & b) which may be accompanied by tortuous defects due to dilated blood vessels. The latter tend to be particularly prominent with haemangioblastomas (Fig. 3.100c).

Intradural masses are outlined in the subarachnoid space which tends to be widened around them as they act like wedges displacing and flattening the spinal cord and/or nerve roots. Such masses are likely to be neurofibromas or meningiomas (Fig. 3.99) (Bull 1953). The latter may be partly calcified and are especially frequent in the dorsal region in middle-aged females. Multiple intradural masses may be neurofibromas or metastases from a malignant neoplasm of central nervous tissue or of systemic origin.

Extradural masses displace the theca away from bones lining the spinal canal and tend to compress the theca and nerve root sheaths. Only by observing any bone and/or soft tissue changes may the traumatic, neoplastic or inflammatory nature of the lesion be determined. A disc protrusion is generally suspected from the acute or recurrent history, and the site of the extradural impression which is often but by no means always anteriorly placed in the canal and opposite a disc space (Fig. 3.101). In the thoracic region especially, calcification is not infrequent within the nucleus pulposus of degenerate discs and may be shown on radiographs and CT both within the disc spaces and in prolapsed nuclear material (McAllister & Sage 1976).

Trauma to the spine may cause cord dysfunction due to fracture, dislocation, disc prolapse or haematoma. If plain X-rays or CT show extensive disruption, myelography is rarely indicated. It will show the degree of deformity or obstruction of the theca at the level of bone and disc damage. Extra-axial haematoma may cause more extreme and diffuse compression. Haematomyelia expands the cord, but cord swelling may occur from contusion also.

Avulsion injuries usually affect an upper limb. The torn roots usually are not visible and the contrast medium extends out into irregular cavities (Fig. 3.102), which may be both within the spinal canal deviating the theca and within and beyond the intervertebral foramina occupied by the avulsed nerve root sheaths (Neuenschwander *et al.* 1980).

Now that protruded and prolapsed disc substance can be demonstrated by CT, there are no neurological indications for spinal venography or discography.

## Computerized myelography

CT after intrathecal injection of non-ionic contrast medium (computerized myelography [CM]) reveals the detailed anatomy of the subarachnoid space; the morphology of the spinal cord, brainstem and cerebellum, including the inferior poles of the tonsils and biventral lobules (Fig. 3.103), the spinal and cranial nerves and the blood vessels traversing the subarachnoid space are all well shown. If CM is used as a definitive procedure a relatively small total amount of contrast medium can be used in low concentration. Frequently CM is used to supplement myelography to elucidate or confirm abnormalities. It is especially useful if contrast density is low as, for example, above or below a partial obstruction.

Focal or diffuse swelling (Fig. 3.104) or atrophy of the spinal cord is evident from change from normal dimensions; mass lesions within the subarachnoid space or encroaching onto it are outlined as filling defects (Fig. 3.99). The relationship of the subarachnoid space to the adjacent structures and displacement or deformity of the theca and compression of the spinal cord or roots are clearly defined. Congruous

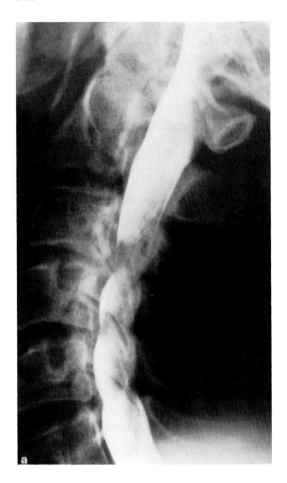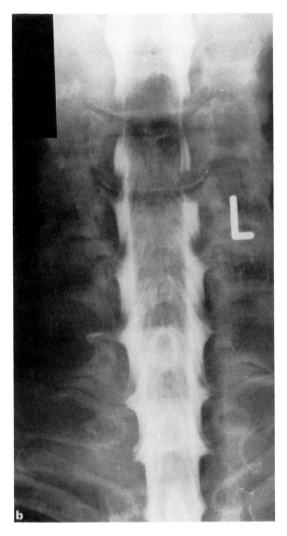

**Fig. 3.101.** Cervical spondylosis with disc protrusion. Iohexol myelogram, (a) lateral, (b) AP, (c) oblique projection. There are impressions on the anterior surface of the theca opposite the C3–6 discs. At the site of the maximum impression, C3–4 level, there are posterior osteophytes and the cord is flattened. The C4–6 nerve root sheaths are occluded. Computerized myelogram, (d) C3–4 level showing that the cord compression has been more marked on the right side and there is considerable cord thinning on this side.

deformity of the spinal cord persists after compression is relieved, as, for example, by changes of posture, and its degree and extent are very well shown by CM (Fig. 3.103).

Cysts or pouches freely communicating with the subarachnoid space, including fissures within the spinal cord, will be opacified immediately; cysts which communicate poorly or have semipermeable walls fill slowly and are best shown between four and twelve hours after intrathecal injection of contrast medium. Arachnoid cysts, syringomyelia and post-traumatic

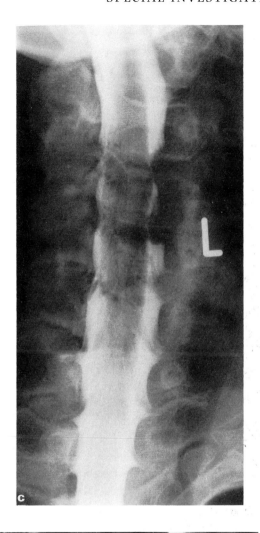

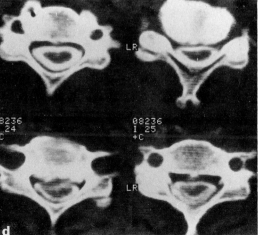

intramedullary cysts (Fig. 3.105) are usually opacified; many tumour cysts also opacify. Diffuse or poorly defined opacification may occur in regions of noncystic myelomalacia following trauma, demyelination and degenerative diseases causing cord damage.

## Spinal angiography

Spinal angiography is essential for the localization of spinal arteriovenous fistulas (Fig. 3.106) and angiomatous malformations diagnosed by or suspected from myelographic or NMR studies. Arteriographic localization of the

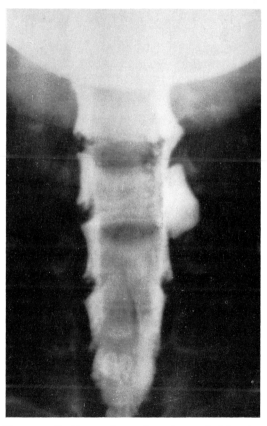

Fig. 3.102. Post-traumatic pseudomeningocoele. Iohexol myelogram. The left 5th and 6th roots are not visible, having been avulsed. The left 6th root sheath has been torn and a walled-off cavity (pseudomeningocoele) communicates with the subarachnoid space at this level.

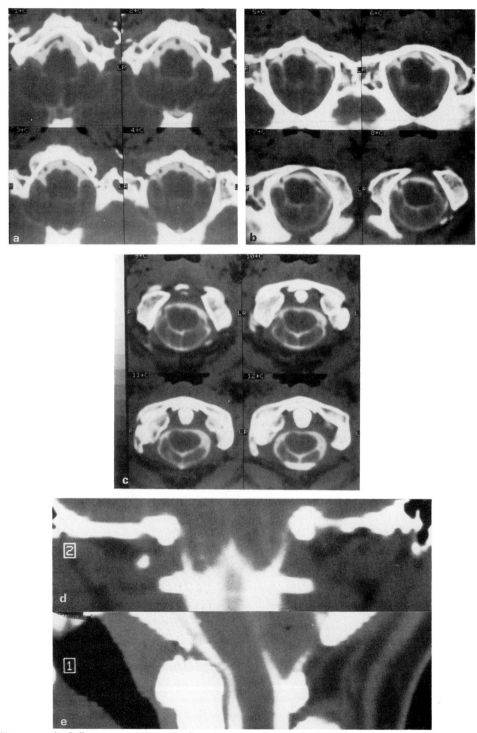

**Fig. 3.103.** Cerebellar ectopia. Computerized myelogram, (a, b, c) axial, (d) coronal, (e) sagittal reformatted sections. The cerebellar tonsils extend below the foramen magnum and the intracranial part of the cisterna magna is small. The spinal cord is slightly flattened by compression against the odontoid peg.

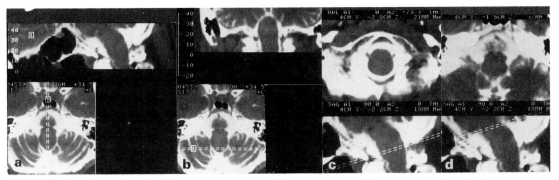

**Fig. 3.104.** Low-grade astrocytoma. Computerized myelogram, cervicomedullary junction, (a) sagittal reformatted section, (b) coronal reformatted section, (c, d) reformatted sections, (c) at cervicomedullary junction and (d) through upper medulla. There is considerable swelling of the medulla and upper cervical spinal cord. The cerebellar tonsils are displaced posteriorly and lie well above the foramen magnum. There is patchy increased density within the swollen cord due to permeation of contrast medium into the intramedullary tumour.

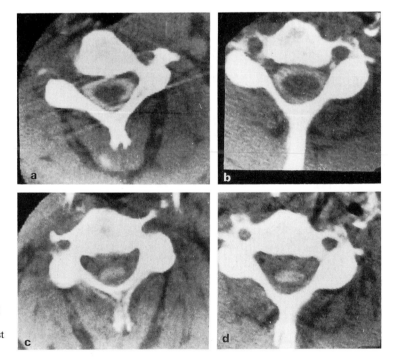

**Fig. 3.105.** Post-traumatic cystic myelomalacia. Computerized myelogram, lower cervical region, (a, b) 1 hour, (c, d) 16 hours after injection of iohexol. The spinal cord is of normal size, but a central cavity fills with contrast medium on the late scans.

site of origin of the arteria radicularis magna reduces the hazards of surgery on the thoracic spine for scoliosis, disc prolapse and extra-axial tumours. Angiography is also useful for the demonstration of haemangioblastoma nodules. This type of tumour may be suspected when myelography shows cord swelling associated with considerable dilatation of intraspinal vessels in the absence of obstruction. Localization of an haemangioblastoma nodule may allow surgical removal through a short laminectomy at the same time as establishing cyst drainage (Fig. 3.107).

Haemangioma of bone is usually an incidental

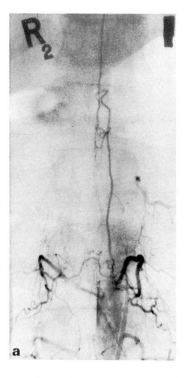
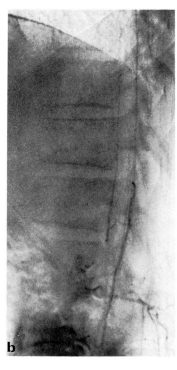

Fig. 3.106. Dural arteriovenous fistula. Left 2nd lumbar angiogram, (a) AP, (b) lateral projection. There is filling of the adjacent and contralateral vessels through paravertebral and trans-spinal anastomoses. There is an arteriovenous fistula in the left L2–3 intervertebral foramen. It drains superiorly to the posterior coronal plexus entering it at D12 level. The plexus is draining mainly superiorly through posterior and anterior spinal veins which outline the surfaces of the spinal cord.

radiological finding, but such tumours can encroach on the spinal canal and cause cord compression. Incision into the highly vascular bone may cause torrential haemorrhage, which can be reduced considerably by pre-operative embolization procedures.

The angiographic technique involves cathet-erization of the arteries supplying the appropriate radiculopial and radiculomedullary vessels (Djindjian *et al.* 1970). In the cervical region the vertebral and costocervical arteries, in the thoracic, lumbar and sacral regions respectively, the intercostal, lumbar and sacral arteries around the level of the lesion are first injected, but in

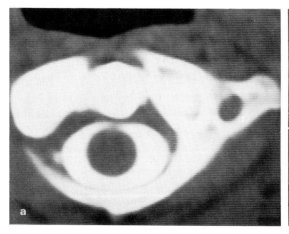
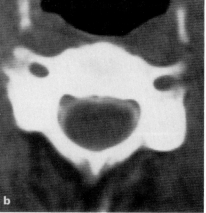

Fig. 3.107. Haemangioblastoma. Computerized myelogram. (a) At C1 level the spinal cord is slightly enlarged, (b) at C4 level the cord is markedly enlarged.

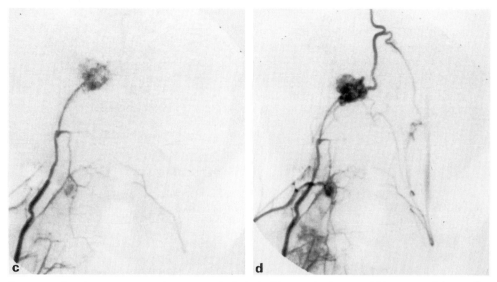

**Fig. 3.107.** Spinal angiogram, serial exposures, (c, d) the highly vascular haemangioblastoma nodule opacifies densely and there is early venous filling from it.

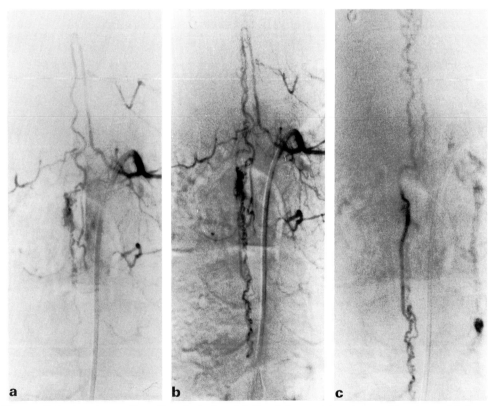

**Fig. 3.108.** Angiomatous malformation of spinal cord. Left 11th intercostal angiogram, (a) early arterial phase. The artery supplies the arteria radicularis magna which enters the anterior spinal artery with the typical hairpin bend at D10 level. The anterior spinal artery supplies an angiomatous malformation on the right side of the spinal cord at D12 level. (b) late arterial, (c) venous phase, the AVM drains superiorly to the coronal plexuses of the spinal cord.

many cases of spinal arteriovenous fistula there is no reliable indication of its site, so that the angiographic procedure may be extensive and may even involve the injection of all the segmental arteries. The hazards of the procedure have been virtually abolished by the introduction of the nonionic contrast media and deterioration during and after spinal angiography is now rare (Kendall 1979).

Arteriovenous fistulas are most common in middle-aged and elderly males. In such cases they are generally related to the dura at or below middorsal level and drain into the coronal plexuses lying on and draining blood from the spinal cord (Fig. 3.106). Increase in the pressure within this plexus causes ischaemic hypoxia of the cord and this precipitates change in cord function. Simple occlusion of the vein draining to the coronal plexus or closure of the dural fistula by surgical excision or embolization often results in considerable functional recovery (Symon et al. 1984).

Arteriovenous malformations within spinal cord substance are less frequent (Fig. 3.108); they tend to occur in younger patients, involve the cervical region and present with subarachnoid haemorrhage. Most of these lesions will be shown if a view of the cervical spine is included in vertebral angiography of patients with negative intracranial, four vessel angiography.

# References

ALEXANDER G.L. & NORMAN R.M. (1960) *The Sturge–Weber Syndrome.* John Wright & Sons, Bristol.
ARNELL S. & LINDSTROM F. (1931) *Acta Radiol.,* **12,** 287.
ASCROFT P. (1960) Unpublished communication to the 61st Meeting of the Society of British Neurological Surgeons.
BABCOCK D.S. & HAN B.K. (1981) *Radiology,* **139,** 655.
BASSI P., ZOINI C., CUSMANO F., & SANNA M. (1985) *Neuroradiology,* **27,** 26.
BRAMWELL B. (1887) *Ed. Med. J.,* **32,** Part 2, 693.
BRANT-ZAWADZKI M., MILLER E.M. & FEDERLE M.P. (1981) *Amer. J. Roentgenol.,* **136,** 369.
BRANT-ZAWADZKI M., GOULD R., NORMAN D., NEWTON T.H. & LANE B. (1982) *Amer. J. Neuroradiol,* **3,** 593.
BRANT-ZAWADZKI M., BADAMI J.P. & MILLS C.M. (1984) *Radiology,* **150,** 435.

BRANT-ZAWADZKI M., KELLY W., KJOS B., NEWTON T.H., NORMAN D., DILLON W. & SOBEL D. (1985) *Neuroradiology,* **27,** 3.
BROMAN T. & OLSSON O. (1948) *Acta Radiol.,* **30,** 326.
BRUIJN G.W. (1959) *Pneumoencephalography in the Diagnosis of Cerebral Atrophy.* Smits, Utrecht.
BULL J.W.D. (1953) *Acta Radiol.,* **40,** 283.
BURROWS E.H. (1963) *Clin. Radiol.,* **14,** 77.
BURROWS E.H. (1981) *Brit. J. Radiol.,* **54,** 195.
BUSSE O. (1921) *Virchows Arch. path. Anat.,* **228,** 178.
CARMODY R.F., SMITH J.R., SEEGER J.F., OVITT T.W. & CAPP M.P. (1982) *Radiology,* **144,** 529.
CARR D.H., BROWN J. & BYDDER G.M. (1984) *Lancet,* ii, 484.
CIRIC I., MIKHAEL M.A., TARKINGTON J.A. & VICK N.A. (1980) *J. Neurosurg.,* **53,** 433.
DANDY W.E. (1918) *Ann. Surg.,* **68,** 5.
DANDY W.E. (1919) *Ann. Surg.,* **70,** 397.
DE LACEY G., GUILDING A., WIGNALL B., REIDY J. & BRADBROOK S., (1980) *Clin. Radiol.,* **31,** 457.
DI CHIRO G., DELAPAZ R.L., BROOKS R.A., SOKOLOFF L., KORNBLITH P.L., SMITH B.H., PATRONAS N.J., KUFTA C.V., KESSLER R.M., JOHNSTON G.S., MANNING R.G. & WOLF A.P. (1982) *Neurology (NY),* **32,** 1323.
DJINDJIAN R.D., HURTH M. & HOUDART R. (1970) *Angiography of the Spinal Cord.* Masson et Cie, Paris.
DU BOULAY G.H. & EL GAMMAL T. (1966) *Brit. J. Radiol.,* **39,** 421.
DU BOULAY G.H. (1980) *Principles of X-Ray Diagnosis of the Skull.* Butterworth, London.
EMERY J.L. & LENDON R.G. (1973) *J. Path.,* **110,** 83.
EPSTEIN B.S. & DAVIDOFF C.M. (1953) *An Atlas of Skull Roentgenograms.* Lea and Febiger, Philadelphia.
EVANS W.A. (1942) *Arch. Neurol. Psychiat.,* **47,** 931.
FALK B. (1953) *Acta Radiol.,* **40,** 220.
FIELD J.R., ROBERTSON J.T. & DE SAUSSURE R.L. (1962) *J. Neurosurg.,* **19,** 775.
FOLEY K.M. & POSNER J.B. (1975). *Neurology,* **25,** 565.
FOLEY W.D., SMITH D.F., MILDE M.W., LAWSON T.L., TOWNE J.B. & BANDY D.F. (1984) *Radiology,* **151,** 651.
FULTON J.F. (1946) *Harvey Cushing: A Biography.* Thomas, Springfield, Illinois.
GADO M., HANAWAY J. & FRANK R. (1979) *J. Comp. Assist. Tomogr.,* **3,** 1.
HAHN F.J.Y. & RIM K. (1976) *Amer. J. Roentgenol.,* **126,** 593.
HARRISON C.R. & LUTTERELL C. (1953) *J. Neurosurg.,* **10,** 205.
HAUGHTON V.M. & HO K.C. (1982) *Radiology,* **143,** 699.
HAUGHTON V.M., ROSENBAUM A.E., WILLIAMS A.L. & DRAYER B., (1980) *Amer. J. Neuroradiol.,* **1,** 527.
HESCHL R (1859) *Vjschr. prakt. Heilkunde. (Prague),* **61,** 59.
HILLEMACHER A. (1982) *Fortschr. Neurol. Psychiatr.,* **50,** 93.
HINCK B.C., CLARK W.M. & HOPKINS C.E. (1966) *Amer. J. Roentgenol.,* **97,** 141.
HINDMARSH T. & GREITZ T. (1977) In: *Computerised Axial Tomography in Clinical Practice.* (Eds. Du Boulay G.H. & Moseley I.F.) pp. 205–12 Springer, Berlin.
HIRASHIMA Y., SHINDO K. & ENDO S. (1983) *Neuroradiology,* **25,** 23.
HUBER P., KRAYENBUHL H. & YASARGIL M.G. (1982) *Cerebral Angiography.* Thieme, Stuttgart.
HUCKMAN M.S., GRAINDER L.S. & CLASEN K.C. (1977) *Semin. Roentgenol,* **12,** 27.
JIMENEZ J.P. & GOREE J.A. (1967) *Amer. J. Roentgenol.,* **101,** 88.

JOHANSEN J.G., ORRISON W.W. & AMUNDSEN P. (1983) *Radiology*, **146**, 391.

KENDALL B.E. (1979) *Metrizamide Myelography.* pp. 147–52. Nyegaard, Birmingham.

KENDALL B.E. & KINGSLEY D. (1978) *Brit. J. Radiol.*, **51**, 171.

KENDALL B.E., REIDER-GROSSWASSER I. & VALENTINE A., (1983) *Neuroradiology*, **25**, 11.

KRAYENBÜHL H. & RICHTER H. (1952) *Die Zerebral angiographie.* Thieme, Stuttgart.

LAREN J.L., SMITH D. & FOSSAN G. (1980) *Acta Radiol.*, **21**, 141.

LAST R.J. & TOMPSETT D.H. (1953) *Brit. J. Surg.*, **40**, 525.

LAZORTHES G. (1961) *Vascularisation a Circulation Cerebrales.* Masson, Paris.

LEEDS N. & SEAMAN W.B. (1962) *Radiology*, **78**, 570.

LINDGREN E. (1950) *Acta Radiol.*, **33**, 389.

LIVERUD K. (1958) *J. Oslo Cy. Hosp.*, **8**, 209.

LONDON D.A., CARROLL B.A. & ENZMANN D.R. (1980) *Amer. J. Neurordiol*, **1**, 295.

LORBER J. (1958) *Acta Radiol.*, **50**, 204.

MACPHERSON P. & TEASDALE E. (1985) *Neuroradiology*, **27**, 214.

MANELFE C. & BONALFE A. (1980) In: *Computerised Tomography.* (Eds. Caille J-M. & Salamon G.) pp. 104–14. Springer, Berlin.

MANI R.H., EISENBERG R.L., MCDONANLD E.J., POLLACK J.A. & MANI J.R. (1978) *Amer. J. Roentgenol.*, **131**, 861.

MCALLISTER V.L. & SAGE M.R. (1976) *Radiology*, **27**, 291.

MILLS C.M., CROOKS L.E., KAUFMAN L. & BRANT-ZAWADZKI M. (1984) *Radiology*, **150**, 87.

MONIZ E. (1927) *Rev. Neurol.*, **34(ii)**, 72.

MUHR C., BERGSTROM K., GRIMELIUS L. & LARSSON S.G., (1981) *Neuroradiology*, **21**, 55.

NAIDICH T.P., MCLONE E.D.G. & HARWOOD-NASH D.C. (1983) *Computed Tomography of the Spine and Spinal Cord.* (Eds. Newton T.H. and Potts D.G.) Clavadel Press, San Anselmo.

NAIDICH T.P., LEEDS N.E. & KRICHEFF I.I. (1977a) *Radiology*, **123**, 631.

NAIDICH T.P., PUDLOWSKI R.M. & LEEDS N.E. (1977b) *J. Comp. Assist. Tomogr.*, **1**, 16.

NEUENSCHWANDER S., BRAUNER M., GILBERT A. & FAURE C. (1980) *Ann. Radiol.*, **23**, 93.

NORLEN G. & WICKBOM J. (1958) *J. Neurol. Neurosurg. Psychiat.*, **21**, 1.

NORTHFIELD D.W.C. & RUSSELL D.S. (1937) *Lancet*, **i**, 377.

PATTEN D.D. & WOOLFENDEN J.M. (1977) *Radiol. Clin. N. Amer.*, **15**, 177.

PERRET G. & NISHIOKA H. (1966) *J. Neurosurg.*, **25**, 98.

PYKETT I.L., NEWHOUSE J.H., BUONANNO F.S., BRADY T.J., GOLD-MAN M.R., KISTLER J.P. & POHOST G.M. (1982) *Radiology*, **143**, 157.

RANSON S.W. & CLARK S.L. (1947) *The Anatomy of the Nervous System*, 8th Edn. Saunders, Philadelphia.

REHNCRONA S., BRISMAR J. & HOLTAS S. (1985) *Neurosurgery*, **16**, 23.

RING B.A. (1962) *Acta Radiol.*, **57**, 289.

ROBERTSON E.G. (1957) *Pneumoencephalography.* Blackwell, Oxford.

ROGERS J.V., SHUMAN W.P., HIRSCH J.H., LANE S.C., HOWE J.F. & BURCHIEL K. (1984) *Amer. J. Neuroradiol.*, **5**, 755.

SAHLSTEDT H. (1935) *Acta Radiol.*, Suppl. **24**, 16.

SCHEIBLE E.W., JAMES S.H.E., LEOPOLD G.R. & HULTON S.W. (1983) *Radiology*, **146**, 743.

SERRATS A.A.F., VLAHOVITCH B. & PARKER S.A. (1968) *J. Neurol. Neurosurg. Psychiat.*, **31**, 379.

SJAASTED O. and NORDVIK A. (1973) *Acta Neurol. Scand.*, **49**, 396.

SOSMAN M.C. (1927) *Radiology*, **9**, 396.

STEVENS J.M. & KENDALL B.E. (1985) *Neuroradiology*, **27**, 390.

STEVENS J.M., OLNEY J.S. & KENDALL B.E. (1985) *Neuroradiology*, **27**, 48.

STEVENS J.M., RUIS J.S. & KENDALL B.E. (1983) *Neuroradiology*, **25**, 71.

STRAIN W.H., PLATT J.T. & WARREN S.L. (1942) *J. Amer. chem. Soc.*, **64**, 1436.

SUGAR R.O., HOLDEN N.L.B. & POWELL C.B. (1949) *Amer. J. Roentgenol.*, **61**, 166.

SUNDERLAND S. (1948) *J. Neurol. Neurosurg. Psychiat.*, **11**, 245.

SYMON L., KUYAMA H. & KENDALL B. (1984) *J. Neurosurg.*, **60**, 238.

SYNEK V. & REUBEN J.R. (1976) *Brit. J. Radiol.*, **49**, 233.

TRESS B.M. (1983) *Radiology*, **146**, 87.

TWINING E.W. (1939) *Brit. J. Radiol.*, **12**, 385, 569.

WALLACE S., GOLDBERG H.I., LEEDS N.E. & MISHKIN M.M. (1967) *Amer. J. Roentgenol.*, **101**, 34.

WEISBERG L., NICE C. & KATZ M. (1984) *Cerebral Computed Tomography.* pp. 117–157. W.B. Saunders, Philadelphia.

WILLIAMS A.L., HAUGHTON V.M., DANIELS D.L. & THORNTON L.S. (1982b) *Amer. J. Neuroradiol.*, **3**, 95.

WILLIAMS A.L., HAUGHTON V.M., MEYER G.A. & HO K.C. (1982a) *Radiology*, **142**, 403.

WULFF J.D., PROFFITT P.Q., PANSZI J.G. & ZEIGLER D.K. (1982) *Neurology*, **32**, 766.

YOUNG I.R., BYDDER G.M., HALL A.S., STEINER R.E., WORTHINGTON B.S., HAWKES R.C., HOLLAND G.N. & MOORE W.S. (1983) *Amer. J. Neuroradiol.*, **4**, 223.

# Chapter 4
# Other investigations—radioisotope, ultrasound and neuroelectrical studies

## J. D. MILLER

Many of the investigations described in this chapter developed in parallel with and as alternative investigations to various procedures in radiology. At a time when most of the latter were invasive, such as air encephalography and myelography, the relatively noninvasive nature of isotope brain scanning and ultrasound echo-encephalography made them attractive preliminary investigations, despite their lower degree of diagnostic precision. The arrival on the scene of computerized tomography and magnetic resonance imaging, which combine high diagnostic precision for virtually the entire range of craniospinal lesions with almost total lack of risk to the patient, has dramatically altered this concept and demands a reappraisal of what isotope and ultrasound studies can offer the neurosurgeon.

Neuroradiological studies are mainly demonstrations of structural change in the nervous system or its coverings. By a skilful choice of isotope tracer, its manner of administration and the equipment used for its detection, the nuclear medicine specialist can now offer a series of studies of the function of the organ in question, and to a certain extent, this applies also to the brain, or at least to its blood supply. In this chapter, the development of isotope scanning of the brain is described together with some of the more recent methods of assessing brain function in patients. In a similar historical way the application of ultrasound studies to neurosurgery is recounted and reference made to the current status and usage of ultrasound based investigations.

From the outset, the detection, amplification and recording of cerebral electrical activity in the form of electroencephalogram (EEG) could be considered as a study of brain function rather than a means of detecting structural abnormalities. For many years, however, EEG has been employed in both ways, and this has been to the detriment of the reputation of EEG as a neurodiagnostic method, for, compared with CT or modern radioisotope studies, the EEG is a time-consuming and inefficient means of detecting a structural lesion of the brain.

The requirement of the neurosurgeon to have information on the level of neurological function in the clinically inaccessible patient who is being artificially ventilated has brought new challenges to the clinical neurophysiologist. Recent developments in electronics and computing, permitting brain electrical activity to be recorded and displayed in a condensed and easily interpreted format in the electrically hostile environments of the operating theatre and intensive care unit, have made this possible and are ushering in a new era of collaboration between the neurophysiologist, the neuroanaesthetist and the neurosurgeon, based upon the assessment of brain function in circumstances where this cannot be determined by a bedside neurological examination.

## Radioisotope studies

The discovery that certain dyes injected intravenously might selectively stain damaged brain tissue and tumours, rendering them visible, was the first step toward brain scanning (Sorsby *et al.* 1942). Moore (1947) found that intravenous fluoroescein rendered tumour tissue visible by its fluoroescence when viewed in ultraviolet light. By using di-iodofluoroescein labelled with the radioactive isotope [131]I, Moore (1953) found it possible

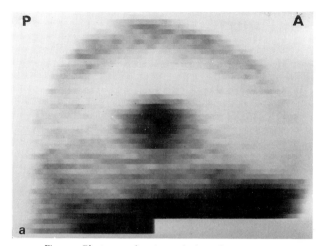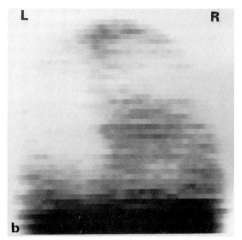

**Fig. 4.1.** Photoscan showing right lateral intraventricular meningioma a) right lateral b) postero-anterior view.

to localize the more intense radiation emanating from a tumour by placing a Geiger–Mueller counter successively over different points on the skull. There followed a whole series of elaborations on this new diagnostic procedure. The invention of the scintillation spectrometer and of collimators increased the sensitivity of detectors and sharpened marginal definition between normal and abnormal activity. Another advance was the construction of scanning apparatus in which the detector system was moved automatically over the head in the anteroposterior and lateral parasagittal planes, indicating detected radioactivity by monotone or coloured ink marks on a paper print-out. An area of abnormality was delineated by the contrasting density or colour of the ink marks. This form of display soon yielded to the photoscan, in which a light signal activates photographic film in place of the ink dot on paper (Fig.4.1). Apparatus was next developed which could 'see' the entire head at one time, and the scintillation from emission of gamma activity from the head was recorded by a gamma camera (Mallard 1963), Anger 1964) (Fig. 4.2).

Many radioisotopes have been tested in the search for any special affinity to penetrate brain tumours; to date, none has been found that is entirely specific to brain tumours, whether benign or malignant. The reasons for choosing a particular isotope include issues of expense and availability, energy of gamma and other emissions, duration of half-life (the time for radioactivity to decay to half of the starting level), rate and specificity of entry into the tumour, and subsequent wash-out, and the capacity to form an appropriate carrier compound.

Certain organs of the body have a particular affinity for certain radioactive compounds, iodine and the thyroid for example, and blocking agents may need to be given before the dose of radioisotope. In addition to, and of more importance than, the physical half-life, attention must be paid to the biological half-life, which relates to the dose of radioactivity delivered to the body and hence to the rate of elimination of the agent from the system. The physical half-life of $^{131}$I as RIHSA is 8 days, but the biological half-life is 180 days, which permits serial scans over a period of days. This method has been used in the past to study the pattern and rate of absorbtion of cerebrospinal fluid.

$^{99m}$Technetium has the much shorter half-life of 6 hours. This means that a higher dose can be given with improvement in contrast and detection of abnormalities, but serial scanning is not possible. Wilke (1970) discussed these aspects of brain scanning and provided a list of

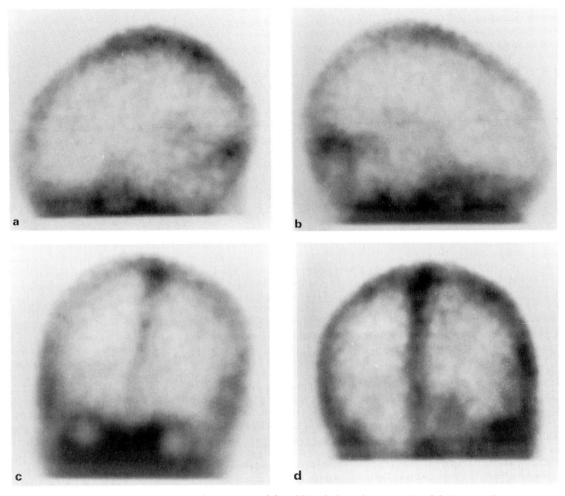

Fig. 4.2. Gamma scan showing right occipital metastasis a) left and b) right lateral view c) AP and d) PA view. (By courtesy of Dr M.V. Merrick.)

the characteristics of a number of radioisotope compounds, of which $^{99m}$technetium remains one of the most favoured.

Why radioisotopes reach a higher level in tumours and other cerebral lesions than in normal brain was a problem examined in detail by Bakay (1967). A low level of penetration from the bloodstream into the brain is observed with a large number of substances; this phenomenon is recognized as the blood–brain barrier (Rapoport 1976). Low grade astrocytomas, which structurally resemble normal brain tissue, attract little or no greater concentration of radioactive tracer than the surrounding brain. Consequently an isotope brain scan is usually negative in such cases. High levels of radioactivity are found in meningiomas and in metastases, tumours of non-neuroectodermal origin which do not have a blood–brain barrier. Glioblastomas, which readily take up isotope, are associated with pathological changes in the capillaries and larger vessels that vitiate the blood brain barrier. The barrier is also defective around infarcts and abscesses and in cerebral contusions, all of which give recognizable foci in isotope brain scans. There is a consensus view that the presence or absence of the blood–brain barrier plays a major role in the differential uptake of radioisotope in and around focal cerebral lesions. Whether the isotope tracer is also actively taken up by tumour cells, and if so, whether metabolic activity is a deciding factor, or whether the isotope remains entrapped in the extracellular space remains a subject of investigation (Raimondi 1964). In vascular tumours some of the high concentration of isotope is due to the excessive local blood volume.

### Indications and reliability

The present indications for isotope brain scanning comprise patients in whom the clinical evidence in favour of a tumour or other expanding lesion is small or negligible, and the test can therefore be regarded as an initial screening procedure. Among these may be some examples of a small tumour, where the surgeon hopes that an early operation will allow a more favourable prognosis. A positive finding would encourage the referring clinician to pursue diagnosis by CT, or if the results of the initial study are equivocal a further isotope scan can be done after a suitable time interval. In practice, patients in this latter category are also referred on for CT in most cases. The reliability of isotope brain scanning as a screening test is limited because only tumours larger than 2 cm in diameter can be detected reliably. A negative isotope scan should not, therefore, be completely reassuring. In about half of patients with proven cerebral astrocytomas the initial isotope scan has been reported negative.

In the differential diagnosis between cerebral infarct and tumour, a single positive scan is of little differentiating value, but a scan repeated some weeks later can be of great value if it shows the partial or complete disappearance of the focus typical of a cerebral infarct.

Planiol (1966) reported positive scan results in 84% of patients with intracranial space-occupying lesions of all types; in meningiomas 93%, glioblastomas 92% and metastases 88%. There was only one negative isotope brain scan in 24 cases of brain abscess, giving 96% positive findings. Similar percentages for successful localization were given by Wilke (1970). Suwanela et al. (1971) reviewed published records of isotope brain scanning in brain abscesses. They found that the examinations had been positive overall in 90% of 180 recorded cases. These authors made the important additional observation that for subdural abscess, notoriously difficult to diagnose by other means, isotope scanning was successful in 100% of cases.

More recently, Rehncrona et al. (1985) have reported favourably on the use of radioactive indium-labelled leucocytes to improve the detection and localization of cerebral abscesses.

### Disorder of the cerebrospinal fluid circulation

Albumen is a normal constituent of ventricular CSF (50–100 mg/L) and lumbar subarachnoid CSF (150–450 mg/L). It is conveyed by bulk flow from the ventricular system over the cerebral convexities and largely absorbed by the arachnoid villi into the blood of the superior sagittal sinus. Consequently, the behaviour of the CSF circulation can be examined by injecting a suitable radioactive tracer into the lumbar or ventricular CSF and following its progress through the CSF pathway by sequential scans, made over a period of 48 hours, or even longer. The most widely used tracer was $^{131}$I-labelled human serum albumen, and the most frequent indication was the investigation of certain cases of hydrocephalus. While this method has certain advantages over the unpleasant procedure of lumbar air encephalography, it was eventually shown not to be very reliable in identifying cases most suitable for surgical treatment by a CSF diversion procedure. That, coupled with a small but significant incidence of meningitic reactions to the RIHSA, has led to the gradual decrease in the use of this investigative technique and its substitution by a combination of CT and measurement of intracranial pressure.

If tracer is injected into the lateral ventricle in a normal subject, radioactivity can be detected in the cistern magna in one hour, over the Sylvian fissures in three hours, at the convexity of the cerebral hemispheres in 12 hours, and by 24 hours the only residual radioactivity should be over the sagittal sinus (Di Chiro 1966). In hydrocephalus the ventricular enlargement is obvious and the tracer remains in the ventricular system for 24 hours or more.

If the tracer is injected into the lumbar subarachnoid space, it ascends to the cervical region in about 15 minutes and thereafter its distribution in space over the convexities and over time are the same as for ventricular injection. Under normal circumstances, no tracer should be able to enter the ventricular system against the flow of CSF. In communicating hydrocephalus the isotope tracer may enter the ventricular system and persist for 48 hours or more. This is always an abnormal finding, but may not always be present in cases of hydrocephalus.

## Perfusion studies of the brain using radioisotopes

When the gamma camera is used, it is possible to follow by rapid serial photoscans the passage through the cerebral circulation of a bolus of radioactive nondiffusible tracer that has been injected intravenously (Fig. 4.3). It can be visu-

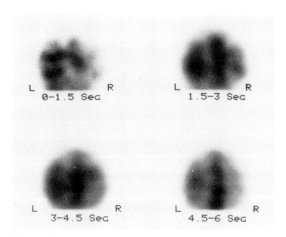

**Fig. 4.3.** Dynamic scan of ischaemic right cerebral hemisphere. (By courtesy of Dr M.V. Merrick.)

ally determined that a carotid artery or major venous sinus has been occluded, or that there is gross ischaemia in one or other cerebral hemisphere.

More precision can be provided for this type of perfusion scan by computing and displaying in colour coded format the transit time of the tracer in each small sector of the brain 'seen' by the gamma camera, termed a pixel (Merrick 1984). This form of data processing measures the velocity, rather than the volume of blood flow through the brain. The two are not quite the same. In a theoretical model of laminar flow of non-Newtonian fluid through a system of rigid tubes (Poiseuille's Law) the velocity of flow is proportional to the square of the radius of resistance vessels, while the volume flow is proportional to the fourth power of the radius. The relationship between the two types of flow ought, therefore, to be described by the nonlinear function $y = x^2$. Experimental evidence supports this theoretical prediction, showing that slow transit times fairly reliably indicate low values of cerebral blood flow, but when blood flow is increased above normal, the transit time method will underestimate volume flow (Rowan *et al.* 1970a). In practice the transit time method tends to provide a rather wide range of both normal and abnormal values, so that in individual cases it may be difficult to determine whether a given transit time obtained in a single patient is definitely abnormal, and what that means in terms of cerebral blood flow (Rowan *et al.* 1970b).

To obtain true volume flow measurements of the cerebral circulation, it is necessary to use freely diffusible, but metabolically inert, tracers. When these are delivered to the brain via the bloodstream, they diffuse rapidly from the blood into brain tissue. Because the tracer is neither consumed nor produced by the brain, the same amount of tracer is available to diffuse out of the brain back into the bloodstream when the brain is subsequently perfused by blood which contains no tracer substance. The rate at which the brain fills with, and is cleared of, the tracer is a function of cerebral blood flow. Kety and Schmidt (1945), working in Philadelphia, devised a method of measuring cerebral blood flow in man by using nitrous oxide inhaled in low concentration as the diffusible, inert tracer substance. By giving this over a period of ten minutes they assumed the brain would become saturated by the tracer, so that cerebral venous blood obtained from the jugular vein would faithfully reflect the brain level; by applying the Fick Principle the value for cerebral blood flow could then be calculated from the brain level divided by the integrated arteriovenous difference in amount of tracer during the period of administration. This method computes blood flow in the whole brain as mls blood/100G brain/minute.

If a radioactive diffusible tracer is used which has definable and characteristic gamma emissions, these can be detected from the brain through the intact skull by multiple scintillation detectors that can each be shielded (collimated) and placed so as to 'see' a defined sector of the brain. The rate of clearance of isotope from the brain can then be used to measure the regional cerebral blood flow, expressed again in ml/100G min (Lassen & Ingvar 1963). The most widely used tracer is now [133]Xenon, administered by inhalation in gaseous form or intravenously dissolved in saline (Mallett & Veall 1965, Obrist et al. 1967, Wyper et al. 1976).

Compact and mobile equipment is now available which permits measurement of regional cerebral blood flow in up to 10 areas of the brain, and more bulky apparatus can allow measurement in over 200 brain regions to create colour coded 'flow maps' of the brain and its circulation. From the latter studies have come dramatic demonstrations of increases in regional CBF in the appropriate brain areas associated with specific brain functions such as speech, motor activity in one limb, local sensory stimulation including vision and audition, and a range of psychological tasks (Stokely et al. 1980).

When CBF is measured, it is important that the measurement of flow is accompanied by measurement of arterial pressure and $PCO_2$, body temperature and other variables known to affect cerebral blood flow, as described in Chapter 2. While valuable information on neurosurgical problems has emerged from single measurements of cerebral blood flow, much more has come from studies in which the response of blood flow to a change in arterial $PCO_2$ (reactivity) or arterial pressure (autoregulation) has been tested. The most valuable clinical uses for the measurement of cerebral blood flow have been in deciding whether an indwelling vacular shunt is needed during carotid endartectomy (Boysen 1973, Sundt et al. 1974), whether permanent carotid ligation is safe (Jennett et al. 1966, Leech et al. 1974, Jawad et al. 1977) and whether induced arterial hypotension during operations to clip an intracranial aneurysm is tolerated without the production of brain ischaemia (Pickard et al. 1980). Other uses for measurement of cerebral blood flow have been to decide when it is safe to withdraw treatment for brain ischaemia associated with cerebral vasospasm following subarachnoid haemorrhage (Mendelow et al. 1986), and in deciding which head injured patients should be treated with barbiturate therapy (Messeter et al. 1986).

**Tomographic methods**

A major limitation of the methods of studying the brain using radioisotope tracers and external detectors that have been described above, has been difficulty in determining whether the observed changes emanate from the cerebral cortex or from underlying deep structures such as the basal ganglia. To overcome this problem and provide better three dimensional localization on radioisotope studies, a tomographic approach was developed by Kuhl et al. in Philadelphia (1975). This has been refined into the technique of single photon emission computerized tomography (SPECT). With this approach and a suitable choice of radiolabelled tracer or ligand, measurements of blood flow in the basal ganglia, or the localization of labelled neuropeptide in deep brain structures are possible (Stokely et al. 1980).

This method is already being superceded by what promises to be the most powerful method yet for using certain radioisotopes to study brain function *in vivo* in man, positron emission tomography (PET). This technique depends upon positron emitting radioisotopes. which have to be produced in a cyclotron and most of which have a short half-life, so that the cyclotron and the PET scanner should ideally be in juxtaposition. When positrons collide with electrons, the annihilation radiation is in the form of two photons which are emitted in opposite directions at an angle of precisely 180° to one another. Using detectors on either side of the head programmed to record counts only on those detectors that are exactly opposite each other, time-of-flight measurements to locate the source of the activity, and by rotating the array of counters around the head with a similar form of data processing to that used for CT, it is possible to generate detailed tomographic images of the brain that are based, not upon structure, but upon some function, the exact nature of which depends upon the isotope and scanning sequence used. It is now possible to measure directly and in any part of the brain, the regional cerebral blood volume and flow, oxygen and glucose metabolism, and the uptake and distribution in the brain of wide range of neurotransmitters, neuropeptides and drugs (Jones 1980, Phelps *et al.* 1982). While the investigative potential of this new neuroscientific tool is enormous, the very high cost of the equipment means that, in the UK, PET will be available in only two or three centres.

## Ultrasound studies

Waves with the physical characteristics of sound, but of a frequency far above the upper limit of audibility (18000 Hz) are termed ultrasound. They comprise rapidly succeeding zones of compression and rebound. In liquid these waves travel in straight lines, but are attenuated, reflected or diverted when they encounter a physical change in the matter they are crossing. They cannot cross a vacuum, and the acoustic interface between air and a solid or liquid is virtually impenetrable to ultrasonic waves. If ultrasonic waves passing through a liquid encounter a solid object they are largely diverted; air within a crack in metal will similarly cause reflection of the ultrasonic waves. If the acoustic interface is exactly perpendicular to the wave the latter is deflected straight back to the source, where it will be recorded as an 'echo' of the original wave. This is the principle underlying echo sounding, as used for underwater detection and finding flaws in metal castings. Ian Donald, a Glasgow obstetrician, was the first to borrow this method for medicine, using a modified ultrasound metal flaw detector to examine the abdominal and pelvic contents of pregnant women instead of X-ray. Leksell (1955) applied the technique to neurosurgery and used it for detecting lateral displacement of normally midline intracranial structures, thereby obtaining indirect evidence of an intracranial space-occupying lesion.

The temporal echogram depicts the midline echo. The site of application of the probe lies in the area of scalp above the ear. All air must be excluded between the face of the probe and the scalp; this is achieved by application of a coupling medium, such as electrode jelly. The probe is directed toward the opposite side of the skull, its axis pointing slightly upwards and posterior (Jefferson & Hill 1966). The final position of the probe is adjusted to obtain the best echo from the opposite side of the head and from the midline. The test is then repeated on the other side. The recorded echo traces are displayed on the oscilloscope one above the other. By convention the right trace, emanating from the probe over the right side of the head, is placed uppermost with the echo deflections upward; the left trace is displayed underneath with its echo deflections directed downward. Under normal circumstances the midline echo deflections should be in line with one another.

### The normal echoencephalogram

Three groups of complexes of echo deflections can usually be identified (Fig. 4.4). The near

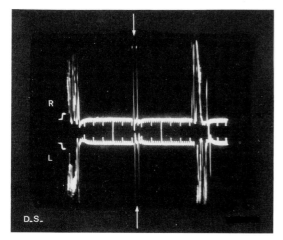

**Fig. 4.4.** Normal echogram.

**Fig. 4.5.** Echogram showing 1.0 cm right to left midline shift.

complex, seen at the left of the trace, is produced from the scalp and skull directly underlying the probe, and there is a similar but lower amplitude echo from the far side of the skull produced by the dura and inner table of the skull. The third echo lies somewhere between the two skull echoes, both in amplitude and position; it may be a simple deflection or it may be notched on its descending limb, and it may exhibit a pulsatile change in amplitude. The rest of the trace is usually flat, though small deflections are sometimes noted on either side of the midline echo,

arising possibly from the lateral ventricles or the Sylvian fissure. The origin of the midline echo was for long a matter for conjecture. Leksell (1958) expressed the view that the pineal gland was responsible, but ingenious experiments by Lithander (1961) provided convincing evidence that the midline echo might arise from the falx, septum lucidum, wall of the third ventricle, pineal body or aqueduct (Fig. 4.5). Jefferson and Hill believed that the midline echo most often arose from the walls of the third ventricle. The appearance of a double midline echo in cases of

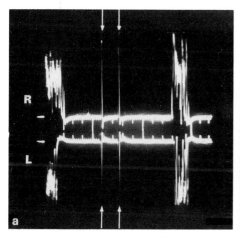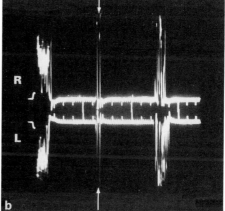

**Fig. 4.6.** Hydrocephalus due to aqueduct obstruction:
a) preoperative echogram; double arrows indicate the separated walls of the dilated third ventricle.
b) postoperative echogram; following ventricular CSF shunting and return of third ventricle to normal width.

hydrocephalus and its disappearance following CSF shunting lends strong support to this contention (Fig. 4.6).

## The abnormal echoencephalogram

Displacement of the midline echo is the most, some might say the only, important abnormality in this investigation, for it provides strong presumptive evidence of a unilateral space-occupying lesion or of a swollen cerebral hemisphere, due, for example, to a tumour, oedema or a swollen contusion. A shift of 3 mm or more is regarded as significant. In an extensive review of several large reported series of cases, Jefferson and Hill (1966) calculated the failure rate of ultrasound detection of midline shift, the combination of false–positive, false–negative and doubtful results, to be 11%.

In most neurosurgical centres the echoencephalogram has been entirely supplanted by CT, but it may still be of value when an adequate history cannot be obtained or the patient is already in coma and CT is not available, yet an intracranial haematoma or abscess is suspect. Identification of midline displacement can then be followed by angiography on the appropriate side to achieve more accurate localization if time will permit.

## Ultrasound scanning

In obstetrics it has been possible for some time to use ultrasound in a mobile scanning mode, moving the scanning head to produce multiple echoes so as to build up detailed images of the pelvic contents, including the uterus and the developing fetus, even to make an antenatal diagnosis of hydrocephalus. This form of ultrasound B-mode scanning has been extended to the premature newborn, to examine the skull contents and determine ventricular size (London et al. 1980). With maturation, however, the skull soon becomes impervious to the ultrasound waves, and investigators now require an 'acoustic window' through which to scan and image the skull contents using ultrasound. This can be provided for a limited time and to a limited extent by the fontanelles (Babcock & Han 1981).

With progressive refinement of ultrasound scanning equipment the scanning head has now become small and mobile enough to be taken into the operating theatre, draped by sterile covers and used to examine the spinal cord and brain via a laminectomy, a craniotomy or even a burr hole. This method is now finding ready application in the location and biopsy of intramedullary tumours and small, deeply placed brain tumours, and in the location and cannulation of small ventricles (Rogers et al. 1984).

## Doppler ultrasound studies

It is possible to measure the direction and velocity of blood flow in larger vessels by placing an ultrasound probe over the vessel in question and using the Doppler effect to detect the rate at which the column of blood is moving. Until recently, this external noninvasive method was limited for the neurosurgeon to examination of flow in the carotid arteries and branches of the external carotid, including anastomoses between the superficial and the middle cerebral arteries (Spencer et al. 1979). While the method was refined to provide imaging of the interior of neck vessels, this was of value only in examining the carotid bifurcation for the detection of carotid stenosis. This has been superceded by digital venous subtraction angiography which provides a more accurate image and can detect ulceration in an atheromatous plaque, which is not possible with ultrasound methods.

In the last few years, however, it has become possible to measure the velocity of blood flow in intracranial arteries, although this is still limited to the major vessels. For example, changes in blood flow through the proximal part of the middle cerebral artery induced by vasospasm, carotid artery occlusion and changes in arterial $PCO_2$ can now be demonstrated by application of a small, hand-held probe to the side of the head (Aaslid *et al.* 1982, Bishop *et al.* 1986). This will greatly extend the value of such studies to neurosurgeons, for whom they had previously been of only limited interest.

## Neuroelectrical recording

The electrical activity of the brain was discovered in this country by Caton (1875) and independently by Danilevsky in Russia and by Beck in Poland shortly afterwards. At that time Victor Horsley was still studying anatomy and physiology at University College, and William Macewen, having read the work of Hughlings Jackson on cerebral localization, was preparing to operate upon his first brain abscess. Progress in this new field was initially slow, awaiting improvements in the detection, amplification and recording of the minute fluctuations of electrical potential, of the order of 1.0 to 100.0 microvolts, when recorded from the scalp. Hans Berger is said to have begun in 1902 to verify the original observations by Caton, but he first published on this topic in 1929 (Walker 1957, Brazier 1960). The clinical possibilities of the new method rapidly became apparent, and in 1935 Gibbs, David and Lennox described the three second spike and wave abnormality that characterizes petit mal epilepsy.

Caton's work was performed on the exposed surface of the brain in animals; recording from the exposed human cortex was not undertaken until 1934, by Foerster and Altenburger (1935), and by Adrian and Matthews (1934) who carried out this procedure at the London Hospital, during an operation by Cairns for a glioma in the pariental lobe. Electrocorticography is now most often carried during operations for the relief of epilepsy. The need to detect electrical events that occur in the depths of the brain, and their temporal relationship to those occurring in the cortex and elsewhere has led to procedures for the insertion of fine electrodes into deep brain structures. Bickford and Cairns were the first to show the feasibility of this way of extending the electroencephalogram (Woltman 1953).

The neurosurgeon now looks less to EEG for help in the detection and localization of intracranial space-occupying lesions or in the differential diagnosis of abscess from other inflammatory conditions, save perhaps encephalitis, but it continued to play a crucial role in the investigation of a case of epilepsy in which surgical treatment may be thought desirable. See Chapter 17.

With increasing use of artificial ventilation in neurosurgical intensive care units, in which patients receive both sedative and relaxant drugs so that neurological evaluation is not possible, there is a clear need to obtain records of brain electrical activity as an index of brain function and to detect seizure activity which would for the same reason not be clinically overt. Numerous modifications in data acquisition, processing and display have led to a pronounced resurgence of neurosurgical interest in recording of brain electrical activity. It is therefore worthwhile to know something of the basis of EEG recording, from which the subsequent methods have evolved.

The EEG recording represents the amplified summation of postsynaptic potentials from large numbers of neurons, probably originating mainly from the fifth layer of the cerebral cortex. The generation of such electrical potentials depends for its energy upon generation of adenosine triphosphate; this is derived almost entirely from the oxidative metabolism of glucose (Prior 1985).

**Electrode connections**

One line, trace or channel of an EEG records the greatly magnified fluctuations of electrical potential arising between two points on the scalp. Electrical contact with the scalp is effected by silver–silver chloride electrodes stuck by adhesive to the scalp, or as platinum–iridium needles inserted into the scalp. Precautions must be taken to ensure that contact with the scalp remains satisfactory, otherwise electrical artifact will make the record useless; the impedance of the electrodes should be less than 5 kilohms. It is common practice to apply a number of scalp electrodes sufficient to 'feed' 8 or more channels, so as to ensure that recording of electrical activity from both sides of the head is available. It is well to bear in mind that only one fifth of the cerbral cortex can be sampled electrically from the scalp; the remainder includes the medial and basal parts of the cerebral cortex and the depths of the sulci. The international standard pattern of electrode placement employs 18 electrodes in four symmetrical rows from before backwards, a medial and a lateral one on each side and three in the midline over the vertex; they conform also to transverse rows. In any row the electrodes should be an equal distance (about 7 cm) apart. The electrodes are connected to the EEG recording machine by flexible leads; internal switching allows the technician to select from a wide range of combinations of electrical activity (montages) for display. If each channel is fed by two adjacent electrodes this is bipolar recording, reflecting the relative changes in potential between these neighbouring electrodes. Since each intermediate electrode feeds two channels, this permits detection of the important EEG sign of phase reversal. In this situation if electrode B becomes electronegative to the adjacent electrodes A and C the deflection becomes negative in channel AB and positive in channel BC; if the negative focus is precisely under electrode B the two opposite deflections are equal in amplitude and this provides topographical location of the cerebral abnormality. Alternatively, the channels can be formed by linking each of the scalp electrodes to a single reference electrode located usually on the ear or the mastoid process. This is unipolar recording which displays simultaneously the rise and fall of potentials recorded at multiple points on the scalp and compared to the reference electrode. By using a computer, it is possible to average a number of sweeps of scalp activity from the electrodes. Since spontaneous activity is random, this process of averaging produces a straight line, but if each sweep is triggered to a specific stimulus of the visual, auditory or somatosensory systems, then any

electrical activity specifically linked to these stimuli can emerge from the averaged EEG record. This is the principle upon which the recording of averaged evoked potentials is based. For further information on the technical aspects of recording EEG or evoked potentials appropriate textbooks should be consulted (Cooper *et al.* 1980, Tyner *et al.* 1983, Chiappa 1983).

The electrical signal is converted to a graphic record by means of a stylus or ink jet playing upon paper moving at a constant speed, usually 3.0 cm/sec. The rise and fall of electrical potential is observed as a wave with simple or complex characteristics, possessing amplitude and period (length). Complexity of the waveform derives from the superimposition of several waves of different amplitude and periodicity. The complex waveform can be resolved into these different component by means of Fast Fourier Analysis using a small computer.

The height or amplitude of a wave is determined by the strength of the electrical signal and the degree to which the recording system can magnify the signal. Gain controls are provided in the recording system that allow this magnification to be adjusted and prevent extreme deflections of the trace. The rate of response of the apparatus to sudden changes in electrical potential is adjustable and determined by the time constant, the time taken by the signal to fall to 37% of its original height. Fast electrical activity can be modified or even ignored by the use of filters; this important device can be used to eliminate from the record 50 Hz mains interference.

### The electroencephalogram

The EEG record comprises a variety of waves of simple or complex form, of different amplitude and frequency; waves of similar form may, however, recur at regular intervals and this generates a rhythm; others occur only irregularly, at random intervals. Certain waveforms are characteristically picked up from certain areas of the scalp, others betoken abnormality. Waves of

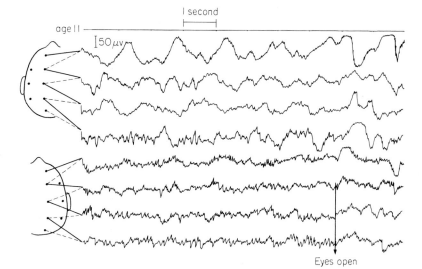

**Fig. 4.7.** Patient with left frontal abscess; EEG shows polymorphic delta activity with phase reversals between channels 1 and 3, reduction of ipsilateral fast (beta) activity and some reduction of alpha activity posteriorly. Note blocking response to eye opening.

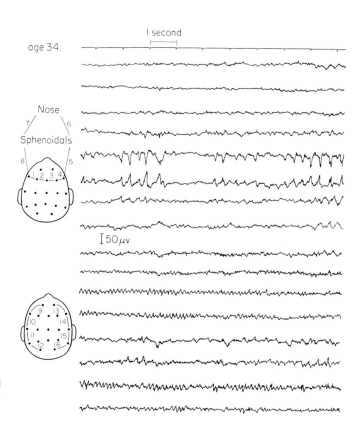

**Fig. 4.8.** Patient with right temporal lobe epilepsy: focal spike discharges seen predominantly from right-sided sphenoid electrodes with phase reversals.

similar shape which appear in different channels at the same time are described as synchronous. 'Reading' an EEG consists of recognizing the most important wave components by means of their periodicity, frequency and amplitude and assessing their rhythmicity, or irregularity, and their topography. The eye has to scan not only horizontally, but also vertically over the 8 or 16 channels to note whether similar abnormalities appear simultaneously in different channels, and if in adjacent channels, the nature of any phase relationships. With practice common patterns of abnormality become instantly recognizable, but the process is a complex one; computer analysis of EEG records virtually always requires that the electrical data are reduced into a much simpler form before analysis can proceed.

Although the waves which appear in an EEG extend through a wide range of frequencies, from one to 50 Hz, the frequencies are for convenience divided into bands or groups to which Greek letters have been assigned (Fig. 4.7).

Alpha waves occur in a frequency range of 8–13 Hz; they are a prominent feature in the temporal, parietal and occipital regions, and were the waves first described by Hans Berger. They recur regularly as a rhythm at 9–10 Hz as a rule, and are distinguished by appearing when the eyes are shut and the subject relaxed. They are in phase, synchronous in the appropriate channels and symmetrical on both sides of the head. If the subject opens his eyes or concentrated his thoughts upon a particular problem, the alpha waves subside and may entirely disappear. This phenomenon is known as the 'blocking' response to eye-opening.

Beta waves occur at a frequency of 13 Hz or more and provide rhythmic electrical activity over most of the head, but most marked in the frontal and central regions. The amplitude is less

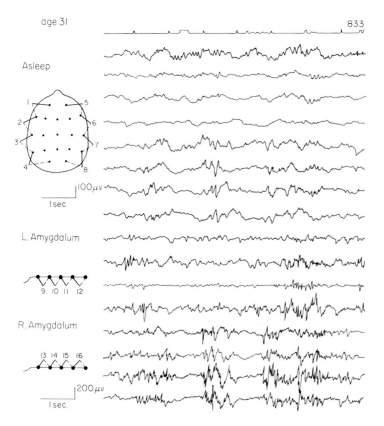

Fig. 4.9. Patient with right temporal lobe epilepsy: high voltage focal spike discharges obtained from intracerebral electrodes (right amygdalum – channels 13 to 16). Note that discharges are also seen from the right temporal scalp leads (channels 5 to 8) but at much lower voltage, as indicated by the higher gain for the scalp electrode recording.

than alpha activity as a rule, but increases when the patient is tense or has had barbiturate drugs (Brazier & Finesinger 1945). This response provides a test of normally active cerebral cortex and its reduction or absence in a particular area can provide evidence of a local organic lesion (Pampiglioni 1952). The expression 'fast activity' is a common synonym for beta activity.

Gamma waves have been defined as waves with a frequency greater than 30 Hz, but in practice such activity is usually included in the beta band.

Delta waves are those at the slow end of the frequency spectrum, less than four per second, occasionally as prolonged as 2 Hz. They are seen in the normal adult EEG only during sleep, but are common in organic lesions of the brain, particularly when these are acute, in raised intracranial pressure, in coma and epilepsy. In the latter they may be closely associated with spikes to form a complex and characteristic paroxysmal discharge.

Theta waves occur at 4–7 Hz, lying between alpha and delta frequencies. They are to be seen sporadically in normal records, particularly in the frontotemporal regions, but when frequent and obvious they are of pathological significance.

Spikes are pointed waves rising and falling abruptly on a narrow time base (15–60 msec) and attaining an amplitude of up to several hundred microvolts, as compared with the average amplitude of 50 microvolts for alpha waves. They occur as isolated events or in runs, often linked with delta waves, and are not seen in a normal record. They constitute the typical abnormality of epilepsy: during a fit, as part of the epileptic discharge, between fits at random intervals (Fig 4.8). They may, however, be seen in the record of a patient who has never had seizures, and they may be absent from the record of an epileptic patient (Fig 4.9). Spikes which are caused by a lesion of the subjacent cortex usually arise from a background of slow waves. Those derived from a distant source tend to arise from a normal background.

### The EEG in childhood

In infants no rhythmic activity is seen and much of the record is virtually flat, interrupted by irregular runs of slow waves (1–5 Hz) of low voltage. Rhythms appear at 4–6 months of age, with delta prominent at first, then theta up to the age of five years. Alpha rhythm is established by the age of 10 years. Maturation of the record results in development of beta activity and the corresponding subsidence of slower activity. The age at which the static normal adult pattern is attained is usually between 18 and 20 years (Hill & Driver 1962). As a generalization, the EEG of the child is complex and unstable and the diagnosis of pathological changes requires skill and much experience.

### Activation of the EEG

The EEG reacts quickly to certain changes in the environment, a simple example being the response of alpha rhythm to opening and closing of the eyes. Certain techniques have been evolved that take advantage of this delicate reactivity of the EEG because they exaggerate an abnormality in the record. The methods are usually employed in the study of epileptic discharges, although they can also evoke latent slow wave activity to indicate a local lesion. Hyperventilation is used a part of the routine examination; the patient is asked to breathe deeply and fast for three minutes and there is slowing of the EEG wave activity, probably as a result of the reduction of cerebral blood flow that follows this manoeuvre. The EEG also changes considerably during physiological sleep, to an extent that depends upon the depth of sleep.

### The EEG in intracranial space-occupying lesions

It is usually possible to recognize two patterns of disturbance. One is localized to the portion of brain that contains or is compressed by the lesion; the other is of a general character, comprising changes in the normal rhythms and abnormal waves of wide distribution. The size of the mass, its invasiveness, its rapidity of growth, the degree of associated oedema, internal herniation and increased intracranial pressure are all factors that determine the balance between local and generalized neuroelectrical disturbances. A small frontal meningioma may for a long time show only a local abnormality of the EEG, whereas a large glioblastoma can cause so much generalized disturbance as to submerge any localized changes. The potentials recorded from the scalp EEG are derived directly from cortical neurons, although this activity may be influenced or controlled by impulses from deeper lying structures. A localized EEG abnormality is more likely to develop if the cortex is directly involved by the tumour or the pressure effects from it. A deep tumour causes less local disturbance but is more likely to cause a generalized upset in the EEG record. Extreme examples are tumours in the ventricular system and in the posterior fossa. No particular form of EEG activity can be attributed to the cerebellum, although neuroelectrical activity can be recorded from this structure if electrodes are placed directly upon its surface.

### Local EEG signs

The earliest and most important neuroelectrical sign of a tumour is localized slow wave activity. At first these are in the theta range and may easily escape detection, later they are in the delta range. These may occur singly or in groups varying in frequency, shape and in amplitude; because of such irregularity this type of abnormal record is often referred to as 'polymorphic' delta activity. Phase reversal is additional evidence of a localized subjacent lesion, but no great reliance can be placed upon accuracy of localization. Electrical activity can arise only from living neurons, and tumours are electrically inert. Oedema and vascular changes vary considerably in the surrounding brain. The scalp and the skull act as a spatial averager of electrical activity, trans-

mitting those components common to, and synchronous over, a large area of cerebral cortex (Cooper *et al.* 1965).

Although slow waves are the usual focal response to a tumour, in the region of the central fissure localized exaggeration of the fast, beta activity may appear, occasionally in a form likened by some to the teeth of a comb, called 'mu rhythm'. Localized depression of the normal background rhythms is an occasional sign of a subjacent mass, and may be seen in cases of chronic subdural haematoma. Total loss of electrical activity is not seen, even with large lesions because potentials from adjacent active neurons can be conducted across volumes of tumour tissue, CSF or cyst fluid. In cases of hemispherectomy, even when the large pool of CSF in the area of resection has been replaced by air, EEG activity can still be detected from the affected side (Cobb & Sears 1960).

Paroxysmal discharges provide an important local sign. Spikes and sharp waves occurring singly or in short runs, often mixed with slow waves, may be a pointer to a mass lesion in the vicinity, although these discharges will be arising from the brain adjacent to the mass and not from tumour or haematoma itself. The incidence of epilepsy as a symptom of tumour is high, and it might therefore be anticipated that paroxysmal abnormalities in the EEG would be frequent in such cases. This is not the case.

### Diffuse and generalized EEG signs

In cases of expanding intracranial lesions the alpha rhythm becomes reduced in amplitude, first on the ipsilateral side, then on both sides. The blocking response on eye opening becomes impaired, and then completely lost. This applies particularly to posterior or deep lesions. Theta waves are said to be the commonest abnormality on the EEG, whatever the cause. Delta waves as an indication of a local disturbance have been described; when they arise as a distant reaction to a deep lesion they are usually frontal, regular and bilaterally synchronous.

## Subdural haematoma

It might be thought that in surface haematomas, extradural and subdural, the interposition of a thick layer of blood between the cortex and the skull would result in an isoelectric EEG; in fact this is rare. The fluctuations in cortical potential are conducted through the haematoma. Reduction in amplitude of normal rhythms may occur, but can be difficult to detect because of obscuration by abnormal slow wave activity. The latter, in the form of diffuse bilateral theta or delta, is usually the predominant feature in such cases. The abnormal slow wave activity may be of lower amplitude on the affected side, sharing in the local depression of electrical activity. Rodin *et al.* (1955) found an ipsilateral delta focus in two thirds of their cases of subdural haematoma, and noted reduction in the amplitude and frequency of alpha activity on the affected side in half the patients.

## Raised intracranial pressure

It is doubtful whether any specific pattern of EEG disturbance can be identified with the state of intracranial hypertension. Fischer-Williams *et al.* (1962) found that increased intracranial pressure was nearly always present when there was generalized disorganization of the record with dominant irregular slow wave activity. In most cases with benign intracranial hypertension, which may in this context be regarded as an example of pure uncomplicated raised intracranial pressure, the EEG is entirely normal.

When the EEG is diffusely abnormal in a patient with elevated intracranial pressure, osmotherapy may reduce the diffuse abnormality to reveal localized EEG abnormalities associated with the causative lesion. It is likely that the diffuse EEG disorganization and delta activity associated with raised intracranial pressure arises in two ways, by reductions in cerebral blood flow and by brain distortion and shift, affecting brain stem structures. In the presence of an expanding lesion the cortical circulation, with which we are mainly concerned in relation to the EEG, is protected from the first increases in intracranial pressure by autoregulatory mechanisms, and fails only at a relatively late stage. This may account for the recording of a normal EEG in patients with unequivocally high intracranial pressure. Observations during cardiac surgical procedures have shown that transient reductions in cardiac output can be monitored by the EEG which rapidly responds by the appearance of slow activity within seconds of a fall in arterial pressure. Similarly, in patients undergoing temporary carotid occlusion as a preliminary to permanent carotid ligation, or insertion of a vascular shunt for endarterectomy, EEG slow wave activity appears within 20 seconds of carotid occlusion if this manoeuvre is associated with an abrupt fall in cerebral blood flow (Leech *et al.* 1974).

Expanding intracranial lesions cause internal herniations, and compression and deformity of the brain stem. In such cases raised intracranial pressure is likely to be accompanied by anatomical disturbances in diencephalic and brain stem structures that may also adversely affect the EEG (French & Magoun 1952).

## Brain ischaemia

When cerebral blood flow decreases to the point that neurotransmitter synthesis is adversely affected and the first signs of failure of energy metabolism appear there is a decline in the proportion of alpha and beta activity with a corresponding increase in the proportion of slow activity; a burst suppression pattern then appears, followed by complete EEG silence if the brain ischaemia continues. This stage is reached at mean blood flow levels of 20 ml/100G/min, representing a reduction in flow to 40% of the normal value. Even when the blood flow reduction is uniform, due for example to a fall in arterial pressure, the EEG changes may not be entirely uniform, with the earliest changes appearing in the interarterial boundary zones.

## Cerebral death

Brain damage from the anoxia of temporary cardiac or respiratory arrest may be so severe that the patient remains in deep coma until death, days or weeks later. The neurosurgeon encounters this problem usually in cases of sudden severe intracranial hypertension complicating head injury or spontaneous intracranial haemorrhage; respiratory arrest occurs, artificial ventilation is instituted and cardiac action restored but the neurological status remains unimproved. For how long should this state of assisted existence be maintained? In the United Kingdom, the diagnosis of brain death is made entirely upon clinical grounds, dependent on the verification of absence of spontaneous respiration, response to painful stimuli and brain stem reflex activity. The neurosurgeon can be aided in this decision by the EEG. In pronounced degrees of cortical damage from anoxia, an isoelectric EEG record is obtained. Persistence of EEG activity is therefore evidence of less severe damage; it has been found possible to correlate the degree of EEG abnormality with prognosis for neurological recovery (Binnie *et al.* 1970). It must, however, be emphasized that in the UK at least, the diagnosis of brain death must be made on clinical grounds, and an isoelectric EEG can be regarded only as nonmandatory supporting evidence. The stricture that the clinical assessment of brain death cannot be carried out when the patient is under the influence of sedative drugs applies equally to the EEG recording.

## EEG data reduction and display

When EEG monitoring is required over a prolonged period some form of data reduction is necessary, but a form in which the key elements are preserved. Two main approaches are used to this problem. The first is frequency domain analysis, in which the spectrum of the relative amounts of activity in each of the major frequency bands is analysed and displayed serially for successive epochs of EEG recording so as to show in an easily understandable form a shift in the EEG frequency spectrum towards faster or slower rhythms (Bickford *et al.* 1973, Myers *et al.* 1977). The second form of condensed recording is a continuous recording of EEG wave

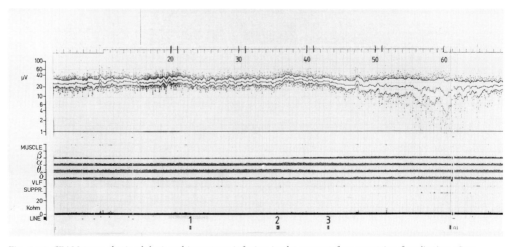

**Fig. 4.10.** CFAM trace obtained during thiopentone infusion in the course of an operation for clipping of an intracranial aneurysm. At marker 1 the thiopentone infusion starts, at 500 mg/hr; at 2 the rate is increased to 1000 mg/hr, and at marker 3 to 1500 mg/hr. Beta band activity begins to increase at 38 minutes, but burst suppression, indicated by widening of the amplitude analysis, is not achieved until 50 minutes. The aneurysm was clipped at 61 minutes, the infusion stopped and the EEG analysis returns to normal over the next 5 minutes (By courtesy of Dr J. L. Jenkinson.)

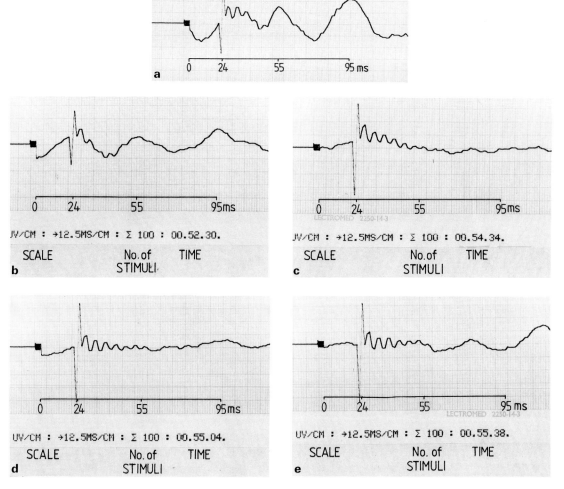

**Fig. 4.11.** CFAM in evoked potential mode during an operation for resection of a thoracic intramedullary tumour. The stimulating electrode placed over posterior tibial nerve for recording somatosensory response.

a) Base line record showing P55 and P95 waves.

b) Myelotomy started at 52 minutes 30 seconds; both waves still obvious.

c) At 54 minutes both waves disappear as the spinal cord is opened.

d) At 55 minutes both waves still absent.

e) Both P55 and P95 waves begin to return at 55 minutes 38 seconds, but with increased latency so that they come in at 75 and 106 ms respectively. The patient showed no increase in neurological deficit after operation, probably because the duration of loss of evoked response was so short (the critical period of loss of response appears to be about 20 minutes).

(By courtesy of Dr J. L. Jenkinson).

amplitude plotted against time, as in the cerebral function monitor (Maynard *et al.* 1969). A more recent development combines this form of analysis with a simultaneous display of the relative amounts of beta, alpha, theta and delta activity. This is the cerebral function analysing monitor (CFAM) (Fig. 4.10; Maynard & Jenkinson 1984).

### Evoked neuroelectrical potentials

With repetitive sensory stimulation, electrical potentials occur and are propagated in anatomically defined pathways through the spinal cord and brainstem to the cerebral cortex. These potentials are of low voltage and are normally 'buried' in the random electrical activity recorded from scalp electrodes. By repeating the stimuli at regular intervals several hundred times, and by using a trigger mechanism and a small computer to average the time-locked trains of electrical activity for the short time period following each stimulus, a recognizably uniform response can be discerned from the scalp recording electrodes, consisting of a series of positive and negative waves occurring at predictable time intervals from the stimulus, and named as such. Thus the N5 wave refers to the negative wave that occurs five milleseconds after the stimulus (Chiappa 1983).

The sensory stimuli can be applied to the visual, the auditory and the somatosensory systems, and the measurement of evoked responses can be used to test the integrity of the appropriate anatomical pathways in the spinal cord and brain. The visual response travels from the optic nerves and chiasm along the length of the cerebral hemisphere via the optic radiation to the visual cortex, over which it is detected from appropriately placed scalp electrodes. The auditory evoked response travels from the cochlea and eighth nerve through the brain stem via the cochlear and superior olivary nuclei, the lateral lemniscus, the inferior colliculus and the medial geniculate body before reaching the auditory cortex. The early waves in the auditory evoked response, the first five occurring in the 10 ms

period from the stimulus, are thought to emanate from the defined stations in the brain stem. The somatosensory response to median nerve stimulation travels in the posterior columns of the spinal cord through the brain stem to the thalamus and the sensory cortex. The response can be recorded over the upper cervical spine and from the scalp over the postRolandic cortex. The time difference between the two latter recording sites is about five ms and is designated the central conduction time (Hume & Cant 1978).

Multimodality evoked potentials have been used in patients with head injury to indicate which patients have brain stem dysfunction and which have damage confined to the cerebral hemispheres, and to detect the occurrence of secondary ischaemic and hypoxic insults in patients in the intensive care unit (Greenberg *et al.* 1977). EEG and evoked potentials have also been used to detect brain insults in patients undergoing open heart surgery (Branthwaite 1975) and carotid artery surgery (Markand *et al.* 1984; Fig. 4.11). Recording of somatosensory evoked potentials can be of value during complex spinal surgery, and visual evoked potentials during removal of tumours around the optic chiasm, such as craniopharyngioma. The central conduction time increases in a predictable manner with cerebral ischaemia, and may therefore be helpful as a monitor of brain circulation during operations in which temporary clamping of major cerebral arteries may be needed.

## References

AASLID R., MARKWALDER T-M. & NORNES H. (1982) *J. Neurosurg.*, **57**, 769.
ADRIAN E. D. & MATTHEWS B. H. C. (1934) *Brain*, **57**, 355.
ANGER H. O. (1964) *J. nucl. Med.*, **5**, 515.
BABCOCK D. S. & HAN B. K. (1981) *Radiology*, **139**, 655.
BAKAY I. (1967) *J. Neurosurg.*, **27**, 239.
BICKFORD R. G., BRIMM J., BERGER L. & AUNG M. (1973) In *Automation of Clinical Electroencephalography* (Eds. P. Kellaway, I. Peterson) Raven Press, New York.
BINNIE C. D., PRIOR P. F., LLOYD D. S. S., SCOTT D. F. & MARGERISON J. H. (1970) *Brit. med. J.*, **3**, 265.
BISHOP C. C. R., POWELL S., INSALL M., RUTT D. & BROWSE N. L. (1986) *Lancet*, **1**, 710.

Boysen G. (1973) *Acta neurol. Scand.*, **49**, Suppl 59.

Branthwaite M. A. (1975) *Thorax*, **30**, 258.

Brazier M. A. (1960) *Epilepsia*, **1**, 328.

Brazier M. A. B. & Finesinger J. E. (1945) *Arch. Neurol. Psychiat.*, **53**, 51.

Caton R. (1875) *Brit. med. J.*, **2**, 278.

Chiappa K. H. (1983) *Evoked Potentials in Clinical Medicine.* Raven Press, New York.

Cobb W. & Sears T. A. (1960) *EEG clin. Neurophysiol.*, **12**, 371.

Cooper R., Ossleton J. W. & Shaw J. C. (1980) *EEG Technology*, Third edition. Butterworth Medical, London.

Di Chiro G. (1966) *Acta radiol.*, **5**, 988.

Fischer-Williams M., Last S. L., Lyberi G. & Northfield D. W. C. (1962) *Brain*, **85**, 1.

Foerster O. & Altenberger H. (1935) *Deutsch Nervenheilk*, **135**, 227.

French J. D. & Magoun H. W. (1952) *Arch. Neurol. Psychiat*, **68**, 591.

Gibbs F. A., Davis H. & Lennox W. G. (1935) *Arch. Neurol. Psychiat.*, **34**, 1133.

Greenberg R. P., Becker D. P., Miller J. D. & Mayer D. J. (1977) *J. Neurosurg.*, **47**, 163.

Hill D. & Driver M. D. (1962) In *Recent Advances in Neurology and Neuropsychiatry*, 7th edn. (Ed. Brain L.) p. 169. Churchill, London.

Hume A. L. & Cant B. R. (1978) *EEG clin. Neurophysiol.*, **45**, 361.

Jawad K., Miller J. D., Wyper D. J. & Rowan J. O. (1977) *J. Neurosurg.*, **46**, 185.

Jefferson A. & Hill A. I. (1966) In *Progress in Neurological Surgery* (Eds. H. Krayenbuhl, P. E. Maspes & W. H. Sweet) Karger, Basel.

Jennett W. B., Harper A. M. & Gillespie F. C. (1966) *Lancet*, **2**, 1162.

Jones T. (1980) *Brit. med. Bull.*, **36**, 231.

Kety S. S. & Schmidt C. F. (1945) *Amer. J. Physiol.*, **143**, 53.

Kuhl D., Reivich M., Alavi A., Nyari I. & Sdtaaumm M. M. (1975) *Circul. Res.*, **36**, 610.

Lassen N. A. & Ingvar D. H. (1963) *Arch. Neurol.*, **9**, 615.

Leksell L. (1955) *Acta Chirurg. Scand.*, **110**, 301.

Leksell L. (1958) *Acta Chirurg. Scand.*, **115**, 255.

Lithander B. (1961) *J. Neurol. Neurosurg. Psychiat.*, **24**, 22.

London D. A., Carrol B. A. & Enzmann D. R. (1980) *Amer. J. Neuroradiol.*, **1**, 295.

Leech P. J., Miller J. D., Fitch W. & Barker J. (1974) *J. Neurol. Neurosurg. Psychiat.*, **37**, 854.

Mallard J. R. (1963) *Proc. roy. Soc. Med.*, **56**, 680.

Mallett B. L. & Veall N. (1965) *Clin. Sci.*, **29**, 179.

Markand O. N., Dilley R. S., Moorthy S. S. & Warren C. J. (1984) *Arch. Neurol.*, **41**, 375.

Maynard D. E. & Jenkinson J. L. (1984) *Anaesthesia*, **39**, 678.

Maynard D. E., Prior P. F. & Scott (1969) *Brit. med. J.*, **4**, 545.

Mendelow A. D., Dharkar S., Patterson J., Nath F. & Teasdale G. M. (1986) *J. Neurol. Neurosurg. Psychiat*, **49**, 35.

Merrick M. V. (1984) *Essentials of Nuclear Medicine.* Churchill Livingstone, Edinburgh.

Messeter K., Nordstrom C-H, Sundbarg G., Algottson L. & Ryding E. (1986) *J. Neurosurg.*, **64**, 231.

Moore G. E. (1947) *Science*, **106**, 130.

Moore G. E. (1953) *The Diagnosis and Localisation of Brain Tumours.* Charles C. Thomas, Illinois.

Myers R. R., Stockard J. J. & Saidman L. J. (1977) *Stroke*, **8**, 331.

Obrist W. D., Thompson H. K., King C. H. & Wang H. S. (1967) *Circul. Res.*, **20**, 124.

Pampiglioni G. (1952) *EEG. clin. Neurophysiol.*, **4**, 79.

Phelps M. E., Mazziotta J. C. & Huang S. C. (1982) *J. cereb. blood. Flow. Metabol.*, **2**, 113.

Pickard J. D., Matheson M., Patterson J. & Wyper D. J. (1980) *J. Neurosurg.*, **53**, 305.

Planiol T. (1966) In *Progress in Neurological Surgery* (Eds. H. Krayenbuhl, P. E. Maspes, W. H. Sweet). Karger, Basel.

Prior P. F. (1985) *Brit. J. Anaesth.*, **57**, 63.

Raimondi A. J. (1964) *Arch. neurol.*, **11**, 173.

Rapoport S. I. (1976) *Blood Brain Barrier in Physiology and Medicine.* Raven Press, New York.

Rehncrona S., Brismar J. & Holtas S. (1985) *Neurosurgery*, **16**, 23.

Rodin E. A., Bickford R. G. & Svien H. J. (1955) *Arch. Neurol. Psychiat.*, **69**, 743.

Rogers J. V., Shuman W. P., Hursch J. H., Lanje S. C., Howe J. F. & Burchiel K. (1984) *Amer. J. Neuroradiol.*, **5**, 755.

Rowan J. O., Harper A. M., Miller J. D., Tedeschi G. M. & Jennett W. B. (1970a) *J. Neurol. Neurosurg. Psychiat.*, **33**, 733.

Rowan J. O., Cross J. N., Tedeschi G. M. & Jennett W. B. (1970b) *J. Neurol. Neurosurg. Psychiat.*, **33**, 739.

Sorsby A., Wright A. D., Elkeles A. (1942) *Proc. roy. Soc. med.*, **36**, 137.

Spencer M. P. & Reid J. M. (1979) *Stroke*, **10**, 326.

Stokely E. M., Sveinsdottir E., Lassen N. A. & Rommer P. (1980) *J. Comput. Ass. Tomogr.*, **4**, 230.

Sundt T. M., Sharborough F. W., Anderson R. E. & Michenfelder J. D. (1974) *J. Neurosurg.*, **41**, 310.

Suwanela C., Poshyachinda V. & Poshyachinda M. (1971) *Acta Neurochir.*, **25**, 165.

Tyner F. S., Knott J. R. & Mayor W. B. (1983) *Fundamentals of EEG Technology.* Raven Press, New York.

Walker A. E. (1957) *J. Neurophysiol*, **20**, 435.

Wilcke O. (1970) *Acta Neurochir*, **23**, 285.

Woltman H. W. (1953) *Proc. Mayo Clin.*, **28**, 145.

Wyper D. J., Lennox G. & Rowan J. O. (1976) *J. Neurol. Neurosurg. Psychiat.*, **39**, 141.

# Chapter 5
# Malignant intracranial tumours

## J. S. GARFIELD

The diagnosis and management of patients with these conditions forms the largest part of general neurosurgical practice. Perhaps due to the nature of the lesion, and the absence of the 'magic bullet' for cancer in general, neurosurgical attitudes are rarely enthusiastic in terms of attempted treatment and research, compared to many other rarer conditions. The past twenty years have seen great advances in method of diagnosis, particularly in radiology, but although there has been much activity in the form of chemotherapeutic trials, overall prognosis has not improved significantly. However more critical pathological classification and evaluation of therapeutic trials, often multicentre, are developments which have provided a firmer basis for management advances when they arrive. With so much uncertainty, decisions about the management of the individual patient have become no easier, vain attempts at therapy may do no more than prolong suffering, and the indiscriminate use of chemotherapy, unless it is part of a correctly structured trial, is hardly justified. These daily practical problems should not be overlooked in any general text of neurosurgery.

In this chapter on malignant neoplasms the approach will be:

General definition of malignancy
Primary malignant neoplasms in general
(a) histological classification
(b) incidence
The supratentorial primary malignant neoplasm
(a) classificiation
(b) clinical features related to site
(c) management: differential diagnosis, degree of urgency and methods of investigation
(d) surgical management

The infratentorial primary malignant neoplasm
(a) classification
(b) clinical features
(c) methods and urgency of investigation
(d) surgical management

## General definition of malignancy

The histological criteria of malignancy are generally applicable to the primary malignant intracranial neoplasms (*see* below), but the gradation and severity of the histological appearances and subsequent deductions about the degrees of malignancy and behaviour of a tumour in an individual patient give rise to considerable difficulties. Due to the confined space in the intracranial compartments and especially in the posterior fossa, a tumour which is relatively 'benign' or which has only a few of the histological criteria of malignancy, may behave in a malignant fashion in the sense of threatening life. Conversely a neoplasm in the supratentorial compartment which is histologically more malignant may behave in a more benign fashion, with slow evolution of the clinical features over the course of months or even years. Therefore prognosis and management must be guided by a combination of the clinical status and age of the patient, and the site and histological appearances of the tumour; those factors may well conflict. These problems of classification of severity arise even with some of the metastases such as lymphoma.

# Primary malignant neoplasms

## (a) Systems of histological classification

With the exception of the meningeal sarcoma (or malignant meningiomas), the primary malignant neoplasms arise from *neuroectodermal* (neuroepithelial) tissue and are generally classified according to the apparent cell of origin or degree of differentiation towards certain identifiable cells. The history and evolution of the histological classification of the neuroectodermal tumours is of considerable interest, and is of importance if the current difficulties with classification are to be understood. The use of the term 'glioma' has led to some confusion: historically the word has been used to include all neuroectodermal tumours but in recent years, at least in surgical usage, it has tended to be reserved for tumours arising from neuroglia, that is the astrocytomas, ependymomas and oligodendrogliomas.

The classification of the glioma has been the subject of much controversy and a fascinating and important historical review is given by Scherer (1940) on which the following brief summary is based. Although Virchow created the term 'glioma', such tumours had already been described under other names. He distinguished two kinds of brain tumour, glioma and sarcoma. The former were of slow evolution, often very large, showing no clear limitation, not necessarily destroying the normal architecture; some were tough tumours and in these microscopic examination revealed a proliferation of glial fibres; others were soft and found to be largely cellular. This description applies to astrocytomas. Virchow's sarcoma was described as rounded, often having to the naked eye definite boundaries and frequently infiltrated with haemorrhage; microscopically the tumour was highly cellular, the cells of irregular shape and size; it was vascular and liable to fatty degeneration (necrosis). Although written one hundred years ago, this clearly defines the glioblastoma multiforme. Scherer then emphasised the contribution of Stroebe at the end of the last century when the techniques of microscopy had improved. Within the 'glioma' nerve cells and fibres are often conserved though not in 'sarcoma'; leptomeninges are not invaded by the 'glioma' but frequently by 'sarcoma'; both tumours my be present in one growth; the common occurence of cysts in 'glioma'; glial fibres are common in 'glioma' but absent in 'sarcoma'; mitoses and polymorphism are absent in the former but characterize the latter; 'gliomas' infiltrate nerve fibre pathways which may exert a mechanical influence upon the shape of the tumour cell. Scherer (1940) states that the next variety of brain tumour to be identified (as distinct from the previous two) was that now called an ependymoma, by Storch in 1899. High regard is paid by Scherer to the work of Tooth (1912) because this was the first study of gliomas to be based on a large amount of material, to pay adequate attention to clinical aspects and to make use of neurosurgical experience. Thereafter the classification of gliomas became dominated by the histogenic hypothesis of Ribbert, namely 'the origin of gliomas from slumbering embryonal mother cells.... This finds its most dogmatic expression in Bailey and Cushing's work (1926)'. This preoccupation with histogenesis is considered to have been unfortunate except that it stimulated interest in these tumours. Scherer (1940) pays tribute to Bailey and Bucy for identifying the oligodendroglioma and to Bailey and Cushing for identifying the medulloblastoma and the cerebellar astrocytoma. But he gives point to the argument by emphasizing that the last two tumours were recognized by reason of a broad biological approach. Scherer came to the conclusion that preoccupation with cytology and the rigidity imposed by the histogenetic doctrine were detrimental to the study of gliomas and embarked on examinations of the whole brain containing its tumour and correlated pathological findings with clinical details.

Purely expansive growth is exhibited only by the ependymoma. All other gliomas are infiltrative, though varying in degree. In some the growth zone (for example, advancing margin) is narrow, though microscopic spread can be detected beyond the naked eye edge; this margin may be accentuated in some cases by softening around the mass which makes enucleation deceptively easy, but glioma cells have infiltrated beyond so that enucleation splits the growth zone and recurrence is explained. Grey matter delays invasion, so that a glioblastoma may 'flow' below the surface of a gyrus and escape detection at operation; large association bundles provide a pathway for spread. The ventricle may mould some gliomas without the wall being infiltrated, while others spread along the ependymal wall. Diffuse infiltrative growth is characteristic of many glioblastomas which appear compact to the naked eye and yet microscopic examination reveals tumour cells at a very considerable distance around nerve cells and between their fibres; this accounted for the high percentage of bilateral growths in Scherer's series. Primary diffuse growth is a term applied to a widespread infiltration by glioma without the formation of a lump and without marked destruction of pre-existing tissue, as typified by the astrocytoma.

Multicentric growth is seen particularly in the glioblastoma. The resemblance between tumour cells and glial counterparts, mature and immature, forms a convenient basis for nomenclature. Anaplasia, or dedifferentition of the cell types due to some unknown cause is held responsible. Areas of further dedifferentiation may occur in slowly growing gliomas, explaining the tendency of the astrocytoma to develop into a glioblastoma. Apart from this example many gliomas are composed of more than one type of cell. Classification rests not only upon a study of the individual tumour cells, but also upon the architecture of the tumour, its stroma, the extent and nature of vascular proliferation and occlusion, necrosis and haemorrhage.

In an attempt to correlate histological diagnosis with malignancy, to take into account anaplastic tendencies and to bring classification of the gliomas into line with that of tumours elsewhere in the body, Kernohan *et al.* (1949) introduced a modification of the glioma groupings. They applied the Broders system of grading

**Table 5.1.** The gliomas. Classification of neuroectodermal tumours.

| | *Russell & Rubinstein (1977)* | *Kernohan* et al. *(1949)* | | *Weller & McLellan (1983) adapted from WHO (1979)* |
|---|---|---|---|---|
| | astrocytoma | astrocytoma | grade 1 | *astrocytic tumours* |
| | astroblastoma | astrocytoma | grade 2 | astrocytoma |
| | polar spongioblastoma | deleted | | glioblastoma multiforme and anaplastic astrocytoma |
| *Glial series* | oligodendroglioma | oligodendroglioma | grades 1–4 | *oligodendroglial tumours* |
| | ependymoma | ependymoma | grades 1–4 | oligodendroglioma |
| | subependymoma | ependymoma | grades 1–4 | mixed oligo-astrocytoma |
| | papilloma choroid plexus | papilloma | | anaplastic (malignant) oligodendroglioma |
| | colloid cyst | colloid cyst | | *ependymal tumours* |
| | glioblastoma multiforme | astrocytoma | grades 3–4 | anaplastic (malignant) ependymoma |
| | | | | *embryonal tumours* primitive neuroectodermal tumour |
| *Pineal series* | pineoblastomas | pineoblastoma | | medulloblastoma |
| | pineocytoma | pineocytoma | | *choroid plexus tumours* choroid plexus papilloma |
| | medulloblastoma | medulloblastoma | | anaplastic (malignant) choroid |
| | medulloepithelioma | ependymoma | grade 4 | plexus papilloma |
| *Neuron series* | neuroblastoma | neuroastrocytoma | grades 2–4 | *malformative lesions* |
| | ganglio-neuroma and -glioma | neuroastrocytoma | grade 1 | colloid cysts of the 3rd ventricle |

tumours according to the degree of malignancy as judged by cytology. There are four grades and they dispensed with certain terms.

In more recent years great efforts have been made to formulate a classification and nomenclature which will indicate a broad histological appearance with which pathologists and surgeons are familiar, and at the same time indicate a degree of malignancy which can be correlated with prognosis, with or without treatment. The World Health Organization classification (Zülch 1979) has gradually replaced the Kernohan grading, perhaps more so in continental Europe than in Britain, but especially in evaluation of chemotherapy in multicentre trials. The evolution of the systems of classification are illustrated in Table 5.1 which allows comparison between three partly differing classifications, the last being an adaption (Weller & McLellan 1983) of the WHO classification.

## (b) Incidence

Certain general characteristics of the gliomas need comment before dealing in detail with each variety. Their incidence is not equally divided between the sexes; in the astrocytoma and glioblastoma groups Penman and Smith (1954) calculated that between the ages of 25 and 54 (at onset of illness) the ratio of males to females is 1.86 to 1. An even greater preponderance of males suffer from medulloblastoma. The age incidence of gliomas varies for the different groups; the medulloblastoma is largely a tumour of children, the glioblastoma is common in middle aged persons, while the astrocytoma has two age peaks, in children most frequently in the cerebellum and in adults most frequently in the cerebral hemispheres. Penman and Smith also confirmed previous observations that the left cerebral hemisphere is more frequently affected than the right. When due allowance is made for the relative volumes of the several lobes of the cerebrum they found that the temporal is the most common site. Ask-Upmark (1938) considered that gliomas of the parietal and temporal lobes

together far out-numbered those of the frontal lobe, though the surface area of the frontal lobe equals the combined area of the parietal and temporal lobes. Ostertag (1952) correlates the type of growth and its location in the brain by noting that tumours of more primitive cell type tend to occur more frequently in phylogenetically older parts of the brain. In order to determine whether hereditary influences play any part in the occurrence of gliomas, Van der Wiel (1960) studied 100 subjects with glioma and all their living relatives in the Netherlands. He came to the conclusion that status dysraphicus predisposes to gliomas. There are many curious features about age, sex, location and heredity predilections for which no answer is forthcoming. Such problems are not unique for gliomas amongst the tumours in general, and somewhat similar problems are presented for instance by the selective variability of the response of neurons to differing degrees of hypoxia and of ischaemia, and the greater vulnerability of certain anatomical groups of cells (Schadé & McMenemey 1963).

## (c) Distant metastases

Although at one time it was generally believed that a glioma never spread to distant parts of the body, sufficient and well documented cases have now been recorded to prove the error of this view. It is again the medulloblastoma which provides most of the examples. Glioma metastases have been recorded in bones, lymph nodes, liver, lungs and kidneys; infiltration of the tissues at the site of the previous operation is often extensive and subcutaneous nodules an important clinical finding. Osseous metastases are the commonest and intractable limb pain in a child treated for a medulloblastoma should suggest this possibility; the latter may cause considerable osteosclerosis.

## The pathology of primary supratentorial malignant neoplasms

### (a)  Classification

Reference has already been made to the systems of classification which have evolved, the most acceptable at present being the WHO classification of the neoplasms in the supratentorial compartment, even within the broad heading of malignancy, is often of more practical value if it is primarily *anatomical* rather than histological, as shown in Table 5.2.

Not only is the site of the lesion the most important consideration in the planning of investigations and primary treatment, but the different sites of the same cell-type (for example, astrocytoma) tend to be associated with a higher or a lower degree of histological malignancy. Thus the hemisphere astrocytomas, when they present clinically, are usually of a high grade of malignancy (for example, glioblastoma multiforme and anaplastic astrocytoma), whereas astrocytoma of the optic nerves and chiasm are always histologically relatively benign. A further value of anatomical classification is that certain cell types tend to favour or eschew certain anatomical sites. Thus oligodendrogliomas and

Table 5.2. Anatomical classification of primary supratentorial malignant neoplasms.

A  Neuroectodermal
    1  hemisphere tumours:
        frontal
        temporal
        parietal
        occipital
    2  corpus callosum
    3  basal ganglia, thalamic and para-third-ventricular
    4  para- and intralateral ventricular
    5  hypothalamic
    6  optic nerve and chiasm
    7  pineal recess

B  Meningeal sarcoma/malignant meningioma
    1  parasagittal
    2  convexity or cortical
    3  sphenoid ridge
    4  parasellar
    5  falcine
    6  tentorial (superior surface)

ependymoma are rarely seen in tumours growing primarily in the corpus callosum, and tumours clearly restricted radiologically to the pineal recess are very rarely 'gliomas', unless they have arisen in the superior vermis of the cerebellum.

The *histological* classification follows the WHO system described, the Kernohan numerical grading still being used, although clear differentiation between grade 3 and grade 4 is often imprecise, and between grade 2 and grade 1 often meaningless in terms of prognosis. The added difficulties are:

(a)  supratentorial tumours often show a mixture of histological features some of which are characteristic of an astrocytoma and others of an oligodendroglioma;
(b)  the biopsy tissue, especially if limited, may not be representative of the whole tumour;
(c)  biopsies at different times may reveal a change usually towards a more malignant pattern;
(d)  unless immunoperoxidase staining for glial fibrillary acidic protein (GFAP) is used, and if necessary, electron microscopy, the true glial nature of a tumour may not be determined;
(e)  the need for uniform critical pathology review is now obligatory for all meaningful studies of glioma therapy, such are the difficulties for the individual pathologist.

## Tumour types

### Astrocytoma

*Macroscopic appearances*

This tumour and the glioblastoma multiforme are the most commonly occurring gliomas. An astrocytoma may arise in any part of the brain though its histological appearance may be modified by the structure of the areas which it inhabits. So long as anaplastic changes do not supervene it is characterized by slow growth and the average preoperative duration of symptoms

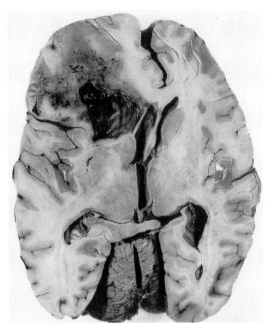

**Figure. 5.1.** Anaplastic astrocytoma of left frontal lobe. Tumour expands the gyri and destroys their normal configuration: grey and white matter cannot be distinguished. The margin of tumour merges imperceptibly with brain tissue. Small haemorrhages, small areas of necrosis and small cysts are present in its substance and on its deep aspect there is a large cyst separated from the frontal horn by a thin septum. The lobe is greatly expanded and its medial surface is marked by herniation under the falx. The lateral ventricules are compressed and displaced across the middle line. Male aged 33 years: 3 months headaches, unsteady gait, papilloedema, terminal attacks of opisthotonus.

is nearly three years (Elvidge *et al.* 1937). Occasionally the interval is many years, and a partial removal of the tumour may be followed by years of useful existence. It has a predilection for the cerebrum in adults with a maximum incidence between the ages of 30 and 40 years and for the cerebellum in children, where it reaches a peak in those aged 5 to 10 years.

In the cerebral hemispheres the tumour commonly forms a mass with an ill defined edge which merges imperceptibly with the surrounding brain and its colour may be little different from white matter or it may be somewhat yellow (Fig. 5.1.). The tissue is avascular. Its consistency is firm, fibrous or rubbery and it

is by this feature that it is usually detected. It may contain fine deposits of calcium which impart a grittiness to its texture. Martin and Lemmen (1952) studied the frequency of calcification in intracranial tumours and detected microscopic deposits in 16% of astrocytomas occurring above the tentorium; in approximately half, the deposits were sufficient to be detected radiologically, a proportion which held good for other tumours. A similar figure for radiologically visible calcium was noted by Gol (1961). These figures for calcification visible on plain radiographs of the skull are considerably lower than those for calcification visible on computerized tomography (*see* Chapter 3).

Where the tumour approaches the cortex, the gyri become broadened and flattened and on first being exposed after reflection of the dura they are paler than healthy brain, though later they become hyperaemic. If the astrocytoma infiltrates the cortex, the gyri become distorted and their normal pattern destroyed. To palpation the cortex feels firmer than normal. Cysts form in about half the cases. They vary in size; part of the tumour may be honeycombed by microcysts, or there may be one large cyst at the margin of the tumour. Such a cyst may be so large as partially to envelop the tumour, which may then form a nodule protruding into the cyst from its wall, the so-called mural nodule. The cysts contain yellow usually clear fluid which readily clots after aspiration. They are of clinical importance, because the fluid may accumulate rapidly thereby accelerating the rate of evolution of intracranial hypertension and neurological deficit. When the fluid accumulates slowly, the signs of neurological deficit which might otherwise be anticipated by a solid mass of similar size are frequently absent. This is probably because the cyst is expansive and not infiltrative.

Less commonly encountered are astrocytomas which appear to be more discrete and rounded, of a greyish almost translucent appearance, soft and homogeneous in texture and sometimes slightly vascular. Because they are soft they will not be detected when an exploring brain cannula passes through them. The cortex over such a

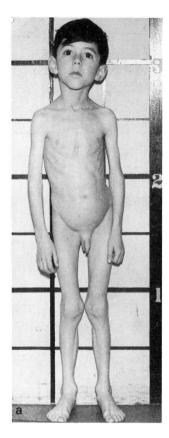
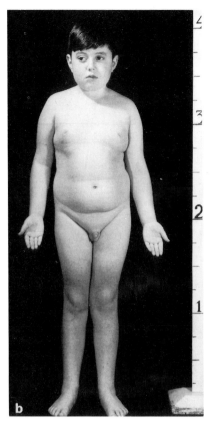

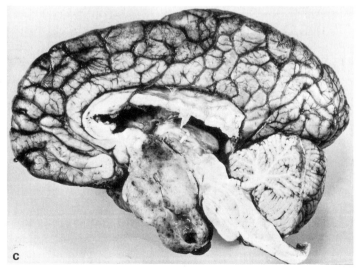

**Fig. 5.2.** Example of diencephalic wasting which started at the age of 6 months.
(a) Aged 3 years; weight 28 lb (average for age 32 lb, for height 35 lb). No neurological abnormality, skull X-rays normal, A.E.G. showed poor filling of anterior end of 3rd ventricle.
(b) Five years later, obese, diminutive genitalia, nearly blind from papilloedema and atrophy. Died soon after date of this photograph.
(c) Juvenile astrocytoma occupying 3rd ventricle, invading optic chiasma and forming a large mass ventral to pons.

tumour remains soft to the touch. The tumour may present on the surface as a small tell-tale area of grey translucent tissue in sharp contrast to the surrounding brain. It is very fragile, easily damaged and the fine vessels coursing on its surface readily bleed.

The variation in macroscopic appearances within the same tumour is characteristic of the astrocytomas, some parts being relatively avascular, pale, firm and diffuse features, but other areas being soft, necrotic and haemorrhagic, which is consistent with the more anaplastic astrocytoma and glioblastoma multiforme. These variations in histological appearance and behaviour can be correlated with growth kinetics shown by *in vivo* and *in vitro* studies (Hoshina 1984).

Some of the gliomas of the basal ganglia are astrocytomas. They form a firm smooth enlargement (Nevin 1938) and may spread bilaterally and into the centrum ovale to merit the term gliomatosis cerebri. A well defined group is found in the anterior part of the third ventricle in children. The tumour forms an apparently circumscribed mass which when large enough entirely fills the third ventricle and may extend as a lobulated mass through its floor into the interpeduncular and pontine cisterns (Fig. 5.2). It also infiltrates the optic chiasma and optic nerves. Within the ventricle and in the lobular extensions in the subarachnoid space the tissue is soft, at times gelatinous of greyish appearance, and of little vascularity. Histologically they are of the piloid variety and because of their age incidence are often qualified as juvenile. They provide a distinct clinical group by reason of the hypothalamic and visual disturbances which their locality determines.

Allied to those tumours by histology, anatomical contiguity, and predominance in young people (75% under 12 years of age; Fowler & Matson 1957) are the gliomas of the optic nerve and chiasma. The fusiform tumour may be entirely restricted to one optic nerve and situated anywhere in its length, though as it increases in size its anterior extremity indents the globe of the eye and its posterior overlaps the chiasma.

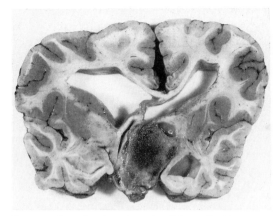

**Fig. 5.3.** Juvenile astrocytoma involving optic chiasma, right hypothalamus, optic tract and basal ganglia, partially filling and compressing 3rd ventricle: female, aged 4 years, who survived ventriculocisternostomy and radiotherapy for 3 years.

In this event the optic canal becomes expanded, though it moulds the tumour to a dumb-bell shape. Ultimately it infiltrates the chiasma and the other optic nerve, extends into the third ventricle and there forms a mass similar to one which arises, primarily in the ventricle. Sometimes, however, the tumour uses the optic pathway as a bridge to attain and infiltrate the lateral wall of the ventricle and the basal ganglia, (Fig. 5.3). The biological behaviour of this group of slowly growing gliomas of the basal ganglia, (excluding, of course the glioblastoma) of the anterior third ventricle, and of the optic nerve and chiasma are thus somewhat similar.

*Histology*

Although in the past much was made of the different histological appearances of the astrocytoma, a more recent view is to accept variation between different tumours, and likewise different areas of the same tumours, as a continuum of the same disease. There is, however, some correlation between the different appearances and certain clinical syndromes, particularly in those tumours which do not show pronounced histological features of malignancy. The histological types of astrocytoma have been well summarized by Weller and McLellan (1983).

*Protoplasmic* astrocytomas often have a soft, gelatinous consistency and are composed of cells which extend a few delicate processes to form a cobweb-like structure between the cell bodies. Few, if any, intracytoplasmic glial fibrils are present in the processes and the cells are often separated by microcystic cavities. There is some variation in nuclear shape and size but usually the cells have moderately regular, round nuclei. *Fibrillary* astrocytomas may also be soft in consistency and similar to protoplasmic astrocytomas but their processes contain more glial fibrils. Some tumours are firm and rubbery and composed of tightly packed spindle-shaped astrocytic cells containing large numbers of intracellular glial fibrils. Such tumours are often called *pilocytic* astrocytomas and may contain thickened, brightly eosinophilic processes (Rosenthal fibres). In some astrocytomas, the tumours cells are plump with abundant eosinophilic cytoplasm and eccentric nuclei; they superficially resemble hypertrophic reactive astrocytes seen in areas of brain damage. Such gemistocytic cells form the majority of the tumour in *gemistocytic* astrocytomas and they are seen to a greater or lesser extent in other astrocytic tumours.

The tumours arising in association with tuberose sclerosis have features of the gemistocytic astrocytoma; although usually histologically benign, they may undergo malignant change. Electron microscopy may enable glial fibrils to be identified within the cytoplasm. The degree of differentiation and ease of identification of astrocytes in these tumours is one of the features upon which the degree of malignancy can be judged; the pilocytic astrocytoma, which may be considered histologically benign very rarely occurs above the tentorium except in children in the region of the third ventricle, but it is found characteristically in the child's cerebellum (*see* below). Gliomas of the optic nerve and chiasm, with their characteristically indolent clinical course have been considered to be a mixture of oligodendroglioma and piloid and stellate astrocytes (Russel & Rubinstein 1977), but a more recent series (Packer *et al.* 1983) considered the tumours to be simply low grade astrocytomas. Changes towards higher malignancy may also occur in low grade tumours which, after many years suddenly undergo anaplastic changes. *Anaplastic* astrocytomas must not be confused with tumours reproducing precursors of astrocytes, such as polar spongioblastomas or astroblastomas. The concept of anaplasia implies the production of atypical, aberrant, often genetically abnormal lines of cells and not reversion to a more primitive stage of the normal line of development.

## Anaplastic astrocytoma and glioblastoma multiforme

Although there are histological features which may allow differentiation between these tumours, this may be difficult, pathologists may differ in their views upon the same tumour and, as yet, there is no more than a suggestion that there is any correlation with prognosis (Brucher 1984). Macroscopic differentiation is not possible, and the behaviour of these tumours and the management of the patients is similar. Furthermore glioblastoma multiforme may be regarded as an extreme form of the anaplastic astrocytoma, which in its turn has a higher degree of malignancy occurring in the whole or part of the astrocytoma already described. The majority occur in the frontal or temporal lobes, some 20% in the parietal region, but relatively few are truly occipital. The tumour may be encountered in any part of the brain, but most frequently in the cerebrum and particularly the centrum ovale. It forms a firm pink fleshy mass often rounded and apparently circumscribed. It expands the brain, often exciting considerable oedema, transgresses deep fissures such as the Sylvian, readily passes through the corpus callosum to the opposite hemisphere (Fig. 5.4) or spreads across the internal capsule to involve basal ganglia (Plate 1). Arising in the latter it may bulge into the ventricle, spread out into the capsule

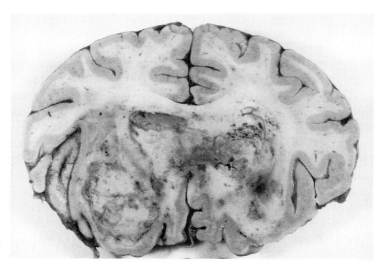

**Fig. 5.4.** Glioblastoma of frontal lobes and corpus callosum.

or extend caudally into the brain stem. Deeply set arteries may first be displaced by it but later are engulfed. The texture of the tumour varies. In places it is tough and fibrous, trabeculae carrying large blood vessels; elsewhere the tissue may be homogeneous, soft and a translucent pinkish grey; cavities may contain opaque creamy fluid which simulates pus, the walls of the cavity being shaggy and necrotic. Apart from these areas the tumour is vascular and spontaneous haemorrhage into its substance may be the cause of death. At necropsy the cut surface presents a variegated appearance as a result of necrosis and of altered blood pigment of varying ages. Vascularity extends beyond the macroscopic borders of the tumour and pervades the surrounding brain tissue, which is commonly much softened and even diffluent. This peripheral zone of softened white matter provides an apparent line of cleavage, rendering a removal of the mass relatively easy. But this line of cleavage is deceptive, for it has already been infiltrated by the growing edge of the tumour. When the tumour approaches the cortex it frequently spreads out to infiltrate the subcortical white matter much further than is apparent to the naked eye; the growing edge of the tumour may be diverted for a time by the basal masses of grey matter, though both are eventually overrun. When a glioblastoma presents on the surface of the brain it

appears at one or more places as a red fleshy mass or as a greyish pink translucent zone. There are many adventitial vessels (both arterial and venous) coursing over the tumour and gradually blending with the peripheral cortical vessels. The existence of abnormal arteriovenous shunts may be inferred from observation of 'red veins', containing fully oxygenated blood, shunted through the vascular of the tumour without transcapillary extraction of oxygen. The structure is delicate and readily bleeds and the loss of extravascular support when the dura mater is opened may precipitate spontaneous rupture of superficial or deep vessels. The tumour may invade the surface of adjacent dura mater, the adhesions being firm and vascular. Unlike the less malignant astrocytoma, these tumours do not have cysts containing clear yellow fluid, but the cysts are the result of necrosis of the centre of the tumour. Satellite nodules may occur in the cerebral hemisphere at some distance from the main tumour mass.

*Histology*

The term 'glioblastoma' is unsatisfactory in a term based on histogenesis as there is no cell called 'glioblast'. Nevertheless the term serves a useful purpose in designating a tumour in which anaplasia has reached such a high degree that the origin of the tumour cells cannot be identified with certainty. Corresponding to the gliosarcoma of early writers and recognized by them as a highly malignant tumour it was renamed spongioblastoma multiforme by Globus and Strauss (1925). Its present title was adopted in order to avoid confusion with the spongioblastoma polare, a much less common glioma, which runs a more favourable course. There is however, no class of glial cells which can be called a glioblast, whereas the spongioblast is a well recognized stage in the development of the astrocyte, though its blastomatous counterpart may be an infrequent member of the cell population of a glioblastoma.

These tumours, more than any other intracranial tumours exhibit the general features of malignancy which are: variation in size and shape of cells, variation and abnormal nuclear patterns and hyperchromasia, many and abnormal mitotic figures, giant cell formation, pseudopalisade arrangement of cells with hyperchromatic nuclei round areas of necrosis, and an increase in the number of capillaries in the infiltrating zone of the tumour, with capillary endothelial proliferation in the more central areas. In the presence of such anaplasia it may be difficult to identify the original cell type of the tumour; only the identification of GFAP by immunoperoxide staining or immunofluorescence of GFAP fibrils by electron microscopy may achieve this (Plates 2 and 3). There is some evidence from careful autopsy studies that the aggressions of these tumours is related to a predominance of small anaplastic cells (Giangaspero & Burger 1983). In some tumours bizarre giant multinucleate cells may predominate, all the component cells being large; this tumour became known as a giant celled or monstrocellular glioblastoma, and despite earlier suggestions, there is insufficient evidence to consider this a sarcoma (Russell & Rubinstein 1977). All glioblastomas are invasive, their demarcation from surrounding tissue is indistinct and tumour cells extend deeply into the adjacent cerebral structures. Even at some distance from identifiable neoplastic tissue scattered glial cells may be found which exhibit irregularity of nuclear structure suggestive of neoplastic, and not of reactive, changes. Superficial glioblastomas tend to invade the leptomeninges and obliterate the subarachnoid space. They may become adherent to the dura mater but hardly ever invade or transgress it, with the exception of small herniations through perivenous lacunae most frequently seen in the floor of the middle fossa. Tumours abutting on the ventricular surface may invade and breach the ependyma, encroach upon the ventricle and sometimes fill it completely.

Considering the high degree of malignancy of glioblastomas they metastasize surprisingly rarely. The common pathway of dissemination is the cerebrospinal fluid and tumour seedlings may be found in the subarachnoid space and on the ependymal surface of the ventricles. Extensive spread through the spinal subarachnoid space may lead to encasing of the cord in a sheath of solid tumour. Extracranial metastases are exceptional; distant spread to the lungs or bones is usually facilitated by surgical interference, though cases of spontaneous metastasis have been recorded (Rubinstein 1967).

## Oligodendroglioma

*Macroscopic appearances*

The characteristic features of this glioma were defined by Bailey and Bucy (1929). It is a tumour usually of adults, with the highest frequency between 30 and 50 years. It affects the cerebral hemispheres, particularly the frontal lobes; approximately one-third are frontal, and less than one-tenth infratentorial. Rate of growth varies considerably, the duration of symptoms extending from a few months to 20 years. Of all brain tumours the oligodendroglioma is the most likely to contain calcareous deposits which can be demonstrated radiologically in about 40% of cases.

The tumour forms a rounded, often well circumscribed, greyish pink mass and is to the naked eye indistinguishable from some astrocytomas; its margin often seems well defined. The consistency of the tumour varies; it is frequently gritty with calcium deposits and in places gelatinous as a result of mucinous degeneration; necrosis and cyst formation are not common. Although they are usually not particularly vascular tumours at operation, spontaneous haemorrhage is more common in them than in astrocytoma and may be fatal. They may bleed into the ventricle and hence provide an unusual cause for subarachnoid haemorrhage. Although the tumour usually occupies the centrum ovale a minority bulge into the lateral ventricle and the bulk of the tumour may lie within that cavity. As a result, there is a propensity for these tumours to spread over the wall of the ventricle and to be disseminated throughout the cerebrospinal fluid pathway.

*Histology*

A typical oligodendroglioma consists of a continuous sheet of small, round, densely packed cells interrupted only by a remarkably regular network of small blood vessels (Fig. 5.5). The nuclei resemble those of normal oligodendrocytes, although not infrequently they are somewhat larger. They are round, darkly staining with a compact chromatin pattern. The cytoplasm is scanty and indistinct unless it has undergone a degenerative change known as acute swelling; it then becomes clear and colourless and the appearances of the cells are those of nuclei placed in the centres of empty circular membranes. These tumours are usually compact and well demarcated from the surrounding brain tissue. Sometimes, however, otherwise typical oligodendrogliomas infiltrate the cerebral parenchyma diffusely; in these, instead of solid sheets, strands of oligodendroglial cells, sometimes arranged in parallel rows separate the fibres of the white matter and the nerve cells of the cortex.

Deposition of calcium salts starts as pericapillary droplet calcification which progresses to the formation of solid mineral tubes around

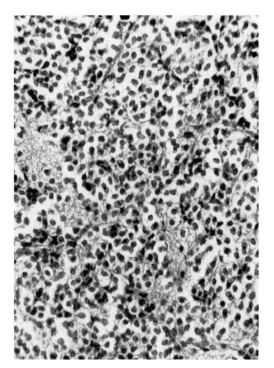

**Fig. 5.5.** Oligodendroglioma: typical appearance with clear cytoplasm surrounding small dense nucleus. H. & E. × 300.

the vessels and grows to form laminated calcospherites. These may become confluent and form the bulk of the tumour with only small groups of viable cells scattered in the clefts between the stones (Fig. 5.6).

Pure oligodendrogliomas are rare. Even in predominantly oligodendroglial tumours scattered astrocytes can be demonstrated and in some tumours they may be abundant. Conversely, scattered oligodendroglial cells are not infrequently seen in otherwise typical astrocytomas. Tumours in which some areas are purely or almost purely, oligodendroglial and others astrocytic also occur.

Anaplastic changes may be found. The cells become more irregular, often oval, and variable in size and the density of their chromatin pattern. Bizarre cells may appear, mitoses which may be found also in benign variants become abundant and often atypical, vascular proliferation may occur and areas of necrosis become prominent. As anaplasia progresses the appearances merge

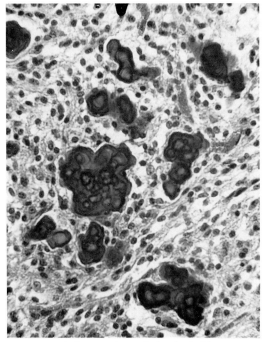

**Fig. 5.6.** Calcification of typical oligodendroglioma. H. & E. × 300.

the substance of the cerebral hemispheres, the presentation being similar to other supratentorial hemisphere gliomas. Nevertheless they are rare in the supratentorial region, and more likely to be related to the ventricular system and lie within the third or lateral ventricles. Whereas the more common infratentorial ependymomas occur mainly in children, the supratentorial tumours occur mainly in young adults. They may extend outwards in the hemisphere having insignificant relationship to the lateral ventricle, or the reverse may be the case so that the tumour occupies and expands the ventricle. Macroscopically the ependymomas are relatively well circumscribed tumours, especially when they lie mainly within a ventricle; when they extend onto the surface of the brain there is a remarkably distinct border, the tumour appearing as a large plaque spreading outwards from its area of origin.

*Histology*

Ependymomas consist of ependymal cells and a glial stroma in various proportions. The ependymal elements form a low cuboidal epithelium lining small tubules and rosettes with a distinct lumen; sometimes they line larger clefts or spaces and may be thrown into folds imparting a papillary appearance to the tumour. Groups of ependymal cells may also form small solid clusters with irregular outlines, resembling the obliterated central canal of the spinal cord. Normal ependymal cells are ciliated but cilia are not often recognizable in tumours, except by electron microscopy. On the other hand their corresponding intracellular organelles, the blepharoplasts, are frequently demonstrable by appropriate staining techniques. The stroma which consists of subependymal glia is predominantly astrocytic and contains abundant glial fibrils forming a dense network. Oligodendroglial elements may also be present. A characteristic feature of ependymal tumours is the formation of perivascular pseudorosettes with cell-free zones around blood vessels con-

with those of glioblastoma. Some malignant oligodendrogliomas consist of uniform aggregations of dark, round or oval nuclei with numerous mitotic figures and no distinguishing features other than small islands of more typical oligodendroglial cells. These appearances may be difficult to distinguish from the primitive neuroectodermal tumours (*see* below). Unlike the anaplastic astrocytoma and glioblastoma multiforme the equivalent malignant changes in oligodendrogliomas do not carry so grave a prognosis. In the presence of anaplasia identification of surface markers or the electron microscopic pattern will allow the tumour to be characterized.

**Ependymomas**

Although their name suggests that these tumours are derived from the cells lining the ventricular system, they may also occur within

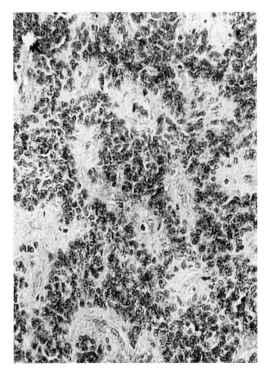

**Fig. 5.7.** Ependymoma: solid type with clear zones around blood vessels. H. & E. × 240.

sisting of thin, tapering processes converging on the vessels (Fig. 5.7). Poorly differentiated ependymomas show nuclear pleomorphism and hyperchromasia, and have a greater propensity for spread through the CSF pathways, and recurrence at the site of previous tumour removal.

## Ganglionic tumours

This very small group of tumours is usually subdivided into ganglioneuromas and gangliogliomas. In both, neurons form an essential part of the tumour tissue and both contain supporting glial elements. In ganglioneuromas the glia resembles the normal supporting tissues of the central nervous system; in gangliogliomas it has undergone neoplastic change and resembles one of the various types of astrocytoma though oligodendroglial areas may be also found. Ganglion-celled tumours are said to be more frequent in young people and to be more commonly situated in the floor of the third ventricle though they occur anywhere. Their rate of growth is generally slow.

### Histology

It is essential for the diagnosis of ganglion-celled tumours that the neurons in the tumour should be both ectopic and abnormal. They must be found in areas where neurons of the type encountered do not normally occur and they must exhibit structural abnormalities, such as multiple nuclei or irregular, bizarre processes. The features of malignancy depend upon the characteristics of the glial component which appears to dictate the clinical behaviour of the tumour.

## Primitive neuroectodermal tumours or embryonal tumours

Despite the considerable controversy over the nature and origin of this group of tumours, and the view that medulloblastoma (see below) is an entirely separate entity, a more rational view is now gaining ground that medulloblastoma is but one of a larger group of primitive neuroectodermal tumours. These develop from primitive multipotential cells, which in the course of their growth produce tumours with histological features of malignancy, and some evidence of neuronal differentiation of a primitive type (Plate 4).

These tumours are very rare in the supratentorial region, and occur almost exclusively in children below the age of ten years and very rarely up to the age of 20 years. The supratentorial tumours, which are remarkable for the great size they can reach before obvious symptoms occur, are either within the frontal or parietal lobes, or related to the ventricular system; they appear macroscopically as well circumscribed firm round masses, either causing gross hemisphere displacement, dilatation of one lateral ventricle, or hydrocephalus. Although space-occupying rather than purely invasive, these tumours metastasize readily through the CSF pathways, and also recur frequently at the site of the previous surgical removal.

Histologically the tumours resemble peripheral neuroblastoma, hence one apellation being cerebral neuroblastoma or medulloblastoma, with, in some cases, differentiation to ganglion cells and often the formation of a striking fibrous tissue stroma (Horten & Rubinstein 1976, Russell & Rubinstein 1977). As with medulloblastoma survival is related to age, and it has not proved possible to establish by controlled trial the place of radiotherapy, overall survival after surgery and radiotherapy being 60% at 3 years (Berger & Edwards 1983, Bennett & Rubinstein 1984).

### Microglioma: primary malignant lymphoma

There has been considerable dispute and uncertainty about the incidence and particularly the origin of these tumours, and it is only in recent years with the development of immunological methods of identification of lymphomas, that their classification as a primary malignant lymphoma of the brain has been established. The presentation is similar to that of the more slowly growing astrocytoma, or of degenerative conditions, and macroscopically there may be no more than mild diffuse swelling and softening in a cerebral hemisphere without any clear demarcation from normal brain. Histologically there may be a diffuse infiltration by lymphoid cells, with proliferation of microglial cells, hence the earlier name for this tumour; there may also be considerable formation of reticulin. The pathological and surgical aspects of primary lymphoma of the central nervous system have been reviewed by Helle *et al.* (1984).

## Clinical presentation of supratentorial malignant neoplasms

As with so much of medicine, the accurate clinical diagnosis of intracranial tumours depends more upon an accurate, carefully recorded and dissected *history*, than upon abnormal *physical signs*. Sadly it is this aspect of clinical medicine which often receives scant attention, particularly in this age of increasingly sophisticated investigations. Major errors in management of patients arise more from failure to obtain an accurate history than from lack of investigation. Indeed if the history suggests the presence of raised intracranial pressure or a focal neurological lesion, the absence of relevant abnormal physical signs should never, in itself, be allowed to vitiate that diagnosis.

Supratentorial neoplasms may present in one of several ways, which can be conveniently classified as:

1  raised intracranial pressure;
2  focal neurological disturbances;
3  disorders of the mind and intellect;
4  systemic disorders.

*Raised intracranial pressure* is dealt with in Chapter 2.

*Focal neurological disturbances* can be conveniently divided into (a) abnormal paroxysmal neuronal activity, and (b) loss of neuronal or fibre tract function.

(a) Abnormal paroxysmal neuronal activity. This is manifest as an epileptic fit, the result perhaps of disturbance of the nutrition of the neurons and brought about by local pressure, by interference with blood supply, by cellular invasion or possibly by oedema. Fits due to tumours do not differ from those due to other causes and their patterns may be as complex. During the interictal periods neurological function may be entirely normal, though if after a fit which for example has caused clonic movements of a group of muscles, there is a persistent weakness and if after repeated fits, there is each time a further lessening of power, it must be concluded that structural changes occurred and this would be strong evidence in favour of a neoplasm. Todd's post-epileptic paralysis is a well-known phenomenon, but normal function is totally restored in a few hours or rarely days. The electroencephalograph (EEG) may reveal abnormalities different from those in epilepsy due to causes other than a tumour even when there is no interictal disturbance of function (Chapter 4). Epilepsy is a frequent and important symptom of brain tumour, although brain tumour is not the commonest cause of epilepsy.

The fits associated with a brain tumour may be generalized or they may be localized disturbances of cortical function in accordance with the portion of the brain in which the 'sudden excessive rapid and local discharges of the grey matter' originate (Jackson 1873). Accurate observation of the events comprising a fit may provide important clues to the diagnosis and the significance of focal epilepsy and the diverse patterns which may be encountered are considered below, taking each lobe separately. Generalized and focal attacks may occur in the same patient and the focal attacks may be of more than one pattern; though each pattern tends to be stereotyped, fits may change to a different pattern during the course of the illness. Generalized convulsions have no localizing value though they are more frequent when the tumour is deeply situated in the frontal lobe.

Not only is epilepsy an important symptom of a brain tumour, for the dramatic and often frightening experience invariably prompts the patient to seek medical advice, but it is often the earliest symptom. It was the first symptom in 50% of the cases of parietal tumour causing epilepsy, 78% of the frontal and 93% of the temporal (Lund 1952). Long periods of time may elapse between the onset of epilepsy and the development of other symptoms; in Lund's series it was less than two years in 46% of cases with epilepsy and over five years in 30%. The incidence of epilepsy varies considerably with the histological nature of the tumour as well as its situation and a long history of fits is particularly common in certain tumours; ten years or more is by no means unusual.

(b) Loss of neuronal or fibre tract function. The effect is not necessarily one of simple motor or sensory deficit, but it may reveal itself by complex disturbance such as dysphasia or a partial visual field deficit or by release phenom-

ena (such as grasp reflex, involuntary movements or spontaneous conjugate deviation of the eyes) or the deficit may declare itself as faulty memory or intellectual deterioration. The abnormal signs revealed by examination will be the result not only of the local anatomical and physiological damage wrought by the tumour, but also of the raised intracranial pressure and accompanying herniations (if present). In the exercise of diagnosis the various signs must be related to the appropriate cause, so that a complete picture is obtained of the abnormal processes active within the cranium.

*Disorders of the mind and intellect* may occur as part of the symptomatology of raised intracranial pressure (*see* Chapter 2) or as a disturbance of a specific cerebral area as in the frontal or parietal lobe syndromes (*see* below). Loss of intellect is such a common disorder of pathological states and of ageing that it is easily overlooked by patient and physician, especially if, as is often the case, it does not fit the pattern of a specific lobar lesion. Furthermore, the slow and insidious progress of the deficit may make even close family members unaware of the deterioration for a very long time.

*Systemic disorders* comprise abnormalities of growth, of physical habitus, of sexual functions and of vegetative and metabolic processes. They may result from the direct effect exerted by the tumour on endocrine secretions or on their normal control as a result of pressure, infiltration or ischaemia or in some instances they arise indirectly, for example the dehydration secondary to vomiting.

## Specific syndromes of supratentorial tumours

Clinical diagnosis of the localization of a supratentorial lesion is aided by a knowledge of syndromes which may in part, or whole, be associated with particular regions of the cerebral hemispheres and deep structures, although the lesion may usually involve more than one region. These syndromes form the basis of much of clinical neurology. However it has to be admitted that with improved methods of investigation, and especially CT scanning and, more recently nuclear magnetic resonance imaging, syndromes can no longer be ascribed with such confidence to lesions in particular anatomical sites. In addition hydrocephalus, be it obstructive or communicating (normal pressure) and whatever its cause, will add clinical features which can mimic the traditional neurological syndromes.

**Frontal lobe**

The posterior boundary of the frontal lobe is the central sulcus, consequently tumours affecting the posterior part of the frontal lobe abut upon the precentral gyrus or its projection fibres traversing the white matter to join the corona radiata and internal capsule. Involvement of these pathways gives rise to contralateral spastic weakness with reflex changes appropriate to upper motor neuron damage. If the tumour is situated deeply in the white matter where the projection fibres converge, a relatively small lesion will be sufficient to cause a hemiplegia; if the tumour is close to the cortex, subcortical or lying on the cortex where the representation of movements is spread over a wide area it may be larger and yet cause weakness of much lesser extent. Localization of the lesion will be in accordance with the distribution of representation of muscular activity in the motor cortex. In this respect lesions of the superior and medial part of the lobe, the paracentral lobule, produce severe weakness of the foot, while lesions in the lower part on the dominant side, cause dysphasia affecting predominantly the expressive aspect and dysarthria. The more restricted in extent and intense in degree the weakness, i.e. the more focal are the abnormal signs, the closer to the cortex and the smaller the tumour is likely to be. An estimate of the posterior limit of the tumour will be derived from the results of testing of discriminative types of sensory perception; if these are affected, then the sensory projection fibres

to the postcentral gyrus are involved, by invasion or by pressure ischaemia.

Focal (Jacksonian) motor epilepsy is commonly due to tumours in this part of the brain, whether glioma or meningioma. Theoretically the seizure may start in any group of muscles but experience shows that they usually originate in the hand, the face and the foot in that order of frequency. The attacks may be of the simple pattern of spreading clonic convulsions, or of the adversive variety, or they may exhibit more complex postures of the limb, described fully in Chapter 17.

Tumours involving the cortex anterior to the precentral gyrus may give rise to a grasp reflex. This is usually found in the hand but occasionally it may be evoked in the foot, in which case the tumour is situated nearer the midline. Tonic innervation, an inability to relax a voluntary contraction, may also occasionally be encountered. A grasp reflex may also be found in chronic hydrocephalus. Frequency, urgency and precipitant micturition may be encountered with tumours and other lesions of this part of the frontal lobe, distinct from the incontinence of dementia (Nathan 1963, Andrew & Nathan 1965).

Massive tumours of the frontal lobe or deeply situated in its posterior part not infrequently give rise to tremor, contralateral or bilateral. The tremor may mimic Parkinsonism though it is rarely as severe and rarely does it affect the fingers so as to produce the so-called pill-rolling movement. Not infrequently and not necessarily accompanied by tremor, the tone of the limbs increases, so that a Parkinson-like rigidity develops. A satisfactory explanation for these disturbances of the extrapyramidal motor system is not forthcoming; in many cases the tumour does not invade the basal ganglia, and indeed it may be a convexity meningioma, but in all cases the tumour is a large one. It may be that size, causing displacement of basal ganglia or their blood supply, is more important than invasion and extensive interruption of nervous activity.

Apart from epilepsy, tumours of the anterior and basal portion of the frontal lobe give rise to little or no focal clinical disturbance until they reach a large size. Destruction of a sufficient quantity of frontal lobe leads to impairment of the mental faculties. In its mildest form this is seen as impairment of memory, lack of concentration, rapid and excessive fatigue. In the family circle it may pass unnoticed, but may declare itself at work by a slowing of activity leading to a diminished wage if this depends upon piece work, or by a poor performance compared with workmates. The housewife finds difficulty in keeping abreast of her daily routine duties. As these symptoms progress they become obvious and merit the term dementia. In the early stages impairment of intellect may not be apparent and work of a repetitive nature may be possible, but careful psychological tests often show a deficit which superficial examination fails to reveal. Sooner or later deterioration of personality declares itself by lack of initiative, disregard for self and for others, slovenly behaviour, lack of personal cleanliness, apathy, slowness at meals and later inability to feed oneself and incontinence of urine and faeces. The affect becomes disturbed. In the early stages there may be a heightened sense of well-being coupled at times with undue jocularity, known as *Witzelsucht*; insight is eventually lost. Later the emotions are dulled; there is little or no reaction to stimuli and the face becomes expressionless.

These symptoms are those which are now recognized as due to frontal lobe deficit, from whatever cause. They arise from lesions in either frontal lobe, and their severity depends upon the intensity and upon the geographical extent of the white matter destruction. The operation of leucotomy and its various modifications has greatly stimulated the study of the functions of the frontal lobe, for long regarded as a 'silent' area, but 'silent' only because appropriate tests were not employed. Elsewhere this subject is taken up in more detail, but it is relevant to the diagnosis of frontal lobe tumours that in patients who have had leucotomy carried out the more severe degrees of dementia and of personality change are seen in those patients in whom the leucotomy has been made in a plane too posterior and exten-

sive brain necrosis has occurred beyond the limits of the leucotomy. Tumours arising in the depths of the posterior part of the frontal lobe more readily produce these symptoms than those situated anteriorly, nearer the pole, when psychometric and neurological tests may fail to expose any deficit. An assessment of mental deterioration is important in order to determine whether the tumour is intrinsic (a glioma or a metastasis) or extrinsic (meningioma). In the former, disintegration is usually rapid and severe unless the glioma is very slowly growing, such as an astrocytoma or oligodendroglioma, in which case there may be extensive 'felting' or induration of the white matter without the interruption of neuronal pathways that is caused by a glioblastoma multiforme. A meningioma may reach a large size, slowly indenting the brain, but without affecting the mental faculties so much, though when papilloedema and oedema of the brain around the tumour develop, mental deterioration proceeds more rapidly though rarely to the extent seen with intrinsic tumours.

Tumours involving the orbital surface of the frontal lobe may cause disturbance of the sense of smell, if they abut on the olfactory bulb or tract. If there has been no severe or long standing rhinitis, anosmia is a valuable sign, for the region of the olfactory plate of the ethmoid is a common site for a meningioma; when it is small the anosmia will be unilateral, when large the tumour compresses both olfactory tracts. A glioma may also impair the sense of smell by pressure upon or by invasion of the olfactory pathways. A distorted sense of smell is rarely caused by tumour and epileptic olfactory hallucinations are caused by lesions further posterior, in the parolfactory area.

## Parietal lobe

Tumours involving the anterior part of the parietal lobe interfere with those varieties of sensibility represented in the post-central gyrus. These are discriminative and include joint sense, vibration sense, tactile localization, light touch, two-point discrimination, stereognosis and *Zahlenschreibenerkenntnis*. The degree to which these diverse qualities are individually affected varies; they are not necessarily equally affected. Where there is some uncertainty as to the presence of abnormality, it is important to test more than one. The distribution of the sensory deficit will be in accordance with the regional cortical representation running parallel with the cortical representation of motor activity. The demonstration of weakness of the part affected by the sensory loss suggests that the tumour has transgressed the central fissure, but it is necessary to distinguish between weakness due to impairment of the motor pathways in which the appropriate reflex changes will be found and weakness due to clumsiness resulting from loss of postural (joint) sensibility. Severe loss interferes greatly with the normal execution of voluntary movements. The tone of the affected limb is diminished and involuntary movements (pseudo-athetosis) may be seen or may be evoked if the patient voluntarily moves the unaffected limb against resistance. Lesions of the postcentral gyrus cause marked muscular wasting of the affected limbs and if the lesion was present in childhood leads to asymmetry of growth (Penfield & Robertson 1943). Extensive subcortical tumours may give rise to impaired appreciation of painful cutaneous stimuli but parietal tumours do not commonly cause analgesia and the mechanism remains obscure. Subcortical lesions may give rise to the suppression of stimuli from the contralateral side of the body, when both sides are stimulated simultaneously at similar points, 'sensory extinction' (Critchley 1949). This is a valuable localizing test, for suppression may be revealed when other sensory deficits are lacking or are equivocal; also known as inattention and perceptual rivalry it may affect the visual fields. When a stimulus (a moving finger) is presented at similar places simultaneously, in both homonymous visual fields the patient perceives the moving finger only in the 'healthy' half field, though unilateral stimulation reveals no hemianopia.

When the tumour occupies a more posterior part of the parietal lobe and if it extends sufficiently deeply, it will involve the upper part of the optic radiation as this emerges from the posterior limb of the internal capsule. These fibres are sweeping lateral to the vestibule of the lateral ventricle, to terminate in the upper lip of the calcarine fissure. Their interruption gives rise to blindness in the lower half of the opposite visual fields, an inferior contralateral homonymous quadrantanopia. Usually the loss does not extend quite to the fixation area and small defects, sector or peripheral, will not be detected unless a careful examination is made on a Bjerrum screen. Careful examination of the visual fields is particularly important in the diagnosis of cerebral tumours, an importance perceived and repeatedly emphasized by Cushing (1921) in a series of papers which still deserve study. The neurosurgeon should learn the technique and become proficient at it; the examination also affords him an opportunity of assessing the patient's concentration and intelligence.

Tumours of the postero-inferior part of the parietal lobe of the dominant hemisphere give rise to dysphasia and to disturbance of the allied activities of reading (dyslexia), writing (dysgraphia) and calculation (dyscalculia).

When the dysphasia is mild it is particularly noticeable in the receptive aspects, so-called sensory dysphasia but when the lesion is extensive the dysphasia becomes global and results in jargon speech; comprehension may be so impaired that communication is virtually extinguished. Gerstmann (1940) described a syndrome which he believed was constantly due to a lesion of the left (i.e. dominant) angular gyrus. It comprised four elements; dysgraphia, dyscalculia, finger agnosia (an inability to identify any of the digits of both hands) and failure to discriminate between right and left, subjectively or objectively. Although it is agreed that these disturbances arise from lesions at the parieto-occipital junction in the dominant hemisphere, the constancy of the four elements and of the relationship to the angular gyrus has been called into question (Critchley 1966).

Other more complex disturbances may be

encountered in tumours which involve the posterior part of the parietal lobe where it joins the temporal and occipital lobes. These include agnosia, a disorder of awareness, or of appreciating the nature of a task; apraxia, a disorder of performance without there being accountable weakness or sensory loss. When marked the resultant disabilities are usually obvious though their analysis may require special knowledge and tests; when slight they easily escape detection or they may be ascribed to obtuseness or to intellectual impairment. A particular form of apraxia is the patient's difficulty to put on his clothes; of agnosia, the neglect by the patient of himself and of extrapersonal space. Neglect of the limbs of one side, of stimuli within the half fields on one side becomes evident to the acute observer in the course of a neurological examination which reveals no coarse abnormal signs to account for it. Failure to discriminate between right and left has been mentioned and allied to this is loss of topographical memory: the patient loses himself in familiar surroundings, for instance his own home and cannot describe a well known route. In general, lesions in the dominant posterior parietal lobe cause bilateral disorders, whereas those in the nondominant hemisphere cause effects limited to the contralateral side.

Epilepsy occurs in about 60% of cases of parietal lobe tumour and as in cases of frontal lobe tumour the nearer to the central sulcus the tumour is situated the more likely it is to cause fits. In Lund's series (1952), epilepsy occurred in 70% of tumours involving the precentral or postcentral gyri, while the incidence for tumours elsewhere in the parietal lobe was 54%. Penfield and Erickson (1941) gave 71% and 68% respectively for tumours in these sites. In about half the cases the epileptic seizure is of a focal sensory nature, comprising sensations of tingling, pins and needles, numbness, pain or burning. The arm, leg and face are the regions most often affected, in that order of frequency, but face, arm, and leg is the order of frequency for motor seizures. Lund's detailed analysis of the localization of tumours giving rise to focal motor and to focal sensory fits gives numerical emphasis to

what is common clinical experience, that focal seizures are not invariably accurate indicators of the site of the tumour. Precentral tumours may give rise to sensory and post-central tumours to motor phenomena and tumours in other parts of the cerebrum may occasionally cause focal seizures of a motor or sensory nature. Generalized convulsions may occur as a result of a tumour anywhere in the cerebrum and afford no help in localization, except to the extent that they are more likely to occur if the tumour is situated deeply, or in the frontal lobe. But the deeper the tumour is situated the less frequently does epilepsy develop and it may be said in general that the incidence falls as the distance from the sensorimotor cortex increases in any direction. An easy fallacy may creep in here, however, as the deeper neoplasms are more rapidly growing and this may account for the low incidence of seizures (Penfield & Erickson 1941).

### Occipital lobe

The outstanding feature of tumours in the occipital lobe is the loss of contralateral (homonymous) fields of vision and the extent and the situation of the loss will depend upon the location and size of the tumour. Involvement of the upper or the lower lip of the calcarine fissure will cause an inferior or superior quadrantic loss respectively. A tumour must be relatively small if it is to spare the opposing lip and it is likely to be a meningioma arising from the falx. Intrinsic tumours usually affect the whole of the optic radiation as it reaches the deep surface of the visual cortex and the hemianopic defect is then total, reaching to the fixation point. If the tumour is situated more laterally, that is near the convexity, the fixation area is spared. Tumours of the extreme tip of the lobe, the occipital pole, will particularly affect those fibres derived from the macula and if small enough will produce a scotoma of hemianopic shape (this is a rare finding in expanding lesions but common in gunshot injuries). The patient is often unaware of the loss of vision, except that he complains of a liability to collide with objects in the affected half field. A left hemianopia may cause difficulty in reading (quite apart from the dyslexia which results if the tumour extends into the parietal lobe in the dominant hemisphere) because the word beginning each line cannot be easily identified as the eyes scan the printed page. A right hemianopia causes no such difficulty.

Epilepsy occurs less commonly in tumours of the occipital lobe. Lund (1952) cites 33%, Penfield and Erickson (1941) 32% and Tönnis (1962) 11.6%. The seizure may take the form of abnormal visual sensations and hallucinations and comprise crude or unformed disturbances in the appropriate half field of light, colour, or dimness. Similar disturbances may occur in tumours involving the posterior (i.e. contiguous) parts of the parietal and temporal lobes, although in the latter the hallucinations are more likely to be highly organized and associated with other disturbances described below. Penfield and Rasmussen (1950) reported that visual hallucinations of an unformed nature were evoked in 22 patients as a result of stimulation, and in all it was occipital cortex that was stimulated; such strict localization is not the case when the epileptic response is due to tumour. Cairns (1939) observed visual hallucinations in 10 cases of occipital tumour and 21 of temporal tumour and in his opinion they could occur as a result of a tumour anywhere in the cerebrum.


## Temporal lobe

Tumours of the temporal lobe may remain clinically 'silent' until raised intracranial pressure enforces medical aid, or they may give rise to outspoken localizing symptoms, according to their position in the lobe and to its dominance. Tumours situated in the anterior extremity (pole) of the lobe may reach a considerable size and remain silent; meningiomas arising from the outer and middle third of the sphenoid ridge, whether right or left, are difficult to diagnose clinically. The same applies to tumours in the inferior part of the lobe (and consequently to the infrequent meningiomas arising from the floor of the middle fossa). But when the tumour is large enough to encroach upon the upper part of the lobe (or when it originates there) it will involve the inferior part of the optic radiation (Meyer's loop), resulting in a homonymous upper quadrantanopia. This is in sharp contrast to the inferior quadrantic defect produced by parietal lobe lesions. Cushing (1922) drew attention to the nature of these visual field defects (present in 33 of 39 cases) and emphasized the importance of careful examination of the visual fields. A tumour in this situation in the dominant hemisphere also gives rise to nominal dysphasia, and if extensive, to the more severe and global disturbances of speech and allied functions described earlier (parietal lobe tumours).

Tumours in the deep (medial) part of the temporal lobe may cause severe loss of memory for recent events, sufficient to bring about a state of dementia; the patient may confabulate and present the syndrome of Korsakov's psychosis. This may be due to involvement of the hippocampus and its connections.

Mental disturbance of a different character may be encountered, such as occurs in some patients with so-called temporal lobe epilepsy though when caused by a tumour, epilepsy may not occur or may not be a prominent symptom. Emotional instability with a particular inclination to bad temper and an exaggerated reaction to slight or imagined offence which may lead to aggressiveness; continuing carping criticism; a paranoid outlook; an unreasonable attitude and intolerance of opposition or contrary advice; these qualities may render the patient a very difficult member of the family.

Epilepsy is a frequent symptom of a tumour in the temporal lobe; in Lund's analysis it occurred in 63% of cases, nearly as frequent as in Rolandic tumours. But Tönnis (1962) puts the incidence as low as 37%, and Penfield and Erickson (1941) 48%. It is likely that the highest figure is most accurate, when the incidence of small, unsuspected tumours revealed at operation undertaken for temporal lobe epilepsy is taken into consideration. There is a great diversity of pattern in the seizures which may be encountered. They may be focal motor (12% in Lund's series arose from temporal lobe tumours) affecting usually face, arm or leg. Hallucinations of taste are more commonly due to tumour in the temporal lobe than elsewhere and out of 21 cases with such attacks, the temporal lobe was involved in 14 and in 10 of these tumours had directly involved the hippocampus or 'had come very close to that structure'. Hallucinations of smell also occur; the temporal lobe was involved in 13 of 18 patients with this type of seizure. Although paroxysms of abnormal sensations of taste or smell are not common when compared with other epileptic manifestations, constituting 12% of all cases of tumour with epilepsy, the symptom is valuable in indicating that the temporal lobe and probably its deep surface is implicated. Focal seizures are of much greater localizing value as an initial symptom than when they arise in the later stages, when herniation of the uncus and hippocampus may be the cause. Visual hallucinations of a crude, unorganized nature may be evoked by tumours in the temporal lobe usually in the posterior part where the lobe merges with the adjoining parietal and occipital lobes. They have already been discussed. Unorganized auditory hallucinations (not to be confused with tinnitus of labyrinthine origin) are rare symptoms in these patients. Paroxysmal disturbances of speech may occur in tumours of the temporal lobe (and with about equal frequency in those of the frontal and parietal lobes). There is an inability to speak, sometimes initiating the attack, or developing during or after other accompaniments; the speech centres are temporarily paralysed for 'words are never produced by electrical stimulations and do not occur as a positive manifestation of epileptic discharge' (Penfield & Erickson 1941). Such attacks usually arise as a result of a lesion in the dominant hemisphere, though they occasionally occur with lesions in which is presumed to be the non-dominant hemisphere.

Of greater significance are certain bizarre epileptic patterns which have a much higher incidence in tumours in the temporal lobe than elsewhere. They comprise *déjà vu* dreamy states, psychical illusory states, highly organized auditory hallucinations and organized dream-like visual hallucinations. They may be accompanied or preceded by gustatory and olfactory hallucinations and by disturbances of autonomic activities, salivation, flushing, sweating and abdominal rumblings. Careful observations often reveal slight automatic movements such as smacking of lips, chewing and swallowing and sometimes a more prolonged period of complicated purposeful but inappropriate automatic behaviour ensues. In Lund's series there were 35 patients with dreamy states (used as a broadly inclusive term and including other accompanying seizure patterns) and in 29 the temporal lobe was involved.

## Corpus callosum

Considerable attention has been paid to the functions of the corpus callosum in recent years, by studying the effects of its partial and total division in animals and in man. Natural destructive lesions in man usually involve neighbouring portions of the cerebrum on one or both sides and the effects of these may overshadow those of callosal interruption.

Tumours originating in and confined to the corpus callosum are uncommon, though extension into it from either hemisphere is frequent Bull (1967) analysed autopsy records of 200 cases of cerebral astrocytoma and found that the corpus callosum was involved in 72 (36%). The commissure affords a bridge whereby gliomas can spread to the opposite cerebrum and those arising within the corpus callosum may spread symmetrically so that a horizontal section of the brain displays a butterfly-shaped mass of growth; thus in large tumours the symptoms and signs depend upon the portion of the hemispheres invaded.

When the middle third is affected, early bilateral signs of motor and sensory disturbance develop as a result of invasion of the adjacent motor and sensory pathways, in which the lower limbs may be more affected than the upper; the deficit is rarely symmetrical, nor are the feet predominantly affected as in bilateral para-sagittal meningiomas. In the posterior part of the corpus callosum, a particularly uncommon situation, the tumour will give rise to little obvious disability until it spreads deeply in either parieto-occipital region and before that happens the mass may cause severe symptoms of intra-cranial hypertension by obstructing the posterior part of the third ventricle; in this coronal plane the falx has considerable depth so that there is little space between its free edge and the third ventricle and upper brain stem to accommodate a mass of tumour. Disturbances of ocular move-ments, particularly upward gaze, may be caused by pressure downwards on the superior colliculi, mimicking a pineal tumour. When the tumour arises in the anterior part of the corpus callosum where the falx is narrow, there is plenty of room and the tumour may reach a large size before causing much disturbance of intracranial pres-sure. Indeed, as these tumours are commonly infiltrative gliomas in elderly subjects, it is a fre-quent surprise at post-mortem examination that such a large tumour should have given such a short history. The chief symptoms are pro-gressive dementia (Harrison 1984) and per-sonality changes, though from the size of tumour revealed at post-mortem examination, it is clear that these symptoms do not become manifest until the tumour has spread laterally into the frontal lobe, so that the symptoms are as likely to be due to frontal lobe deficit as to loss of the commissure. Thus most tumours of the corpus callosum present no specific clinical picture but should be suspected when progressive dementia is an outstanding feature and when there are signs of bilateral hemisphere involvement. Spec-ific callosal syndromes will be detected only if the tumour is relatively small and appropriate tests are made.

Evidence of the relief of epilepsy by section of the corpus callosum in whole (i.e. from anterior to posterior commissure) or in part is conflicting, varying from modest reduction especially in falling seizures but not in general and focal seiz-ures (Rayport 1983, Gates *et al.* 1984) to favour-able reduction in seizures when prior depth electrode recording determines the area of cal-losal section (Bouvier & St Hilaire 1983). Sur-prisingly in most patients there are few detectable adverse neurological effects, but the minutiae of so-called disconnection syndromes have been reviewed extensively by Geschwind (1965).

## Basal ganglia and thalamus

Although these structures are frequently invaded by neighbouring gliomas, tumours arising within them are not common. Their chief symp-toms relate to involvement of the internal capsule, with consequent contralateral motor, sensory and hemianopic defects. In the early stages the hemiparesis may only be evident to the examiner and is more frequent than the sensory impairment. The latter may involve all varieties of sensation or some may be preserved intact. It is unusual for these patients to experience the syndrome of spontaneous pain and dysaesthesia of Dejerine and Roussy (1906) but distortion of cutaneous sensation amounting to discomfort is more frequent. Tremor may occur but complex involuntary movements are rare and other stri-atal disturbances such as waxy muscular rigid-ity, akinesia and bradykinesia are normally ter-minal features. Ataxia and nystagmus may be present and with the tremor these signs may suggest a cerebellar localization. Pupillary inequality, impairment of reaction and impaired conjugate movement may also occur (McKissock & Paine 1958). Ataxia and ocular disturbances are due to involvement of midbrain structures by pressure or infiltration.

Epilepsy was present in one-fifth of the cases reported by Tovi *et al.* (1961) and in some it resembled the clinical pattern of petit-mal, but a diversity of attacks occurs, and there is no localizing significance.

When mental symptoms occur, including dull-ness, intellectual slowing and overt dementia, they are more likely to be due to expansion of the tumour medially causing compression of the third ventricle and thereby hydrocephalus, than to any more specific localized lesion such as the dorsomedial nucleus of the thalamus (Arseni 1958).

## Lateral ventricles

Gliomas arising in the centrum ovale and in the basal ganglia frequently extend as a lobulated mass into the lateral ventricle, the para-ventricular glioma. There they may grow to a size which causes surprise at necropsy, but the pattern of clinical disturbance which they evoke is largely that due to the portion within the brain tissue itself. The tumours now to be considered are those which, while they arise from tissues forming the walls of or contained within the ventricle, are situated virtually entirely within the cavity of the ventricle and invade brain tissue not at all or only to a negligible degree. Negligible, that is, so far as the production of neurological disturbance is concerned; from the point of view of surgical removal, a slight extension into the wall of the ventricle may render the procedure hazardous. Provided a lateral ventricle tumour does not extend into the third ventricle it may reach a large size, moulding itself to the ventricular cavity; cerebrospinal fluid passes around its surface to reach the third ventricle. Symptoms and signs are largely due to direct pressure on structures in or adjacent to the walls of the ventricle. The tumours encountered are glioma, meningioma, choroid plexus papilloma and epidermoid. The history is usually predominantly of intracranial hypertension due to the size of the tumour over a period of several years, with sometimes vague symptoms or episodic disturbance of sensory and motor function of the limbs on one side.

Examination may disclose no localizing signs but sometimes there is a mild motor and sensory hemiparesis and in most cases of meningioma a hemianopia, perhaps because these tumours commonly occupy the vestibule of the ventricle where the optic radiation sweeps around its lateral surface. In the case of the choroid plexus papilloma of infants the presentation is one of hydrocephalus with papilloedema.

### Third ventricle and hypothalamus

The commonest tumour is glioma and these tend to occupy the middle or posterior parts of the cavity. Colloid cyst and craniopharyngioma arise in the anterior part. Other tumours are choroid plexus papilloma, epidermoid cyst and teratoma. Tumours arising in the pineal body invaginate themselves into the posterior part of the ventricle.

Hydrocephalus dominates the picture; the symptoms of intracranial hypertension may be acute and fulminating, remittent, slowly progressive or virtually absent. In the last two groups, great enlargement of the lateral ventricles may give rise to dementia and disorders of the motor system. Headache is often aggravated by straining and certain positions of the head, though this feature is not by any means restricted to cases of third ventricle obstruction. A characteristic symptom is sudden and transient loss of tone of the limbs, so that the patient without warning abruptly falls, without loss of consciousness. The anteriorly placed tumours and those invading the floor of the ventricle are liable to cause disturbances attributable to interference with hypothalamic specialized functions, namely hypersomnia, stupor, transient disturbances of consciousness, diabetes insipidus and mellitus, obesity, endocrine disturbances and autonomic upsets. Tumours in the posterior extremity of the third ventricle may cause neurological signs indicating a lesion of the superior colliculi and tegmental portion of the midbrain; consequently the distinction from pineal tumour and midbrain tumour may be difficult.

The 'juvenile' astrocytoma of the third ventricle arises anteriorly so that early in its evolution it may infiltrate the optic chiasm and hypothalamic centres.

On account of its anatomical position the earliest symptoms relate to vision and to disturbance of hypothalamic function. Infiltration of the optic chiasma gives rise to the chiasmal syndrome but, because the subjects are usually young, detailed analysis of the visual failure may not be possible. Vision is impaired so insidiously that only at a late stage do the parents appreciate that the child is becoming blind. In older subjects in whom acuity and visual fields can be accurately assessed, visual loss is usually asymmetrical and the fields of an irregular pattern. Primary optic atrophy is present.

Gliomas invading the floor of the third ventricle infiltrate the tuber cinereum and, like craniopharyngiomas in this region, give rise to diabetes insipidus, and to lack of sexual development if the patient is old enough. In both tumours, the chiasm may or may not be affected at the time the patient present for treatment and obstructive hydrocephalus develops sooner or later. In consequence their clinical distinction may be impossible.

Gliomas in the tuberal part of the third ventricle may give rise to precocious puberty. Bauer (1954) reviewed the literature of hypothalamic disease and found 60 cases in which necropsy had been performed; pubertas praecox was present in 24 and the commonest lesion was a glioma. Such gliomas are usually astrocytomas, firmer in texture than the usual juvenile type just discussed, but ependymoma and ganglioglioma have also been described.

The intraventricular ependymoma usually occupies the posterior part of the third ventricle, where it is well placed to obstruct the mouth of the Sylvian aqueduct, giving rise to obstructive hydrocephalus.

### Optic nerve and chiasm

Glioma restricted to one optic nerve usually arises within the orbit and gives rise to progressive failure of vision of that eye and to proptosis. Only when the glioma has extended into the chiasm is vision of the other eye affected, consequently accurate measurement of the visual acuity and charting of the fields are of great importance. Since these tumours are

common in children this information may be difficult to obtain. The tumours grow slowly, so that diagnosis may at first be uncertain and only repeated examinations reveal the progressive nature of the lesion. The typical pattern of field disturbance is a scotoma in the first instance, central or paracentral, subsequently breaking outwards to form a loss in the periphery. A central scotoma causes marked loss of acuity although the peripheral field remains normal while a paracentral scotoma may easily escape detection. A concomitant squint, due to the amaurosis, is a common early finding. The proptosis is usually painless, without deviation of the globe which retains its mobility until the tumour reaches a large size. Unilateral failure of vision in association with proptosis in a child renders the diagnosis fairly certain, for meningioma, aneurysm and other causes of this symptom complex occur in a much older age group. On occasion defective vision may precede the proptosis for a long time. Primary optic atrophy is commonly present, though papilloedema may occur and if the tumour impinges on the back of the globe the optic disc may become more prominent by invagination. A careful search should be made for evidence of von Recklinghausen's disease, in the patient or in a relative; *café au lait* patches are present in about 20% of the patients. Extension of the tumour backwards through the optic foramen expands the latter and radiological examination of the optic foramina is an essential investigation. Many years may elapse before the tumour involves the chiasm, a development that is revealed by a defect in the visual field of the other eye. Spread of the tumour into the other optic nerve causes enlargement of its foramen.

Gliomas arising in the optic chiasm disturb vision in both eyes, though in the early stages the field defects tend to be irregular and incongruous. Extension into both optic nerves causing enlargement of both optic foramina occurs at an early stage in contrast to the glioma of the optic nerve. 75% of these tumours occur in children under the age of twelve (Matson 1969) and the tumours may grow very slowly over the course of many years, which is consistent with the relatively benign histological features of what are almost always low grade astrocytic gliomas.

## Management of supratentorial malignant gliomas

### Introduction

Management includes clinical diagnosis, differential diagnosis, decisions concerning degree of urgency of investigation, this proceeding to therapy which may include surgery, radiotherapy and chemotherapy. Syndromes related to specific supratentorial regions have already been described, but it is necessary to add some more general remarks about the presentation of the tumours, and the order of decisions which need to be made in the management of an individual patient. Particular attention will be drawn to problems of differential diagnosis, danger signals and pitfalls which include the dangerous assumption that the patient has an inoperable or untreatable lesion. Radiology has been covered elsewhere (*see* Chapter 3) but comments will be made about limitations of radiology in management.

### General presentation

Owing to their slow growth, the astrocytomas and the oligodendrogliomas provide some of the longest histories amongst intracranial tumours. The average duration of symptoms before diagnosis is some 3–4 years, though the range extends from a few months to 30 years (Reymond & Ringertz 1950, Levy & Elvidge 1956). Epilepsy is the symptom which may for so many years antedate progressive neurological deficit and raised intracranial pressure, manifestations leading to a definitive diagnosis of tumour. In his analysis of 'Epilepsy in association with intracranial tumour', Lund (1952) found that its frequency was as shown in Table 5.3.

In those cases in which the lesion lay in the

Table 5.3. Frequency of epilepsy in association with intracranial tumours (Lund 1952).

| Tumour | Percentage |
| --- | --- |
| oligodendroglioma | 81 |
| vascular malformation | 79 |
| astrocytoma | 66 |
| glioblastoma | 42 |
| meningioma | 40 |
| metastasis | 19 |

vicinity of the central sulcus this order was maintained with the exception that vascular malformations headed the list. When epilepsy occurred it was the initial symptom in a very high percentage, for example oligodendroglioma 95%, astrocytoma 81% and meningioma 65%. The significance of epilepsy as an early symptom of a slowly growing glioma is also underlined by the records of the Montreal Neurological Institute (Rasmussen & Blundell 1961). During a period of 30 years, when 1108 operations for epilepsy were performed, a tumour was encountered in 171 cases. Of these, the tumour was a glioma in 127, (74%), the astrocytoma being much the most frequent (in 77 cases, 44%). The Montreal experience also confirms Lund's Scandinavian figures, that a long history of epilepsy is more likely to be due to a glioma than a meningioma; there were only 15 meningiomas (9%) among the 171 cases with tumour. Numerical evidence is also brought out by these analyses and by Tönnis (1962) confirming general clinical 'impressions' that a glioblastoma is the least likely glioma to produce epilepsy. At variance with these findings are those of Penman and Smith (1954) for in their series of gliomas epilepsy occured with virtually equal frequency in glioblastoma (47%) and in astrocytoma (43%). The reason for this discrepancy is not apparent.

The chronological sequence of other and more definite manifestations of a slowly growing glioma of the cerebral hemispheres varies considerably. If the tumour is situated in an 'eloquent' part of the brain, for instance the paracentral lobule, so that disturbance of neurological function is obvious to the patient, this is usually the next (or in the absence of epilepsy, the first) symptom to develop. But evidence of this kind, due to infiltration and disorganization of nervous tissue by the slowly infiltrating glioma may escape the patient's notice. Many patients are unaware of a quadrantanopia, though when fully developed a hemianopia is brought to their attention by collisions with objects on the blind side. Failing memory and intellect and personality disturbances may be coupled with lack of insight and more apparent to others than to the patient and their development without epilepsy and without symptoms of raised intracranial pressure may lead to the false assumption that they are psychogenic rather than organic. But although the gliomas invade and destroy brain tissue, the diffuse, low-grade astrocytoma may attain a considerable bulk yet the enveloped neural elements still function; in this event intracranial hypertensive symptoms may precede paralytic signs. The glioblastoma and anaplastic astrocytoma often provide the reverse of this; widespread and rapid neurological deficit with little evidence of raised intracranial pressure. The propensity for astrocytomas to become cystic adds an unpredictable variant to chronological sequence and thereby makes diagnosis more difficult. The formation of a cyst may occur at any time during the growth of an astrocytoma, that is to say when the tumour is small so that it may have given rise to few or no symptoms, or when it is already large and has caused symptoms for perhaps several years. A small cyst is of no significance, but if a large amount of fluid collects rapidly the evolutionary pattern changes dramatically. Rapid expansion of the mass gives rise to rapidly increasing intracranial pressure, at a speed which may threaten life within days or weeks.

Notwithstanding the anomalies revealed by analysis restricted to necropsy studies, there is no doubt that the outstanding characteristic of the glioblastoma is its rapid and destructive growth, whether it develops primarily as such, or by anaplasia in a pre-existing astrocytoma. The duration of symptoms prior to admission to hospital is commonly only two or three months

(Krayenbühl 1959) and is often as short as two or three weeks. As noted earlier, the peak of incidence is at a later age than for other gliomas, rising and falling abruptly over the period of 50–70 years. Because of this late age incidence there is often little or only terminal evidence of raised intracranial pressure, the somewhat shrunken brain of elderly people providing more room for the expanding tumour than would be the case in the younger patient. The infiltrative and destructive nature of this tumour is also in part responsible for this characteristic clinical picture, for a considerable amount of brain may be entirely replaced by the growth with relatively little increase in bulk. The vascular hyperplasia and endothelial proliferation which is such a striking feature of its histology may be associated with episodic deterioration due to spontaneous haemorrhage, thrombosis and necrosis. The illness may terminate abruptly as a result of a massive haemorrhage. Because of an abrupt onset and of rapid deterioration a diagnosis of cerebral thrombosis is not infrequently made early in the illness; such a diagnosis is partially correct in the sense that a vascular 'accident' has occured, but incorrect, or rather incomplete, in that this is but a complication arising in a tumour, the diagnosis of which becomes clearer as deterioration progresses. The rapidity and invasiveness of its spread, its destructiveness, the size this tumour can attain, and the frequency with which it arises in the frontal and temporal lobes, account for certain common clinical features. In an analysis by Krayenbühl (1959) of 422 cases of glioblastoma, three-quarters were frontal or frontoparietal, temporal or temporoparietal or corpus callosum in situation. Extensive replacement of brain by tumour in these regions should result in outspoken mental disturbance or paralytic signs, or both. In fact the commonest sign was paresis (in 348 patients) and the next commonest was mental disturbance (in 326 patients). Headache was the commonest symptom (in 319 patients). Papilloedema was absent in rather more than half the patients.

To summarize, the glioblastoma is characterized by a short illness of only a few weeks or months, which may develop insiduously but inexorably, or may be marked by step-like episodes of deterioration; headache is frequent though papilloedema as often as not is absent; evidence of neurological disorder is manifest by progressive obfuscation, dementia and by such coarse paralytic signs as hemiparesis, both motor and sensory, hemianopia and dysphasia. Epilepsy may occur but it is less common than in other forms of glioma.

Certain features may lead to particular difficulties in management. There is great variation in the presence of the classical symptom and signs of raised intracranial pressure, even between patients with seemingly similar mass lesions. Despite the traditional description of the headache of raised intracranial pressure being dull, throbbing, generalized, worse on awakening and aggravated by coughing and stooping, none of these features can be relied upon. The safest criterion is that for a particular patient, headache of whatever character, is a new or changed symptom. Why the headache of raised intracranial pressure should be episodic with remissions of days or even weeks, is not understood. Shift and displacement of brain may for a time relieve symptoms of raised intracranial pressure, only for it to rise again as tumour expansion continues. Slowing of the pulse, and a rise in blood pressure are relatively late signs of raised intracranial pressure, as is overt deterioration in level of consciousness. Papilloedema is present in only 30% of patients immediately prior to surgery for intracranial mass lesions (Garfield, personal observation).

Finally, tumours in certain areas may become very large before they produce either focal neurological disturbance or severe symptoms of raised intracranial pressure. These 'silent areas' are the anterior temporal region, especially in the non-dominant hemisphere, the frontal pole, the subfrontal region, the corpus callosum, the septum pellucidum, and the space within the lateral ventricles.

## Decision in clinical management

When the neurologist or neurosurgeon is faced with a patient who may have a malignant supratentorial tumour he must rapidly consider:

1 The degree of urgency of investigation;
2 Anatomical localization, and in particular whether the lesion is above or below the tentorium;
3 The differential diagnosis.

### The degree of urgency of investigation

This depends primarily upon the severity of raised intracranial pressure and the likelihood of uncal herniation at the tentorial hiatus (coning). Danger signals include overt deterioration of level of consciousness, bouts of very severe headache with vomiting, episodic or sustained impairment of visual acuity, and pronounced bradycardia. Even if papilloedema is absent or only mild, these danger signals are no less important. If the patient has had a lumbar puncture during the preceding hours, the dangers of coning are greater. The assumption of intracranial malignancy, however strong, should not diminish the importance of the warning signs.

### Anatomical localization

For purposes of immediate management the main clinical localization needed is the differentiation between a lateralized supratentorial and an infratentorial mass lesion; to that should be added the rare case of acute chiasmal compression. Cardinal localizing signs for supratentorial lesions are focal epilepsy, dysphasia and homonymous visual field defect. It is unusual for an infratentorial lesion to produce a hemiparesis and virtually impossible for it to produce a homonymous field defect, and it cannot ever produce dysphasia. With the advent of CT scanning, more precise clinical localization is not required, at least in the initial management of an acute situation.

*Differential diagnosis*

The most important differential diagnoses of the supratentorial malignant tumour, with their particular difficulties, can be classified as follows:

(a) *other mass lesions*: Intracranial abscess and especially the more chronic cerebral abscess may mimic a malignant tumour, and in particular the anaplastic astrocytoma, glioblastoma and metastases. The absence of fever or any evidence of sepsis elsewhere including the middle ear or paranasal sinuses, with normal haematology and erythrocyte sedimentation rate, do not exclude an abscess and make the diagnosis very difficult; some 30% of abscesses are of unknown aetiology (Garfield 1969).

*Chronic subdural haematoma* may also mimic a supratentorial tumour, although strongly lateralized hemisphere signs are not common with a haematoma. *Benign tumours* and especially the meningioma, may sometimes present with a short history, indistinguishable from that of a malignant tumour.

(b) *Vascular lesions*: The stroke-like presentation of malignant (and also benign) hemisphere tumours is well known, but poorly understood. Occasionally haemorrhage may occur and produce a significant *intracerebral haematoma* exerting mass effect, but this is rare. The presence of very small and even microscopic haemorrhages is not sufficient explanation for the stroke-like evolution of these tumours. The explanation is more likely to be *ischaemic*, either through pressure of the tumour, and its surrounding brain swelling (oedema), upon arteries, especially branches of the middle cerebral or it is related to thrombosed vessels frequently seen macroscopically within the tumours at surgery. The exponential relationship between the volume of a mass and intracranial pressure means that although pressure may rise little at first, in the late stages sudden surges of intracranial hypertension can reduce perfusion pressure abruptly to cause cerebral ischaemia.

Conversely a major *cerebral or cortical infarction* may mimic a malignant tumour when, not infrequently, the history is one of steady progression and not of sudden onset or step-wise progression.

*Inflammatory diseases*: Although relatively rare, the indolent course of *tuberculous meningitis*, especially in the elderly, may mimic a malignant tumour, and is easily overlooked even when investigations have not revealed a tumour. The very rare *tuberculoma*, rare at least in European practice, may mimic exactly the lateralized supratentorial malignant tumours, especially the low-grade astrocytoma and oligodendroglioma; a *syphilitic gumma* will also mimic a glioma. *Sarcoidosis*, a diagnosis which is difficult to substantiate even with biopsy of arachnoid, may also be confused with a malignant brain tumour. Occasionally *viral encephalitis* may mimic a malignant tumour, although usually the course of this disease is shorter and the patient more acutely and generally ill, with nuchal rigidity in addition to the other signs.

Of the *degenerative conditions*, the *pre-senile* and other *dementias* may mimic tumours (Marsden & Harrison 1972) especially the intrinsic frontal tumour and those of the corpus callosum (Harrison 1984), as may the rare, and often disputed, cases of cerebral *multiple sclerosis*.

## Investigations

With the increasing availability in recent years of noninvasive methods of investigation, especially CT scanning, there is less reluctance to submit patients to intracranial investigations, even when neurological symptoms and disability are mild. The issue of clinical differential diagnosis, at least in the nonurgent circumstances, might seem, therefore, to have become less important. By the same token, the elderly are no longer spared the neurosurgeon's attention, something that is not always to the benefit of the patient. However, many medical and surgical centres do not have access to CT and careful clinical differential diagnosis and assessment *before* investigation encourages the surgeon to manage the patient rather than the CT scan appearances; nowhere is this more important than in dealing with patients with malignant tumours.

## General medical investigations

Certain of these are especially relevant. All patients should have a *chest radiograph*, not simply as part of the search for a primary or metastatic growth, but also to exclude tuberculosis, and as a guide to fitness for major surgery. *Anaemia* needs investigation and correction, a raised *sedimentation rate* may suggest generalized malignancy or an intracranial abscess, but the *white blood count* usually does little more than exclude a leukaemia, or raise suspicion of a lymphoma. The realities of hospital practice rarely allow the rapid diagnosis of neurosyphilis, which is fortunately a very rare, albeit eminently treatable, differential diagnosis.

## Electroencephalography (EEG)

For a variety of reasons the value and use of EEG in the diagnosis and management of patients with brain tumours has declined in recent years, *pari passu* with the advances in radiological imaging. It is rare for a careful history not to clarify whether episodic attacks are or are not epileptic. Apart from the occasional difficulties with circulatory disturbances and hysteria, recourse to the EEG usually implies inadequate history taking from the patient and relatives. Furthermore, a normal EEG never excludes epilepsy. EEG localization of tumours is now less important. It is often inaccurate, and changes on serial EEG are not an acceptable guide to the need for further investigations. Indeed unless epilepsy is known to have been present from an early age, the diagnostic label of 'idiopathic' is now largely without meaning. Only after full investigation by CT scanning, nuclear magnetic resonance imaging and above all after a sufficient period of negative follow-up, can epilepsy be said to be truly idiopathic; even then the low grade astrocytoma may not declare its presence in any other way.

## Radiology

This has been dealt with fully in Chapter 3. Reference here will be made only to a few practical points. As with absence of papilloedema, so also the absence of evidence on plain skull radiographs of raised intracranial pressure can never exclude that condition. Conversely, skull radiographs may occasionally provide valuable evidence of long standing increased pressure with few, or none of the clinical features, which may be helpful in the diagnosis of benign intracranial hypertension in the presence of a normal CT scan. In an emergency, especially when a CT scan is not immediately available, the position of the calcified pineal or choroid plexus seen on skull radiographs may differentiate rapidly between supratentorial and infratentorial mass lesions; for the hydrocephalus of the latter an immediate burr hole for lateral ventricular drainage without further radiology may be life-saving. For a supratentorial lateralized mass lesion, as with all other lesions, *CT scan* is the ideal method of investigation; but if it is not available, the older investigations of *carotid angiography* or *isotope scanning* may yet be useful. The clinician should be aware that CT may not be able to differentiate between abscess and tumour, and magnetic resonance imaging does not clearly define the margins of a glioma. When there is neither clinical nor plain skull radiograph evidence of a lateralized supratentorial mass, and CT scanning is not available, positive contrast ventriculography may delineate a tumour accurately if it is related to the ventricular system. Even in this era of noninvasive imaging, neurosurgeons should be able to do a ventriculogram and give radiographic advice.

# Surgery of supratentorial malignant gliomas

## Introduction

Despite the increasing accuracy of pre-operative diagnosis due mainly to advances in radiology, decisions about surgery for the individual patient may still be very difficult. In every case a series of questions arises, to many of which the answers can only be a matter of personal opinion and speculation, often swayed by the views, understandably emotional, expressed by the patient and the family (Garfield 1980). Points for consideration are:

1   the need for histological diagnosis;
2   the hazards and accuracy of limited biopsy by craniotomy or burr hole and the place of stereotactic biopsy;
3   the relief of symptoms;
4   the influence of tumour removal upon the longterm survival;
5   the influence of surgery upon quality of life.

### The need for histological diagnosis

The answer to this question lies in the accuracy and reliability of radiology, and the availability of 'treatment', if the diagnosis is confirmed; as a corollary it is assumed that non-malignant lesions, such as meningioma and abscess are both treatable and curable. Despite the great advances in radiology, and especially CT scanning, confusion between glioma and abscess still occurs; when it is more widely available, MRI may reduce these errors. But while patients still have to be managed with imperfect radiological techniques, it remains a wise counsel that 'no patient should be allowed to die without the pathology being established'. Clearly this maxim must be tempered depending upon the site of the lesion; thus a tumour infiltrating the corpus callosum, and fanning out into one or both cerebral hemispheres is not amenable to surgery, and the radiological appearances can only be those of a malignant primary tumour, so that it may be reasonable to forgo histological verification. Similarly a thalamic mass, with or without contrast enhancement on CT, may be suitable only for stereotactic biopsy (see below), a technique not necessarily available in every neurosurgical department. In those circumstances it may be considered reasonable to accept the presumed histological diagnosis, deal with the hydrocephalus and give radiotherapy. However, in general, it is unwise to embark upon radiotherapy without histological verification of the tumour; few radiotherapists would accept such a course (see below). This becomes even more important when chemotherapy is contemplated, because of the toxic nature of the treatment. Finally, if any form of trial of therapy is to be conducted histology is essential, preferably from several areas of the tumour.

### Methods of biopsy

The traditional, somewhat nihilistic approach is the simple *burr hole biopsy*, in which a cannula is passed into the brain, usually in several directions and vigorous suction is applied when a tumour, or more realistically a change in resistance to the exploring cannula, is felt. In experienced hands, the histological specimen usually gives the diagnosis, provided the pathologist is also experienced in immediate examination of small amounts of tissue by smear or frozen section. However the morbidity and mortality of this method of biopsy are significant because haemorrhage due to the exploring cannula cannot be controlled. Therefore this method is acceptable only if (a) an experienced pathologist is immediately available to confirm or refute the expected diagnosis of a malignant tumour for which there is no indication for an attempt at total or partial removal, or (b) the surgeon can proceed without delay to craniotomy if the diagnosis is not established, or a benign tumour is present, especially if there is any deterioration in the patient's level of consciousness following the biopsy.

As well as its hazards, burr hole biopsy has considerable limitations in its accuracy. Reactive gliosis and perivascular cuffing occur in association with malignant tumours, but they may also occur in the neighbourhood of cerebral abscess, benign tumours and infarcts. Necrotic tissue without any identifiable tumour cells is often present at the centre of the more malignant gliomas (glioblastoma multiforme and anaplastic astrocytoma), but the tissue may not permit accurate identification or characterization of the lesion, and it may be confused with an infarct. Finally the tissue obtained may not be representative of the overall grade of malignancy which may vary from one part of the tumour to another, and upon which a rational approach to treatment should be based.

*Biopsy at craniotomy* avoids most of the hazards and limitations of burr hole biopsy, but by its very nature may lead the surgeon to be more aggressive than is warranted in the light of the malignancy and location of the tumour and the prospects of survival with disability and distressing deficit.

*Stereotactic biopsy* is a technique which has gained ground in recent years, and avoids much of the hazards of 'free hand' burr hole biopsy, while achieving accuracy without the need for open craniotomy; it is particularly suitable for deeply situated lesions, including those in the thalamus and midbrain. The technique requires the placement of a stereotactic frame in conjunction with localization by CT. The safety of the procedure allows multiple biopsies to be taken from different parts of the lesion, and the histological appearances can, to some extent, be correlated with the different CT scan characteristics (Daumas-Duport *et al.* 1983). A variety of sterotactic frames are available (Thomas *et al.* 1984, Kleihues *et al.* 1984) and the proportion of positive histological diagnoses is high. That permits wider use of radiotherapy for deep-seated lesions such as thalamic and brain-stem gliomas, whereas in the past there was a natural reluctance to embark upon such therapy.

*Relief of symptoms by tumour removal*

With those gliomas which form space-occupying lesions rather than producing infiltration without mass effect, distressing symptoms of raised intracranial pressure such as severe headache, vomiting and failing visual acuity may be relieved by removal or reduction of the tumour mass. Clearly this is acceptable only if it does not produce disabling focal deficit. Sites of tumour which are particularly suitable for these major internal decompressions are (a) frontal lobe, especially at the frontal pole; (b) anterior, and particularly nondominant, temporal lobe; (c) occipital. Even if the tumour extends beyond the limits of a standard lobectomy, for example more than 8 cm posterior to the pole on the medial surface of the frontal lobe, or more than 6 cm posterior to the temporal pole, it is reasonable to perform lobectomy with further extension of tumour removal provided the surgeon confines himself strictly to removal of tissue which macroscopically is obviously tumour. Alternatively with a posterior frontal tumour, especially if it is cystic, it is reasonable to evacuate the cyst, and 'debulk' the tumour, without the formal manoeuvre of a lobectomy. Indeed this may avoid some of the technical problems with venous drainage of the hemisphere medially, and the arterial supply from branches of the anterior cerebral and pericallosal vessels. An occipital lobectomy will produce a homonymous hemianopia, but that deficit is usually present already. Although theoretically attractive, frontal or temporal lobectomy for relief of intracranial pressure due to more diffuse or widespread tumours is ineffective. Thus many years ago there was a progressive movement away from external decompression (Horsley 1893, Macewen 1893, Cushing 1905), to lobectomy and internal decompression (McKenzie 1936), the latter becoming more selective. It has yet to be proved whether recent technical aids such as the ultrasonic surgical aspirator or the laser have improved the immediate results of internal decompression.

Relief of focal neurological deficit by tumour

removal is a matter for debate, and is difficult to foretell in the individual patient. Traditionally, severe and distressing focal deficits, such as aphasia, have been regarded as a contra-indication to attempts at tumour removal. However if removal does not stray beyond the obviously malignant or necrotic parts of the tumour, deficit may be improved, even with large dominant hemisphere lesions (Tandon 1984). A useful guide is the clinical response to pre-operative steroid therapy; if focal deficit is ameliorated it is likely that tumour excision will be successful in alleviating signs of dysfunction.

*The influence of tumour removal upon longterm survival*

On the basis of the first principle that reduction of tumour bulk should improve survival and allow more effective additional therapy, it was always the hope that extensive removal of supratentorial gliomas would improve prognosis, beyond the immediate relief of raised intracranial pressure. It soon became clear that prognosis was related more to type of tumour and grade of malignancy than to any other single factor, including extent of tumour removal. This is well illustrated by the earlier large series of patients treated surgically before the advent of radiotherapy, but the progressive lowering of operative mortality over the years must be taken into account before applying these figures to current practice. Cushing (1932) with craniotomy and attempted radical removal, for glioblastoma multiforme had an operative mortality of 24%. For 145 cases of protoplasmic and fibrillary astrocytoma following surgery, operative mortality was 11%; 20% of patients survived 5 years and 13% survived 10 years (German 1961). It is difficult to assess the true value of macroscopically total or subtotal removal of tumour in studies since the availability of radiotherapy; clinicians have become increasingly reluctant to deny patients radiotherapy even though the benefits of radiotherapy are limited for the more malignant tumours, and unproven for the less malignant. The difficulty

is increased by the inevitable selection of the younger and less disabled patients for aggressive surgery, radiotherapy and, more recently, chemotherapy (*see* below). Frankel and German (1958) found that following 'total' removal of *glioblastoma multiforme*, 45% of patients were alive at six months, whereas only 20% were alive after partial removal; at 1 year the figures were 22% and 7%, but at 2 years they were 7% and 4%, and finally at 36 months both were 2%. The figures show a similar but declining advantage for lobectomy which creates a generous internal decompression. However these figures are not corrected for the factors of age and functional status as rated by the Karnofsky index. What is more revealing are the curves for survivors from the time of onset of the illness, which show an unimpressive advantage for the treated group (178) cases) compared to the untreated (30 cases) during the first year.

Similar conclusions were reached by Roth and Elridge (1960), Hitchcock and Sato (1964) and Weir (1973). Without radiotherapy average survival in 76 patients following craniotomy was 3.3 months (Garfield & Dayan 1973). In recent studies (EORTC Brain Tumour Group 1978, 1981) the factors of age below 50 and functional status have been significant, but beyond slight favourability of frontal location of tumour, type and extent of tumour removal, including lobectomy, has not been significant.

The figures for survival following removal of the more differentiated glioma such as oligodendroglioma are considerably more favourable, with average postoperative survival of 7.7 years (Horrax 1951), and 5 and 10 year survival of 85% and 55% (Sheline *et al.* 1964). Patients with the rarer lower grade astrocytomas (for example, Kernohan grade 2) appear to benefit from tumour removal, but survival is generally less favourable than with the pure oligodendroglioma, probably because the apparently favourable grade of malignancy is not representative of the whole tumour. In a very large review of 1454 cases of well differentiated gliomas (Brain Tumour Registry in Japan 1982), decompression produced a 34.3% 5 year survival, partial resection 42.5% and gross total resection 75.5%. However there will always be doubt over the part played by surgery beyond the immediate relief of intracranial pressure in an individual case because of the great variation and unpredictability of the rate of growth of residual tumour. The whole problem of the assessment of the role of surgery in the supratentorial gliomas continues to be a matter of debate and creates dilemmas in the management of patients (Punt 1984).

*Quality of life*

Even more so than prediction of length of survival, prediction of quality of survival in the individual patient is often a matter of speculation. However the more traditional view that surgery in itself will not lessen deficits such as aphasia and hemiplegia, has been challenged (Tandon 1984), and if tumour removal by suction is restricted to obvious tumour tissue even severe deficits may improve. In practice this may be difficult to achieve because inevitably there is a tendency to stray into functioning brain, and to court problems with, in particular, branches of the middle cerebral artery; operative decisions which may often be demanded of the less experienced surgeon are difficult in this respect. Certainly repeated operation very rarely brings functional improvement (Young *et al.* 1981). Where the tumour occupies either frontal pole or the nondominant temporal or occipital pole, surgical treatment is best achieved by a lobectomy. Jefferson (1937) made a study of the effects of removing either frontal lobe and considered that provided Broca's area is respected, the frontal lobe of the dominant hemisphere is not more important to mental functions or personality than its fellow. Care must be exercised to ascertain that the tumour is unilateral, for a frontal lobectomy on one side when the other lobe is involved might seriously reduce the sum total of functioning frontal lobe tissue. If there is reason to suspect such involvement, the lobectomy should start with an inspection of the medial surface and

identification of the medial border of the tumour. Many gliomas of the dominant temporal lobe can be removed by a lobectomy provided the posterior part of the superior temporal convolution and deep white matter are preserved; removal of a large slowly growing glioma, particularly if cystic, from the anterior part of the temporal lobe will often be followed by a marked improvement in the dysphasia it has caused, similar to the resolution of dysphasia when an abscess is successfully treated. A small occipital lobectomy on the dominant side can be accomplished without interfering with speech mechanisms, provided resection of convexity cortex and subcortical white matter is no more than a few centimetres; but an occipital glioma sufficiently small to remove in this way is rare. During the course of a lobectomy, it may be found that the deep part of the tumour extends beyond the line of intended resection. A decision has to be made, guided by the contour and size of the pole of the tumour, whether further brain may be safely resected. Sometimes the projecting portion of tumour is merely bulging into the ventricle and by opening the ventricle its removal is easily performed. But inspection of the ventricle may reveal that tumour is extending plaque-like over its wall, rendering macroscopically complete extirpation impossible. In the frontal region tumour may unexpectedly infiltrate the caudate nucleus, the posterior orbital surface, or spread under the depths of the Sylvian fissure into the temporal lobe. When extensions make radical removal impracticable, this decision should be made promptly and only the main mass should then be removed; completion of a formal lobectomy is often the quickest way of achieving this. Because of their size and situation, the majority of hemisphere gliomas do not lend themselves to removal by lobectomy. Some are too small or too far removed from the pole of the brain to warrant the ablation of so much brain; in these a local removal, including a rim of apparently healthy brain, is all that can be attempted. If the tumour is tough it can be removed by blunt dissection, if soft by suction from within outwards. In both cases the wall of the resultant cavity can be denuded of a further 5–10 mm by suction in an endeavour to move the zone of microscopic infiltration, though recurrence is likely, perhaps not for years. Where an apparently discrete tumour involves motor and sensory cortex or pathways, removal of its visible margin is justifiable; there will be residual neurological deficit but this is usually less severe ultimately than that caused by the tumour, providing haemostasis is perfect and no arteries supplying distant healthy cortex are damaged. The degree of recovery of function which may occur after the loss of portions of the pre- and postcentral convolutions is often surprising, so that the final disability may be relatively small and the sacrifice well worth making if the period of survival is several years. Where a diffuse astrocytoma has created a large mass and caused a considerable increase of pressure, part of the tumour should be removed in order to reduce bulk and consequently the intracranial pressure. When the tumour mainly occupies motor, sensory or speech areas, removal is impracticable and a biopsy is taken, either with a wide bore cannula or through a small incision in the cortex.

Gliomas arising within the basal ganglia occur at all ages, although more frequently between 10 and 40 years; they are uncommon, probably no more than 0.5% of all intracranial gliomas. The duration of the illness varies in accordance with the nature of the glioma, from a few weeks to several years. Epilepsy is a rare event; the tumours may be asymptomatic until they encroach upon the internal capsule and produce a hemiparesis, which is usually sensory as well as motor. Involvement of the optic radiation in the posterior part of the internal capsule gives rise to homonymous hemianopia. The extent to which signs of striatal disorder develop varies, but they are often absent. The syndrome of spontaneous pain, thalamic dysaesthesiae, so common a sequel of ischaemic lesions, is rarely caused by a tumour. Raised intracranial pressure occurs late, and is usually due to obstruction of the third ventricle or foramina of Monro, and requires CSF shunting. Stereotactic biopsy followed by radiotherapy is the preferred man-

agement, and, unlike the hemisphere glioma, survival may be surprisingly long, on occasion a matter of years.

With tumours of the third and lateral ventricles direct open surgery and attempted removal usually requires a significant proportion of tumour to project into the ventricle, which allows access through the body of a dilated lateral ventricle and if necessary through the foramen of Monro. A generous opening in the septum pellucidum improves access and post operative communication of CSF between the lateral ventricles. Unfortunately although gliomas may project into a lateral ventricle and appear radiologically to be essentially intraventricular tumours, at surgery they are often found medially to be infiltrating deeply without any clear line of demarcation.

Surgical access to gliomas in the *hypothalamic and suprasellar regions* is usually limited. The decision to attempt open surgery depends upon the radiological evidence in favour of an extrinsic or intrinsic tumour, and it may be impossible to differentiate earlier between craniopharyngioma and glioma. In the presence of hydrocephalus, unless the tumour is clearly projecting upwards through the foramen of Monro and is accessible by the transventricular route, preliminary CSF shunting is advisable, to be followed at a later stage by a subfrontal suprasellar approach for biopsy and attempted tumour removal. Alternatives are stereotactic biopsy, or, in the lateral ventricles, ventriculography and biopsy.

The surgery of *gliomas of the optic nerve or chiasm* is often a matter for debate, especially when there is still reasonable preservation of vision in one or both eyes, and when the evolution has been very gradual. Clearly when vision has already been totally lost, or very severely impaired in one eye only, and at subfrontal exploration the tumour is unequivocally anterior to the chiasm, total excision of the intracranial and intra-orbital tumour by optic nerve section is desirable, and may result in a true cure. However the lowgrade tumour may already have extended backwards microscopically to involve the chiasm, and therefore the prognosis is uncertain;

preservation of vision for up to 21 years has been recorded (Matson 1969). Reports which deal with survival and not preservation of vision contribute little guidance to the problems of management, the benefits of radiotherapy remain unproven and 'an unbiased view of the results of therapy for optic nerve gliomas is virtually impossible to obtain' (Tenny *et al.* 1982).

## Radiotherapy of supratentorial malignant gliomas

In the presence of an inevitably fatal disease for which surgery can usually provide no more more than a temporary respite, and only an occasional longterm survival, it is to be expected that, by extrapolation from other fields of cancer, radiotherapy would be part of the standard treatment for malignant supratentorial gliomas. Unfortunately the precise role of radiotherapy, and the prediction of its effectiveness is still far from clear, despite therapeutic trials going back to the 1960s. In current practice, including the protocols of some current studies, the place of radiotherapy has become accepted to the point where some clinicians regard it as unethical to deny their patients this treatment. Indeed it is doubtful whether a controlled randomized study of radiotherapy versus no radiotherapy for glioblastoma multiforme and anaplastic astrocytoma would obtain the approval of protocol review committees on ethical grounds.

Before summarizing the 'best results' of radiotherapy, some of the factors which may vitiate the results of trials, or at least make assessment difficult, will be considered. Pathology review may reveal errors of initial histological grading of malignancy when unexpectedly favourable results are recorded. Results must be corrected for favourable prognostic factors such as age under 50, and Karnofsky index of function of 70 or better; although total as opposed to partial tumour removal may not have any significant effect upon free interval and survival, frontal site of tumour does (EORTC 1981). Finally steroids (dexamethasone) in high dosage, if used indis-

criminately, without control or recording, may favourably influence the effects of radiotherapy. The evidence that exists for beneficial effects of radiotherapy is relevant only to the more malignant tumours, glioblastoma multiforme, anaplastic astrocytoma, astrocytoma grade 3 and 4, malignant oligodendroglioma and ependymomas. In the management of intracranial ependymoma, surgery followed by aggressive radiotherapy has produced encouraging results with 10 year survival rates of 75% for low grade and 67% for high grade tumours, using combined craniospinal irradiation for all high grade and all posterior fossa tumours (Salazer *et al.* 1983). There is no convincing evidence that radiotherapy is effective in well differentiated oligodendroglioma and in low grade astrocytoma (Kernohan grade 2), for which a fully randomized study is currently being formulated by the EORTC.

Using external megavoltage radiotherapy in doses of up to 6000 rads over the course of six weeks following surgery 'best results' have included 18%, 22% and 7.9%, 5 year survival (Capra 1980) and mean duration of free interval of 30 weeks and survival of 44.5 weeks (EORTC Brian Tumour Group 1983).

Despite these modest overall results there are a small number of patients who, after radiotherapy, survive for many years, and in whom there are no favourable prognostic factors which can be identified. Methods of interstitital radiation have received attention in recent years, but the results are not yet convincing. Delayed radiation necrosis of the cerebrum is well documented (Brismar *et al.* 1976) and may mimic recurrent tumours (Safdari *et al.* 1984), but is very rare with photon therapy provided radiation dosages do not exceed 5,000 or 6,000 rads in six weeks.

## Chemotherapy of supratentorial malignant gliomas

Despite intensive activity in laboratory studies and in clinical trials of potential chemotherapeutic agents during the past twenty years or more, no single agent or combination of agents has as yet significantly changed the overall outlook in terms of survival or free interval following surgery and radiotherapy. Factors which make the assessment of the results of radiotherapy so difficult (*see* above) are even more relevant when gauging the true effects of chemotherapy. With the added difficulties of delivery of drugs to the tumour in the face of the peculiarities of the cerebral circulation and the blood–brain barrier, and the great variation in the growth kinetics of gliomas (Hoshina 1984), it is not surprising that so little therapeutic progress has been made. Attempts have been made to predict the clinical effects of agents depending upon their effects upon tumours grown *in vitro*. Methods of administration have included systemic, intracarotid, intracavitary, intraventricular and intrathecal. The types of agents used have included cell-cycle specific drugs (for example methotrexate) non cell-cycle specific drugs (for example the alkylating agents) and radiosensitisers (for example misonidazole). In some studies clinical response, albeit temporary, has been reported especially with recurrent tumours. In the face of a vast literature one can do no more than refer the reader to articles which contain reviews of this very complex and changing field (Levin 1980, Kelly 1984). Practical guidance to clinicians could currently include the following simple points:

1   There is no evidence of any beneficial effect of chemotherapy upon the lower grade tumours.
2   The beneficial effects upon the more malignant tumours (for example glioblastoma multiforme and anaplastic astrocytoma) are at best transient, and always unpredictable.
3   There is no obligation, at least on a scientific basis, for the clinician to advise chemotherapy.
4   Chemotherapy schedules, which may be prolonged, may engender some hope in patients, but they may also cause distress and curtail the remaining comfort and support within a devoted family.
5   In the light of continuing attempts to improve therapy, it is right that patients should be entered into properly conducted and formulated trials. It is not acceptable that patients should be given haphazard chemotherapy at the whim of the individual clinician.
6   If advances are to be achieved, as in other fields of cancer, they are likely to be slow and step-wise. Significant progress is more likely to originate from laboratory (cellular) work than from extensive clinical trials.

# Infratentorial primary malignant neoplasms

## Classification

Reference has been made already in the general classification to the major infratentorial neoplasms. The incidence of the different histological types shows an especial relationship to age which is rare with the supratentorial tumours. Thus in childhood medulloblastoma is the predominant tumour, followed by cerebellar astrocytoma of varying grades of malignancy; ependymoma and brain stem glioma are less common (Matson 1969). Difficulties arise in the classification of the astrocytoma because the differentiation between the benign and malignant growth is at times uncertain, and only prolonged follow-up can provide the correct answer. Whether a solid noncystic cerebellar astrocytoma can be regarded as benign as the mural nodule (Kernohan grade 1) of a cystic cerebellar astrocytoma of childhood is still a matter of neurosurgical debate.

## Medulloblastoma

The characteristics of this clearly defined tumour were set out by Bailey and Cushing (1925) when they suggested its name. In their paper they included a small number of tumours of the cerebrum which they considered histologically similar to the much larger number of cerebellar tumours. Nowadays the cerebral examples are

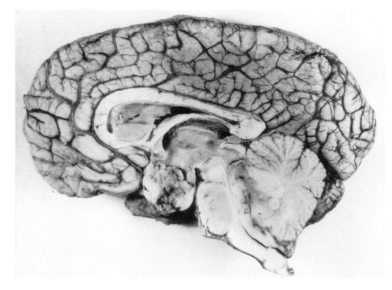

**Fig. 5.8.** Medulloblastoma. The tumour fills the fourth ventricle, adherent to the floor in one area, diffusely invades the cerebellum; the third ventricle and upper aqueduct are dilated: the hypothalmic portion of the third ventricle is filled with a large transventricular deposit.

regarded as neuroblastomas, or primitive neuro-ectodermal tumours.

The medulloblastoma is a highly malignant tumour of the cerebellum, particularly common in children. The curve of its incidence against age rises to a sharp peak at about five years and falls nearly as rapidly, continuing at a low level into adult years. The majority of the tumours in children are situated in the midline; in older patients they are usually in the lateral lobes.

The tumour usually forms an ovoid mass filling the fourth ventricle or its caudal portion and replacing much of the vermis, which to the surgeon's eye is broadened and bulges between the lateral lobes (Fig. 5.8). When large, the tumour protrudes through the foramen of Magendie and is visible in the cisterna magna; a lobule often thrusts upwards into a dilated aqueduct. Although blending with the roof and lateral walls of the fourth ventricle, it may be little or not at all adherent to the floor until at a later stage tumour invades the medulla and pons. The consistency is usually soft so that suction easily removes it, but the tumour is often permeated by a fine meshwork of tough strands. Its margin is poorly defined and cannot be identified by blunt dissection, and macroscopic removal must include a rim of surrounding brain. Although

other gliomas may occasionally spread in the subarachnoid space by seeding, this phenomenon is common in the medulloblastoma. A small separate greyish-pink plaque may be seen on the surface of the brain, and may be found within the lateral and third ventricles. Occasionally the tumour infiltrates the cerebellar cortex and in continuity spreads into the subarachnoid space. Such areas are sometimes quite firm as a result of leptomeningeal fibroblastic reaction and belie the true nature of the tumour. Laterally situated tumours in older patients often appear more circumscribed and are firmer growth than the typical medulloblastoma; occasionally they form lobulated masses denting the surface of the cerebellum. The prognosis for survival after removal of these laterally placed firmer tumours of later years is generally considered to be more favourable than for the midline tumours in children. They also have a modified histological appearance. For these reasons some authorities classify them separately as arachnoidal sarcoma of the cerebellum (Kernohan & Uihlein 1962). The arguments against this view, maintaining that the particular histological appearances are due to manner of spread and local reaction have been fully reported by Rubinstein and Northfield (1964).

*Histology*

Typical tumours of this group are homogenous, highly cellular with a sparse vascular stroma. The cells are closely packed, have prominent oval nuclei with a dense chromatin pattern and scanty cytoplasm. Mitotic figures are abundant (Fig. 5.9). In some tumours, cells are arranged in circular rosettes around cellfree areas; these contain delicate argyrophilic fibres suggestive of neuroblastic differentiation. Further transitional stages between neuroblasts and mature neurons are seen occasionally. Other tumours show spongioblastic differentiation and occasionally typical oligodendroglioma areas. Reticulin fibres are absent in some parts of the tumour and form dense networks in others (Fig. 5.10). These connective tissue fibres are found in areas where the neoplasm invades the leptomeninges. They are particularly prominent in tumours arising from the cerebellar hemispheres which only involve the superficial layers of the

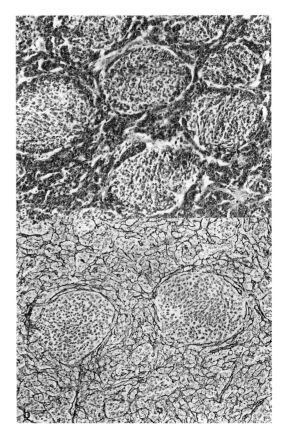

**Fig. 5.10.** 'Desmoplastic' variety of medulloblastoma with scattered islands free from connective tissue.
(a) H. & E. × 110
(b) Reticulum. × 110

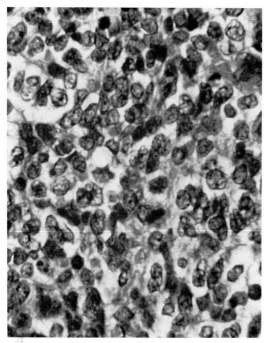

**Fig. 5.9.** Medulloblastoma. The uniform high cellularity with abundant mitotic figures is characteristic of the 'typical' tumour. H. & E. × 650.

cortex and spread extensively into the subarachnoid space ('desmoplastic medulloblastomas'). They are less abundant in midline tumours which grow largely into the lumen of the fourth ventricle. The tumour cells are cytologically identical in all parts of the tumour although they may be compressed by the connective tissue and arranged into tightly packed parallel rows of darkly stained cells.

The biological behaviour of all medulloblastomas irrespective of differentiation is similar, although the 'desmoplastic' tumours of the cerebellar hemispheres are often more circumscribed. They all tend to metastasize widely through the cerebrospinal fluid pathway and to form secondary deposits within the ventricles and in the subarachnoid spaces, particularly around the spinal cord. Distant metastases occur more frequently than in any other type of intracranial tumour.

*Other tumours*

The *astrocytomas* of the posterior fossa arise in the cerebellum and in the brain stem, particularly the pons. The histological features have much in common with the supratentorial astocytomas, but with a greater tendency towards the more benign or less malignant types. The *ependymomas* of the posterior fossa, as with the supratentorial tumours, vary in degrees of malignancy, the most benign type being the subependymoma, usually found closely related to the fourth ventricle and cisterna magna into which this relatively firm tumour may project. All three types of tumour in the posterior fossa (medulloblastoma, astrocytoma, ependymoma) have their greatest incidence in the early years of life; this is particularly so for the medulloblastoma, the incidence age curve rising steeply to a maximum during the ages of 5–10 years; the peak for the astrocytoma is broader and covers the period of 5–15 years; for both tumours the curve falls sharply beyond 15 years of age, but a few cases occur up to middle age. The highest incidence for the ependymoma is at 5 years, but the curve falls more slowly (Zülch 1965). In a child, a glioma is much more likely to occur in the cerebellum than in the cerebrum, but this ratio becomes reversed in adults. Penman and Smith (1954) concluded from their studies that up to the age of 9 years an infratentorial glioma is about four times more probable than a supratentorial one; during the next ten years the chances are about equal; over the age of 20 years supratentorial gliomas are about twenty times more frequent than infratentorial ones. It is this inverse relationship which accounts for the fact that in a child an intracranial tumour is about twice as likely to be below the tentorium as above it; whereas in adults the reverse is the case.

## Clinical features

*Tumours of the brain stem*, using this term to include midbrain, pons and medulla, can conveniently be grouped together for consideration of the clinical syndromes they produce, as they have certain features in common. They all give rise in due course to a progressive contralateral spastic hemiparesis, hemisensory loss and an ipsilateral involvement of one or more of the cranial nerves which emerge from the brain stem, from the third nerve downwards. This 'crossed paralysis' is the hall mark of a brain stem lesion and the identification of the affected cranial nerve indicates the level and extent of the tumour. Eponymous names have been bestowed upon the syndromes according to the cranial nerves predominantly affected at the differing anatomical levels. Progression of the tumour across the breadth of the brain-stem brings bilateral involvement, although the ultimate neurological picture is rarely symmetrical. The rate of progress varies with the histological nature of the tumour; they are mostly gliomas, more commonly seen in children or young adults and the total history may be weeks or many years. On occasion the early signs suggest an encephalitis or disseminated sclerosis and the true diagnosis may only become evident as fresh signs develop and fill in the picture more clearly. The higher in the brain stem the tumour the more frequent do episodic disturbances seen to occur and these may be associated with attacks of decerebrate rigidity. The brain stem is densely packed with highly important nuclei and neuronal pathways. Consequently, considerable neurological damage can be caused by a tumour of quite small size, too small by size alone to bring about an elevation of the intracranial pressure. For this reason brain-stem tumours often run their whole course without causing any elevation of the intracranial pressure or even hydrocephalus. This is particularly true of the invasive and more rapidly growing gliomas. Slowly growing tumours eventually deform the aqueduct and obstruct the passage of cerebrospinal fluid and those of the pons may reach sufficient size to embarrass its flow through the basal cisterns, though they rarely obstruct the fourth ventricle.

The midbrain is only about 2 cm in length and may be invaded by tumour extending downwards from the cerebrum or upwards from the pons; occasionally tumour arises within it. When the tumour originates in the ventral part it interrupts the crus and produces spastic weakness and sensory loss on the contralateral side and sooner or later involves the emerging third nerve fibres, or more dorsally its nucleus. When the tumour originates in the more dorsal portion (tegmentum), coarse tremor occurs as a result of interruption of red nucleus connections; chorea and hemiballismus suggests an extension towards the subthalamic nucleus. These involuntary movements are contralateral. Tumour of the cerebellum when situated high up under the tentorium may also give rise to tremor, due to involvement of the superior cerebellar peduncle, but tremor from a tumour in this situation is ipsilateral. Occasionally in tumours of the midbrain, postural reflexes of Magnus and de Kleijn can be evoked; the arm on one side is flexed and the leg extended when the head is turned to that side; when it is turned to the other side these limbs relax and the other arm and leg adopt the posture. Involvement of the midbrain dorsal to the aqueduct (tectum) will affect the colliculi. The superior pair take part in the control of the size of the pupils and invasion by tumour leads to inequality of enlargement and to lack of reaction to light. There may be paralysis of upward (and it is said also of downward) conjugate eye movement, and ptosis. These abnormal signs may also be caused by downward pressure upon the superior colliculi, as a result of tumours arising in the pineal body and of brain herniation due to distant lesions, for example hydrocephalus, chronic subdural haematoma.

Within the pons gradual extension of intrinsic tumours may involve cranial nerve nuclei, especially the 6th, 5th and 7th, producing an uncrossed diplopia, trigeminal paraesthesiae and sensory loss, and facial spasms prior to a lower motor neuron facial weakness. Tumours, such as medulloblastoma and ependymoma arising in

or deep to the floor of the fourth ventricle may produce vomiting as a very early and isolated symptom and thereby mislead the paediatrician; only later will the sinister features of dysphagia with nasal regurgitation, dysphonia due to vocal cord paralysis, dysarthria and wasting and fasciculation of the tongue indicate the presence of an extensive intramedullary lesion.

With cerebellar tumours symptoms of raised intracranial pressure are often prominent. Headache is severe, often located in the suboccipital region and aggavated by coughing, change of posture and by neck movement. Rigidity and tenderness of the neck muscles occur, perhaps as a reflex mechanism to guard against movement and probably related to tonsillar herniation. The head may be tilted and rotated to one side. This position is sometimes adopted so as to avoid the diplopia due to weaknes of an ocular muscle, but in that case it is usually of a simple rotation; tilting (lateral flexion) is thought to be due to interference with labyrinthine pathways affecting the relationship between muscle tone and the position of the head. The drowsiness and mental obfuscation seen in expanding processess above the tentorium are often absent, or deferred to a late stage. In adults and particularly after middle age, progressive dementia may occur as a result of the hydrocephalus. Disturbances of vision due to posterior fossa mass lesion are of particular significance. The so-called 'transient amblyopic attacks' in which the patient may describe the 'greying-out' of vision with the preservation of outlines only, many indicate incipient coning of the cerebellar tonsils at the foramen magnum, with acute rises of intracranial pressure and severe hydrocephalus. If not urgently relieved, permanent severe impairment of visual acuity may result, even though the patient may be otherwise well after surgery. In these, and in about half of all patients with posterior fossa tumours, papilloedema is striking.

The prominence of vertigo, ataxia and incoordination, and nystagmus varies greatly. The time-honoured features of truncal ataxia with vermis lesions and lateralized ataxia incoordination and nystagmus with cerebellar hemisphere lesions are very variable, and the latter are more striking when the cerebellar peduncles are most affected.

Tumours of the cerebellum may give rise to 'false' localizing signs which may lead to the mistaken diagnosis of tumour of the pons or medulla. The commonest is a sixth nerve paresis, particularly if this is bilateral. Weakness of other cranial nerves, as a result of compression of the brain stem, rarely impairment of postural sense and of pain and temperature sense and signs of pyramidal involvement may occur with large tumours, with those extending into the spinal canal or causing severe tonsillar herniation. But such signs are usually only slight relative to the disturbance of cerebellar function and late in appearance, whereas in pontine and medullary tumours cranial nerve paralysis is an early and prominent feature, while hydrocephalus is slight or absent. It is not rare for a lateralized cerebellar lesion to be mistaken clinically for a contralateral frontal lesion and vice versa.

In the terminal stages of cerebellar tumours, attacks of decerebrate rigidity are liable to occur, so-called cerebellar seizures. As described elsewhere these are usually attributed to transient ischaemia of the brain stem as a result of upward herniation of the vermis through the tentorial hiatus. Neck stiffness and head retraction due to impaction of the cerebellar tonsils sustained, may be mistaken for signs of meningeal inflammation; if a clinical diagnosis of meningitis is erroneously made, and lumbar puncture done, fatal coning at the foramen magnum may be precipitated with abrupt arrest of respiration without prior deterioration in level of consciousness. It is unusual for these events to occur without a history of severe and often episodic headache, during which the child, in particular, may cry out and hold his head with his hands.

### Investigations

With lesions of the posterior fossa, decisions concerning the urgency of investigation are paramount; neurological exercises in precise clinical localization of lesions should not be allowed to waste precious hours or even minutes when coning at the foramen magnum may be imminent. In such circumstances the surgeon's relatively fundamental clinical approach is more appropriate.

The danger signals with posterior fossa mass lesions are:–

severe episodic headache
a child who clutches his head
neck stiffness and head retraction
impaired visual acuity, transient or sustained
opisthotonus, episodic or sustained
irregular or slow respiration
impaired consciousness
severe papilloedema

The radiological investigations have been described fully in Chapter 3. However in the presence of any of the danger signals listed above, the clinican must be aware of some important practical points. If a lumbar puncture has been done (unwisely) during the preceding hours, the risks of fatal coning are greater. Therefore any delay beyond the half hour in obtaining the definitive investigation of a CT scan may put the patient, and especially the child, at great risk. In those circumstances where the clinical diagnosis of a posterior fossa mass is probable, there may be time for no more than skull radiographs in the adult to exclude the presence of a laterally displaced calcified pineal before directly making burr holes (frontal or posterior parietal) in order to tap the ventricles, relieve the acute rise in intracranial pressure, and set up external ventricular drainage. Thereafter CT can be done as soon as possible. As an alternative a little time may be 'bought' by immediately controlling respiration while awaiting CT. Steroid therapy may also be valuable in reducing raised intracranial pressure, even when hydrocephalus is the major cause. Older neurosurgeons will know that if the CT apparatus fails, ventriculography remains a valuable and rapid method of localization of an infratentorial mass, and they will not hesitate to use it in those special circumstances.

## Surgery and postoperative treatment

The accuracy of preoperative diagnosis depends upon radiology (*see* Chapter 3), but in practice, conventional radiology (CT scan) of the posterior fossa does not provided total certainty of the pathological diagnosis, with the exception of acoustic schwannoma and cerebellar haematoma. Therefore prior to surgery, despite probabilities, there usually remain the differential diagnoses of: medulloblastoma, metastases, astrocytoma, ependymoma, haemangioblastoma, abscess, meningioma and the very rare choroid plexus papilloma, dermoid cyst and epidermoid (cholesteatoma).

Attention has already been drawn to the indications for urgent action, and relief of acute hydrocephalus. Posterior fossa exploration should not be delayed long after relief of hydrocephalus, because shifts of the posterior fossa mass may cause increase pressure upon the brain stem, although a true 'upward cone' is very rare. The objectives of surgery can be summarized as:

1   establishment of pathological diagnosis;
2   reduction of a mass lesion and permanent relief of CSF obstruction;
3   total removal of a lesion and thereby surgical cure.

Operative details are beyond the scope of this account, but some general points of guidance can be given. Anaesthesia during posterior fossa surgery should be with controlled ventilation. It may be lengthy, and requires expertise if signs such as changes in blood pressure, pulse and ECG patterns are to guide the surgeon when approaching the brain stem. The position (for example sitting, lying, 'park bench' etc.) is a matter of custom, surgical comfort, ease of access and safety, and still, therefore, of some debate. For cerebellar hemisphere, vermis, fourth ventricle and cisternal and tentorial lesions the sitting position gives superb access, view, and operative field conditions, but the hazards of air embolism, although reduced by sonic monitoring and measures to maintain the cerebral venous pressure above zero, persist. Therefore the sitting

position has generally given way to the alternatives. With the uncertainties of preoperative diagnosis, the exposure must always be sufficient to deal with the unexpected and the benign, and therefore, posterior fossa craniectomies should be generous, exposing the margin of the lateral sinus above and usually including the margin of the foramen magnum below. Removal of the arch of the atlas improves the approach to low cerebellar and fourth ventricle tumours. It is not always easy to determine from CT the site of origin of tumours, the major error being to mistake an extrinsic laterally placed mass for a more medially placed cerebellar hemisphere lesion. The approach to any lesion which is not clearly centred on the midline must allow a good view of the lateral extremity of the posterior fossa and the cerebellopontine angle. Finally, a wise precaution is to have a posterior parietal burr hole through which the lateral ventricle can be tapped either during or at any time after posterior fossa surgery.

### Medulloblastoma

It has long been recognized that attempts to extirpate this tumour by operation alone fail (Bailey & Cushing 1925). It is, however, initially the most radiosensitive of all intracranial tumours and early and efficient irradiation is the most effective method of treatment at present available. Nevertheless operation plays an important role by relieving hydrocephalus and in providing biopsy material so that the true nature of the tumour can be ascertained. At operation, which in young children can be carried out through a median incision, the tumour may be seen protruding through the foramen of Magendie or it may be concealed within a bulging vermis. On occasion the nature of the tumour is evident by opaque greyish patches of disseminated tumour in the leptomeninges. The tumour is exposed by a vertical incision in the vermis or if necessary by excision of the overlying vermis and sufficient removed to free the cavity of the fourth ventricle. Having obtained immediate confirmation of histology by frozen section or smear, the objective is to remove as much as possible of the tumour mass, and thereby relieve the obstruction to CSF flow and improve the efficacy of postoperative treatment (Park *et al.* 1983), but without producing neurological disability. Even using newer surgical technology such as the laser or ultrasonic aspirator, to continue attempts at tumour removal when the cerebellar peduncles and the floor of the fourth ventricle are involved may be unwise. However in all cases the bulk of what is often a surprisingly large and relatively avascular mass filling a ballooned fourth ventricle can be removed, allowing the CSF to gush forth from the dilated and shortened aqueduct. Landmarks in the surgery of these tumours include Cushing's (1932) operative mortality of 33%, Olivecrona's (1967) of 28.6% for radical surgery and 44% for partial removal. In Matson's (1969) series of 130 children with cerebellar medulloblastoma there were 22 postoperative deaths but only 4 after 1954. In Toronto (Park *et al.* 1983) the operative mortality in 144 cases was 11.1% but without any deaths since 1973, while Choux and Lena (1982) achieved a mortality of 11.3% in 44 patients after 1970. Although some earlier works advocated very limited tumour removal, improvements in anaesthesia and postoperative care have allowed more extensive excision of tumour, within the technical limitations already described.

The question of pre-operative definitive CSF shunting, as distinct from urgent external ventricular drainage, has been debated recently (Albright 1983, McLaurin 1983, Park *et al.* 1983), as have so many aspects of the management of this disease in the immediate and the long term, including the incidence of extracranial metastases (Campbell *et al.* 1984). Representative figures for the incidence of metastases are: spinal 12.5%, supratentorial 14.6% and systemic 9.7%, the majority being skeletal, less commonly peritoneal and rarely in lymph nodes. With pre-operative ventriculoperitoneal shunting without a millipore filter the incidence of systemic metastases was 17.2% (Park *et al.* 1983).

It is difficult to determine the common practice, but certainly in Britain pre-operative shunting is not used routinely. However postoperative problems of CSF flow due to basal cistern adhesions are common, and ventriculoperitoneal shunting is often required later.

The postoperative management including radiotherapy and chemotherapy has been the subject of many trials, which have varied in their conditions and objectivity. Cushing's first 13 patients were treated by operation only, and the maximum survival was 21 months, the average 7 months (Bailey & Cushing 1925). Radiotherapy was first employed in 1919, and its value could be estimated within 10 years (Bailey *et al.* 1928). At first only small doses were given, exclusively to the tumour site, and recurrence at the site or elsewhere was treated as it became evident. When the biological habits of the tumour became known, more extensive irradiation was carried out; the beneficial effects were reported by Cutler *et al.* (1936). Planned treatment of the whole neuraxis through a series of accurately matched separate fields was a considerable and logical advance. But it has the disadvantage that free tumour cells may be carried by movements of the cerebrospinal fluid from one field to another, and thus escape irradiation. Paterson and Farr (1953) introduced a method whereby the whole neuraxis is irradiated simultaneously. Although there is still debate about the role of chemotherapy, the effectiveness of radiotherapy to the neuraxis is accepted. The dosage in recent series (Choux & Lena 1982) has become standardized as: posterior fossa 50–55 grey, spinal 30–36, cerebrum 30. The adverse effects of retardation of growth and intellect (Hirsh 1979), endocrine deficiencies and haematopoietic marrow suppression are real, but vary considerably in different series, and may well be related to the care with which the techniques of radiotherapy are applied. These complications are not sufficiently severe or frequent to invalidate the use of radiotherapy in view of the proven prolongation of life, although in current studies reduction of cerebral radiation is one objective. Unfortunately, as yet, the place of chemotherapy is not clear. Vinca alkaloids, methotrexate, and nitrosoureas, cyclophosphamide and other agents have been used in various trials, in combination with the course of radiotherapy, and as subsequent repeated courses of chemotherapy. Although initially hopes were raised by an apparent response of recurrent tumours to chemotherapy, larger cooperative studies have not yet produced statistically significant evidence of prolonged survival. Nevertheless there are sufficient grounds for cooperative studies to be pursued, as they are by the Société Internationale d'Oncologie Pediatrique (SIOP). Irrespective of chemotherapy recent representative figures for overall survival following surgery and radiotherapy in children include: at one year 88% (Bloom *et al* 1982), 73% (Choux & Lena), 73% (Park *et al.* 1983); at five years 51% (Bloom *et al.* 1982), 37% (Choux & Lena 1982), 47% (Park *et al.* 1983). Because of these figures, there are always grounds for some optimism in the individual case, and a small number of patients survive for 10 years or more. Favourable factors include age over 5 years, absence of brain stem involvement, total macroscopic removal, desmoplastic cell type (not confirmed by Choux & Lena 1982). The observation (Packer 1983) that overall survival rate was 70% with tumours which did not show cellular differentiation compared to 32% with tumours which showed differentiation along glial, ependymal and neuronal lines suggests that radiotherapy is also an important factor. These factors and the early postoperative neurological status give a less certain guide to the longer term quality of life. It is the potential distress of severe disability to parents and child that continues to perplex the surgeon in the management of this malignant condition.

## Astrocytoma

In the cerebellum the astrocytoma may lie in the midline, or in a lateral lobe. It is usually a rounded mass with a well defined discrete margin, tough, yellowish or pink, or of greyish translucent tissue. It is usually more vascular than the surrounding white matter. The overlying folia are broadened and on occasion the tumour may force its way to the surface. The majority are cystic and the tumour may be only a nodule in the wall of the cyst. According to its position the tumour bulges into the roof of the lateral aspect of the fourth ventricle, compressing and obliterating it. Tumour or cyst may attain remarkable dimensions, occupying virtually the whole of a lobe, or the central one half of the cerebellum so that when removed the floor of the fourth ventricle lies widely exposed at the bottom of a shallow gutter, bordered either side by the compressed lateral lobe. Occasionally the tumour extends into the middle cerebellar peduncle and thereby gains a foothold in the pons, rendering that portion of it irremovable. Less frequently access to the pons is through the inferior peduncle. In the German literature these tumours are commonly classified as spongioblastomas. Russell and Rubinstein (1977) emphasize the diversity of the histological appearances, and that anaplastic changes may occasionally be present (in 9% of their series). Prognosis of cerebellar astrocytoma is largely dependent upon the degree of malignancy determined histologically. The truly benign cystic cerebellar astrocytoma of childhood, one of the most favourable intracranial tumours, characteristically occurs within the cerebellar hemisphere, the circumscribed benign (grade 1 astrocytoma) tumour nodule projecting into an often very large cyst containing clear pale yellow fluid. Medially the cyst wall may be no more than a thin curtain separating the cyst from the cavity of the fourth ventricle. Cure can be achieved by total removal of the mural nodule alone.

The histologically malignant astrocytomas, albeit of different grades, vary in the degree to which they are macroscopically circumscribed. They are usually relatively firm and avascular, pale grey tumours, surrounded by firm cerebellar white matter. Unfortunately they may involve the cerebellar peduncles medially without any clear line of demarcation, and the surgical difficulties are much as with medulloblastoma. Extension into the brain stem is not common. Provided the tumour is macroscopically confined to the cerebellar hemisphere or vermis, it is reasonable to attempt a total removal, in order to improve the prognosis, whatever the grade of malignancy. Sometimes the tumour may be impossible to differentiate operatively from cerebellar white matter and in those circumstances surgery may have to be restricted to obtaining a generous biopsy, and doing only sufficient to allow free flow of CSF from the aqueduct and fourth ventricle. When there is infiltration of the inferior vermis and a cerebellar tonsil, tumour removal should not be allowed to damage the posterior inferior cerebellar artery. With the rarer multi-locular cystic tumours, the grade of malignancy is higher, and there is not the favourable mural nodule. Figures for the overall prognosis of the malignant cerebellar astrocytomas are not easy to obtain, despite comprehensive reviews in the past (Gol & McKissock 1959), and more recent studies (Steinberg et al. 1985). The difficulties are consistent with the observation that after partial removal of these tumours sequential CT evidence of residual tumour may continue for years in patients who remain asymptomatic until later clinical recurrence. Certainly survival is generally longer than after surgery for supratentorial tumours of similar histology. In the light of these observations, the place of postoperative radiotherapy is still a matter of debate in the management of the individual patient. It may be accepted that radiotherapy has no part to play in patients with grade I and grade II tumours, but for the most malignant tumours radiotherapy to the posterior fossa and the spinal neuraxis is usually given.

## Ependymoma

Ependymoma is often indistinguishable in its presentation, from medulloblastoma. The tumour may attain a great size as its occupies the dilated fourth ventricle, with remarkably few localizing signs, the main features being vomiting, due to early involvement of the floor of the fourth ventricle, and raised intracranial pressure. At operation the tumour may present between the cerebellar tonsils in the cisterna magna, and extend downwards over the upper cervical spinal cord. Alternatively it may lie entirely within a ballooned fourth ventricle, with a variable degree of attachment to the medial aspects of the cerebellar peduncles and to the floor of the fourth ventricle. Frequently the final attachment of the tumour is to the medulla at the obex. The ependymomas are more common in children than adults, and in children account for about 20% of all posterior fossa tumours (Matson 1969). Because the tumour may be sensitive to radiotherapy the overall prognosis is somewhat better than for medulloblastoma, although it is difficult to predict outcome in the individual patient after surgery and neuraxis radiotherapy (Salazar et al. 1983).

Unfortunately these tumours seed through the CSF, and tumours of the cauda equina may follow or even precede the presentation of the posterior fossa lesion.

The much rarer subependymoma (Fig. 5.11) sometimes seen as an incidental finding in the fourth ventricle and also known as subependymal astrocytoma, consists almost entirely of subependymal glia and may exhibit prominent perivascular pseudo rosettes. True ependymal elements, if present at all, are scanty and may represent fragments of the normal ependymal lining included in the tumour. Their separation from true ependymomas is somewhat arbitrary as all intermediate stages may be observed between tumours consisting almost exclusively of subependymal glia and those consisting predominantly of ependymal cells. Both subependymomas and the stroma of true ependymomas may contain fine, granular deposits of calcium. Although it may appear histologically benign, even after apparently total macroscopic removal from an origin that is often similar to that of the ependymoma, these tumours tend to recur at the same site after an interval of many years. Operatively the tumour may be a firm well circumscribed globular mass, which resembles a choroid plexus papilloma of the fourth ventricle.

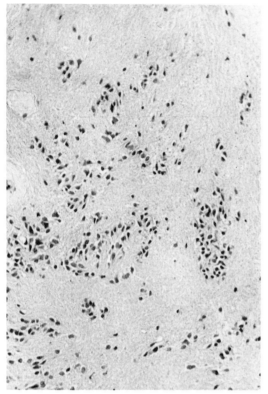

**Fig. 5.11.** Subependymoma: clusters of cells scattered in fibrillary glial stroma. H. & E. × 240

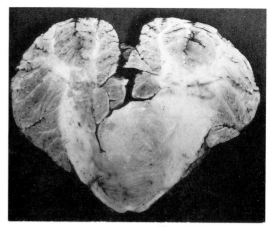

**Fig. 5.12.** Astrocytoma of pons extending into left middle cerebellar peduncle, lower midbrain and upper two thirds of medulla: the clinical picture was a cerebellopontine angle syndrome.

Radiotherapy is not indicated after removal, whether total or partial.

## Intrinsic brain stem tumours

In the brain stem the common variety of glioma is astrocytoma, although there are often areas of anaplasia which assume the appearance of glioblastoma. The tumour may produce a diffusely swollen appearance, such as is seen in the pons when in some specimens the basilar artery and its branches are engulfed in deep grooves. The floor of the fourth ventricle is elevated by the tumour (Fig. 5.12). Rarely the tumour remains confined to a particular area, causing only a local obstruction, say to the aqueduct of the Sylvius (Fig. 5.13) or may extend as a lobulated mass into the cisterna magna though

its almost pedunculated attachment to the medulla will reveal the true nature of its origin. Cases may be followed by many years of useful survival. Brain stem gliomas are thought to be more frequent in young people; Russell and Rubinstein (1977) reported that in 18 of 25 examples, death occurred below the age of 20 years. Barnett and Hyland (1952) found the

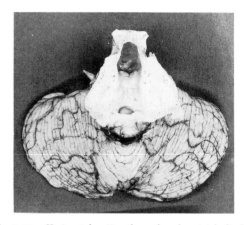

**Fig. 5.13.** Horizontal section through 3rd ventricle displays its enlargement and (in the upper part of the picture) great thinning of the floor: in the posterior part of the 3rd ventricle is seen the dilated mouth of the aqueduct occluded by a dome of the tumour which caudally terminated at the junction of the aqueduct and 4th ventricle. An astrocytoma with only slight spread into periaqueductal tissue.

average age in a series of 90 lay in the fourth decade, the range being from 3 to 58 years. The management of these tumours continues to perplex neurologists and neurosurgeons. Advances in radiology (*see* Chapter 3), and especially CT and MRI now allow more certain diagnosis in terms of pathology and precise localization and extent of the tumour. Nevertheless there may still be difficulties in differentiating radiologically between tumour and encephalitis, demyelination or even angioma. In most cases, however, this problem does not arise, and therefore in the management of the patient there are three fundamental questions

1   Is histological verification necessary?
2   Is radiotherapy advisable with or without histological verification of what is probably an astrocytoma (of lower rather than higher grade of malignancy) or an ependymoma?
3   What are the indications for an attempt at (partial) tumour removal?

The literature does not yet provide a clear answer to any of these questions for the individual patient, largely because, until the recent advent of stereotactic methods of biopsy, antemortem histological verification was rare. Furthermore, although at least in children (Matson 1969) the majority of patients die within a year of onset of symptoms, much longer survival without radiotherapy was sometimes recorded (Olivecrona 1967) and Bouchard (1966) reported that 38% of patients lived for at least 5 years after radiotherapy.

The question of attempts at tumour removal is in some ways the easiest to resolve. If CT indicates a significant cystic element, and if the mass, solid or cystic, projects backwards beyond the line of the floor of the fourth ventricle, the tumour can be approached from below between the tonsils, through the fourth ventricle. Having entered the cyst or solid tumour, the use of the operating microscope and the ultrasonic aspirator may allow reduction of the mass and representative histological diagnosis. Unless an unusually clear line of demarcation between tumour and brain stem appears, the hazards of attempting anything approaching a complete removal are great. The higher, and therefore the more pontine, rather than medullary the tumour, the less the indication for surgery.

In those circumstances stereotactic biopsy is the least hazardous method for verifying the pathology. Unfortunately until these newer techniques have led to studies of sufficiently large numbers of cases to allow a meaningful correlation between verified pathology, radiotherapy and outcome, the use of radiotherapy without histological verification will remain a matter of opinion rather than reasoned judgement.

# References

ALBRIGHT A. L. (1983) *Clin. Neurosurg.,* **30**, 278.
ANDREW J. & NATHAN P. W. (1965) *Proc. roy. Soc. Med.,* **58**, 553.
ARSENI C. (1958) *Arch. Neurol. Psychiat.,* **80**, 18.
ASK-UPMARK E. (1938) *Acta Med. Scand.,* **94**, 392.
BAILEY P., SOSMAN M. C. & VAN DESEL A. (1928) *Amer. J. Roentgenol,* **19**, 203.
BAILEY P. & BUCY P. (1929) *J. Path. Bact.,* **32**, 735.
BAILEY P. & CUSHING H. (1925) *Arch. Neurol. Psychiat.,* **14**, 192.
BAILEY P. & CUSHING H. (1926) *Tumours of the Glioma Group.* Lippencott, Philadelphia.
BARNETT H. J. & HYLAND H. H. (1952) *Quart. J. Med.,* **21**, 265.
BAUER H. G. (1954) *J. clin. Endocrin,* **14**, 13.
BENNET J. P. & RUBINSTEIN L. J. (1984) *Ann. Neurol.,* **16(1)**, 21.
BERGER M. S., EDWARDS M. S. B., *et al.* (1983) *J. Neurosurg.,* **59(3)**, 418–23.
BLOOM H. J. G. THORNTON H. & SCHWEISGUTH O. (1982) In *Paediatric Oncology* (Eds. Raybaud C., Clement R. & Le Breuil G.) *Exc. Med. Int. Cong. Series,* **570**, 309.
BOUCHARD J. (1966) *Radiation Therapy of Tumours and Diseases of the Nervous System.* Kimpton. London.
BOUVIER G., ST. HILAIRE G. M., *et al.* (1983) *Appl. Neurophysiol.,* **46 (1–4)**, 52.
BRAIN TUMOUR REGISTRY IN JAPAN (1982) *Brain Tumour Registry in Japan,* **4.** National Cancer Centre, Tokyo.
BRISMAR J., ROBERSON G. H., *et al.* (1976) *Neuroradiol.,* **12**, 109.
BRUCHER J. M. (1984) Personal Communication to Brain Tumour Cooperative Group of European Organization for Research and Treatment of Cancer (EORTC).
BULL J. W. D. (1967) *Clin. Radiol.,* **18**, 2.
CAIRNS H. W. B. (1939) *Brit. med. J.,* **2**, 361.
CAMPBELL A. N. *et al.,* (1984) *Cancer,* **15 53(4)**, 974.
CAPRA L. G. (1980) In *Brain Tumours, Scientific Basis, Clinical Investigation and Current Therapy.* (Eds. Thomas and Graham) pp. 322–43. Butterworth, London.

CHOUX M. & LENA G. (1982) Neurochirurgie, 28, Suppl 1, 1.
CRITCHLEY McD. (1949) Brain, 72, 538.
CUSHING H. (1905) Surg. Gynec. Obstet., 1, 297.
CUSHING H. (1921) Brain, 44, 341.
CUSHING H. (1932) Intracranial Tumours, Thomas, Springfield, Illinois.
CUTLER E. C., SOSMAN M. C., & VAUGHAN W. W. (1936) Amer. J. Roentgenol., 35, 429.
DAUMAS-DEPORT C., MEDER J. F., MONSAINGEON V., et al. (1983).
DEJERINE J., ROUSSY G. (1906) Rev. Neurol., 14, 521.
ELVIDGE A., PENFIELD W. & CONE W. (1937) Res. Pub. Ass. nerv. ment. Dis., 16, 107.
EORTC Brain Tumour Group (1978) Europ. J. Cancer, 14, 851.
EORTC Brain Tumour Group (1981) J. Neurosurg., 55, 27.
EORTC Brain Tumour Group (1983) Europ. J. Cancer, 19(1), 39.
FRANKEL S. A. & GERMAN W. J. (1958) J. Neurosurg., 15, 489.
FOWLER F. D. & MATSON DD. (1957) J. Neurosurg., 14, 515.
GARFIELD J. S. (1969) Brit. Med. J., 2, 7.
GARFIELD J. S. & DAYAN A. D. (1973) J. Neurosurg., 39, 315.
GARFIELD J. S. (1980) In Brain Tumours, Scientific Basis, Clinical Investigation and Current Therapy., (Eds Thomas and Graham) pp. 301–21. Butterworth, London.
GATES J. R., et al. (1984) Epilepsia, 25(3), 308.
GERMAN W. J. (1961) Clin. Neurosurg., 7, 1.
GERSTMANN J. (1940) Arch. Neurol. Psychiat., 44, 398.
GESCHWIND N. (1965) Brain, 88, 585.
GIANGASPERO F. & BURGER P. C. (1983) Cancer, 52(12), 2320.
GLOBUS J. H. & STRAUSS I. (1925) Arch. Neurol. Psychiat., 14, 139.
GOL A. (1961) J. Neurosurg., 18, 501.
GOL A. & McKISSOCK W. (1959) J. Neurosurg., 16, 287.
HARRISON M. J. (1984) Postgrad. Med. J., 60(703), 321.
HELLE T. L., BRITT R. H. & COLBY T. V. (1984) J. Neurosurg., 60, 94.
HIRSCH J. F., RENIER D. & CZERNICHOW P. (1979) Acta Neurochir., 48, 1.
HITCHCOCK E. & SATO F. (1964) J. Neurosurg., 21, 497.
HORRAX G. & WU W. Q. (1951) Neurosurg., 8, 473.
HORSLEY V. (1893) Brit. Med. J., 2, 1365.
HORTEN B. C. & RUBINSTEIN L. J. (1976) Brain, 99, 735.
HOSHINA T. (1984) J. Neurosurg., 61, 895.
JACKSON H. (1873) The Selected Writings of John Hughlings Jackson, (Ed. Taylor J. 1931) vol. 1, p. 100. Hodder and Stoughton, London.
JEFFERSON G. (1937) Brit. Med. J., 2, 199.
KELLY K. A. (1984) Cancer Treatment Reviews, 11(1), 1–26.
KERNOHAN J. W., MABON R. E., SVIEN H. J., et al. (1949) Proc. Mayo Clin., 24, 71.
KERNOHAN J. W. & UIHLEIN A. (1962) Sarcomas of the Brain. Thomas Springfield, Illinois.
KLEIHUES P., et al. (1984) Acta Neurochir., (suppl) 33, 171–81.
KRAYENBÜHL H. (1959) Acta Neurochir. (Suppl), 6, 31.
LEVIN V. A. & EDWARDS M. S. (1984) In Brain Tumours, Scientific Basis, Clinical Investigation and Current Therapy. (Eds Thomas and Graham) Butterworth, London.
LEVY L. F. & ELVIDGE A. R. (1956) J. Neurosurg., 13, 413.
LUND M. (1952) Acta Psych. Neurol. Scand., Supplement 81.
McKENZIE K. G. (1936) Arch. Neurol. Psychiat., 36, 542.

MACEWEN W. (1893) Brit. med. J., 2, 1367.
McKISSOCK W. & PAINE K. W. E. (1958) Brain, 81, 41.
McLAURIN R. L. (1983) Clin. Neurosurg., 30, 286–92.
MARSDEN C. D. & HARRISON M. J. G. (1972) Brit. med. J., 1, 249.
MARTIN F. & LEMMEN L. J. (1952) Amer. J. Path., 28, 1107.
MATSON D. (1969) Neurosurgery of Infancy and Childhood. 2nd edition. pp. 410, 449, 461. Thomas, Springfield, Illinois.
NATHAN P. (1963) Neurologia Med. chirurg., 5, 9.
NEVIN S. (1938) Brain, 61, 170.
OLIVECRONA H. (1967) Handbuch der Neurochirurgie. Springer, Berlin.
OSTERTAG B. (1952) J. nerv. ment. Dis., 116, 726.
PACKER R. J., et al. (1983) Childs Brain, 10(6), 393.
PACKER R. J., SUTTON L. N., et al. (1984) J. Neurosurg., 61, 296.
PARK T. S., HOFFMAN H. J., HENDRICK E. B., et al. (1983) J. Neurosurg., 58(4), 543.
PATERSON E. & FARR R. F. (1953) Acta Radiol., 39, 323.
PENFIELD W. & ERICKSON T. C. (1941) Epilepsy and Cerebral Localization. Bailliere, Tindall and Cox, London.
PENFIELD W. & RASMUSSEN T. (1950) The Cerebral Cortex of Man. Macmillan, New York.
PENFIELD W. & ROBERTSON J. S. M. (1943) Arch. Neurol. Psychiat., 50, 405.
PENMAN J. & SMITH M. C. (1954) Spec Rep. Ser. Med. Res. Can. (Lond.), 284.
PUNT J. (1984) In Dilemmas in the Management of the Neurological Patient. (Ed. Warlow and Garfield) pp. 158–67. Churchill Livingstone. Edinburgh.
RASMESSEN T. & BLUNDELL J. (1961) Clin. Neurosurg., 7, 138.
RAYPORT M., FERGUSON S. M. & CORRIE W. S. (1983) Appl. Neurophysiol., 46(1–4), 47.
REYMOND A. & RINGERTZ N. (1950) Schweiz. Arch f. Neurol., 65, 221.
RUBINSTEIN L. J. & NORTHFIELD D. W. C. (1964) Brain, 87, 379.
RUBINSTEIN L. J. (1967) J. Neurosurg., 26, 542.
RUSSELL D. S. & RUBINSTEIN L. J. (1977) Pathology of Tumours of the Nervous System. 4th edition, p. 310. Edward Arnold, London.
ROTH J. G. & ELVIDGE A. R. (1960) J. Neurosurg., 17, 736.
SAFDARI H., et al. (1984) Surg. Neurol., 21 (1), 35, 41.
SALAZAR O. M., CASTRO-VITA H., et al. (1983) J. Neurosurg., 59, 652.
SCHADÉ J. P. & McMENEMEY W. H. (1963) Selective Vulnerability of the Brain in Hypoxaemia. Blackwell Scientific Publications, Oxford.
SCHERER H. J. (1940) J. Neurol. Psychiat., 3, 147.
SHELINE G. E., BOLDREY E., et al. (1964) Radiology, 82, 84.
STEINBERG G. K., SHUER L. M., et al. (1985) J. Neurosurg., 62, 9.
TANDON P. N. (1984) J. Neuro-Onocol., 2, 279.
TENNY R. T., LAWS E. R., et al. (1982) J. Neurosurg., 57, 452.
THOMAS D. G. T., ANDERSON R. E., et al. (1984) J. Neurol. Neurosurg. Psychiat., 47, 9.
TÖNNIS W. (1962) In Handbuch der Neurochirurgie. (Eds Olivecrona H. & Tönnis) p. 244. Springer-Verlag, Berlin.
TOOTH H. H. (1912) Brain, 35, 99.
TOVI D., SCHISANO G. & LILJEQUIST B. (1961) J. Neurosurg., 18, 730.
VAN DER WIEL H. J. (1960) Inheritance of Glioma. Elsevier, Amsterdam.
WEIR B. (1973) J. Neurosurg., 39, 448.

WELLER R.O., McLELLAN D.L. (1983) *Clinical Neuropathology*, p. 107. Springer Verlag, Berlin.

YOUNG B., OLDFIELD E.H., *et al.* (1981) *J. Neurosurg.*, **55**, 917.

ZÜLCH K.J. (1965) *Brain Tumours: Their Biology and Pathology*, 2nd edn. Heinemann, London.

ZÜLCH K.J. (1979) *Histological typing of tumours of the central nervous system—International Histological Classification of tumours*. World Health Organization, Geneva.

# Chapter 6
# Cysts and other space-occupying lesions

J. S. GARFIELD

## Choroid plexus papilloma

Although linked by ancestry, the papilloma of the choroid plexus and the ependymoma are quite distinct in appearance and behaviour. Conflicting opinions are expressed on the age incidence of papillomas; this is probably a consequence of insufficient numbers and of selection according to the hospital practice on which the report is based. Bohm and Strang (1961) recorded only 6 cases below the age of 15 years in a series of 25; Ringertz and Reymond (1949) stated that they usually occur in childhood and adolescence, while Posey (1942) found that 50% recorded at that time were in patients under the age of 20 years. It is generally agreed, however, that the lateral ventricle tumour is much commoner in children than in adults and conversely an infratentorial situation is the rule in adults. In the 25 examples of Bohm and Strang there were 15 in the fourth ventricle and the ages of the patients were from 18–60 years. The renewed interest taken in infantile hydrocephalus in recent years and the more extensive use of air studies is responsible for disclosing increasing numbers in the lateral ventricles in children; Cushing (1932) with an experience of over 2000 intracranial tumours encountered only 12 papillomas, of which 6 were midline in the fourth ventricle and 3 were situated laterally, mimicking an acoustic tumour.

Within the lateral ventricle, which the tumour may not fill, it occurs as a rounded dark pink mass with a finely granular or nodular surface (Fig. 6.1). It is firmer than normal brain and often stringy; it may be gritty from calcification and usually very vascular. It might be confused macroscopically with an intraventricular men-

ingioma, which however generally has a smooth surface, though it may be lobulated and its texture is tougher and rarely gritty. Both are attached to the choroid plexus, usually in the vestibule, whence the tumours derive their major blood supply and consequently may be identified by angiography. In the third and fourth ventricles the tumour is of the same texture but usually fills the cavity and may extrude through its communications. Ordinarily the tumour is clearly separable from surrounding white matter. Russell and Rubinstein state that malignant papillomas are rare; they had only two examples, both in the lateral ventricles in children, the tumour invading brain tissue; the cells showed malignant characteristics. The experience of Bohm and Strang (1961) seems to have been less fortunate, for they state that three-quarters of the lateral ventricle tumours were malignant, though all those in the fourth ventricle were benign.

In 1952 Kahn and Luros reported that after the removal of a papilloma hydrocephalic symptoms were relieved. This experience has been repeatedly confirmed by many neurosurgeons and there is now no doubt that choroid plexus papilloma can cause hydrocephalus even when its situation is such that its bulk does not obstruct the flow of cerebrospinal fluid. Alternative causes for the hydrocephalus should be considered. Meningeal fibrosis may occur as a result of recurrent subarachnoid bleeding to which these tumours are prone, or of the leptomeningeal dissemination of papilloma cells. Tumour seeds of macroscopic size may also occur, in the ventricles and in the subarachnoid spaces (Russell & Rubinstein 1959).

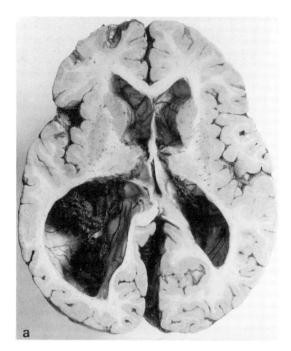

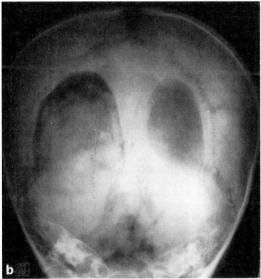

Fig. 6.1 (a) Papilloma of choroid plexus in vestibule of left lateral ventricle: hydrocephalus: note that ventricle around the tumour is more dilated than elsewhere. Infant aged 11 months. Several months of vomiting: early papilloedema: death followed suboccipital craniotomy for presumed medulloblastoma.
(b) Typical appearance in ventriculogram.

## Histology

The benign papilloma resembles closely the structure of normal choroid plexus. It consists of branching fronds, each surrounded by a sparse connective tissue stroma and lined by a single layer of cuboidal epithelium devoid of cilia and blepharoblasts. In some instances the epithelium may be tall columnar and rarely it may show evidence of mucus production, typical goblet cells being scattered among the columnar cells (Fig. 6.2) (Matsushima 1983).

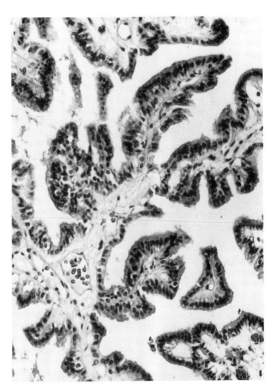

Fig. 6.2 Papilloma of choroid plexus. H. & E. × 240

## Malignant forms

These rare tumours are virtually confined to the lateral ventricles of young children. The histological appearances are bizarre.

In some parts the papillary structure and the relation to blood vessels are preserved, but the lining epithelial cells include atypical forms with giant hyperchromatic nuclei and mitotic figures. Other parts of the tumour form solid sheets of undifferentiated cells indistinguishable from other anaplastic gliomas. These tumours invade the cerebral parenchyma and may metastasize widely through the cerebrospinal fluid pathway.

*Diagnosis in wet film preparations*

The fragmented papillae seen in films are in many cases indistinguishable from pieces of normal choroid plexus frequently seen in biopsies (obtained by needling) particularly of the temporal lobes. Diagnosis of malignant tumours depends on the finding of papillary structures lined by obviously abnormal cells. The presence of papillary fronds in a malignant glial tumour may only indicate invasion of the choroid plexus by a glioblastoma. Malignant papillary tumours in adults are almost invariably secondary carcinomas.

**Diagnosis and treatment**

In children the diagnosis is rarely more precise than hydrocephalus, for there are no symptoms of particular significance (Matson 1969). But unlike the hydrocephalus due to congenital abnormalities, the infant usually develops normally in every respect for the first year or so and when hydrocephalus occurs, papilloedema is often detected (Laurence *et al.* 1961). This would be an unusual sign in infantile hydrocephalus. In the majority of cases the cerebrospinal fluid is xanthochromic and its protein content elevated; this is a highly suggestive finding if the fluid is taken from the lateral ventricle. Precise diagnosis can be obtained by ventriculography, but sufficient air or positive contrast medium must be introduced to enable the lateral ventricles to be fully examined. Ventriculography has now been almost completely replaced by CT scanning, but in the absence of CT scan, ventriculography should remain in the neurosurgeon's armamentarium.

The management of the supratentorial choroid plexus papilloma is surgical excision. The most common area of origin is related to the trigone or immediately anterior to the trigone in the floor of the body of the lateral ventricle. The approach is therefore through a midparietal craniotomy centred above the ear; the dilated ventricle is entered and the tumour mobilized. The major surgical problems are related to the venous drainage of the tumour and unwary surgeons may find themselves in difficulties which increase as the internal cerebral vein is approached. It may be difficult to differentiate surgically between the true base of the tumour and normal choroid plexus. Postoperative disappointments include the failure of normal CSF circulation to be established, either due to fibrosis within the ventricular system or to inadequate CSF pathways at the tentorial hiatus and over the cerebral hemispheres. Choroid plexus papillomas of the third ventricle (Jooma & Kendall 1983) are rare and are approached by the transventricular route, either from the frontal convexity or the anterior corpus callosum.  In 5 of the cases of Matson and Crofton (1960) the tumour was histologically malignant and had invaded the wall of the ventricle; this was considered to be the chief cause of postoperative death.

In the posterior fossa the papilloma commonly fills the fourth ventricle and may protrude through the foramen of Magendie, its papillary surface providing a means of recognition by the surgeon. On occasion the tumour extends outwards through a foramen of Luschka into the cerebellopontine angle, where it causes symptoms and signs which simulate an acoustic tumour. The length of history may extend from a few months to several years and the clinical picture provides no clue as to the nature of the tumour, but X-ray of the skull may reveal calcification. Deposits of calcium are rare in other tumours in the posterior fossa. Bohm and Strang (1961) found calcification in 6 of 15 fourth ventricle tumours.

Unfortunately problems of CSF flow due to adhesions at the exit foramina of the fourth ventricle, the cisterna magna and the prepontine and ambiens cisterns, often make postoperative CSF shunting necessary.

## Pineal tumours

Tumours arising in the region of the pineal body are often loosely dubbed 'pineal' although many are not of pineal origin. Because of their anatomical relationships they give rise to similar and characteristic clinical disturbances and to similar CT and ventriculographic appearances, but reviews of published cases based on necropsy and biopsy bear witness to the diversity of these tumours. The current trend of treatment is towards relief of hydrocephalus by CSF shunting, followed by radiotherapy. The place of excision, attempted excision, partial removal or simply biopsy is still a matter of debate. Stereotactic biopsy offers a less dangerous course in establishing the histology, as may examination of centrifuged lumbar CSF. McGovern (1949) analysed 236 cases and considered less than one-fifth were truly pineal, the lesions in the others being teratomas, gliomas, 'hypertrophies' and cysts. A similar study by Haldeman (1927) of 113 cases gave the following result: sarcoma 24, teratoma 22, cyst 14, glioma 11, pinealoma 10, adenoma 4, hyperplasia 4, and miscellaneous 24. This profusion of names is evidence of uncertainty of classification and this is aggravated by the few cases encountered except in the largest clinics. Zülch's (1965) enormous series of 6000 brain tumours contained only 25 pinealomas and 14 teratomas; how many of the latter were in the region of the pineal is not stated. The classification of Russell and Rubinstein (1959) is here adopted:

1 teratoma (a) typical (b) atypical;
2 pinealoma (a) pineoblastoma (b) pineocytoma;
3 glioma;
4 cyst.

### 1 (a) Teratoma: typical

Teratomas of the brain nearly always occur in the median plane and the pineal region is the commonest site. Pineal teratomas occur largely in males. The tumour forms a firm mass, its consistency and texture depending upon the degree to which such elements as cartilage, bone, etc. have been formed. Cysts may be present, often containing pearly or porridge-like material. The well differentiated tumours are benign, and usually easily separated from brain tissue, but where there is contact with leptomeninges or with large blood vessels a considerable reactive fibrosis is excited. It is this which renders their removal difficult and dangerous, for they may be firmly bound to the upper brain stem and to the internal cerebral veins.

*Histology*

These tumours, like benign teratomas in other parts of the body, consist of a mixture of well differentiated tissues derived from various germinal layers and arranged to form easily recognized organoid structures, such as skin with appendages, bone, cartilage, muscle and many others (Fig 6.3). Some tumours appear to replace the pineal, others are parapineal and only displace or compress the intact gland. Less differentiated examples have also been recorded in which unidentifiable epithelial tubules are scattered among tissues of mesenchymal origin. These are described as 'teratoid' and may be malignant. They sometimes contain foci of tissue resembling atypical teratoma. The rare chorioncarcinomas of this region may also form part of teratoid tumours.

### 1(b) Teratoma: atypical

The largest group of tumours, generally known as pinealoma (or germinoma) was regarded by Russell as an atypical teratoma. This view was based upon the morphology of the cells, the pres-

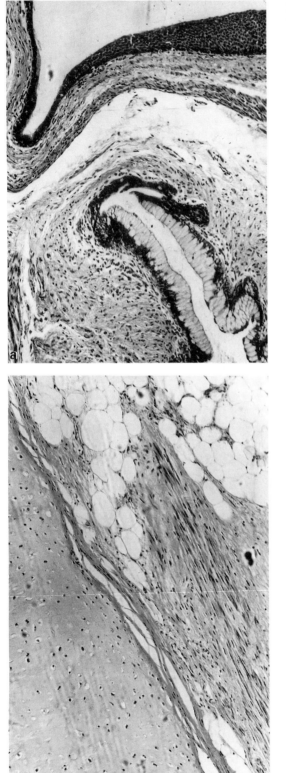

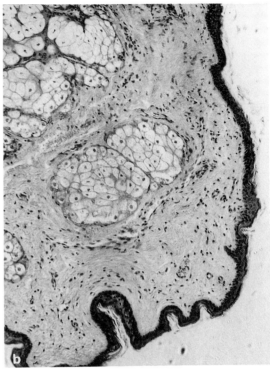

Fig. 6.3 Benign teratoma of pineal. (a) Two cysts, one lined with transitional, the other with mucus-producing columnal epithelium.
(b) Keratinized squamous epithelium and sebaceous glands.
(c) Cartilage, smooth muscle and adipose tissue.
V.G. × 240

ence of other tissues in some 'pinealomas' and of 'pinealoma' areas in tumours in this region generally accepted as atypical teratomas and the cytological similarity to spheroidal-celled carcinoma of the testicle, a tumour regarded by many as an atypical teratoma. Cases occur in which tumours of this histological type arise in the third ventricle or its vicinity but in which the pineal body itself is clearly not involved; they have been termed 'ectopic pinealomas'. If they are atypical teratomas, their presence in these sites will occasion no surprise since typical teratomas also occur here. The liability of the hypothalamus to invasion by these tumours explains the high incidence of pubertas praecox in recorded cases of pineal tumour (14% in Haldeman's series) and of diabetes insipidus. In those cases in which it develops in the pineal region vision deteriorates as a result of papilloedema due to hydrocephalus. In the infrequent case in which the tumour starts in the anterior part of the third ventricle vision deteriorates as a result of invasion of the optic chiasm and primary optic atrophy supervenes. Dayan *et al.* (1966) have made an extensive and critical review of this tumour.

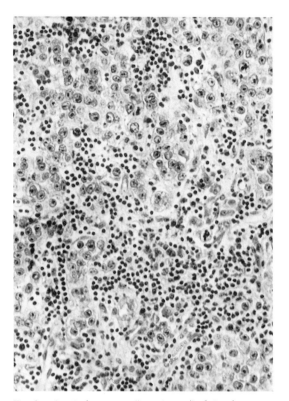

**Fig. 6.4.** Atypical teratoma ('germinoma') of pineal. Juxtaposition of groups of large round tumour cells and small lymphocytes. H. & E. × 240

*Histology*

The characteristic feature of these tumours is the intermingling of tumour cells with inflammatory elements (Fig. 6.4). The tumour cells are round, with a fairly large nucleus, a distinct chromatin pattern and scanty eosinophilic cytoplasm. They resemble those seen in testicular seminomas and ovarian dysgerminomas. They usually lie in loose clusters surrounded by inflammatory cells, mainly lymphocytes, but also histiocytes which in some cases may form epithelioid-cell granulomas with giant cells closely resembling the lesions of sarcoidosis. The inflammatory elements may overshadow the neoplastic ones, which in some cases may be reduced to a few isolated cells embedded in granulation tissue, an important point in the interpretation of diagnostic biopsies. Atypical teratomas are malig-

nant tumours which spread extensively through the cerebrospinsal fluid pathway. Tumour tissue may coat the ependymal lining of the ventricles and the choroid plexuses or fill the ventricular cavities. It may invade the brain parenchyma, most commonly the corpus callosum and the quadrigeminal plate. It may disseminate through the subarachnoid space, particularly of the spinal cord and the cauda equina. In rare instances it may transgress the dura mater and invade the base of the skull, vertebral bodies and the sacrum. Distant haematogenous metastases have also been reported.

Atypical teratomas can be diagnosed in wet film preparations where the tumour cells display a characteristiclly bizarre pattern of nuclear chromatin (Dayan *et al.* 1966). The small round cells of the inflammatory stroma are also present in variable numbers.

## 2 Pinealoma

Although Russell and Rubinstein interpret the majority of pineal tumours as atypical teratoma, a view not shared by Zülch though given qualified approval by Willis, they agree that there remains a small group of tumours which should be regarded as arising from the parenchyma of the pineal. These are the pinealomas.

### Histology

(a) *Pineoblastoma.* This exceedingly rare tumour consists of closely packed, undifferentiated cells with dark nuclei and barely visible cytoplasm. In their appearance they closely resemble medulloblastomas. Occasionally better differentiated examples are seen which tend to reproduce the lobular 'mosaic' pattern of the fetal pineal.

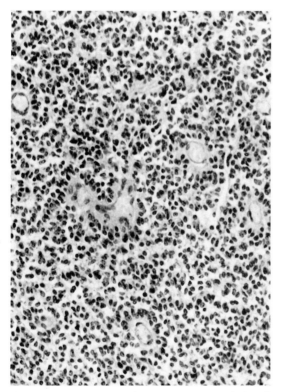

**Fig. 6.5.** Pineocytoma: a uniform tumour composed of small cells of a single type in places arranged in perivascular pseudorosettes. H. & E. × 240

These tumours are malignant, but too few examples have been described for valid observations on their growth and spread.

(b) *Pineocytoma.* This uncommon neoplasm consists of fully differentiated, mature pineal cells (Fig. 6.5). These cells contain round nuclei with a coarse chromatin pattern, scanty cytoplasm and short processes demonstrable by appropriate silver impregnations. The tumours are moderately cellular and contain abundant blood vessels which divide the cell groups into lobules or palisaded rows. Both true rosettes and perivascular pseudorosettes may be prominent. Little is known of the biological behaviour of this tumour but it appears to be a growth of slow evolution and low degree of malignancy.

## 3 Gliomas

Since the pineal body contains glial tissue it is not surprising that some tumours are gliomas, though it may be impossible to determine in a given case whether the glioma arose within the pineal, or invaded and destroyed it. Ringertz *et al.* (1954) found astrocytoma, spongioblastoma, ependymoma, papilloma of choroid plexus and glioblastoma to be responsible for about one-fifth of their pineal tumours. Jooma and Kendall (1983) recorded three patients who proved to have pineal gliomas in a series of 35 pineal tumours.

## 4 Cysts

Cysts in the pineal may be dermoid, epidermoid, or possibly due to degeneration of glia.

### Diagnosis

The clinical manifestations of pineal tumours fall into three groups; those due to hydrocephalus, those due to involvement of the quadrigeminal plate and those due to invasion of the hypothalamus. The symptoms and signs of raised intracranial pressure due to hydrocephalus, the result of obstruction of the posterior end of the third ventricle or the upper end of the aqueduct have no special features and usually precede other symptoms. Consequently at this stage the differential diagnosis includes all causes of obstructive hydrocephalus, particularly a high cerebellar tumour or aqueduct stenosis, and only ventriculography, CT scan or NMR identifies the condition, though an excessively dense and large pineal calcification makes the diagnosis likely.

The local disturbances due to mass lesions in the region of the pineal recess, including defects of vertical gaze and small but unequal pupils with reduced reactions to light, which are loosely referred to as Parinaud's syndrome (Parinaud 1883), occur in the majority of cases, especially with germinoma and teratoma. There may also be defects of downward gaze, disconjugate eye movements, and truncal ataxia with a tendency to topple forwards. The clinical differential diagnoses include: carrefour meningioma, aneurysm of the Great Vein of Galen, and superior vermis tumours. Chronic subdural haematoma, when it causes large shifts of the hemispheres and mid brain, may mimic mass lesions in the pineal region.

Pubertas praecox (precocious purberty) is the most dramatic evidence of hypothalamic disturbance and naturally figures prominently in the literature, but is probably not as common as some reports suggest. The patients are nearly always males (Ringertz *et al.* 1954). Diabetes insipidus is perhaps a more common finding and may at times escape detection; other signs of hypothalamic involvement are hypopituitarism, hypersomnia and visual failure due to invasion of the chiasm. When these features occur in a patient presenting the 'local signs' of a pineal tumour, they are the result of its direct spread or its seedling, across the floor of the third ventricle (Fig. 6.6). There is a group of cases in which hypothalamic manifestations occur without (or prior to) clinical evidence of a 'pineal' tumour, and the presentation is of a tumour of the anterior part of the third ventricle. This syn-

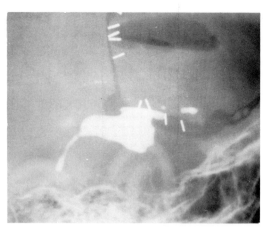

**Fig. 6.6.** Atypical teratoma: anterior and posterior ends of third ventricle contain tumour which obliterates the normal recesses: calcification in the pineal body is unduly large and is separated from the posterior end of the ventricle by a considerable interval. A considerable interval also separates the anterior limit of the ventricular air from the sella and an AEG had suggested a mass in the suprasellar region.

drome can be caused by an atypical teratoma arising primarily in the hypothalamic region and often referred to as ectopic pinealoma. A feature which distinguishes it to some extent from other tumours in this region (glioma, craniopharyngioma, pituitary adenoma, epidermoid cyst) is the early occurrence of diabetes insipidus.

### Treatment

The management of patients with pineal mass lesions has varied over the years as neurosurgery has evolved, and particularly as the efficacy of radiotherapy for pineal germinomas has become recognized. CT scanning and, more recently, NMR have allowed accurate pre-operative diagnosis. Histological verification can be obtained by examination of the CSF, and tumour markers may provide strong evidence of the type of tumour. In addition the management of obstructive hydrocephalus by CSF shunting has become commonplace, although not without its complications and technical failures. Ventriculo-cisternostomy (Torkildsen 1948) has progressively given way to ventriculo peritoneal shunting; but it should be remembered that the reestablishment of a purely intracranial and more normal CSF pathway may have fewer complications, especially when the pineal mass responds to radiotherapy. This, and other drainage procedures have been associated with an overall early mortality of less than 5% and 5 year survival rates of 60% to 75% and up to 85% for germinomas (Rao *et al.* 1981). Dandy (1921), the greatest and bravest pioneer in the history of neurosurgery, devised an occipital supratentorial approach to the pineal, but which proved difficult and to some extent hazardous due to interference with the internal cerebral veins. An alternative is the infratentorial suboccipital approach (Stein 1971) but this has generally found less favour unless the tumour is clearly projecting downwards into the posterior fossa.

Although the surgical approach by the supratentorial medial occipital route is now associated with a very low mortality (Jooma & Kendall 1983) there is still considerable debate amongst neurosurgeons about the indications for surgery in the individual case. Although practice varies, a reasonable approach is as follows: following demonstration by CT scan of a pineal tumour associated with obstructive hydrocephalus, hydrocephalus is first relieved by CSF shunting. If there is any question of a vascular lesion such as an aneurysm of the Great Vein of Galen, vertebral angiography is done. Rarely vascularity of a tumour indicative of its malignancy may be helpful. Following CSF shunting, lumbar CSF should be centrifuged and examined freshly for the presence of neoplastic cells which may confirm the diagnosis of germinoma or pineablastoma. If the alphafetoprotein level is raised, this is specific for teratoma. Beta-human chorionic gonadotropin may be secreted by germinomas and teratomas if they contain elements of choriocarcinoma.

If the evidence overall favours the diagnosis of germinoma external radiation (5000 rads) is given; a dramatic and early reduction in size of the mass on repeated CT scan effectively confirms the presumptive diagnosis, and radiotherapy is the definitive treatment, with survival extending to many years (Kahn 1961, Rubin and Kramer 1965, Jooma & Kendall 1983). If there is no evidence to support the diagnosis of germinoma the choices of management are (a) a therapeutic or diagnostic trial of radiotherapy; (b) direct surgery and attempted removal; (c) stereotactic biopsy as a guide to open surgery or radiotherapy. Stereotactic implantation of radioactive gold seeds is rarely used now. Clearly removal of the very rare dermoid or epidermoid or the unsuspected carrefour meningioma (a formidable procedure) is the treatment of choice; but the overall benefits of aggressive surgery are unproven and remain a matter of debate (Hide 1975, Jooma & Kendall 1983). Stereotactic biopsy is the most significant recent advance, and this in combination with improved definition of CT scanning and NMR, will deter the surgeon from embarking upon fruitless and damaging surgery when the lesion is an unresponsive tumour (for example, malignant glioma) which is infiltrating the midbrain or superior cerebellar vermis. Thus the grounds for direct surgery for pineal tumours are already diminishing, and as soon as really effective chemotherapy is available, they will diminish even more.

## Colloid cyst of third ventricle

Although these cysts are often placed in the same group as ependymomas and papillomas they are in no way similar to them or indeed to any other neoplasm of the brain; in some respects they resemble the mucous enterogenous cysts of the spinal canal. Sjovall (1910) who first described the colloid cyst, suggested that it may derive from the paraphysis, a glandular structure found in the brain of lower vertebrates but vestigial in humans, though present in the embryo. This structure develops from the roof plate of the diencephalon in common with the tela choroidea of lateral and third ventricles and the pineal body, and in appropriate sections can be seen lying contiguous and immediately dorsal to the lamina terminalis. It is note-worthy that in some animals it is an actively secreting organ. Kappers (1955) considers that the majority of the cysts are ependymal in origin, though admits that some may be paraphysial: in the literature they are not infrequently referred to as ependymal cysts.

The position of the colloid cyst of the third ventricle is constant: it is situated in the anterior part of the ventricle applied to its roof just behind the foramen of Monro where it is attached to the tela choroidea. It may be quite small, asymptomatic, and a chance finding at post-mortem examination (as was the case in Harvey Cushing's brain; Fulton 1946). In such cases it may be only a few millimetres in diameter and occupies little space in the upper part of the ventricle. Specimens which cause symptoms are 2–3 cm in diameter, spherical, obstruct the foramina of Monro and block the cavity of the third ventricle; they may elevate its roof so that a characteristic filling defect is seen in the floor of the lateral ventricle (Figs. 6.7 and 6.8). The wall of cyst is smooth and thin, transmitting the colour of its contents; the fluid is glairy (hence the name) or mucoid, olive green or yellow in colour. It is usually clear and contains no cholesterol crystals, which for the surgeon is a significant point of difference from the fluid derived from a

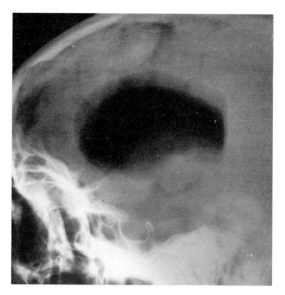

**Fig. 6.8.** A colloid cyst is clearly outlined as a rounded filling defect in the upper anterior part of the third ventricle: it juts into the floor of the lateral ventricle which is markedly dilated.

craniopharyngioma or glioma. The former usually, the latter occasionally contains such crystals, which lend a sparkling or glittering opalescence to the fluid. The cyst is lined by epithelium; there is no solid portion. It gives rise to a remarkable diversity of clinical syndromes

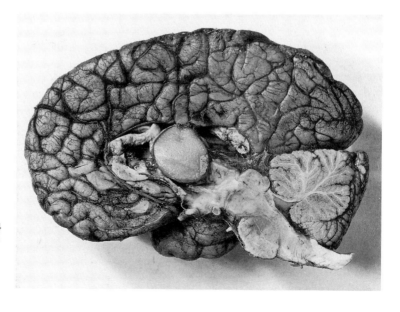

**Fig. 6.7.** Large colloid cyst of third ventricle. Patient aged 14 years had complained of visual difficulties for a year, no cause found: 2 days of progressively severe headache terminated in respiratory arrest.

as a result of hydrocephalus and of pressure upon the lateral walls of the third ventricle. No example of malignant change has been recorded.

*Histology*

Colloid cysts of the third ventricle consist of an outer fibrous capsule lined by a layer of epithelium (Fig. 6.9). The epithelium may vary in appearance from low cuboidal to tall columnar

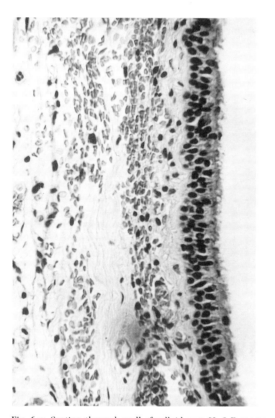

**Fig. 6.9.** Section through wall of colloid cyst. H. & E. × 420

and may be defective in parts of the cyst. If well preserved it is usually ciliated. In about one third of the cases it contains droplets of mucin and typical goblet cells are occasionally seen. The contents of the cyst consist of a homogeneous mucoid material and epithelial debris.

**Diagnosis**

Although the first known successful removal of a colloid cyst was performed by Dandy in 1921, they had been recognized as a cause of hydrocephalus for many years. In his monograph on third ventricle tumours, Dandy (1933) tabulates details of 31 cases derived from the literature, the first of these being by Wallmann in 1858. The operation in 1921 marked a great technical advance for two reasons. Firstly, the diagnosis of such a lesion by ventriculography, only three years after its introduction. Although the technique and the radiography were not sufficiently advanced to outline the cyst, the argument given in the account of the case and which led him to operate was illuminating in its logicality. The right ventricle only was tapped and air injected, revealing on the film its great distension and its medial boundary extended into the left hemicranium; as much of the ventricle was on the left side as the right. This was then a new finding in ventriculography. It was quite evident that there was closure of the right foramen of Munro. Some days later the left ventricle was tapped and air injected, and the X-rays revealed a similar appearance: 'it was a mirror image of the other'. Dandy correctly deduced that a tumour must block both foramina of Monro, thereby preventing air from passing from one side to the other. He courageously decided to operate and the successful result provides the second reason for regarding this case as a landmark in neurosurgery.

In his analysis of his own and other recorded cases Dandy drew attention to the major symptoms of colloid cysts, as we recognize them now. Foremost are those due to raised intracranial pressure from hydrocephalus and which of themselves provide no clue as to the cause. But important features are present in some cases. Symptoms may arise abruptly and progress precipitously to a fatal issue within 24 hours. The symptoms may remit completely, only to return after an interval of many years. In Cairns and Mosberg's (1951) series, this happened in 9 out of 10 cases, the intervals of freedom extending up to 10 years.

Considerable emphasis has been placed by many writers on the tendency for the headache to be aggravated by sudden change in posture, for example, to be made worse by stooping down. But this is also encountered in patients with tumours elsewhere and is by no means pathognomonic of a colloid cyst, though it may be more frequent in such patients. This fluctuation of headache has been ascribed to movement of the cyst within the third ventricle so that the cyst becomes jammed against the foramina of Monro. Such an explanation is mechanically attractive, but post-mortem examination of specimens large enough to cause hydrocephalus shows that their size then is such that change in posture could have had no effect and their momentum can be very little different from surrounding tissues. Only the smallest and therefore asymptomatic cysts could swing freely in the third ventricle.

Remission for long periods is even more difficult to explain and may be due to spontaneous necrosis and performation of the wall of the cyst when the pressure of its contents becomes very high, resulting in discharge of contents and partial collapse. The walls of some are so fragile that this seems possible.

A symptom of acute hydrocephalus from any cause, but particularly common in this condition, is sudden weakness of the legs, causing the patient to fall without warning, though unaccompanied by loss of consciousness or by vertigo. These drop attacks were noted by Dandy and by many since.

If hydrocephalus develops very slowly in an adult it may cause dementia (without evidence of raised intracranial pressure) as described by Riddoch (1936).

Although ventriculography has been superceded by the noninvasive investigations of CT scan and NMR, it should not be forgotten that ventriculography can provide precise diagnosis. The typical appearance is marked dilatation of the lateral ventricles, and a thin crescent of contrast or air which outlines the bulging anterior extremity of the third ventricle, its concave posterior margin being caused by the cyst. If the foramina of Monro are completely blocked, the cyst is usually large enough to create a midline rounded indentation in the floors of the lateral ventricles in the AP projection. Indeed in the absence of satisfactory sagittal reconstructions of high definition, CT scan may fail to differentiate clearly between an intrinsic irremovable third ventricle glioma infiltrating upwards into the base of the septum pellucidum and into the floor of the lateral ventricles, and an 'extrinsic' and removable colloid cyst. Such diagnostic difficulties were rarely experienced with ventriculography. Management is surgical, the objective being total removal of the lesion. The transventricular approach is facilitated by the presence of hydrocephalus through a short cortical incision in the right posterior frontal region, passing through the white matter to enter the dilated lateral ventricle in line with the foramen of Monro. Insertion of two selfretaining retractors along the track of the incision is helpful; alternatively, the anterior part of the corpus callosum can be traversed to enter the lateral ventricle just above the foramen of Monro.

The cyst is seen through the dilated foramen of Monro, which may be enlarged if necessary away from the anterior pillar of the fornix; it is aspirated, in order to diminish its size and to exclude an aneurysm, seized with forceps and gently withdrawn from the third ventricle and its attachment to the choroid plexus divided after clipping or coagulation. Haemorrhage from the plexus or neighbouring terminal vein is the hazard. The operative mortality is relatively low. Only one of Dandy's 5 patients died, the cause of death being stenosis of the aqueduct; Cairns and Mosberg (1951) reported 2 deaths in 11 cases in which the cyst was removed and in the 50 cases of McKissock (1965) there were 8 deaths; coma at the time of the patient's admission carried a bad prognosis. On the whole the late results of operations have been gratifying; memory defects and dementia may persist, though often these symptoms improve sufficiently to allow of employment; epilepsy occasionally develops.

An alternative to total removal of the cyst is aspiration either using the ventriculoscope or by a CT stereotactic method (Rivas 1985). However it will require much longer periods of follow-up than are available so far, before the incidence of recurrence can be assessed after these methods, although it can be claimed that they can be repeated with negligible mortality and morbidity. That claim presupposes that the recurrence does not present with sudden acute obstruction or death.

## Dermoid and epidermoid cysts

These epithelial lined cysts are rare, providing 1.0% or less of intracranial tumours. They are considered together since their natural histories are similar and their identification often depends entirely upon the microscopical appearances of the cyst wall. They are derived from epiblastic cells predestined to form skin which have become detached from their neighbours and included in mesenchyme at about the third to the fifth week of fetal life, when the neural tube is closing. Their situation in the central nervous system will depend upon the fortuitous position of this epithelial rest relative to the rostrocaudal axis of the neural tube, to its coverings and to the primary elements of the developing brain.

Critchley and Ferguson (1928) provided a fascinating historical review of the early literature on these tumours which have excited attention because of their rarity and their unique appearance. The outstanding contributions are those of Verattus who in 1745 described an intraventricular mass containing hair; LePrestre in 1828 who used the word 'pearl' in describing the appearance of the tumour. In 1829 Cruveilhier introduced the term 'pearly tumour' and showed that this appearance was due to cholestrol and stearine-like material. The name 'cholesteatoma' was given in 1838 by Müller, and von Remak in 1854 and Boström in 1897 put forward the view now generally accepted that these tumours have an embryological origin. Mahoney (1936) also reviewed the literature, listing the chief details of 142 cases (all epidermoids) and added 5 from Foerster's clinic. Although they may give rise to

symptoms at all ages, the maximum incidence occurs between the ages of 30 and 60 years.

*Extracranial* dermoid cysts are relatively common pea-like subcutaneous swellings, usually noticed in childhood, lying in a depression in the skull and occurring along the lines of fusion of the facial processes and in the sagittal plane of the scalp. Deeper inclusion between the lateral nasal and the maxillary processes accounts for their presence within the orbit; lying in its upper and outer part they cause proptosis, the globe being displaced downwards and inwards. *Cranial* pearly tumours may arise within the bone in the diploë; they erode the tables, the inner more than the outer, so that the dura mater may be exposed and impressed but rarely penetrated. These tumours are commonly classified in the literature as diploic, and 23 of the 142 listed by Mahoney were so situated. Those arising in the skull vault usually give rise to a painless external boss; only occasionally is the outer table destroyed and the swelling soft and fluctuating and then the intracranial pulsations may be transmitted through it; the absence of transillumination will exclude a meningocele. They may occur in the frontal bone behind the superciliary ridge and when the erosion of bone is near the frontal sinus may be mistaken for a mucocele of the sinus or for chronic osteitis. A small but interesting group was described by Jefferson and Smalley (1938) arising in the middle portion of the petrous bone and produce a painless progressive facial palsy; the cleanly-cut destruction of bone is easily demonstrated radiologically. Tumours in this situation are not to be confused with the cholesteatomas of chronic middle ear disease which have a different aetiology. Epidermoid cysts may also give rise to destruction of the apex of the petrous bone, in association with signs of a cerebellopontine angle syndrome. As mentioned later, such cysts may occur within this angle lying intradurally and causing no erosion of bone. It is likely that those which cause bone erosion are primarily extradural, arising in the apex of the petrous bone, though they may insinuate themselves forwards to the optic chiasma and backwards to the pons (Baumann & Bucy 1956).

*Intracranial.* A more frequent situation for these tumours is within the dura mater. Of 240 published cases and of 100 cases provided by members of the Société de Neurochirurgie de Langue Française, Lepoire and Pertuiset (1957) estimated that 80% were intradural. They tend to be situated primarily in the subarachnoid cisterns of the base of the brain, though by expansion may bury themselves in brain tissue. Parapontine—including the cerebellopontine angle—form the largest group and parapituitary or chiasmal the second common situation. A considerable number occur within the lateral ventricles, usually in the temporal horn or vestibule, occasionally in the fourth ventricle. A few arise within the Sylvian fissure embedding themselves in the temporal lobe or spreading forwards to the chiasm and they may also lie between the cerebral hemispheres in a 'supracallosal' position (Pattison 1937).

In their outstanding review Lepoire and Pertuiset offer an ingenious hypothesis to explain the seemingly haphazard anatomical distribution of the intradural tumours. They consider that the epiblastic inclusions are carried to their final destinations by the developing network of cerebral arteries. On this basis they classify location according to the major arterial territories: carotid (chiasmal and parasellar, frontal, supracallosal and Sylvian), vertebrobasilar (cerebellopontine angle, prepontine, cerebellar), choroidal (intraventricular).

## Pathology

The wall of an epidermoid cyst is so thin as to be transparent, transmitting the characteristic appearance of its contents, which are creamy-white and glistening. The latter quality is imparted by the crystals of cholesterol. The contents are firm, crumbly, flaky or amorphous with a greasy texture and comprise the products of degeneration of the desquamating stratified epithelium which lines the cyst. Externally the tumour has a nodular surface and though clearly demarcated from brain tissue, its capsule is usually firmly adherent to blood vessels, leptomeninges or choroid plexus, with which it may be in contact. The tenuous nature of the wall and firm adhesions to these tissues makes its total removal often impossible. The tumour insinuates itself into the various subarachnoid recesses and cisterns, expanding them and displacing and burrowing into the neighbouring brain. Although it may reach a large size and extend for example from the chiasma to the pons yet the rate of growth and therefore the rate of displacement of nervous structures is so slow that symptoms develop insidiously and signs are often much less than might be anticipated.

Dermoid cysts are much less frequent, may have a thicker tougher wall than epidermoids and their true nature suspected by the presence of hairs in their contents, which are otherwise similar to the contents of the epidermoid, but may be softer and even fluid. A particular and important variety occurs in the middle line of the posterior cranial fossa. It may lie in the cerebellar vermis or in the fourth ventricle or it may be extradural. Not infrequently it is connected to the overlying skin by a fibrous cord which obliquely penetrates the occipital bone. This cord may contain a patent canal lined by epithelium, the external orifice forming a minute sinus in the region of the external occipital protruberance. This form of dermoid cyst provides an exact counterpart to the sacral dermal sinus. Both are a potential source of meningitis due to bacterial invasion of the dermal sinus. Meningitis may also complicate the course of the illness by the escape of cyst contents into the ventricle or subarachnoid space; it is the cholesterol which is held responsible for this chemical irritation (Greenfield 1932). The episode may be relatively mild and transient, but occasionally a massive leak of cyst contents causes a fulminating and rapidly fatal illness. Material spilt at the time of operation may cause a low grade meningitis and delay recovery.

Anaplasia in the wall of these cysts is very rare. Davidson and Small (1960) found only 5 cases in the literature, and reported one of a frontal lobe epidermoid in which an optic nerve was invaded by carcinoma.

## Histology

*Epidermoid cysts* consist of an inner lining of heavily keratinized stratified squamous epithelium supported by an outer collagenous layer (Fig. 6.10). The contents of the cyst consist of desquamated keratin and a variable amount of cholesterol crystals. Escape of cyst contents into the surrounding tissue leads to a localized granulomatous inflammation in which foreign body giant cells are prominent. Where the cyst is adjacent to brain tissue it may produce a glial reaction.

*Dermoid cysts* differ from epidermoids in that

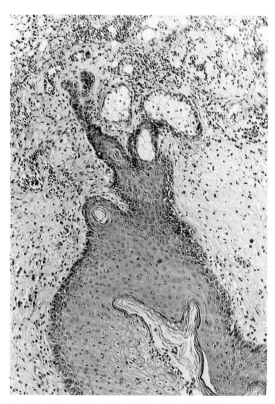

Fig. 6.11. Dermoid cyst: the lining of keratinized squamous epithelium is surrounded by a layer of connective tissue containing skin appendages (hair follicles and sebaceous glands). H. & E. × 240

in their more thick walled parts the epithelium is supported by a well formed dermis containing skin appendages, usually hair follicles with sebaceous glands, less frequently sweat glands (Fig. 6.11). They are often connected by a fibrous stalk to a dimple on the overlying skin. Microscopically this stalk may contain a narrow canal lined with squamous epithelium. If patent this may be the pathway of pyogenic infections of the cysts. Rupture of the cyst leads to spread of inflammation into the neighbouring tissues, the nature of which depends on the contents. If sterile, foreign-body type granulomas are produced while infected contents may set up a suppurative meningitis.

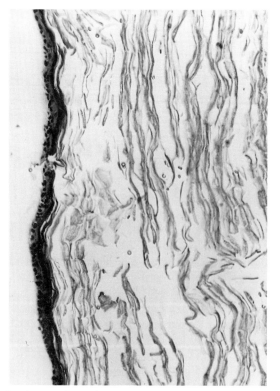

Fig. 6.10. Epidermoid cyst: the cyst wall consists of a thin layer of keratinized squamous epithelium only; the lumen contains lamellae of desquamated keratin. H. & E. × 240

## Diagnosis

*Extradural* epidermoids can usually be diagnosed by the radiological appearances. Those in the diploe produce a clearly defined osteolysis often with a dense scalloped margin; a tangential view shows that the tables are 'expanded'. Those arising in the frontal bone and causing proptosis may be mistaken for chronic osteitis or for mucocele of the frontal sinus; the long history, the absence of pain and of symptoms of sinusitis usually permit a correct diagnosis. Epidermoids arising in the petrous bone form two clinical groups and both are characterized by tell-tale bone destruction. The one group as described by Pennybacker (1944) arise in approximately the middle one-third where they compress the facial nerve and for which reason the patient seeks medical advice. Hearing may or may not be affected. The other group destroy the apex of the petrous bone and may expand into the middle fossa and backwards into the posterior fossa; in this way they may implicate cranial nerves from the second to the eighth and even lower. A similar clean-cut destruction of the apex of the petrous bone is also seen in trigeminal neurofibroma but in which the neurological disturbance is much more limited; acoustic tumour and meningioma do not produce this type of osteolysis. Carcinoma of the nasopharynx may destroy the apex of the petrous but usually at the same time invades the contiguous sphenoid and basi-occiput. Chordoma may give rise to extensive cranial nerve palsies but the sphenoid is usually the site of erosion.

The *intradural* dermoids give rise to symptoms and signs in accordance with the various sites of predilection, with the proviso that their growth is slow (the average duration of symptoms is about 5 years) and their ramifications liable to be so extensive that the neurological picture is bizarre and diagnosis obscure. Disseminated sclerosis is a common early diagnosis. Involvement of the optic nerves and chiasma leads to visual failure from primary optic atrophy, the pattern of the visual fields suggesting a compressing lesion. Endocrine function is generally unimpaired and the pituitary fossa normal. Epidermoid cysts in the cerebellopontine angle often cause trigeminal neuralgia. Olivecrona (1949) noted that such patients were usually young, that the pain was generally confined to the mandibular division and that the corneal reflex was often impaired; in these circumstances he considered that an air-encephalogram should be carried out in order to display any abnormality in the cisterna pontis and its lateral extensions. Larger cysts in this region cause signs indistinguishable from those of an acoustic tumour; absence of erosion of the internal porus, a normal value of protein in the cerebrospinal fluid and retention of hearing and of vestibular function would be suggestive of an epidermoid cyst. Bilateral cranial nerve palsies of irregular pattern may be encountered in those cysts which spread ventral to the pons.

Epidermoids within the cerebral hemispheres, like other tumours, give rise to epilepsy and for many years this may be the only symptom; a duration of 30 years has been recorded (Keville & Wise 1959). A high incidence of mental symptoms (Mahoney 1936) and an absence of papilloedema in half the patients (Tytus & Pennybacker 1956) are features which make diagnosis difficult.

The dermoid cysts in the posterior cranial fossa usually give rise to symptoms in childhood, though they may be silent for many years; the true nature of the lesion is evident if examination of the occiput reveals a dermal sinus, although this is easily overlooked as its orifice may be minute and hidden by scalp hair. Recurrent meningitis is a feature in young patients in whom there may be little or no clinical evidence of a cerebellar mass unless it becomes infected and forms an abscess. Matson and Ingraham (1951) reported on 10 cases of congenital dermal sinus; in 8 there was intracranial infection, 5 presenting as primary meningitis. In adults the clinical and radiological evidence of a dermal track may be present without a history of recurrent meningitis and the picture will be that of a midline cerebellar tumour.

As noted above, recurrent episodes of men-

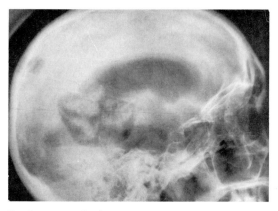

**Fig. 6.12.** An epidermoid cyst (cholesteatoma) occupying the vestibule of the lateral ventricle: it also extended into the brain stem, thereby obstructing the aqueduct and causing hydrocephalus. Note great distension of the third ventricle which straddles the sella, whose dorsum is intact. The flaky nature of cyst contents is revealed by the air.

ingitis may punctuate the history of cases of epidermoid; the meningitis is of bacterial or of chemical origin. On occasion the leak is massive and death rapidly occurs.

## Radiological investigation

X-rays of the skull may reveal the nonspecific changes due to prolonged raised intracranial pressure and very rarely calcification in the cyst. The various patterns of focal bone erosion have already been described; the extradural epidermoids are usually betrayed by the radiological examination, but except for the occipital groove or channel transmitting a dermal sinus the intradural cysts give no specific evidence of their presence.

## Treatment

Although epidermoid and dermoid cysts are histologically benign, the feasibility of total removal depends upon their situation. The diploic cysts present no particular difficulty; the wall of the cyst can be removed from the excavation in the bone by vigorous curettage, or by

craniectomy. If the wall is too firmly adherent to dura mater to be dissected from it, the dura mater should be excised and the defect filled with a fascia lata graft or nonirritating synthetic substitute. Cysts in the petrous bone can be dealt with radically, care being taken to avoid damage to the facial nerve, which however frequently does not recover its function and an inlay nerve graft may be considered necessary. The rare cysts which arise at the apex of the petrous bone (paratrigeminal) are usually too extensive to be totally removed.

The intradural cysts are often too large, their ramifications too devious and their walls too firmly adherent to important structures to allow extirpation. The most that can be achieved is a careful evacuation of their contents. In the series of Tytus and Pennybacker (1956) removal was incomplete in about one half of the intradural cases. Recurrence of symptoms after thorough removal of the contents occurs only after many years. During operation, care should be taken to prevent contamination of the field with the cholesteatomatous debris and to empty the cyst entirely. Postoperative chemical meningitis (and occasionally bacterial) is a common complication and may persist for months. Meningeal fibrosis may be severe leading to hydrocephalus needing operative relief.

The dermoid cysts of the posterior fossa present a somewhat different problem. If the patient, usually a child, presents with a pyogenic meningitis without evidence of cerebellar mass, the meningitis should first be treated and the dermal sinus and cyst excised later. If the meningitis fails to respond to treatment, or if the cyst is already giving rise to raised intracranial pressure and signs of cerebellar disorder, the cyst and dermal sinus must be promptly excised under appropriate antibiotic cover; it is in effect an abscess and will maintain the meningeal infection. Dermoid cysts in this situation lend themselves more readily to total removal and when death occurs this is usually due to meningitis, either in its acute phase or as a result of subsequent meningeal fibrosis causing hydrocephalus.

# Arachnoid cysts

Cerebrospinal fluid may be trapped in the sub-arachnoid space to form cyst-like cavities at various points around the brain. Some truly merit the description cyst, in that they are closed cavities entirely shut off from the fluid in the neigh-bouring subarachnoid space: the wall of the cyst appears everywhere to be intact. Others are local distentions of the subarachnoid space due to mul-tiple adhesions from leptomeningeal fibrosis; some may be likened to pouches since they com-municate by a narrow neck with the general subarachnoid space.

## Arachnoidal cyst

This lies within the subarachnoid space and has its own wall consisting of a tenuous transparent membrane similar in every respect to the arach-noid which covers it. Careful examination at oper-ation will reveal the identity of the two mem-branes around its margin, although over its superficial and its deep surfaces the cyst wall may be fused with the covering arachnoid and the adjacent pia mater respectively. The contents are clear and watery, resembling normal cere-brospinal fluid; the interior of the cyst wall is smooth and glistening. The adjacent brain is impressed by the cyst but otherwise appears normal and the overlying skull may be thinned and bulging. There are three likely sites, none can be called common: over the convexity of a hemisphere, in the cisterna chiasmaticus (Hoffman et al. 1982) and in the cistern magna. In the latter situation it separates the cerebellar tonsils and lobes, obstructs and opens up the foramen of Magendie, so that the surgeon may perceive the floor of the fourth ventricle through the pellucid layers of arachnoid and cyst wall. It is easy to overlook the cyst wall and to mistake the condition for a distended cisterna magna due to communicating hydrocephalus; conversely, an example of distention of the cisterna magna or of the Dandy–Walker malformation may be mistakenly described as a cyst.

Those cysts and loculated distentions of the subarachnoid space which occur in the middle fossa deserve special mention (Sato et al. 1983, Go et al. 1984). The collection of fluid distends the mouth of the Sylvian fissure, displaces the temporal pole backwards: sometimes the neigh-bouring frontal lobe and the opercula are dis-placed so that the insula is uncovered. It is likely that the collection always develops in childhood because of the accompanying changes in the skull. The temporal squame and the great wing of the sphenoid are thin and bulge outwards, the roof of the orbit and the sphenoidal ridge are elevated and displaced forwards and the posterior wall of the orbit is thrust forwards thus forming an unusually capacious middle fossa. There may be slight proptosis and asymmetry of the face and a prominence of the temple. The radiological changes were first described by Davidoff and Dyke (1938) who noted them in four cases in which there had been recent head injury and in some a more remote injury. In each a subdural haematoma was evacuated and the authors ascribed the bone changes to an earlier hae-matoma which had persisted and in which fresh bleeding had occurred. They named the con-dition *relapsing juvenile chronic subdural haema-toma.* Robinson (1964) had personal experience of 9 cases, examined the brain of a tenth and reviewed the literature. He concludes that the basis of the condition is a failure of the temporal lobe to develop fully, and that the 'cyst' in the anterior part of the middle cranial fossa is a localized 'external' hydrocephalus. He proposed the name of *temporal lobe agenesis syndrome*, and recognized the susceptibility of these patients to subdural haematoma which is regarded as a complication, not a cause. Whatever may be the correct interpretation of the cause of this curious condition, Robinson makes the important point that operation is not necessarily required. Cases occur in which the radiological changes are found by chance. Only if there are symptoms of a progressive lesion or of raised intracranial pressure is operative exploration necessary and this usually for the evacuation of a haematoma, within the 'cyst' or as an entirely separate entity.

## Parasitic cysts

### Hydatid cyst

Hydatid disease is geographically related to sheep-raising. The worm, *echinococcus granularis*, ordinarily resides in the intestines of dogs and ova in the faeces infect pastures. The embryos penetrate the intestinal mucosa of grazing sheep, gain the lymphatics and the portal circulation and lodge in lymph nodes, liver and lungs, where they become encysted. Human beings are infected from dogs either by the contamination of food or from the fingers as a result of handling the dogs. If an embryo successfully traverses the capillary filters of the liver and lungs, it passes into the systemic circulation and in about 2% of cases of hydatid disease lodges in the brain. Such a hydatid cyst is solitary and the mode of infection is called primary. Very rarely multiple cysts occur in the brain; they arise as a secondary or metastatic spread, due to the rupture of a cyst in the myocardium. In this country the disease is rare, less so in Wales (Langmaid & Rogers 1940), but South American countries, Australia and New Zealand have a much higher incidence. An authoritative account of the disease was given by Dew (1928).

Cerebral hydatid cysts are much more common in children than in adults; in the cases of Arana-Iniguez (1961) 81% were children, in those of Phillips (1948) 93% were under the age of 17 years. Dew (1928) found that in children the brain was affected in 4.3% and in all cases regardless of age 0.6%; in both groups the liver was infested in 76%. The cyst rarely occurs in the cerebellum (only once in the 29 cases of Phillips) and most commonly lies in the posterior half of the cerebral hemisphere, in the territory of the middle cerebral artery (in only 2 of that series was the cyst frontal). Phillips makes the point that although in the literature the commonest site is said to be the parietal lobe, the cyst is often so large that it extends beyond the confines of a single lobe. In one of his cases, the cyst had a capacity of 20 ounces and Arana-Iniguez and Julian (1955) illustrate one of 10 cm

diameter which weighed 628 g. They estimate that a cyst takes 3–4 years to reach the size when treatment becomes necessary.

In the brain a hydatid cyst produces compression of the surrounding tissue, displaces blood vessels and when large is covered by only a thin film of cortex, but it remains free from adhesions to the brain, a feature of paramount value in its removal. Its wall is usually likened to grey wash-leather, of moderate strength and several millimetres thick. The outer layer of the wall is of fibrous tissue, the intermediate of laminated chitinous material and the inner a germinal layer. To this layer are attached brood capsules containing scolices, the embryonic worm heads. The fluid in the cyst is commonly watery and colourless, containing a fine deposit of scolices and sometimes daughter cysts; occasionally it is yellow. The scolices are usually living and contamination of the operative field leads to widespread and therefore ineradicable secondary infestation. In the cranial form of the disease, the bone is gradually eroded by the spread of numerous small cysts imparting a honeycomb appearance; it is restricted to the base of the skull.

*Diagnosis*

The duration of symptoms is usually 1–2 years and the clinical picture is one of raised intracranial pressure which usually provides the earliest symptoms, with signs of a cerebral deficit; hemianopioa and hemiparesis commonly predominate. The high incidence of the cyst in the posterior part of the hemisphere renders hemianopia an important sign, but it is often difficult to elicit in young children. The long tract signs are often insignificant compared with the size of the cyst and the degree of raised intracranial pressure. This is presumably due to the slow rate of expansion of the cyst and the gradual displacement of axons in contrast to their invasion and destruction by gliomas. Phillips drew attention to tremor and signs of cerebellar disturbance (contralateral to the lesion) which may be seen if the cyst is large and which frequently lead to faulty localization. Radiological examination of the skull confirms the presence of intracranial hypertension and the calvarium over the site of the cyst may be thin and bulging. Calcification of the cyst wall is very rare; formerly angiography provided the best means of diagnosis of both the localization and the nature of the lesion. Vessels are markedly displaced and pursue a curved course, stretched and approximated circumferentially around an area lacking vessels. There are no pathological vessels. Ventriculography should be avoided at all costs because of the likelihood of puncturing the cyst and the consequent dissemination of scolices, formerly a common cause of secondary infestation and death. CT is now the radiological investigation of choice. There is general agreement among those with extensive experience of intracranial hydatids that such special tests as Casoni's and complement-fixation are usually negative and eosinophilia rarely occurs. Dew (1928) stated that in 80% of cases of cerebral hydatid cysts, the liver also contained cysts. This is not borne out by neurosurgical experiences, and as Phillips pointed out, those patients who survive the removal of a hydatid cyst from the brain usually live for many years.

*Treatment*

In order to avoid contamination of the operation field with living scolices, it is necessary to be familiar with the CT or angiographic appearances and to recognize immediately the external surface of a hydatid cyst if one is unexpectedly encountered, so that appropriate measures can be taken to avoid opening it. Although Phillips had good results by injecting formaldehyde into the cyst, waiting 10 minutes, collapsing the cyst by aspirating its contents, and then withdrawing its wall, other methods have rendered this obsolete. But when a cyst has been incised because its nature has not been recognized, formaldehyde should be used, although the risk that scolices in the spilt fluid will be implanted remains high.

Arana-Iniguez and Julian (1955) recommend that the craniotomy should be large and the cyst wall exposed by a series of radiating cortical incisions, a technique ascribed by them to Dowling. The head is then placed so that the cyst is dependent; in this position its weight causes its spontaneous extrusion, helped by gently irrigating with saline between the cyst and the brain. This simple technique is possible because of the absence of adhesions between the adventitia of the cyst wall and its bed. In those rare cases in which the disease involves the cranium, the same authors state that the affected area of bone must be removed.

*Prognosis*

Provided the cyst is removed without spilling its contents, the results appear to be excellent. All 13 patients of the series of Arana-Iniguez and Julian survived, though the duration of follow-up is not stated. Of the 29 reported by Phillips, culled from the Australasian literature and including 5 of his own, approximately one-half died of the operation or of a subsequent recurrence; amongst the survivors were two who were alive and well 20 years later.

*Cysticercosis*

This disease is caused by the presence in various organs and tissues of the encysted larvae of the human tape worm, *taenia solium*. It is usually the pig which is affected, but occasionally man forms the intermediate host, by ingesting the ova of his own worm or those of another host in contaminated food and water. The embryos are liberated by the digestive juices, penetrate the wall of the intestine and are distributed to various parts of the body. Human cysticercosis is relatively common in some Eastern European countries and in Central and South America. In this country the disease is rare, but a unique, compact and limited group of cases occurred among British soldiers who were stationed in

India. It has been estimated that the incidence was between 1 and 2 per 1000 of the men serving in India during the the period 1921–37 (Dixon & Lipscomb 1961).

The cyst is a small round or oval body rarely more than 10 mm in diameter, white or yellowish-grey, firm and often gritty, anchored by fibrosis in the surrounding tissue, in the brain by a varying degree of gliosis. Its wall is thin, distended with clear fluid and presenting on its inner surface a nodule which is the scolex. During the time it remains alive the parasite gives rise to a minimum of local reaction, a state of balance which has been likened to symbiosis, but when it dies degenerative products cause intense reaction. The cyst enlarges as a result of increase in its fluid content and gives rise to a local inflammatory response. In the brain there arise oedema, endarteritis and thrombosis if the parasite happens to have lodged in the vicinity of a vessel and marked ependymitis and leptomeningitis and subsequent fibrosis if it is near the ventricle and subarachnoid spaces. Subcutaneous nodules become evident and later disappear. All the embryos do not die at the same time, so that the clinical manifestations of the disease fluctuate.

The literature on cysticercosis is largely concerned with those dramatic cerebral manifestations of the disease which bring the patient to a neurosurgical centre. The review by Dixon and Lipscomb (1961) redresses the balance and permits such cases to be seen in proper perspective; it comprises an analysis and long term follow-up of 450 cases. Autopsies were performed in 55; in 47 the disease was confirmed and was wholly or partly the cause of death in 35. Cysts were found in the cerebrum in 44, in the meninges in 22 (but in another 22 the records were uninformative) and in the muscles in 18 (absent in 10 and unrecorded in 19). There were isolated examples of cysts in the spinal cord, heart, eye, lung, parotid and peritoneum; the liver was infected in only one case in this series.

The brain may be studded with several hundreds of cysts, or there may be only a few. They commonly lie in the cortex, or at the junction of grey and white matter, in basal nuclei, but rarely in white matter. Frequently they lie in the subarachnoid space, on the convexity or in the basal cisterns where severe leptomeningeal fibrosis leads to hydrocephalus. Isolated cysts may be deposited under the ependyma of the ventricles and may be seen as a filling defect in a ventriculogram. Inflammatory reaction may completely block the ventricular pathways. Sometimes the cysts lie relatively free within the fourth ventricle, the cisterna magna, or the basal cisterns. In these situations the cysts are rather larger than those within the substance of the brain, thin walled and held together by filmy adhesions like a bunch of grapes. This is the racemose form, of which there were only 3 examples in the 450 cases of Dixon and Lipscomb but provides a much higher proportion of cases of cysticercosis coming to operation. Although the cysts appear loose and can be withdrawn at operation, they are associated with dense leptomeningeal fibrosis which is probably more responsible for the hydrocephalus than are the cysts.

*Symptoms*

Clinical manifestations can be related to the presence of cysts causing focal lesions, to the intense inflammatory reactions which punctuate the history and to the hydrocephalic sequelae. These reactions are thought to have an allergic basis and may also give rise to systemic disturbances after operation in which cyst contents or debris may have been spilt. Difficulties in diagnosis arise in some instances from the long duration and fluctuation of the illness, from the complexities of the clinical picture as a result of multiplicity of lesions and from the failure to consider cysticercosis because of its rarity. Three syndromes can be distinguished and all may occur at different times in the same patients. Epilepsy is the commonest and all patterns may be encountered; it was present in over 90% of the cases of Dixon and Lipscomb and in three-quarters it was the first symptom. It is of importance that in nearly one-third it remained the only manifestation. In neurosurgical series the incidence of epilepsy is lower, about 40%. The syndrome next in frequency is of raised intracranial pressure; Dixon and Lipscomb found it in only 6.4% of their cases but as might be anticipated the proportion is much higher amongst neurosurgical admissions; in 80% of the cases of Stepien and Chorobski (1949), Arseni and Samitca (1957) and of Obrador (1962). The symptoms of raised intracranial pressure may be associated with evidence of a focal cerebral lesion, so that the picture is similar to that of a cerebral tumour. About half the cases with the intracranial hypertension present in this manner. The other moeity comprises those in which the picture is one of obstructive hydrocephalus sometimes accompanied by cerebellar or cerebellopontine angle signs. This group includes cases of racemose cysts and of occlusion of ventricular and of leptomeningeal pathways. Mental disturbance is a common feature of cysticercosis of the nervous system and may be found in all three groups. It may vary from mild impairment of memory and intellect to profound dementia, behaviour disorders, confusional and hallucinatory states. Although the picture is one of gradual worsening, there may be periods of acute exacerbation and of spontaneous improvement. Obrador (1948) suggested that mental symptoms are pronounced in some cases because of involvement of the diencephalon.

## Diagnosis

The presence of subcutaneous nodules is of great value; although the parasite is deposited in muscles, after some years the nodule feels to be beneath the skin. They are usually painless and the patient may be unaware of their presence. Biopsy should be performed. Radiological examination of the muscles and of the skull may reveal calcified cysticerci, though their absence does not exclude the diagnosis. Dixon and Lipscomb consider that the minimum interval between infection and calcification in muscle is 5 years

and in the brain 10 years. Calcification was radiologically demonstrable in muscle in 87% and within the cranium in 36% of cases. These figures are much higher than those from other sources doubtless because a more careful search was made. CT scan is now the radiological investigation of choice. Ventriculography or angiography is seldom necessary. In the supratentorial lesions they will show evidence of a localized mass, or of small ventricles with little or no displacement; this appearance is similar to that seen in intracranial benign hypertension.

Specific tests may be helpful; in this country the results have often been negative, but in others much reliance is placed upon them. The cerebrospinal fluid shows a pleiocytosis and an increase in the protein content during an active phase of the disease and an eosinophilia in fluid and in blood is highly significant.

## Treatment

There is general agreement that operation is rarely if ever advisable for the treatment of the epilepsy, because of other undetected lesions and of the risk that operation may evoke a sensitivity reaction. Operation is necessary for the relief of raised intracranial pressure, for which it can often be very successful though carrying a considerable risk. The aim is palliation and not cure. In the case of cysts in the cerebral hemispheres, the hypertension is due to intense oedema surrounding a localized group, the syndrome of a tumour; or to generalized oedema simulating the state of benign intracranial hypertension. A large decompressive osteoplastic flap in the former and bilateral subtemporal decompressions in the latter have been recommended. Where obstructive hydrocephalus is demonstrated a posterior fossa exploration is usually carried out and obstructive fibrous lesions excised or racemose cysts removed. It is clear from the literature that these operations have a very high mortality and that relapse often occurs. This is probably due to the persistence of hydrocephalus as a result of leptomeningeal fibrosis. The insertion of a ventriculoperitoneal shunt and the avoidance of exploration of the posterior fossa would appear to be a more logical measure.

## Sarcomas

Both the classification and the histogenesis of these uncommon tumours remain highly controversial. In their monograph Kernohan and Uihlein (1962) subdivide them into fibrosarcomas, giant cell sarcomas, circumscribed sarcomas of the cerebellum, diffuse meningealsarcomatosis, haemangiopericytomas and sarcomas of the reticulo-endothelial system. There is a substantial body of opinion which includes the giant celled sarcomas and those of the cerebellum among neuroectodermal tumours, as monstrocellular glioblastomas and desmoplastic medulloblastomas respectively. Haemangiopericytomas form a subgroup of angioblastic meningiomas and are discussed elsewhere.

Most intracranial sarcomas are of meningeal origin, only a minority originating in the substance of the brain where they arise from the vascular adventitia or the perivascular pial sheath. While most of them tend to be invasive, some remain remarkably circumscribed while others tend to spread diffusely. Diffuse leptomeningeal spread may lead to coating of the entire brain and spinal cord with tumour, the site of origin of which may become unidentifiable. This is diffuse meningeal sarcomatosis, a term which refers to the type of spread rather than to cellular structure, through admittedly only the more anaplastic forms tend to spread in that fashion. The degree of differentiation of the tumour forms the basis of Christensen and Lara's (1953) classification into three types: fibrous, spindle celled and polymorphocellular. The first group represents a low grade tumour of moderate cellularity with formation of abundant collagen fibres. spindle celled sarcomas are more densely cellular with scanty fibres, but the cells still retain the morphological characteristics of fibroblasts. The polymorphocellular tumours are totally anaplastic, contain a great variety of cell

types including giant forms and their fibroblastic properties express themselves only in the formation of a fine reticulin stroma.

As primitive mesenchymal cells are multipotential occasional variants have been recorded in which the tumours, or parts of them, differentiate in a direction other than fibroblastic. these include chondrosarcomas, osteosarcomas, rhabdomysarcomas and malignant mesenchymomas; all of these are excessively rare. When sarcomas invade brain tissue they provoke a glial reaction which in most cases is purely hyperplastic. On rare occasions however, a neoplastic change takes place in the glia and produces a mixed tumour. These must be distinguished from the far commoner perivascular fibrosarcomas arising in malignant gliomas or from the rare 'collision tumours' in which two independent tumours accidentally come into contact.

For practical purposes of prognosis and management, the gliosarcoma may be regarded as a variant of the malignant glioma. these tumours respond very poorly, if at all, to radiotherapy.

## Metastatic tumours

The wide variation in the incidence of intracranial metastatic tumours, can be related to the practice of particular departments, the vigour with which the search for metastases is conducted, the improved accuracy of CT scanning and more recently NMR, and the thoroughness of autopsy examinations. A representative figure from a neurosurgical department prior to the introduction of CT scanning was that of Richards and McKissock (1963) who recorded that metastases accounted for 10% of all intracranial tumours. A more recent autopsy study (Costigan & Winkerlman 1985) suggests a figure nearer 20%, while in nonsmall cell lung carcinoma, up to 33% of patients have been found to have CNS metastases at autopsy (Budinger 1958). In individual cases the use of CT scan will reveal intracranial metastases more readily than earlier methods of investigation, and that is reflected in the reduction of surgery because of the demonstration of multiple lesions (Sharr 1983). There is general agreement that the commonest origin is bronchogenic carcinoma with carcinoma of the breast a close second; stomach and kidney come next and every organ liable to malignant growth occasionally provides a source. Lower bowel carcinoma being more common than upper, the incidence of such intracranial metastases is higher than from carcinoma of the stomach. Of increasing importance is truly metastatic lymphoma, with more accurate general diagnosis, and more favourable results of general and intracranial treatment, as distinct from primary cerebral lymphoma ('microglioma'). Prostatic intracranial metastases are rarely reported (Baumann *et al.* 1984).

## Pathology

The dura mater may be studded with secondary deposits forming irregular modules and plaques on its inner surface. These are due to invasion of the dura mater by deposits in the adjacent skull. Involvement of the dura mater may be complicated by pachymeningitis interna haemorrhagica (Russell & Cairns 1934). The veins and capillaries of the outer, dense layer of the dura mater become permeated by cancer cells, causing congestion and dilatation of the capillaries on the inner surface. The leptomeninges may be diffusely infiltrated by carcinoma cells and it may be difficult to find a macroscopic nodule in the brain from which the tumour may have spread. Tumour cells form a sheet lining the leptomeningeal spaces and spreading into the Virchow–Robin spaces; choroid plexus and ventricular ependyma may or may not be invaded. The arachnoid may not appear abnormal to the naked eye, though at times it is obviously opaque, grey and thickened. There is marked hydrocephalus. The stomach is a much more frequent cause for carinomatosis of the leptomeninges than for the nodular type of metastatic disease.

Metastases occur anywhere within the brain; they may be solitary in which case the tumour may reach a large size, 5–6 cm, or several of different sizes, or they are innumerable and dot the cut surface of the brain. Small nodules are often found at the junction of white and grey matter and easily escape detection. The tumours tend to preserve a round shape and to appear circumscribed. Superficial ones become adherent to the overlying dura mater and, like a glioblastoma, provoke a meningioblastic reaction which renders them at the surgeon's first sight similar in appearance to a meningioma. The cut surface of the tumour is often firm, homogeneous like a potato, usually pinkish-grey and rarely vascular. Necrosis often occurs so that they contain milky fluid; this fluid looks like pus and may lead the surgeon to believe that he has encountered an abscess. This diagnosis may seem valid in some patients with a short history, particularly if a radiological shadow in the lung appears to be an abscess. Microscopical examination of the fluid from a necrotic metastasis reveals only amorphous debris. The cut surface of some metastases exudes stringy mucoid material due to the presence of mucin-secreting tumour cells. Secondary growths often provoke an intense and widespread oedema of the brain, which accelerates the speed at which the clinical picture evolves and intensifies internal herniations. The extent of the oedema often bears no relation to the size of the tumour which may be quite small. The softening of the brain around the tumour renders them easily removable, but histological examination across this apparently discrete margin reveals infiltration with tumour cells.

## Presentation and diagnosis

Patients with solitary or multiple intracranial metastases can be categorized for purposes of diagnosis and management as: (a) those with a proven extracranial malignancy; (b) those without evidence, proven or unproven of extracranial malignancy, in whom therefore, the differential diagnosis is that of any intracranial space-occupying lesion.

The intracranial symptoms are little different from those already discussed in earlier sections. Because of the usually rapid growth of metastases, the intracranial history is generally measured in weeks rather than the months or more of the malignant glioma. Exceptions are metastases from carcinoma of the breast, which, like the parent tumour, may remain relatively static for many months, and on occasions for a year or more, although the metastases may advance more rapidly than the primary tumour which may be occult. In the presence of multiple intracranial metastases the clinical picture may be confusing, especially when there is the combination of signs attributable to both supra- and infratentorial lesions, and the temptation is to ascribe the findings to cerebrovascular disease. The true incidence of multiplicity of intracranial metastases is very difficult to estimate; with improvements in radiology and especially CT scanning, the demonstration of multiple small lesions increases, so that figures from earlier reports are now of little value, as Sellwood (1972) emphasized. When autopsy studies are taken into account, the incidence of truly solitary metastases is lower than 20%. It is too soon to say whether NMR will lower this figure further, particularly with metastatic malignant melanoma in which the individual deposits may remain undetected unless they are responsible for spontaneous intracranial haemorrhage and small focal haematomas. Within the limits of radiological methods, and without autopsy studies, supratentorial metastases occur only twice as frequently as infratentorial, at least as judged by reports of surgical management, a surprisingly low figure in view of the relative size of the supra- and infratentorial structures.

The interval between diagnosis of the primary tumour and the presentations of the intracranial metastasis is capricious and bears little relationship to the type of tumour, with the exception of the breast especially in the older patients in whom the intervals tend to be of years rather than months. Claims that a longer latent period, or a long duration of intracranial symptoms carry a better prognosis have not been confirmed (Sharr & Garfield 1978). Because of the difficulties of clinical diagnosis of the primary tumour, it is not surprising that hypernephroma often remains occult at the time of presentation of the metastasis; but it is surprising that bronchogenic carcinoma may remain occult for up to two years after the intracranial metastasis has been treated. In the presence of proven extracranial malignancy, differential diagnosis is more limited than in its absence. When only a solitary intracranial lesion has been demonstrated, it can never be assumed, however probable, that the lesion is metastatic, but when multiple lesions have been demonstrated the assumption is usually acceptable for purposes of management. In the absence of proven extracranial malignancy, the most important and potentially remediable lesion to exclude is intracranial abscess, solitary or, multiple, the latter being a particularly difficult diagnosis. CT scanning may fail to differentiate between multiple metastases and abscesses. The presence of multiple cranial nerve, and especially oculomotor and facial nerve lesions is highly suggestive of a carcinomatous meningitis.

**Investigation and management**

Intracranial investigations will follow the procedures described in other sections. In the absence of a known extracranial malignancy and the demonstration of a solitary brain lesion, the breasts, thyroid gland and testes must be carefully examined and general radiology need be no more than a chest radiograph. If that is normal, management will be as for a primary brain tumour. When *multiple lesions* are present, the search for a primary extracranial tumour should be more assiduous, and should include intravenous urography, upper gastrointestinal and large bowel endoscopy and radiology, isotope bone scan, bone marrow histology, sputum cytology, examination of the urine for melanins, and selected whole body CT scan. In the presence of multiple intracranial lesions, the demonstration of the primary tumour will obviate the necessity for intracranial surgery; but there may well be a place for general treatment of lymphoma, cranial irradiation for bronchial or renal metastases, and removal of a primary renal or large bowel tumour.

When the search for a primary tumour fails, there is still a place for biopsy of the most accessible of the intracranial lesions, specifically to exclude the diagnosis of multiple abscess, tuberculoma, or lymphoma.

The management of the patient with a *solitary intracranial lesion*, and a known or radiologically demonstrated primary cancer continues to be a matter for debate. The results of intracranial surgery in the individual patient are unpredictable, but overall, in recent series, they have been disappointing, despite anecdotal reports of long survival. Figures for mean survival after removal of a seemingly solitary supratentorial metatases may be 6.3 months for bronchial, 10.3 months for breast, 4.8 months for melanoma, 4.9 months for gastrointestinal and 11.5 months for renal carcinoma. With the exception of breast carcinoma (12.3 months) the mean survival was less after posterior fossa operations (Sharr & Garfield 1978). When the figures for three neurosurgical units were combined the overall results were similar, there being no improvement following the introduction of CT scanning (Sharr 1983). This suggests that even if more patients with multiple lesions are excluded from surgery, the results are no better. Unless the tumour is responsive to specific chemotherapy, as is lymphoma, there is no evidence so far that chemotherapy for intracranial carcinoma improves the prognosis.

There is some evidence that postoperative cranial irradiation improves survival (Galicich *et al.* 1980), and elective brain irradiation in patients with nonsmall cell lung cancer who showed neither clinical nor radiological evidence of an intracranial lesion, reduced the incidence of CNS metastases, and prolonged the metastasis-free interval; but it did not prolong survival, death being due to extracranial disease (Umsawasdi *et al.* 1984). Bronchial carcinoma being the most common site of origin of intracranial metastases, the following scheme is suggested for the man-agement of a patient who presents with a solitary supra- or infratentorial lesion. If the chest radiograph is normal the management proceeds on the basis that the lesion is not a metastasis.

If the chest radiograph is suggestive of a parenchymal tumour an immediate thoracic surgical opinion is sought. On the basis of tomography, and bronchoscopy it is likely that the pathology and operability of the thoracic tumour can be established. For a more peripheral lesion needle biopsy may suffice.

If the thoracic lesion is deemed to be operable, and there is no evidence of widespread extracranial metastases, the degree of supratentorial neurological deficit is acceptable, and the solitary intracranial metastasis is surgically accessible, then excisional supratentorial or infratentorial surgery is appropriate. If those criteria cannot be met, no more than symptomatic relief, albeit temporary, is usually justified, which may include CSF shunting for obstructive hydrocephalus, Dexamethasone, and radiotherapy, provided that malignancy has been histologically verified. Finally it must be stressed that it is the common everyday problems such as this which call for more wisdom and compassion in management, than do the rarer and more dramatic situations with which the life of the neurosurgeon is so popularly identified.

# References

ARANA-INIGUEZ R. (1961) *Second Int. Cong. Neurol. Surg.*, Exc. Int. Cong. Series No. 36, E.15.

ARANA-INIGUEZ R. & JULIAN J.S. (1955) *Neurosurg.*, 12, 323.

ARSENI C. & SAMITCA D.C. (1957) *Acta Psychiat. Neurol. Scand.*, 32, 389.

BAUMANN C.H.H. & BUCY P.C. (1956) *J. Neurosurg.*, 13, 455.

BAUMANN M.A., et al. (1984) *Cancer*, 54 (8), 1723–5.

BOHM E. & STRANG R. (1961) *J. Neurosurg.*, 18, 493.

BUDINGER J.M. (1958) *Cancer*, 11, 106–16.

CAIRNS H. & MOSBERG W.H. (1951) *Surg. Gynec. Obstet.*, 92, 545.

CHRISTENSEN E. & LARA D.E. (1953) *J. Neuropath. exp. Neurol.*, 12, 41.

COSTIGAN D.A. & WINKELMAN M.D. (1985) *J. Neurosurg.*, 62, 227.

CRITCHLEY McD. & FERGUSON F.R. (1928) *Brain*, 51, 332.

CUSHING H. (1932) *Intracranial Tumours*. Thomas, Springfield, Illinois.

DANDY W. E. (1921) *Surg. Gynec. Obstet.*, **33**, 113.

DANDY W. E. (1933) *Benign Tumours in the Third Ventricle of the Brain.* Bailliere, Tindall & Cox, London.

DAVIDOFF L. M. & DYKE C. G. (1938). *Bull. Neurol. Inst. New York*, **7**, 95.

DAVIDSON S. I. & SMALL J. K. (1960) *J. Neurol. Neurosurg. Psychiat.*, **23**, 176.

DAYAN A. D. & MARSHALL A. H., *et al.* (1966) *J. Path. Bact.*, **92**, 1.

DEW H. (1928) *Hydatid Disease.* Australiasan Medical Publishing Co. Ltd., Sydney.

DIXON H. F. B. & LIPSCOMB F. M. (1961) *Spec. Rep. Ser. med. Res. Coun. (Lond.)*, 299.

FULTON J. F. (1946) *Harvey Cushing: A Biography.* Thomas, Springfield, Illinois.

GALICICH J. H., SUNDARESAN N., *et al.* (1980) *J. Neurosurg.*, **53**, 63.

GALLUZI S. & PAYNE P. M. (1956) *Brit. J. Cancer*, **10**, 410.

GO K. G., *et al.* (1984) *J. Neurosurg.*, **60** (4), 803.

GREENFIELD J. G. (1932) In *Cytology and Cellular Pathology of the Nervous System*, (Ed. Penfield W.) vol 3, p. 1221. Hoeber, New York.

HALDEMAN K. O. (1927) *Arch. Neurol. Psychiat.*, **18**, 724.

HIDE T. A. H. (1975) *Abstract, Fifth Congress of European Association of Neurosurgical Societies.*

HOFFMAN H. J., *et al.* (1982) *J. Neurosurg.*, **57** (5), 597.

JEFFERSON G. SMALLEY A. A. (1938) *J. Laryng. Otol.*, **53**, 417

JOOMA R. & KENDALL B. E. (1983) *J. Neurosurg.*, **58**, 654.

JOOMA R., *et al.* (1983) *Childs Brain*, **10**(4), 242.

KAHN E. A. (1961) *Clin. Neurosurg.*, **7**, 79.

KAHN E. A. & LUROS J. G. (1952) *J. Neurosurg.*, **9**, 59.

KAPPERS J. A. (1955) *J. comp. Neurol.*, **102**, 425.

KERNOHAN J. W. & UIHLEIN A. (1962) *Sarcomas of the Brain.* Thomas, Springfield, Illinois.

KEVILLE F. J. & WISE B. L. (1959) *J. Neurosurg.*, **16**, 564.

LANGMAID C. & ROGERS L. (1940) *Brain*, **63**, 184.

LAURENCE K. M., HOARE R. D. & TILL K. (1961) *Brain*, **84**, 628.

LEPOIRE J. & PERTUISET B. (1957) *Les Cystes Epidermoides Cranio-encephaliques.* Masson, Paris.

LEWIS P. (1967) *Brain*, **90**, 177.

McGOVERN V. J. (1949) *J. Path. Bact.*, **61**, 1.

McKISSOCK W. (1965) *J. Neurol. Neurosurg. Psychiat.*, **28**, 461.

MAHONEY W. (1936) *Zsch. ges. Neurol. Psychiat.*, **155**, 416.

MATSON D. D. & INGRAHAM F. D. (1951) *Pediatrics*, **8**, 463.

MATSON D. D. & CROFTON F. D. L. (1960) *J. Neurosurg.*, **17**, 102.

MATSON D. D. (1969) *Neurosurgery of Infancy and Childhood.* Thomas, Springfield, Illinois.

MATSUSHIMA T. (1983) *J. Neurosurg.*, **59** (6), 1054.

MEYER P. C. & REAH T . G. (1953) *Brit. J. Cancer*, **7**, 438.

OBRADOR S. (1948) *Arch. Neurol. Psychiat.*, **59**, 457.

OBRADOR S. (1962) *Acta Neurochirurg.*, **10**, 320.

OLIVECRONA H. (1949) *Acta Psychiat. Neurol. Scand.*, **24**, 639.

PARINAUD H. (1883) *Arch. Neurol. (Paris)*, **5**, 145.

PATTISON A. R. D. (1937) *Lancet*, **2**, 1303.

PENNYBACKER J. (1944) *Brit. J. Surg.*, **32**, 75.

PHILLIPS G. (1948) *J. Neurol. Neurosurg. Psychiat.*, **11**, 44.

POSEY L. C. (1942) *Arch. Path.*, **34**, 911.

ROA Y. T. R., MEDINI E., *et al.* (1981) *Cancer*, **48**, 708.

RICHARDS P. & McKISSOCK W. (1963) *Brit. med. J.*, **1**, 15.

RIDDOCH G. (1936) *Brain*, **59**, 225.

RINGERTZ N., NORDENSTAMM H., *et al.* (1954) *J. Neuropath. exp. Neurol.*, **13**, 540.

RINGERTZ N. & REYMOND A. (1949) *J. Neuropath. exp. Neurol.*, **8**, 355.

RIVAS J. J. & LOBATO R. D. (1985) *J. Neurosurg.*, **62**, 238.

ROBINSON R. G. (1964) *Brain*, **87**, 87.

RUBIN P. & KRAMER S. (1965) *Radiology*, **85**, 512.

RUSSELL D. S. & CAIRNS H. (1934) *Brain*, **57**, 32.

RUSSELL D. S. & RUBINSTEIN L. J. (1959) *Tumours of the Nervous System.* Arnold, London.

SATO K., *et al.* (1983) *Childs Brain*, **10** (5), 301.

SELLWOOD R. B. (1972) *Brit. J. Radiol.*, **45**, 647.

SHARR M. M. & GARFIELD J. S. (1978) *Brit. med. J*, **1**, 1535.

SHARR M. M. (1983) *J. Neuro-Oncol.*, **1**, 307.

SJOVALL E. (1910) *Beitrag. z. Path. Anat.*, **47**, 248.

STEIN B. M. (1971) *J. Neurosurg.*, **35**, 197.

STEPIEN L. & CHOROBSKI J. (1949) *Arch. Neurol. Psychiat.*, **61**, 499.

TORKILDSEN A. (1948) *J. Neurosurg.*, **5**, 249.

TYTUS J. S. & PENNYBACKER J. (1956) *J. Neurol. Neurosurg. Psychiat.*, **19**, 241.

UMSAWASDI T., VALDIVIESO M., *et al.* (1984) *J. Neuro-Oncol.*, **2**, 253.

ZÜLCH K. J. (1965) *Brain Tumours, their Biology and Pathology.* Heinemann, London.

# Chapter 7
# The meningiomas: haemangioblastoma

P. M. FOY

## Meningiomas

### Introduction

Cushing and Eisenhardt (1938) in their mono-graph on meningiomas gave an account of the earliest descriptions of these tumours and of the controversies which have arisen over their nomenclature and histogenesis. Bright (1831) suggested that the tumour was a growth of the dura mater or perhaps of the arachnoid, thus opening a discussion which lasted many years. Schmidt (1902) drew attention to the similarity between the microscopical appearance of the cells of the tumour and those of the arachnoidal villi and it is now accepted that meningiomas arise from the endothelium which lines the lep-tomeningeal spaces. Some meningiomas are so firmly attached to the dura mater that they appear to be arising from it, but it is thought that they are derived from sequestered clumps of arachnoidal cells which occur within the dura mater. Some arise only from the pia mater and these occur mainly in the spinal canal. Intra-ventricular examples owe their origin to the lep-tomeningeal contribution to the tela choroidea and choroid plexus. Russell (1950) drew atten-tion to the diversity of reaction forms which arachnoidal cells exhibit as a result of stimu-lation and which are reflected in the various histological types of tumour. It was Cushing's study of a meningioma which had invaded the sagittal sinus that led him to initiate inves-tigations into the function of the arachnoidal villi and granulations and their relation to the circulation of the cerebrospinal fluid, work which was taken up by Weed. The term 'meningioma' was introduced by Cushing in his 1922

Cavendish Lecture as a 'simple and non-com-mittal designation' and is now universally em-ployed, although many alternatives have been proposed.

### General characteristics

The meningiomas constitute about 15% of all intracranial tumours, roughly a third of the number of gliomas. They are most commonly detected in middle age when there is a clear predominance in women. In childhood and ado-lescence they are uncommon, accounting for only 1.5% of 2620 intracranial childhood tumours reviewed by Mendiratta et al. (1967). Intracranial meningioma in infants under one year is extremely rare, Amano et al. adding the sixteenth case to the world literature in 1980. At the other extreme, meningiomas in the elderly may be more common than is generally supposed. Wood et al. (1957) reported 100 men-ingiomas found incidentally at necropsy, and the peak incidence was in the seventh decade. Inter-estingly, there was no sex dominance in these asymptomatic tumours.

Meningiomas may be multiple and this was defined by Cushing and Eisenhardt (1938) as a condition in which the patient had more than one meningioma and less than a diffusion of them, without signs of neurofibromatosis. Sheehy and Crockard (1983) reported a series of 566 cases of meningioma collected over a 34 year period in which the incidence of multiple meningioma was 1.1% prior to computerized tomographic (CT) scanning, rising to 8% after the introduction of CT scanning. They suggested that the detection rate will continue to rise and approach the 10% found incidentally by Wood *et al.* (1957) at necropsy. Cushing and Eisenhardt believed that in some cases injury to the head was an aetiological factor; amongst a total of 295 intracranial meningiomas there were 23 cases in which the residual local evidence of trauma (for example, a scalp scar) lay over the site of the tumour. Walshe (1961) has recorded further examples. However, Annegers *et al.* (1979) in a prospective study of a community population concluded that head injury was not a significant aetiological factor in meningioma.

Similarly the role of radiotherapy as an aetiological factor in meningioma remains controversial. Iacono *et al.* (1981) reported a case and reviewed 38 cases of meningiomas occurring after radiation and their statistical analysis led them to support the concept of radiation as a cause of the tumours.

In its simplest form, as seen on the convexity of the cerebral hemisphere, the tumour forms a rounded mass, having a precise margin clearly demarcated from the brain in which it is embedded and firmly attached to the overlying dura mater, at times intimately fused with it (Fig. 7.1). Small examples occur as chance findings at necropsy and can be lifted off the brain which is indented to receive it, with little or no damage to the impressed leptomeninges and cortex. Large tumours may attain a diameter approaching 10 cm, causing a remarkable degree of dislocation of the brain and of distant pressure effects, well illustrated by Case 6 (Ida Jones) of Cushing and Eisenhardt. The surface of the tumour may be quite smooth, finely granular, or coarsely lobulated. Its texture is usually firm and fibrous, sometimes friable and sufficiently soft to respond to suction and in such, surface fragments are easily detached during operative removal and left in the brain or may lie in the superficial tissues, a fruitful cause of recurrence and of nodules in the scalp scar. At times the tumour is gritty from calcareous deposits (psammoma bodies) and may even contain bone. Rarely the tumour contains butter-like areas due to lipoid changes. The blood supply of the tumour is for the most part transmitted through its dural

attachment, hence from the external carotid circulation, the angiographic identification of which is diagnostic. To a lesser degree it is derived from adventitious branches of the cortical arteries. Vascularity varies greatly; some tumours have a poor blood supply and on that score give rise to little trouble during removal; in others the blood supply is very rich and in such haemorrhagic shock may still be a cause of death. Much of the venous drainage of the tumour passes through the dural attachment. Small tumours do not cause much atrophy of the indented cortex, and the convolutional pattern may often be detected in the cavity left after the removal of the tumour. In the larger tumours cortex may disappear more or less completely; in these separation of tumour from brain may be difficult and the line of cleavage may easily be lost if the tumour is soft, so that the risk of leaving fragments is very real. Rarely cyst-like accumulations of yellow fluid are encountered between tumour and brain. The presence and degree of oedema of the neighbouring brain varies considerably from case to case and by no means runs parallel with the size of the tumour. Softening of the surrounding brain is common with large tumours, but the massive swelling of white matter often seen around a glioblastoma and a metastasis is not as frequent, although internal herniations are widespread and severe. Henschen (1955) draws attention to the great variation in the duration of symptoms in cases of meningioma, and quotes the case of a patient who died ten hours after a fit; autopsy revealed very extensive oedema around the tumour. At the other extreme symptoms may last for 25 years. He considered the oedema an important controlling factor and it has been widely suspected that meningiomas reveal themselves clinically when they precipitate cerebral oedema. Stevens *et al.* (1983) studied oedema production in 160 cases of meningioma using computerized tomography (CT). Oedema production was positively correlated with tumours of large surface area, anterior parasagittal position, prominent vascularity, involvement of dural sinuses, and with a short clinical history. They suggested that

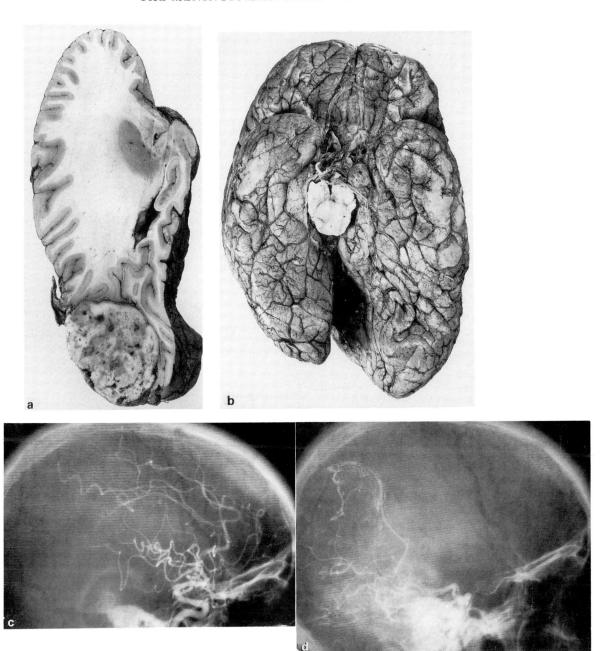

**Fig. 7.1.** (a) Meningioma embedded in convexity of occipital lobe: the cortical pattern is discernible in parts of its bed, but much grey matter has been destroyed: elsewhere the sulci are tightly compressed and convex surfaces of gyri flattened.
(b) The brain stem is displaced to the right, with pronounced herniation of the left uncus and hippocampal gyri.
(c) Left carotid angiogram: the posterior half of the cranium is 'avascular', the branches of the middle cerebral artery are displaced forwards, 'concertinaed'.
(d) Vertebral angiogram: a branch of the posterior cerebral artery supplies the anterior pole of the tumour which is clearly demarcated.

[continued on p. 258]

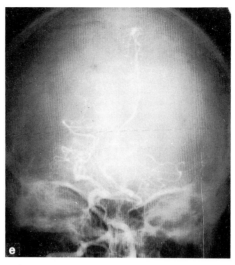

(e) The branch is seen to arise from the left posterior cerebral artery, the proximal part of which is displaced to the right, in conformity with the hippocampal herniation seen in (b).
The patient, a 56-year-old female, had suffered from schizophrenia for 20 years. Over the course of several weeks she had become confused, unsteady and had headache. She was found to have papilloedema and a right motor sensory hemiparesis. She died two days after angiography.

mechanical factors were predominant in producing the oedema which occurs with meningioma. However, Philippon *et al.* (1984) presented electron microscopic evidence of the secretion and excretion of macromolecular material by tumour cells in many meningiomas and the secretory activity was strongly correlated with the extent of peritumoural oedema. They also postulate a potential role for oestrogen and progesterone receptors in oedema production.

A noticeable feature when a meningioma has been removed is the rapidity with which the brain swells and obliterates the cavity occupied by the tumour. This swelling is due in part to vasodilatation in brain previously compressed by tumour and in part to reactionary oedema. This, and the widespread herniations which continue for a time to obstruct the flow of cerebrospinal fluid, are commonly the cause for the slow and stormy recovery from operation and for the bulging of the decompression which may persist for months. Convalescence after the removal of a glioma is often much smoother, because excision of the glioma often includes that portion of brain which harbours it and consequently there is usually more room to accommodate swelling.

Not infrequently the bone overlying the dural attachment of a meningioma shows characteristic changes, which when identified radiographically are of diagnostic importance. The internal surface becomes pitted and the diploe enlarged to accommodate the large venous outflow from the tumour; when the bone flap is separated from the dura mater, these adventitious channels are divided and the outer surface of the dura mater bleeds freely, indicating the site of the tumour. The internal surface is also grooved by enlarged meningeal arteries converging on the tumour; this is particularly well seen when the tumour is situated in the vicinity of the middle meningeal artery. The enlarged meningeal feeding arteries can be identified by angiography. Reactive changes may take place in the bone over a meningioma, to form a lump or hyperostosis. In its simplest form, the inner table, pitted with vascular channels, becomes elevated in sessile or conical shape, denting the dural attachment. In extreme cases the outer table is also involved so as to form a smooth boss. The lump is usually painless and so slowly does it grow that the patient may be unaware of it. The hyperostosis varies in texture; it may be spongy and softer than the surrounding bone, or sclerosed and much harder. Occasionally the central area of the internal prominence, the enostosis, is excavated by soft tumour tissue which has transgressed the dura mater and tumour may be encountered under the galea and permeating muscle. The incidence of hyperostosis bears no relationship to the histological nature of the tumour, nor to the size of the tumour, but has an unaccountable predilection for certain sites. The conical enostosis may arise from a tumour anywhere, but large sessile external lumps are particularly frequent with parasagittal tumours and tumours straddling the sphenoidal ridge often cause hyperplastic changes extending to the temporal fossa and the orbit. In these, the intradural tumour may be relatively thin, forming the so-called meningioma-*en-plaque*. Histological examination of a hyperostosis revealed meningioma cells in 21 of 23 cases studied by Rowbotham (1939), although Zülch (1965) stated that there are 'many instances of bony hyperplasia without actual tumour infiltration' Rowbotham suggested that enostosis might be due to the elevation of the dura mater from the bone by the enlarged venous pathways and aggravated by movement of the tumour, and Russell (1950) also thought that a mechanical factor played a part. The 23 cases of hyperostosis studied by Rowbotham occurred in a series of 100 meningiomas, a much higher incidence than the estimate of 4.5% given by Courville (1947).

## Special characteristics

Although meningiomas may arise anywhere they show a strong predilection for certain situations and this distribution bears a loose correlation with that of the arachnoidal granulations. The anatomical location and the biological behaviour of the tumours lead to the recognition of clinical syndromes, characteristic for each group, which are described later in the chapter. In the following list of sites, the percentage figure is derived from Cushing and Eisenhardt (1938).

*Parasagittal and falx (24%)*

In Cushing's series the proportion of parasagittal to falx meningiomas was approximately ten to one; in McKissock's series (Gautier-Smith 1970) it was three to one. The anatomical distinction between the two groups lies in their relationship to the superior sagittal sinus. The former arises from the wall of the sinus, the latter arises from the falx; it may be difficult at operation to determine whether a large tumour with an extensive dural attachment is parasagittal or falcine in origin although there are differences in their clinical behaviour.

The parasagittal tumour is primarily attached to the wall of the superior sagittal sinus, fills the angular interval between the falx and the convexity dura mater and deeply indents the medial surface of the hemisphere. The wall of the sinus may be incorporated in the tumour, the lumen partially or totally occluded. Large tumours spread downwards over the falx, depressing the corpus callosum and the pericallosal artery; they may also spread on to the convexity dura mater, but this is less common; often when the convexity dura mater is reflected in the course of the craniotomy only a narrow rim of tumour is visible separating the medial margin of the hemisphere from the sinus. Indeed, if small the tumour can be overlooked at exploration, particularly if the craniotomy is incorrectly sited.

The falx meningioma only gains a secondary attachment to the walls of the sinus if it is large and widely spread. It forms a bun-shaped mass which deeply indents the medial surface of the hemiphere and depresses the corpus callosum and the terminal divisions of the anterior cerebral arteries. It frequently extends through the thickness of the dural partition so that the tumour is bilateral though rarely symmetrical. Those arising from the posterior part of the falx often spread in nodular fashion on to the tentorium, rendering their total extirpation difficult if not impracticable. At craniotomy no tumour is visible until the medial margin of the hemisphere is mobilized which may require division of important veins to the sagittal sinus; consequently accurate angiographic localization is essential in order to minimize exploration and mobilization of the brain.

The distribution of these tumours is not evenly spaced along the length of the sinus; the greatest number occur within its middle one-third, bringing them into close relationship with the superior extremity of the sensorimotor cortex. The tumours are least common along the posterior one-third of the sinus. Hyperostosis is frequent in the parasagittal meningiomas; they occurred in practically one-quarter of Cushing's series and he emphasized that in these the tumour is often bilateral. No hyperostosis is present in those arising solely from the falx.

*Convexity (18%)*

Convexity meningiomas arise from the dura over the cerebral hemispheres and have no attachment to the superior sagittal sinus or the base of the skull. These tumours tend to lie in the area about the coronal suture. In nearly three-quarters of Cushing's cases, the tumour lay anterior to the central fissure. The overlying bone is often irregularly pitted by increased vascularity and a central spur-like enostosis may develop. The convexity group was the largest (34%) of McKissock's intracranial meningiomas (Gautier-Smith 1970).

*Sphenoidal ridge (18%)*

This term, coined for convenience by neurosurgeons, is given to the sharply edged shelf of bone which, supporting the posterior part of the undersurface of the frontal lobe, provides the boundary between the anterior and middle cranial fossae. Its inner two-thirds is provided by the lesser wing of the sphenoid, terminating medially in the anterior clinoid process; its outer one-third by the greater wing and its conjunction with the temporal, parietal and frontal bones,

the pterion. Meningiomas arising from the dura mater clothing the ridge cause clinical syndromes which vary according to their situation along the length of the ridge. The tumour spreads over the dura mater covering the anterior fossa, downwards over that of the anterior wall of the middle fossa and in massive tumours may extend along the floor of the fossa over the tentorium and medially into the cavernous sinus. Nager (1964) has described cases in which the tumour invaded the petrous bone bilaterally. The growth may gain the orbit by penetrating the superior orbital fissure or the optic canal. In some cases the tumour is a thin nodular layer on the dura mater, the so-called meningioma-*en-plaque*. In others it forms a dome-shaped mass straddling the ridge, pressing upwards into the under surface of the frontal lobe, opening up the Sylvian fissure and displacing backwards the tip of the temporal lobe. Those arising from the inner one-third overlap and press upon the optic nerve and then the optic chiasm, a relationship which gives them significance as a clinical group. These and large examples of the middle-third group, also impinge upon the internal carotid artery and its terminal branches, displacing them and sometimes partially or totally engulfing them, a matter of major surgical importance. Hyperostosis is particularly common and its radiological detection of great value in diagnosis. The anterior clinoid process becomes club-like; the sharp edge of the ridge is rounded and its upper surface elevated and thickened; these changes may involve the orbit and temporal fossa to a degree sufficient to cause facial disfigurement. The bone may be soft and vascular, or sclerosed and harder than normal. The meningioma-*en-plaque* is particularly prone to occur at the outer end of the ridge and to excite widespread hyperostosis.

*Olfactory groove (10%)*

These tumours, sometimes of great size, take origin at first from the dura mater covering the lamina cribrosa of the ethmoid on one side. As they enlarge they involve a greater area of dura mater, bilaterally, and eventually form an approximately spherical midline mass deeply buried in the inferior surface of both frontal lobes. The site of origin causes destruction of one olfactory bulb or tract, sometimes both and anosmia is an important sign. The tumour may depress or destroy the olfactory plate; posteriorly the floor of the anterior fossa may develop an irregular hyperostosis. The posterior surface of the tumour may bulge backwards sufficiently to exert a downward pressure upon the optic nerve and chiasm, though a thin layer of brain may intervene and the anterior extremity of the third ventricle may be displaced backwards. The relationship to the anterior cerebral arteries is of great importance as the arteries and their branches are at risk during removal of the tumour.

### Suprasellar (10%)

The tumour is midline and arises from the tuberculum sellae, between the optic foramina and occasionally forms a hyperostosis. As it enlarges it overhangs the diaphragma sellae over which it may spread and engage the optic nerves and the chiasma in the manner of a pituitary adenoma and with similar consequences, though the sella turcica remains of normal size. These tumours are rarely large because of the relatively early development of visual failure. The arch of the anterior cerebral and anterior communicating arteries is elevated by the tumour and may indent it so that the tumour may be dumb-bell shaped, a larger anterior and a smaller posterior portion. The arterial arch is at risk during operation, for incautious traction on the tumour may tear the artery if it is engaged in a groove in the tumour.

Although it is convenient to recognize the olfactory groove and tuberculum sellae meningiomas as two distinct groups, in some cases it is difficult to determine the precise site of origin and the clinical pictures merge.

Less common situations for meningiomas in the supratentorial compartment of the cranium are the floor of the middle fossa, the cavernous sinus, the tentorium, the sheath of the optic nerve and the ventricles.

### Posterior fossa (8%)

Relatively few meningiomas arise below the tentorium and they can be divided into ventral or basal and convexity groups. The former group comprises midline tumours attached to the clivus, those situated laterally along the lines of the sigmoid groove and bulging into the cerebellopontine angle and those arising from and straddling the margin of the foramen magnum, partly within the cranium and partly intraspinal. For the most part these are sessile tumours, having a granular surface and enveloping the cranial nerves at or even within their foramina of exit. They displace the major arteries, vertebral and basilar, in accordance with their situation. The convexity tumours rise from the dura mater enveloping the cerebellar lobes or from the undersurface of the tentorium, usually situated laterally, forming a globular mass and are rare. The tentorial tumour may also extend as a bilobed mass upwards into the cerebral hemisphere and downwards into the cerebellum (Fig. 7.2).

### Histology

The microscopic appearances of meningioma fall into a variety of different patterns which have led to a multiplicity of classifications and confused terminology. A widely accepted scheme is that of Courville (1945) who classified meningiomas into five basic types: (1) syncytial, (2) transitional, (3) fibrous, (4) angioblastic, (5) malignant. A variety of secondary changes may occur in any of these types.

The *syncytial* or endotheliomatous meningiomas consist of polygonal, poorly defined cells, arranged in sheets, separated by vascular trabeculae (Fig. 7.3). The cytoplasm is usually homogeneous, the nuclei round or oval with sparse chromatin and two or three small nucle-

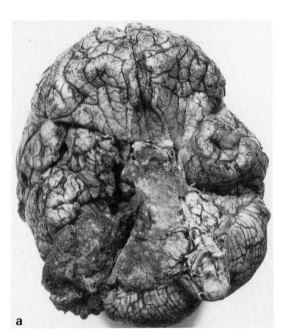
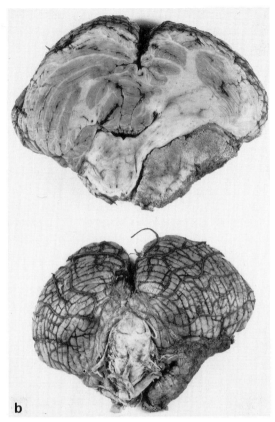

**Fig. 7.2.** Meningioma of cerebellopontine angle extending forwards on clivus to diaphragma sellae, through the tentorial hiatus to indent the temporal lobe and gain attachment to the floor of the middle cranial fossa. The patient was a 68-year-old. There had been deterioration of personality for 'some years', confusion and unsteadiness of gait in recent weeks, with drowsiness, frequent motor seizures and circulatory failure.

oli. Collagen and reticulin fibres are confined to the fibrovascular trabeculae.

The *transitional* type is characterized by the formation of cellular whorls (Fig. 7.4a). These consist of a small central core of two or three polygonal cells wrapped in concentric layers of flattened cells, resembling the structure of an onion bulb. Sometimes the whorls contain a small central vessel. The intervening tissue consists mainly of strands of spindle cells, but syncytial sheets may also be formed. The central parts of the whorls may undergo hyaline degeneration with subsequent deposition of calcium salts. These calcified, concentric, psammoma bodies form a characteristic feature of many transitional meningiomas (Fig. 7.4b).

There is no justification for separating these tumours into a separate group of psammomatous meningiomas.

The *fibroblastic* or fibrous type consists of interlacing bundles of long, thin spindle cells, with elongated nuclei (Fig. 7.5). There is some tendency to formation of loose whorls, less compact than those seen in the transitional variety. Fibroblastic tumours contain abundant reticulin and collagen fibres between individual cells.

It is important to emphasize that these three types do not represent different tumours, but only variable patterns within a single type of neoplasm. It is therefore not surprising to find two or more patterns in the same tumour, often shading into each other.

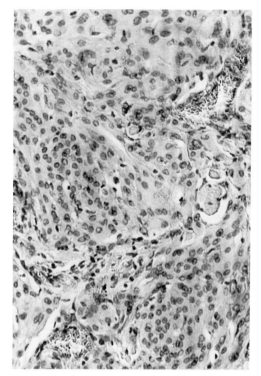

**Fig. 7.3.** Meningioma: syncytial type. H. & E. × 240.

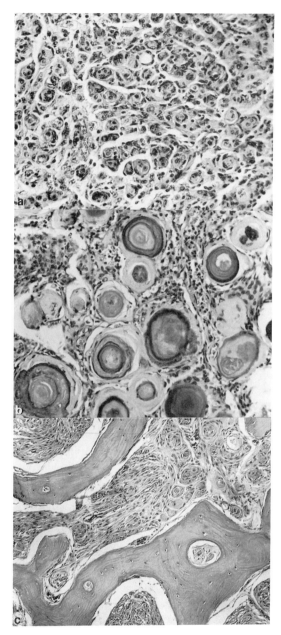

**Fig. 7.4.** Meningioma.
(a) Transitional type with whorls. H. & E. × 180
(b) Transitional type with psammoma bodies. H. & E. × 180
(c) Transitional type filling marrow spaces of vault of skull. H. & E. × 90

Angioblastic meningiomas comprise a less well defined and probably less homogeneous group. Their histogenesis and classification is still highly controversial, some authorities treating them as a single group with some variation in pattern and ascribing to them a meningeal, predominantly pial, origin, while others consider these tumours a mixture of unrelated entities, some of meningeal, some of primary vascular origin. Their common feature is the predominance of vascular channels in their structure, separated by sheets, columns or trabeculae or extravascular cells (Fig. 7.6). Some of these tumours resemble cerebellar haemangioblastomas and consist of sheets and nests of homogenous polygonal cells, many of them containing abundant lipid droplets. Others consist of highly cellular columns, sometimes arranged radially around vessels, with an abundant reticulin stroma separating individual cells and usually containing mitotic figures. These tumours resemble haemangiopericytomas which may occur in various parts of the body.

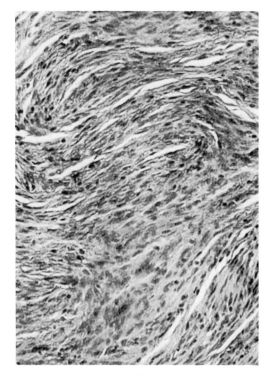

**Fig. 7.5.** Meningioma: fibroblastic type. H. & E. × 240

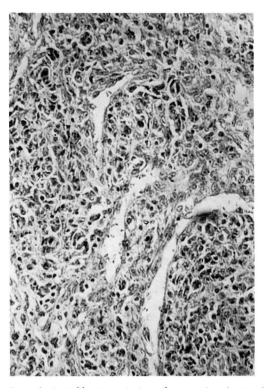

**Fig. 7.6.** Angioblastic meningiona (haemangiopericytoma). H. & E. × 240

Whether these tumours are considered variants of a single type or subdivided into haemangioblastomas, haemangiopericytomas and angioblastic meningiomas proper would be largely of theoretical interest were it not for the difference in their biological behaviour. The 'haemangiopericytoma' type is, in distinction to the others, a malignant tumour, though often of fairly low grade.

*Other variants of meningioma*

Xanthomatous changes may occur in all types of meningioma. Patches of foam cells containing sudanophilic lipid may be scattered through otherwise unremarkable tumours.

Melanotic meningiomas are found occasionally in the posterior fossa and region of the upper cervical cord where the normal leptomeninges are frequently pigmented. Apart from the pres-

ence of abundant melanin granules these tumours do not differ from other meningiomas.

Calcification may occur in the whorls of transitional meningiomas as psammoma bodies, or it may be deposited in hyalinized walls of blood vessels or in the stroma of the tumour. Some of these calcified structures may undergo ossification, but osseous as well as cartilaginous metaplasia may occur independently of any degenerative changes. These changes may permit identification of the tumour on plain skull radiographs.

Myxomatous change occurs occasionally in the stroma with the production of abundant connective tissue mucin.

*Malignant changes and metastases*

Most meningiomas are benign both in their histological structure and their biological behav-

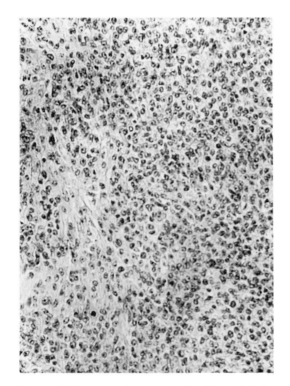

**Fig. 7.7.** Malignant meningioma showing high cellularity and lack of definite pattern. H. & E. × 240

iour. Occasional malignant tumours occur, particularly among recurrent meningiomas. The demarcation of malignant meningiomas from meningeal sarcomas is somewhat artificial and arbitrary. The concept of a malignant meningioma implies malignant change in a previously benign meningioma, while a meningeal sarcoma is a malignant tumour *ab initio*.

The criteria of malignancy in a meningioma are based on increasing dedifferentiation on the one hand, and invasiveness on the other. As the tumour acquires malignant characteristics on successive recurrences it tends to lose its typical structure and the cells become arranged in ill-defined sheets and cords (Fig. 7.7). The cell density increases and mitotic figures, some of them atypical, appear. Cellular pleomorphism by itself is not a criterion of malignancy as some benign meningiomas contain numerous large nuclei. In some malignant tumours the pattern becomes

even more undifferentiated and resembles that of a spindle celled sarcoma.

Invasiveness of meningiomas requires some qualification. Transgression of the dura mater is a common occurrence in benign tumours and does not indicate malignancy. Benign tumours commonly penetrate into, and may occlude, the dural venous sinuses. As the dura forms the internal periosteum of the skull tumours growing on both sides of the dura freely penetrate the inner table (Fig. 7.4c) and the diploe of the skull, sometimes eroding the bone, sometimes causing a hyperostotic reaction. Benign tumours, however, do not penetrate through the external periosteum of the skull. Invasion of the galea aponeurotica and of the scalp indicates malignancy. On its inner aspect a benign meningioma compresses the brain, but remains clearly demarcated from it. Invasion of the brain and subsequent reactive gliosis indicate a malignant trend (Fig. 7.8). Extracranial metastases are distinctly rare and

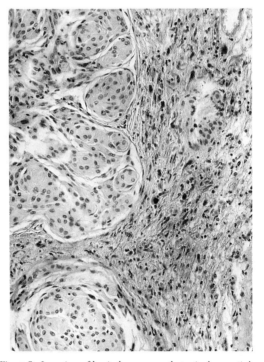

**Fig. 7.8.** Invasion of brain by apparently typical syncytial meningioma must be considered evidence of malignancy. The invaded brain tissue (pons) contains Rosenthal fibres. H. & E. × 210

dissemination via the cerebrospinal fluid pathways even rarer. Cushing and Eisenhardt had a remarkable patient, Dorothy May Russell, who underwent 17 operations for her intracranial meningioma and was found at autopsy to have pulmonary metastases. Histology of the metastases showed a papillary meningioma and this rare type of tumour has been given a separate classification in the World Health Organization Scheme (Zülch 1979).

*Diagnosis in wet-film preparations*

Meningiomas smear badly and instead of spreading evenly break up into clumps of cells of various sizes. These clumps usually consist of groups of uniform, oval or polygonal cells with oval nuclei and abundant homogenous cytoplasm. The presence of whorls, which usually remain intact, makes the diagnosis unequivocal. In their absence occasional difficulties may be encountered in distinguishing meningiomas from some secondary carcinomas which tend to spread similarly. The nuclei however are usually different, those of carcinoma cells being more pyknotic and pleomorphic.

**Diagnosis and treatment**

*Parasagittal and falx*

Meningiomas arising from the anterior third may give little or no clinical indication of their localization. Headache is the predominant symptom, preceding papilloedema by a year or more. Impairment of memory, intelligence and personality develop insidiously, though not to the degree seen in invasive tumours of the frontal lobe. Guillaume *et al.* (1957) found such changes in 30%, but in only 5% of middle-third and in 22% of posterior-third meningiomas. Gautier-Smith noted a high proportion with severe dementia in the anterior group. Olivecrona (1934) drew attention to the occurrence of frequency and of incontinence of urine in patients

with preserved personality. Ataxia, tremor and ipsilateral facial pain may accompany a massive frontal lobe tumour and thus indicate erroneously a posterior fossa lesion. Epilepsy, usually of a nonfocal type, occurs in about one-quarter of the cases (Lund 1952).

Middle-third tumours are characterized by motor or sensory focal epilepsy as an initial symptom of several years' duration. It occurred in three-quarters in Lund's analysis and a higher incidence is recorded by Cushing; it is more likely to develop if the tumour is parasagittal. The seizure commences in the foot, as a convulsive movement or as paraesthesia, sometimes painful, and usually shows a typical Jacksonian march. Later the foot and leg develop a spastic weakness; the dorsiflexors of the foot are most affected, as a result of the pressure against the paracentral lobule. Loss of discriminative sensibility occurs in the more posterior tumours; in these the weakness may be flaccid and the 'foot-drop' simulates a lateral popliteal nerve lesion. Tumours situated anterior to the paracentral lobule may give rise to epilepsy in and weakness of the upper limb owing to the forward obliquity of the motor strip. Symptoms of raised intracranial pressure are commonly less marked in middle-third compared with anterior-third tumours, because the focal symptoms and signs compel earlier attention. Bilateral tumours may rarely give rise to bilateral disturbances and the resulting paraplegia may be fruitlessly investigated by myelography.

Posterior-third meningiomas, the least common variety, have one characteristic localizing sign, a homonymous hemianopia. Its pattern depends upon the size and location of the tumour; when this is large the entire half-field is lost, when situated further forward so as to lie above the calcarine fissure the inferior quadrant is more affected and correspondingly when near the tentorium the upper bank of the calcarine fissure may be spared and the field defect is then upper quadrantic. A slowly developing hemianopia is often not noticed by the patient, consequently the symptoms of raised intracranial pressure and of impaired mental processes, like the anterior one-third tumours, are more marked

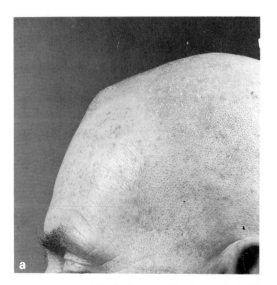

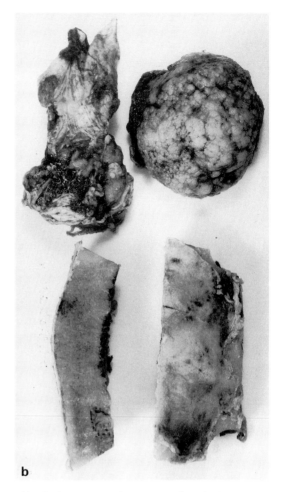

Fig. 7.9 (a) Insignificant midline boss at the hairline caused by the hyperostosis of a parasagittal meningioma.
(b) Radiological rarefaction was demonstrated at the hyperostosis and to the naked eye the texture of the bone
is less dense than at either end of the specimen. The inner surface of the bone is pitted by the tumour invasion,
the outer surface is smooth. The tumour was bilateral and the sagittal sinus was invaded and was excised.
Nodules of tumour cover the outer surface of the dura mater of the sinus specimen. This 44-year-old male had
experienced focal motor epilepsy in left lower limb for 3 years and for a few weeks noticed increasing weakness
of dorsiflexion of left foot.

than in middle-third tumours. Epilepsy is uncommon.

The most valuable evidence of a parasagittal meningioma is the presence of a hyperostosis (Fig. 7.9), often not noticed by the patient, or not declared because it is not associated with the symptoms. At times obvious, it usually has to be sought, for it may be only an insignificant boss and even unrecognized until the head is shaved.

With big tumours there may be dilated scalp vessels. Meningioma of the falx produces no hyperostosis. Radiographs of the skull show direct evidence of a meningioma in about half the cases of parasagittal tumour, but not when the tumour is restricted to the falx thereby not involving the endosteal layer of the dura mater. The hyperostosis is recognized by the new bone which forms external to the outer table and suitably

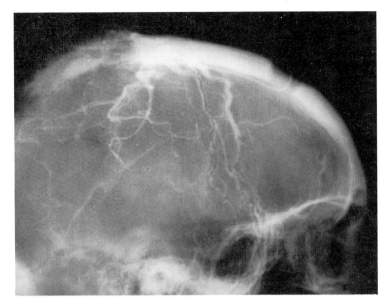

Fig. 7.10. Sinogram in a case of parasagittal meningioma. The catheter (containing opaque medium) has been inserted through a burr hole over the sinus. The sinus is totally obstructed at the point where the bone is invaded. There is retrograde filling of cortical veins anterior to the block. The middle meningeal veins also fill, identified by sinuous thread-like negative contrast due to accompanying unfilled meningeal arteries.

projected films may show radial spicules, the sunray effect. The inner table may be thickened and careful tangential views may reveal a conical spur. The bone may be sclerosed, or may in parts show destruction by the tumour (Fig. 7.10). Increased vascularity around its margin and enlargement of the middle meningeal channels differentiate it from a sessile ivory osteoma. Occasionally calcification or even bone subjacent to the hyperostosis will indicate the precise position of the tumour. CT scanning has essentially replaced other neuroradiological investigations in the diagnosis of intracranial tumours of all types and is particularly sensitive in the case of meningiomas. Characteristic features of meningioma on CT scanning include a high density, homogenous mass with well-defined rounded borders and striking enhancement with contrast medium (Fig. 7.11). Hyperostosis, bone destruction, calcification within the tumour and surrounding brain oedema can also be demonstrated. Of great importance is the fact that small tumours approaching one centimetre in size may be detected.

Although the CT scan is of immense benefit in diagnosis and precise tumour location, angiography is also necessary to demonstrate vascular relationships, both arterial and venous,

prior to surgery. The phlebogram may reveal that the cortical veins are numerous and abnormal, suggestive that the sinus is obstructed;

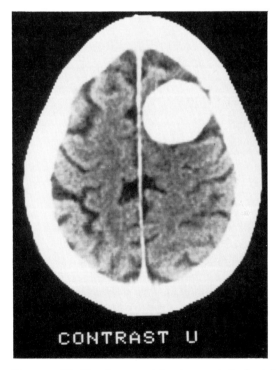

Fig. 7.11. CT with enhancement showing a posterior frontal meningioma.

a sinogram (Fig. 7.10) should be performed in middle and posterior-third tumours in order to make certain, for the state of the sinus is of great importance surgically.

The removal of a parasagittal meningioma is technically difficult and presents several hazards. One is haemorrhage 'the most important single cause of death' (Olivecrona 1947): from the scalp, from the highly vascular bone, from the tumour and dura mater and from the sagittal sinus, particularly in the region of the torcula. Another is the hyperostosis; when this is large and infiltrated by tumour, it cannot be incorporated in the bone flap because anchorage to the tumour prevents the elevation of the flap, or if this is forced, transmits violence to the underlying brain. The hyperostosis may be removed piecemeal by burr and bone forceps as described by Cushing, or by isolating it circumferentially and reflecting an adjacent bone flap, which provides access to the undersurface of the hyperostosis so that its attachment to the growth can be divided. The final hazard is the removal of the tumour which is rendered immobile by its attachment to the sinus and falx.

There are two broad techniques for removing the tumour. The first is to divide its dural attachments, separate it from the surrounding brain and remove it in one piece. This technique can only be applied to sinus tumours by cutting through tumour close to the sinus and the falx, removing the main mass in one piece and then dealing with the residual base. The second and preferable technique which is advocated by Logue (1975) is to reduce the bulk of the tumour by exenteration and then retract the capsule away from the brain so that the last manœuvre is freeing of the tumour from the falx and sinus. The treatment of the sinus has been a matter of controversy. The anterior third of the sinus may be resected without serious risk and is justifiable if thereby a total extirpation of the tumour can be obtained, but resections of the sinus from the level of the Rolandic veins backwards are liable to give rise to serious and permanent cerebral damage, particularly on the opposite side, from interference with cortical venous drainage. If the sinus is already totally obstructed by tumour and a prior sinogram may have ascertained this, its resection is necessary and likely to be safe, though anastomotic veins in front and behind should be carefully preserved. Grant (1947) reported the excision of up to 15 cm of the invaded superior and inferior sagittal sinuses and intervening falx without subsequent paralysis. If tumour invades but does not obliterate a sinus, it may be possible to open the sinus or excise part of it to achieve total tumour removal and then repair the sinus by suturing or using a patch graft (Logue 1975). It is generally felt that a patent sagittal sinus in its posterior two thirds should never be sacrificed if it can possibly be avoided. Radiological investigation may have made it clear that the tumour extends bilaterally, or invasion of the falx may reveal its extension to the other side, but in every case this possibility should be borne in mind. A window cut in the falx allows exploration of its other side. A decision may be made to deal with a large extension at a separate session, from the opposite side, though it is usually easily accessible from the side of the major mass, provided the exposure has been planned accordingly by taking the bone flap across the middle line.

Meningiomas of the falx do not present the operative technical difficulties of the hyperostosis and the attachment to the sinus, but they provide other problems. They do not present at the medial margin of the hemisphere and they may lie deep in the longitudinal fissure, consequently it may be difficult to locate the tumour. Division of the cortical veins entering the sinus may cause swelling of the neighbouring hemisphere, further hampering access and increasing postoperative disability. Cushing recommended approaching them through an incision in the cortex. They are often bilateral; the pericallosal arteries lie immediately beneath and are thus at risk during the dissection.

The operative mortality in Cushing's series varied between 11% for the parasagittal tumours with hyperostosis, to 56% for falx tumour. Many of these operations were carried out in multiple stages, before the introduction of surgical endothermy and when blood transfusion was frugal. The influence of a generous supply of blood is seen in Olivecrona's figures. During the years 1924–46 there were 26 operative deaths and loss of blood was the cause in six. During the years 1947–54 there were eight deaths and none was due to loss of blood. The average mortality was 12.3%, anterior one-third parasagittal meningiomas carrying the least risk (5.4%) and falx meningiomas the greatest at 20%. Almost precisely similar figures were reported by Guillaume *et al.* (1957). In the more modern series of Logue (1975) the mortality rates were 4.4.% for parasagittal meningiomas and 2.4% for falx meningiomas.

*Convexity*

The distinction between a slowly growing glioma and a meningioma arising from the convexity dura mater is usually difficult by clinical methods alone. Both give rise to focal epilepsy, with increasing frequency the nearer the tumour lies to the central fissure; both gradually produce the disturbance of neurological function characteristic of the area of brain involved. In the case of meningioma, symptoms of raised intracranial pressure, often for a year or more, usually precede the development of focal signs; by contrast, the focal signs indicating impairment of neurological function and due to infiltration of brain by glial tumour, usually precede raised intracranial pressure and are relatively more severe. Radiological changes in the overlying bone often provide the clue to correct diagnosis and comprise localized increase of vascularity, enlargement of the neighbouring meningeal vessel grooves and new bone formation. External hyperostosis is less common than with parasagittal meningiomas, but an enostosis is frequently to be found. CT scanning. and angiography usually confirm the diagnosis and the angiogram may show characteristic tumour circulation and feeding meningeal vessels.

The removal of a convexity meningioma offers fewer problems than elsewhere. Haemorrhage

during the various stages may be considerable but can be controlled step by step. The hyperostosis is rarely of a size to render reflection of the bone flap difficult. The dura mater is opened by an incision encircling the attachment of the tumour, haemostasis of the vascular edges being secured as the incision progresses and the blood supply of the tumour is thus greatly diminished during the stage in which it is exposed. The tumour can then be removed by exenteration and great care taken in dissecting the capsule from the cortex so that a minimum of damage is inflicted and no tumour fragments are left behind.

The operative mortality in the Cushing series was unusually high, 21%; modern techniques have lowered the mortality very considerably, that of Guillaume *et al.* (1957) being 8%, and Logue (1975) 2.4%.

*Sphenoidal ridge*

It is customary to follow Cushing's description which distinguished three groups, those arising from the inner, the middle and the outer third of the sphenoidal ridge. This is an artificial separation, in that there is no natural tendency for them to be so grouped (Cushing's numbers were 13, 11, 16 respectively) and large tumours may extend along the whole ridge; but the value of this classification lies in emphasizing the varying clinical pictures which are evoked according to the position of the tumour relative to neighbouring anatomical structures. It was for this reason that Cushing so grouped them. But it is those tumours which arise from the inner end of the ridge, on or close to the anterior clinoid process, which manifest a well defined syndrome, whereas the other two groups merge one with another and are less easily distinguished. Henderson (1938) divided 'ridge' meningiomas into two groups, inner and outer. This description is preferred and will be adopted.

The inner sphenoidal ridge (or clinoidal) meningiomas owe their importance to the closely adjacent optic nerve, which early suffers compression with consequent gradual loss of vision in that eye. The history of uni-ocular visual failure may be of many years' duration. Primary optic atrophy develops and examination of the visual fields may reveal a central scotoma which, if extensive, breaks out to the periphery, usually on the temporal side; ultimately only a residual crescent of visual field may remain. In other cases there is a nasal hemianopia, due to pressure on the lateral border of the optic nerve, or occasionally a temporal hemianopia, due to notching of the medial border of the optic nerve by the inner margin of the optic canal, against which the nerve is displaced. A temporal hemianopia in the field of the other eye indicates that the tumour is pressing on the optic chiasma; at this stage the ipsilateral eye may already be blind. Anosmia on the side of the tumour is common, due to compression of the olfactory tract. Spread of the tumour into the cavernous sinus or into the superior orbital fissure can cause paralysis of the third nerve and sometimes of the fourth and of the sixth nerves; the ophthalmic division of the trigeminal nerve may also be involved, causing numbness of the forehead on that side. Exophthalmos is frequent, due either to impairment of venous drainage of the orbit or to spread of tumour into the orbit. Headache and pain are absent in the early stages, but symptoms of raised intracranial pressure develop if the ocular manifestations are ignored. Papilloedema develops in the contralateral eye for the arachnoid sheath of the ipsilateral optic nerve has been closed by the pressure of the overlying tumour and the nerve is atrophic. This characteristic syndrome, of primary optic atrophy in one eye and papilloedema in the other, described by Paton (1909) and more fully by Foster Kennedy (1911) and now carrying the latter's name, may be produced by any tumour arising in proximity to one optic nerve. Foster Kennedy's 6 cases included meningioma, glioma and an immense frontal abscess; in 5 the optic atrophy was associated with a central scotoma.

The outer ridge meningiomas can be divided into two clinical groups, though cases occur which combine the characteristics of both. In the one are those which give rise to inconspicuous or no localizing symptoms and signs, the patients presenting with raised intracranial pressure and often with considerable papilloedema; the symptoms develop insidiously, usually within a year. These tumours are large rounded masses, lying astride the ridge, opening up the Sylvian fissure and they are notable for their 'silence' except for epilepsy (see below). The second group comprises those patients with a marked and extensive hyperostosis. In the course of years proptosis gradually develops, the temple becomes prominent and the orbital margin thickened. The eyeball may remain normally mobile except that the proptosis is irreducible by pressure; it is not pulsatile. The eyelids are commonly oedematous, in advanced cases markedly so and then the conjunctiva is also oedematous and may be congested. Vision in the eye is retained unless tumour has invaded the orbit. The course of the illness is usually painless and prolonged. The tumour is frequently of the *en plaque* type, in which case the intracranial pressure is not raised. Epilepsy may occur in any of the ridge meningiomas, as with other brain tumours, but those that impinge upon the temporal lobe, either by opening up the Sylvian fissure or by spreading into the middle fossa, are liable to produce those special patterns of seizure, that originate in the temporal lobe.

Radiological examination is of the greatest importance, for the detection of a hyperostosis may provide the only clue to diagnosis. The anterior clinoid process is usually thickened in the inner-ridge tumours (though rarely it is absorbed) and the sella turcica shows signs of raised intracranial pressure. The hyperostosing pterional tumours are obvious, the bone changes being widespread and the density such as to be mistaken for an osteoma or a fibrous dysplasia. Increased width of meningeal channels and the stippling due to vascularity may be detected if the bone is not too dense. In the absence of a hyperostosis, the differential diagnosis will include pituitary adenoma, aneurysm of the internal carotid artery, epidermoid cyst, craniopharyngioma and glioma. CT scanning and angiography will usually clarify the diagnosis, and provide information about the situation of the major arteries. Vessel displacements depend upon the situation of the tumour and its direction of growth. The internal carotid artery and its bifurcation may be depressed backwards and medially if an inner ridge tumour overlaps them; or the carotid artery may be stretched upwards if the tumour expands below it, giving the anterior and middle cerebral arteries an arch-like curve concave downwards. The more lateral tumours elevate the stem of the middle cerebral artery so that its transverse portion takes an upward and backward curve away from the ridge and the sharp angle between the transverse course and the Sylvian branches is flattened or lost. A pathological circulation may clearly outline the mass. *En plaque* tumours may show no abnormality on the angiogram.

The removal of a sphenoidal-ridge meningioma is often a matter of great difficulty, particularly one from the inner third. It is deeply placed, firmly attached, in close proximity to, or even enveloping, major arteries, while the optic apparatus lies hidden under its deepest aspect. It is in such deeply placed tumours that modern neuroanaesthesia and aids such as steroids and osmotic diuretic agents have proved their value, by diminishing the bulk of the brain and reducing haemorrhage. The approach is by a frontolateral flap, identifying the tumour by exploring along the ridge. The tumour is usually removed piecemeal, excavating its interior so as to diminish its bulk and progressively dividing its dural attachment, thereby diminishing its blood supply. As the tumour becomes mobile and its bulk diminishes, its relation to the optic nerve and chiasma and to the internal carotid and its branches is made possible and it can be gradually delivered, bearing in mind that deep processes may surround these vessels. Not uncommonly a fringe of the tumour spreads around the nerve and the artery and over the diaphragma sellae.

The introduction of microsurgical techniques has greatly facilitated the dissection and removal of these difficult tumours. Additional aids such as the surgical laser and the ultrasonic surgical aspirator are also beginning to prove of value. However, tumour infiltrating the cavernous sinus usually must be left and it may not be feasible to remove the tumour that is intimately involved with the optic nerve or major arteries. Laterally placed tumours do not present the same difficulty of access, but their removal may be complicated by the thickening of the bone. This is best removed by multiple burr holes and with rongeurs before opening the dura mater, a slow and painstaking manœuvre well illustrated in Cushing's monograph. This may necessitate removing part of the roof and posterior wall of the orbit which will afford an orbital decompression and relieve exophthalmos. When normal bone is reached the dura mater is opened and the portion attached to the tumour divided by an encircling incision. This mobilizes the tumour and interrupts most of its blood supply; its interior is then excavated and it is gradually removed.

Pterional tumours *en plaque* with widespread thickening of the bone grow very slowly and operation is not always indicated. If proptosis is slight operation may be deferred though if severe, operation devised as an orbital decompression may be advisable. Cushing quotes the case of a patient who had had slowly increasing exophthalmos for 31 years, who refused operation and in whom at the age of 73 years there had been little change in the condition for the previous 6 years. Of 25 patients of Olivecrona with this type of tumour, there were 10 who were not operated on; a conservative attitude to these tumours is recommended and 'surgical measures should be considered only as a last resort' (Castellano *et al.* 1952).

The mortality of these operations varies greatly according to the situation and size of the tumour. In Cushing's series of ridge meningiomas the overall figure was 16% ranging from 6% for the pterional *en plaque* to 30% for the pterional massive tumours. Guillaume *et al.* (1957) reported a mortality of 22%. Prognosis depends upon the completeness of removal, but even when this is incomplete the residual tumour may grow so slowly that the patient lives an active life for many years; such was the case for over 15 years and over 25 years in two of Cushing's patients.

*Olfactory groove*

It might be thought that anosmia would be a common presenting feature of olfactory groove meningiomas but even if present the patient rarely complains of this and may be unaware of it. The sense of smell should be tested but Symon (1977) reported that 50% of his massive bilateral tumours had a normal sense of smell pre-operatively. Epilepsy of the grand mal type is a common feature, 30% in Symon's series, and when it occurs is usually the first feature. Symptoms of raised intracranial pressure develop late and in the more anteriorly situated tumours failing vision from chronic papilloedema is the presenting symptom, while uni-ocular visual failure from direct pressure atrophy slowly develops if the tumour is situated slightly more posteriorly. In these tumours the Foster Kennedy syndrome may be encountered but is uncommon, the symmetry and central situation of the tumour being such that both optic nerves are pressed upon, though the vision in one eye is usually much worse than in the other. The visual field defects vary, including central scotoma, peripheral constriction, and hemianopia; a common finding is blindness of one eye and a temporal hemianopia in the other. A history of defective vision in one eye for as long as 10–15 years is by no means uncommon. Although these tumours may reach a large size, 5–7 cm in diameter indenting the undersurfaces of both frontal lobes, mental deterioration is rarely marked, in contrast to the dementia produced by a glioma of comparable size; such changes are usually no more than impaired memory, euphoria and lack of concentration. Tremor of the hands is not uncommon as in the other slowly growing massive tumours of the frontal lobe, but the absence of abnormal neurological signs apart from the anosmia and the visual changes is typical. Differential diagnosis includes meningioma of the anterior clinoid process and the tuberculum sel-

lae (but even at operation it may be difficult to tell the precise site of origin in some cases); frontal lobe glioma; glioma of the optic nerves and chiasm occur in a much younger age group; pituitary adenoma, craniopharyngioma and epidermoid cyst give rise to primary optic atrophy but endocrine and radiological investigations usually clearly distinguish them. Hydrocephalus from stenosis of the aqueduct may give rise to primary optic atrophy, anosmia and mental impairment.

Radiological examination of the skull may show erosion of the cribriform plate and a hyperostosis in front of the tuberculum sellae, neither signs easily detected except in high quality films (Fig. 7.12). CT scanning (Fig. 7.13) and angiography are essential investigations for diagnosis and surgical planning. The arterial supply to the tumour generally comes from the ophthalmic circulation via ethmoidal perforating branches and pathological circulation in the tumour may be visible. The anterior cerebral arteries are characteristically displaced backwards, and the pericallosal and callosomarginal branches displaced upwards, so that combined they form a high arc concave forwards. According to the situation of the tumour the vessels of both sides may remain in the median plane or may be displaced somewhat to one side.

The approach to an olfactory groove meningioma is usually by a frontal craniotomy, on the right side if the tumour is median, or on the side of the tumour if it is predominantly unilateral. It is common practice to carry out a polarfrontal lobectomy to 5–7 cm behind the pole in order to uncap the tumour. The interior of the tumour is gutted, its dural attachment divided, and the mobilized tumour thus diminished in size gradually removed. If the tumour is bilateral the mass on one side is first removed in this way, thus providing room for manœuvre so that the remaining half can be dislodged from the medial and undersurface of the opposite frontal lobe. The anterior cerebral arteries and their branches and the terminations of the internal carotid arteries are at risk though they may be protected by a thin layer of brain. Sometimes a nodule of

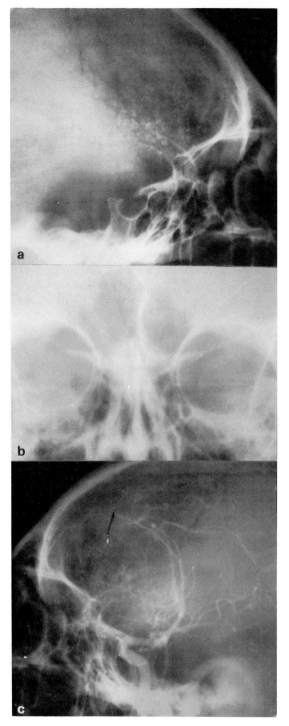

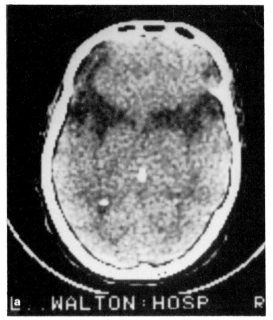

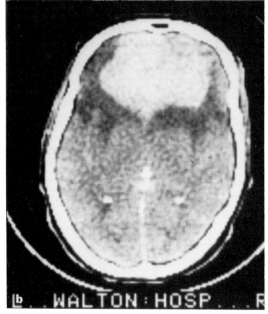

**Fig. 7.12.** Olfactory groove (or anterior basal) meningioma.
(a) Speckled calcification above the floor of the anterior cranial fossa, absence of olfactory plate and hyperostosis in the region of the tuberculum sellae.
(b) Midline thickening of bone of floor of anterior fossa.
(c) Termination of the internal carotid artery depressed, anterion cerebral arteries displaced backwards, pericallosal arteries displaced backwards and upwards. 52-year-old male: 3 months failing vision, euphoric, slightly defective memory, dull countenance, bilateral anosmia, bilateral primary optic atrophy, blind right eye, hand movements only with left eye. Two years after removal of tumour, vision R = 2/60, L = 6/9.

**Fig. 7.13.** CT before (a) and after (b) contrast enhancement. Large olfactory groove meningioma with oedema of the frontal lobes.

tumour is wedged under a major vessel. In this danger area deep to the mass hasty dissection or clumsy manipulation will rupture the vessel. The optic nerves and chiasma lie under the deepest part of the tumour and consequently their identification is not possible until late in the dissection, their immediate recognition being rendered more difficult by their compression. Constant reference to such bony landmarks as the sphenoidal ridge leading up to its clinoid process, and the crista galli help orientation; the anterolateral margin of the optic foramen gives immediate evidence of approach to the optic nerve, but its recognition is often difficult or delayed because pressure atrophy makes the bone edge paper-thin. The invaded dura mater can be excised or coagulated and a hyperostosis should be coagulated. The olfactory groove may be perforated by tumour, so that the roof of the nose is entered when the tumour is totally extirpated; the opening must be sealed by a fascia–lata graft. An alternative approach to the median tumour is obtained by a bifrontal bone flap, division of the anterior end of the sagittal sinus and falx so that the frontal dura mater can be reflected backwards to uncover both frontal poles, which are then separated from one another to expose the tumour (Henderson 1938). This avoids a lobectomy, but access is much restricted and damage is inflicted on both frontal lobes by retraction and by division of their veins to the sagittal sinus; it is not as good a method.

The dangers of operation in this and the next group of cases relate to haemorrhage from deeply placed and important arteries, to infarction of vital areas of brain, particularly the hypothalamus, by interruption of small arterial twigs from the anterior arch of the circle of Willis, and to oedema and necrosis of the frontal lobes by operative trauma. Cushing's mortality was high, one-third of the patients dying and frequently after multiple-stage operations. He pays tribute to a report by Olivecrona of only 2 deaths in 18 cases.

*Suprasellar*

Suprasellar meningiomas arising from the tuberculum sellae are situated only a centimetre or so posterior to olfactory meningiomas, but this distance is sufficient to evoke a quite different clinical pattern. Early in their growth they come into contact with the optic chiasma and being at that stage relatively small and ventral to the chiasma, elevate it and like a pituitary tumour give rise to bitemporal hemianopia, though rarely symmetrical. It was this tumour which led Cushing to describe the syndrome of the chiasmal lesion without enlargement of the pituitary fossa (1922 and 1930); meningiomas in this situation were also described by Holmes and Sargent (1927). The absence of anosmia, papilloedema, headache and of any mental deterioration distinguishes them from olfactory groove and ridge meningiomas; lack of endocrine disturbance from pituitary tumours, craniopharyngioma, and glioma of the optic chiasma (the latter rare in adults). Radiographs of the skull may reveal no abnormality, or at the most erosion of the posterior clinoids from pressure at a distance, but no enlargement of the sella or of the optic foramina. The pathognomonic sign is sclerosis and thickening of the tuberculum sellae, though it is present only in a minority of patients. With small lesions close to the base of the skull the value of CT is probably less than in most other situations, particularly when older scanners are being used. Additional information may be obtained by coronal and sagittal reconstructions and by the introduction of contrast material into the cerebrospinal fluid pathways and outlining the chiasmal cistern. Angiography may reveal arch-like elevation of the anterior cerebral arteries, but a small tumour may cause no arterial displacement and provide no shadow of pathological circulation. Air encephalography has been largely abandoned but still has some advantages.

Operation is carried out as for a subfrontal approach to a pituitary adenoma but amongst other problems the tougher nature of the tumour makes removal more difficult, whereas intracapsular evacuation of a soft adenoma is easily performed. Its finely granular surface and prolonged slow growth renders its separation from the optic nerves and chiasma more tedious and the chiasm in particular is more easily damaged, because it has borne the brunt of the thrust by the tumour. There may be a constriction around the tumour, caused by the arch of the anterior cerebral arteries: behind this the deep portion may be tightly impacted and its removal difficult and hazardous, or the arterial arch may be torn before this relationship has been recognized.

Because these tumours primarily affect vision and do so at an early stage, they rarely reach the size of other anterior basal meningiomas and operation carries a somewhat lower mortality. But prognosis for recovery of vision is poor; in only a quarter of Cushing's patients were the fields restored to normal. An eye which is already blind or virtually so prior to operation will not recover useful vision. This means that operation is imperative to preserve and possibly to improve vision in the better eye. In large tumours there is an appreciable risk that operation will worsen vision as a result of damage to an already tenuous chiasma. Division of the nerve of a blind eye is justifiable if this renders the removal of the tumour easier and less likely to damage the rest of the optic apparatus. The possibility should be foreseen and discussed with the patient before the operation. In these, as in other meningiomas, the surgeon may have to be content with a partial removal with the reassurance that survival for 28 years has been recorded (Grant & Hedges 1956) so slow may be the growth of this tumour.

Before concluding this section on meningiomas which directly compress the optic apparatus, the importance of an accurate diagnosis of the cause of failing vision must be stressed. Inaccurate diagnosis, or no diagnosis and procrastination are still liable to be the fate of a patient complaining of gradual loss of sight in one eye, though when the second eye becomes affected, the diagnosis of a compressing chiasmal lesion becomes obvious. At this stage, however, vision in one eye has usually been irretrievably damaged and the tumour is of a size to render its

removal a matter of considerable risk. Most of these meningiomas affect one eye first; progress is so slow that it may be imperceptible without repeated examination and the essential field test may not be undertaken because optic atrophy may be absent or slight (Hobbs 1962). The duration of visual symptoms is usually many years and a 30 years' history has been described (Grant & Hedges 1956). If a convincing ocular cause cannot be found a tentative diagnosis of optic nerve compression should be made, and every endeavour made to prove it radiologically. During a 5 year period, 310 patients attended the Mayo clinic for mainly unilateral loss of vision. Of these 38 had a tumour (Uihlein & Weyand 1953, Uihlein 1958). If no other cause for progressive unilateral visual failure can be found, operative exploration should be recommended, even if radiological investigation is negative, for this is the only method whereby certainty can be assured. Radiological methods may not demonstrate very small tumours, some of which nestle under an optic nerve and may not be easily detected even at operation (Craig & Gogela 1950).

*Lateral ventricle*

Lateral ventricle meningiomas are relatively rare, 50 cases having been recorded by 1942 (Abbot & Courville) and this number increased only to 175 by 1965 (Delandsheer). They do not present a striking clinical picture; mild intermittent symptoms of raised intracranial pressure often for several years are followed by mild global disturbance of the function of one hemisphere, namely minimal sensorimotor impairment, visual hallucinations, hemianopia and dysphasia if the dominant hemisphere is the seat of the tumour. Such signs may also be caused by a glioma, but such an anatomically widespread disturbance is unusual in a glioma unless it is rapidly growing and thereby causing a dense deficit. It is this discrepancy, and extensive but mild disturbance which is characteristic of the lateral ventricle meningioma. Jefferson and Jack-

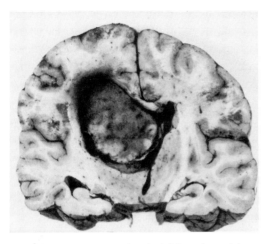

**Fig. 7.14.** Meningioma within the left lateral ventricle: female aged 28 years.

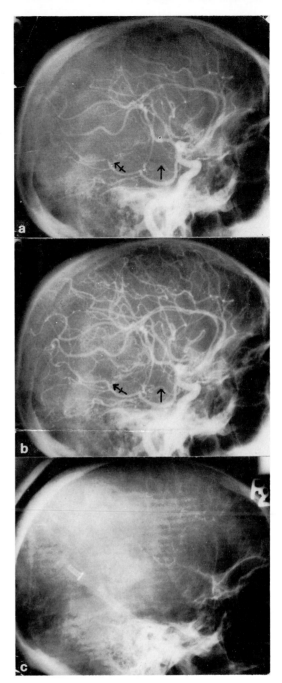

son (1939) draw attention to the long history in some patients, 10 years in their first. They are more frequent in females and in the left ventricle (Fig. 7.14). Other features which have received emphasis are variation in the symptoms during change of posture (Gassel & Davies 1961) and ataxia (Wall 1954).

Diagnosis is by radiological investigation which, according to Mani *et al.* (1978) in their review of 22 cases, should be CT followed by carotid and vertebral angiography. The unenhanced CT scan characteristically shows a high density lesion with discrete borders. Ventricular dilatation will be demonstrated and the CT scan may detect tumour calcification that can not be seen on plain skull radiographs. The majority of meningiomas enhance strongly after intravenous injection of contrast material. Carotid angiography may show typical abnormalities which comprise enlargement of an anterior choroidal artery, abnormal vessels and depression of the great cerebral veins of Galen (Fig. 7.15) (Huang & Araki 1954). Vertebral angiography may demonstrate large posterior choroidal vessels and a tumour circulation. Ventriculography and pneumo-encephalography are no longer recommended.

Various surgical approaches to lateral ventricle meningiomas have been proposed. Rarely,

**Fig. 7.15.** Intraventricular meningioma.
(a) Delay in filling of cortical arteries in temporoparietal region compared with frontal: a pathological circulation is developing, to be seen in the 'bare area' between the temporal area and the posterior cerebral artery, being fed by the anterior (1) and posterior (2) choroidal arteries. The posterior cerebral artery is of primitive pattern, arising as a direct branch of the internal carotid artery and in the first part of its course it is markedly displaced downwards, suggesting transtentorial herniation.
(b) The arterial phase of tumour circulation is now well developed and cortical arteries are better filled.
(c) Capillary phase of tumour circulation (the 'blush'). Anteroposterior angiograms showed the pathological circulation to be situated deep in the hemisphere.

the tumour may be in the frontal horn and the approach to this is the simplest and most direct, through an incision in the frontal lobe. More commonly the tumour is situated in the trigone or the temporal horn and can be reached by resection of the occipital lobe, or incisions through the middle temporal gyrus, the parietal lobe or through the splenium of the corpus callosum. If the tumour is in the non-dominant hemisphere and an inferior parietal incision is made a contralateral homonymous hemianopia may be the only permanent deficit. However, the majority of these tumours are in the left ventricle and too large an incision placed too near the supramarginal and angular gyri will also cause severe dysphasia, dyslexia and dysgraphia. An incision in the middle temporal convolution provides poorer access, but is less liable to damage speech. Fornari *et al.* (1981) advocate a sagittal paramedial cortical incision, 3–4 cm from the interhemispheric fissure, in order to minimize damage to the optic radiation. The transcallosal approach was described by Kempe and Blaylash (1976) but may lead to a disconnection syndrome (Levin & Rose 1979). The operative mortality in a large group of cases from various sources was 20% (Delandsheer 1965).

*Posterior fossa*

There are several classifications of posterior fossa meningiomas according to their sites of dural attachment and the following simplified version is derived from Logue (1979):

| | |
|---|---|
| Cerebellopontine angle | 43% |
| Cerebellar (including tentorial) | 36% |
| Clivus and basi-occiput | 8% |
| Foramen magnum | 6% |
| Others (for example, intra-ventricular, no dural attachment, or extensive attachment) | 7% |

Their evolution is slow, the average duration of symptoms in 71 patients of Olivecrona being 4 years (Castellano and Ruggiero 1953).

1. *Cerebellopontine angle tumours* arise from the posterior surface of the petrous bone and form the largest group. They simulate an acoustic nerve tumour by reason of the frequent involvement of the cranial nerves in this region. In 30 cases of the Swedish series, the acoustic nerve was involved in 24, the trigeminal in 19 and the facial in 16. Meningioma provides about 10% of all cerebellopontine angle tumours and is the next in frequency to the acoustic schwannoma. It is often impossible to differentiate between the two, but an unusual mode of evolution should raise a question. Marked involvement of the fifth and of cranial nerves below the eighth, with sparing of some function of the eighth, would be unusual in an acoustic tumour. Petit-Dutaillis and Daum (1949) found that bilateral trigeminal involvement is more common in meningioma. Plain radiography usually does not help to distinguish the two tumours, for both may cause erosion of the petrous bone, and hyperostosis only occasionally occurs in this region (Bager 1944). Meningiomas may arise within the internal auditory meatus or outside it, and may lie predominantly within the petrous bone or within the posterior fossa.

2. *Cerebellar convexity tumours.* In this group the tumour arises from the tentorium or from the dura mater lining the lateral and posterior surfaces of the posterior fossa. It includes those which are sometimes described as arising in the 'lateral recess', viz. posterior to the sigmoid sinus. This is an unfortunate use of a term which anatomists give to the pointed lateral prolongation of the fourth ventricle which terminates in the foramen of Luschka. The absence of cranial nerve involvement distinguishes this group from the others; the cerebellar signs are trivial. A long history of headache and relative slightness of the localizing signs should raise the suspicion of an extrinsic tumour; painful stiffness of the neck and trigeminal pain and impairment of the corneal reflex, a false localizing sign, are additional frequent pointers. Some tentorial tumours may extend upwards into the temporal or occipital lobes, so that there may be epilepsy, visual hallucinations and hemianopia to confuse the diag-

nosis. A few tumours cause compression of the colliculi, simulating a pineal tumour; these project forwards from the junction of the tentorium and the falx, the 'carrefour falcotentoriel' of French writers.

3. *Clivus and basi-occiput meningiomas* form a small group and are rare tumours. Clivus tumours were defined by Castellano and Ruggiero as arising from the dura of the superior part of the clivus. They grouped tumours arising from the lower half of the clivus (basi-occiput) with those arising from the foramen magnum because of the similarity in their clinical and surgical aspects.

The clivus tumours spread laterally and involve the intermediate cranial nerves at their exit from the skull, the median position of the tumour being apparent only when cranial nerves of both sides are affected. Johnson (1953) found that an abducens palsy was of particular significance, due to direct involvement, and not a false-localizing sign. Pontine compression gives rise to nystagmus, ataxia, pyramidal tract signs and to spinothalamic loss. Russell and Bucy (1953), who analysed a large series of recorded cases, and others have drawn attention to the risk of mistaking a clivus tumour for a pontine glioma. A long history (one third of their cases had symptoms for over 3 years) and intracranial hypertension would be unusual for a pontine glioma. Chordoma, aneurysm of the basilar artery, epidermoid, disseminated sclerosis and syringobulbia must also be included in the differential diagnosis.

4. *Foramen magnum meningiomas*, sometimes described as craniospinal (or spinocranial if the tumour started in the spinal canal) produce a clinical picture which is shared by other tumours occurring at this site and by malformations both congenital and acquired; they may simulate tumours at a distance and certain intrinsic diseases of the brain-stem and spinal cord. Love *et al.* (1954) analysed 74 cases of tumour at this level; amongst them were 26 meningiomas, 16 astrocytomas, 14 ependymomas, 4 medulloblastomas, 3 neurofibromas, 2 oligodendrogliomas, an intramedullary glioma and

an aneurysm of the vertebral artery. A subsequent paper was devoted to the meningiomas and neurofibromas (Dodge *et al.* 1956) of which equal numbers appeared to have developed above or below the foramen and about two-thirds lay anterior or anterolateral. Symonds and Meadows (1937) in a critical review describe in detail 4 cases of meningioma, and 1 of each of neurofibroma, of separation of the odontoid process and of aneurysm of the vertebral artery. A variety of malformations and deformations occur at this level which give rise to a somewhat similar clinical picture and are described elsewhere (Arnold–Chiari malformation, basilar impression, assimilation of the atlas and atlantoaxial subluxation). Pain in the back of the head and in the neck is a common initial symptom in cases of tumour; it is often aggravated by change in posture and by movement of the neck and for this reason the head is held stiffly. Pain may precede other developments by many months. Spastic weakness, numbness, pain and paraesthesiae in the ipsilateral upper limb develop next; movement of the head often aggravates the paraesthesiae and there may be a hyperpathic response to cutaneous stimuli. Weakness spreads to the ipsilateral leg, then the opposite leg and finally the opposite upper limb. Occasionally the contralateral upper limb is affected before the legs. At the stage of motor and sensory loss confined to the limbs on one side, a false diagnosis of a cerebral lesion is easily made. Depending upon the precise situation and extent of the tumour above the foramen magnum, examination can reveal involvement of the vagus, spinal accessory and hypoglossal nerves, dysphagia and respiratory obstruction occur, nystagmus in about half the cases (Dodge *et al.* 1956) and signs of interference with the cervical sympathetic supply (Horner syndrome) and disturbance of trigeminal sensation due to compression of the descending sensory root may be present. Wasting of the distal muscles of the upper limb and in particular of the intrinsic muscles of the hand may be so pronounced as to direct the search for a lesion lower in the cervical cord, or to lead to a diagnosis of syringomyelia.

The wasting is thought to be the result of pressure upon the anterior spinal artery, which provides the main blood supply to the cervical cord as far down as the reinforcing radicles which join it at about the seventh cervical segment. Sensory loss is dissociated; spinothalamic loss is present over at least part of the ipsilateral arm and over a 'jacket' area or over the whole of the opposite side; posterior column loss occurs in the arms, the legs are usually spared.

Radiological examination plays an important role in the localization of meningiomas in the posterior fossa. Plain skull radiographs may show specific abnormalities such as tumour calcification, erosion of the petrous tip or porus acousticus, hyperostosis, erosion of the clivus or destruction of the occipital bone. However, they are more often normal. In the 30 cases reported by Grand and Bakay (1975) they rarely revealed the presence and location of the tumour. CT has become the single most important investigation, being capable of showing the location and size of the tumour, distortion of the brain stem and cerebellum, and the presence of hydrocephalus. Yaşargil et al. (1980) commented that the value of CT scanning in the diagnosis of posterior fossa meningiomas cannot be overestimated and that its diagnostic accuracy approaches 100%. Angiography is valuable and may reveal vessel displacement and abnormal vascularity (Krayenbühl & Yaşargil 1965). Ventriculography and pneumoencephalography are no longer routinely used but myelography is still extremely valuable in delineating foramen magnum lesions. Most recently, magnetic resonance imaging is proving to be the most informative and definitive study of all.

The removal of a convexity cerebellar meningioma usually present no surgical problems unless it is attached to the tentorium or to a major sinus. Supratentorial extensions are best approached above the tentorium through a posterolateral osteoplastic craniotomy, but correct and precise regional diagnosis is essential. If a lateral sinus is invaded it can be resected, but the torcula Herophili should be preserved.

The three main intradural approaches to cerebellopontine angle meningiomas are the frontotemporal Sylvian, the subtemporal and the lateral suboccipital. The frontotemporal Sylvian approach developed by Yaşargil et al. (1980) involves splitting the Sylvian fissure, retracting the temporal lobe and dividing the tentorium. This approach allows resection of any middle fossa extension and earlier and easier identification of the basilar artery and the third, fourth and fifth cranial nerves. Disadvantages include working at a depth through a narrow space with late exposure of the seventh and eighth cranial nerves and difficulties in getting lower than these nerves. The subtemporal approach gives similar exposure of blood vessels and nerves to the frontotemporal but at less depth and with a wider space. However, this is offset by the problems of temporal lobe retraction with the possibility of postoperative swelling and hemiparesis, and dysphasia if on the dominant side. The subtemporal approach has been modified by Morrison and King (1973) using the translabrynthine–transtentorial route, and by Hakuba et al. (1977) with a transpetrosal–transtentorial approach. The lateral suboccipital route is favoured by many neurosurgeons using the sitting or lateral positions, according to preference. With this approach the arachnoid cisterns can be drained at an early stage and retraction damage to the cerebellum lessened. The lower cranial nerves can be identified earlier and preserved more easily, but this does not apply to the upper cranial nerves and basilar artery. There, a combined supratentorial and suboccipital approach in appropriate cases may give the best chance of total tumour excision.

Cerebellopontine angle meningiomas are difficult tumours to eradicate, most series reporting a high proportion of incomplete removals and a high mortality. Castellano and Ruggiero (1953) reported an operative mortality of over 40% and maximum survival of 20 years. The results have improved over the years and Sekhar and Jannetta (1984) reported 22 cases with no operative mortality and minimal morbidity, although 8 of these cases had incomplete removals. An impressive series of 30 cases with total tumour excision and no operative mortality was reported by Yaşargil et al. (1980).

Clivus meningiomas are among the most inaccessible of all intracranial tumours. They may be approached from one side, as described for angle tumours, choosing the side with greater cranial nerve involvement. In addition a variety of anterior approaches to the clivus have been developed and may be usefully adopted for extirpation of clivus meningiomas. Through an incision in the neck, Stevenson et al. (1966) mobilize the pharynx so as to expose the base of the skull; removal of the anterior rim of the foramen magnum and the occipital bone in front of this provides a window through which a midline tumour can be attacked. A transoral approach to the same area has been devised by Mullan et al. (1966). Rougerie et al. (1967) proposed a low rhinoseptal transphenoidal approach for clivus chordomas, this approach being a variant of that used for pituitary adenomas. Clivus meningiomas are formidable lesions and traditionally carry an extremely high operative mortality. However, Hakuba et al. (1977) reported a series of 6 cases with total tumour excision and with one operative death. The best results to date are those of Yaşargil et al. (1980) who reported 20 cases, 7 of which had total tumour removal with no operative mortality, and 13 who had subtotal excisions with an operative mortality of 13%.

Foramen magnum tumours are exposed through a midline incision which allows for a small suboccipital craniectomy including a generous opening of the foramen magnum and a hemilaminectomy of the upper two or three cervical vertebrae on the appropriate side. If the tumour is situated anterior or anterolateral to the spinal cord and medulla it may be completely hidden from view until division of the ligamenta denticulata and upper two or three posterior cervical roots allows sufficient gentle displacement of the cord to bring it into sight. Its relationship to the spinal accessory nerve and to the vertebral artery must be determined and the nerve may need to be divided. Partial exenteration of the tumour diminishes its size, so that its full extent

can be estimated; total fragmentary removal may then be possible. The liability to respiratory failure in these patients has been emphasized in the excellent paper by Dodge et al. (1956). This alarming complication is aggravated by flexion of the neck and by placing the patient in the seated position for the operation. Controlled respiration provides the advantages of low venous pressure and the prone position can be more safely used. Stein et al. (1963) describe the results of operation on 23 patients with meningioma of the foramen magnum; 5 died from recurrence and 12 were living for periods up to 18 years with little or no neurological disability. Yasargil et al. (1980) reviewed the literature; of 117 operated foramen magnum meningiomas collected, there were 7 operative and 8 postoperative deaths with 79 good, 9 fair and 11 poor results. The Mayo clinic experience of 102 benign tumours of the foramen magnum operated upon between 1924 and 1982 was reported by Meyer et al. (1984). There were 78 meningiomas, 23 neurofibromas and 1 teratoma, with an operative mortality of 5%, mainly due to large anteriorly placed tumours.

*Meningiomas of the optic nerve*

Meningiomas of the optic nerve are much less frequent than gliomas in the proportion of 1 to 6 (Mathewson 1930) and Schwannoma is even rarer (Vincent & Hartmann 1937). The tumour surrounds the nerve as a fusiform mass, at times of cartilaginous consistency, and by the time the patient presents for advice it often extends from the globe to the optic foramen. Cushing and Eisenhardt (1938) had only one case and a review of the literature at that time led them to doubt whether an isolated meningioma of the optic nerve within the orbit ever occurred. Cushing was impressed by the manner in which intracranial meningiomas in the vicinity of the optic foramen insinuate themselves through the foramen along the sheath of the optic nerve and by the frequency of recurrence of an 'orbital' tumour when excised via the orbit, flush with the optic foramen. But he quotes a case of neurofibromatosis in which post-mortem examination revealed an isolated meningioma of the optic nerve within the orbit which did not extend as far as the foramen (Shapland & Greenfield 1935). As Jefferson (1940) put it, there is 'no *a priori* reason why a tumour should not for a time be confined to the nerve in the orbit'. Hudson (1912) accurately described the morbid anatomy of these tumours and their histological appearance. The nerve is surrounded and compressed by the tumour but is not invaded by it; its sheath is distended and broken up by the tumour, which spreads into the orbital fat, engulfs the ciliary arteries and nerves and may follow them through the sclera into the globe. He notes the similarity between the microscopic appearance of the tumour cells and the arachnoidal endothelial cells, which led him to believe that the tumour originated from the arachnoidal sheath of the optic nerve. Occasionally meningiomas arise primarily within the orbit separate from the optic nerve. Craig and Gogela (1949) encountered 8 such cases; during the same period of time they also found 9 arising from the optic nerve sheath, and 35 which had spread into the orbit from neighbouring intracranial tumours. There are several points of distinction between meningiomas and gliomas of the optic nerve. Meningiomas occur evenly at all ages; vision usually fails late in the course of the disease, after the development of exophthalmos; movement of the eyeball is usually greatly restricted and there may be pain in the eye. Fundus changes are not dissimilar in the two tumours. Valuable investigations include high resolution CT, angiography and orbital ultrasonography. As with gliomas of the optic nerve, investigation should be aimed at detecting any evidence of intracranial extension of the meningioma and whether the orbital tumour is derived from a larger mass arising from the floor of the anterior fossa, for example olfactory groove, tuberculum sellae, anterior clinoid process.

The treatment of meningiomas of the optic nerve is excision. The standard approach is by transfrontal exploration which allows thorough examination of the apex of the orbit, the optic canal and the neighbouring intracranial area. In this way total excision is most likely to be achieved. Other approaches by lateral and medial orbitotomy have been employed, depending upon the precise location of the tumour. Maroon and Kennerdell (1984) reported their experience with over 300 orbital tumours including 30 optic nerve meningiomas and described the various surgical approaches. Occasionally the cause of slowly progressive failure of vision can not be detected despite detailed investigation; operative exploration of the region of the optic chiasma and nerves should then be undertaken. Optic nerve sheath meningiomas may occur in the mouth of the optic foramen, too small to identify radiologically, and indeed may even escape detection by the surgeon if a careful search is not made (Dandy 1922, Craig & Gogela 1950).

**Recurrence of meningioma**

Although meningiomas are ordinarily regarded as benign tumours and the great majority have a benign histological appearance, their sites of origin and their tendency to spread over the surface of the dura mater and through that membrane into dural sinuses and bone make total extirpation at times impossible and all too frequently uncertain. The consequent likelihood of recurrence places a premium upon surgical judgement in these cases, problems already considered in the appropriate sections. Recurrence is also encountered when tumours in anatomically favourable situations have been apparently totally removed. Occasionally the recurrence may assume a frankly sarcomatous appearance, or may at the most show increased mitoses and a papillary appearance. Zülch (1965) considers malignant dedifferentiation very rare; he suggests that meningiomas with sarcomatous change form a link with fibrosarcoma of the dura. If the tumour is rapidly growing but still encapsulated he classifies it as a malignant (sarcomatous) meningioma and if it is infiltrating, a fibrosarcoma.

An excellent review of recurrence was published by Simpson (1957) who studied a series of 339 patients with meningioma. He grouped them according to the extent of the operation. In group 1, the tumour was considered to be totally removed; this included its dural attachment (and sinus) and any involved bone. In this group there were 9% recurrences (a similar proportion is reported by Schäfer 1965) at time intervals of from 13 months to 13 years. In group 2, the tumour was totally removed and its dural attachment coagulated by endothermy; there were 19% recurrences, a maximum interval being 13 years. When the tumour was macroscopically totally removed but dural attachment or sinus or bone not treated, the recurrence rate was 29%. He found that any of the commonly accepted histological types of tumour might recur, although as it happened the angioblastic tumours in his series had not recurred. There were 5 tumours which showed many mitoses and an unorganized architecture, described as undifferentiated; only one patient survived, three having died of rapid recurrence and 1 after a partial removal. Of the 19 cases of recurrence after apparently total extirpation (groups 1 and 2), 2 were regarded as malignant because they gave rise to haematogenous metastases, though this may also occur with histologically benign tumours. In 4 the appearances were malignant. In the remaining 13 microscopic appearances were banal and scrutiny of the notes led Simpson to believe that in these recurrence was due to residual nests of tumour cells. These may be undetected (invisible) infiltration of dural septa, minute fragments adherent to brain, surface fringes and minute multiple foci. Recurrence from invaded bone rarely occurred. Crompton and Gautier-Smith (1970) reviewed the pathology of 181 parasagittal and falcine meningiomas and concluded that syncytial meningiomas are most likely to recur and that the presence of mitotic figures, focal necroses and cerebral infiltration are pointers to recurrence. It is now generally accepted that the thoroughness of surgical removal is the most important factor in determining tumour recurrence and in the

114 cases analysed by Adegbite et al. (1983) it was the only factor of statistical significance. The lesson to be learnt from these critical reviews is clear. The surgeon must be fully acquainted with the biological characteristics of the tumour and with the considerable power of survival and growth which even small nests of meningioma cells appear to possess. Total resection must include all areas of dural attachment with a generous margin. Separation from the brain must be carried out with meticulous care so that no minute fragment of tumour is detached from the main mass to form an implant in the cavity. The most careful judgement is necessary at times to decide whether such radical surgery carries an unjustifiable risk to life or too great a consequent neurological deficit. Palliative partial removal of meningiomas may be followed by many years of symptomatic relief. (See also Morello et al. 1963.)

The value of irradiation in the treatment of meningiomas is difficult to assess. There are no statistics comparable to those now available for gliomas. In Simpson's series it was given to 28 patients and he found 'little evidence of permanent benefit'. Jones (1960) describes the case of a large anterior basal angioblastic meningioma treated by irradiation. The patient died 10 years later of a glioma; autopsy revealed that the meningioma had greatly shrunken in size and its histological appearance changed to a psammomatous type. In practice, many neurosurgeons agree with the conclusions of Carella et al. (1982) that irradiation has an established role in the treatment of incompletely excised, recurrent, or malignant meningiomas.

## Haemangioblastoma

The terminology of tumours and malformations of blood vessels is liable to cause confusion. The name 'angioma' is often applied indiscriminately to any of these conditions; when used for the tumour now being considered the distinguishing qualification 'capillary' is added. Cushing and Bailey (1928) introduced the term 'haemangioblastoma' to emphasize its neoplastic origin from blood vessel tissues; the synonym 'angiorecticuloma' was invented by Roussy and Oberling (1930) because of the similarity between the tumour cells and reticuloendothelial cells. The occurrence of cysts in the cerebellum, often accompanied by a tumour, sometimes quite small and vascular in appearance, has been observed since the latter part of the last century. Possibly the first recorded case of cerebellar haemangioblastoma was that of Jackson (1872). A careful study of cystic tumours of the cerebellum was undertaken by Lindau (1926) based upon recorded cases and upon his own material of 16 cysts with an 'angioma' in the wall, 8 in conjunction with a glioma and 2 simple cysts the cause of which was not apparent. His notable contribution was to point out that in a proportion of cases a haemangioblastoma was also present in the retina (von Hippel disease, *see* Collins 1930), that the tumour might also occur elsewhere in the hind brain and in the spinal cord and that there might also be cysts in the pancreas and liver and a hypernephroma. Lindau (1930) stated that 25% of cases of von Hippel disease have cerebral complications and 20% are familial. There is great variation in the recorded incidence of retinal tumour in patients with cerebellar haemangioblastoma. There was only one example in the 70 cases reported by Olivecrona (1952) but roughly one-tenth of the patients of Krayenbühl and Yaşargil (1958) had retinal tumours. In both series only a few families were affected. In a family reported by Möller (1944) 10 members of 3 generations were affected; 5 had cerebellar, 3 had retinal and cerebellar and 1 had retinal haemangioblastomas. Other features of the tumour have considerable biological interest. Syringomyelia may accompany a spinal cord haemangioblastoma, and the cavitation may extend for nearly the whole length of the cord. The tumour rarely occurs in the cerebrum; Tomasello *et al.* (1980) reported a case and reviewed 39 other cases in the literature. The relationship between the haemangioblastoma and the angioblastic type of meningioma is a matter of controversy among neuropathologists, and is discussed at length by Russell and Rubinstein (1977). Carpenter *et al.* (1943) reported polycythaemia in 2 cases of cerebellar haemangioblastoma; since then other observers have recorded similar experiences, and have confirmed that the haemoglobin concentration and red cell count return to normal after removal of the tumour. Waldman *et al.* (1961) studied such a case in detail and by animal experiment showed that the cyst fluid contained an erythropoietic factor; it has also been found in plasma and in the tumour (Boivin *et al.* 1965). It is of interest to note that Roussy and Oberling identified erythroblasts in their specimens; although Cushing and Bailey anticipated that immature blood cells might be present in these tumours they were unable to detect them. Other tumours elsewhere in the body are now known to produce erythropoietin (Penington 1965).

It is generally accepted that the haemangioblastoma of the cerebellum is a tumour arising in the vascular mesenchyme as a result of some dysgenetic abnormality, that in a proportion of cases similar tumours occur elsewhere in the nervous system with a predilection for the retina and may be associated with cysts in abdominal viscera and that a hereditary factor sometimes determines its incidence. Van der Hoeve (1932) included Lindau disease amongst the phakomatoses (phakos being a mother spot) with Bourneville disease (tuberose sclerosis) and von Recklinghausen disease.

The haemangioblastoma of the cerebellum is exceptionally rare below the age of 10 years and is most common in middle age. This is of importance in diagnosis, for if the meningiomas and acoustic tumours be excluded, then in the later years of life when the incidence of glioma of the cerebellum diminishes, that of haemangioblastoma increases and surpasses it. There is a preponderance in males. The tumour usually occurs in a lateral lobe (in 80% of Olivecrona's cases) but may be midline and involve the floor of the fourth ventricle. The tumour is cystic in the majority of cases and the tumour may then be so small as to form only a small nodule in the wall of the cyst; it may then easily escape detection by the surgeon. The cyst fluid is yellow and Cumings (1950) states that its composition is such as to suggest that it is formed by diffusion from the blood and not as a result of the degeneration of tumour cells. The tumour appears as a discrete rounded mass, apparently well demarcated from the brain (though this is not necessarily the case microscopically) and varying in colour from pink or purple to yellow (depending upon the preponderance of haemangiomatous or of xanthomatous tissue). The nodule of tumour is usually close to or involving the cortex and may be lightly adherent to the overlying dura mater. Russell (1950) identified direct continuity of tumour with pia in two thirds of her specimens. An important characteristic of these tumours is an obvious excessive vascularity of the surface of the cerebellum overlying the tumour. There may be several enlarged cortical arteries and the draining veins are distended and may contain red blood. The appearance then mimics that of an angiomatous malformation and is not seen in other tumours of the cerebellum: it is of diagnostic importance to the surgeon. Tonsillar herniation is often severe and if a large cyst is present it may occupy the tonsil of that side and distend it downwards into the spinal canal. It is this which gives rise to the rapid deterioration and sudden respiratory failure which is liable to occur in these patients.

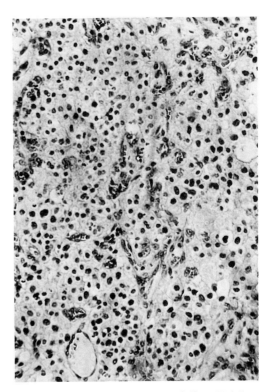

**Fig. 7.16.** Haemangioblastoma of cerebellum. H. & E. × 240

### Histology

The tumour consists of a mesh-work of blood spaces separated by a cellular stroma (Fig 7.16). The blood spaces are thin-walled channels of various sizes ranging from capillaries to large sinuses. All the blood spaces are lined by endothelium separated from the stromal cells by a basement membrane.

The stroma consists of islands and columns of plump, polygonal cells with uniform spheroidal nuclei. Their cytoplasm may be either pale and homogenous or may be distended by abundant droplets of sudanophilic lipid. Reticulin impregnation clearly outlines the basement membranes

of the vascular channels. In the stroma the reticulin network may be abundant, separating individual cells, or sparse, surrounding groups or clusters of cells.

Cysts, where present, lie outside the tumour and their walls are lined by fibrillary glia, frequently containing Rosenthal fibres.

### Diagnosis

There is great variation in the duration of symptoms, from a few weeks up to 2 years, though the majority of patients present for treatment within a year. It is well recognized that pregnancy may aggravate the symptoms of brain tumour; Robinson (1965) noted that half his female patients with this tumour had their first symptom during pregnancy and quotes one case with a remittent history of 28 years duration. In many cases the symptoms are those of a posterior fossa tumour with cerebellar signs more marked on one side because the tumour is usually situated in one lobe and the clinical picture thus provides no clue to the pathological diagnosis. Mondkar *et al.* (1967) draw attention to the sudden onset of headache, suggestive of subarachnoid haemorrhage. The process of elimination may be helpful, for the absence of signs of a cerebellopontine angle lesion and of other cranial nerve palsies will make an acoustic tumour and a meningioma unlikely and the older the patient the less likely is the tumour to be a glioma, though it may be a metastasis. A careful enquiry may bring to light evidence of a family history of brain tumour and the finding of a retinal tumour (often difficult to detect as they usually lie in the peripheral part of the retina), exudative retinitis, or polycythaemia makes the diagnosis certain. Patients with a cerebellar haemangioblastoma, particularly if the tumour is cystic, may rapidly deteriorate and in the older writings sudden death was frequently described. Tonic seizures occurred in 14 of the 70 patients of Olivecrona, bulbar symptoms in 2, and 4 died suddenly soon after admission. These events are due to tonsillar herniation, commonly severe because the cyst is liable to expand into the tonsil and herniate it through the foramen magnum. Compression of the underlying restiform body by the tonsil or by the tumour may give rise to interruption of posterior column tracts, causing impaired discriminative and postural sensibility and astereognosis. These signs may be falsely interpreted as due to a parietal lesion and were described by Cushing and Bailey (1928) in their cases 19 and 20. In the latter it led to a negative exploration of the parietal lobe; subsequent ventriculography corrected the diagnosis. Such false localizing signs may of course be caused by any tumour in this situation. Radiological investigations should include CT and vertebral angiography. A CT scan may show a markedly enhancing lesion and any associated cyst. Vertebral angiography is characteristic (Fig. 7.17) showing either a dense nodule or a tangle of vessels—in either case there may be an associated translucent area due to cyst formation. In

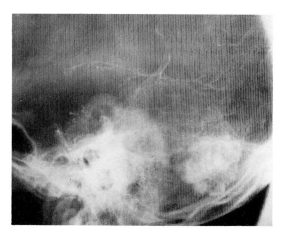

**Fig. 7.17.** Tumour circulation of a cerebellar haemangioblastoma.

the series reported by Jeffreys (1975) pre-operative angiography was carried out on 14 patients and the correct diagnosis made in every case. In addition CT and angiography allow the detection of multiple tumours.

### Treatment

The great majority of these tumours are satisfactorily treated by operation: abnormal vessels over the cerebellar cortex provide the clue to the situation of the tumour and those which appear to be arteries should be secured before the veins. When a cyst is present it should be widely opened so that its interior can be scrutinized and the tumour nodule removed; if the nodule is not found and excised the cyst will refill. It may be necessary to cut a small free bone flap, over the lateral sinus which is then displaced upwards, in order to remove large tumours involving the superior surface of the cerebellum. The rare tumours which involve the medulla are usually irremovable, though Bird and Mendelow (1960) describe a case of multiple tumours one of which involved the medulla, and removal of this tumour enabled the patient to make a good recovery. Very massive and highly vascular tumours may be irremovable and radiotherapy has proved beneficial in these cases.

## Prognosis

The mortality of the operation is still rather high. Cushing obtained a case mortality of 25%, many of the patients having more than one operation. Olivecrona's figure was 17% and Pennybacker's 8% (1954). Jeffreys (1975) reported 67 cases with an operative mortality of 15%, and more recently Ferrante et al. (1984) described 61 cases with an operative mortality of 8%. Many follow up statistics are of little value in ascertaining the incidence of recurrence, because these may be delayed for many years; in a case reported by Vinas and Horrax (1956) 22 years elapsed. The majority of patients have no further trouble, but recurrence of the tumour may take place at the site of the previous lesion or remote from it indicating that it is a fresh tumour. Recurrences occurred in 14% of McKissock's series (Mondkar et al. 1967) and one patient suffered 5. Pennybacker describes 6 patients with recurrences, an incidence of 12%, and emphasizes the difficulties of diagnosis. This may arise because deterioration is insidious and occurs at an age when cerebral atherosclerosis is developing and may be considered an adequate explanation, particularly as the decompression may not bulge. He strongly recommends angiography, which will indicate whether the tumour is too extensive or too vascular to warrant a further exploration. In one patient the recurrence invaded the dura mater and the muscle; a bruit was present. A helpful point in diagnosis is the polycythaemia which may occur with a recurrence as with the primary tumour; this occurred in one half the patients with recurrent tumour reported by Cramer and Kinsey (1952).

# References

ABBOTT K.H. & COURVILLE C.B. (1942) Bull. Los Ang. Neurol. Soc., 12, 7.

ADEGBITE A.B., KHAN M.I. PAINE K.W.E. et al. (1983) J. Neurosurg., 58, 51.

AMANO K., MIURA N., TAJIKA Y. et al. (1980). J. Neurosurg., 52, 829.

ANNEGERS J.F., LAWS E.R., KURLAND L.T. et al. (1979) Neurosurgery, Vol 4, No. 3, 203.

BAGER C.C. (1944) Acta Psychiat. Neurol. Scand., 19, 23.

BIRD A.W. & MENDELOW H. (1960) Brit. J. Surg., 47, 173.

BOIVIN P., BOUSSER J., BRION S. & GUIOT G. (1965) Presse Méd., 73, 2799.

BUSCH E. (1939) Acta Chirurg. Scand., 82, 282.

CAMPBELL E. & WHITFIELD R.D. (1948) J. Neurosurg., 5, 131.

CARELLA R.J., RANSOHOFF J., NEWALL J. (1982) Neurosurgery, Vol. 10, No. 3, 332.

CARPENTER G., SCHWARZ H. & WALKER A.E. (1943) Ann. intern. Med., 19, 470.

CASTELLANO F. & RUGGIERO G. (1953) Acta Radiol. Suppl., 104, 177.

CASTELLANO F., GUIDETTI B. & OLIVECRONA H. (1952) J. Neurosurg., 9, 188.

CHERRINGTON M. & SCHNECK S.A. (1966) Neurology, 16, 86.

COLLINS E.T. (1930) Proc. Roy. Soc. Med., 24, 372.

COURVILLE C.B. (1945) Pathology of the Central Nervous System, 2nd edn. Pacific Press Publishing Association, Mountain View, California.

COURVILLE C.B. (1947) Bull. Los Ang. Neurol. Soc., 12, 6.

CRAIG W. McK. & GOGELA L.J. (1949) Amer. J. Ophth., 32, 1663.

CRAIG W. McK. & GOGELA L.J. (1950) J. Neurosurg., 7, 44.

CRAMER F. & KINSEY W. (1952) Arch. Neurol. Psych., 67, 237.

CROMPTON M.R. & GAUTIER-SMITH P.C. (1970) J. Neurol. Neurosurg. Psychiat., 33, 80.

CUMINGS J.N. (1950) Brain, 73, 244.

CUSHING H. (1922) Brain, 45, 282.

CUSHING H. (1930) Arch. Ophth., 3, 505 and 704.

CUSHING H. & BAILEY P. (1928) Tumours Arising from the Blood Vessels of the Brain. Thomas, Springfield, Illinois.

CUSHING H. & EISENHARDT L. (1938) The Meningiomas. Thomas, Springfield, Illinois.

DANDY W.E. (1922) Amer J. Ophth., 5, 169.

DELANDSHEER J.M. (1965) Neurochirurgie, 2, 1.

DODGE H.W., LOVE J.A. & GOTTLIEB C.M. (1956) J. Neurosurg., 13, 603.

EL-BANHANWY A., SHELDON P.W.E. & PENNYBACKER J. (1963) J. Neurol. Neurosurg. Psychiat., 26, 462.

FERRANTE L., CELLI P., FRAIOLO B., et al. (1984) Acta Neurochir., 71, 283.

FORNARI M., SAVOIARDO M., MORELLO G., et al (1981) J. Neurosurg., 54, 64.

GASSEL M.M. & DAVIES H., (1961) Brain, 84, 605.

GAUTIER-SMITH P.C. (1970) Parasagittal and Falx Meningiomas. Butterworth, London.

GRAND W. & BAKAY L., (1975) Acta Neurochir., 32, 219.

GRANT F.C. (1947) Surg. Gynaec. Obstet., 85, 419.

GRANT F.C. & HEDGES T.R. (1956) Arch. Ophth., 56, 163.

GUILLAUME J., BILLET R., CARON J-P. & CUCCIA D. (1957) Les Méningiomes. Presse Universitaires de France, Paris.

HAKUBA A., NISHIMURA S., TANAKA K., et al (1977) Neurol. Med. Chir. (Tokyo),, 17, 63.

HENDERSON W.R. (1938) Brit. J. Surg., 26, 124.

HENSCHEN F. (1955) In Handbuch der Speziellen Pathologischen Anatomie und Histologie. 13/3, Nervensystem (Ed. Lubarsch O., Henke F. & Roessle R.) Springer, Berlin.

HOBBS H. (1962) Brit. med. J., 2, 255.

HOESSLY G.F. & OLIVECRONA H. (1955) J. Neurosurg., 12, 614.

HOLMES G & SARGENT P. (1927) Brain, 50, 518.

HUANG Y.S. & ARAKI C. (1954) J. Neurosurg., 11, 337.

HUDSON A.C. (1912) Roy. London Opth. Hosp. Reps., 18, 317.

IACONO R.P., APUZZO M.L.J., DAVIS R.L., et al (1981) J. Neurosurg, **55**, 282.

JACKSON H. (1872) Medical Times and Hosp. Gaz., **2**, 541 (quoted by Sargent P. 1930. Proc. roy. Soc. Med., **24**, 372).

JANE J.A. & McKISSOCK W. (1962) Brit. med. J., **2**, 5.

JEFFERSON G. (1940) Proc. roy. Soc. Med., **33**, 692.

JEFFERSON G.J. & JACKSON H. (1939) Proc. roy. Soc. Med., **32**, 1105.

JEFFREYS R. (1975) J. Neurol. Neurosurg. Psychiat., **38**, 105.

JOHNSON R.T. (1953) Proc. roy. Soc. Med., **46**, 737.

JONES A. (1960) Ann. Roy. Coll. Surg. Eng., **27**, 310.

KEMPE L.G. & BLAYLOCK R. (1976) Acta Neurochir., **35**, 233.

KENNEDY F. (1911) Amer. J. Med. Sci., **142**, 355.

KRAYENBÜHL H. & YAŞARGIL M.G. (1958) Schweiz. med. Wschr., **88**, 99.

KRAYENBÜHL H. & YAŞARGIL M.G. (1965) Die Zerebrale Angiographie, 2nd edn. Thieme, Stuttgart.

LEVIN H.S. & ROSE J.E., (1979) Neurosurgery, **4**, **2**, 168.

LINDAU A. (1926) Acta Path. Microbiol. Scand., **Suppl. I.**

LINDAU A. (1930) Proc. roy. Soc. Med., **24**, 363.

LOGUE V. (1975) In Krayenbühl H. (ed) Advances and Technical Standards in Neurosurgery, Vol. 2, pp. 171. Springer Verlag, Wien and New York.

LOGUE V. (1979). (In Rob C., Smith R., eds.) Operative surgery. Fundamental International Techniques, 3rd ed. Vol. II: Head and Neck. (S.P. Wilson, Editor) pp 128–173. Butterworths, London and Boston.

LOVE J.G., THELEN E.P. & DODGE, H.W. (1954) J. Int. Coll. Surgeons, **22**, 1.

LUND M. (1952) Acta Psych. Neurol. Scand., **Suppl. 81.**

MANI R.L., HEDGCOCK M.W., MASS S.I., et al. (1978) J. Neurosurg., **49**, 249.

MARKHAM J.W., FAGER C.A. HORRAX G. & POPPEN J.L. (1955) Arch. Neurol. Psychiat., **74**, 163.

MAROON J.C. & KENNERDELL J.S. (1984) J. Neurosurg., **60**, 1226.

MATHEWSON G.A. (1930) Amer. J. Ophth., **13**, 880.

MENDIRATTA S.S., ROSENBLUM J.A., STROBOS R.J. et al. (1967) Neurology, **17**, 914.

MEYER F.B., EBERSOLD M.J. & REESE D.F. (1984) J. Neurosurg., **61**, 136.

MÖLLER H.U. (1944) Acta Psych. Neurol. Scand., **19**, 275.

MONDKAR V.P., McKISSOCK W. & ROSS RUSSEL R.W. (1967) Brit. J. Surg., **54**, 45.

MORELLO G., MIGLIAVACCA F. & BERTAZOLLI A. (1963) Second European Congress of Neurological Surgery. Excerpta Medica International Congress Series No. 60, 74.

MORRISON A.W. & KING T.T. (1973) J. Neurosurg., **38**, 382.

MULLAN S., NAUNTON R., HEKMATPANAH J. & VAILATI G. (1966) J. Neurosurg., **24**, 536.

NAGER G.T. (1964) Meningiomas involving the Temporal Bone. Thomas, Springfield, Illinois.

OLIVECRONA H. (1934) Die Parasagittalen Meningiome. Thieme, Leipzig.

OLIVECRONA H. (1947) J. Neurosurg., **4**, 327.

OLIVECRONA H. (1952) J. Neurosurg., **9**, 317.

PATON L. (1909) Brain, **32**, 65.

PENINGTON D.G. (1965) Proc. roy. Soc. Med., **58**, 488.

PENNYBACKER J. (1954) Zbl.f.Neurochir., **12**, 63.

PETIT-DUTAILLIS D. & DAUM S. (1949) Rev. Neurol., **81**, 557.

PETIT-DUTAILLIS D. & PERTUISET B. (1955) Neurochirurgie, **1**, 29.

PHILIPPON J., FONCIN, J.F., GROB R., et al (1984) Neurosurgery, **14**, 3, 295.

ROBINSON R.G. (1965) Arch. Neurol. Scand., **41**, 372.

ROUGERIE J., GUIOT G., BOUCHE J., et al. (1967) Neuro-Chirurgie, **13**, 559–570.

ROUSSY G. & OBERLING C. (1930) Presse Med., **38**, 179.

ROWBOTHAM G.F. (1939) Brit. J. Surg., **26**, 593.

RUSSELL D.S. (1950) J. Clin. Path, **3**, 191.

RUSSELL D.S. & RUBINSTEIN L.J. (1977) Pathology of tumours of the nervous system. 4th edition. Arnold, London.

RUSSELL J.R. & BUCY P.C. (1953) Surg. Gynaec. Obstet., **96**, 183.

SCHÄFER E.R. (1965) Acta Neurochirurg., **13**, 186.

SEKHAR N. & JANNETTA P.J. (1984) J. Neurosurg., **60**, 500.

SHAPLAND C.D. & GREENFIELD J.G. (1935) Trans. Oph. Soc. U.K., **55**, 257.

SHEEHY J.P. & CROCKARD H.A. (1983) J. Neurosurg., **59**, 1.

SIMPSON D. (1957) J. Neurol Neurosurg. Psychiat., **20**, 22.

STEIN B.M., LEEDS N.E., TAVERAS J.M. & POOL J.L. (1963) J. Neurosurg., **20**, 740.

STEVENS J.M., RUIZ J.S. & KENDALL B.E. (1983) Neuroradiology, **25**, 125.

STEVENSON G.C., STONEY R.J., PERKINS R.U. & ADAMS J.E. (1966) J. Neurosurg., **24**, 544.

SYMON L. (1977) In (Krayenbühl H. ed.) Advances and Technical Standards in Neurosurgery, Vol 4, pp. 67–91. Springer Verlag, Wien and New York.

SYMONDS C.P. & MEADOWS S.P. (1937) Brain, **60**, 52.

TOMASELLO F., ALBANESE V., IANNOTTI F. et al. (1980) J. Neurosurg., **52**, 578.

TÖNNIS W. & SCHÜRMANN K. (1951) Zbl. Neurochir., **11**, 1.

UIHLEIN A. (1958) Brit. J. Ophth., **42**, 157.

UIHLEIN A. & WEYAND R.D. (1953) Arch. Ophth., **49**, 261.

VAN DER HOEVE J. (1932) Trans. Oph. Soc. U.K., **52**, 380.

VINAS F.J. & HORRAX G. (1956) J. Neurosurg., **13**, 641.

VINCENT C. & HARTMANN E. (1937) J. Belge. Neurol. Psychiat., **37**, 455.

WALDMAN T.A., LEVIN E.H. & BALDWIN M. (1961) Amer. J. Med., **31**, 318.

WALL A.E. (1954) J. Neurol. Neurosurg. Psychiat., **17**, 91.

WALSHE F.M.R. (1961) Lancet, **2**, 993.

WOOD M.W., WHITE R.J. & KERNOHAN J.W. (1957) J. Neuropathol. Exp. Neurol., **16**, 337–340.

YAŞARGIL M.G., MORTARA R.W. & CURCIC M. (1980) In Krayenbühl H. (ed.), Advances and Technical Standards in Neurosurgery, Vol. 7, pp. 3–115. Springer Verlag, Wien and New York.

ZÜLCH K.J. (1965) Brain Tumours: Their Biology and Pathology. Heinemann, London.

ZÜLCH K.J. (1979) Histological typing of tumours of the Central Nervous System. World Health Organization, Geneva.

# Chapter 8
# Schwannoma and neurofibroma

P. M. FOY

## Introduction

Benign encapsulated tumours arise on cranial, spinal and peripheral nerves and may be solitary or multiple; in the latter case they constitute the chief feature of von Recklinghausen disease. A great variety of names has been applied to these tumours: neurofibroma, neurinoma, perineural fibroblastoma, schwannoma, neurolemmoma, peripheral glioma. This diversity of nomenclature has depended upon the interpretations placed upon the histology of the tumours, the identity of their cells and upon opinions regarding their embryological origin, whether mesodermal or ectodermal. In addition to the microscopical appearance of the tumours, due regard must be paid to two other important features of von Recklinghausen disease. A variety of other lesions often accompanies neurofibromatosis, of which the following are the more common: meningioma, glioma, stenosis of the aqueduct, skeletal deformity, spinal bifida and skin pigmentation, the tell-tale café-au-lait patches. Secondly, the disease is inherited. A succinct account of the history, pathology and various manifestations of von Recklinghausen disease was given by Robb-Smith and Pennybacker (1952). Solitary tumours of nerves, as exemplified by that of the acoustic nerve, can however occur without the other manifold lesions of neurofibromatosis and without any familial tendency. Comparison of the appearances of the solitary tumours with those of neurofibromatosis reveals macroscopical as well as microscopical differences. The solitary tumour is circumscribed, rounded, its nerve of origin incorporated in its capsule and applied to one aspect of the tumour. In von Recklinghausen disease the affected portion of nerve is commonly diffusely swollen in spindle fashion, with irregular nodular enlargements; a considerable length of nerve and its branches may be enlarged to form a plexiform mass. The nerve fibres are incorporated in the tumour. It is now widely accepted that in both varieties the essential neoplastic cell is derived from the cells forming the sheath of Schwann (Russell & Rubinstein 1977). The solitary tumour may be regarded as a simple and localized neoplasm of these cells occurring at a point in the course of the nerve and possessing a special architecture. Neurofibromatosis arises as a result of an inherited fault affecting Schwann cells diffusely; according to Robb-Smith and Pennybacker it is an 'inherited dysgenesis of the neural crest characterized by an irregular elongation of certain neurites in a nerve trunk, with consequent proliferation of the nerve sheath elements'. Solitary tumours are now most commonly called 'schwannoma'. The term 'neurofibroma' introduced by von Recklinghausen is hallowed by use and serves a purpose in emphasizing its structural difference from the schwannoma and in identifying a widely ranging inherited disorder. But the link between the two varieties of nerve tumour is illustrated by the frequent presence in neurofibromatosis of tumours which are clearly schwannomas, and a schwannoma may be found within a neurofibroma.

Although many of the cranial nerves may be affected in neurofibromatosis, the acoustic nerve complex is the most common site for the schwannoma. The trigeminal nerve occasionally develops such a tumour, and the lower cranial nerves very rarely. Females are more frequently affected than males.

## Histology of nerve sheath tumours

Typical schwannomas form well encapsulated tumours lying in close apposition to the nerve from which they originated, without invading it (Fig. 8.1). They consist of Schwann cells which may be arranged in two entirely different patterns (Antoni 1920). Type A tissue consists of strands, shoals and whorls of closely packed spindle cells with elongated, darkly staining nuclei which show a tendency to grouping and even to striking palisading, usually more conspicuous in spinal and peripheral tumours than in the common acoustic schwannomas. Type B tissue consists of loosely arranged stellate cells, the processes of which form a fine meshwork. The two types of tissue are usually intermingled, although clearly demarcated from each other, one or the other pattern predominating. The stroma of the tumour consists of fine reticulin fibres, collagen being scanty. In some long-standing tumours however, strands of collagen fibres,

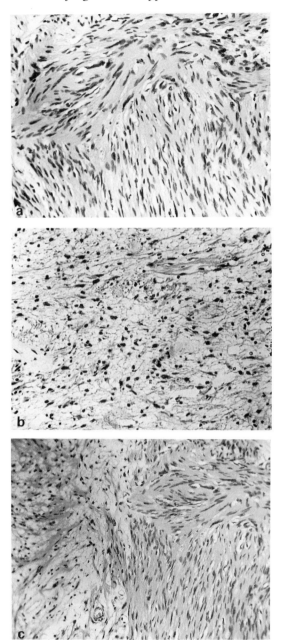

**Fig. 8.1.** (a) Antoni type A tissue. H. & E. × 180
(b) Antoni type B tissue. H. & E. × 180.
(c) Juxtaposition of type A and type B tissue. H. & E. × 130.

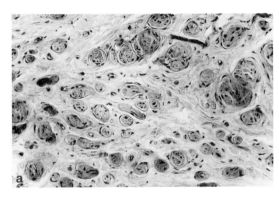

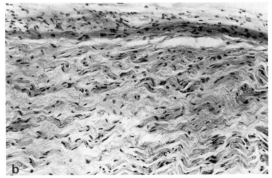

**Fig. 8.2.** Neurofibroma.
(a) Proliferation of Schwann cells in 'onion-skin' pattern around widely separated nerve fibres. H. & E. × 180
(b) Widely separated nerve fibres, wavy collagen fibres in a sparsely cellular matrix. The 'capsule' is formed by the perineurium. H. & E. × 180.

sometimes hyalinized, may be abundant. Other degenerative changes include intracellular deposition of lipid leading to formation of xanthomatous areas and frequent aggregations of iron pigment, a residue of old haemorrhages.

By contrast, neurofibromas are diffuse tumours expanding the nerve trunk and separating its fascicles as well as individual fibres (Fig. 8.2). They are sparsely cellular and consist of thin long spindle cells arranged along bundles of stout, wavy, collagen fibres, separated by a loose matrix, often mucoid in character. Apparently intact nerve fibres can be seen running through the tumour. This basic pattern is subject to numerous variants, commonly seen in the lesions of von Recklinghausen disease.

*Malignant forms.* Both malignant schwannomas and neurofibromas can develop either as solitary tumours or in the context of von Recklinghausen disease. They occur mainly on peripheral nerves, the common cranial nerve or spinal root tumours remaining almost invariably benign. The malignant forms are characterized by increased cellularity, atypical cell forms, presence of mitoses and invasiveness. The better differentiated tumours regain some of the characteristic features of schwannomas and neurofibromas respectively. The anaplastic forms are highly pleomorphic spindle cell sarcomas, the neural origin of which can only be surmised on circumstantial evidence.

## Acoustic schwannoma

The incidence of acoustic schwannoma among intracranial tumours is about 8%. The tumour forms a smooth rounded sometimes slightly lobulated fleshy mass, commonly 3–4 cm in diameter; occasionally it may be no longer than a pea and Cushing (1917) recorded one of 7 cm; the patient survived a decompressing operation for over three years and as Cushing pointed out this great size was doubtless permitted by the decompression. The tumour possesses a capsule of variable toughness, a point of practical importance to the surgeon who may wish to use it for traction. Arachnoid bridges the gap between tumour and neighbouring brain; it is often thickened and may be distended with yellow fluid to form a cyst capping the tumour. Cushing thought that such a loculus might be fed by the tuft of choroid plexus which protrudes through the foramen of Luschka and that intermittent drainage of the loculus might explain fluctuation of symptoms. The tumour is firmly attached to the petrous bone by the fusion of its capsule with the dura mater around the margin of the internal porus acousticus, which it fills and it usually extends into the internal ear. Small tumours occupy the porus without expanding it and without acquiring firm adhesions to the dura mater, but large tumours expand the porus so that its mouth may measure a centimetre or more across. This gives rise to the radiological appearance of a large 'trumpeting' of the meatus. The medial aspect of a large tumour indents and displaces the pons medially and dorsally, the middle cerebellar peduncle being particularly affected (Fig. 8.3); the displacement also affects the crura and medulla but to a lesser degree and rarely is either structure indented. The overlying lateral cerebellar lobe is also impressed by the tumour, tonsillar herniation develops and the lower part of the aqueduct and the fourth ventricle can be compressed and displaced. If the tumour is very large, its upper pole may be above the edge of the tentorium and its lower pole may nearly reach the margin of the foramen magnum. Although these tumours conform generally to the description given, they vary somewhat in their relation to the pons. Some extend more in a ventral direction so that part comes to lie anterior to the pons, which is displaced dorsally as well as medially; others lie entirely lateral to the pons, which is thrust medially and little or not at all dorsally. Variation in the direction of thrust probably accounts in part for differences in the clinical picture. The firm nature of the tumour, its slow growth and its anchorage to the petrous bone and dura gives rise to much deformity of the neighbouring cranial nerves (Fig. 194 of Cushing 1917 shows this admirably). The superior or inferior vestibular components of the eighth nerve disappear into the capsule at the porus and only occasionally at post-mortem examination can its proximal end be identified. The auditory component can usually be separated from the capsule. The facial nerve maintains continuity, though much flattened and thinned and adherent to, or incorporated in, the capsule. It pursues a course around the tumour on its ventral and anterior surface, that is to say during operation it lies on the deepest aspect of the tumour. The much flattened trigeminal nerve is carried upwards and forwards by the upper pole of the tumour so that as it leaves Meckel's cave it is often found to be kinked forwards towards the clivus and then it sweeps medially and backwards around the tumour to reach the pons. The extensibility of these two nerves compatible with near normal function is remarkable. Henschen (1955) states that each measures about 2 cm in length, in the case of the facial nerve about 1 cm lying within the porus and in large tumours the trigeminal nerve may be lengthened to 5 cm. Although at operation the fourth nerve is often seen after the upper pole of the tumour has been removed, it appears to escape direct pressure. The sixth nerve lies central and usually medial to the main mass of the tumour and after the tumour has been removed is seen in the floor of the cavity applied to the petrous bone as it passes forwards to penetrate the dura. Cushing stated that it never came into direct contact with the tumour, an opinion derived from the study of hardened specimens. But it is seen so regularly after total removal of large tumours that observation on post-mortem specimens must be misleading, particularly as the distal end of nerves becomes displaced. The abducens palsy which Cushing considered common may be due to compression of the distal part of the nerve against the petrous bone or traction as the pons is displaced. The glossopharyngeal, vagus and accessory nerves are rarely displaced, though commonly the lower pole of the tumour rests against them as they converge on their point of exit. Occasionally the medullary roots of the glossopharyngeal and vagus take a slightly

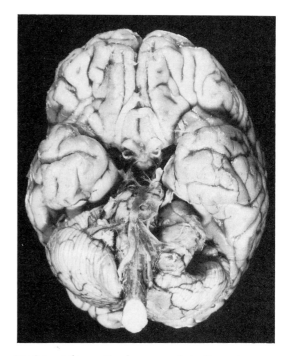

**Fig. 8.3.** Left acoustic schwannoma indenting and displacing the brain stem. There is a lateral cystic collection between the tumour and cerebellum. The trigeminal nerve is seen stretched over the upper part of the tumour. Male aged 58 years with an 18 month history of ataxia, incoordination and dementia. Died after an ethiodan ventriculogram.

downward course as they pass laterally below a large tumour.

The texture of an acoustic schwannoma varies considerably. Some are tough, relatively avascular, fibrous and withstand the grip of forceps. Others are soft, friable, vascular and more difficult to handle; the larger vessels run on and just under the capsule, though a few large ones are found in the depths. Fatty and cystic degeneration often occur, gratifying to the surgeon who can then easily evacuate the interior of the tumour by suction, thus quickly diminishing its bulk.

The blood supply to the tumour consists of small twigs derived from the pontine branches of the basilar artery, from cortical vessels of the cerebellum and larger branches from the anterior and posterior inferior cerebellar arteries. The anatomy of the two inferior cerebellar arteries is

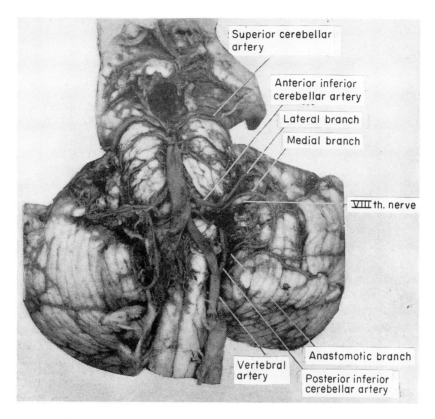

**Fig. 8.4.** Showing anatomy of the anterior and posterior inferior cerebellar arteries, and the relationship of the anterior to the eighth nerve (from Atkinson 1949).

of great importance in the surgery of the cerebellopontine angle and particularly in the removal of an acoustic tumour. The posterior usually lies near the lower pole of the tumour, often overlapped by it, and any nutrient branch enters the tip of the pole or its deep (ventral) surface. The anterior inferior cerebellar artery normally crosses ventral to the eighth nerve as it passes from the basilar artery to reach the cerebellum (Fig. 8.4). Consequently it will lie on the deep (ventromedial) surface of the tumour and between it and the pons. Atkinson (1949) has shown that an anastomosis links this vessel with the posterior inferior cerebellar artery, thus providing a collateral flow if either the anterior or the posterior artery is unusually small or if its circulation is impeded. This may be of vital importance because the anterior inferior cerebellar artery supplies a large portion of the teg-

mentum pontis, infarction of which is usually fatal. According to Atkinson, Greenfield had noticed that post-mortem examination on patients who had died after the removal of an acoustic tumour frequently revealed occlusion (surgical or thrombotic) of the anterior inferior cerebellar artery and infarction of that side of the pons (Fig. 8.5). This problem was studied by Atkinson who demonstrated the paramount need to preserve the integrity of this artery.

As long ago as 1910 Henschen (1955) drew attention to the fact that acoustic tumours appear to originate in the distal part of the nerve, within the porus, and probably from the vestibular portion; he was the first to report that enlargement of the porus could be demonstrated radiologically. Henschen's views have been upheld by the observations of other workers; histological examination of macroscopically

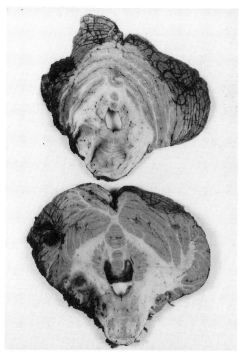

**Fig. 8.5.** Haemorrhagic infarction of lateral aspect of pons, middle cerebellar peduncle and cerebellar cortex following removal of right acoustic schwannoma: post-mortem examination revealed 'clip' on right anterior inferior cerebellar artery. During the operation, after the tumour had been removed there was troublesome bleeding from a small vessel at the junction of the pons and middle peduncle: a 'clip' successfully controlled bleeding after failure for half an hour using other methods. Death occurred 3 days after operation, shortly after vomiting. No food was found in the lungs, but this may have been aspirated at bronchoscopy.

oping eighth nerve growing towards the pons carries with it for a short distance only its sheathing of Schwann cells; proximally, their place is taken by a glial sheath which grows out from the pons. Why the vestibular division should be more prone is unexplained. Bilateral tumours (without other evidence of von Recklinghausen disease) are rare. Cushing (1932) encountered none in a series of 176 patients with acoustic tumours and Olivecrona only six in a total of 310 patients. They are of course common in patients with neurofibromatosis.

*Diagnosis*

Cushing states that the term cerebellopontine angle was introduced by Henneberg & Koch (1902) when describing a case of bilateral acoustic tumours. Although clumsy, the expression has remained in use for it draws attention to a neurological syndrome which, with variations in evolution and in detail, can be produced by many different tumours. The adjacent ventral surfaces of the pons and the cerebellum form with the posterior surface of the petrous bone a somewhat wedge shaped space, which constitutes the lateral extension of the pontine subarachnoid cistern and into which cerebrospinal fluid leaks from the foramen of Luschka. It is traversed by the fifth, sixth, seventh and eighth nerves. Tumours in this situation may involve these cranial nerves, the long tracts and nuclei in the lateral part of the pons and the cerebellum, by pressure and by infiltration. The variants of the syndrome depend upon the precise site of origin of the tumour, so that the chronological sequence of events is of particular importance in distinguishing the intrinsic from the extrinsic tumour.

The frequency and variety of other tumours which may be found in the cerebellopontine angle is indicated by the following list derived from Rembold and Tönnis (1956):

acoustic schwannoma   234 (unilateral)
meningioma                        28

normal petrous bones has revealed minute schwannomas deep in the internal porus and in the majority of cases arising from the vestibular division (Fowler 1936a, Hardy & Crowe 1936). In some cases auditory and vestibular functions were known to be normal. Similar tiny tumours have been found in the 'normal' ear of patients with an obvious acoustic tumour in the other ear (Scott 1938). That the tumour arises from the vestibular nerve is supported by the clinical observation, underlined by Cushing, that vestibular function fails before, or more severely than, auditory function (Dix & Hallpike 1958). Henschen attributed this peripheral origin of the tumour to an embryological factor; the devel-

'arachnoiditis' of
   angle          28
epidermoid      15
glioma          9
haemangioblastoma  3
metastasis      3
sarcoma        1
vascular
   malformation   1
hypoglossal nerve
   tumour       1
unclassified tumour  1

In his monograph on *Tumours of the Nervus Acusticus*, Cushing (1917) suggested that the first recorded description of a post-mortem examination was that of Sandifort in 1777. Cruveilhier gave a full clinical account of a case and the post-mortem findings; this is documented with much detail, and the illustrations of the brain and of the accompanying changes in the skull are so beautiful, that Cushing fortunately reproduced them in full. He pointed out that accuracy in diagnosis had to wait for the discoveries of the functions of the cerebellum, which were made towards the end of the last century, but by 1904 Stewart and Holmes were able to discuss the differential diagnosis of intra- and extracerebellar tumours, a contribution full of valuable clinical observation. Cushing set out the characteristic features of the tumour emphasizing the pattern of evolution and it is as valuable a survey today as it was almost 70 years ago.

The earliest symptoms are due to disorder of the eighth nerve: deafness, tinnitus and vertigo. Patients unfortunately frequently ignore deafness and indeed are often unaware of its gradual onset when unilateral until a chance event reveals it. The patient may notice difficulty in recognition of speech before hearing loss and this is particularly evident when using the telephone. Tinnitus is rarely severe enough to be troublesome. Vertigo is less tolerated, though the violent episodes which are encountered in Ménière disease, are not common in acoustic schwannoma. Hallpike (1959) gives a useful summary of the differential diagnosis between Ménière disease, cerebellopontine angle tumour, vestibular neuronitis and 'positional nystagmus of benign paroxysmal type', all of which give rise to the triad of deafness, tinnitus, and vertigo. Trigeminal symptoms may be next to arise or they may not appear until later. They take the form of numbness or paraesthesiae in the face, or occasionally of paroxysms of pain so severe that a preliminary diagnosis of trigeminal neuralgia may be made. Weakness of the facial muscles is not appreciated by the patient and is usually a late sign. Recurrent tic-like spasms of the facial muscles may occur, however, and were described in Cruveilhier's case. They may be incorrectly diagnosed as focal epilepsy. Eighth nerve symptoms may persist for years before the development of disturbed coordination of movement due to pressure on the cerebellum and pons. Ataxia of gait and of arm are complaints which drive the patient to a doctor; they are usually ipsilateral and contralateral signs of pyramidal tract involvement also occur, due to indentation of the pons. Symptoms of raised intracranial pressure arise at about the same time, sometimes following the development of ataxia. Headache is often occipital and unilateral, around and behind the affected ear, aggravated by straining and similar to that caused by a meningioma at the foramen magnum. The raised intracranial pressure is caused by obstruction to the flow of cerebrospinal fluid due either to the compression of the fourth ventricle or to the blockage of the tentorial opening. Hydrocephalus develops and may give rise to impairment of mental faculties. In the final stages slurring of speech and dysphagia make their appearance. Although they have been ascribed to pressure upon the lower cranial nerves, it is more probably that they are due to compression of the medulla, or to interference with its blood supply from pressure on the anterior and posterior inferior cerebellar arteries. With attacks of decerebrate rigidity, they are encountered in the terminal stages of any posterior fossa tumour.

The physical signs provoked by an acoustic schwannoma depend upon its size, although what may be regarded as typical signs may be absent even in a large tumour. Lundborg (1952) made a detailed study of 300 cases from Olivecrona's clinic. He grouped the tumours according to size; 250 were larger than a walnut. Leaving for later consideration tests of eighth nerve function, the relationship of certain abnormal signs to the size of tumour was as follows:

|                        | Small tumours (per cent) | Large tumours (per cent) |
|------------------------|:------------------------:|:------------------------:|
| Nystagmus present      | 12                       | 97                       |
| Corneal reflex absent  | 62                       | 92                       |
| Facial weakness        | 25                       | 63                       |
| Cerebellar signs       | 0                        | 86                       |

It follows that clinical diagnosis may be relatively easy late in the disease, when there is a full chronological pattern and abundant abnormal signs, but will be correspondingly more difficult at an early stage when the 'typical' cerebellopontine angle syndrome has not evolved. The problems of early diagnosis are considered later.

*Tests of auditory function*

Deafness of varying degree was present in 98% of the cases reviewed by Lundborg in 1952 while Edwards and Patterson (1951) found deafness to be total in 63% and partial in 36% of their series. Conversely, normal or nearly normal hearing does not exclude the diagnosis of acoustic schwannoma.

Developments in the field of audiology have led to many improvements of the clinical tests of hearing. The purpose of audiological testing is to assess the degree of hearing loss and to give an anatomical location to the pathological process. Pure tone audiometry, both by air and bone conduction, will quantify the hearing loss and give a gross differentiation between conductive and sensorineural deafness. The deafness of a subject with an eighth nerve tumour is sensorineural in type and special auditory tests have

been devised in an attempt to differentiate between lesions in the cochlea, within the inner ear, and lesions behind the cochlea involving the auditory nerve itself. Loss of speech discrimination is an early sign of an acoustic tumour and speech audiometry classically reveals very poor discrimination scores (Ballantyne *et al.* 1978). Fowler (1936b) described the phenomenon of loudness recruitment which is characteristic of cochlear disorders. In unilateral deafness the phenomenon is best revealed by means of the Alternate Binaural Loudness Balancing procedure used by Fowler. At or near to threshold values the intensity levels which yield equal sensations of loudness at the two ears will be separated by the amount of the deafness. At high intensities however, this separation will be abolished and sounds of equal intensity will give sensations of equal loudness. This is the loudness recruitment phenomenon. It occurs in nearly 100% of cases of perceptive deafness due to Ménière or other diseases which affect the hair cells or Corti's organ, i.e. end-organ deafness. As shown however by Dix *et al.* (1948) it is generally absent in cases of perceptive deafness due to affections of the cochlear nerve fibres, i.e. nerve fibre deafness, and this holds for 90% of cases of acoustic nerve tumour. The occurrence of loudness recruitment, partial or complete, in a small proportion of cases has been attributed by Dix and Hood (1953) to interference by tumour pressure with the blood supply of the cochlear end organs.

The short increment sensitivity index test is another test of loudness recruitment and is designed to measure the ability to detect a very small increase in sound intensity in the impaired ear. In cochlear lesions the vast majority of the increases are heard, whereas in retrocochlear lesions less than 30% of the increases are detected.

Bekesy audiometry, introduced in 1947, has been superseded by the tone decay test. This test measures the ability to maintain perception of a tone presented at an intensity slightly above the hearing threshold. Subjects with normal hearing or with a conductive hearing loss can hear this tone for a prolonged period. In the presence of a cochlear lesion there is a slow and relatively small decay in audibility of the tone, whereas in retrocochlear lesions there is a rapid and much more pronounced decay.

In the past 15 years or so more objective tests of auditory function have evolved, including the acoustic reflex test, the measurement of auditory brain stem evoked responses and electrocochleography. These tests are particularly sensitive to changes in the retrocochlear system and offer the prospect of early diagnosis of acoustic schwannoma. The acoustic reflex test is based upon reflex contraction of the stapedius muscle induced by intense sound and measuring the subsequent change in acoustic impedance. The acoustic reflex threshold is determined by increasing the intensity of the sound stimulus until a change in impedance is observed. The acoustic reflex may be absent in either conductive or sensorineural deafness. The point of diagnostic importance is that in retrocochlear lesions when the acoustic reflex is present there is characteristic rapid reflex decay.

Auditory brain stem evoked responses are electrical potentials of minute amplitude that occur in response to a sound stimulus. They can be recorded from scalp electrodes by extracting background electroencephalographic activity by using computer averaging techniques. Retrocochlear lesions cause delay, distortion, separation and absence of characteristic wave forms. The measurement of brain stem evoked responses is the best technique for detecting retrocochlear lesions and its specificity may be increased by the use of electrocochleography in combination (Eggermont *et al.* 1980). Electrocochleography by itself appears to be of limited value.

No single auditory test is sufficiently specific or sensitive in isolation and the accuracy of anatomical location of an auditory lesion is considerably enhanced by employing a battery of tests. It must also be borne in mind that all audiological tests are unreliable in the presence of marked hearing loss. Many patients with acoustic tumours show a mixed pattern of cochlear and retrocochlear hearing loss and in a small number of cases the picture is that of a cochlear lesion alone. Johnson (1977) analysed audiometric patterns in a large number of patients with acoustic tumours and in only about 50% of cases were the results consistent with a retrocochlear lesion.

### Tests of vestibular function

The investigation of vestibular function is also of great importance. As already indicated, tumours of the eighth nerve have their origin in and their major impact upon the vestibular branch of the nerve. Nevertheless it is important to note that at any rate in the early stages of tumour development the clinical manifestations of vestibular damage tend to be very insidious. This arises from the fact that the destructive process is a slow one and that with it keep pace the central processes of vestibular compensation. Thus it is by no means rare to encounter patients in whom the vestibular damage has advanced to the point of complete abolition of the caloric responses with very little vertigo or indeed any symptomatic evidence of vestibular disease.

It follows that in the early or so called otological stage in which the tumour is for the most part confined to the internal auditory canal, its diagnosis qua vestibular function is chiefly dependent upon the results of objective tests. Of these the most valuable is the Caloric Test of Barany modified according to the method described by Fitzgerald and Hallpike (1942). The test is carried out with the patient supine upon a couch. The head is raised 30° above the horizontal thus bringing the horizontal canals into the vertical plane their position of maximum sensitivity to thermal stimuli. These are provided by successive irrigation of the meatuses with water; first, at 30°C, then at 44°C. The temperatures, equidistant from body temperature, are calculated to bring about equal and opposite cupular deflections.

The nystagmic reactions are observed with the eyes open and visual fixation maintained and their durations measured. The caloric response is always absent in large tumours but with very small tumours it may be present (Dawes & Hankinson 1984). In the later or neurological stage of its development the tumour expands beyond the internal auditory canal and meatus and presses upon the brain stem. Of this the most familiar and important result is nystagmus. This is attributable to derangement of the vestibular nuclei and other brain stem mechanisms which have to do with the control of conjugate deviations of the eyes. As described by Dix and Hallpike (1966) the nystagmus has a number of special characteristics of high diagnostic significance. For its study and evaluation the eye movements require to be accurately recorded using modern electronystagmographic equipment as developed and described by Hallpike *et al.* (1960a and b).

In the majority of cases, the diagnosis of an acoustic schwannoma can be established by clinical methods, but difficulty arises in about one-third of the cases (Revilla 1947, Lundborg 1952, Edwards & Patterson 1951), owing to an unusual pattern. Shephard and Wadia (1956) made a special study of atypical cases. They stressed the importance of seeking deafness in patients in whom the diagnosis of an intracranial tumour was obscure. Symptoms of acute hydrocephalus dominated the picture in one group of cases and mental symptoms ascribed to chronic hydrocephalus in another. Long tract signs and episodes of disturbed consciousness due to compression of the pons were prominent and unusual features in a third group.

The diagnosis of an acoustic nerve tumour when it is still small and has not protruded from the internal porus sufficiently to compress the trigeminal nerve or the cerebellum and pons, is a matter of great difficulty. In otological practice, an acoustic tumour is only occasionally the cause of deafness; McKenzie (1965) found only two in a series of 300 patients whose deafness led to detailed examination. Nevertheless, in view of the technical problems of removing the average-sized tumour and of the relatively high morbidity this carries even in expert hands, early diagnosis

should be sought so that modern techniques can be applied and a lowering of mortality and morbidity achieved. Elliott and McKissock (1954) described four such cases in which the decision to operate was based largely upon the abnormal results of eighth nerve function tests. In each case a small tumour was successfully removed. They made the interesting observations that even with tumours too small to impinge upon the trigeminal nerve or upon the cerebellum and pons, there may be depression of the corneal reflexes and unsteadiness of gait. The former they ascribed to interference with the facial nerve and the latter to disturbance of the vestibular nerve.

*Cerebrospinal fluid*

In the great majority of cases of acoustic schwannoma there is considerable elevation of the amount of protein in the lumbar spinal fluid. Edwards and Patterson (1951) found the protein content normal in only 3% of the cases in which the fluid was examined. A common figure is 2–4 G/L and it may reach over 10 G/L. The examination is valuable in the differential diagnosis from meningioma, where the figure is seldom as high, and epidermoid cyst, glioma and disseminated sclerosis in which the figure is usually normal. The conjunction of impaired eighth nerve function with an elevation of the cerebrospinal fluid protein strongly supports a diagnosis of tumour. However, with the availability of screening tests to detect small tumours, routine estimation of cerebrospinal fluid protein is no longer employed in diagnosis.

*Radiological investigations*

Enlargement of the internal auditory meatus is virtually pathognomonic of an acoustic schwannoma and demands a high standard of technique and definition for its radiological demonstration. In Towne's projection the plane of the posterior surface of the petrous bone should be seen in profile and the mouth of each meatus with least distortion. If the routine angle of tilt does not provide clear definition, further films should be exposed with varying degrees of tilt. Tomograms in the coronal plane also reveal erosion of the petrous. In Stenver's projection, the central ray passes through the petrous bone of one side, perpendicular to its posterior surface. Each petrous bone is X-rayed separately and compared. The meatus is seen as a C-shaped area of translucency, the closed end of the limbs corresponding to the sharply defined lateral lip of the meatus. In the routine P–A skull projection, the apex of the petrous bone may be somewhat translucent when a large acoustic schwannoma is present. The destruction of the apex produced by a tumour of the trigeminal nerve or by an extradural epidermoid is more severe, its margin is clearly defined and lies in a vertical plane. Meningioma may erode the bone but usually in an irregular manner and the destruction is not confined to the meatus. Unequivocal enlargement of the internal meatus can be detected in about two thirds of the cases; in

Lundborg's (1952) analysis the meatus was considered normal in only about 15%, but in few of these patients was the tumour small.

Computerized tomographic (CT) scanning with contrast enhancement has become the workhorse of the diagnostic evaluation of acoustic tumours (Harner & Laws 1981). Tumours which protrude more than one centimetre outside the auditory canal are readily detected (Figs. 8.6 and 8.7) but smaller lesions may not be seen on the routine contrast-enhanced scan. Acoustic tumours are usually of brain density on CT and show moderate enhancement after the infusion of contrast material. With large tumours the CT may also show widening of the ipsilateral pontine cistern, shift of the fourth ventricle and hydrocephalus. The diagnostic yield for tumours with an extracanalicular extension of less than one centimetre can be increased by using thin, overlapping slices, slow scan speed, continuous infusion of contrast material and high-resolution images. CT with air or oxygen introduced into the cerebellopontine angle as contrast (Fig. 8.8)

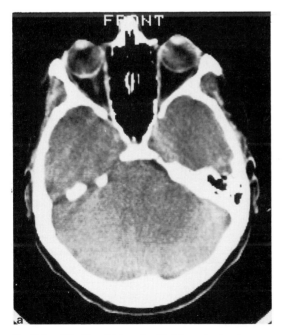
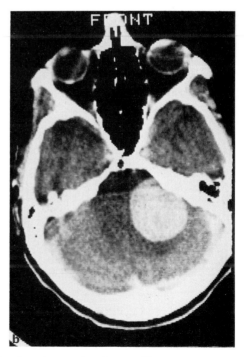

**Fig. 8.6.** CT without (a) and with (b) contrast enhancement showing a large, enhancing acoustic schwannoma.

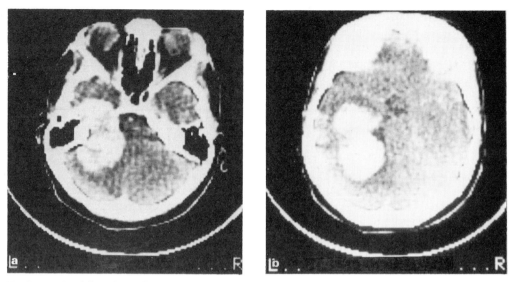

**Fig. 8.7.** (a) and (b) Enhanced CT scans showing an enormous acoustic tumour with petrous bone destruction and supratentorial extension. Tumour removed by combined supratentorial and posterior fossa approaches.

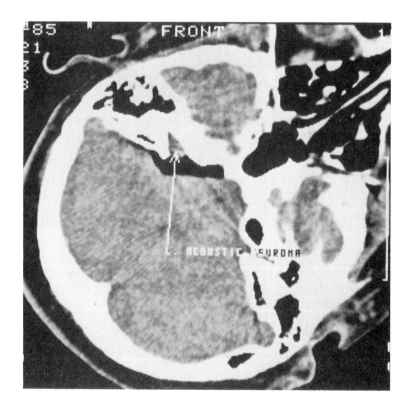

**Fig. 8.8.** CT air meatogram demonstrating an intracanalicular acoustic tumour.

can detect purely intracanalicular tumours (Valavanis *et al.* 1982). With the advent of magnetic resonance imaging (MRI) it has become possible to detect purely intracanalicular acoustic schwannomas without any invasive procedure (Young *et al.* 1983).

Vertebral angiography is not useful in detecting small tumours but with large lesions vessel displacement may be demonstrated as well as tumour circulation. The anatomy of the anterior inferior cerebellar artery is of particular importance with large tumours (Atkinson 1949).

In patients with raised intracranial pressure but without tell-tale enlargement of the meatus, ventriculography formerly helped to establish the diagnosis. Hydrocephalus could be demonstrated, with the fourth ventricle compressed, displaced dorsally towards the opposite side, and rotated so that the lateral recess on the side of the tumour is displaced more dorsally than that of the opposite side (Twining 1939). If there were no symptoms of raised intracranial pressure, spinal insufflation gave more useful information, for the air outlined the tumour in the cerebellopontine angle. In the search for small tumours, opaque medium may be used as in myelography: the patient is prone and the head manipulated to allow the contrast material to flow into the cerebellopontine angle and into the internal auditory meatus (Scanlan 1964).

## Treatment

The treatment of an acoustic tumour is to remove it; a decompression may temporarily relieve the symptoms of raised intracranial pressure but they return as the growth progressively compresses the aqueduct and the fourth ventricle and obstructs the tentorial hiatus. Decompression fails to relieve neurological disability which steadily progresses. There is no evidence that the tumour is sensitive to conventional radiotherapy, but stereotactic radiosurgery may prove of value with small tumours, particularly when these are bilateral. Its situation under the cerebellar lobe and its relationship to the brain stem render it 'one of the most difficult to enucleate of all brain tumours' (Cushing 1917). The first recorded successful operation was by Ballance in 1894 (Ballance 1908) although Cushing thought that the tumour might have been a meningioma. Thereafter sporadic successes occurred and the development of the methods of access was traced by Cushing (1917). He favoured a full bilateral exposure of the cerebellum and for the most part contented himself with as thorough a removal of the tumour as was possible within the confines of its capsule, the so-called intracapsular removal. This subtotal removal was usually preferred in order to avoid damage to blood vessels ramifying on the capsule and to the pons. The facial nerve may frequently be spared and in a few patients Cushing thought that hearing was slightly improved. The term 'intracapsular removal' must be recognized as synonymous with incomplete removal, although in Cushing's hands the amount of residual tumour must have been small because his rate of symptomatic recurrence was low. If too much tumour is left behind the result is poor because hydrocephalus is not relieved and pontine compression persists. 'There is danger in doing so much as to damage fatally the adjacent vital centres; there is danger in doing too little to relieve the patient's symptoms' (Pennybacker & Cairns 1950).

Total removal of the tumour was brought back into favour by Dandy (1925, 1934) who evolved a technique which has become the basis of the modern operation. He recommended a unilateral exposure of the cerebellum; he considered bilateral exposure an unnecessary burden for the patient. Unnecessary, because the room needed for manipulations could be obtained by resecting the lateral part of the cerebellar lobe which covers the tumour ('uncapping': Dandy states that Frazier suggested this in 1905), by tapping the ventricle and by releasing fluid from the cisterna magna. Uncapping the tumour was also regularly practised by Cushing after an operation in 1928 when it was forced upon him by intense swelling of the cerebellum. Horrax and Poppen

(1939) favoured total removal through a uni-lateral small osteoplastic flap which uncovered the lateral sinus. This provides good access to the upper pole of the tumour along the under-surface of the tentorium. But the flap is cum-bersome and cutting it time consuming; it is unnecessary provided unilateral craniectomy exposes the lower margin of the lateral sinus and bone removal is taken out to the mastoid air cells. If these are unusually well developed they should be sacrificed, but they must be carefully sealed with wax or muscle, otherwise cere bro-spinal fluid may leak into the middle ear and drain into the pharynx through the Eustachian tube, providing a pathway for infection and men-ingitis at some later date. The tumour is exposed by retracting or excising the overlying portion of cerebellum. Cushing apparently restricted resec-tion to the lower and outer portion of the cer-ebellum and German (1961) suggests that too radical a resection might damage the dentate nucleus, but this fear is probably unfounded as the nucleus will be displaced out of the field by the tumour. The amount of resection depended upon the size of the tumour, as estimated by the surgeon during his preliminary inspection of the angle. The lateral one-third to one-half of the lobe can be safely removed and the line of the resection should be practically vertical, cutting the upper border so that the tentorium is exposed and the lower border opposite the lateral margin of the foramen magnum. In this manner, both upper and lower poles of the tumour are exposed and no retraction of brain is necessary during the removal of the tumour. This is usually effected by a preliminary intracapsular piecemeal removal, by detachment from the meatus which mobilizes the tumour and by gradual dissection around the lateral and ventral aspects of the tumour, alternately easing out the upper and lower poles. Fragments of tumour within the meatus must be removed, or the interior of the canal cauterized. The minutiae of the classical operation can be studied in the writings of Cushing (1917), Oli-vecrona (Givré & Olivecrona 1949), German (1961) and Northfield (1970). It is now possible with the aid of microsurgical techniques to remove totally the largest tumour without excis-ing any of the cerebellum and with minimal retraction. Details of the microsurgical approach are given by Yaşargil *et al.* (1977).

Total removal of tumours of the size which heretofore have comprised the bulk of the neuro-surgeon's experience usually results in complete and permanent facial palsy. When the tumours are small, an infrequent experience, or do not enter the meatus the nerve can be spared and Cairns reported three such cases in 1931. Olivecrona was able to preserve the facial nerve in approximately one-third; but he points out that in this group were the more favourable cases and that the higher mortality following extirpa-tion without saving the facial nerve was in part due to increased operative trauma resulting from the attempt to spare the nerve. Eradication of tumour remnants in the meatus irretrievably damages the nerve, unless the canal is opened and microdissection is employed. Recently impres-sive results have been achieved in preserving not only the facial nerve but also in some instances the cochlear and vestibular nerves. Yaşargil *et al.* (1977) reported a series of 171 cases with anatomical preservation of the facial nerve in 86% and functional preservation in 82%. In this series there were 137 cases of large tumours and only 28 of the patients developed a facial palsy. Interestingly, objective hearing was preserved in only one case and in a further five there was some preservation of hearing for a few days postoperatively to be replaced by tinnitus. Wanx-ing (1981) reported restoration of hearing after total removal of a large acoustic tumour. Lye *et al.* (1982) achieved anatomical preservation of the facial nerve in 83% of their cases and in 70% with large tumours. Delgado *et al.* (1979) suggest that intraoperative monitoring of facial muscle evoked responses may help to identify and preserve the facial nerve. Occasionally the pontine stump of the facial nerve has been sal-vaged and linked by a free graft to the facial nerve extracranially (Dott 1958) or to the stump in the internal meatus (Drake 1963). A faciohypoglossal anastomosis provides a fair aesthetic result, the improvement in facial tone lending a nearly normal appearance when the face is at rest and some patients who practice associated movement before a mirror acquire a surprisingly good ultimate result.

The trigeminal nerve is only lightly or not adherent to the tumour; consequently, provided great care is exercised in removing the upper pole of the tumour, the nerve usually escapes damage. It is most vulnerable near its pontine insertion where it is usually most flattened and fragile and least easy to identify and to protect. Loss of the corneal reflex combined with a facial paralysis always leads to keratitis; a tarsorrhaphy is advisable for three months, after which time the adhesion may be partially divided and the state of the eye carefully observed. Corneal abrasion occurs so readily in patients who have had an acoustic tumour removed that occlusion of the lids as a routine for the first postoperative week is a wise precaution.

Damage to the pons, by direct bruising or by ischaemia due to occlusion of small arteries, results in varying degrees of nystagmus, impaired conjugate deviation of the eyes to the ipsilateral side, ataxia and sensorimotor hemiparesis. Provided a major vessel such as the anterior inferior cerebellar artery or its anastomotic branches has not been damaged, considerable recovery can be anticipated particularly with the aid of efficient physiotherapy. Progress is slow and most patients with average-sized tumours require six months for rehabilitation. Severe degrees of pontine damage are accompanied by coma, pyrexia, unstable blood pressure (often a peak of hypertension occurs during the time of deep occurs during the time of deep dissection in these patients), profuse pulmonary secretions and impaired ventilation and disturbance of coughing and swallowing mechanisms. Pontine infarction is the commonest cause of death (Olivecrona 1967). Tracheostomy and vigilant care of the airway, postural drainage and maintenance of an adequate blood pressure and feeding by gastric tube are essential requirements and test nursing care to the uttermost. In the past some surgeons carried out tracheostomy prophylactically after every operation for the removal of large tumours, but such a decision must depend upon the quality of routine postoperative observation and care. Swallowing mechanisms however are so frequently disturbed that clear fluids should be first introduced with the help of the speech therapist, and if there is any doubt at all about swallowing gastric tube feeding for a few days is a wise precaution.

*Translabyrinthine operation*

Cushing (1917) stated that in 1904 Panse suggested an approach through the petrous bone and the method was attempted on several occasions by other surgeons. It was also combined with a unilateral suboccipital craniectomy. Both operations were in due course abandoned; largely because of inadequate surgical facilities at that time and because of faulty diagnosis or because the tumour was too large. Cushing considered that too little stress was placed 'upon what may happen to cerebellum and brain stem as the result of manipulation of the tumour in a restricted field'. But he prophesied that 'it is however within the realm of possibility that in the case of a very early and minute tumour largely limited to the internal canal the translabyrinthine operation may in time become the operation of choice, but this will necessitate far more precocious and more exact diagnoses than we as yet are capable of'. Seventy years later this possibility is being realized, for otological tests and other diagnostic procedures have become so refined that a small tumour can now be detected. But the responsibility for early detection rests upon the otologist to seek for a tumour in cases of unilateral deafness. The technique described by House (1964) provides a method of removal whilst preserving the facial nerve. The approach is through the mastoid process to the middle ear where the prominence due to the underlying facial nerve is identified and using the nerve as a guide, bone is removed posterior to it until the internal auditory meatus is reached. The opening is enlarged to expose the dura mater, above as

far as the superior petrosal sinus and below to
the sigmoid sinus and jugular foramen. The operation is performed under a dissecting microscope
using a high speed burr and continuous
irrigation. The tumour is separated from the
facial nerve by microdissection, working from its
lateral extremity and even large tumours can be
totally removed by this route. Large tumours
may also be dealt with successfully by a two
stage operation; translabyrinthine resection of
the lateral portion of the tumour followed by a
posterior fossa removal of the main mass. An
alternative method is removal of the posterior
wall of the internal auditory canal through a
unilateral posterior fossa exposure and microdissection of the portion in the canal before
dealing with the main tumour (Rand & Kurze
1965). However, King and Morrison (1980)
reported a series of 150 cases and concluded that
the translabyrinthine approach with a transtentorial extension, could achieve total removal
of acoustic tumours of all sizes. Their mortality
and morbidity compared well with the best posterior fossa reports.

*Results*

The mortality achieved by Cushing (1932) still
sets a standard difficult to surpass. His overall
operative mortality was 11.4% but the figures
for the last three consecutive groups of 50 cases
were 15.6%, 11.3% and 3.4%, demonstrating
how important a part is played by the acquisition
of surgical skill and judgement (*see also* the analysis by Northfield 1970). Nearly all these operations were intracapsular and therefore partial
removals, but the late results (*see* below) show
that his partial removal was thorough. The
results from other sources are listed in Table 8.1.
The results reported in more modern series with
total tumour removal are very impressive. King
and Morrison (1980) had a mortality of 2% in
150 cases and Yaşargil *et al.* (1977) a mortality
of 2% in 171 cases with no mortality in the last
104 patients.

Whether the tumour should be totally

**Table 8.1**  Operative mortality.

|  | *Overall (per cent)* | *Total removal (per cent)* |
|---|---|---|
| Horrax (1954) | 13.3 | 11 |
| Hullay & Tomits (1965) |  | 4 |
| Jefferson (1950) | 26 | 8.8 |
| Northfield (1970) | 27 | 24 (1st series) |
|  |  | 15 (2nd series) |
| Olivecrona (1967) | 20 | 19 |
| Pennybacker & Cairns (1950) | 20 | 16 |

removed, or whether only an intracapsular (i.e.
partial) removal should be performed depends on
several factors. The mortality figures suggest that
complete removal is less dangerous than a partial
one; but they are misleading. The group of cases
in which the tumour was completely removed
included the small tumours in which technical
difficulties and the risk of pontine softening are
less; the decision to limit the operation to a partial
removal is often made because the tumour is
large or is presenting great technical difficulties,
or because the patient is old or in poor condition.
Relative inexperience in the type of tumour is a
factor which should also influence the surgeon's
decision.

Intracapsular removals have serious disadvantages, of which recurrence is the most
obvious. A second operation may be undertaken
but it carries an even higher mortality rate. The
decision to re-operate is often deferred because
of the risk, because deterioration is insidious and
the diagnosis uncertain and therefore delayed.
The patient is older, and adhesions resulting from
the first operation may distort anatomy and
hinder recognition of structures. Recovery of functions such as balance and coordination is often
not as satisfactory as after total removal. In
Olivecrona's series recurrence occurred in 50%
within four years of the first operation. When
account was taken of the enhanced dangers of a
second operation, 60% of patients were dead
within four years either from operations or from

recurrence (Givré & Olivecrona 1949). The recurrence rate was not so high in Cushing's experience and his 182 cases have been reviewed by German (1961). At the end of the first five years it was 24%, and six years later it had risen to 28%; there were 24 patients alive 30 years after their first operation. Some of Olivecrona's patients also lived for many years after a partial removal, and 'the conclusion that some acoustic tumours grow imperceptibly or cease to grow after incomplete removal is inescapable' (Olivecrona 1950). Cairns' results were somewhat similar to Cushing's, for 18% of the survivors of the first operation required a second operation within four years, with a mortality of 50%.

Disability after the removal of an acoustic schwannoma may be severe. Facial palsy in a woman (less often in a man) may give rise to much distress; if associated with loss of corneal sensation a tarsorrhaphy may be necessary for a long time with consequent loss of binocular vision. Unsteadiness of gait may never completely recover but is moderate to severe in only about one-tenth of the cases (Northfield 1970); general asthenia, loss of confidence and a state of invalidism is more likely to occur in the older patients, in great contrast to the ability of young people to overcome these handicaps. Horrax (1950) estimated that useful survival occurred in 25% of Cushing's patients. In a series of his own cases of total extirpation, useful survival occurred in 62%. 'Useful' he defined as a return to some sort of work, including housework. A return to work in 50% following both partial and total removals was reported by Pennybacker and Cairns (1950) and by McKenzie (1965) in total removals. In the series reported by Hullay and Tomits (1965) 94% 'returned to their professions'. Of the 171 patients in the series of Yaşargil et al. (1977) 147 were said to remain in good to excellent condition (self sufficient and working unless unable to work on account of age).

Summarizing, total removal of an acoustic schwannoma is the operation of choice, particularly in young patients, but special circumstances may sometimes render an intracapsular operation advisable, such as bilateral tumours. Preservation of the facial nerve is desirable, but only if this can be achieved without adding to the risk of the operation. The operative risks both to life and to the facial nerve largely depend upon the size of the tumour; they can be greatly reduced by earlier diagnosis. In the past, although a firm diagnosis may have been made, the advice of some neurosurgeons has been that operation should not be undertaken until there is evidence that the tumour impinges on the pons or causes raised intracranial pressure. In the light of our present knowledge of this tumour and of modern advances in surgical and anaesthetic techniques this attitude of procrastination can no longer be justified. In about two-thirds of the cases the evolution of symptoms is typical and in these, radiological and otological investigations are able to provide a diagnosis before the tumour has extended much beyond the internal auditory meatus. At this stage, the operation of total removal carries only a small risk, with excellent prospects of saving the facial nerve, and even of preserving some auditory function.

## Trigeminal schwannoma

Schwannomas of the trigeminal nerve are rare, only three or four occurring for every 100 of the acoustic nerve. In consequence, most neurosurgeons cannot expect to encounter more than a few during their professional lifetime; this makes the contributions of Jefferson (1955), Olive and Svien (1957), Schisano and Olivecrona (1960) and Benedittis et al. (1977) particularly valuable. They describe personal experiences of a total of 49 cases; Jefferson's paper is profusely and beautifully illustrated. The tumour more commonly arises in the gasserian ganglion forming a predominantly middle fossa mass; in other cases it arises behind the ganglion on the root and projects into the posterior fossa. Occasionally the tumour is dumb-bell shaped; a narrow neck in Meckel's cave connects a middle-fossa and a posterior-fossa mass. Krayenbühl (1936) examined the published records of 54 cases of primary tumour of the trigeminal nerve and in only 29 was it possible to be certain of its exact origin; in 26 it was of the ganglion and in three of the root. In Olivecrona's series the disparity was not so marked; 11 originated in the ganglion and four in the root. Jefferson makes the point that probably most of these tumours are to some extent dumb-bell shaped, though one end may be much larger and clinically predominant. It is surgically important to be aware of this possibility. Schwannoma of the trigeminal nerve has the same age incidence as that of the acoustic nerve, but the duration of symptoms may be much longer. In Olivecrona's series, no patient had a history of less than one year and in one-third it was of 10–14 years.

The ganglion tumour forms an ovoid mass in the middle fossa, bulging out from the cavernous sinus, which it compresses. It is covered by a thin sheath of dura mater and the ganglionic tissue is compressed and lies on the periphery of the tumour. Large tumours extend forwards to the superior orbital fissure, and may surround the internal carotid artery and elevate the optic nerve and chiasma. As noted above, its posterior extremity may protrude from Meckel's cave under the tentorium. Occasionally the tumour extends into the three branches of the ganglion but this is uncommon. Although the cavernous sinus is so closely related to the medial aspect of the tumour, severe ophthalmoplegia is uncommon. Marked erosion of bone is an important consequence of tumour pressure; it affects the apex of the petrous bone, the root of the great wing of the sphenoid, the lateral aspect of the sella turcica and in large tumours the ipsilateral anterior clinoid process. The root schwannoma occupies and distends Meckel's cave (eroding the apex of the petrous bone) and bulges out as a rounded somewhat lobulated mass, occupying the cerebellopontine angle and thereby resembling the acoustic schwannoma. It lies however somewhat higher and further forward and may hug the clivus or dorsum sellae. It indents and displaces the upper part of the pons and the crus cerebri and on occasion the displacement is sufficient to press the contralateral crus against the opposite margin of the tentorium. The tri-geminal root is incorporated in the capsule, but the seventh and eighth nerves curve around the caudal pole of the tumour.

*Diagnosis*

The commonest and usually the earliest symptoms are of disturbed sensory functions, whether the tumour is of the ganglion or of the root. These may take the form of vague numbness or paraesthesiae within the area of the trigeminal distribution and in the early stages may be transient. Trigeminal pain is frequent in the ganglion tumours and may be that of paroxysmal neuralgia, or may be dull and continuous. Krayenbühl drew attention to the distinction that pain rarely occurs if the tumour involves the root, and this view is supported by Benedittis *et al.* who reported no pain with their root tumours. However, Arseni *et al.* (1975) reported 6 tumours solely of the root which did produce facial pain and Yonas and Jannetta (1980) added a further two cases. Hyperaesthesia instead of hypoaesthesia may occasionally occur (Jefferson 1955). Sooner or later impairment of superficial trigeminal sensation, in one or in all divisions, can be demonstrated in nearly all cases. Wasting and weakness of the masticatory muscles occurs in about half the cases. Diplopia is frequent, though the degree of ophthalmoplegia is not severe in spite of the proximity of the tumour to the third, fourth and sixth nerves. In other respects, apart from evidence of raised intracranial pressure which is often absent, the ganglion and the root tumours give rise to ipsilateral proptosis and occasionally to optic atrophy and visual field defects indicating pressure upon the optic nerve or chiasma. Extension of a root tumour into the cerebellopontine angle gives rise to that syndrome. Involvement of the facial and the acoustic nerves simulates an acoustic tumour. Nystagmus, ataxia of the ipsilateral limbs and pyramidal signs are frequent; the latter are usually contralateral but they may also be ipsilateral due to the pressure of the opposite cerebral peduncle against the tentorium.

Typical radiological changes can be demonstrated in nearly all cases and their recognition is so important for diagnosis that they should be sought assiduously. The commonest finding is a cleanly-cut erosion of the tip of the apex of the petrous bone; it can be well seen in a postero-anterior half-axial skull X-ray film if the upper border of the petrous bone is projected across the middle of the orbit. Erosion of the medial part of the great wing of the sphenoid and enlargement of the foramina ovale and rotundum occur in ganglion tumours which may also destroy the side of the body of the sphenoid. Jefferson draws attention to Guillaume's observation (Guillaime *et al.* 1949) that the destruction of the floor of the middle fossa and of the apex of the petrous expose to view in the lateral film a much greater downward extent of the dorsum sellae and clivus. Destruction of the margins of the superior orbital fissure may occur as in other slowly growing retro-orbital masses. Further radiological investigations are as for acoustic schwannoma and should include CT scanning and angiography. The carotid angiogram characteristically shows anterior, medial and inferior displacement of the proximal part of the carotid syphon and if there is a large posterior fossa extension of tumour then the vertebral angiogram may show contralateral displacement of the basilar artery and upward displacement of the posterior cerebral artery.

As in the case of the acoustic schwannoma, if the chronological sequence of symptoms, the clinical findings and the bone changes are characteristic, diagnosis is straightforward. Alternative middle fossa lesions which must be considered are subclinoid giant carotid artery aneurysm, meningioma, chordoma and malignant growths of the base of the skull. The latter include sarcoma of the sphenoid, carcinoma of the ethmoid and sphenoidal air sinuses and nasopharyngeal carcinoma and reticulosarcoma. These malignant tumours have a particular importance for neurosurgeons because of the striking neurological disturbances they cause when they invade the cranium. Godtfredsen (1941, 1944) and Jefferson (1953) have

been especially interested in this subject. Jefferson points out that the tumour can enter the cranial cavity along several routes. From the retropharyngeal space to the carotid sheath which guides it upwards through the foramen lacerum. Through the pterygomaxillary fossa and the foramina ovale and rotundum, and by direct spread through the wall of the sphenoidal air sinus. All these pathways lead to the cavernous sinus and the gasserian ganglion and provide an anatomical explanation for their neurological complications. The commonest are trigeminal pain with loss of sensation and paralysis of masticatory muscles, ophthalmoplegia, deafness (from obstruction of the eustachian tube) and blindness (due to invasion of the optic nerve from the anterior end of the cavernous sinus or from direct spread through the wall of the sphenoidal sinus). Other cranial nerves may be involved as the tumour spreads over the dura mater of the posterior cranial fossa. The distinction from a trigeminal schwannoma can usually be made by reason of the greater intensity of the neurological symptoms and signs, some of which may be bilateral. The pain is severe and continuous, often extending beyond the boundary of the trigeminal nerve as a result of malignant invasion and the loss of sensation and masticatory paralysis is dense, rarely so in the case of a benign tumour. Ophthalmoplegia is often total and loss of vision exceptional in a schwannoma (in Case 2 of Olive and Svien 1957, one eye was totally blind). The radiological changes in malignant invasion are ill defined and ragged at their margins, in contrast to the smooth edged erosions produced by the schwannoma. Very rarely malignant trigeminal schwannomas are encountered; Levy *et al.* (1983) reported two cases bringing the total in the literature to five.

The alternative diagnosis in a case of trigeminal tumour whose main mass is in the posterior fossa cover a range of lesions quite different from the middle fossa tumour. An acoustic schwannoma may be closely mimicked, but the deafness is usually only mild and labyrinthine function impaired but not abolished. The pattern of bone erosion should make the distinction clear. Meningioma, epidermoid cyst and aneurysm of the basilar artery must be considered; the elevation of protein content of the cerebrospinal fluid is high in the first and normal or nearly so in the other two; radiological examination should prove decisive. Although a glioma pontis may appear to be likely on clinical grounds in cases with a short history, radiological examination will correct this impression. More commonly the long history, fluctuating facial paraesthesiae, pyramidal signs, ataxia and nystagmus lead to a clinical diagnosis of disseminated sclerosis until definite cranial nerve palsies develop.

*Treatment*

Ganglion tumours and those dumb-bell tumours in which the posterior fossa mass is small can be excised by a middle fossa approach through a temporal craniotomy. The temporal lobe is elevated in order to expose the tumour and opinions vary as to whether the dura mater should be stripped from the floor of the fossa until the tumour is reached, or whether the dura mater be opened at the margin of the craniotomy, an entirely intradural approach. In the former case the brain is somewhat better protected against retraction, in the latter a better exposure is obtained. But if access is limited the inferior margin of the temporal lobe may have to be resected; the final degree of trauma to the brain is likely to be less than that due to excessive retraction, which affects a wider volume of tissue. The tumour is incised and its interior evacuated. Small tumours can be totally extirpated, though great care is necessary to avoid damage to the ocular motor nerves in the cavernous sinus. Intracapsular subtotal removal is advisable in massive tumours. The posterior end of the tumour can be reached if the tentorium is divided, thus exposing the upper part of the cerebellopontine angle. Those tumours which have their main mass in the posterior fossa are approached as for an acoustic tumour. The tumour will be identified as arising from the fifth and not from the eighth nerve by recognizing the seventh and eighth nerves crossing the caudal pole of the tumour to reach the internal porus. The surface of the tumour is usually smooth, rounded or lobular, whereas the meningioma is finely nodular with a broad sessile attachment to the dura mater. If the facial and acoustic nerves are to be preserved the surgeon has only a small amount of room above them in which to manœuvre and at a greater depth than in a case of acoustic tumour. In consequence the exercise is even more difficult, though the anterior inferior cerebellar artery seems to be less of a hazard because of the higher level of the tumour. If the tumour is found to extend deeply into the eroded apex of the petrous bone, this portion should be treated cautiously as the internal carotid artery is in close proximity. In the case of malignant schwannoma Levy *et al* (1983) recommend radiotherapy in addition to surgery.

*Results*

In spite of the size to which these tumours may grow, and of the technical difficulties, the mortality is less than that for the acoustic schwannoma, and the long term results of partial removal rather better. Of the 40 cases of Jefferson, Olivecrona and Svien referred to above, in two no operation was performed; in the others a partial or total removal was carried out with four deaths, an operative mortality of 10%. Benedittis *et al.* (1977) had no operative mortality in their 9 cases and a total removal was achieved in four patients. In one of Jefferson's patients a partial posterior fossa removal proved satisfactory for nearly 20 years, when a second operation was necessary for recurrence; thereafter the patient remained well and working during the next six years. In three of the cases reported by Schisano and Olivecrona, subtotal removal was followed by over 20 years of active life.

## Jugular foramen schwannoma

Schwannomas involving the jugular foramen are very uncommon. Maniglia *et al.* (1979) reported a case, bringing the total in the literature at that time to 56 cases. This makes the series of Pluchino *et al.* (1975) and Kaye *et al.* (1984) particularly valuable as they describe personal experiences of a total of 25 cases. Kaye *et al.* (1984) observed three main patterns of tumour growth and postulated that the position of the tumour depends on the point of origin from the nerves as they pass through the pars nervosa of the jugular foramen. More distal lesions expand inferiorly from the base of the skull, whereas more proximal lesions will enlarge into the posterior fossa and tumours arising in the mid region will tend to expand primarily into the bone. These patterns of tumour growth give rise to different modes of clinical presentation. Those tumours with a large intracranial component present with deafness, vertigo and ataxia and there may be only minimal deficits of the jugular foramen nerves. The deafness is sensorineural in type and the presentation mimics that of acoustic schwannoma. Occasionally with large tumours there is evidence of raised intracranial pressure, facial weakness or there may be decreased corneal reflex. In contrast those tumours growing primarily within bone or extracranially show earlier and more marked involvement of the lower cranial nerves viz. hoarseness, difficulty in swallowing and weakness of the sternomastoid and trapezius muscles. Diminished taste sensation over the posterior third of the tongue and glossal hemiatrophy may also be present. These tumours are often misdiagnosed pre-operatively as glomus jugulare tumours, epidermoids or chordomas.

Plain radiographs and tomography may demonstrate erosion and widening of the jugular foramen with smooth distinct margins. This is in contrast to glomus jugulare tumours which typically cause enlargement of the jugular foramen with irregular indistinct margins. However, schwannomas growing primarily within the bone can show considerable destruction of bone. Angiography generally demonstrates an avascular or only slightly vascular mass whereas a glomus jugulare tumour is usually highly vascular. CT scanning is the most useful radiological investigation, showing the intracranial and extracranial extent of the tumour as well as associated bony changes. This information is essential for the pre-operative planning of the surgical approach.

The object of surgical treatment of jugular foramen schwannomas, as for acoustic tumours, is total removal. Those tumours which are mainly intracranial are approached sub-occipitally and the technique is essentially the same as that for acoustic tumours. However, tumours growing mainly in bone or extracranially pose particular technical problems and are best dealt with by a combined posterior fossa and otological approach. An infralabyrinthine approach is indicated if the internal auditory canal is not involved and hearing is preserved. This technique involves dissection of the internal carotid artery, internal jugular vein and lower cranial nerves at the base of the skull and mobilizing the facial nerve by a complete mastoidectomy. The jugular bulb is exposed and the tumour can be delivered from the skull base. If there is radiological evidence of tumour involving the internal auditory meatus and bone superiorly then a more radical translabyrinthine transcochlear approach is indicated. Any intracranial extension of tumour can be removed via the suboccipital route. Operative details of the otological approaches to the skull base are given by Fisch and Pillsbury (1979). If the vagus nerve is divided during tumour resection, microscopic anastomosis or nerve grafting may prove successful. Cerebrospinal fluid fistula can be a problem and may be prevented by a fascial or free fat graft where indicated.

### Results

Removal of jugular foramen schwannomas is generally accompanied by damage to the lower cranial nerves, particularly if there is a large intracranial extension. Some degree of sputum retention and aspiration are almost invariable and may pose serious postoperative problems. Pluchino *et al.* (1975) reported an operative mortality of 16% and there was an overall mortality of 9% in their review of the literature. Kaye *et al.* (1984) reported no mortality in their series and they attributed this to modern improvements in diagnosis, microsurgical techniques and combined suboccipital-otological surgical approaches.

### Facial schwannoma

Schwannomas of the facial nerve are rare tumours. They may arise from any part of the facial nerve and as with jugular foramen schwannoma there are three groups, intracranial, intratemporal and extratemporal, according to the point of origin along the nerve and subsequent tumour extension. Friede (1977) states that the majority of facial schwannomas occur within the facial canal or beyond and that the intradural portion of the nerve is an exceptional site of origin of the tumour. This view is also taken by Isamat *et al.* (1975) who consider the intracranial tumours to have arisen from the intrapetrous portion of the facial nerve in the region of the geniculate ganglion and then extended into the middle fossa or less commonly into the cerebellopontine angle. The intracranial variety of facial schwannoma is extremely rare; Murata *et al.* (1985) reported two cases bringing the total in the literature to 21 cases compared to more than 160 reported cases of intratemporal schwannoma. These rare intracranial tumours are in the province of the neurosurgeon and they present a well-defined clinical picture. The initial symptoms in the 21 reported cases were progressive facial weakness in 19 cases and hearing loss in 13 cases. The facial weakness is often complete or severe in contrast to the minimal facial signs in acoustic schwannoma or other cerebellopontine angle tumours even in those that have reached a large size and where there is a long history. The superior petrosal nerve

and chorda tympani may be affected producing diminution in tear secretion and loss of taste over the anterior two thirds of the tongue with reduced salivation. Hemifacial spasm can also be an initial symptom as in one of the cases of Isamat *et al.* (1975). Interestingly, these intracranial tumours do not involve cranial nerves other than the acoustic and neither cerebellar signs nor intracranial pressure are features.

Intratemporal schwannomas most commonly arise from the vertical part of the facial nerve: 44 cases compared to 8 arising from the tympanic segment of the nerve in the review of Isamat *et al.* (1975). These schwannomas tend to destroy the facial canal and to invade the middle ear and the mastoid. Occasionally the tumour is seen as a polyp at the external auditory meatus. In the series of Fisch and Rüttner (1977) two of their 9 intratemporal tumours extended extratemporally through the stylomastoid foramen. The typical symptom in the majority of these lesions is a slowly progressive facial weakness, but the palsy can be sudden in onset or even intermittent as reported by Castro (1977). Hearing loss is a constant finding and may be the first symptom thus mimicking an acoustic tumour. As these tumours arise distal to the geniculate ganglion the superior petrosal nerve is usually spared but this is not the case with the chorda tympani. Extratemporal schwannomas usually present with a peripheral facial weakness as the initial symptom (Jackson *et al.* 1980).

Fisch and Rüttner (1977) in their series of intratemporal tumours involving the facial nerve reported 37 benign lesions including 9 schwannomas of the facial nerve, 12 cholesteatomas, 9 haemangiomas, 1 arachnoid cyst and 3 each of meningiomas and glomus jugulare tumours.

Investigations are as for acoustic schwannomas. Plain radiographs and tomography of the petrous bone will show bony erosion and destruction according to the site of the tumour. CT scanning and angiography are important in differential diagnosis and in demonstrating the presence of any intracranial extension.

An intracranial facial schwannoma with a

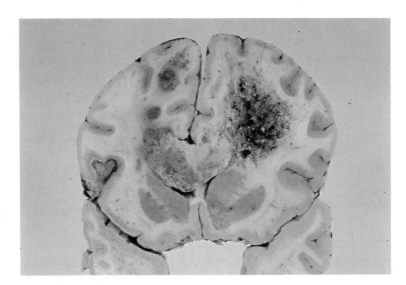

**Plate 1.** Coronal brain slice showing malignant astrocytoma of 'butterfly' configuration. (Courtesy of Dr A. Gordon.)

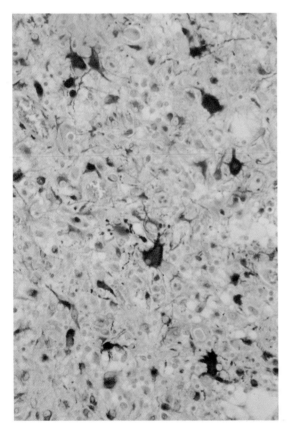

**Plate 2.** Section of malignant astrocytoma stained for glial fibrillary acidic protein (GFAP). (Courtesy of Dr J. E. Bell.)

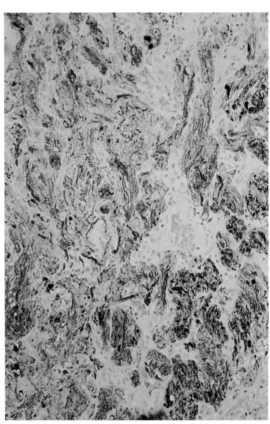

**Plate 3.** Section of cerebellar astrocytoma stained for GFAP. (Courtesy of Dr J. E. Bell.)

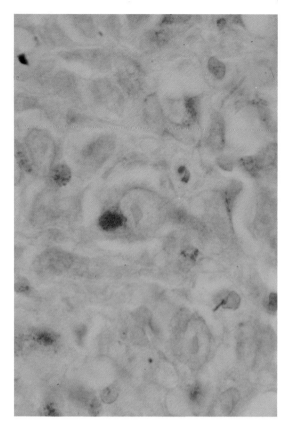

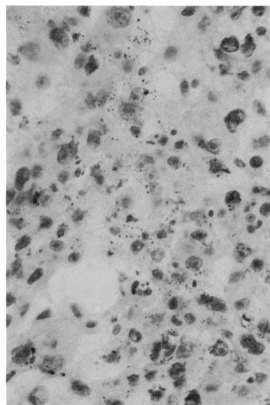

**Plate 4.** Primitive neuroectodermal tumour (PNET) stained for GFAP. (Courtesy of Dr J. E. Bell.)

**Plate 5.** Frozen section of haemangioblastoma stained for fat. (Courtesy of Dr A. Gordon.)

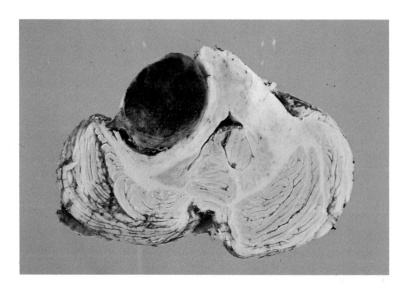

**Plate 6.** Large haemorrhagic acoustic neurinoma showing indentation of cerebellum and brain stem and distortion of fourth ventricle. (Courtesy of Dr A. Gordon.)

middle fossa extension is approached surgically by a subtemporal craniotomy. A cerebello-pontine angle extension may be approached as for an acoustic tumour via the sub-occipital route or using the translabyrinthine approach with modifications as necessary. With the appropriate surgical approach and the use of microsurgical techniques total removal of the tumour can be achieved.

### Schwannomas of oculomotor, trochlear and abducent nerves

Solitary schwannomas arising from the nerves to the extraocular muscles are exceedingly rare. Okamoto *et al.* (1985) reviewed the literature and collected 16 reported cases of tumours arising from these nerves: 9 from the oculomotor nerve, 5 from the trochlear nerve and only 2 from the abducent nerve. In oculomotor schwannoma the initial symptoms are due to oculomotor palsy but there is often accompanying visual loss due to optic nerve compression and occasionally proptosis from intraorbital extension of the tumour. The tumour may also involve the trochlear, trigeminal and abducent nerves in the parasellar region and when the tumour is large it may not be possible at surgery to identify the nerve of origin.

Ho (1981) reported a case of trochlear nerve schwannoma found incidentally at autopsy and reviewed the two previously reported cases. These two tumours were located at the tentorial incisura and in addition to palsy of the fourth nerve there was involvement of the trigeminal nerve. In one of the cases of Leunda *et al.* (1982) a trochlear nerve palsy was associated with an incomplete oculomotor palsy.

## References

ANTONI N. (1920) *Ueber Rückenmarkstumoren und Neur-ofibrome*, Bergmann, Munich.
ARSENI C., DUMITRESCU L., CONSTANTINESCU A. (1975) *Surg. Neurol.*, **4**, 497.

ATKINSON W. J. (1949) *J. Neurol. Neurosurg. Psychiat.*, **12**, 137.
BALLANCE C. A. (1908) *Some Points in the Surgery of the Brain and its Membranes*, 2nd edn., p. 283. Macmillan, London.
BALLANTYNE J. C., GROVES J., EDWARDS C. H. & DOWNTON D. (1978) *A Synopsis of Otolaryngology*. John Wright & Sons Ltd, Bristol.
BENEDITTIS G. DE., BERNASCONI V. & ETTORRE, G. (1977) *Acta Neurochir.*, **38**, 37.
CASTRO D. (1977) In Fisch U. (ed) *Facial Nerve Surgery*, Kugler Medical Publications BV Panel Discussion No 15 463.
CUSHING H. (1917) *Tumours of the Nervus Acusticus*. Saunders, Philadelphia.
CUSHING H. (1932) *Intracranial Tumours*. Thomas, Springfield, Illinois.
DANDY W. E. (1925) *Surg. Gynaec. Obstet.*, **41**, 129.
DANDY W. E. (1934) *Arch. Surg.*, **29**, 337.
DAWES J. D. K. & HANKINSON J. (1984) In Ballantyne J., Groves J. (eds). *Scott-Brown's Diseases of the Ear, Nose and Throat*. Fourth edition. **Vol 2**. *The Ear*. pp. 639 Butterworths, London.
DELGADO T. E., BUCHHEIT W. A., ROSENHOLTZ H. R. & CHRISSIAN S. (1979) *Neurosurgery*, **Vol 4 No 5**, 418.
DIX M. R. & HALLPIKE C. S. (1958) *Proc. roy. Soc. Med.*, **51**, 889.
DIX M. R. & HALLPIKE C. S. (1966) *Acta Otolaryng.*, **61**, 1.
DIX M. R., HALLPIKE C. S. & HOOD J. D. (1948) *Proc. roy. Soc. Med.*, **41**, 516.
DIX M. R. & HOOD J. W. (1953) *J. Laryng. Otol.*, **47**, 343.
DOTT N. M. (1958) *Proc. roy. Soc. Med.*, **51**, 900.
DRAKE C. G. (1963) *Arch. Otolaryngol.*, **78**, 456.
EDWARDS C. H. & PATTERSON J. H. (1951) *Brain*, **74**, 144.
EGGERMONT J. J., DON M. & BRACKMANN D. E. (1980) *Ann. Otol. Rhinol. Laryngol.*, **89**, suppl 75, 1.
ELLIOTT F. A. & McKISSOCK W. (1954) *Lancet*, **ii**, 1189.
FISCH U. & PILLSBURY H. C. (1979) *Arch. Otolaryngol.*, **105**, 99.
FISCH U. & RUTTNER J. (1977) In Fisch, U. (ed) *Facial Nerve Surgery* Kugler Medical Publications BV 448.
FITZGERALD G. & HALLPIKE C. S. (1942) *Brain*, **65**, 115.
FOWLER E. P. (1936a) *Laryngoscope*, **46**, 616.
FOWLER E. P. (1936b) *Arch. Otolaryng.*, **24**, 731.
FRIEDE R. L. (1977) In Fisch, U. (ed) *Facial Nerve Surgery*, Kugler Medical Publications BV 470.
GERMAN W. J. (1961) *Clin. Neurosurg.*, 7, 21.
GIVRÉ A. & OLIVECRONA H. (1949) *J. Neurosurg.*, **6**, 396.
GODTFREDSEN E. (1941) *Arch. Psychiat. Neurol.*, **16**, 47.
GODTFREDSEN E. (1944) *Acta Otolaryngol.*, Suppl. **59**.
GUILLAUME J., ROGÉ R. & MAZARS D. (1949) *Rev. Neurol.*, **81**, 225.
HALLPIKE C. S. (1959) In *Lectures on the Scientific Basis of Medicine*, Vol. 7, p. 1. The Athlone Press, University of London.
HALLPIKE C. S., HOOD J. D. & TRINDER E. (1960a) *Confin. Neurol.*, **20**, 232.
HALLPIKE C. S., HOOD J. D. & TRINDER E. (1960b) *Proc. roy. Soc. Med.*, **53**, 1059.
HARDY M. & CROWE S. J. (1936) *Arch. Surg.*, **32**, 292.
HARNER S. G. & LAWS E. R. (1981) *Neurosurgery*, **Vol 9. No 4.**, 373.
HENNEBERG & KOCH M. (1902) *Arch. Psychiat.*, **36**, 251.
HENSCHEN F. (1955) In *Handbuch der speiziellen Pathologischen*

*Anatomie und Histologie*, 13/3, (ed. Lubarsch, O., Henke, F. & Roessle, R.) p. 845. Springer, Berlin.

Ho K. L. (1981) *J. Neurosurg.*, **55**, 132.

Horrax G. (1950) *J. Neurol. Neurosurg. Psychiat.*, **13**, 268.

Horrax G. (1954) *New Eng. J. Med.*, **250**, 981.

Horrax G. & Poppen J. L. (1939) *Ann. Surg.*, **110**, 513.

House W. F. (1964) *Arch. Otolaryng.*, **80**, 731.

Hullay J. & Tomits G. H. (1965) *J. Neurosurg.*, **22**, 127.

Isamat F., Bartumeus F., Miranda A. M., Prat J., Pons L. C. (1975) *J. Neurosurg.*, **43**, 608.

Jackson C. G., Glassock M. E., Hughes G., Sismanis A. (1980) *Laryngoscope*, **90**, 1581.

Jefferson G. (1950) *J. Neurol. Neurosurg. Psychiat.*, **13**, 279.

Jefferson G. J. (1953) *Trans. Oph. Soc. U.K.*, **73**, 117.

Jefferson G. J. (1955) *Clin. Neurosurg.*, **1**, 11.

Johnson E. (1977) *Arch. Ololaryngol.*, **103**, 152.

Kaye A. H., Hann J. F., Kinney S. E., Hardy R. W. & Bay J. W. (1984) *J. Neurosurg.*, **60**, 1045.

King T. T. & Morrison A. W. (1980) Translabyrinthine and transtentorial removal of acoustic nerve tumours. *J. Neurosurg.*, **52**, 210.

Krayenbühl H. (1936) *Brain*, **59**, 337.

Leunda G., Vaquero J., Cabezudo J., Garcia-Uria J. & Bravo G. (1982) *J. Neurosurg.*, **57**, 563.

Levy W. J., Ansbacher L., Byer J., Nutkiewicz A. & Fratkin J. (1983) *Neurosurgery*, **13**, 572.

Lundborg T. (1952) *Acta Otolaryngol.*, Suppl. **99**.

Lye R. L., Dutton J., Ramsden R. T., Occleshaw J. V., Ferguson I. T. & Taylor I. (1982) *J. Neurosurg.*, **57**, 739–46.

McKenzie W. (1965) *Proc. roy. Soc. Med.*, **58**, 1076.

Maniglia A. J., Chandler J. R., Goodwin W. J. & Parker J. C. (1979) *Laryngoscope*, **89**, 1405.

Murata T., Hakuba A., Okumura T. & Mori K. (1985) *Surg. Neurol.*, **23**, 507.

Northfield D. W. C. (1970) *Proc. roy. Soc. Med.*, **63**, 769.

Okamoto S., Handa H. & Yamashita J. (1985) *Surg. Neurol.*, **24**, 275.

Olive I. & Svien H. J. (1957) *J. Neurosurg.*, **14**, 484.

Olivecrona H. (1950) *J. Neurol. Neurosurg. Psychiat.*, **13**, 271.

Olivecrona H. (1967) *J. Neurosurg.*, **26**, 1.

Panse R. (1904) *Archiv. Ohrenhk.*, **41**, 251.

Pennybacker J. & Cairns H. (1950) *J. Neurol. Neurosurg. Psychiat.*, **13**, 272.

Pluchino F., Crivelli G. & Vaghi M. A. (1975) *Acta Neurochir.*, **31**, 201.

Rand R. W. & Kurze T. L. (1965) *J. Neurol. Neurosurg. Psychiat.*, **28**, 311.

Revilla A. G. (1947) *Bull. John Hopk. Hosp.*, **83**, 187.

Rembold F. & Tönnis W. (1956) *Dtsch. Z. Nervenheilk.*, **175**, 329.

Robb-Smith A. H. T. & Pennybacker J. (1952) In *The British Encyclopaedia of Medical Practice*, ed. Lord Horder, vol 10 p. 549.

Russell D. S. & Rubinstein L. J. (1977) *Pathology of Tumours of the Nervous System*, 4th edition. Arnold, London.

Scanlan R. L. (1964) *Arch. Otolaryngol.*, **80**, 698.

Schisano G. & Olivecrona H. (1960) *J. Neurosurg.*, **17**, 306.

Scott P. (1938) *Proc. roy. Soc. Med.*, **31**, 1417.

Shephard R. H. & Wadia N. H. (1956) *Brain*, **79**, 282.

Stewart T. G. & Holmes G. (1904) *Brain*, **27**, 522.

Twining E. W. (1939) *Brit. J. Radiol.*, **12**, 569.

Valavanis A., Dabir K., Hamdi R., Oguz M. & Wellaver J. (1982) *Neuroradiology*, **23**, 7.

Wanxing C. (1981) *J. Neurosurg.*, **54**, 268.

Yaşargil M. G., Smith R. D. & Gasser J. C. (1977) In Krayenbühl H., (ed.) *Advances and Technical Standards in Neurosurgery*, Vol 4, pp. 93–129. Springer-Verlag, Wien and New York.

Yonas H. & Jannetta P. J. (1980) *Neurosurgery*, **6**, 3, 273.

Young I. R., Bydder G. M., Hall A. S., *et al.* (1983) *Amer. J. Neuroradiol.*, **4**, 223.

# Chapter 9
# The pituitary adenomas and craniopharyngioma

R. V. JEFFREYS

## Pituitary adenomas

### Introduction

The story of tumours of the pituitary gland may be said to have started when Marie (1886) described in detail 'deux cas d'acromegalie: hypertrophie singuliere non congenitale des extremities, inferieures et cephalique'. He proposed the name because he considered the enlargement of the extremities to be the initial phenomenon and the most characteristic trait. He found a few examples in the literature, the first being reported by Saucerotte to the Academie de Chirurgie in 1772. He refers to the case described by Henrot in 1887 in which at post-mortem examination a tumour 42 × 30 mm replaced the pituitary body; it was bounded in front by the optic chiasm which was flattened to a ribbon 1–2 mm thick. Marie made no special reference to these findings and admitted that the cause of acromegaly was unknown. Minkowski (1887) noted visual failure in a case of acromegaly and described alterations in the visual fields corresponding to bitemporal upper quadrantic defects. Since enlargement of the hypophysis had been found *post mortem* in other cases, he interpreted the visual failure in his case as the result of chiasmal compression by pituitary enlargement. This is probably the first recorded example of the diagnosis of a pituitary tumour by detecting a chiasmal syndrome. Minkowski considered the hypophyseal mass to be significant in the genesis of acromegaly. Several years later Marie and Marinesco (1891) published the results of histological examination of the various tissues and organs in acromegaly, and used the phrase 'l'hypertrophie constante de la glande pituitaire'

though its role remained unknown. It is of historical interest to note that in this paper the term 'pituitary gland' is employed, whereas in his previous paper Marie only wrote of the 'pituitary body', a change which perhaps reflects the evolution of an idea. That a mass in or compressing the pituitary gland was not necessarily associated with acromegaly and indeed might cause other systemic disturbances was noted by Babinski (1900). For ten years he observed a young girl of average height but who displayed obesity and genital infantilism; she never menstruated and she suffered from headaches, failing vision and epilepsy. Post-mortem examination revealed compression of the optic chiasm by a massive tumour occupying the pituitary fossa and indenting the brain; as a result of histological examination it was designated an epithelioma of the pituitary gland. Doubtless it would now be called a craniopharyngioma. Cushing encountered his 'earliest certified case of hypophyseal disease' in 1901, characterized by obesity and infantilism, in which post-mortem examination revealed a teratoma involving the pituitary gland and third ventricle (case III in *The Pituitary Body*, 1912). This encounter was, by strange coincidence, contemporaneous with the important contribution by Frohlich (1901) which he had not seen. X-ray examination of the skull, first practised by Oppenheim in 1899, was a new stimulus to clinical investigation at this time. Not only did Cushing attract patients in sufficient numbers to acquire a great personal experience, but he instituted a series of experiments in animals to determine the effects of hypophysectomy. He perceived the importance to the neurosurgeon of a critical examination of the visual fields, in which he became particularly interested. Jefferson (1940) wrote 'I have therefore given the chief credit to Cushing for the chromophobe picture because no one before 1912 had seen the problem so clearly or had had so much experience'. The year 1912 marked the publication of Cushing's monograph *The Pituitary Body and its Disorders*. The main patterns of disorder, neighbourhood and systemic, were identified and the monograph remains a superb achievement of clinical observation, experimental research and industry. Cushing's mortality for operations on the pituitary gland during this last ten years was 2.4% (Henderson 1939).

The last fifteen years have witnessed major advances in the diagnosis and management of pituitary tumours, and these will be discussed in the appropriate sections. However, at this stage it is pertinent to introduce some of them. The major endocrinological advance has been the introduction into routine clinical practice of assessment of circulating blood levels of the anterior pituitary hormones by radio-immunassay (RIA). This allows the clinician the facility not only of accurate pretreatment diagnosis, but also allows the facility of assessing endocrinological progress or otherwise. Anatomical diagnosis has been greatly advanced by the introduction of computerized tomography (CT) which not only delineates the size and extent of an adenoma but in the majority of cases is the only specialized radiological study that is necessary.

There have also been major therapeutic advances, both medical and surgical. On the one hand the introduction of pharmacological agents antagonistic to overproduction of certain of the anterior pituitary hormones (for example Bromocriptine) and on the other hand improved replacement hormones for deficiencies in the production of anterior pituitary hormones have proved of great value in controlling the endocrinological status of patients. The most important surgical advances have been the introduction of the operating microscope and intraoperative fluoroscopy which have added a new dimension to both the subfrontal and transsphenoidal operations.

Such advances have helped to produce an exciting era in the diagnosis, management and understanding of pituitary adenomas such that the surgeon can aim at, though not always achieve, leaving a patient without an adenoma but with normal pituitary function.

**Morbid anatomy**

Pituitary adenomas cause symptoms in two main ways: endocrine effects and pressure on adjacent structures. In general the effects of endocrine changes, in particular hypersecretion, tend to occur early when an adenoma is small. As a result of early surgical exploration the topographical distribution of hypersecretory microadenomas (less than 10 mm in diameter) has been assessed by Hardy (1979) (Fig. 9.1). Histochemical and immunofluorescent studies have further confirmed the same localization of these pools of cells in normal pituitary gland. Therefore it would seem that hypersecretory adenomas arise in these areas, enlarge and start to compress

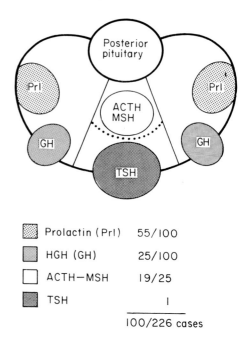

| | Prolactin (Prl) | 55/100 |
| | HGH (GH) | 25/100 |
| | ACTH—MSH | 19/25 |
| | TSH | 1 |
| | | ——— |
| | | 100/226 cases |

**Fig. 9.1.** Position of hypersecretory microadenomas (smaller than 10 mm diameter). After Hardy 1979.

the rest of the gland, though the mechanism that initiates this process is not known. The mode of origin of nonsecretory adenomas (functionless or chromophobe) is far less certain, though recently it has been suggested (Klibanski *et al.* 1983) that these are in fact hypersecretory adenomas producing only a part of the appropriate hormone (the alpha subunit) which is biologically inert.

As an adenoma enlarges it displaces the pituitary gland to form an eccentrically placed mass at the periphery; not infrequently the surgeon encounters such a remnant immediately under the attachment of the pituitary stalk and should be alert for this. It is recognizable by its creamy white colour, in contradistinction to the red purple colour of the gland. Expansion of the adenoma leads to pressure resorption of the bone of the fossa particularly in a downward direction. Lateral expansion broadens the fossa, the medial wall of each cavernous sinus bulges and in turn displaces the internal carotid arteries laterally. Backward pressure erodes the dorsum sellae, which in large adenomas inclines backwards or may be radiologically invisible. The pituitary capsule is a separate covering of the developing adenohypophysis and not a derivative of either the dura mater or pia-arachnoid (Chi & Lee 1980). Previously it was supposed that the diaphragma sellae isolated the pituitary fossa within the skull except for the passage of the pituitary stalk through a small opening. However, in 10% of 250 cases at post-mortem, without recognized pituitary disease, the structure was too thin to serve as a reliable barrier (Bergland *et al.* 1968). This may explain why some adenomas erupt early out of the fossa and into the cranial cavity without enlarging the fossa first. However, in the majority of cases the diaphragma sellae is elevated and remains as a thin covering over the adenoma. The pituitary stalk usually lies behind the dome of the adenoma, in the midline or displaced to one side.

Elevation of the dome of the adenoma above the plane of the clinoid processes brings it eventually into contact with the optic chiasm. The degree of elevation required depends upon the individual position of the chiasm. From a study of air-encephalograms in patients without pituitary disease Bull (1956) found the chiasm to lie 10–13 mm above a line drawn through the nasion and the tuberculum sellae in 58% of films examined. The extremes were 4 mm and 17 mm. Jefferson (1940) considered that the dome must extend 10–20 mm above the normal limit of the diaphragma before seriously implicating the chiasm. The optic chiasm varies not only in its height above the sella, but also in its relationship to the dorsum in an anterioposterior direction. The dissections of Schaeffer (1924) showed that in about 90% of individuals the anterior edge of the chiasm lies approximately in the same coronal plane as the dorsum sellae. In about 5% the optic nerves are so short that the chiasm lies anterior to the dorsum, *prefixed*; in the other 5% optic nerves are long and the chiasm lies on a plane posterior to the dorsum, *postfixed*. In his radiological study Bull estimated lengths of the optic nerves: in rather more than half they were 15–18 mm, and extremes were 10 and 23 mm. These variations determine the relationship of the optic nerves and chiasm to the expanding adenoma, and account for variations in disturbances of the visual acuity and fields. In the majority of cases much of the adenoma lies anterior to the chiasm which itself is displaced upwards and backwards. The undersurface of the brain comprising the anterior part of the third ventricle and the posterior extremities of the gyri recti are indented by any further expansion of the adenoma (Fig. 9.2). A prefixed chiasm directs the adenoma backwards and it bulges upwards behind the chiasm and indents the floor of the third ventricle (Fig. 9.3). On occasion the adenoma breaks through the stretched capsule. This may occur at any point and when it does the structure immediately adjacent will adhere to the adenoma tissue.

Some adenomas continue to expand well beyond the sella turcica and are often described as large adenomas with 'extrasellar' extensions (*see* Fig. 9.7). There is no arbitrary line of demarcation between an 'average' sized adenoma and one with extrasellar extension; indeed every

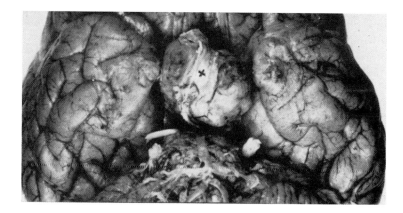

**Fig. 9.2.** indentation of chiasm and undersurface of brain by large suprasellar extension.

adenoma which impinges on the optic apparatus must have some degree of extrasellar extension; but the term is valuable in drawing attention to adenomas which in consequence of their size and extensions present special clinical features and pose difficult problems for treatment. Recently Symon and Jacobowski (1979) proposed the separation of 'giant' adenomas from those with less severe degrees of extrasellar extension. 'Giant' adenomas were selected on the basis of surgical findings and radiological evidence of extrasellar extension more than 40 mm above the planum sphenoidale, or less than 6 mm from the highest point of the adenoma to the foramen of Monro, or multidirectional spread. Such giant adenomas

occurred in 13.6% of cases with extrasellar extensions. The common direction for the adenoma to extend is upwards between the frontal lobes, either symmetrically or off to one side. In cases with a normal or postfixed chiasm the bulk of the adenoma lies anterior to it. Mental retardation, confusion, dementia and epilepsy may so colour the clinical picture that the true diagnosis may not easily emerge. With a prefixed chiasm an upward extension of the adenoma passes behind the chiasm which is displaced upwards and forwards and into the third ventricle which may be completely obliterated. Compression of the tuber cinereum and other hypothalamic structures leads to such disorders

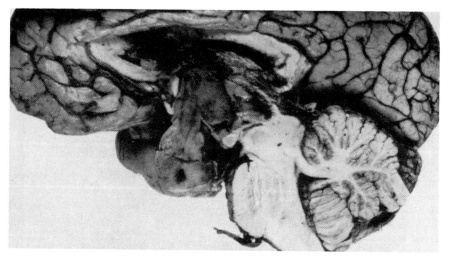

**Fig. 9.3.** Extension into obliteration of third ventricle by large suprasellar extension.

as obesity, diabetes insipidus and hypersomnia. Obstructive hydrocephalus can occur and give rise to raised intracranial pressure, but papilloedema will only occur if the adenoma has not already occluded the leptomeningeal sheath of the optic nerve.

Less commonly the adenoma breaks through its capsule in a lateral direction, usually below the terminal portion of the internal carotid artery (already elevated by the dome of the adenoma) and embeds itself in the medial aspect of the temporal lobe. In its lateral passage it may compress the lateral aspect of the optic tract producing a homonymous hemianopia.

Occasionally the adenoma invades the cavernous sinus on one or both sides and this often leads to multiple ocular palsies and to pain, paraesthesiae and sensory loss in the territory of the trigeminal nerves. The dissections of Trumble (1951) reveal the manner of spread of these adenomas into the cavernous sinus. The medial wall of the cavernous sinus comprises in its upper part the sella turcica and in its lower part the body of the sphenoid. Expansion downwards of the cavity of the sella brings the adenoma into direct relationship with a much more extensive area of cavernous sinus, so that the floor of the sella lies below the siphon of the internal carotid artery. The adenoma now has a broad surface of sinus against which to thrust and to find a weak spot, above or below the artery. Jefferson (1940, 1954) made a particular study of these extrasellar extensions and considered that trigeminal involvement was pathognomic of an invasive adenoma. Evidence that an adenoma has broken through its confining capsule into the cavernous sinus is of great importance for treatment; operation can no longer eradicate it and in that sense it is a malignant, or 'invasive', adenoma: the term that Jefferson later preferred to use since histologically there is no real evidence of malignancy. Scheithauer et al (1986) have documented the rate of invasion of pituitary adenomas of all types to be 35%.

Although not of similar grave significance, extension of the adenoma in a downward direction must be mentioned. Destruction of the anterior and inferior walls of the sella allows the adenoma to herniate into the sphenoidal air sinus. Occasionally, several months after treatment by irradiation, a spontaneous cerebrospinal rhinorrhoea may develop. Even if the floor of the sella remains intact it may become extremely thin, a state of affairs that will be seen and utilized if the transsphenoidal approach is used for direct surgical attack on the adenoma.

The capsule of the adenoma is usually well defined and sufficiently tough to be 'handled' by the surgeon, particularly helpful if the subfrontal approach is used; the exception to this being nodular excrescences where the capsule is deficient. The consistency of adenomas tends to vary with endocrinological type: growth hormone (GH) and prolactin (PRL) producing adenomas tend to be creamy white/yellow in colour and soft in consistency, ACTH producing adenomas vary from red through to white and are often rather rubbery, and nonsecretory adenomas are usually red or purple, often rather vascular and soft. Degeneration leads to necrosis of part of the adenoma; when the surgeon incises the capsule creamy material flows out which might be mistaken for pus. Cystic degeneration occurs in about 10% of large adenomas. The fluid in a cyst is commonly turbid and yellow, but may also be haemorrhagic. Spontaneous haemorrhage into an adenoma occurs in up to 16% of cases (Wakai et al. 1981); the severity of the haemorrhage ranging from headache through to symptoms suggestive of subarachnoid haemorrhage and even on occasions acute chiasmal compression. This latter complication represents a neurosurgical emergency and requires immediate surgical intervention.

### Histology

Pituitary adenomas arise from the cells of the adenohypophysis and reproduce the cell types normally present in that gland. Previously adenomas were classified by the staining reactions of the granules within their cytoplasm to haematoxylin and eosin: eosinophil (acidophil) staining red or orange, basophil staining blue or magenta and chromophobe not staining at all. Early in the history of pituitary histopathology it was found that eosinophil adenomas gave rise to acromegaly, basophil to Cushing disease and chromophobe adenomas were often associated with hypopituitarism. These early attempts to correlate histopathological findings with endocrinological changes paved the way for more recent developments, such as electron microscopy and immunohistochemical staining for individual hormones. Before discussing the various histopathological techniques now available it would perhaps be advantageous to clarify what exactly it is that the neurosurgeon expects from his neuropathological colleague when he sends a specimen to him. The histopathological findings can relate either to an overall view of pituitary adenomas or to a particular case. In the former the findings become part of scientific research into pituitary adenomas. In the latter the neurosurgeon is looking for confirmation as to whether or not the specimen is a pituitary adenoma, the degree of activity both in terms of cell growth and hormone production, and correlation with the pre-operative endocrinological diagnosis. The neuropathologist cannot arrive at a prognosis, since it is only the neurosurgeon who can deduce this by relating the pre-operative radiological findings to the completeness or otherwise of removal of the adenoma.

At the present time there is not only some confusion regarding the classification of an individual adenoma but also differing classifications may be added together; for example an adenoma may be described as a mixed growth hormone producing adenoma; this means that the pre-operative endocrinological tests showed a rise in growth hormone and that on H&E staining there were both eosinophilic and chromophobe cells and the immunostaining showed growth hormone in the granules of the adenoma cells. For this reason the techniques available to the neuropathologist will be described first, and a functional hormonal classification follows.

*Histopathological techniques*

1  *Conventional sections.*  The fresh adenoma tissue is fixed in formalin, embedded in paraffin wax, microtomed and stained with haematoxylin and eosin (H&E) or more complex stains such as Mallory's acid fuchsin–anilin blue, Slidder's orange fuchsin–green or Herlant's tetrachrome (*see* Plates 7–14). All these stains have the merit of colouring the nuclei and granules of the cells and demonstrating the architecture of the adenoma. The cells of adenomas may be arranged in two patterns: diffuse and sinusoidal. In the diffuse pattern, which is more common, the cells are arranged in solid sheets, groups or clusters of uniform polygonal cells separated by a vascular stroma. Their nuclei are round and centrally placed, their cytoplasm will be clear in the case of chromophobic adenomas and may contain a varying number of coloured granules in the case of hypersecretory adenomas. In the sinusoidal pattern there will be festoons of cells draped around the blood vessels and lining narrow cleft-like spaces.

Adenomas, particularly large ones, may undergo a variety of changes: necrosis, haemorrhage and cyst formation being the common ones. Small areas of calcification may also be found. Mitoses are seen only occasionally, even in 'invasive' adenomas. True malignant carcinomas are exceedingly rare and differ from benign adenomas in their nuclear pleomorphism, presence of mitoses, evidence of true invasiveness of other surrounding structures and of distant metastases.

2  *Electron microscopy.*  Specimens require rapid fixation in either osmium tetroxide or glutaraldehyde and are then treated with a variety of techniques (Landolt 1975), the complexities of which are beyond the scope of this book. A great deal of information has accrued over the years from a study of the ultrastructure of the cells of both the normal pituitary gland and of pituitary adenomas, but perhaps the most useful information to the neurosurgeon relates to the secretory process, which is similar in all pituitary cells. The different hormones are synthesized in

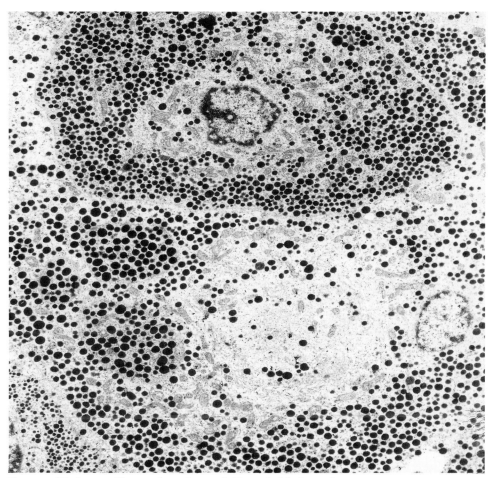

**Fig. 9.4.**   GH adenoma. Electron photomicrograph. Two cells full of granules.

the cisterns of the endoplasmic reticulum and transported to the Golgi cisterns where they are condensed and packed into vesicles forming the granules which grow by fusion and ripen beneath the cell membrane before extrusion takes place (Landolt 1975) (Fig. 9.4). There is general agreement that adenomas associated with hypersecretion contain granules, but in the case of nonsecretory adenomas the findings have not been so uniform. Landolt (1975) found that most of these adenomas showed evidence of secretory processes (including granule formation) whereas Jeffreys and Buxton (1984) found this to be the case in only 30% (Fig. 9.5).

  3   *Hormone staining.*   All six hormones of the

anterior pituitary can be looked for in sections of adenoma. The sections are prepared in the same way as for convential microscopy until the stage of staining. Only one hormone may be stained on each section. The method used is an immunological one in which antiserum to the specific hormone (raised in an experimental animal, usually a rabbit) is added to the section. The attached rabbit protein is then identified by another antiserum and this reaction is identified by the peroxidase–antiperoxidase method and finally stained with either aminoethylcarbazole or diaminobenzidine tetrahydrochloride. Thus any cell which contained the appropriate hormone at the time of fixation can be identified.

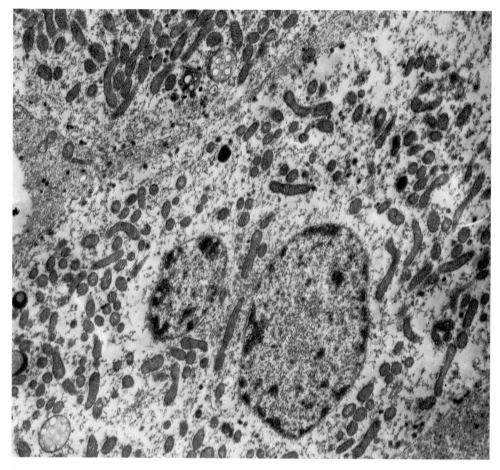

**Fig. 9.5.** Nonsecretory adenoma. Electron photomicrograph. One cell full of mitochondria but only very occasional granules.

This method has confirmed that within the normal pituitary gland there exist pools of cells producing a specific hormone in the same locality as hypersecretory adenomas found at surgery (Hardy 1979). There is however one major problem; not every adenoma associated with a raised blood level of a particular hormone necessarily stains for that hormone on sections (for example Jeffreys & Buxton found that only 50% of adenomas producing acromegaly stained for growth hormone). This may be due to a histological technical error though this is now thought to be unlikely, and Landolt has suggested that as the neurosurgeon manipulates the adenoma 'hormonal diarrhoea' takes place in which there is a sudden discharge of the hormone from the granules into the blood stream. Be that as it may there is no doubt that this method had produced a great deal of new information, some of which will be referred to later (*see* Symptoms and signs, *below*).

## Symptoms and signs

The manifestations of a pituitary adenoma are caused by the space-occupying effects upon surrounding structures and/or disturbances of endocrine function. Since the accompanying endocrine disturbances of nonsecretory adenomas are often very insidious and not apparent to patients it is common for them to present late with disturbances of vision and other space-occupying effects. On the other hand the endocrine disturbances of hypersecretory adenomas are more obvious such that patients tend to present earlier when the adenoma is quite small and confined to the sella.

*Endocrine disturbance*

1   *Acromegaly.* Pierre Marie (1886) was responsible for establishing the clinical and pathological changes and for inventing the term acromegaly. Cushing (1912) stated that Marie attributed it to 'diminution' of pituitary function, though he later wrote to Cushing that it was perhaps less a question of 'quantity' of secretion and more one of 'modification'. When Cushing published his monograph *The Pituitary Body and its Disorders*, the view that acromegaly was due to hypersecretion of the eosinophilic cells was relatively recent and was by no means universally accepted; the isolation of a growth factor by Evans and Long in 1921 and the production by Putnam *et al.* (1929) of an acromegalic state in dogs by the injection of this growth factor provided the necessary proof. Now it is fully accepted that acromegaly is exclusively due to overproduction of growth-hormone by either an adenoma or hyperplasia of the pituitary gland.

Fully developed acromegaly is obvious, an appearance unusual even to the layman, though some patients may develop acromegaly so insidiously that some years may elapse before they present to a doctor. The changes in bones render the supraciliary ridge prominent; aggravated by enlargement of the frontal sinuses, the facial skeleton becomes heavy. An increase in the size of the mandible causes the chin to project, the lower incisors to occlude in front of the uppers and to become separated. Hands and feet enlarge particularly in their width and the digits become blunt. The skin darkens, coarsens, thickens, enlarges and an excess of subcutaneous tissue throws it into folds; in this hypertrophy the nose,

ears, tongue and scalp may share. The skin is greasy and may sweat excessively and the hair increases and coarsens. The voice becomes hoarse and deepens in pitch because the larynx is involved; 50% of acromegalics have small airway narrowing (Harrison *et al.* 1978) and pulmonary function tests show that most acromegalics have some degree of hypoxaemia. In addition the thorax deepens and osteoporosis can lead to kyphosis which can also have a deleterious effect on pulmonary function. Osteoarthritis is common and many acromegalics experience pain in their joints. Median nerve compression in the carpal tunnel is common. Systemic hypertension may occur and on occasions can be severe. Cardiac hypertrophy has been found to be common and often occurs in patients without clinical evidence of hypertension or without correlation with the presence or severity of hypertension, suggesting that the cardiomegaly is peculiar to acromegaly (Jadresic 1983). There is a high incidence of diabetes mellitus (27% in the experience of Jadresic *et al.* 1982) which can prove refractory to treatment. Klein *et al.* (1982) have found an increased frequency of colonic polyps.

The patient may be unaware of his changed appearance; his special complaints are of headache, lack of energy, physical weakness, musculoskeletal pains and symptoms due to the systemic upsets from hypertension and diabetes mellitus. The usual several years' delay in establishing the diagnosis may contribute to the development of complications. Greene (1951) states unequivocally that the expectation of life is shortened and that death usually occurs from cardio- or cerebrovascular disease or from intercurrent infection, aggravated by diabetes mellitus. A long term review of 194 acromegalic patients by Wright *et al.* (1970) supports this statement and emphasizes the need to treat acromegaly early, and not to await the further development of symptoms.

Acromegaly is the reaction of the adult to hypersecretion of growth hormone. Occasionally a pathological hyperactivity takes place in the child and growth is so active that the child is literally head and shoulders above its contemporaries. A growth chart (which should be recorded when such a diagnosis is under consideration) reveals the curve steadily climbing beyond the norm, though consideration should be paid to the stature of predecessors. After puberty acromegaly become evident. Hypersecretion in the child seems to be disproportionately more intense than in the adult so that the adenoma produces little or no enlargement of the sella and compression of the optic chiasm does not occur. The early diagnosis of gigantism can be difficult and requires expert paediatric endocrinology in order to effect early treatment.

*2  Cushing disease.*  The bodily disturbance which has been given the eponymous title of Cushing syndrome is due to excessive secretion of cortisol. It can come about in one of three ways: firstly, from an adenoma of the pituitary gland producing excess ACTH thereby causing the adrenal glands to secrete excess cortisol (often now called Cushing disease); secondly, from an adenoma or carcinoma of the adrenal gland; thirdly, from some malignant neoplasms elsewhere in the body (for example carcinoma of the bronchus) producing ectopic ACTH thereby stimulating otherwise normal adrenal glands. Cushing (1932) became interested in the condition and, finding a basophil adenoma of the pituitary gland in some patients, considered that the disorder was due to an abnormal influence of the basophil cells and called the disease basophilism.

The disease may affect children or adults and when fully developed the physical appearances are striking. The onset is insidious though usually more rapid than acromegaly. Obesity is nearly always present though not normally severe; its rapid development may cause the skin to be thin and fragile and purple striae appear around the trunk. Subcutaneous fat is deposited particularly on the face, neck, cervicothoracic junction and trunk. The skin becomes a characteristic plum or purple colour, most marked in the face. The discoloration is due to vaso-dilatation and stasis, and spontaneous bruising may

occur. The skin is greasy, acne is common and facial hair excessive most noticeably in women. Fatigue and physical weakness can occur; concomitant with these are wasting and flaccidity of muscles which is due to a myopathy. Osteoporosis occurs commonly and can be so severe that spontaneous fracturing of vertebrae and long bones leads to further deformities. Systemic hypertension is common and occasionally can be severe. Severe psychiatric disorders may arise during the illness and occurred in more than one-quarter of the patients seen by Mason (1971). Virtually all the psychiatric disorders are of the affective type, the majority being depressive (Cohen 1982). Untreated, Cushing disease is fatal; the mortality rate is four times that of the general population matched for sex and age (Ross & Lynch 1982).

Some patients with Cushing disease have been treated by bilateral adrenalectomy and skin pigmentation is common in such patients. Of more serious import is the development of a secondary pituitary adenoma which can be aggressive in both its rate of growth and invasion of surrounding structures (Nelson syndrome, first described in detail by Nelson *et al.* 1960). The incidence of such a problem varies from 9% (Ernest & Ekman 1972) to 30% (Besser *et al.* 1972). In such patients the serum level of ACTH is high and there is a tendency for patients with larger pituitary fossae to have the higher levels of ACTH (Besser *et al.* 1972).

*3  Prolactinoma.*  A pituitary adenoma may cause excessive prolactin secretion by two different mechanisms: thus it may interfere with the normal hypothalamic inhibition of prolactin secretion by distortion of the pituitary stalk and/or hypothalamus, and it is not alone in this, since raised serum prolactin has been found in patients with craniopharyngiomas (Frantz *et al.* 1972) and meningiomas in the supra- and parasellar regions (Lundberg *et al.* 1981). On the other hand, the cells of a pituitary adenoma may be the source of the excess prolactin, and it is now common practice to refer to such adenomas as prolactinomas. These tumours may be small (less than 1 cm) or larger but confined to the sella, or they may be very large with a supra or lateral extrasellar extension. A significant number of patients with acromegaly have been found to have a raised serum prolactin as well as having demonstrable prolactin on immunostaining of the adenoma. In such cases it is still customary to refer to the diagnosis as acromegaly. The term prolactinoma is reserved for a pituitary adenoma exclusively secreting excess amounts of prolactin. In the past (before RIA of prolactin became commonplace), it is likely that a number of nonsecretory adenomas causing anterior hypopituitarism and diagnosed as chromophobe adenomas were in reality prolactinomas.

Hyperprolactinaemia leads to hypogonadism in both sexes and may also cause galactorrhoea in women. Amenorrhoea and infertility occur in women, such that it is standard practice in infertility clinics to estimate the serum prolactin. In men the presenting endocrinological symptom is impotence. However it must be appreciated that there are a number of drugs which can raise the serum prolactin: phenothiazines, methyl-dopa, oestrogens and many others (Thorner & Besser 1978). It is vital in such patients that an enquiry is made of any possible medication.

4 *Hypopituitarism.* Severe failure of all the hormones secreted by the adenohypophysis gives rise to a dramatic clinical picture first described by Simmonds (1914) and later studied by Sheehan and Summers (1949). Destruction of the gland to this degree is usually the result of shock, as for example in postpartum haemorrhage; the infarct is comparable to that produced by hypophyseal stalk section and is due to failure of circulation in the portal vessels (Daniel 1963) as a result of low blood pressure. The advanced degree of panhypopituitarism which characterizes Simmonds disease is only rarely caused by a pituitary adenoma. Although pituitary hypofunction is present, in most cases, by the time that vision becomes affected, a superficial examination may easily fail to detect it. All the endocrine secretions are not equally depressed and as Hubble (1952) has described it

there is a selective failure comparable to Franklin's 'order of sacrifice' (1951). Fraser (1970) puts the order of susceptibility to ischaemia and other insults as follows: GH, FSH & LH, ACTH, TSH.

In nonsecretory adenomas the commonest and earliest sign of hypofunction is amenorrhoea; if the adenoma arises after the menopause this piece of evidence is missing. In men failure of libido and potency occur but cannot be so accurately dated as can amenorrhoea in women. Examination of the testes reveals atrophy. Although the secretion of growth hormone is highly susceptible to the adverse affects of compression of the pituitary gland, stunted growth is not often encountered because nonsecretory adenomas are rare during childhood and adolescence (which is in sharp contrast to craniopharyngioma).

Exposed skin is pallid or sallow in colour, and soft or scaly in texture. Hair is thinned or lost from the eyebrows, axillae, pubes and trunk. Men often find that they need to shave only two or three times a week to appear respectable. In men particularly the pallor and smoothness of the skin and the rounding of the contours tends to produce a somewhat youthful appearance. Clinical hypothyroidism is manifested by physical sluggishness, a preference for warmth and a dislike of cold. In severe cases there may be frank myxoedema with subnormal body temperature and torpor. Depression of adrenocortical function is seldom clinically overt and symptoms develop insidiously. Lack of energy, undue fatiguability, muscular weakness and low blood pressure are among the more common symptoms. Acute failure may be precipitated by intercurrent infections, in which case patients become acutely ill with vomiting, poor tissue perfusion and confusion which can deteriorate to altered levels of consciousness. Jefferson (1957), in tracing a series of patients with non-secretory pituitary adenomas and craniopharyngiomas who had eventually died, found that in nearly one-half death seemed to have been due to secondary adrenal failure.

5 *Excess TSH and gonadotrophin secretion.*

Considering that there are six hormones secreted by the anterior part of the pituitary gland it is remarkable that only three types of adenoma with hypersecretion occur commonly (GH, ACTH and PRL). However, cases of hypersecretion of the other three hormones are being reported. TSH-producing adenomas that cause a pituitary dependent hyperthyroidism do occur rarely (Hill *et al.* 1982), such that rigid critieria for their diagnosis must apply. Benoit *et al.* (1980) suggested five necessary criteria: raised serum T3 and/or T4, raised serum TSH, a pituitary adenoma that shows evidence of TSH on immunostaining, undetectable longacting thyroid immunoglobulins and absence of infiltrative ophthalmopathy.

FSH and LH-producing adenomas are rare, but recently cases have been reported (Trouillas *et al.* 1981). Finally, some 'non-secreting' pituitary adenomas may be producing endocrinologically inactive precusor fragments of hormones.

*Space-occupying affects*

*Symptoms.* *Failure of vision* is the commonest first symptom as an adenoma expands upwards out of the sella. In the early stages it may be no more than a transient indistinctness, later progressing to a permanent impairment of vision. One eye may be affected alone, or before the other. The description of a greyness or a shadow interrupting the outer part of the field of view is clearly that of a hemianopia. At times vision seems only slightly affected for some months and then abruptly worsens within days. Visual hallucinations, perhaps confined to the more affected eye occasionally occur, described as 'dazzles' or unformed lights, and when associated with pain over that eye may be misinterpreted as migraine. The duration of impaired vision may be as short as a few weeks and in about one-half of patients it is no more than one year. Vision may worsen during pregnancy and improve after parturition.

*Headache* is not a common and rarely a severe symptom in patients with a nonsecretory adenoma; it may be frontal or bitemporal and may be localized above one eye, usually the one with the worse vision. Headache is more common in acromegaly and may be sufficiently severe to drive a patient to seek advice without there being visual symptoms. It is often of many years duration. In Cushing's 67 cases of acromegaly (Henderson 1939) headache was severe in 55, in 13 of whom vision was unaffected. No satisfactory explanation has been offered for the discrepancy of the severity of headache in acromegaly and nonsecretory adenomas, though it may relate to the expansion of the facial skeleton and forehead in acromegaly. Pain in the face, usually in the ophthalmic division of the trigeminal nerve, is an occasional complaint; the symptom should be distinguished from headache, for it may betoken spread of the adenoma into the cavernous sinus.

*Diplopia*, usually transient, occurs in about one-quarter of patients with large adenomas (Wise *et al.* 1955) but examination reveals a weakness of the ocular muscles in only a few. The following explanation for diplopia without muscle weakness is offered by Lyle (1961): as bitemporal hemianopia develops the width of the area of the superimposed visual field in which stereoscopic vision is still available steadily narrows; in order to widen this limited stereoscopic field the eyes diverge, thus interfering with the normal register of the images on the two retinae.

*Mental symptoms* of considerable diversity and degree may develop over a period of several years. They are frequently insidious and the patient may not connect them with visual symptoms; they may be obvious to relatives and colleagues and not to the patient. Undue fatigue, lack of interest and of drive and a general slowing of mental and physical activities are common; the relief of these symptoms after treatment impresses the patient if he is able to recall his earlier state. Failing memory, deterioration of personality and frank dementia passing into bouts of confusion and stupor are the more severe effects of large adenomas.

*Epilepsy* suggests a large adenoma extending

into the frontal or temporal lobes of the brain. The seizures often have no other localizing value.

*Signs.* *Primary optic atrophy* is present in the majority of patients who have an adenoma which affects vision. The optic disc is pale, paper-white in advanced cases, sharply defined and with a deep cup in which the lamina cribrosa is often clearly seen. The degree of atrophy usually corresponds with the severity of loss of vision and the length of history. Occasionally, however, vision may be severely affected and yet the optic discs appear normal. McConnell and Mooney (1938) found that this occurs if the adenoma is retrochiasmal, when they may be little or no direct pressure upon the optic nerves and chiasm. The visual acuity of each eye, with and without correcting lens, should be tested with Snellen types.

*Visual field* examination is of the greatest importance; every neurosurgeon should learn and practise the technique so that he can plot visual fields accurately. His knowledge of pituitary adenomas, his study of the patient and the radiological examinations particularly qualifies him to appreciate the significance of the deformations of the visual fields. The techniques are described fully in Traquair (Scott 1957) and by Hughes (1954). The peripheral field is examined on a perimeter with a 10 mm white object. Each field is examined on either the Bjerrum or Friedman screen. If visual acuity is badly affected large test objects will be necessary. Of particular importance is the detection and plotting of scotomas. The blind spot is a physiological scotoma corresponding to the optic nerve head and it enlarges with the swelling of the nerve head due to papilloedema. Pathological scotomas may be central, occupying the area of fixation or macular vision, or paracentral. The shape of the scotoma may be circular or irregular arcuate, comma-like and eccentric. The scotomas due to chiasmal and optic nerve compression are usually central or paracentral and may occupy part of a field with a clear cut vertical or horizontal edge, thus qualifying for the description of hemianopic or quadrantanopic scotoma. They

may present in the field of one or both eyes, and be homonymous or heteronymous. Careless examination is unlikely to detect a small scotoma and a large hemianopic scotoma can be mistaken for a total field defect because of the failure to detect the narrow rim of field skirting and outlining the peripheral field of the scotoma. If the patient's complaint of failing vision is confirmed by the detection of a poor acuity in either eye and if this cannot be improved by correcting a refractive error and there is no intraocular cause, then a central scotoma is almost certain to be present and every effort should be made to display it.

The disturbances of the visual fields produced by pituitary adenomas conform to two general patterns. They may be hemianopic or scotomatous. Scotomas may affect one or both eyes, to the same or dissimilar degrees; central and circular or with a sharp vertical margin passing through or just skirting the fixation area. Hemianopias may be partial (quadrantic) or complete, bitemporal (heteronymous) or homonymous, and symmetrical though commonly more advanced in one eye (Fig. 9.6 a–h).

*Bitemporal hemianopia* is the commonest pattern, occurring in 65% of Cushing's cases (Henderson 1939). The defect involves the superior temporal quadrants at first and progresses until only each nasal field remains, sharply demarcated by the vertical meridian through the fixation point. Excessive growth of an adenoma to one side may also jeopardize the optic nerve on the side, vision in that eye being completely lost.

*Homonymous hemianopia* occurred in 10% of Cushing's cases. Its presence should lead to the suspicion of a temporal lobe extension of the adenoma, though pressure of the adenoma on the lateral aspect of the chiasm or optic tract will also cause it. Henderson (1939), commenting on Cushing's cases, stated that in the case of an adenoma extending into the temporal lobe the homonymous defects were usually incomplete (quadrantic), whereas if the adenoma compressed the optic nerve and/or tract vision in the eye on that side was severely affected.

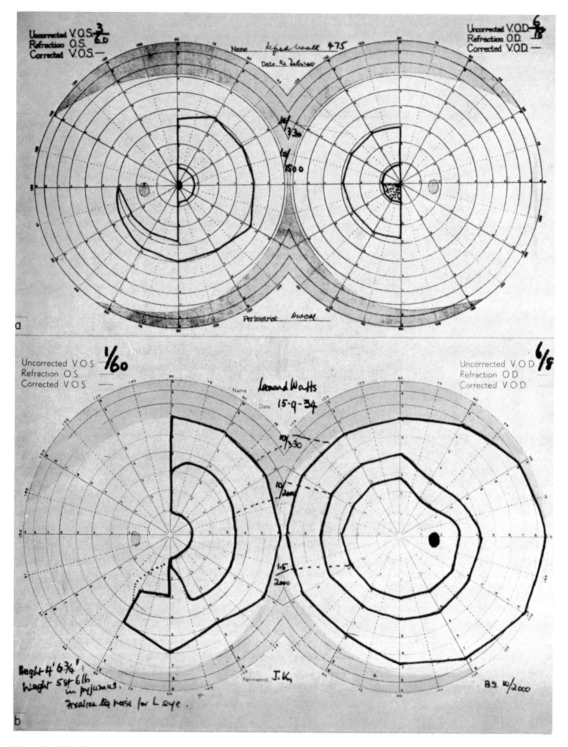

**Fig. 9.6.** (a)–(h) Examples of visual field deficits due to pituitary adenomas with suprasellar extensions.

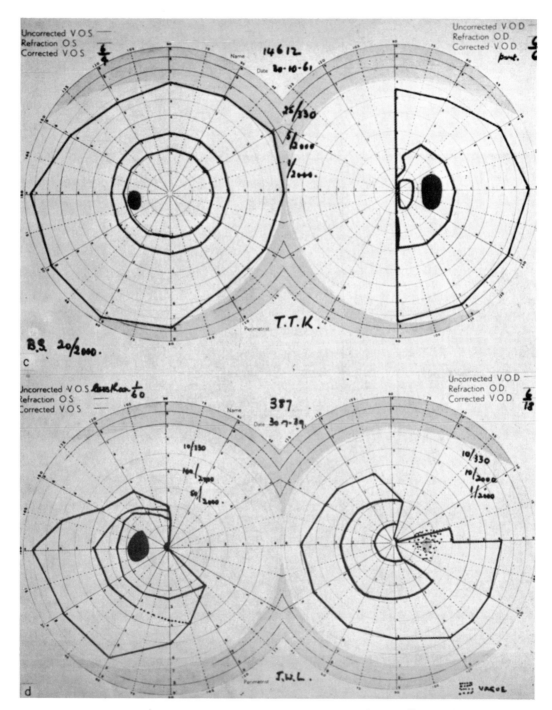

**Fig. 9.6.** (a)–(h) Examples of visual field deficits due to pituitary adenomas with suprasellar extensions.

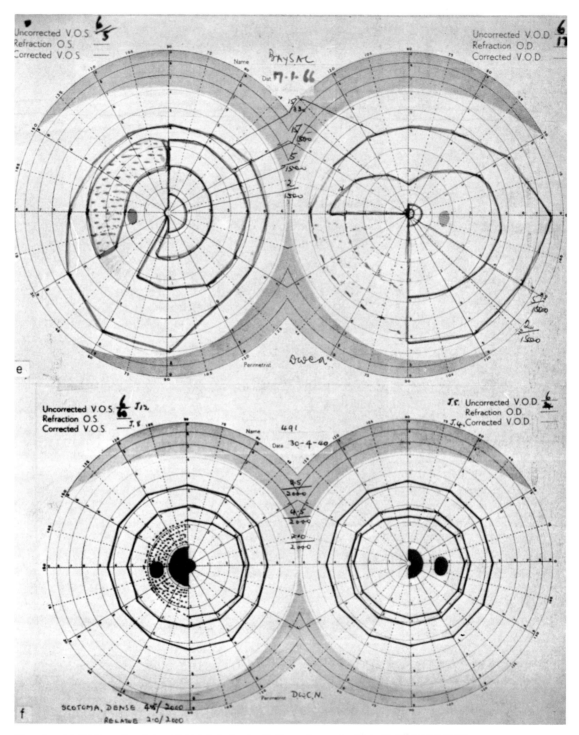

**Fig. 9.6.** (a)–(h) Examples of visual field deficits due to pituitary adenomas with suprasellar extensions.

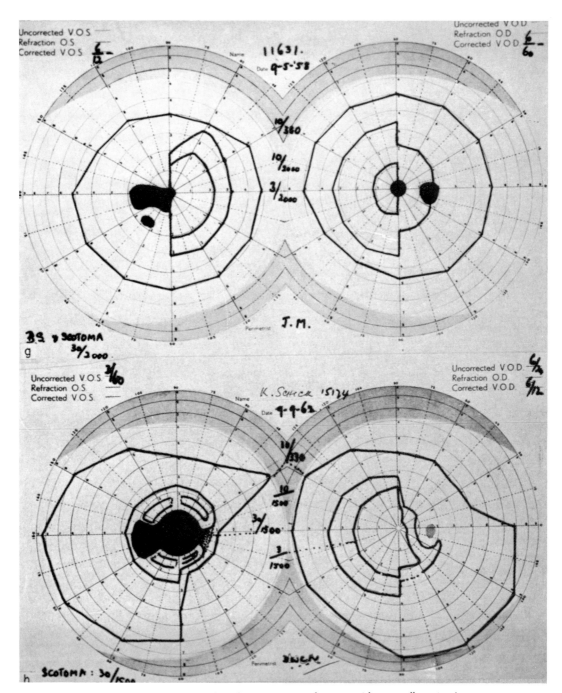

**Fig. 9.6.** (a)–(h) Examples of visual field deficits due to pituitary adenomas with suprasellar extensions.

*Scotoma* was found in one or both eyes in 6% of Cushing's cases. It was Cushing's view that bilateral central scotomas were more common with retrochiasmal adenomas and Henderson points out that this relationship is likely to occur with a prefixed chiasm. He also makes the point that in these patients there may be little or no pallor of the discs. Bitemporal (and unitemporal) scotomas of hemianopic shape are fairly common, and because the macular portion of the field is only bisected, do not interfere much with acuity, though they may make it difficult for the right eye to scan the line of letters from left to right. It is easy to fail to find such scotomas but their presence is as pathognomonic of a chiasmal lesion as a bitemporal hemianopia; as long ago as 1897 Nettleship described central scotoma as an early symptom of chiasmal compression.

*Loss of vision* is one eye may be apparently complete, though careful testing with a large object may reveal a residual rim of vision in the periphery of the field. Discovery of such a small residuum is important for it will reveal whether the pattern is heteronymous or homonymous, the significance of which has already been emphasized.

*Papilloedema* is a rare accompaniment of a pituitary adenoma, occurring in 2 cases of 314 reported from the Mayo Clinic (Love 1952). That it happens so rarely is presumably due to the regularity with which the enlarging adenoma engages the optic nerves and obliterates their arachnoid sheaths. Papilloedema may be due to an extension which has emerged from the sella by a narrow stalk, thereby sparing to some extent the optic nerves, to form a large intracerebral mass. Of the 14 cases of cavernous sinus extension described by Jefferson (1955) papilloedema was present in four; this he ascribed to blockage of the sinus.

*Ocular palsies* occur in about 10% of patients and they are generally considered to be evidence of involvement of the cavernous sinus. The third nerve is the most commonly affected, in 23 of Jefferson's 312 pituitary adenomas. Cairns (1938) was of the opinion that the nerve was compressed by the adenoma against the interclinoid ligament. An isolated third nerve palsy cannot be considered incontrovertible evidence of an extension into the cavernous sinus, though involvement of the fourth and sixth nerves makes it very probable. The ophthalmoplegia may be bilateral. Occasionally an ocular palsy is the presenting symptom of a pituitary adenoma (Weinberger *et al.* 1940, Symonds 1962).

*Trigeminal nerve* disturbance may be evidenced by facial pain; the ophthalmic division is most commonly affected. Careful examination may reveal impairment of cutaneous sensibility, in which event Jefferson considered that the adenoma had indubitably invaded the cavernous sinus.

*Mental changes* have been mentioned above. In the majority of patients there is no evidence of disturbance of mental faculties. In large adenomas, tests may reveal in some a loss of the power of concentration and slowing of activity. In more advanced cases, usually with hydrocephalus, there is an obvious memory defect, impairment of intellect and even frank dementia.

*Pituitary apoplexy*

Spontaneous haemorrhage may occur from pituitary adenomas (particularly nonsecretory and acromegaly) giving rise to a misleading clinical picture. In its most severe form, the illness is characterized by sudden severe headache, often followed by transient or more prolonged loss of consciousness, vomiting, neck stiffness and positive Kernig's sign; there may be fever. The condition is thus similar to spontaneous subarachnoid haemorrhage from a ruptured intracranial aneurysm, and a lumbar puncture should be performed in order to sample the cerbrospinal fluid. Paralysis of one or more of the ocular nerves is often bilateral. Commonly there is a sudden deterioration of vision ranging from amaurosis to more minor disturbances of visual acuity and fields. An accurate history from the relatives, the physical signs of endocrinological change and radiological changes in the sella should suggest the diagnosis, though angiography may still be necessary to exclude an aneurysm. Small haemorrhages are frequent, for traces of such, sometimes of different ages, within an adenoma are often encountered by the surgeon. Some of these may have been asymtomatic to the patient, though in others they may account for unexplained sudden headache or minor sudden changes in visual function. In severe cases the haemorrhage not only causes acute distension of the adenoma, but it may precipitate acute adrenocorticosteroid failure due to sudden extra pressure on the remnants of the pituitary gland or on its stalk.

The incidence of this complication varies in the reported literature from 1.5% to 27.7%; however, recently Wakai *et al.* (1981) in a review of 560 cases all undergoing surgery found an incidence of 16.6%: 7.5% were clinically asymtomatic and the evidence for previous haemorrhage came at surgery, but 6.8% had major disturbances of the type described above and 2.3% experienced more minor symptoms.

The diagnosis of such problems has been considerably eased by CT scanning since this technique will not only demonstrate the pituitary adenoma but in many cases will also detect the haemorrhage or cysts remaining from previous haemorrhage. The initial management should consist of supporting the pituitary or adreno-cortical axis with hydrocortisone; large swellings or haematomas causing major neurological disturbance will require urgent surgical decompression. In the case of more minor disturbances it is better to wait, though careful and sequential observation of vision will be necessary.

### Differential diagnosis

As discussed earlier, patients with pituitary adenomas present with space-occupying and/or endocrinological effects. The differential diagnoses of endocrinological symptoms are beyond the scope of this book, and lie within the compass of an endocrinologist with whom it is essential that a neurosurgeon collaborates. The great majority of patients that have a neurological deficit, present with defective vision. Investigations in most cases reveal the correct diagnosis, but their choice can be made more intelligently and their number limited to the most useful, if the likely alternative diagnoses have been considered.

The *chiasmal syndrome*, a term which embraces those patterns of abnormality of the visual fields which indicate a lesion of the optic chiasm, can be produced by a variety of conditions other than pituitary adenoma. When the field defects are bitemporal the cause is likely to be midline, thus limiting the possibilities and a predominance of loss in the upper or lower segments indicates encroachment on the chiasm from below or above respectively. Misleading defects may occur as a result of counter pressure against normal anatomical structures, for example the anterior cerebral arteries. Homonymous haemianopia and asymmetrical visual failure, which in its severest form causes a blind eye, indicate that the mass predominates on one side and thus increases the number of alternatives. Bizarre field defects of rapid or sudden onset, affecting both eyes, suggest other causes. The differential diagnosis of chiasmal compression was the subject of a classical paper by Cushing (1930).

*Craniopharyngioma* is the commonest tumour to mimic a pituitary adenoma and if it arises within the sella the pathological diagnosis may only be established at operation. Age of the patient is important, for its peak incidence is much earlier and delayed growth and sexual maturation are more frequent and more obvious. If craniopharyngioma develops in an adult, hypopituitarism is usually more marked than with a pituitary adenoma and signs of hypothalamic involvement (diabetes insipidus, obesity, hypersomnia) more frequent. Enlargement of the sella may occur but it is with the pituitary adenoma that gross erosion is seen; in the craniopharyngioma the sella is often open and flattened and the dorsum stunted. Calcareous deposits in or above the sella are seen or plain X-ray in half the cases, whereas calcification in a pituitary adenoma is rare.

*Meningiomas* may arise from the tuberculum sellae and indent the chiasm, providing a pattern of visual field defect indistinguishable from that due to a pituitary adenoma. There is no enlargement of the sella but there may be hyperostosis at the point of origin of the tumour. Often there are symptoms and signs of anterior hypopituitarism.

*Glioma* of the optic nerve or chiasm is mostly a disease of children, the average age being 14 years. It is likely to produce bizarre field changes with asymmetry together with reduction of visual acuity. When extensive the neoplasm invades the hypothalamus and third ventricle causing hydrocephalus and disorders of growth. The sella may be enlarged in some cases, though the most characteristic sign is an excavation under the anterior clinoid processes. If the optic nerves are invaded the optic canals may enlarge and proptosis may also be present. About one-third of cases have an associated von Recklinghausen's neurofibromatosis (Oxenhandler & Sayers 1978).

*Aneurysms* of the anterior part of the circle of Willis may reach a size large enough to compress the optic nerves and/or the chiasm. They may arise from the internal carotid artery close to the origin of the ophthalmic artery, or from the anterior communicating complex. In the case of the former the picture is one of asymmetric visual failure as first the ipsilateral optic nerve is compressed and later the chiasm. Structures within the cavernous sinus may be involved, giving rise to ophthalmopareses and to trigeminal pain. The history is usually of episodic or fluctuating visual failure. On occasions the sella may be enlarged, thus rendering the diagnosis more difficult. Aneurysms of the anterior communicating complex may impinge upon the upper surface of the chiasm causing symmetrical bitemporal hemianopia. Anterior hypopituitarism can occur from aneurysms at either site.

*Neoplasms* of the sphenoid (chordoma, sarcoma and carcinoma arising from the sphenoid air sinus) occasionally cause chiasmal compression. Chordoma is of slower growth and ophthalmopareses usually accompany such a neoplasm. The malignant neoplasms are more rapid in evolution, involve neighbouring structures, cause pain and somtimes bloody nasopharyngeal discharge. *Sphenoid sinus mucoceles* present with frontal and orbital pain, visual failure, ophthalmopareses and pre-existing sinusitis (Nugent *et al.* 1970). Since they expand and erode the base of the skull plain X-rays usually reveal their presence.

*Epidermoids* can occur anywhere along the base of the skull and the anterior cranial fossa is no exception. They tend to insinuate around neighbouring structures and lead to problems by distortion rather than compression. Occurring near the midline they may lead to visual failure and minor degrees of anterior hypoputuitarism.

*Empty sella syndrome* was first described by Busch (1951) when he applied it to cases in which the pituitary gland formed only a thin layer of tissue at the bottom or side of a sella which therefore appeared empty apart from cerebrospinal fluid. Obrador (1972) reviewed the syndrome and listed the causative agents, though it would be true to state that considerable debate occurs amongst neurosurgeons both as to the validity of theories of aetiology as well as to treatment. However there is agreement that the syndrome can be divided into two main groups: *primary* when there are no obvious pathological causative factors and *secondary* as a result of either chronically raised intracranial pressure (for example in obstructive hydrocephalus) or subsequent to treatment (either surgery or radiotherapy) of large pituitary adenomas. An empty sella may be associated with cerebrospinal rhinorrhoea and/or visual failure as a result of displacement of the chiasm or hypothalamus into the sella.

*Granulomas* may involve the sellar and parasellar regions. Tuberculomas at these sites can lead to visual failure and anterior hypopituitarism, but there is nearly always evidence of infection elsewhere in the body. Sarcoidosis may affect the structures below the hypothalamus and visual failure and hypopituitarism may result (Harriman 1976). Wegener's granulomatosis involves the triad of respiratory tract, arteries and kidneys with an acute necrotizing arteritis, and the central nervous system can be involved (Drachman 1963). In particular the parasellar region may be affected by direct extension from nasal and paranasal granulomata, such that ophthalmopareses and visual failure will result.

*Pituitary abscess* is a rare phenomenon. By 1977 only 50 cases had been reported (Domingue & Wilson 1977). It can develop rapidly in a normal gland or a pituitary adenoma, and leads to meningitis, visual failure and hypopituitarism. It is a lethal condition unless diagnosed and treated rapidly.

*Acute demyelinating disease* of the optic nerves and chiasm occasionally gives rise to diagnostic difficulty. The failure of vision is usually rapid and may become bilateral; peripheral vision is preserved and the loss of acuity is due to a large central scotoma. Such a problem may mimic a pituitary apoplexy or sudden swelling in a pituitary adenoma, though usually other evidence, often radiological, will make the diagnosis clear.

## Investigations

### Radiology

*Plain X-rays.* Measurements of the sella turcica in normal radiographs reveal considerable variation. The average anteroposterior diameter at the widest point is 11 mm, the average vertical diameter (perpendicular from plane of mouth of sella to its floor) 8 mm, and its coronal diameter (across superior margin of dorsum sellae) 13 mm, according to Di Chiro and Nelson (1962). These authors also emphasize, as others have done, that the pituitary gland occupies but 50–80% of the fossa. The sella also varies in shape, being commonly oval. Enlargement due to an intrasellar adenoma usually causes the fossa to acquire a rounded or ballooned outline and the dorsum sellae a curve concave forwards, compatible with this general shape. The posterior clinoid processes maintain their identity for a long time, though they and in particular the anterior clinoid processes may become sharpened and elevated by the upward drag of the diaphragm sellae. The integrity of the posterior clinoids is important in distinguishing enlargement due to a pituitary adenoma from that due to hydrocephalus, in which the posterior clinoid processes and the dorsum sellae become eroded from above downwards (the clinical distinction may occasionally be difficult because prolonged hydrocephalus can cause hypopituitarism). Further enlargement of the fossa leads to tilting backwards of the dorsum and its gradual destruction, erosion of the floor and extension of the cavity forwards. Massive adenomas remove all trace of the sella, leaving the anterior clinoid processes as overhanging points of bone. The sphenoidal air sinus may contain adenoma and its shadow may encroach upon the contrasting air of the nasopharynx. On occasion the adenoma may expand asymmetrically causing loss of one anterior clinoid process. The floor of the fossa may present a double contour. The capsule of adenoma may occasionally calcify showing as a curvilinear opacity simulating that seen in an aneurysm. Pathological calcification within the substance of an adenoma is very rare, an important point of distinction from a craniopharygioma.

All these radiographical changes can be seen in three X-rays, namely a lateral and posteroanterior skull X-ray and a coned lateral X-ray of the sella. Sella tomography has been advocated by many workers but recently doubts have been expressed as to its value. Hall (1981) feels that the reasons for these doubts are threefold: variations in the normal sella are common, observer variations are appreciable and false positive results are common, such that 22% of normal people, with no clinical evidence of a pituitary adenoma, can show tomographic features suggestive of a small adenoma (microadenoma). In addition, with tomography, there is a not inconsiderable dose of X-irradation to the eyes. For these reasons many workers feel that there is no place for tomography in the investigation of pituitary adenomas, and that the

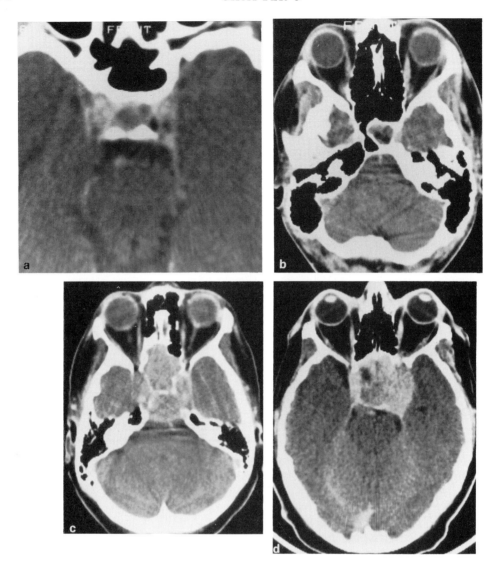

**Fig. 9.7.** Ct scans, all with contrast.
(a) Two micro-adenomas causing excess PRL secretion.
(b) GH adenoma extending downwards into sphenoidal air sinus.
(c) Nonsecretory adenoma eroding planum spenoidale and extending into ethmoidal air cells.
(d) Nonsecretory adenoma extending into right cavernous sinus. A small cyst can also be seen on the left.

three X-rays listed above are more than sufficient in the initial radiological investigations.

*CT scan*  It would be no exaggeration to state that CT scanning has revolutionized the investigation of patients with suspected pituitary adenomas and other sellar and parasellar lesions.

It has the great merit of being noninvasive and harmless to the patient; previously air-encephalography and ventriculography often upset the patient, at times considerably. Moreover these latter techniques could only show a mass lesion, whereas in many cases the CT scan can provide the diagnosis as well delineating the site and

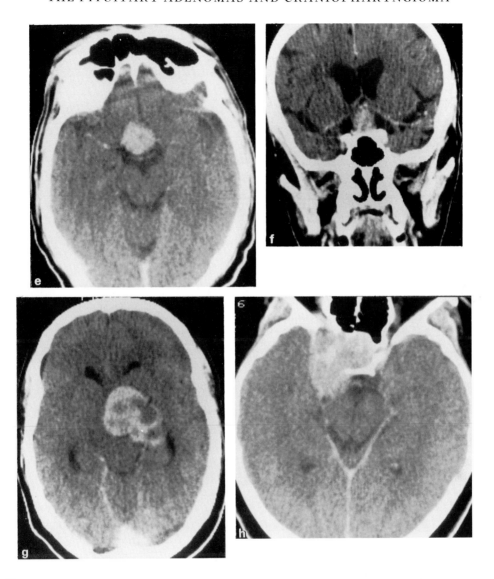

**Fig. 9.7.**
(e) GH adenoma with suprasellar extension.
(f) Same as (e). Coronal CT showing extension into third ventricle.
(g) Nonsecretory adenoma. Massive suprasellar extension into third ventricle and also lifting up right frontal lobe.
(h) FSH and LH adenoma. Extension into left cavernous sinus and left middle fossa.

extent of the lesion. The interpretation of a CT scan has always to be made in the light of the clinical and biochemical findings. Five basic points need to be looked for (Hall 1981). Firstly, the size of the sella and the slope of the floor must be assessed and coronal cuts may be of help.

Secondly, the density of the lesion in or near the sella must be gauged, looking for very high density suggestive of blood or calcification, or other grades of density ranging from hyperdense to hypodense (suggestive of cysts). Thirdly, the degree of enhancement after intravenous iodine-

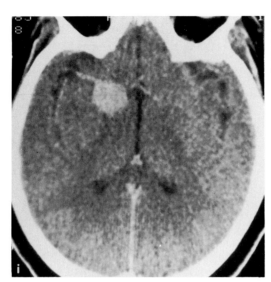 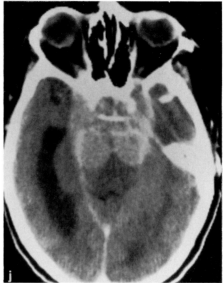

**Fig. 9.7.**
(i) Same as (h). Extension around bifurcation of left internal carotid artery and into Sylvian fissure.
(j) Nonsecretory adenoma. Two extensions into interpeduncular fossa. Also extensions into both cavernous sinuses.

containing contrast medium must be assessed. Pituitary adenomas are usually more dense than brain but show mottled enhancement, meningiomas enhance strongly as may giant aneurysms, and craniopharyngiomas show variable degrees of enhancement. Fourthly, the skull surrounding the sella needs to be assessed, since hyperostosis would strongly favour a meningioma. Fifthly, the brain must be looked at, and in particular the ventricular system, for hydrocephalus or distortion of the third ventricle. An empty sella can also be detected by finding CSF within the sella.

The majority of these processes can be seen easily on basal projections of the CT scan; however coronal reconstructions can provide extra information, in particular the upward and lateral extent of a lesion (Fig. 9.7 a–j).

*Magnetic resonance imaging.* This new investigation provides precise and valuable information on midline cerebral lesions and is particularly well suited for the diagnosis of pituitary tumours, especially those with suprasellar extensions.

*Angiography.* Since an aneurysm of the anterior part of the circle of Willis can simulate a pituitary adenoma both clinically and on CT scan, this alternative diagnosis may need to be excluded and the only way to do so reliably is by angiography. The main clinical items which make angiography advisable are recurrent pain, whether ocular, trigeminal or diffuse, asymmetrical visual fields particularly if one eye is blind and signs of cavernous sinus involvement. The main radiological indication is an enhancing lesion on CT above a sella which on plain X-ray is of normal size. In addition to providing a diagnosis, angiography can also reveal the distortions of the anterior part of the circle of Willis which may occur with a large pituitary adenoma. Finally, it should be remembered that there is a small incidence of intracavernous aneurysm of the carotid artery in patients with pituitary tumours (Fig. 9.8). Intravenous digital

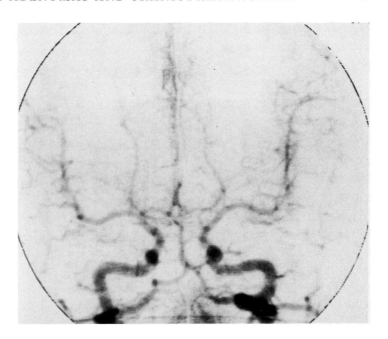

**Fig. 9.8.** ACTH adenoma. Normal digital vascular angiogram by the intravenous method.

subtraction angiography is useful for these diagnostic studies.

*Cisternography.* It is possible for a patient to have a small lesion in the suprasellar cistern and

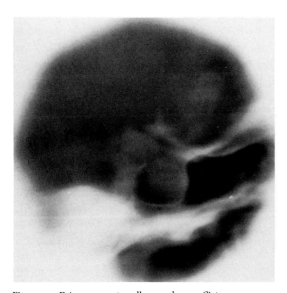

**Fig. 9.9.** Primary empty sellar syndrome. Cisternogram showing sella approximately 80% full of contrast material (i.e. CSF).

for the CT scan to be negative, though this is less likely with fourth generation CT scanners which can produce much thinner slices than was previously the case. If the CT scan is equivocal and yet there is a strong clinical suspicion of a lesion then a cisternogram can be helpful (Hall 1981). A water soluble iodine containing compound is injected into the CSF pathways, usually by cisternal puncture, and the basal cisterns examined by either plain radiology or the CT scanner. Cisternography can also be of help in fully establishing the diagnosis of an empty sella, once the suspicion has been raised on CT scan (Fig. 9.9).

*Cavernous sinus venography.* This procedure has application in two circumstances. Firstly, if there are clinical symptoms and signs which suggest an extension into the cavernous sinus a venogram may well demonstrate the degree of distortion. Secondly, if transsphenoidal surgery is contemplated in a patient who may have atheromatous internal carotid arteries venography will reveal their position; normally the two arteries are separated by at least 8 mm (Fijii *et al.* 1979) which is sufficient to allow the surgeon access, but some atheromatous arteries bulge medially in which case there is either insufficient access or the surgeon may encounter the arteries at operation.

*Endocrinology*

The subject of endocrinology has so expanded recently that it has rightly acquired the status of a special branch of medicine closely linked with the intricate field of biochemistry. Tests of endocrine function have multiplied to an extent that collaboration with an endocrinologist is essential for the proper management of patients with pituitary adenomas. His advice should be sought as to the appropriate tests for assessment, since choice to some extent depends on the clinical findings; and some dynamic endocrine tests are not without risk.

*Hypopituitarism*   It is crucial to note that progression from failure of one to more than one hormone may not occur at all, or may take many years; and that if there is progressive failure hormone loss usually occurs in the following order: GH, LH & FSH, ACTH, TSH and PRL (Abboud & Laws 1979). However in pituitary apoplexy any pattern of hormone loss may occur. Pituitary function can be assessed directly for all its hormones by specific RIA, or indirectly by determination of the function of the target endocrine glands.

1   GH axis. Serum GH is measured by RIA, but the sensitivity of the RIA is such that it cannot distinguish between low–normal and low levels. In normal individuals GH is secreted in a series of pulses; these are brief and between these GH levels are often immeasurably low and random blood samples will not distinguish between normal and hypopituitary patients. Thus a provocative test is necessary; the most commonly used one is insulin hypoglycaemia, since this will also be of use in assessing ACTH reserve (*see* below); the test should not be performed if the patient has cardiac disease or epilepsy. If the GH does not rise during such a provocation then it

can be concluded that there is a low GH production. In practical terms this axis is less important in an adult than in a child or teenager where it is of vital import, as for example in patients with craniopharyngiomas.

2   LH & FSH–gonadal axis. It is usual to assess gonadal function first and follow this with estimations of LH and FSH later. In premenopausal women menstrual and conceptual history is all important and this can then be followed by gynaecological assessments and completed by analyses of the ovarian hormones (oestrogen and progesterone) measured at appropriate times in the menstrual cycle. In men the history of sexual potency or otherwise can be followed by seminal analysis and serum testosterone estimations. If gonadal function tests prove the patient to be hypogonadal then assessment of the gonadotrophins is necessary; this is performed by measuring the levels of LH and FSH at 20 and 60 minutes after an injection of gonadorelin (a synthetic hypothalamic gonadotrophin releasing hormone). High levels of LH and FSH indicate primary gonadal failure, whilst low levels of these hormones indicates a pituitary or hypothalamic cause.

3   TSH–thyroid axis. Thyroid function can be assessed by measurement of the serum total and free thyroxine (T4) and tri-iodothyronine (T3). Since the T3 can be decreased in other diseases, the T4 becomes very important in the diagnosis of hypothyroidism. If this is low, measurement of the TSH is necessary; a high TSH indicating primary thyroid failure and a low TSH pituitary or hypothalamic failure. However, it must be appreciated that some patients with hypothalamic or pituitary hypofunction have inappropriately elevated TSH levels as measured by RIA, but when measured by sensitive bioassay the TSH activity is appropriately low.

4   ACTH–adrenal axis. To document a normal pituitary–adrenal axis it is necessary not only to demonstrate that a patient can produce adequate levels of cortisol for normal living, but that he can increase cortisol production optimally during periods of stress (Abboud & Laws 1979). Plasma levels of cortisol fluctuate widely due to

circadian rhythm and it is usual to measure the level at the times of expected maximum in ACTH and cortisol secretion, namely 8–9.00 hours. If these are low one can assume a low cortisol reserve and it is only necessary to perform a provocative test if the levels are near normal and yet one has reason to suppose that the reserve may yet be insufficient to respond to stress. The most commonly used test being an insulin tolerance test; a normal rise during the test indicating a normal axis, and vice versa.

5   PRL axis. In the majority of cases a random estimation of the serum prolactin is sufficient; if the level is normal then an adequate prolactin axis may be assumed. In fact in many pituitary adenomas the prolactin level may be high. If the level is low then a provocative test can be carried out using TRH, since this also has the merit of assessing TSH at the same time.

*Acromegaly.*   The majority of patients with the clinical features of acromegaly will have a high serum basal level of GH, but since GH levels vary widely in the normal, especially women, it is customary to perform a suppression test: the oral glucose tolerance test (GTT). A normal patient will show suppression of the serum GH to low or undetectable levels, whereas the acromegalic patient may show no suppression or more likely a paradoxical rise during the test. 80% of acromegalic patients show a paradoxical rise in GH following an injection of TRH; this can be of help in borderline cases and is of special help in assessing whether residual adenoma exists after surgery which has led to a reduction in GH to near normal levels. In addition 5–10% acromegalic patients also show hyperprolactinaemia, which may be due either to a mixed adenoma producing both GH and PRL, or due to pituitary stalk dysfunction particularly if there is suprasellar extension of the adenoma. Thyroid disorders are also common in acromegaly, and must be looked for.

*Prolactinoma.*   A random serum PRL estimation is the single most useful test. It is generally agreed that a level in excess of 2000 mU/l is almost always due to a pituitary adenoma; however it is also important to stress that a level between 700–2000 mU/l does not exclude the presence of a prolactinoma and in such an event radiological investigations assume great importance. Certain provocative tests such as TRH stimulation, and suppression tests such as with bromocriptine were initially thought to be helpful in the differential diagnosis of hyperprolactinaemia, but sadly experience has shown this not to be the case (Abboud & Laws 1979). Assessment of the other pituitary hormones must always be carried out, in particular thyroid function tests, as clinically mild hypothyroidism may present with hyperprolactinaemic reproductive disturbance and galactorrhoea.

*Cushing syndrome.*   There are two stages in the investigation of patients suspected, on clinical grounds, of suffering from Cushing syndrome; firstly the presence of Cushing syndrome has to be demonstrated, then the anatomical cause must be found. The common laboratory tests used are serum cortisol, urinary 17-hydroxysteroids and 17-ketosteroids, and urinary free cortisol. No single test can reliably diagnose Cushing syndrome and it is necessary to test the hypothalamic–pituitary–adrenal axis. The normal axis is suppressed by high levels of corticosteroids, whereas in Cushing syndrome the axis is resistant to suppression. A short overnight dexamethasone suppression test can exclude Cushing syndrome, but failure of suppression is not diagnostic. For this a low dose dexamethasone suppression test is necessary and failure of suppression establishes the diagnosis, and the anatomical cause may now be sought. Cushing syndrome due to a pituitary adenoma (Cushing disease) will have high levels of circulating ACTH and will suppress only with a high dose dexamathasone suppression test. An ectopic ACTH-producing neoplasm will also have high levels of ACTH but will fail to suppress. In adrenal neoplasms and hyperplasia the levels of ACTH are low and there will be no suppression.

*Diabetes insipidus.* The diabetes insipidus (DI) syndrome can result from dysfunction of the neurohypophysis or kidney, or from primary polydipsia. Neurohypophyseal DI is due to partial or complete lack of antidiuretic hormone (ADH), whereas nephrogenic DI is due to congenital or acquired renal resistance to ADH. Primary polydipsia is due to compulsive water drinking. Since there is no reliable method of estimating ADH the investigation of these disorders centres around the assessment of serum and urine osmolalities. A hyposmolar urine with a hyperosmolar serum indicates either hypophyseal or nephrogenic DI, of which only the former responds to administration of ADH or one of its synthetic analogues-DDAVP. The importance of accurate fluid balance charts and measurements of the specific gravity of the urine cannot be stressed enough. The neurosurgeon is most likely to encounter DI in the postoperative phase of management of patients with diagnosed pituitary adenomas and such observations form a crucial part of the care of such patients.

## Treatment

The treatment of pituitary adenomas must be decided in accordance with the nature of the disturbance they are producing. Those with space-occupying signs (failing vision, ocular palsy and extensions into the brain) present a different problem from those with secretory hyperfunction and with little or no neurological disturbance. In the first group treatment is principally concerned with a mass, at times of considerable size, in which the chiasmal syndrome dominates the picture in the majority of cases. In the second group the aim of treatment is to eliminate the hypersecretory state yet leave the pituitary gland with normal function. Some patients combine both problems and one line of treatment may be satisfactory for both.

The earliest operations for pituitary adenoma were by frontotemporal craniotomy; Caton and Paul (1893) made the first attempt, though the operation was limited to a decompression. At

that time intracranial surgery was insufficiently advanced to permit such difficult manoeuvres and the operation had a forbidding mortality. A direct approach to the sphenoid avoided some of these problems and within a few years and with some ingenuity suitable techniques were evolved (Landolt & Strebel 1980). In the early transnasal operations the nose was mobilized and an approach made through the ethmoid. This was abandoned because of the mutilation to the face. Kanavel (1909) suggested a more inferior route, by resecting the nasal septum and this was elaborated by Hirsch (1910). Halstead (1910) used a sublabial incision in order to expose the septum and this was the operation adopted by Cushing as the standard procedure until 1925. By this time neurosurgical techniques had developed sufficiently to allow a return to frontal craniotomy. Cushing switched his allegiance to this operation, though he never publicly explained why (Rosegay 1981). Many neurosurgeons followed suit; however, Dott, a pupil of Cushing, returned to Edinburgh and continued successfully with the transsphenoidal approach for many years. Guiot from Paris, following a visit to Dott, took up this approach with enthusiasm and applied the new techniques of operative microsurgery and intraoperative fluoroscopy. He then imparted his knowledge to a younger generation of neurosurgeons, amongst whom was Hardy (Rosegay 1981). Over the past 20 years the subfrontal and the transsphenoidal operations have been the cornerstones of pituitary surgery.

When confronted with a patient with a pituitary adenoma the neurosurgeon, in collaboration with his endocrinological colleague, must firstly decide which single method or combination of methods are applicable. Available to the treatment team are surgery, pharmacotherapy and radiation therapy. Most neurosurgeons recommend radiation therapy either when surgery has been unsuccessful in fully obliterating a pituitary adenoma or routinely in the postoperative phase to minimize the possibility of recurrence (Symon & Jacobowski 1979). However, some neurosurgeons feel that routine postoperative radiotherapy is unnecessary if radical surgery is undertaken (Jeffreys 1984). Jefferson (1978) has advocated radiation as the prime treatment in patients with massive adenomas and in poor general health. It is probably true to state that at the present time the arguments concerning radiation treatment are unresolved.

Various pharmacological agents have been tried in attempts to counteract the effects of hypersecretory states, though only two have had any success: *bromocriptine* and *metyrapone*. Bromocriptine has proved fairly successful in the treatment of hyperprolactinaemia, and some workers favour it as the treatment of first choice provided there is no suprasellar extension of a prolactinoma though others still favour surgery in the first instance. Newer, more potent, ergot derivatives include pergolide and mesulergine (Grossman & Besser, 1985). It is generally agreed that the initial treatment of acromegaly is by surgery though bromocriptine has a part to play if the postoperative levels of GH remain high. The initial treatment of Cushing disease is surgery but metyrapone is of help in stabilizing a patient pre-operatively.

*Choice of operation*

With the advent of better endocrinology (in particular biochemical tests) there has been a change in emphasis in the surgery of pituitary adenomas, such that neurosurgeons have been operating more for small hypersecretory adenomas than for large space-occupying ones. Guiot (1978) performs 90% of his operations by the transsphenoidal route and only 10% by the intracranial approach. The choice of approach is in part relative and in part absolute. The intracranial route is absolutely indicated when an adenoma has traversed the diaphragm and produced intracranial extensions that are separated from the sella portion by a constricted neck (Guiot 1978), when there are extensions around the anterior and/or middle cranial fossae, and when there is doubt concerning the nature of a suprasellar lesion (for example meningioma). The transsphenoidal route is absolutely indicated under two circumstances; when the adenoma protrudes down into the sphenoidal air sinus without upwards extensions and when the patient is so ill or frail that the intracranial route would be hazardous. All other choices are relative but the majority of neurosurgeons now favour the transsphenoidal route if possible, reserving the intracranial route for those occasions when there are absolute indications as listed above. It is essential that the operating microscope is used with either approach.

*Transfrontal operation*

The operation is started by making either a bilateral coronal skin incision at the hair-line or a unilateral frontal incision usually on the right. A small unilateral osteoblastic flap is raised, the anterior limb of which is cut along the supraciliary ridge. This may traverse the frontal air sinus, and should this occur the mucosa should be reflected back into the sinus and the hole in the bone repaired with a free dural or temporal fascia graft. A low craniotomy provides a more direct approach to the adenoma and lessens the need for retraction of the frontal lobe. The dura is opened and the operating microscope brought into play. If the patient's head is extended the frontal lobe falls away from the orbit and only a small amount of retraction is necessary with a self-retaining retractor. A careful assessment of the clinical and radiological findings should have given the surgeon a shrewd idea of the shape and size of the adenoma and he will have formulated his plan of operation accordingly. After opening the arachnoid covering the ipsilateral optic nerve and the dome of the adenoma the surgeon examines the anatomy and in particular makes an attempt to visualize the contralateral optic nerve before making an incision in the capsule of the adenoma in front of the chiasm. Evacuation of a cyst greatly eases local tension. The capsule is widely incised and adenoma within the sella evacuated with rongeurs, curettes and sucker. The capsule is then slowly and gently disengaged from the optic nerves and chiasm, made possible by the diminution in size of the adenoma resulting from the preliminary intracapsular evacuation. As the capsule is mobilized it is drawn away from the chiasm towards the sella where there is now room. In repeated stages more adenoma is removed from within the capsule and more capsule loosened and removed. Throughout the dissection the optic nerves and chiasm should be kept under observation in order to prevent manipulation unless absolutely necessary. As the retrochiasmal part of the adenoma is brought into view careful watch should be kept for the pituitary stalk. This may be in the midline though displaced posteriorly, or it may be displaced to one side. As much capsule as possible is removed, but the attachment of the stalk indicates the limit of this excision. The interior of the sella is cleared of adenoma. Under the operating microscope the pituitary gland can be seen as dark red and contrasts with the colour of the adenoma which may either be purple or grey, or creamy white or yellow. In some cases the capsule is firmly adherent to the optic nerves and chiasm and its removal might damage these structures or interfere with their blood supply. Only experience can teach the neurosurgeon what is safe and practicable; if in doubt it is wise to restrict the operation to as thorough an intracapsular removal of adenoma as possible, since this will relieve the tension on the visual apparatus and radiation therapy can be given postoperatively. However, any adenoma under the hypothalamus must be removed from within the capsule, since if this is left it may swell in the early postoperative phase and cause hypothalamic compression.

In the course of the removal extensions of the adenoma are dealt with so far as it is possible and appropriate. Subfrontal extensions may be easily removed, though on occasions if exposure requires undue brain retraction then it is better to resect a small portion of the frontal pole. Extension into the cavernous sinus may be detected when exenterating the intrasellar portion of the adenoma, or alternatively may be detected by bulging of the dura mater lateral to the internal carotid artery. The more superficial part of such an extension can be dealt with by making a fresh incision into the capsule lateral to the optic nerve and medial to the artery on the ipsilateral side, though this is impossible on the contralateral side. The deeper part of such an extension will be left since to enter the cavernous sinus may damage the oculomotor nerves to say nothing of the disastrous haemorrhage that may ensue.

What should be done if the adenoma is largely retrochiasmal or if there is extreme prefixation of the chiasm? A useful manoeuvre is to reflect a small flap of dura covering the tuberculum sellae forwards from between the optic foramina, to remove the underlying bone, to displace any sphenoid sinus mucosa and thus gain access to the enlarged sella anterior and ventral to the chiasm.

During the operation haemorrhage may be encountered in differing ways and can be worrying to the inexperienced. Pituitary adenomas are often vascular and there is a steady capillary ooze throughout the intracapsular dissection and which only ceases when all the adenoma has been removed, so much so that if the cavity within the sella continues to ooze it is essential to recurette it. Brisk venous haemorrhage indicates a hole into the cavernous sinus and once the site is identified can be occluded with surgicel or gelfoam. Brisk arterial haemorrhage can arise from tearing small arterial branches out of the internal carotid and anterior cerebral arteries; in the majority of cases this can be controlled by wrapping the artery with surgicel or, failing this, a circumferential arterial clip. Haemostasis must be meticulous; postoperative haematomas in this site drive upwards into the hypothalamus and are catastrophic.

*Transsphenoidal operation*

The details of the operation were described by Cushing (1914) though many neurosurgeons have their own minor modifications. The two

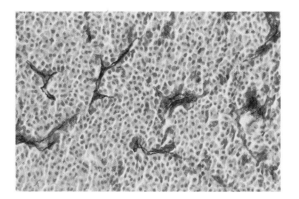

**Plate 7.** Nonsecreting pituitary adenoma stained with haematoxylin and eosin.

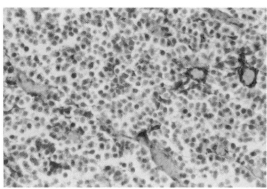

**Plate 8.** Nonsecreting pituitary adenoma. Slidder's stain.

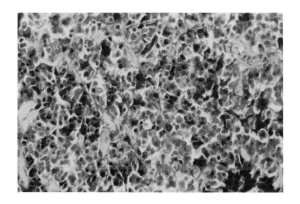

**Plate 9.** Growth hormone secreting pituitary adenoma. Slidder's stain.

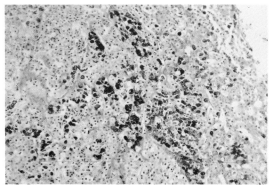

**Plate 10.** ACTH secreting pituitary adenoma. Slidder's stain.

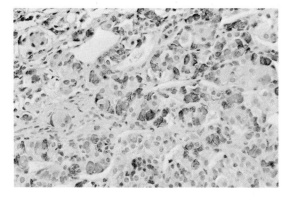

**Plate 11.** Growth hormone secreting pituitary adenoma. Immunoperoxidase staining for GH.

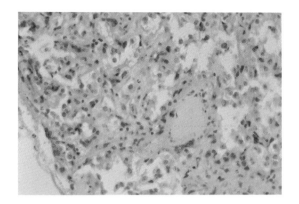

**Plate 12.** Prolactin secreting pituitary adenoma. Immunoperoxidase staining for PRL.

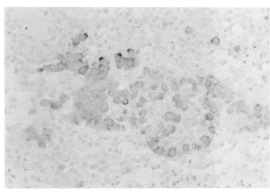

**Plate 13.** Adrenocorticotrophic hormone secreting adenoma. Immunoperoxidase staining for ACTH.

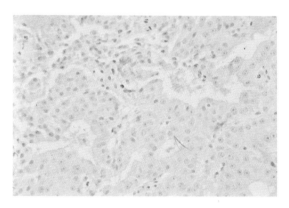

**Plate 14.** Thyroid stimulating hormone secreting pituitary adenoma. Immunoperoxidase staining for TSH.

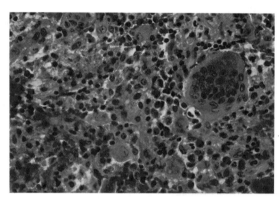

**Plate 15.** Eosinophilic granuloma of skull, stained with toluidine blue and eosin showing giant cells and eosinophils with macrophages. (Courtesy of Dr J. E. Bell.)

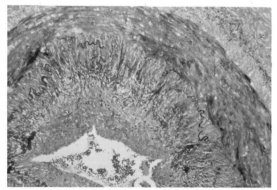

**Plate 16.** Temporal arteritis. Hart–Masson technique used to show characteristic disruption of internal elastic lamina (wavy black line) and exuberant inflammatory infiltrate. (Courtesy of Dr J. E. Bell.)

major advances in recent years have been the operating microscope and intraoperative radiological control with image intensification. The former has allowed the neurosurgeon to operate on small (micro) adenomas with preservation of the pituitary gland, and the latter allows the neurosurgeon to check the position of his tools, particularly important when he goes beyond the confines of the sella. An up-to-date account has been given by Hardy (1971).

Through an incision under the upper lip a submucous resection of the nasal septum is carried out; special bivalved speculae compress the turbinates and provide a tunnel of about 2 cm diameter. Its axis runs parallel to the posterior border of the vomer which forms a convenient landmark, leading one to the undersurface of the sphenoid and to its air sinus. Removal of the alar of the vomer can be of help. The mucosa of the air sinus is removed, and at this stage the operating microscope is brought into play. A window is made in the floor of the sella with a drill and punch forceps. The pituitary capsule will be seen to bulge downwards into the air sinus. A cruciate incision is made into the capsule and the leaves shrunk with coagulation. From this point on the technique will vary according to the size of the adenoma.

For small adenomas confined to a sella or normal or slightly enlarged size and associated with hypersecretion, an incision through the capsule may immediately enter them. In which case tissue is taken for histopathological examination before removing the adenoma by suction and curettage. In some cases, however, the adenoma does not present immediately to the surgeon, and the contents of the sella will have to be systematically explored. This is best performed, with minimal damage to the normal pituitary gland, by making parallel incisions into the sella contents in the sagittal plane. If the adenoma is found then the surgeon proceeds as above. If no adenoma is encountered the surgeon will have to decide whether or not to remove the anterior pituitary gland. This is obviously a radical step and most surgeons would favour so doing only for cases of Cushing disease, and

aborting the operation at this point in cases of acromegaly and prolactinoma.

In the case of large adenomas with a suprasellar extension tumour tissue is first removed from within the sella before tackling the tissue within the suprasellar extension. At all times the surgeon must take care to remain within the capsule and also check the position of the end of his tools with the image intensifier. All easily removable tissue is taken and the surgeon can judge whether or not he has been successful in achieving an adequate decompression by seeing the downward descent of the diaphragma or furthermost pituitary capsule.

The two most common complications that can occur are a CSF leak and venous haemorrhage. The former usually occurs due to rupture of arachnoid that lies within the sella anteriorly, and must be repaired with muscle, fascia lata or some other such material. The latter occurs either from holes in venous sinuses lying within the capsule or from the cavernous sinus itself. Small venous sinuses can usually be coagulated with bipolar coagulation. Holes in the cavernous sinus are not so easily dealt with and need packing with surgicel or muscle; if this event occurs early in the operation and cannot easily be controlled it may be necessary to abandon the operation and return later.

*Pre- and postoperative care*

Once the diagnosis has been made and the decision to operate taken, the next issue to be resolved is the question of supportive corticosteroid cover. If there has been time to investigate fully the endocrinological status the cortisol response to stress will be known. If this is defective the patient will require hydrocortisone both pre- and postopertively. If it is decided to administer dexamethasone to reduce raised intracranial pressure this will be sufficient cover for stress and hydrocortisone need not be given. However, so harmless is the administration of hydrocortisone for short periods and so devastating the effects of insufficient cortisol cover that when in doubt it is wise to give hydrocortisone, and continue until such time as it may be withdrawn; usually 4–5 days in the case of patients with an adequate pre-operative stress response or until the patient's endocrinological status can be reassessed, usually one month postoperatively.

Oral or parenteral prophylactic antibiotics are unnecessary though it is wise to attempt to sterilize the nasal cavities pre-operatively in those patients who are to undergo transsphenoidal surgery; the usual method being to instil an antibiotic cream into the nostrils for 3–4 days pre-operatively.

In the case of patients with hypersecretory adenomas and who are taking antagonistic drugs many surgeons continue with these through the operation though they may also just as well be withdrawn; in fact, although bromocriptine does not appear to have deleterious effects during surgery, metyrapone may produce bizarre cardiovascular changes which can be alarming.

In the postoperative phase a careful watch must be kept on fluid balance with particular regard to the development of diabetes insipidus. If there is more than 1 litre of negative balance coupled with a urinary specific gravity less than 1005 then DDAVP will required; in the acute phase this can be given parenterally, though later it can be taken as a nasal spray.

All patients will require full endocrinological reassessment postoperatively; since the tests are expensive and pituitary function takes a while to become fully re-established it is sensible to perform the reassessment no sooner than one month after surgery.

*Medical treatment*

Medical treatment of pituitary adenomas centres around two main issues: replacement of deficiencies in either pituitary hormones or hormones in target glands, and the reduction of hyper-

secretion of specific pituitary hormones. At no stage, as has been made clear above, must surgical and medical treatment be thought of as separate entities, but must be integrated in the mind of the clinicians when planning the treatment of a particular patient. For this reason close collaboration must exist between the neurosurgeon and the endocrinologist. Full details of medical treatment will be found in endocrinological treatises (Belchetz 1984), but a brief account follows below.

The longterm replacement of hormone deficiencies is based on the results of the endocrinological assessment. The single most important deficiency is that of cortisol and it is essential that this is replaced with hydrocortisone, the usual maintenance dose in an adult being 20 mg in the morning and 10 mg at night; however it is essential that the patient is warned that the dose must be doubled in the event of any physical stress such as an intercurrent infection. Patients must carry a steroid card at all times.

Thyroid deficiency is treated with thyroid replacements, of which there are various types, the most common being thyroxine in a dose of between 0.1 and 0.2 mg daily. Gonadotrophin deficiencies are treated with testosterone esters in men, and in women with oestrogen and/or progestogens, though this is required only in the premenopausal era. It is felt that GH deficiency in the adult does not require treatment, though in the prepubertal child it requires active treatment (*see* below under Craniopharyngioma). PRL deficiency is never treated. Shortage of the posterior pituitary ADH is treated with the synthetic preparation DDAVP, which has the great merits of being short acting and capable of being taken as a nasal spray, allowing the patients to treat themselves at home.

All three of the common hyprsecretory pituitary adenomas, namely acromegaly, prolactinoma and Cushing disease, can be treated medically with antagonistic agents; though it must be clearly understood that only surgery can adequately tackle any space-occupying effects of such adenomas. Therefore the indications for medical treatment are either to suppress any continuing hypersecretion after surgery for large adenomas, or as the primary or secondary treatment for small adenomas.

At the present time it is generally accepted that the primary method of treatment of acromegaly is surgery. If surgery is unsuccessful in totally reducing GH to a normal level (less than 5 mU) bromocriptine is given orally, starting in small doses of the order of 7.5 mg daily in divided doses and working up to, if necessary, doses of 50 mg daily. Due to the propensity of bromocriptine to cause gastrointestinal upsets the drug should be taken during meals. The control of such treatment must be by serial estimations of GH together with a stimulation test (*see* above). While GH is usually reduced, the levels are seldom within normal limits.

The primary treatment of hyperprolactinaemia due to a prolactinoma is a more vexed problem. Bromocriptine was introduced specifically as a PRL antagonist and as such it has had considerable success, so much so that some clinicians feel it the primary treatment for prolactinomas wholly confined to the sella. Bromocriptine frequently brings PRL levels down dramatically, often to normal. It has a good safety record, even during pregnancy and to date it appears to have no teratogenic effects (Krupp & Turkalj 1984). However it is likely that patients will have to take the drug indefinitely and some surgeons feel for this reason that surgery should be the primary treatment and reserve bromocriptine for continuing hyperprolactinaemia (Faria & Tindall 1982). Bromocriptine has also been reported to shrink a proportion of large adenomas permitting medical treatment to be followed by radiotherapy. In such cases assessments of visual fields and acuity must be repeated regularly, every few days. More experience is needed to resolve this question.

The results of medical treatment for Cushing disease (*see* below) are not as successful as those for acromegaly and prolactinoma. It is the consensus at the present time that surgery should be the primary treatment and that metyrapone the secondary one; in a patient with severe Cushing disease it is wise to minimize the more severe endocrinological effects for a few weeks before surgery, by giving metyrapone.

*External radiation*

The earliest reliable and convincing evidence on a large scale of the value of radiotherapy on nonsecretory pituitary adenomas was provided by Henderson (1939) in his study of Cushing's cases; recurrence after the transsphenoidal operation alone was 68.2%, but in those patients who in addition had X-ray therapy this was reduced to 34.7%; the comparable figures for patients who had had a subfrontal operation were 42.5% and 12.9%. A stringent criterion of the value of irradiation alone is the improvement in the visual fields; one of the earliest papers recording this important proof was that of Evans and Picciotto (1948). Further evidence is provided by the occurrence of cerebrospinal rhinorrhoea after radiotherapy, an occasional sequel to the shrinkage of the adenoma if it has previously eroded through the floor of the sella into the sphenoidal air sinus. The 'empty sella' syndrome gives further proof; in this syndrome vision may deteriorate several years after surgery and radiotherapy, and investigations (*see* above) indicate that the sella contains only a small pituitary gland or residual adenoma, and the rest of the space within the sella is taken up by CSF or prolapsing optic nerves and chiasm (*see* above).

The decision to irradiate a pituitary adenoma involves two questions: whether to irradiate as the primary treatment, and whether to recommend postoperative radiotherapy. Regarding the former, Jefferson (1978) has advocated irradiation as the primary treatment for pituitary adenomas that are so large as to render operation unsafe or that occur in patients who are unfit for major surgery. Whilst this approach can be used in a limited number of cases, the consensus opinion among neurosurgeons is that (transsphenoidal) surgery should be used first whenever possible. The question of routine postoperative radiation therapy is difficult to answer, since opinion is divided, though it is clear that such treatment is given to prevent recurrence. It is important, therefore, to define what is meant by recurrence: this can either mean recurrence of symptoms or recurrence of adenoma, and these two are not synonymous. It is incorrect to discuss the recurrence of an adenoma that was known to be partially removed at surgery; the term should be reserved for those cases in whom the surgeon feels that he has undertaken a radical removal of an adenoma, though there may be a few cells left which later develop into another adenoma. Symon and Jakobowski (1979) routinely irradiated postoperatively in their series of 101 pituitary adenomas with suprasellar extension and had no recurrences, although they admit that only 60% of cases had a follow-up of more than four years. On the other hand Jeffreys (1984) found a 4% recurrence rate in 46 cases that were not irradiated. The question is not resolved at the present, though it would be wise to irradiate cases in which the surgical treatment is known to be incomplete; and to do this early in the postoperative period rather than waiting until symptomatic recurrence has developed.

## Results and prognosis

The treatment of pituitary adenomas is directed both towards the relief of any space-occupying effects and to the re-establishment of normal pituitary endocrinological function; these aspects need separate consideration.

### Pituitary adenomas with space-occupying effects

Pituitary adenoma with extrasellar extension poses a greater surgical problem than one without extension. Cushing's mortality for hypophysectomy during his last ten years was 2.4% (Henderson 1939), but the surgical mortality in patients with very large suprasellar extensions was much greater. All mortality figures have to be seen against a background of operability rate,

that is to say how many cases did and did not undergo operation. In 1979 Symon and Jakobowski reported a mortality rate of 1% for adenomas with suprasellar extensions, rising to 3.4% in cases with giant adenomas. In a recent series of 52 cases with large suprasellar extensions leading to visual failure Jeffreys (1984) found that as a result of surgery by the subfrontal route 50% of patients regained normal vision, 43% were improved to functional vision and 1% were unchanged; for Symon and Jakobowski (1979) the equivalent figures were 50%, 38% and 9% respectively. Postoperative frontal lobe swelling may be a sequel to the subfrontal route, occurring as a transient phenomenon in 11% of Jeffreys' series. Postoperative epilepsy occurs in 3.8% of patients operated on by the subfrontal route (Foy et al. 1981). The recurrence rate in patients in Symon's series who had routine postoperative radiotherapy was 0%; in Jeffreys' series where radiotherapy was not used the recurrence rate was 4%.

Improvement in vision can also be expected after transsphenoidal surgery (Teasdale 1983).

### Endocrinological results

#### Acromegaly

The aim of treatment is to reduce the serum GH level to below 5 mu/l and yet leave the patient with otherwise normal pituitary endocrinological function. Recently Baskin et al. (1982) reviewed their results in treating 102 cases of acromegaly for whom transsphenoidal surgery was the primary therapy; they found that 78% of patients obtained complete remission of acromegaly after surgery alone, though this rate rose to 94% after radiotherapy. There were no deaths, 8% had minor surgical morbidity and 5% had postoperative hypopituitarism. However, of patients subsequently irradiated, 71% eventually developed hypopituitarism. These results are in keeping with other recent large series. All the operative failures had pre-operative GH levels in excess of 50 mu/l and suprasellar extension of the adenoma. If bromocriptine is used without surgery approximately 50% achieve normal GH levels on continuous dosage (Thorner & Besser 1978). In a recent series (Eastman *et al.* 1979) conventional external X-irradiation produced a cure in 73% of cases by the end of five years after treatment, though the incidence of hypopituitarism was 60%. It would therefore seem that for the present, transsphenoidal surgery can produce the best results, both in terms of eliminating excess growth hormone secretion and preserving normal pituitary function.

*Prolactinoma*

Although prolactinomas occur in either sex, most workers in evaluating results have tended to concentrate on women; perhaps because potency in men is such an intangible and complex phenomenon whereas menstruation and fertility are so much easier to record. The pre-operative PRL level relates closely to the results, so that most workers report their series in two groups: patients with PRL levels less than 2000 mu/l and those with PRL levels in excess of 4000 mu/l. For example Faria and Tindall (1982) found that of the former, 78% regained normal menstrual cycles and 76% had return of the PRL to normal levels; whereas of the second group only 39% resumed normal menstruation and 46% achieved a normal PRL level. They also found, as have other workers, a good correlation between the size of the adenoma and the pre-operative PRL level. In assessing fertility Laws *et al.* (1983) found that of 90 women of childbearing age and with a prolactinoma 84% became pregnant after surgery, though 11% required postoperative bromocryptine in addition.

*Cushing disease*

Cushing disease is lethal unless treated, though treatment is often difficult and fraught with problems. The reasonable approach (Burke 1977)

is to institute treatment with metyrapone, and follow this with surgery and radiation therapy, and reserve adrenalectomy for cases in which the cortisol remains high in spite of all other treatments. Fahlbusch (1981) was able to achieve a remission of the disease in 66% of 62 patients, but failed to control the disease by surgery in 34%. Some adenomas are macroscopically aggressive and reports are now appearing of cases with extracranial metastases (Kaiser *et al.* 1983).

*Non-secretory adenomas*

As explained earlier most of these adenomas present as space-occupying lesions with either normal or reduced function of the anterior pituitary. The results of treatment regarding the space-occupying effects have been discussed above, and attention must now be given to the endocrinological aspect. In their series of large pituitary adenomas treated by transfrontal surgery and external irradiation Symon and Jakobowski (1979) found that only 2% of patients regained normal function of the anterior pituitary gland. Jeffreys (1984) found that with surgery alone 29% of patients regained normal function, 23% suffered from a lack of the cortisol response to stress and 42% required replacement with hydrocortisone and thyroid. The reason for the major differences between these two recent series would seem to lie in the damage to the residual pituitary gland by X-irradiation.

Diabetes insipidus may occur after surgery. Jeffreys (1984) found that this happened for a few days in 30% of patients undergoing surgery for large adenomas by the transfrontal route; only 6% needed long term replacement with DDAVP; the comparable figures from Symon's (1979) series were 50% and 13% respectively.

# Craniopharyngioma

## Introduction

'This admittedly somewhat cumbersome term has been employed, for want of something more brief, to include the kaleidoscopic tumours, solid and cystic, which take their origin from epithelial rests ascribable to an imperfect closure of the hypophyseal or craniopharyngeal duct.' Thus Cushing (1932) justified the adoption of this inaccurate word introduced by McLean (1930) to designate a well-defined group of tumours. Inaccurate, because Rathke's pouch arises from the buccal ectoderm and not the pharyngeal endoderm. Synonyms are suprasellar cyst, adamantinoma and Rathke pouch tumour. Although they may give rise to several widely differing yet clearly recognizable clinical entities, these syndromes depend upon the precise anatomical point of origin, age of onset and rapidity of expansion and not upon any morphological variant. Russell and Rubenstein (1977) held the view that they are closely affiliated to the epidermoid cysts of other sites, and included them in the chapter on 'Congenital Tumours of Maldevelopment Origin'. Clinical considerations make it desirable to deal with them here in proximity to the pituitary adenomas. Whether craniopharyngiomas arise from remnants of Rathke's pouch, in accordance with the Cohnheim hypothesis of neoplasia developing in rests of embryonic cells, is now disputed. Small groups of squamous epithelial cells can be found in otherwise normal pituitary glands as high as the pars tuberalis in the newborn and in adults (Erdheim 1904, Goldberg & Eshbaugh 1960). What determines the neoplastic transformation and its timing is unknown. The synonym adamantinoma has been applied to the histologically similar tumour occurring in the jaw which is thought to arise from the epithelial enamel organ. Sprawson (1937) and Willis (1948) regarded both as epidermoid carcinoma. Craniopharyngiomas can occur at all ages, though nearly one half of patients present with symptoms in the first 20 years of life. There is sex equality. Large pituitary adenomas are three times as common as craniopharyngiomas.

## Morbid anatomy

The site of the tumour is of importance in determining the pattern of clinical disturbance; in a series from the London Hospital (Northfield 1957) 3 were intrasellar, 15 were subtuberal and 31 were tuberal, or tuberal and within the third ventricle. They do not apparently occur within the third ventricle without involving the tuber cinereum to some extent, an anatomical feature of significance in surgical treatment. The majority of tumours are cystic, hence the descriptive term formerly adopted, suprasellar cyst. However, tumours without macroscopic cysts occur. When a cyst occurs it is often much larger than the solid portion and can even bulge into the lateral ventricle. The cyst fluid is commonly yellow and sparkling with cholesterol crystals. The solid portion is usually pale, often crumbly and may contain minute crystals, pearly debris, and deposits of calcium. In a few cases the tumour is entirely intrasellar, and like a pituitary adenoma causes ballooning of the fossa with a varying degree of dome-like elevation of the diaphragma sellae and compression of the pituitary gland. As Hardy (1971) has noted, a craniopharyngioma associated with an enlarged sella can be assumed to have originated within the sella, the implication of which is important to surgeons considering the transsphenoidal route.

A considerable number of craniopharyngiomas appear to arise in an intermediate position, between the pituitary gland below and the brain above. They are conveniently described as subtuberal. Pressure downwards causes the diaphragma sellae to be indented; the pituitary stalk may be so attenuated as to be unrecognizable, or the tumour may be separate from it. As it expands the tumour impinges on the floor of the third ventricle, invaginating it without invading it and as it bulges forward compresses the optic chiasm (Fig. 9.10). Very occasionally the tumour may appear within the chiasm

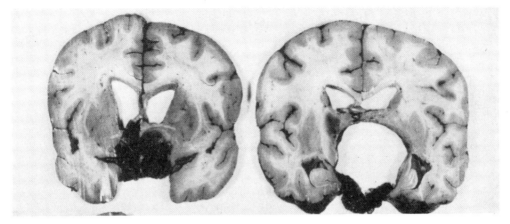

**Fig. 9.10.** Haemorrhagic solid part of craniopharyngioma replacing the hypothalamus, and large cyst filling and expanding the third ventricle.

causing it to expand. Cystic or solid extensions may overhang the dorsum sellae and fill the interpeduncular fossa, and may extend laterally towards the Sylvian fissures and into the temporal lobes. Not infrequently it is the cyst which insinuates itself into the ramifications of the chiasmatic cistern and its communications, closely enveloping all the structures. The wall is frequently transparent and tenuous, so that it is impossible to remove it completely; solid nodules may occur at different points.

The tuberal tumours are characterized by their intrinsic relationship to the floor of the third ventricle. At autopsy large tumours are seen to have replaced the whole of the floor and anterior wall of the third ventricle and occupy most if its

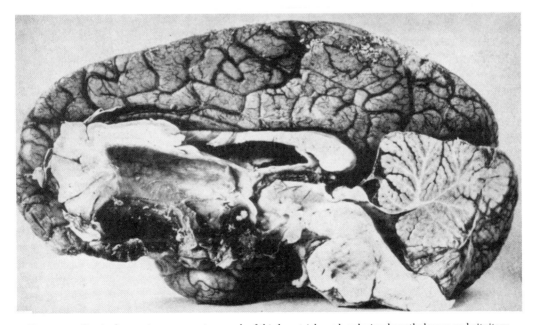

**Fig. 9.11.** Craniopharyngioma occupying much of third ventricle and replacing hypothalamus and pituitary gland.

cavity, making the area of origin impossible to determine (Fig. 9.11). Smaller specimens, or those with a large intraventricular cyst arising from a small solid basal portion, fuse with the tuber cinereum. Tumours arising in this situation may destroy the tuber and thereby the vascular and neural connections of the hypophysis. Extension of the tumour or cystic expansion occupies the third ventricle thereby causing hydrocephalus. The optic chiasm may thus escape compression until a later stage. Anatomical relationships in this group are thus distinct from those of large pituitary adenoma and though there may be manifestations of disturbance of pituitary function hydrocephalic symptoms predominate, an unusual event in pituitary adenomas. As with the subtuberal group, these tumours may send extensions into the frontal lobes. A no less important aspect of these tumours which involve the floor of the third ventricle is their microscopical relationship to brain tissue. At the periphery of the tumour are outlying and apparently isolated islands of epithelium, which give rise to an intense gliosis; it is this fusion of tumour and brain which may render their total surgical removal impracticable.

### Histology

Craniopharyngiomas are epidermoid tumours. The term adamantinoma occasionally applied to them has little justification, as they do not arise from the enamel organ and bear no more than a superficial resemblance to tumours of that structure. They are epitheliomas composed of both basal and squamous cells and may arise from small nests of squamous cells commonly found in the pars tuberalis of the pituitary gland which invests the pituitary stalk and the anterior aspect of the tuber cinereum.

Craniopharyngiomas may be predominantly solid or predominantly cystic. The solid examples consist of a lattice-work of irregular epithelial trabeculae. The cells which form the bulk of the trabeculae are predominantly squamous in character, while the outer layer which rests on a basement membrane consists of typical basal cells. The interstices between the trabeculae are filled with a loose, sparsely cellular connective tissue stroma (Fig. 9.12). The squamous epithelium is particularly prone to degenerative changes. The cells may become loosened and dissociated by oedema and acquire a stellate appearance which gives them a resemblance to the enamel organ. Within the walls of the cysts the epithelium may keratinize and desquamate leading to accumulation of debris similar to the contents of epidermoid cysts. Indeed large cysts may be indistinguishable from epidermoid cysts, but through search usually reveals a more solid part of the cyst wall which has preserved its typical trabicular pattern.

The contents of small or large cysts are usually filled with greenish or yellow mucoid fluid in which shimmering cholesterol crystals are clearly seen under the operating microscope. They may attract the deposition of calcium salts and heavy calcification, occasionally ossification, is a common feature of these tumours. Escape of cyst fluid into the stroma leads to an inflammatory reaction similar to that seen in the walls of epidermoid cysts.

The relationship of craniopharyngiomas to the adjacent brain is of considerable interest. These tumours are not encapsulated and are not separated from the cerebral parenchyma by a layer of leptomeningeal connective tissue. The tumour tissue lies in close apposition to the cerebral parenchyma in which it produces an intense glial reaction, sometimes associated with the formation of Rosenthal fibres. Tongues of tumour may extend into the brain tissue and may permeate not only the tuber cinereum and the floor of the third ventricle, but also other parts of the hypothalamus. Whether this represents true invasion and is thus an expression of low-grade malignancy is a debatable point, and does not receive support from the cytological structure of the intracerebral exclusions.

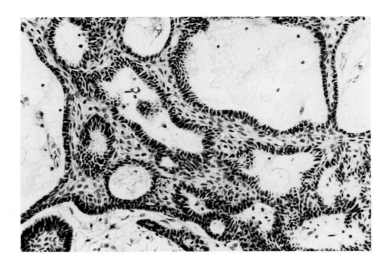

**Fig. 9.12.** Solid and cystic craniopharyngioma. H. & E.

## Symptoms and signs

The common clinical manifestations fall into four groups: raised intracranial pressure, failing vision, endocrine disturbance and mental impairment. These are determined by the site of origin and direction of tumour growth, as described above; though the age of the patient modifies the effects of endocrinological disturbance. In the large majority of patients the presenting symptoms are headache and vomiting, or impairment of vision. Although endocrine disturbances are evident to the skilled observer in about three-quarters, they occur slowly and are often unnoticed by the patient or relatives. Visual failure may be due to papilloedema, optic atrophy (primary or secondary) and to defective visual fields. In only 6% of the London Hospital series of 49 patients (Northfield 1957) were the optic pathways clinically normal. Mental impairment was present in over one-third; it varied in degree from dullness and impaired memory to frank dementia. Set out in Table 9.1 is a list of symptoms and signs and their frequency in Northfield's series.

*Raised intracranial pressure* is particularly common in children. In an analysis of 32 patients, all but 4 of whom were children, Matson (1964) found that headache occurred in 28, vomiting in 19 and papilloedema in 19.

Although a subtuberal tumour with a large cyst may be the cause, more commonly these symptoms signify that there has been encroachment upon the third ventricle with subsequent obstruction to the flow of CSF. In young children this usually causes enlargement of the head and a 'cracked pot' note is emitted when the skull is percussed.

*Impairment of vision* may be due to papilloedema, to chiasmal compression, or to a

**Table 9.1.** Frequency of symptoms and signs in 49 patients with craniopharyngioma (Northfield 1957).

| Presenting symptoms | | |
|---|---|---|
| Headache | | 23 |
| Impairment of vision | | 22 |
| Diplopia | | 2 |
| Severe dementia | | 1 |
| Epilepsy | | 1 |
| | | |
| **Symptoms and signs** | | |
| Endocrine disturbance | | 31 |
| Defects of visual fields | | 26 |
| Papilloedema | | 20 |
| Primary optic atrophy | | 19 |
| Mental impairment | | 14 |
| Hallucinations | | 9 |
|    optic | 5 | |
|    olfactory | 2 | |
|    gustatory | 2 | |
| Epilepsy | | 7 |
| Shivering | | 3 |
| Emotional instability | | 2 |
| 'Falling attacks' | | 2 |

combination of both. The latter may be suspected when the swelling of the optic disc is mild, and when vision has deteriorated to a degree disproportionate to the papilloedema. This combination is usually found in children in whom visual field examination may be difficult. Papilloedema is rare in adults even when the third ventricle is obstructed, probably because the tumour has been present long enough to cause optic atrophy and obliteration of the optic sheaths. The chiasmal syndrome occurs in over half the cases. The patterns of field defect are similar to those produced by pituitary adenomas, except that in the early stages inferior bitemporal quadrantic loss may occur, indicating that the pressure is on the upper instead of the lower aspect of the chiasm. Jefferson (1954) considered that homonymous defects were more common in cases of craniopharyngioma than in those with pituitary adenoma. Visual acuity and field defects may fluctuate spontaneously to a remarkable degree, probably due to variations in tension of fluid within the cyst.

*Endocrine function* is disturbed in the majority of patients and Table 9.2 sets out an analysis of its effects.

Clinical features were recognizable at the first examination in 27 clinical cases and became

Table 9.2. Endocrine disturbance in 31 patients with craniopharyngioma.

| | | |
|---|---|---|
| Hypogonadism | | 24 |
| severe | 15 | |
| moderate | 6 | |
| mild | 3 | |
| | | |
| Stunting in growth | | 17 |
| severe | 4 | |
| moderate | 5 | |
| mild | 8 | |
| | | |
| Diabetes insipidus | | 21 |
| spontaneous | 13 | |
| postoperative | 8 | |
| | | |
| Obesity | | 8 |
| | | |
| Hypothyroidism | | 7 |
| | | |
| Low blood pressure | | 15 |

manifest later in another 4. The age of the patient at the time when the tumour encroaches upon the hypothalamic–hypophyseal mechanisms significantly modifies the clinical picture. It is because these tumours may start before adulthood is attained that they create such dramatic effects upon the whole person.

When a craniopharyngioma develops in childhood to a size sufficient to interfere with hypothalamic–hypophyseal mechanisms it causes infantilism; the fully developed condition producing the Levi–Loraine dwarf. Skeletal growth slows down and the stunted stature becomes more noticeable at puberty when the child's contemporaries grow more rapidly (Fig. 9.13). The

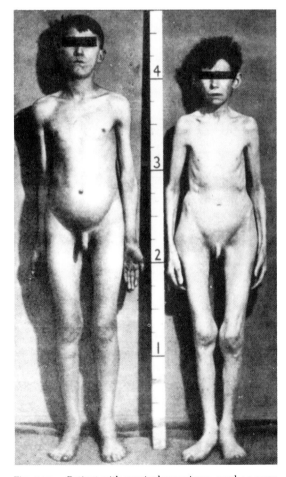

**Fig. 9.13.** Patient with craniopharyngioma, aged 43 years (right), compared with normal boy, aged 10 years (left).

gonads and the secondary sexual characteristics fail to develop. Lack of sex hormones delays closure of the epiphyses, so that limbs are long in proportion to the trunk; the hands and feet are slim and the fingers long and tapering. The skin is thin and pale; the scalp hair remains fine and silky and body hair does not appear. The boy's voice retains its treble pitch. The girl has poor mammary development, mainly flattish pads of fat. The body contours remain rounded; muscular development is poor. Thus adulthood may be attained with the retention of an infantile physique and a timid personality. In the male the lack of a robust and aggressive attitude to life is in part attributable to lack of androgens, but in both sexes psychcological reactions to the realization of the differences from their contemporaries are also important. The fully developed picture described above does not always occur. As in the other causes of hypopituitarism all the pituitary hormones are not depressed necessarily to the same degree. When assessing stature and physique comparison with parents and siblings can be helpful, as will be a period of observation with a growth chart. In the course of a few years a state similar to premature old age may be impressed upon the infantile appearance, and overt hypothyroidism become apparent.

Obesity has often been regarded as a characteristic of these patients, but this is not always so. Only 8 patients of Northfield's series (1957) were excessively fat and in all these the tumour involved the tuber cinereum directly or by pressure.

In an adult, endocrine failure due to a craniopharyngioma is essentially similar to that due to a pituitary adenoma, though it is often more severe and careful review of the patient's medical history will often demonstrate that the symptoms are of longer duration.

Diabetes insipidus occurs spontaneously in about one-quarter of the patients, and in degree and duration it is quite unpredictable. It may come and go, or may persist continuously for many years unless treated. In this respect the tumour behaves very differently from a pituitary adenoma, which rarely causes diabetes insipidus. This is attributable to the anatomical predilection of the tumour; craniopharyngioma, as with any tumour of the floor of the third ventricle, is liable to disrupt ADH secretion without necessarily interfering with the production of ACTH by the adenohypophysis.

A blood pressure persistently below the norm was found in 30% of patients of all ages in Northfield's series, and is perhaps due to hypothalamic dysfunction rather than a feature of anterior hypopituitarism. Certain other features which occur in patients of all ages can be attributed to interference with the connections of the hypothalamus; episodes of hypothermia and hyperthermia, shivering, skin rashes and flushes, and attacks of drowsiness and hypersomnia. Detailed reviews of these manifestations of hypothalamic disorder and their counterparts evoked by animal experimentation in this primitive part of the brain are provided by the writings of Le Gros Clark et al. (1938), Hess (1954), Harris (1955 & 1960), Strom (1960), and Glees (1961). Hess emphasizes that the diencephalon should be regarded as an *area* of integration and not a *centre* which is a 'device to establish connections ... to attribute the central function of organization to a circumscribed structure, even to a conglomeration of cells or a nucleus, is a concept which must be rejected'.

Recurrent symptoms suggestive of meningitis are sometimes encountered and are thought to be due to leakage of the contents of cysts into the CSF pathways, thereby causing a chemical meninigitis.

Hallucinations are not infrequent. Olfactory and gustatory are the least common and may be due to the lesion exciting the entorhinal cortex. More frequent are visual hallucinations; these may be of vivid colours or highly organized, comprising animals and humans, sometimes of horrifying shapes. These may occupy the blind half field. These are similar to the peduncular hallucinosis described by Lhermitte (1932), who emphasized two other characteristics, the dreamlike associated state and the silence of the hallucination.

Impairment of mental processes is present in a considerable proportion of patients, nearly one-third of Northfield's series. It varies from dullness to severe dementia. Patients with irremovable tumours and under observation for many years may show gradual deterioration whilst vision and physique are relatively well preserved. Endocrine failure plays a part, for substitution therapy may noticeably brighten the behaviour. Obstructive hydrocephalus also plays a part since some, though by no means all, patients are improved by ventricular drainage operations. In other cases extension into the frontal lobes is an additional handicap. But even when allowances are made for these complicating factors, there remains impressive evidence that tumours invading the third ventricle cause dementia and particularly interfere with memory. Williams and Pennybacker (1954) draw attention to the memory defect; in 32 patients with craniopharyngioma they found some degree of loss of memory in three-quarters of the 21 in which the tumour involved the third ventricle, whereas in 11 in which the tumour had produced a chiasmal syndrome without evidence of third ventricular involvement there was none with defective memory.

### Investigations

*Endocrine tests* are discussed in the section on pituitary adenomas. Features suggesting infantilism need critical examination; previous photographs and records of height and weight are helpful and assessment of stunted growth should pay regard to familial influences. Radiological examination of epiphyses provides valuable information concerning bone age. The presence or otherwise of diabetes insipidus should be sought by fluid balance charts and by measurement of the specific gravity of the urine. Many patients still present acutely ill, and special attention must be paid to the state of hydration and electrolyte balance.

*Radiological examination* should commence with X-rays of the skull because of the frequency with which calcium is deposited within these tumours. The incidence is variously estimated at 50–80%. It may be present at birth, or more commonly become visible later. The calcification may be within the sella or above it, and is granular, irregular in outline and may be so dense as to suggest bone; it may be curvilinear, suggesting a portion of the wall of a cyst. Calcification following healed tuberculous meningitis may present a similar appearance. The sella turcica is normal in nearly half the cases, but in the others may present a variety of changes. It may have a flattened saucer shape, with a stunted dorsum and concave upper surface to the posterior clinoid processes. The sella may be moderately ballooned like that due to an enlarging pituitary adenoma, but the total destruction of the dorsum and the extreme excavation seen in large pituitary adenomas rarely occurs. Minor degrees of enlargement and rarefaction of the dorsum and the posterior clinoids are indistinguishable from the effects of raised intracranial pressure. In children there may be separation of the sutures and copper beating.

*CT scan* can be diagnostic in the majority of cases. In the case of children under the age of five years and in the case of demented adults it may be necessary to perform this examination under general anaesthesia. A conventional CT scan with basal cuts with and without iodine enhancement is performed initially, and if there is evidence of a mass arising above the sella a coronal scan can be of great help in planning treatment. Calcium deposits are particularly well seen on the unenhanced scan and may be aggregated together or appear as the wall of a cyst. Cyst contents are hypodense with respect to brain, and may be more or less dense than CSF. The prolongations and extensions of a craniopharyngioma are well seen on CT scans, as is the relationship of solid to cyst within the tumour (Fig. 9.14 a–d).

As with large pituitary adenomas *angiography* is only necessary for two reasons: to reveal the arterial displacements in subtuberal tumours and to exclude an aneurysm. In the case of the latter it is very rare for aneurysms to calcify in children and adolescents.

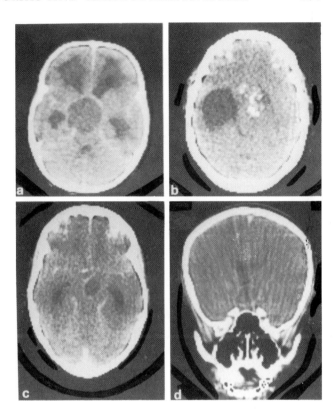

**Fig. 9.14.** CT scans.
(a) Contrasted CT showing large cystic craniopharyngioma with enhancing rim in expanded third ventricle and causing hydrocephalus.
(b) Uncontrasted CT showing large cystic craniopharyngioma extending into left lateral ventricle, with patchy calcification in third ventricle.
(c) Enhanced CT scan showing craniopharyngioma within third ventricle. This was excised only for patient to return with expansion of another craniopharyngioma within the chiasm (see d).
(d) Enhanced CT (same patient as c). Craniopharyngioma within optic chiasm.

## Differential diagnosis

*In children and adolescents* with endocrine disturbance and suprasellar calcification the diagnosis is rarely in doubt; if calcification is absent hypothalamic glioma or ependymoma is the likeliest alternative. Most difficulty arises in children with hydrocephalic symptoms and papilloedema, too young for visual field examination. Such a picture may be caused by a midline cerebellar tumour, aqueduct stenosis, subdural effusions and occasionally tumours of the hemisphere or within the supratentorial ventricular system. However CT scan should easily be able to differentiate these.

*In adults* the two most common difficulties are to distinguish a craniopharyngioma from a pituitary adenoma and a giant aneurysm in the suprasellar region. In the case of the former the presence or absence of calcification can be of great help, since it is very rare for pituitary adenomas to calcify. However, it must be admitted that on occasions it is only at operation that the diagnosis is made. It is of course essential that a surgeon knows whether or not he is dealing with an aneurysm before operating. Large aneuryms arising from the basilar artery or anterior part of the circle of Willis may bulge into the third ventricle and angiography is necessary in those cases in which the CT scan has shown a mass above a sella of normal size.

## Treatment

The treatment of craniopharyngioma is fraught with difficulty and disappointment and demands from the neurosurgeon mature judgement. It subdivides into two main areas: the treatment of the mass lesion with any coincidental raised intracranial pressure, and the treatment of any associated endocrinological disorder. For the former the neurosurgeon has available a variety of direct and indirect surgical procedures together with external radiation; the latter demands close collaboration with an endocrinologist. When considering the nature of operation the surgeon must take account of the natural history of the tumour so far as it can be forecast; partial removal may provide a normal life expectancy in an adult past middle age, whereas in a child, due to the greater growth propensity of craniopharyngioma in this age group (Shapiro *et al.* 1979), this manoeuvre will almost certainly result in early recurrence. Extirpation requires the highest level of skill and ability in this respect should qualify the surgeon's judgement. Matson (1964) and Matson and Crogler (1969) urged radical excision as a primary procedure in the young, and this should be the aim today, reserving other procedures for those patients in whom this is impossible. In a follow-up of Matson's series Katz (1975) was unable to produce predictive criteria to determine which tumours are amenable to radical surgical excision. The skilled neurosurgeon can only embark on radical surgical excision in an individual patient, and if this fails, fall back on the other procedures. Endocrine disturbance is not an indication for operation and requires replacement therapy.

*Direct surgery*

In cases in which the position of the tumour appears to be mainly subtuberal the operative approach and manoeuvres are similar to that for a large pituitary adenoma. When the mass is identified, aspiration of large cysts immediately relieves local tension and improves access so as to allow of an assessment of the local morbid anatomy. Although an 'intracapsular' removal of tumour by 'morcellement' reduces its bulk, the epithelial remnants remain to give rise to recurrence; the removal of the wall of the tumour and of its cysts is essential for total extirpation. The cyst wall is in places tenuous, transparent, friable and adherent; it is difficult to see and remove; not infrequently recurrence some years after an apparently radical excision proves that

epithelial fragments escaped detection and excision. The solid parts of the tumour are often deepest, adherent to the tuber and perhaps posterior to the basilar artery. Dissection has to be of the gentlest, with an acute awareness of the surrounding structures. Judgement is required to decide whether total excision is technically possible and the answer to this question should be decided as early in the operation as possible. Nothing is gained by the meticulous dissection of cyst wall from important vessels with accompanying risk of haemorrhage, if in the final stages a mass of tumour has to be left *in situ* because of its firm union to the floor of the third ventricle. In some cases the tumour sends a prolongation into the third ventricle; it may be possible to remove it by an incision into the lamina terminalis. Extensions of the tumour underneath the hypothalamus and along the body of the sphenoid are extemely difficult to remove completely, but may be approached either in front of a prefixed chiasm or alternatively underneath the temporal lobe.

Tumours within the third ventricle can be approached either through the lateral ventricle or through the corpus callosum, using the presence of hydrocephalus to facilitate the approach. In the case of the former an opening is made into the frontal horn. The tumour can be seen through the dilated foramen of Monro, which can be enlarged if necessary by dividing the anterior pillar of the fornix. Any cysts are emptied, and the tumour loosened from the walls of the ventricle; this is often easy for its dorsal portion, but its ventral and deeper portion is usually firmly adherent due to gliosis. In the case of the transcallosal approach a 2–3 cm incision is made in the corpus callosum and then entry is gained to the third ventricle, when the operation is continued as above.

*Indirect surgery*

There are two main methods for indirectly controlling craniopharyngiomas: cyst drainage and ventricular drainage operations. If it is felt that direct surgery is inadvisable either because of the patient's poor general condition or because the mass is too extensive for radical excision, and provided there is a large cyst, then the volume of the mass may be reduced by drainage operations. The best method is to insert a catheter into the cyst and connect this to a subcutaneous reservoir, so that subsequent intermittent aspiration can be carried out with minimal upset to the patient. Hydrocephalus, either continuing after attempts at radical excision or continuing spontaneously, can be controlled by ventricular drainage operations. If the third ventricle is occluded by tumour a bilateral procedure will be necessary, either in the form of Torkildsen's ventriculocisternostomy or bilateral ventricular catheters connected to a common peritoneal shunt.

*Pre- and postoperative care*

If the patient's state will allow, a full endocrinological assessment needs to be performed under the care of an endocrinologist; the appropriate substitution therapy can then be commenced prior to surgery. However some patients will be in a poor general state as well as deteriorating from pressure effects. Under these circumstances rapid attempts must be made to correct fluid and electrolyte imbalance and the patient must be given steroid cover in the form of hydrocortisone.

Postoperative complications relate to the degree and extent of the damage inflicted upon the hypothalamus and its hypophyseal connections, which when severe usually end fatally. Stupor demands the careful nursing care common for all unconscious patients. Depression or elevation of the temperature, shivering and restlessness are treated symptomatically. Diabetes insipidus must be looked for by carefully noting input and output on fluid balance charts, specific gravity of the urine, and estimations of the serum and urine osmolality. When it occurs it should be treated with DDAVP. It is much better to attempt to stay ahead of problems, but

it must be admitted that complex metabolic disorders can develop which require expert help from not only an endocrinologist but also a clinical chemist. When the patient has recovered, reassessment of endocrinological function will be necessary. Repeat CT scans are performed to assess the completeness or otherwise of (radical) excision, as well as assessing the size of the ventricular system.

*Radiation therapy*

Radiation offers some hope in craniopharyngiomas deemed irremovable, either totally or partially. Recent series have advocated a course of postoperative external radiation for all patients with evidence of craniopharyngiomatous tissue (Shapiro *et al.* 1979, Cabezudo *et al.* 1981), basing this on the evidence that the recurrence rate is lower after such treatment. Cabezudo *et al.* (1981) recommend a course of 5000–6100 rads given over 5–7 weeks, but point out that there are risks of radionecrosis of the brain and optic apparatus, as well as decreased mental performance and retarded growth. However skilled radiation therapy given in small fractionated doses may minimize these adverse effects.

Patients with large cysts would be helped if the cyst could be prevented from refilling with fluid. Attempts to prevent refilling have been made using the installation of radioactive-phosphorus ($P^{32}$) and gold ($Au^{198}$) have been employed (Klar 1953, Talairach *et al.* 1961, Mundinger & Riechert 1962, Spiegel & Wycis 1962). However the results have been disappointing.

*Medical treatment*

The medical treatment of patients with craniopharyngiomas centres around replacement therapy for deficiencies in the hormones of both the anterior and posterior pituitary gland. The replacement of hydrocortisone, thyroid and ADH is along the same lines as that described in the section on pituitary adenomas. In the adult the gonadotrophins are replaced with testosterone or oestrogens as appropriate, but in the child or adolescent these are held back whilst the effects of growth hormone substitution are tried. In the United Kingdom a trial of GH substitution therapy has been supervised by a working party of the Medical Research Council (Milner 1979). It was noted that deficiencies in TSH occurred in 67%, ACTH in 52%, ADH in 43% and gonadotrophins in 97%; and since entrance to the trial depended on GH deficiency this was obviously present in all of the 61 patients in the report of 1979. The response to GH substitution therapy was encouraging, though the report commented that too many children were entering the trial too late to obtain the maximum benefit; these findings reinforce the argument for the early involvement of not only an endocrinologist but also a paediatrician in the management of these difficult cases. GH treatment has recently been suspended due to the rise of transmission of neurotropic viruses. Synthetic GH is now available, however.

### Results and prognosis

In earlier series radical excision of craniopharyngiomas carried a high mortality rate of 30–50% (Cushing 1932, Morello et al. 1962, Northfield 1957, Olivecrona 1963), and this was almost certainly a consequence of inadequate adrenocortical support being available. More recently the operative mortality rate has dropped sharply and varies between 0 and 8%. (Matson & Crogler 1969, Sharpiro et al. 1979, Cabezudo et al. 1981). The quality of survivors in a longterm follow-up of Matson's series (Katz 1975) varies, 68% were doing well (41% excellent, 27% good), though all the survivors suffered from major hypopituitarism. The recurrence rate following attempted radical excision varies from 17% (Matson & Crogler 1969) to 30% (Cabezudo et al. 1981), however this last group of workers reduced the recurrence rate to 6% by giving

external irradiation. In patients treated by surgery that was not radical the recurrence rate is much higher; 78% in Shapiro's series and 71% in Cabezudo's series.

The other aspect of the results of treatment relates to the success or otherwise of endocrine replacement therapy, particularly with regard to growth. In the MRC trial (Milner et al. 1979) when children were started on treatment early the longterm results were satisfactory: out of 30 children with GH deficiency due to craniopharyngioma 18 (60%) achieved a height above the third centile. Many of those who failed to reach this level were commenced on replacement therapy at very late bone ages; it is therefore essential that any child or adolescent is assessed by an endocrinologist once surgery and/or radiation therapy has been completed.

## References

ABBOUD C. F. & LAWS E. R. (1979) J. Neurosurg., 51, 271.
BABINSKI M. J. (1900) Rev. Neurol., 8, 531.
BASKIN D. S., BOGGAN J. E. & WILSON C. B. (1982) J. Neurosurg., 56, 634.
BELCHETZ P. E. (1984) (Ed) Management of Pituitary Disease. Chapman & Hall, London.
BENOIT R., PEARSON-MURPHY B. E. & ROBERT F. (1982) Clin. Endocrin., 12, 11.
BERGLAND R. & RAY B. S. (1969) J. Neurosurg., 31, 327.
BERGLAND R. M., RAY B. S. & TORACLE R. M. (1968) J. Neurosurg., 28, 93.
BESSER G. M., RATCLIFFE J. G., CRYER J. G. & SCOTT A. P. (1972) In Cushing's Syndrome, Diagnosis and treatment (Ed. Binder C. & Hall P.) Heineman, London.
BULL J. W. D. (1956) Acta. Radiol., 46, 72.
BURKE C. W. (1977) In Recent Advances in Endocrinology and Metabolism (Ed. O'Riordan J. L. H.) Churchill Livingstone, Edinburgh.
BUSCH W. (1951) Arch. Path. Anat., 320, 437.
CABEZUDO J. M., VAQUERO J., AREITIO E., MARTINEX R., GARCIA DE SOLA R. & BRAVO G. (1981) J. Neurosurg., 55, 371.
CAIRNS H. (1938) Trans. Oph. Soc. U.K., 58, 464.
CATON R. & PAUL F. T. (1893) Brit. Med. J., 2, 1421.
CHI J. G. & LEE M. H. (1980) J. Neurosurg., 52, 667.
COHEN S. I. (1982) Brit. J. Hosp. Med., 27, 548.
CUSHING H. (1912) The Pituitary Body and its Disorders. Lippincott, Philadelphia.
CUSHING H. (1914) J. Amer. Med. Ass., 63, 1515.
CUSHING H. (1930) Arch. Ophth., 3, 505 and 704.
CUSHING H. (1932) Bull. Johns Hopk. Hosp., 50, 137.
CUSHING H. (1932) Intracranial Tumours. Thomas, Springfield, Illinois.
DANIEL P. M. (1963) In Scientific Basis of Medicine, Annual Reviews, page 83. The Athlone Press, London.

Di Chiro G. & Nelson K. B. (1962) *Amer. J. Roetgenol.*, **87**, 989.

Domingue J. N. & Wilson C. B. (1977) *J. Neurosurg.*, **46**, 601.

Drachman G. (1963) *Arch. Neurol.*, **8**, 145.

Eastman R. C., Gorden P. & Roth J. (1979) *J. Clin. Endocrin.*, **48**, 931.

Erdheim J. (1904) *Sitzungsb. Kon. Wissensch. Wien.*, **113**, Abt. 3537.

Ernest I. & Ekman H. (1972) *Acta Endrocrin* (Copenhagen), **69**, suppl 160, 3.

Evans H. & Long. J. (1921) *Anat. Records.*, **21**, 62.

Evans W. G. & Picciotto G. (1948) *Brit. J. Radio.*, **21**, 330.

Fahlbusch R. (1981) In C. Beardwell, R. L. Robertson (Eds.) *The Pituitary*, Butterworth, London.

Faria M. A. & Tindall G. T. (1982) *J. Neurosurg.*, **56**, 33.

Fijii K., Chambers S. M. & Rhoton A. L. (1979) *J. Neurosurgery*, **65**, 733.

Foy P. M., Copeland G. P. & Shaw M. D. M. (1981) *Acta. Neurochir.*, **55**, 253.

Frantz A. G., Kleinberg D. L. & Noel G. L. (1972) *Recent Progress in Hormone Research.*, **28**, 527.

Fraser R. (1970) *Brit. Med. J.*, **4**, 449.

Frohlich A. (1901) *Wien. Klin. Rundschau.*, **15**, 883.

Glees P. (1961) *Experimental Neurology*. Clarendon Press, Oxford.

Goldberg G. H. & Eshbaugh D. E. (1960) *Arch. Path.*, **70**, 293.

Greene R. (1951) *Practice of Endocrinology*. Eyre & Spottiswoode, London.

Grossman A. & Besser G. M. (1985) *Brit. Med. J.*, **290**, 182.

Guiot G. (1978) In *Treatment of Pituitary Adenomas* (Eds. Fahlbusch R. & Werder K. V.) Thieme, Stuttgart.

Hall K. (1981) In *Advanced Medicine* (Ed. Tunbridge W. M. G.) Pitman Medical, London.

Halstead A. E. (1910) *Surg. Gynae. Obstet.*, **10**, 494.

Harriman D. G. F. (1976) In *Neuropathology* (Ed. Blackwood W. & Corsellis J. A. N.) Arnold, London.

Harris G. W. (1955) *Neural Control of the Pituitary Gland*. Arnold, London.

Harris G. W. (1960) *Handbook of Physiology*. Section 1, Neurophysiology. 2, 1007. Waverley Press, Baltimore.

Harrison B. D., Millhouse K. A., Harrington M. & Nabarro J. D. (1978) *Quart. J. Med.*, **47**, 517.

Hardy J. (1971) *J. Neurosurg.*, **34**, 582.

Hardy J. (1979) In *Functional Neurosurgery* (Ed. Rsamussen T. & Marino R.) Raven Press, New York.

Henderson W. R. (1939) *Brit. J. Surg.*, **26**, 811.

Hess W. R. (1954) *The Diencephalon*. Heinemann, London.

Hill S. A., Falko J. M., Wilson C. B. & Hunt W. E. (1982) *J. Neurosurg.*, **57**, 515.

Hirsch O. (1910) *J. Amer. Med. Ass.*, **55**, 772.

Hubble D. (1952) *Lancet*, **1**, 1123.

Hughes B. (1954) *The Visual Fields*. Blackwell, Oxford.

Jadresic A. (1983) *J. roy. Soc. Med.*, **76**, 947.

Jadresic A., Banks L. M. & Child D. R. (1982) *Quart. J. Med.*, **51**, 189.

Jefferson A. (1978) In *Treatment of Pituitary Adenomas* (Ed. Falhbusch R. & Werder K. V.) Thieme, Stuttgart.

Jefferson G. (1940) *Proc. roy. Soc. Med.*, **40**, 419.

Jefferson G. (1954) *Trans. Oph. Soc. U.K.*, **65**, 262.

Jefferson G. (1955) *The Invasive Pituitary Adenomas*. The Third Sherrington Lecture. Liverpool University Press.

Jeffreys R. V. & Buxton. P. (1984) *J. Neurol. Neurosurg. Psychiat.* **47**, 46.

Jeffreys R. V. (1984) In *Management of Pituitary Disease* (Ed. Belchetz P. E.) Chapman & Hall, London.

Kaiser F. E., Orth D. N., Mukai K. & Oppenheimer J. H. (1983) *J. Clin. Endocrin.*, **57**, 649.

Kanavel A. B. (1909) *J. Amer. Med. Ass.*, **53**, 1704.

Katz E. L. (1975) *J. Neurosurg.*, **42**, 86.

Klar E. (1953) *Arch. klin. Chirurg.*, **276**, 117.

Klein I., Parveen G., Gavaler J. S. & Vanthiel D. H. (1982) *Ann. int. Med.*, **97**, 27.

Klibanski A., Ridgway E. C. & Zervas N. T. (1983) *J. Neurosurg.*, **59**, 585.

Krupp P. & Turkalj I. (1984) In *Prolactinomas and Pregnancy* (Ed. Harrison R. F., Bonnar J. & Thompson W.) MTP Press, Lancaster.

Landolt A. M. (1975) *Acta Neurochir.*, Supplement 22.

Landolt A. M. & Strebel P. (1980) In *Advances and Technical Standards in Neurosurgery* (Ed. Krayenbuhl H.) Springer-Verlag, Wien.

Laws E. R., Fode N. C., Randall R. V., Abboud C. F. & Coulam C. B. (1983) *J. Neurosurg.*, **58**, 685.

Le Gros Clark W. E., Beattie J., Riddoch G. & Dott N. N. (1938) *The Hypothalamus*. Oliver & Boyd, Edinburgh.

Lhermitte J. (1932) *Encephale.*, **27**, 422.

Love J. G. (1952) *Surg. Clin. N. Amer.*, **32**, 1005.

Lundberg P. O., Osterman P. O. & Wide L. (1981) *J. Neurosurg.*, **55**, 194.

Lyle K. (1961) *Proc. roy. Soc. Med.*, **54**, 611.

McLean A. J. (1930) *Ztschr. ges. Neurol. Psychiat.*, **126**, 639.

McConnell A. A. & Mooney A. J. (1938) *Brain.*, **61**, 37.

McGregor A. M., Scanlon M. F., Hall R., Cook D. B. & Hall. K. (1979) *Brit. Med. J.*, **2**, 700.

Marie P. (1886) *Rev & Med.*, **6**, 297.

Marie P. & Marinesco G. (1891) *Arch. Med. exp. Anat. Path.*, **3**, 539.

Mason A. S. M. (1971) *Proc. roy. Soc. Med.*, **64**, 749.

Matson D. D. (1964) *Clin. Neurosurg.*, **10**, 116.

Matson D. D. & Crogler J. F. (1969) *J. Neurosurg.*, **30**, 377.

Milner R. D. G. (1979) *Clin. Endocrin.*, **11**, 15.

Minkowski O. (1887) *Berl. klin. Wsch.*, **24**, 371.

Morello G., Migliavacca G. & Frera C. (1962) *Neurochirurgie.*, **8**, 309.

Mundinger F. & Riechert T. (1962) *Confin. Neurol.*, **22**, 190.

Nelson D. H., Meakin J. W. & Thorn G. W. (1960) *Ann. Intern. Med.*, **52**, 560.

Northfield D. W. (1957) *Brain.*, **80**, 293.

Nugent E. R., Sprinkle P. & Bloor B. M. (1970) *J. Neurosurg.*, **32**, 443.

Obrador S. (1972) *J. Neurosurg.*, **36**, 162.

Olivecrona, H. (1963) *Second Europ. Cong. Neurol. Surg. Exc. Med. Int. Cong. Series* No. 60, 66.

Oppenheim O. (1901) *Psychiat.*, **34**, 303.

Oxenhandler D. C. & Sayers M. P. (1978) *J. Neurosurg.*, **48**, 34.

Putnam T. J., Benedict G. B. & Tell H. (1929) *Arch. Surg.*, **18**, 1708.

Rosegay H. (1981) *J. Neurosurg.*, **54**, 448.

Ross E. J. & Lynch D. C. (1982) *Lancet*, **2**, 646.

Russell D. S. & Rubenstein L. J. (1977) *Pathology of Tumours of the Nervous System*. Arnold, London.

Schaeffer J. P. (1924) *Anat. Records.*, **28**, 243.

SCHEITHAUER B. W., KOVACS K. J., LAWS E. R. & RANDALL R. V. (1986) *J. Neurosurg.*, **65**, 733.

SCOTT G. I. (1957) *Traquair's Clinical Perimetry*, 7th edition. Kimpton, London.

SHAPIRO K., TILL K. & GRANT. N. (1979) *J. Neurosurg.*, **50**, 617.

SHEEHAN H. L. & SUMMERS V. K. (1949) *Quart. J. Med.*, **18**, 319.

SIMMONDS M. (1914) *Dtsch. Med. Wochnschogy.*, **40**, 322.

SPIEGEL E. A. & WYCIS H. T. (1962) *Stereo-encephalotomy*, part 2. Grune & Stratton, New York.

SPRAWSON E. (1937) *Brit. Dent. J.*, **62**, 177.

STROM G. (1960) *Handbook of Physiology*, Section 1. Neurophysiology. 2. 1173. Waverley Press, Baltimore.

SYMON L. & JAKOBOWSKI J. (1979) *J. Neurol, Neurosurg. Psychiat.*, **42**, 123.

SYMONDS C. P. (1962) *Bull. Johns. Hopk. Hosp.*, **111**, 72.

TALAIRACH J., SZIKLA G., TOURNOUX P., CONSTANS P., BANCAUD. & BONIS A. (1961) *Second Intern. Cong. Neurol. Surg. Exc. Med. Int. Cong.* series 36.

TEASDALE G. (1983) *Clin. Endocrin. Metabol.*, **12**, 789.

THORNER M. O. & BESSER G. M. (1978) In *Recent Advances in Endocrinology and Metabolism* (Ed. O'Riordan J. L. H.) Churchill Livingstone, Edinburgh.

TROUILLAS J., GIROD C. & SASOLAS G. (1981) *J. Path.*, **135**, 315.

TRUMBLE H. (1951) *Brit. J. Surg.*, **39**, 7.

WAKAI S., FUKUSHIMA T., TERAMOTO A. & SARO K. (1981) *J. Neurosurg.*, **55**, 187.

WEINBERGER L. M., ADLER F. H. & GRANT F. C. (1940) *Arch. Ophth.*, **24**, 1197.

WILLIAMS M. & PENNYBACKER J. (1954) *J. Neurol. Neurosurg. Psychiat.*, **17**, 115.

WILLIS R. A. (1948) *The Pathology of Tumours*. Butterworth, London.

WISE B. L., BROWN H. N., NAFFZIGER H. C. & BOLDREY E. B. (1955) *Surg. Gynae. Obstet.*, **101**, 185.

WRIGHT A. D., HARTIG M., PALETR H., TEVAARWERK G. DOYLE F. H., ARNOT R., JOPLIN G. F. & FRASER T. R. (1970) *Proc. roy. Soc. Med.*, **63**, 220.

# Chapter 10
# Tumours and tumour-like lesions of the skull

## R. V. JEFFREYS

## Osteomas

These may occur anywhere in the skull but Abbott and Courville (1945) distinguish three groups. The *vault* osteoma arises from the outer table to form a very slowly growing sessile mass; X-ray examination reveals a dense homogeneous protrusion merging imperceptibly with the surrounding bone. Thickening of the inner table, spicule formation, rarefaction and vascular markings are all absent; such changes would suggest the hyperostosis of a meningioma. A rare variety of osteoma may arise in the *great wing of the sphenoid* forming a diffuse mass. The third group comprises those which occur in the *paranasal sinuses*. They are the most important because of the serious intracranial complications to which they may give rise and because of the technical difficulties which may be encountered during their removal. *Orbito-ethmoidal* osteomas grow rather more rapidly than those elsewhere in the skull. They may possess a partial cap of cartilage and are pedunculated; the point of origin may be difficult to determine and if this is not completely removed the tumour is likely to recur. They usually arise from the labyrinth of the ethmoid and it has been suggested that this predilection is due to the presence of cartilagenous rests and to the complicated pattern of fusion of the ethmoid with the frontal and maxillary bones (Abbott & Courville 1945). Eden (1939) considered that these tumours may be osteochondromas. Small and clinically silent osteomas are not infrequently seen within the frontal sinuses as a chance radiological finding (Fig. 10.1). In a series of 51 osteomas of the paranasal sinuses collected by Hallberg and Begley (1950) 40 originated in the frontal

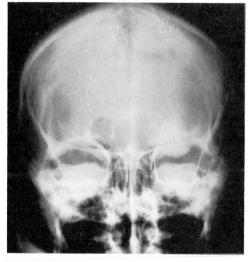

**Fig. 10.1.** Osteoma of lateral compartment of the left frontal sinus, occurring as chance finding on skull radiography.

sinuses, 9 in the ethmoidal and 2 in the maxillary. A large specimen may measure 5 cm or more (Fig. 10.2). It bulges into the medial aspect of the orbit displacing the eyeball laterally and forwards, obstructs the nasal cavity and erodes and protrudes through the floor of the anterior cranial fossa. The dura mater gives way before the osteoma so that it indents the brain which is protected only by leptomeninges and these are often destroyed by pressure atrophy. Frequently a double layer of sinus mucosa is invaginated as a cap over the tumour. If drainage from this diverticulum is imperfect a mucocoele forms between the osteoma and the brain and infection from the nose will lead to suppurative meningitis and to brain abscess. CSF rhinorrhoea, the result of erosion of the bone and of perforation of the dura, is a common complication and adds to the

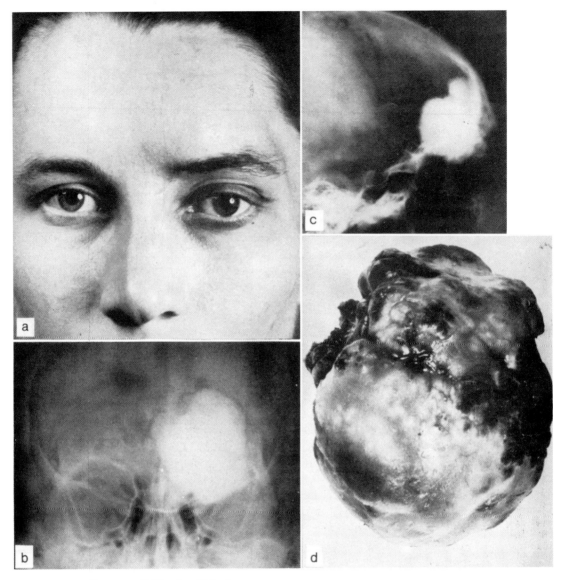

**Fig. 10.2.**  Orbito-ethmoidal osteoma.
(a) left supraorbital prominence, eyeball displaced slightly downwards and forwards.
(b) The tumour is capped by a narrow translucent zone, caused by a covering of cartilage.
(c) The nodularity is well displayed.
(d) The surgical specimen, with cartilage covering the broad surface.

risk of intracranial infection. Occasionally air is forced into the intracranial cavity; it may accumulate extradurally, in the subdural and subarachnoid spaces, in the lateral ventricles, or may create a large cavity within the adjacent frontal lobe, an aerocoele, in which event headaches and hemiparesis may rapidly develop.

Cushing (1927) drew attention to these dangerous complications, which arise spontaneously or attend removal of the tumour, in an account of his experiences in 4 cases. Because of the limited access provided by a direct nasal or orbital route and the impossibility of satisfactorily dealing with the intracranial condition, he introduced the transfrontal approach. The first 2 patients developed CSF rhinorrhoea after the operation and died of meningitis. When the next case presented he sealed the gap in the dura mater with a graft of fascia lata, a manoeuvre which he stated occurred to him in a recent operation for a meningioma. This technique was successful in preventing rhinorrhoea in that and the fourth case and since then has been incorporated into neurosurgical craft. Cushing acknowledged that Dandy had independently devised the same procedure at about the same time. Kessel (1953) has recorded details of 9 cases and Pool *et al* (1962) of 18 cases.

## Mucoceles and pyoceles of paranasal sinuses

Although not tumours in the usual sense of the term, these lesions may behave like neoplasms and produce neighbourhood neurological disturbance. In this context it must be remembered that the sphenoid sinus has the following soft tissue structures adjacent to it: pituitary gland, the first six cranial nerves, the carotid arteries and cavernous sinuses. Obstructed drainage causes the sphenoid sinus to enlarge as a result of retained mucus, which may or may not become infected; the bony walls may be eroded and a cyst-like expansion of the mucosal lining bulges into the cranial cavity. Of 55 cases studied by Lundgren and Olin (1961) the sphenoidal sinus was affected in 40. In analysing 63 reported cases of sphenoidal sinus mucocele Nugent *et al.* (1970) found the clinical features followed a consistent pattern of frontal and orbital pain, visual loss, ocular motor palsies; all these being added to a pre-existing sinusitis. Mucoceles of the frontal and ethmoidal sinuses often erode into the orbit and give rise to proptosis. An osteoma may be the cause of the obstruction and most orbitoethmoidal osteomas are complicated by a

mucocele (or pyocele), though it may be too small of itself to give rise to intracranial complications (Pool *et al.* 1962).

Radiological examination reveals enlargement and opacity of the affected sinus, local erosion of the frontal bone in the case of the frontal sinus and if the sphenoidal sinus is involved there is usually enlargement of the sella turcica in addition to the sinus itself. There is often a lack of a distinct edge to erosion, and a diffuse loss of density of the surrounding bone which might suggest that the lesion is not a benign tumour.

If possible, intracranial operations are to be avoided for fear of precipitating purulent meningitis. In the case of sphenoidal sinus lesions the operation should ideally be performed below the base of the skull either by transsphenoidal drainage or by more radical operations such as those described by Hakuba *et al.* (1975).

## Fibrous dysplasia

This name was introduced by Lichtenstein (1938) in order to distinguish a disease of bone which has a confusing nomenclature. He stated that 'the term osteitis fibrosa was employed in the German literature to include the osseous lesions of hyperparathyroidism, Paget's disease, giant-celled tumour of bone and localized osteitis fibrosa'. In a subsequent paper (Lichtenstein & Jaffe 1942) he stated that 33 other titles had been used in publications describing the same condition. Fibrous dysplasia describes the one common feature, namely a replacement of bone by connective tissue leading to tumefaction, deformity, thinning and expansion of the bone cortex. The rubbery fibrous tissue may be gritty, containing islands of calcification, ossification and cartilage; there may be cysts and small haemorrhagic areas. There is neither generalized osteoporosis nor disturbance of calcium and phosphorus metabolism.

The common variety of fibrous dysplasia affects several bones (*polyostotic*) and the distribution of these lesions is often unilateral. One bone only may be affected (*monostotic*) but Licht-

enstein and Jaffe point out that careful radiological examination of the rest of the limb or of
an adjacent limb often reveals other unsuspected
foci. Albright *et al.* (1937) described a series of
polyostotic cases which were characterized by
patches of brown pigmentation and endocrine
manifestations, particularly pubertas praecox in
female patients. A clear account of this disease
has been given by Fairbank (1950) who considered that *leontiasis ossia* is of a similar nature;
he estimated that the skull is affected in two-
thirds of the cases of Albright syndrome and in
one-third of polyostotic cases. In 10% of monostotic cases the lesion is in the skull (Feiring *et
al.* 1951). There is now general agreement that
fibrous dysplasia of bone is an obscure developmental disorder and Willis (1962) includes it
with such contrasting conditions as solitary cysts
of bone and osteoid osteoma.

Fibrous dysplasia commences in early life,
though it may not be manifest for many years.
Lichtenstein estimated the average age at the
beginning of symptoms to be 10 years. In 46
cases affecting the skull analysed by Leeds and
Seaman (1962), the initial symptom in 21 was
deformity, in 7 ocular disturbance and in 4 a
pathological fracture; in 11 the finding was incidental. In 29 the lesion involved the frontal bone
and in 19 the sphenoid. There was some evidence
that progress in the size of the lesion was limited
to the years of natural growth.

Radiological changes include translucence,
sclerosis and mottling due to both. The vault
lesions often look like a bone cyst forming an
outward bulge, the basal ones diffuse and
sclerosed. At times there may be difficulty in
distinguishing the monostotic variety from a
meningioma; age of the patient is of outstanding
importance, and careful scrutiny of X-rays
should be carried out for those features favouring
dysplasia, for example diffuseness, dense
shadows within the cranium, patches of translucence and absence of vascularity. Leeds and
Seaman (1962) point out the value of a radioactive scan, since the isotope is taken up poorly
in fibrous dysplasia. A thorough clinical and
radiological search for other bone lesions, and

for evidence of cutaneous and endocrine manifestations of Albright syndrome should not be
omitted.

The presence of fibrous dysplasia of the skull
does not necessarily demand operation. Where
diagnosis remains in doubt, and the lesion is
accessible, biopsy is advisable. In some cases the
lesion causes no significant symptoms and can
safely be kept under observation; this is particularly so in adults in whom the lesion may
not materially advance over a period of years. In
others and in young people in whom further
growth may be anticipated, pressure upon the
visual apparatus or eyeball may require relief. In
these radical excision is not necessary and indeed
often impossible. Enough of the mass should be
removed to achieve the object of the operation;
the remnant may never attain a size sufficient to
cause further trouble.

## Chordoma

These tumours, by reason of their distribution
and their morphology, are generally considered
to arise from cell-rests of the notochord. They
occur throughout the neuraxis, from the sphenoid to the coccyx, the majority being at either
extremity. Formerly it was thought that the
sacrococcygeal tumours greatly outnumbered
the spheno-occipital, but more recent figures
reveal that the distribution between these sites
is less uneven; the reason for the original bias
probably being due to the fact that few intracranial lesions were reported since as Zoltan and
Fényes (1960) concluded 'the diagnosis of
cranial chordoma is extremely difficult, its complete removal impossible, and the prognosis is
hopeless'. Forti and Venturini (1960) found that
of 505 published cases 197 were intracranial,
227 were sacrococcygeal and 81 were vertebral.

The cranial portion of the notochord becomes
embedded within the basi-occiput and terminates immediately behind the pituitary fossa
(Fig. 10.3). The sphenoid is prechordal in
development and the dorsum sellae arises as a
separate formation (Keith 1948). Vestiges of

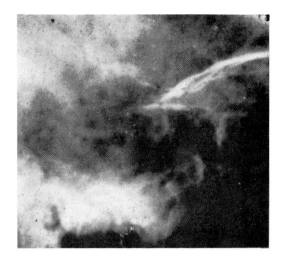

**Fig. 10.3.** Skull X-ray showing extensive destruction of boundaries of sella by chordoma.

notochord may be found occasionally at the base of the dorsum sellae and on the anterior aspect of the coocyx and sacrum (Willis 1962). Willis (1960) states that the earliest example of an intracranial chordoma causing symptoms was recorded by Klebs (1864).

The intracranial chordoma is a tumour which infiltrates and erodes the sphenoid and basi-occiput and may spread into the petrous bones, the paranasal sinuses, the sella turcica and the caverous sinuses. It elevates and perforates the dura mater to form rounded, lobulated masses within any or all of the three cranial fossae. The spread of the tumour is usually asymmetrical and in consequence the signs of cranial nerve involvement tend to be unilateral. Brain tissue is usually not infiltrated but displaced and compressed and arteries and nerves are engulfed by the tumour. In an appreciable number of chordomas, nasal or pharyngeal obstruction is the first symptom (Moya 1960), long preceding evidence of cranial nerve involvement. Whether in these cases the tumour starts in notochordal tissue ventral to the basi-occiput is unknown; their clinical course suggests that the bone is already involved when the patient seeks advice. Falconer *et al.* (1968) subdivided intracranial chordomas into three depending on where the mass of the tumour predominantly lay: *sellar*,

*parasellar* and *clival*. The tumour is usually soft, often mucilagenous, though in parts may be firm like cartilage and gritty as a result of calcareous deposits; it is grey in colour, or red from haemorrhage (often likened to redcurrant jelly), which may give rise to episodes suggestive of a ruptured aneurysm. There may be areas of necrosis. Very rarely they metastasise. A concise and well illustrated account of these tumours was given by Harvey and Dawson (1941), and in a more recent review by O'Neill *et al.* (1985). The latter authors described 34 cases of chordoma occurring during a 50 year period in the Southeast of Scotland, of which 53% were sacrococcygal, 35% intracranial and the remaining 12% in the intervening vertebral column (Table 10.1).

**Table 10.1.** Presenting symptoms and signs of intracranial chordoma.

| |
| --- |
| Cranial nerve palsy 83% |
| Headache 50% |
| Ataxia 17% |
| Papilloedema 17% |
| Endocrine upset 8% |
| Subarachnoid haemorrhage 8% |
| Coma 8% |

Data from O'Neill *et al.* (1985).

### Histology

The microscopic appearance of these tumours is pleomorphic and tends to differ from area to area within the same tumour. It consists of two elements: notochordal cells and a mucoid stroma. Notochordal cells are large polygonal cells which may be arranged in an epotheloid fashion in sheets or cords or may be scattered singly or in small groups in a mucoid matrix. Many of the cells are coarsely vacuolated; some contain a single large vacuole which gives them a *signet ring* appearance, others even more characteristically contain multiple vacuoles and are sometimes called *'physaliphorous'* (bubble-bearing). When scattered in a homogenous mucinous matrix, they resemble the structure of cartilage. Chordomas differ, however, from chondromas or chondrosarcomas through the absence of connective tissue fibres, collagen or reticulin, which are invariably present in cartilagenous tumours.

*Diagnosis and treatment*

Although intracranial chordomas may arise at any age, the majority present between the ages of 20 and 60 years, and more frequently in males. The duration of symptoms varies considerably, from 3 months to 13 years in a series examined by Godtfredsen (1943) and it was more than a year in two-thirds. To some extent this variability will depend upon the inconvenience or severity of the initial symptom, for instance diplopia or deafness contrasted with dysphagia, but the rate of tumour growth seems also to be a variable. The symptoms fall into three categories: headache and vomiting due to raised intracranial pressure, cranial nerve palsies, and nasopharyngeal obstruction; any of these may provide the first symptom (Table 10.1). Involvement of cranial nerves tends to conform with one of two patterns, according to whether the tumour arises anteriorily in the parasellar region, or posteriorily in the basi-occiput. Parasellar tumours are distinguished by the frequency of visual disturbances, which comprise impaired acuity (45%), field defect (22%), ocular palsy (62%), ptosis (26%) and exophthalmos (38%); the percentage incidence is from the review by Moya (1960). Godtfredsen, who made a particular study of the neurological signs of these tumours (1943) and of nasopharyngeal growths (1941), emphasized the frequency of a third or sixth nerve palsy as an early symptom, the sixth twice as commonly as the third. He also noted the occasional involvement of the trigeminal nerve; this was usually restricted to its second division and always in conjunction with a sixth nerve palsy; such anatomical contiguity is found in the lateral wall of the cavernous sinus and the frequent selection of the sixth nerve is doubtless due to the relatively easy pathway for the spread of the tumour to the apex of the petrous bone provided by the foramen lacerum.

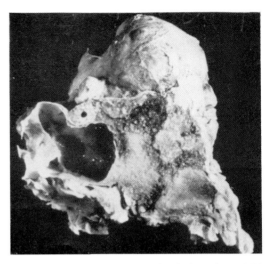

**Fig. 10.4.** Autopsy specimen. Body of sphenoid invaded by chordoma which forms a large rounded mass covered by dura; the pituitary gland is marked by a solid circle; below and in front of the gland is a large sphenoidal air sinus.

Involvement of cranial nerves below the trigeminal indicates a tumour predominantly of the clivus and basi-occiput and in these compression of the pons may give rise to long tract signs and a cerebellopontine angle syndrome may be encountered. Moya (1960) lists facial paralysis (22%), deafness (19%) and hemiparesis (26%).

The radiological demonstration of destructive lesions of the base of the skull can be difficult and necessitates special projections and tomograms in sagittal and coronal planes. In about one-fifth of the cases no bone lesion can at first be detected. In the others, bone destruction, sometimes of great extent, is encountered affecting the sphenoid, basi-occiput and petrous bones, in that order of frequency (Fig. 10.4). The sella may be partially or asymmetrically destroyed, but on occasions is ballooned as though due to a pituitary adenoma. Destruction of the body or greater wing of the sphenoid, together with the apex of the petrous bone, is highly suggestive. Suprasellar calcification was reported in 30% of cases by Kamtin *et al.* (1964). CT scanning will demonstrate the size and extent of a tumour, since chordomas will enhance with iodine contrast; however CT scan cannot by itself give the diagnosis, and the CT scan appearances must be taken together with the changes on plain X-ray. Arising as they do on the floor of the skull, chordomas may distort or even surround the major arteries of the circle of Willis and it is a wise precaution to perform carotid and vertebral angiography before surgical exploration.

In the differential diagnosis of a chordoma, it may be necessary to consider pituitary adenoma and craniopharyngioma, carotid aneurysm, cerebellopontine angle tumours, meningioma, chondroma and intracranial invasion of malignant masopharyngeal neoplasms. Some of these will be excluded by the extent of bone destruction and the information obtained from CT scanning and angiography. When bone erosion is slight or absent the correct diagnosis may only be revealed by surgical exploration.

Treatment of intracranial chordomas has proved generally unsatisfactory. The tumour has often already formed a large mass, or has widely infiltrated the base of the skull by the time the majority of patients seek treatment. Zoltan and Fényes (1960) set out the results of operation in 78 cases reported in the literature: 29 (37%) died and only 6 (7.5%) survived 5 years or more. Whilst agreeing in principle with this gloomy view Falconer *et al.* (1968) felt that worthwhile palliation was achieved by as generous surgical decompression as was feasible, though they also felt that X-irradiation had little to offer. Wold and Laws (1983) reviewed their experience in treating 12 children and young adults with intracranial chordoma and reported that there were 8 (66.6%) survivors, four of whom had been followed up for periods in excess of 5 years. All the survivors had received postoperative X-irradiation. Recently Suit *et al.* (1982) have been treating patients with radical doses of irradiation using a combination of high-energy X-rays (photons) and 160-MV proton beams; since the longest follow-up period was only 26 months it is as yet too early to assess the longterm results of such treatment.

## Chondroma

Tumours of cartilage occasionally arise from the base of the skull (which for the most part ossifies from cartilage). These neoplasms may be either histologically benign (chondroma) or malignant (chondrosarcoma); for reasons of conciseness they will all be referred to as chondroma until treatment and prognosis are discussed. One group of chondromas comprises those arising within the paranasal sinuses; they are only likely to come within the province of the neurosurgeon if they expand upwards and backwards so as to involve the region of the sella and compress the structures in the suprasellar and parasellar regions. The other group arises within the skull, mainly from the region of the foramen lacerum and the synchondroses which converge upon it. According to their point of origin and direction of enlargement they give rise to the neurological disturbance associated with parasellar and cerebellopontine angle tumours. The patients are usually adults and the duration of symptoms varies from months to years. Radiological examination is important because erosion of bone is usually evident and may be extensive; the chondroma commonly calcifies, sometimes densely (Fig. 10.5). A review of such tumours was carried out by Klingler (1950) based upon 26 cases in the literature and 5 of his own; 12 fresh cases were reported by Kleinsasser and Friedmann (1958). In the latter series calcification was detected in 4 of 6 parasellar chondromas, but in none of 3 cerebellopontine angle tumours. These authors state that erosion of the clivus is rare, a point of distinction from chordoma, and enlargement of the internal auditory meatus may not occur with a chondroma of the 'angle' although the apex of the petrous may be eroded. Differential diagnosis is similar to that considered for chordoma.

Operation was performed in the 9 patients with chondroma reported by Kleinsasser and Freidmann (1958) and the tumour partially or totally removed without a death and with good results. In the same paper are the reports of the 3 cases with chondrosarcoma, and the results

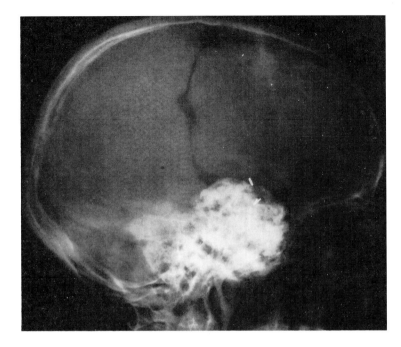

**Fig. 10.5.** Skull X-ray osteochondroma in skull base, which has extensively calcified.

were poor. Recently Suit *et al.* (1982) have advocated radical doses of irradiation using a combination of high-energy X-rays (photons) and 160-MV proton beams; the initial results are a little more encouraging.

## Haemangioma

Whether these vascular lesions should be regarded as malformations or neoplasms seems uncertain. Courville *et al.* (1948) considered them to be neoplastic; Northfield and Russell (1951) grouped them together with the cavernous haemangiomas. They give rise to a slowly growing, often tender, lump on the head and may cause headaches (Rowbotham 1942). The peculiar X-ray appearances were described in detail by Bucy and Capp (1930) who stated that Hitzrot in 1917 was the first to publish an X-ray of an angioma of bone. The characteristic features are erosion of bone with retention, thickening and an increase in density of the trabeculae. In the skull the lesion usually affects the calvarium; the tables may be expanded and spic-

ules of new bone laid down perpendicular to the outer surface, the so-called 'sun-ray' appearance (Fig. 10.6). Bucy and Capp reproduced the photograph of a specimen removed by Cushing which

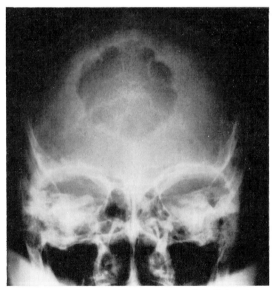

**Fig. 10.6.** Skull X-ray of haemangioma of skull showing typical 'sun-ray' appearance.

illustrates this beautifully. Removal of the tumour may be thought necessary, and if so a small area of surrounding bone should be included in the excision.

## Sarcoma

In a review of osteogenic sarcoma by Cade (1955) based upon a personal experience of 133 cases, in only 2 was the skull the affected bone. He emphasized the importance of age in diagnosis, 78 of the patients were between the ages of 11 and 20 years. Coley (1960) lists 12 (1.2%) affecting the skull in a total of 985 cases of sarcoma of bone. Courveille *et al.* (1962) considered that sarcomatous change in Paget disease (osteitis deformans) provided the majority of cases in adults. They list 36 such examples derived from the literature; the ages of these patients ranging from 42 to 82 years. The tumour causes external and internal swelling, transgresses the dura mater and invades brain.

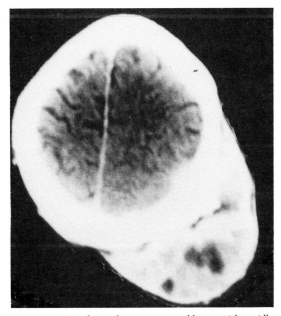

**Fig. 10.7.** CT enhanced scan 20-year-old man with rapidly growing mass over the right parieto-occipital region, which was totally excised and which histology confirmed to be an osteogenic sarcoma.

The X-ray changes are of osteolysis, reactive thickening and radiating spicule formation (Fig. 10.7). Cade (1955) discussed the value of various forms of radiotherapy available at that time, but at that time prognosis for osteogenic sarcoma of the limb was bad though it has improved a little since then. There are too few cases of sarcoma of the skull reported to give an accurate prognosis; since the contemporary treatment for osteogenic sarcoma in limbs is proximal amputation followed by X-irradiation and/or chemotherapy it is clear that the treatment for lesions involving the skull can only be less than adequate. However, if the sarcoma is in the vault of the skull radical excision can be attempted after consultation with an oncologist.

## Histiocytosis

In 1953 Lichtenstein proposed the term *histiocytosis X* to group together 3 syndromes: *eosinophilic granuloma of bone, Hand–Schuller–Christian disease* and *Letterer–Siwe disease*. All these syndromes share the features of infiltration by histiocytes, and he thought that a common aetiological agent might one day be found; such a hope still exists. There is a gradation in severity from the relatively benign eosinophilic granuloma to the rapidly progressive Letterer–Siwe disease which occurs in infancy.

*Eosinophilic granuloma* was first described by Otani and Ehrlich (1940), though Lichtenstein and Jaffe (1940) were making similar and independent observations at about the same time and gave the disease the name by which it is still known. In a later and more extensive account (1944) they pointed out that the granuloma is not always solitary since widespread radiological examination often reveals other and silent foci. The patients are usually children or young adults, and over the course of a month or so a tender bony swelling develops; on the skull it is usually the vault. Plain X-rays demonstrate an area of bone destruction which in some cases may show some reactive sclerosis at its edges (Fig. 10.8). Eosinophilia may be present but

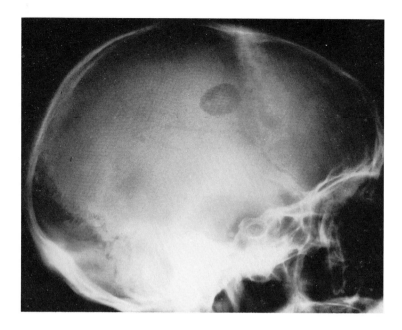

**Fig. 10.8.** Skull X-ray of 8-year-old boy showing an eosinophilic granuloma which was confirmed by excision biopsy.

biopsy may be necessary for diagnosis. The characteristic feature of the granulomatous tissue is the infiltration with eosinophilic leucocytes. The lesion responds well to curettage, but where pain persists radiotherapy may be helpful; in which case 600 rads is usually sufficient (*Lancet* 1977).

*Hand–Schuller–Christian* disease (HSC) may be encountered by neurosurgeons because of the nature of the three most common manifestations, namely exophthalmos, diabetes insipidus and osteolytic lesions. This disease merges into *Letterer–Siwe* (LS) disease, though paradoxically it is the destructive lesions in bone which when present at diagnosis distinguish HSC most clearly from the poorer prognosis of LS (Lancet 1977). HSC disease is one of infants and young children in whom granulomas affect bones, brain, lung, pleura, pericardium, lymph nodes, spleen, liver and skin. The skull bones are prone and the membrane bones in particular. The granulomatous lesions cause destruction without reaction, may be extensive and may involve the full thickness of the calvarium so that there is a bulge transmitting the intracranial pulsations, apt to be mistaken for a variety of cyst. The radiological features are those of osteolysis with clearly defined edges and of irregular outline. Within the skull the granuloma spreads over the subdural endothelial surface and in the subarachnoid space. Exophthalmos results from its direct spread into the orbits and diabetes insipidus from involvement of the pituitary gland, its stalk and the hypothalamus. Damage to these latter structures also accounts for the failure of sexual development and skeletal growth that may occur. The granulomas consist of a yellowish, soft putty-like tissue, due to the presence of histiocytes. Curettage may deal with the skull lesions as may X-irradiation. However, the systemic aspects of the disease, and that of LS disease, will require chemotherapy which may include the use of vincristine, vinblastine, 6-mercaptopurine, cyclophosphamide and prednisolone, either singly or in a variety of combinations (*Lancet* 1977). The hormonal disturbances can be corrected by the appropriate substitution therapy (*see* section on craniopharyngioma, Chapter 9).

## Plasmacytoma

In myelomatosis skull deposits vary in size, are rarely painful (Snapper *et al.* 1953) and only cause a swelling if an individual lesion is very large. On plain skull X-ray the lesions appear similar to those of carcinomatosis: numerous cleanly-cut rounded areas of translucence with no surrounding reactive change (Figs. 10.9, 10.10 & 10.11), though rarely there may be a circumferential zone of sclerosis (Aguayo *et al.* 1964).

Occasionally the skull is the site of an apparently solitary myeloma (or plasmacytoma as it is then usually called). It may reach a large size, creating an external swelling and giving rise to raised intracranial pressure and neurological disturbance. In these circumstances the radiological appearances are somewhat different; the rounded translucent area may be bounded by a denser margin and traversed by retained trabeculae and the tables of the skull are thinned and expanded.

The view is widely held that a solitary plasmacytoma is but the initial manifestation of myelomatosis and that in due course the generalized disease will become evident (Innes & Newall 1961). To accept the solitary nature of a lesion a thorough radiological search must be made, and this can be made either by plain X-rays or $Tc^{99}$-diphosponate bone scan (Fig. 10.12). The reticuloendothelial and immune systems must also be assessed, and in this context it will be wise to enlist the aid of a haematologist.

The neurological complications of cranial and intracranial myelomatosis have been reviewed by Clarke (1954) who noted the frequency with which cranial nerves palsies result from infiltration of the base of the skull. Another feature is proptosis due to the tumour encroaching upon the orbit. Neuropathy also occurs, which may complicate the clinical picture (Victor *et al.* 1958).

Neurosurgical intracranial procedures are rarely warranted in cranial myelomatosis, but the solitary plasmacytoma can be dealt with surgically if accessible. The tumour is often very vascular and haemorrhage constitutes a real

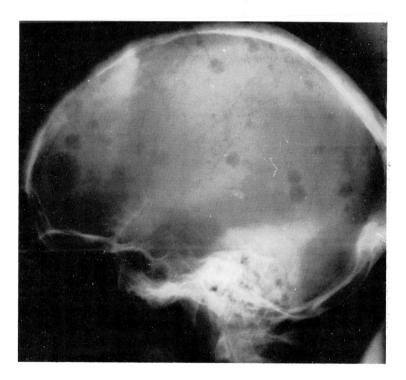

**Fig. 10.9.** Skull X-ray of patient with confirmed multiple myelomatosis. Notice the strong similarities with Fig. 10.10.

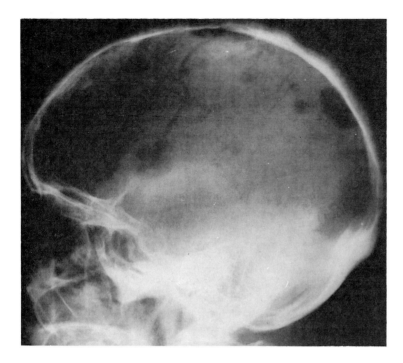

**Fig. 10.10.** Skull X-ray of patient with confirmed multiple metastases from carcinoma of the breast.

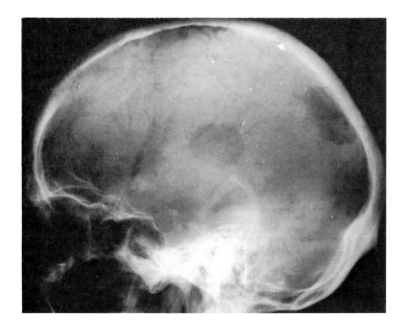

**Fig. 10.11.** Skull X-ray of man with two myelomas of the skull; also see Fig. 10.12.

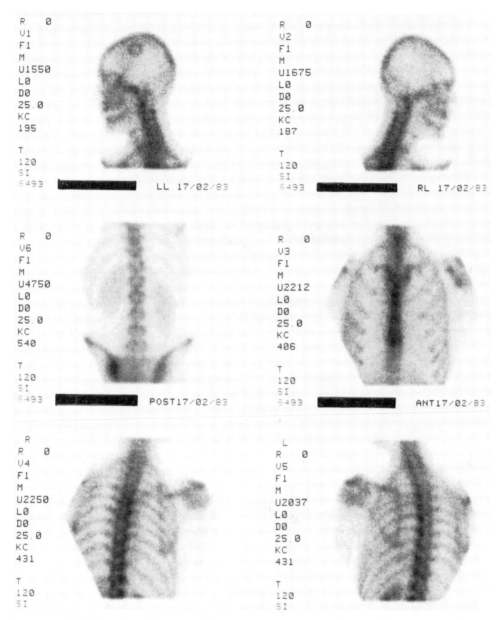

**Fig. 10.12.** Tc$^{99}$-diphosphonate bone scan of same patient as Fig. 10.11. The two skull myelomas can be seen, the parietal more easily; but also note the deposits in the scapulae, some thoracic vertebrae and the 6th right rib.

hazard. More effective treatment is by means of X-irradiation to identified lesions and by chemotherapy for the widespread effects of this disease.

## Glomus jugulare tumour

A small mass of tissue lying in the dome of the bulb of the internal jugular vein was identified and described by Guild (1941) and named by him the glomus jugulare. It is similar in structure to the carotid body and other chemoreceptor organs and like them may give rise to tumours to which the term chemodectoma is applied. More recently histopathologists have grouped together various body tissues which have three features in common: a high content of *Amines*, the capacity for amine *Precursor Uptake*, the presence of amino-acid *Decarboxylase*; for short these cells are called APUD, and tumours that arise from them are called *apudomas*. Carotid body tumours have been recognized since the beginning of the century (Monckeberg 1905) but Willis (1960) states that Bloom (1943) was the first to note similar tumours in other situations. Rosenwasser reported the first case of glomus jugulare tumour in 1945; it presented as a tumour of the tympanic cavity and it became apparent to otologists that vascular polyps often regarded as haemangioma or endothelioma were of this nature (Kramer 1975). Only a thin plate of bone separates the bulb of the internal jugular vein from the tympanic cavity, readily destroyed by a tumour arising in this situation. This accounts for the fact that these tumours often cause otological symptoms in the first instance. They may fill the tympanic cavity, present in the external auditory meatus as a vascular polyp causing deafness, tinnitus (frequently a throbbing synchronous with the pulse and the observer may detect a bruit) and sometimes pain in the ear. Guild (1953) described minute bodies identical with glomus jugulare lying under the mucosa on the medial wall of the middle ear in the course of the tympanic nerve and also found them along the auricular branch of the vagus nerve, and sometimes as far peripherally as the facial canal. It is likely that in some cases the tumour arises from these, which would explain why in about one-half of the recorded cases the tumour remains restricted to the ear (Kramer 1975). Invasion of the petrous bone leads to facial palsy and the tumour may extend into the posterior cranial fossa, reaching as high as the trigeminal nerve and as low as the foramen magnum. Access to the cranial cavity is also provided by the jugular foramen and this may be the route taken by some tumours in which neurological symptoms preceed aural. However, tumours also present with symptoms of a posterior fossa mass without otological symptoms, and in these cases it is more likely that they arise within the cranial cavity rather than within the ear. Tumours may also extend into the neck, into the lumen of the internal jugular vein as a polyp and into the pterygoid fossa.

Glomus jugulare tumours present with maximum incidence between the ages of 40 and 59 years, though the reported age range is 17–85 years (Kramer 1975). There is a strong sex preponderance with tumours occurring five times more frequently in women than men. Bickerstaff and Howell (1953) noted a preponderance of left ear involvement in the ratio of 4:1, especially in men. The tumour usually grows slowly with the average duration of symptoms being 7 years (Kramer 1975). The literature contains reports of cases with multiple glomus tumours, as well as those with a solitary glomus and apudomas elsewhere in the body (Kramer 1975).

Reports have appeared in the literature of distant metastases, though many of them lack histological proof (Kramer 1975); most of these have been to the lungs and liver.

*Histology*

Histologically these tumours are identical with other apudomas such as carotid body tumours. They consist of small nests or trabeculae of solid, tightly packed polygonal cells separated by blood channels which range in size from capillaries to large thin-walled sinuses resembling the blood spaces of a cavernous haemangioma. In order effectively to demonstrate the chromaffin characteristics of the cells it is essential that the surgeon places part of the tumour directly into non-acid dichromate solution for fixation, rather than the usual formalin solution.

*Diagnosis*

The clinical features may show considerable variation, due to the differences in the site of origin and rate of growth. Deafness may be conductive or perceptive; otorrhoea is common and the discharge often bloody. There may be pain in the ear and tinnitus. A bruit may be heard in auscultation over the mastoid process, and auroscopy often reveals a polyp occluding the external auditory meatus or visible through the tympanic membrane. Biopsy will provide a histological diagnosis provided an adequate amount of tissue is obtained and it is fixed in the correct media (*see* above); however, even a biopsy may be rendered difficult by intimidating haemorrhage which yields to packing.

Unilateral progressive paralysis of the fifth to twelfth cranial nerves characterizes progression of the tumour, though cranial nerve palsies do not of themselves signify that the tumour has formed an intracranial mass, for these nerves are at risk to infiltration or compression at various points in their extradural course. Truncal ataxia, limb ataxia, raised intracranial pressure, nystagmus and hemiparesis provide clinical evidence of a posterior mass lesion. Although biopsy of an aural polyp may provide a pathological diagnosis, radiological examination is necessary to define the extent of the tumour. The standard X-rays of the skull should be supplemented by a basal view; features that may be seen include opacification and loss of aeration of the petromastoid air cells, erosion of the petrous bone and enlargement of the jugular foramen. Tomography can be of help in further demonstrating changes in the occipital and petrous bones, and in particular the anatomy of the inner and middle ear; hypocycloidal tomography may demonstrate these structures even more clearly. CT scanning will also demonstrate the anatomy of these structures, but its particular advantage is, after iodine enhancement, to assess the contents of the posterior cranial fossa and delineate the size and extent of a mass lesion (Fig. 10.13).

Carotid angiography may provide a good

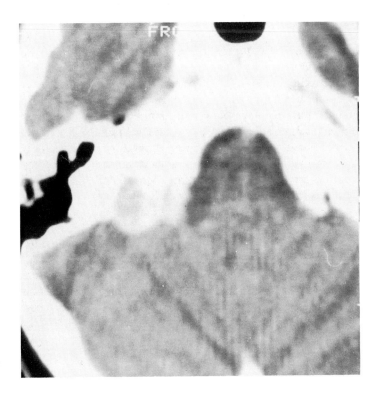

Fig. 10.13. CT enhanced scan of 17-year-old woman with painful deafness in the left ear, showing lesion arising in the petrous bone and beginning to extend into the cerebellopontine angle.

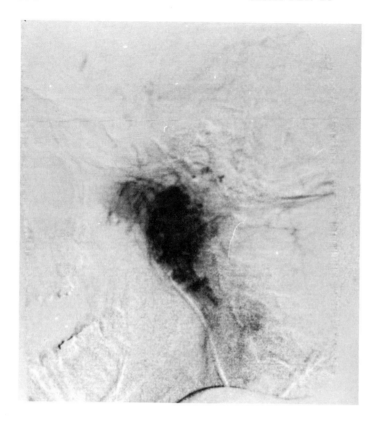

**Fig. 10.14.** Left external carotid angiogram (DVI) of same case as Fig. 10.13, showing large very vascular lesion. This was confirmed histologically as a glomus jugulare tumour.

demonstration of the tumour in its entirety, particularly if allied with subtraction techniques. Tumour circulation is largely derived from the external carotid artery and consequently carotid angiography usually shows no abnormality unless the external branches are well filled (Fig. 10.14). Farrell and Hawkins (1967) have shown that large tumours may acquire a blood supply from the vertebral artery, and they also found jugular phlebography (using the technique of Gejrot & Lauren 1964) helpful in showing obstruction of the internal jugular vein. With this technique it is also possible to demonstrate filling defects due to tumour polyps.

The diagnosis of a glomus jugulare tumour presents considerable difficulties in the earlier stages and it is unlikely to be correct (if indeed thought of) until an aural polyp presents for biopsy or radiological changes can be detected. Occasionally vertigo and vomiting may be sufficiently severe to mimic Ménière disease, or when less so to suggest an acoustic schwannoma. When local cranial nerve palsies follow a long history of aural symptoms the likelihood of a glomus jugulare tumour is considerable. Alternatives are chronic inflammatory disease, carcinoma of the middle ear and those lesions discussed in the differential diagnosis of cerebellopontine angle tumours.

*Treatment*

When the tumour appears to be restricted to the ear, treatment is usually carried out by an otologist and comprises as radical an extirpation as possible by means of a mastoidectomy approach followed by radiotherapy. Mass lesions of the posterior fossa require a neurosurgical approach though not without some trepidation; some of these tumours are extremely vascular. Kempe (1970) has suggested beginning the operation by ligating the external carotid artery, though this may be an unnecessary procedure for some tumours. Opinion is divided on the practical results of X-irradiation (Kramer 1975) though it is usually given in most cases, since even if it does not eliminate the tumour completely it may well reduce its growth potential.

# References

ABBOTT K. H. & COURVILLE C. B. (1945) *Bull. Los Ang. Neurol. Soc.*, **10**, 19.

AGUAYO A., THOMPSON D. W. & HUMPHREY J. G. (1964) *J. Neurol. Neurosurg. Psychiat.*, **27**, 562.

ALBRIGHT F., BUTLER A. H., HAMPTON A. C. & SMITH P. (1937) *New Engl. J. Med.*, **216**, 727.

BICKERSTAFF E. L. & HOWELL J. S. (1953) *Brain*, **76**, 576.

BLOOM F. (1943) *Arch. Path.*, **36**, 1.

BUCY P. C. & CAPP C. S. (1930) *Amer. J. Roentgen.*, **23**, 1.

CADE S. (1955) *J. roy. Coll. Surg. Edin.*, **1**, 79.

CLARK E. (1954) *Brain*, **77**, 61.

COLEY B. L. (1960) *Neoplasms of Bone.* 2nd edition. Hoeber, New York.

COURVILLE C. B., VOGEL R. J. & MURIETTA A. J. (1948) *Bull. Los Ang. Neurol. Soc.*, **13**, 1.

COURVILLE C. B., DEEB P. & MARSH C. (1962) *Bull. Los Ang. Neurol. Soc.*, **27**, 57.

CUSHING H. (1927) *Surg. Gynae, Obstet.*, **44**, 721.

EDEN K. (1939) *Brit. J. Surg.*, **27**, 323.

FAIRBANK H. A. T. (1950) *J. Bone. Joint. Surg.*, **32B**, 403.

FALCONER M. A., BAILEY I. C. & DUCHEN M. B. (1968) *J. Neurosurg.*, **29**, 261.

FARRELL V. J. & HAWKINS T. D. (1967) *Brit. J. Surg.*, **54**, 789.

FEIRING W., FEIRING E. H. & DAVIDOFF L. M. (1951) *J. Neurosurg.*, **8**, 377.

FORTI E. & VENTURINI (1960) *Riv. Anat. Path.*, **17**, 317.

GEJROT T. & LAUREN T. (1964) *Acta Otolaryng.*, **58**, 191.

GODTFREDSEN E. (1941) *Acta. Phychiat. Neurol. Scand.*, **16**, 47.

GODTFREDSEN E. (1943) *Acta. Ophth.*, **21**, 224.

GUILD S. R. (1941) *Anat. Rec. Suppl.*, **2.79**, 28.

GUILD S. R. (1953) *Ann. Oto-rhino-laryng.*, **62**, 1045.

HAKUBA A., KATSUYAMA J. & MATSUOKA Y. (1975) *J. Neurosurg.*, **43**, 368.

HALLBERG O. E. & BEGLEY J. W. (1950) *Arch. Otolaryng.*, **51**, 750.

HARVEY W. F. & DAWSON E. K. (1941) *Edin. Med. J.*, **48**, 713.

INNES J. & NEWALL J. (1961) *Lancet.*, **1**, 239.

KAMRIN R. K., POTANDS J. N. & POOL J. L. (1964) *J. Neurol. Neurosurg. Psychiat.*, **27**, 157.

KEITH A. (1948) *Human Embryology and Morphology.* 6th edition. Arnold, London.

KEMPE L. G. (1970) *Operative Neurosurgery.* Springer, Berlin.

KESSEL F. K. (1953) *Helv. Chirurg. Acta.*, **20**, 83.

KLEBS E. (1864) *Virchows Arch.*, **31**, 396.

KLEINSASSAR O. & FRIEDMANN G. (1958) *D.Z.f. Nernheilk.*, **177**, 378.

KLINGLER M. (1950) *Acta. Neurochir.*, **1**, 337.

KRAMER W. (1975) In *Handbook of Clinical Neurology.* (Ed Vinken P. J. & Bruyn G. W.) **18**, 435.

LANCET EDITORIAL (1977) *Lancet*, **2**, 440.

LEEDS N. & SEAMAN W. B. (1962) *Radiol.*, **78**, 750.

LICHTENSTEIN L. (1938) *Arch. Surg.*, **36**, 874.

LICHTENSTEIN L. & JAFFE H. C. (1940) *Amer. J. Path.*, **16**, 595.

LICHTENSTEIN L. & JAFFE H. C. (1942) *Arch Path.*, **33**, 777.

LICHTENSTEIN L. & JAFFE H. C. (1944) *Arch Path.*, **37**, 99.

LICHTENSTEIN L. (1953) *Arch. Path.*, **56**, 84.

LUNDGREN A. & OLIN T. (1961) *Acta Laryng.*, **53**, 61.

MONCKEBERG J. G. (1905) *Beitrag. Path. Anat.*, **38**, 1.

MOYA G. (1960) *L'Encephale*, **49**, 495.

NORTHFIELD D. W. & RUSSELL D. S. (1951) In *Modern Trends in Neurology.* (Ed. Feiling A.) Butterworth, London.

NUGENT E. R., SPRINKLE P. & BLOOR B. M. (1970) *J. Neurosurg.*, **32**, 443.

OTANI S. & EHRLICH J. C. (1940) *Amer. J. Path.*, **16**, 479.

O'NEILL P., BELL B. A., MILLER J. D., JACOBSON I. & GUTHRIE W. (1985) *Neurosurgery*, **16**, 166.

POOL J. L., POTANDS J. N. & KRUEGER E. G. (1962) *J. Neurosurg.*, **19**, 130.

ROSENWASSER H. (1945) *Arch. Otolaryng.*, **41**, 64.

ROWBOTHAM G. F. (1942) *Brit. J. Surg.*, **30**, 1.

SNAPPER I., TURNER L. B. & MOSCOVITZ H. L. (1953) *Multiple Myeloma.* Grune & Stratton, New York.

SUIT H. D., GOITEIN M., MUNZENRIDER J., VERHEY L., DAVIS K. R., KOEHLER A., LINGGOOD R. & OJEMANN R. G. (1982) *J. Neurosurg.*, **56**, 377.

VICTOR M., BARKER B. R. & ADAMS R. D. (1958) *J. Neurol. Neurosurg. Psychiat.*, **21**, 73.

WILLIS R. A. (1960) *Pathology of Tumours.* 3rd edition. Butterworth, London.

WILLIS R. A. (1962) *The Borderland of Embryology and Pathology.* 2nd edition. Butterworth, London.

WOLD L. E. & LAWS E. R. (1983) *J. Neurosurg.*, **59**, 1043.

ZOLTAN L. & FÉNYES I. (1960) *J. Neurosurg.*, **17**, 888.

# Chapter 11
# Aneurysms

M. D. M. SHAW

Apoplectic death was recognized and recorded in the earliest medical writings but its relation to intracranial haemorrhage was not established until the latter part of the seventeenth century by Wepfer and Brunner who also suggested that cerebral aneurysms might play a part (Walton 1956). Morgagni described a case of bilateral unruptured aneurysms of the posterior communicating arteries and recorded his opinion that rupture of an aneurysm was an important cause of cerebral haemorrhage. It is generally accepted that the first precise description of a case of intracranial aneurysm was recorded by Biumi in 1778; it arose from the intracavernous portion of the internal carotid artery (Bull 1962a). Bull draws attention to the next recorded case, a post-mortem demonstration by John Hunter of bilateral intracavernous aneurysms and which was reported by Blane in 1800. Bull suggests that the earliest recorded case of subarachnoid haemorrhage due to the rupture of an aneurysm was that described by Blackall in 1813; it arose from the terminal part of the basilar artery and it was noted that the ventricles contained blood which had entered at the communication between the third and fourth ventricles. Bartholow (1872) observed a case of aneurysm of the right side of the basilar artery; he noted that the vertebral artery on that side was much smaller than its fellow and made the pertinent suggestion that blood from the larger left vertebral artery impinged with great force against the site of the aneurysm. In this way he was antedating the current interest in anomalies of the circle of Willis and the role that circulatory hydrodynamics may play in the aetiology of cerebral aneurysms. Bartholow also sketched the

clinical picture of the paralytic type of syndrome arising from an aneurysm.

It is of interest that many of the records in the early part of the last century concerned aneurysms of the internal carotid and of the basilar arteries causing compression syndromes, yet in modern practice these form a minority. Interest in the apoplectic results of aneurysm appears to have been a somewhat later development and the papers by Brinton (1852) and Gull (1859) emphasized this aspect, although Brinton thought it only happened in about half. The modern era of knowledge of the natural history of intracranial aneurysms opened with contributions by Fearnsides (1916), Turnbull (1915, 1918) and Forbus (1930) on their clinical aspects; aetiology and pathology by Symonds (1923, 1924); on subarachnoid haemorrhage by Jefferson (1937, 1938) and Dandy (1944) and with the introduction of angiography by Moniz (1927, 1934). For a more detailed historical review Walton (1956) should be consulted; he provides an extensive bibliography. McDonald & Korb (1939) list with references the 1125 cases they could find in the literature.

## Incidence

Increase in the recognition of aneurysms and developments in their surgical treatment have brought about a considerable change in the pattern of neurosurgical work. In 1938, Jefferson stated that 55 cases of intracranial aneurysm had come under his care in the previous 15 years, approximately four a year. Among the neurosurgical centres taking part in the Cooperative Study of Intracranial Aneurysms and Subarachnoid Haemorrhage (Report 1966) nearly one-half had an annual experience of over 20 cases, rising to 160 at one centre. Crawford and Sarner (1965) made a study of the incidence of verified ruptured aneurysms in a well defined population of just over a million; during the year ending August 1963 the incidence was 6 per 100,000 persons under the age of 60 years. One-quarter of the cerebrovascular deaths in the age group 45–59 years were due to ruptured aneurysms. Of these, approximately one-third did not survive long enough for the aneurysm to be diagnosed in life. Pakarinen (1967) found the incidence of a first attack of subarachnoid haemorrhage amongst the inhabitants of Helsinki (population 440,000) to be 15.7 per 100,000 and in three-quarters an aneurysm was the cause; this gives a figure of approximately twice that of Crawford and Sarner. Analysing the records of 461 necropsies in which spontaneous intracranial haemorrhage had been revealed, Russell (1954) found that vascular hypertension was the cause in one-half; ruptured saccular aneurysms came next in frequency, being present in nearly one-quarter, and mycotic aneurysms in 6%.

Although aneurysms are encountered at all ages, they reach their peak between 40 and 60 years as judged by the intitial haemorrhage (Report of Co-operative Study V part I). The proportion of aneurysms which do not rupture is about 10% and these have a similar peak though perhaps more broadly based. Dinning and Falconer (1953) studied the records of 250 consecutive cases of precipitous death due to ruptured aneurysms in which a forensic necropsy had been performed; half occurred in persons between the ages of 50 and 70 years. Ruptured aneurysms are very rare in the early years of life; in the Co-operative Study (V part I) of 2627 cases, there was only one under the age of 5 years and six between the ages of 5 and 10 years. Matson (1965) described 14 cases in childhood, one in an infant of 5 months. Turnbull (1915) found one unruptured in a child of 1 year and 7 months.

There are interesting differences between the sexes in their susceptibility to aneurysmal formation and rupture and in the incidence on the individual cerebral arteries. Unruptured aneurysms are nearly twice as common in women and have a more broadly based peak of incidence. With regard to ruptured aneurysms, under the age of 40 years men preponderate, over the age of 50 years women preponderate to a steadily increasing degree. Crompton (1962, 1967) has drawn attention to differences to be found in necropsy specimens of ruptured aneurysms of the middle cerebral artery in the two sexes; they were nearly twice as common in females, in whom the aneurysm was usually smaller and more sessile, while in males it was more pyriform. No difference was found in the size and the frequency of the medial defects of the cerebral arteries of the sexes. Aneurysms of the internal carotid artery are twice as common in women, whereas those arising from the anterior cerebral artery (including the communicating artery) are somewhat more frequent in men.

There are two characteristic features of intracranial aneurysm. First, they are situated mainly on the circle of Willis and the trunks of the large arteries which supply it; a few arise from its immediate branches but peripherally sited aneurysms are quite rare. Second, the great majority of aneurysms arise at the junction of two vessels, usually at the acute angle. Those which appear to arise from a single artery may have arisen at the site of a minute branch which has disappeared as a result of the enlargement of the sac. The origin of the aneurysm from a point of branching has significance for aetiology, to which reference will be made later; it has significance to the surgeon for it often renders operative obliteration of the sac difficult, whereas a sac arising from a single vessel is usually much easier to deal with.

The site of origin of single aneurysms in the Co-operative Study (V part I) is shown on p. 320.

In two respects these figures vary considerably from other large series of cases. Thus, McDonald and Korb (1939) found that about 20% arose

| | All aneurysms (%) | Ruptured aneurysms (%) |
|---|---|---|
| Internal carotid artery | 41.2 | 38 |
|   at posterior communicating artery | 25.0 | 25 |
| Anterior cerebral artery | 33.5 | 36 |
|   at anterior communicating artery | 28.0 | 30 |
| Middle cerebral artery | 19.8 | 21 |
| Posterior cerebral artery | 0.8 | 0.9 |
| Basilar and vertebral arteries and branches | 4.5 | 4.6 |

from the basilar and vertebral arteries and branches, and Walton (1956) gave a similar estimate. However, most recent series suggest that in a consecutive population coming to vertebral angiography the incidence of aneurysms arising from the vertebrobasilar tree is between 5% (Fortuny et al. 1980) and 8% (Adams et al. 1981) of all aneurysms. Hugenholtz and Elgie (1982) report a higher incidence of 14%. Krayenbühl and Yaşargil (1958) have had a higher incidence of aneurysms of the anterior communicating artery (47.6%).

In a considerable proportion of patients more than one aneurysm is present and it may be difficult to decide which has been the cause of haemorrhage, a diagnostic problem discussed later. McKissock et al. (1964) analysed previous reports and found that multiple aneurysms were revealed in 21–33% of cases of necropsy, and in 5–17% of cases of angiography. In their own series of cases the incidence was 13.7%, diagnosis being made by angiography, operation or necropsy; 624 aneurysms were found in 251 subjects; in one patient there were 7. The incidence in the Cooperative Study (V part 1) was 18.5% based on angiography and 22% based on necropsy findings. It was found that for the inter-

nal carotid and the middle cerebral arteries, two aneurysms were usually symmetrically placed, or on the same vessel.

## Morbid anatomy of the aneurysm

Aneurysms of the intracranial arteries are divided into four groups:

1  saccular, syn: berry, congenital;
2  fusiform, syn: atheromatous, ectatic;
3  mycotic;
4  fistulous: between the internal carotid artery and the cavernous sinus.

Although this classification has a hybrid basis, derived from morphology and pathology, it provides a useful approach to the subject. Nearly all the aneurysms which gravitate to the neurosurgeon are of the saccular variety. Although in the review by Russell (1954) of necropsy findings in intracranial haemorrhage there were 28 examples of mycotic and 92 of saccular aneurysms, this in no way reflects neurosurgical experience, for the patient with a haemorrhage from a mycotic aneurysm is rarely referred to the surgeon. Moreover her review covered the period 1912–52 and antibiotics were available for less than the last quarter of that time; now mycotic aneurysms are very rare indeed and presumably reflect the efficacy of modern antibiotics in the control of pyogenic infection. The older literature gives an additional group of cases, miliary aneurysms. Meadows (1951) states that these are spurious and Russell concludes that they must be very rare; they are of no importance in neurosurgery except as a possible cause of spontaneous intracerebral haemorrhage. The term arteriovenous aneurysm is sometimes used for the lesion better known as arteriovenous malformation; to call it an aneurysm is confusing. Atheroma affecting the whole circumference of a major cerebral artery may lead to its dilatation (ectasia) and lengthening so that it perforce follows a tortuous course; to a minor degree this is not an uncommon finding in angiograms and necropsies of cases of cerebral atherosclerosis. A portion of the internal carotid or of the basilar artery may be so affected that it forms a fusiform aneurysm and may press upon neighbouring structures, the former on the optic nerves and chiasma, the latter upon the pons and lower canial nerves. The interior of a fusiform aneurysm is usually lined with laminated and partly organized thrombus. They form only a small proportion of all intracranial aneurysms; Bull (1962b) gives an incidence of 2% and Courville (1965) of 5%.

Saccular aneurysms are commonly round, berry or pear shaped and attached to the parent vessel by a neck which constitutes the least diameter of the sac. The fundus may be smooth or may show several local bulges which give the sac a multilobular shape (Fig. 11.1). The wall of the sac is thinnest at the fundus, to a degree which may render it transparent when viewed at operation so that swirling blood may be seen through it. Some aneurysms, in paticular those arising from the posterior aspect of the internal carotid at the level of the posterior communicating artery attain a shape resembling a blind tube, measurement of length being several times that of breadth which shows one or more hour-glass like constrictions. A considerable proportion of aneurysms are sessile; the junction of sac and parent vessel cannot be called a neck, being as broad as or broader than other diameters of the sac. Crompton (1962, 1967) found these to be more frequent in women than in men and on the middle cerebral artery than elsewhere. As sessile sacs enlarge they incorporate more of the walls of the parent and of the neighbouring vessels, so that ultimately the main artery enters the sac, and its continuation and its branches arise from the sac. Saccular aneurysms may occasionally attain a great size; Bramwell (1886) recorded one of 3 inches diameter lying under the frontal lobes and du Boulay (1965) one arising from the anterior cerebral artery which measured 6 × 4 cm; the large examples, over 2.4 cm in diameter, usually arise from the internal carotid artery in the region of the ophthalmic artery or from the first part of the anterior cerebral artery. Bull (1969) has made an interesting

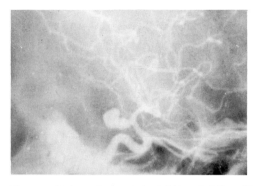

Fig. 11.1. Male aged 40: pain in right temple followed by rapid development of complete third nerve palsy: multilobular pear-shaped aneurysm arising from posterior aspect of right intercranial carotid artery, at or about the origin of the posterior communicating branch (not seen).

study of massive aneurysms. The majority of symptomatic aneurysms measure 7–10 mm across and in the Cooperative Study (IV) this appeared to be a crtical size for rupture. Crawford (1959) found that the majority of necropsy specimens of ruptured aneurysm measured 6–15 mm. Aneurysms found incidentally are usually smaller than 6 mm, although Crawford (1959) points out that minute ones may rupture leaving a hole in the artery.

Microscopic examination reveals a constant picture (Fig. 11.2). At the neck or mouth of the aneurysm the medial muscle of the parent artery ceases abruptly. The internal elastic lamina can be traced for only a short distance into the wall of the sac, becoming attenuated and fragmented before it ceases to exist. The wall of the sac, of variable and uneven thickness, consists of fibrous tissue continuous with the adventitia and the intima of the artery, lacking an endothelial lining. In places the wall may be infiltrated with inflammatory cells, with red cells and haemosiderin may be detected. By some it is thought that these represent areas of seepage of blood or they may reflect the stretching of the sac wall by arterial pulsation, providing a point of weakness and potential rupture (Crompton 1966b). The fundus is usually the thinnest part of the sac; Crawford (1959) in a paper containing beautiful illustrations of macroscopic and microscopic

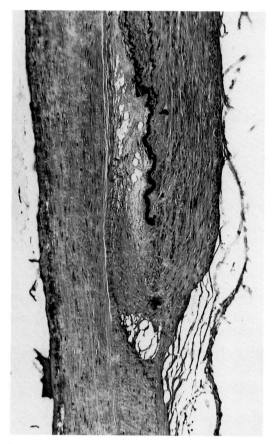

**Fig. 11.2.** Aneurysm: the elastic lamina of the parent vessel comes to an abrupt end at the edge of the aneurysm. Elast. V. G. × 150.

preparations emphasizes the importance of the bubble-like bulges which may protrude from the fundus. These are areas of extreme attenuation, where rupture is likely to take place. The interior of the sac may be smooth or irregular due to plaques of hyperplastic intimal connective tissue or as a result of the organization of thrombus. The cavity may contain a variable amount of thrombus and in large aneurysms is lamellar, suggesting variation in age of the clot. The outer layers of thrombus organize and fuse with the fibrous wall but only if this fusion is universal will spontaneous cure result; recurrent haemorrhage can occur by the dissection of clot from the wall of the sac until an attenuated area is reached. Crompton (1966a) noted that in 166 necropsy

specimens of ruptured aneurysms (nonsurgical) about one-third contained thrombus, which in nearly one-half of these filled the cavity. Where the sac is in contact with leptomeninges, these are thickened by fibrosis and incorporated in the outer surface of its wall. Sometimes a thin layer of fibrin with entangled red cells is seen on the outer aspect of a thin area of wall, compatible with 'weeping' of the aneurysm, but when a clinically evident haemorrhage has occurred, a demonstrable rupture is present, varying from pinhole size to disruption of the sac (Crawford 1959). The hole is plugged with material apparently comprising platelets and Crompton (1959) considers that processes in its formation and organization are important in preventing further haemorrhage. Buckell (1966) has made observations on this point from a different angle which are considered later. Rupture usually occurs through the fundus, in 64% of Crawford's cases (1959) and in 84% of Crompton's (1966b). Only occasionally is it situated at the neck (in 2%). These findings are consonant with surgical experience and are of importance in surgical procedures. When more than one aneurysm arises from an artery or its branches, it is usually the proximal one which ruptures (Jain 1963) and when multiple aneurysms are widely distributed it is generally the largest which gives way (Wood 1964, Crompton 1966b).

Little is known of the factors which promote the fibrous tissue wall of an aneurysm and maintain its thickness. Once the wall of the artery has been breached, the aetiology of which is studied later, the pressure of blood (not necessarily of a pathological degree) and particularly pulsating pressure, stretches the fibrous sac and in due course breaks it. What biological process stimulates fibroblastic reaction so that the wall for a time remains thick enough to withstand the effects of the stretch? In other parts of the body, abnormal movement between structures which ordinarily are immobile relative to one another may result in a local fibroblastic response, and the sac wall may respond similarly to the direct stimulus of pulsating stretch or its focal infiltration with inflammatory and red cells (described above) may be the stimulus. Proliferation of intimal cells within the sac and around its mouth described by Forbus (1930) and regarded by some as early atheromatous change, may be reparative rather than degenerative. On the other hand the connective tissue response which maintains the integrity of the wall might be regarded as the continuing elementary biological response to an injury sustained by the arterial wall, thus bringing it into line with the normal reparative processes of the body. That the area of repair bulges out as a sac is perhaps of no consequence to these bodily processes; but the repairing tissue, the sac wall, contains no blood supply and rapid stretching may overtake the rate of response creating attentuation and rupture. In some aneurysms and certainly in the larger ones, thrombus coats part of or all the wall and its organization will provide reinforcement. Rupture of an aneurysm is increasingly less likely to occur after a certain size has been surpassed; probably reinforcement by organizing layers of thrombus then plays a more important role than increase in the thickness of the wall by interstitial fibroblastic reaction.

## Morbid anatomy of the complications

Because of their position, aneurysms may compress neighbouring structures, brain, nerves, arteries: or as a result of their fragility they may rupture; the haemorrhage causes a variety of lesions and is frequently fatal. These two broad groups of pathological consequences are matched by two patterns of clinical syndrome.

### Compression

Some aneurysms are embedded partially or completely in the brain. The surrounding tissue shows compression atrophy, softening and gliosis, similar to that adjacent to a benign tumour and as with the latter may cause epilepsy (Fig. 11.3) but haemosiderin may be detected betraying a previous effusion of red cells as a

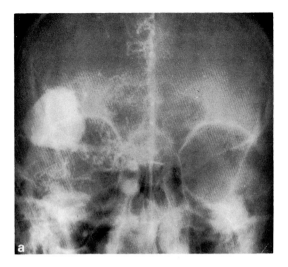

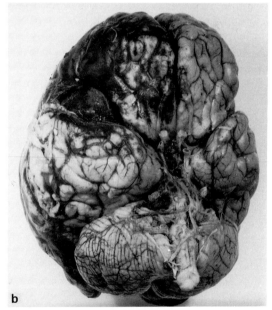

**Fig. 11.3.** Male aged 29 years: 2 years history of epilepsy of temporal lobe pattern: E.E.G. showed progressive abnormality in right temporal area suggestive of an organic focal lesion, for which reason angiography was performed. The massive aneurysm (a) arising from the right middle cerebral artery was accompanied by a smaller one on the left middle cerebral artery: operation was deferred; 6 months later he was admitted in a coma and rapidly died of haemorrhage from the larger aneurysm (b).

result of a frank though perhaps small haemorrhage or 'seepage' through the wall of the aneurysm. Only in a basilar aneurysm is size relative to the neighbouring brain sufficient to give rise to paralysis of function; the pons and medulla may be displaced and indented by a fusiform aneurysm to a degree that mimics a tumour (*see* Fig. 11.9). But abnormal neurological signs due to aneurysm frequently occur as a result of juxtaposition to a cranial nerve. The third nerve is the most commonly affected and may be taken as an example; the clinical aspects of 'paralytic' syndromes are discussed later. Hyland and Barnett (1953) studied the post-mortem findings in 39 cases in which one or more cranial nerves had been affected during life. They found that the palsy might be due to direct contact between aneurysm and nerve, or as a result of haemorrhage affecting the nerve or its nucleus. The two groups were nearly equal in number; the former operated to produce the palsy early in the chronological sequence of events, in the latter the signs were often bilateral and terminal. Not only does an aneurysm compress and thin the nerve, but both become adherent and so firmly that the nerve may be incorporated in the wall of the sac. Any rapid expansion of the sac will then stretch that portion of the nerve, an adequate cause for palsy. Nerve degeneration takes place and in some specimens in which the palsy was of sudden onset Hyland and Barnett found intraneural haemorrhages, presumably the result of infiltration by seepage or by rupture. The aneurysm may also compress and obliterate an adjacent branch of the parent artery provided it is small. Frequently small arteries become adherent to the surface of the aneurysm and when viewed at operation may apparently be arising from the sac. It is important for the surgeon to ascertain the correct anatomy because his procedure is likely to be different in the two arrangements. The use of low-power magnification (microsurgery) has proved very helpful in this respect.

## Haemorrhage

The great majority of aneurysms betray their presence by rupture. This was so in 90% of the

3265 cases of aneurysm reviewed by the Co-operative Study (II). Situated as most of them are, partially or totally within the leptomeninges, blood is injected into the subarachnoid space and the appearance of the brain at post-mortem is unmistakable. The large basal cisterns are distended with clot which extends into the cisterna magna and may be found within the fourth ventricle, laterally into the Sylvian fissure, and as a variable but gradually diminishing film over the convexities. Haemorrhage from a middle cerebral aneurysm often forms a relatively localized collection in the Sylvian fissure and from an anterior communicating aneurysm an interhemispheric collection. These merit the term subarachnoid haematoma and Tomlinson (1959) and Crompton (1962) have drawn attention to their importance; they were found in about 30% of fatal cases. The adjacent cortex becomes damaged by the forceful erruption of blood and local pressure causes its infarction and necrosis; this may allow blood to break into the brain and form an intracerebral haematoma. Linear haemorrhages may be seen in the brain in the immediate vicinity of the aneurysm; they are disposed perpendicular to the surface of the brain and microscopic examination shows that they are perivascular (Tomlinson 1959, Crompton 1962). It is probable that subarachnoid blood is forced into the brain along the perivascular sheaths. In addition to these perivascular extravasations, Crompton (1962) found discrete minute haemorrhages in the hypothalamus sometimes destroying nuclear masses.

Although primary haemorrhage into the subarachnoid space is the typical sequel to rupture of an aneurysm and for many years dominated the literature concerning morbid anatomy and clinical syndromes, of equal, perhaps of more importance is haemorrhage into the brain substance. Earlier writers paid it little more than passing reference. Robertson (1949) was the first to consider this aspect of the disease and its clinical importance in the interpretation of signs, and for treatment. Intracerebral haemorrhage was found at necropsy in 70% of 86 cases of saccular aneurysm; thus in approximately one-

**Fig. 11.4.** Male aged 38 treated by carotid ligation for suspected subarachnoid haemorrhage ascribed to a carotid-posterior communicating aneurysm: 3 years later, dementia, unsteady gait, papilloedema. Ventriculography (a) revealed filling defect in posterior part of third ventricle, thought to be due to pineal tumour and treated by ventriculocisternostomy: deterioration persisted and he died some months later. (b,c) Post-mortem examination revealed a saccular aneurysm arising from the termination of the basilar artery embedded in brain stem and protruding into third ventricle. Aneurysm contained thrombus: surrounding tissues stained with blood.

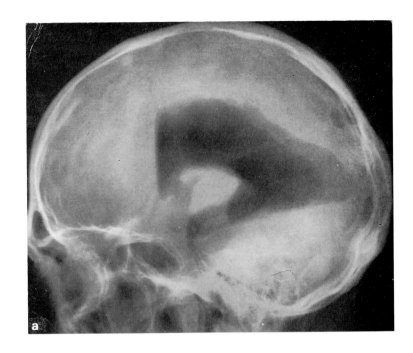

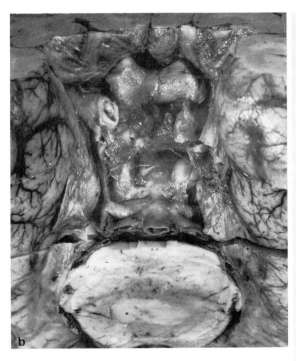

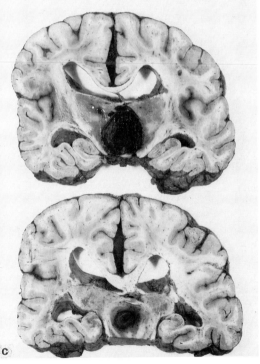

third only was the fatal bleeding entirely sub-arachnoid. Other observers (Tomlinson 1959, Crompton 1962, Courville 1965) and personal experience confirm that haemorrhage into the brain, often of massive extent, is a common post-mortem finding; that it is not inevitably fatal is proved by the frequency with which the neuro-surgeon encounters a haematoma in the course of investigations and operations. Intracerebral rupture occurs when the sac, or part of it, lies embedded in brain, or attached to it by lep-tomeningeal adhesions. Aneurysms of the anterior cerebral, anterior communicating, the carotid bifurcation and the middle cerebral arteries by reason of their position are more frequently the cause of intracerebral rupture. Adhesions which plaster the sac to the brain and obliterate the subarachnoid spread are likely to follow previous small leaks and there is necropsy evidence for this (Crompton 1962). The important deduction follows that a recurrent haemorrhage is likely to be more serious than the previous; this is borne out by clinical experience and as will be seen later, influences decisions concerning treatment. As noted above, blood may also burst into the brain from a subarachnoid haematoma, as a result of laceration or of necrosis of the adjacent cortex. Intracerebral haemorrhage is more frequent into the frontal and into the temporal lobes and from these spreads into the neighbouring lobes. It may be so extensive as to cause death within a few hours. Frontal lobe haematomas are often bilateral, may involve the corpus callosum and the hypothalamus and frequently break into the ventricle. Temporal lobe haemorrhage less often extends into the temporal horn, usually lying below or lateral to it but may dissect deeply into the brain. Aneurysms arising from the terminal bifurcation of the basilar artery may burst into the posterior end of the third ventricle (as is the case described by Blackall in 1813, referred to in the introduction) or by their size cause obstructive hydrocephalus (Fig. 11.4). Rupture into the ventricle, which was found by Courville in about one-third of his necropsy cases, is less frequently fatal than was thought prior to the advent of computerized tomographic scanning. In those coming to post-mortem examination the ventricular system contains a cast of blood and microscopical examination shows extensive damage to the subependymal tissue which in the third and fourth ventricle comprise vital areas.

In addition to subarachnoid and intracerebral collections, blood sometimes escapes into the subdural space; it may be no more than a diffuse film, or it may form a large subdural haematoma. It is not necessarily associated with intracerebral haemorrhage and consequently its recognition and treatment may be life-saving. Clarke and Walton (1953) estimated that subdural collections occurred in 1–2% of cases of subarachnoid haemorrhage but Courville found them in 6% of his necropsy series and clinical experience supports the higher figure. Blood enters the subdural space in 2 ways. The aneurysm may be adherent to the overlying arachnoid which is torn with the rupture of the sac, or the aneurysm lies partly within and partly without the subarachnoid space, as in some examples arising from the internal carotid artery close to the anterior clinoid process. In these blood is injected into both the subdural and subarachnoid spaces. The alternative route is seen in massive intracerebral and subarachnoid haematomas; the force of the haemorrhage is such as to disrupt the overlying cortex and leptomeninges and blood escapes into the subdural space. Clarke and Walton pointed out that in some cases the presentation is such that an aneurysmal origin is not suspected.

## Infarction

A considerable proportion of the damage sustained by the brain as a result of a ruptured aneurysm is due to infarction. The importance of ischaemia as a cause of death and of morbidity in nonfatal cases is now well appreciated. Robertson (1949) drew attention to infarction and Wilson et al. (1954), Tomlinson (1959), Bierse and Tom (1960), Smith (1963), Crompton (1964) and Schneck (1964) have made important contributions. Interest has been stimulated by the uncertainty as to its causation and by the appearances in angiograms, familiar to neurosurgeons and to neuroradiologists, of narrowing of arteries in patients with subarachnoid haemorrhage. Whether this narrowing is due to vascular spasm and is aetiologically related to infarction or whether it has other causes will be discussed later. Estimates of the incidence of infarction depend upon the care with which it is sought and the criterion for size. Crompton (1964) points out that the lesions are usually pale, in the unfixed brain often impalpable and easily pass unrecognized. On the basis of necrosis of at least one-third of the cortical territory of a major cerebral artery, or of ganglionic necrosis of 5 mm diameter or more, he found infarction in 75% of cases and if lesions smaller than these were included, 86% of cases. Infarction of the cortex was present in nearly all, and of the central masses in about one-half. Cortical infarcts are usually restricted to that side of the brain on which the aneurysm lies and often but not exclusively in the territory of the vessels involved in the aneurysm; Schneck found that they were bilateral in about one-third of his cases, but had no example of infarction on the contralateral side only, though Crompton (1964) had several cortical and ganglionic examples. Occasionally the infarction of posterior cerebral territory is secondary to tentorial herniation consequent upon swelling of the brain. Infarction was found most frequently amongst carotid/posterior communicating, and least amongst anterior communicating aneurysms. The hypothalamus is a vitally important area in which infarction may be found. Crompton (1963) made a special study of this region and ischaemic lesions were present in over one-half, in addition to the microhaemorrhages mentioned in the previous section and to massive haemorrhages. Hypothalamic infarction is most frequent with anterior communicating aneurysms.

Smith (1963) has described a different pattern of ischaemic brain damage, which was found in each of 8 brains selected for examination because of their freedom from significant cerebral disruption or clot. In these specimens there were widespread patchy cortical infarcts of microscopic size; all parts of the gyri were affected, not preferentially in water-shed areas. Although the lesions were most plentiful in the territory of the aneurysmal vessels, they were present in all the 6 supratentorial areas served by the anterior, middle and posterior cerebral arteries, except for one case. There was much oedema of the white matter. Bierse and Tom (1960) described microscopic infarcts which may have been identical with the lesions on which Smith concentrated.

Hijdra et al. (1986) studied 18 cases of fatal delayed cerebral ischaemia post mortem and found bilateral infarcts in 14, multiple unilateral infarcts with contralateral swelling in 2, and strictly unilateral pathology in only 2 cases. Of 56 patients who showed clinical deterioration and underwent CT, 47 showed low density lesions in a single (19 cases) or in multiple arterial vascular territories (22 cases) or in both cerebral hemispheres (6 cases). Delayed cerebral ischaemia does therefore appear to be a multifocal or diffuse process in most cases.

Secondary changes occur in the brain as a result of haemorrhage, whether it be subarachnoid, intracerebral or intraventricular and as a result of infarctions. These are the changes which characterize a space-occupying lesion, namely dislocation of brain, obstruction to the flow of cerebrospinal fluid, internal herniations, compression of the brain stem and haemorrhages and haemorrhagic infarctions of the brain stem and of the occipital lobe. The quantity of blood, particularly if it accumulates rapidly, occupies space and so does the oedematous swelling which develops around the necrotic areas of cerebral laceration. Oedema follows infarction and Smith was impressed with the amount of white matter oedema in her cases of diffuse minute ischaemic lesions of the cortex. Where oedema surrounds haemorrhages and necrosis, it can be reasonably assumed to be consequent upon them, but the oedema associated with infarction may be due, at any rate to some extent, to the vascular mechanism which causes the infarct, though after the ischaemic episode oedema will develop or be aggravated as a natural sequential reaction. Blood which occupies the subarachnoid cisterns and the ventricles also delays the passage of cerebrospinal fluid, although massive intraventricular haemorrhage is usually fatal before its obstructive effect can significantly influence hydrodynamics.

## Aetiology of the aneurysm

The pathogenesis of saccular aneurysms has been a contentious subject for the last 65 years and although in the last 25 years a majority opinion has emerged, there are still unanswered questions. Any valid hypothesis concerning intracranial aneurysms must take account of the curve of their age incidence, of their situation predominantly at arterial junctions, of their rarity on the peripheral brain arteries, of their greater frequency in the carotid than in the vertebral network, of their histological structure and of their association (significant or random) with other vascular abnormalities in the brain and conditions elsewhere in the body. To cover such a wide and apparently disparate variety of features by a single aetiological factor may be impossible and indeed this is the modern view.

Priority for the view that in the wall of an artery there may be weak points due to an error of development (congenital) and that such points determine the formation of an aneurysm, is generally attributed to Eppinger (1887). But the 2 cases he described and on which he based his hypothesis have little in common with saccular aneurysms of the brain. They comprised multiple round aneurysms of the arteries of the myocardium in each, and of the mesenteric arteries of one. The illustrations show verrucose arteries, numerous bead-like expansions in the course of the vessels such as are never seen in the brain. Histological examination revealed in some appearances similar to cerebral aneurysms; in other intact muscle but absence of elastica. He considered that a congenital weakness of the elastica was the important factor; his reference to aneurysms of the brain lay in the similarity he found between his specimens and certain brain aneurysms reported in the literature of that time. Bruce et al. (1908) recording a case of ruptured anterior cerebral aneurysm, noted a local defect of the media and suggested that this was of congenital origin. Turnbull (1915, 1918) classified cerebral aneurysms, described their histology and considered that they were due to 'an inherent weakness' at points of arterial junctions. He found one in a child of 1 year and 7 months. He disposed of syphilis as a cause. Forbus (1930) established the existence of defects in the medial muscle (not elastica as Eppinger held) at arterial junctions, in otherwise normal vessels of the brain, the heart and the mesentery, and suggested that they were the result of lack of fusion of the embryonic muscle layer which originates independently in each branch. They also occur much less frequently as fenestrations of the medial muscle in the course of arteries where no branch occurs (Crompton 1966b); here their presence is probably of much greater significance, in the determination of the point of origin of those few aneurysms which do not arise at a fork. The presence of medial defects of developmental origin is now fully accepted; indeed their profusion presents the dilemma that alone they cannot cause aneurysm. Forbus emphasized the all important supportive role played by the elastic layer and considered that his must give way before an aneurysm can develop. Glynn (1940) confirmed the work and the views of Forbus and carried out experiments demonstrating the great strengths of the elastic tissue exposed by medial defects. He pointed out that in the cerebral arteries, by contrast with arteries elsewhere, the elastic layer is entirely limited to the internal lamina, thus rendering these arteries more susceptible to the weakening effects of degeneration. Work along these lines was pursued by Carmichael (1945, 1950) who concluded that the (relatively) occasional development of an aneurysm at the site of the (relatively) common developmental defect of the muscle layer, is due to the acquired fragmentation and dissolution of the elastica at that point. He attributed the degeneration to atheroma and the coincidence to chance. The conjunction of muscle defect and discontinuity of the subjacent elastica is now accepted as the essential prerequisite for the formation of a saccular aneurysm. Whether failure of the elastica is to be interpreted as atheromatous, and whether the coincidental location is determined by chance, are as yet undecided.

There is some evidence that atheroma plays a part in aetiology. Walker and Allegre (1954) found in the necropsies of 39 cases of aneurysm that evidence of hypertension was present at thrice, and generalized atherosclerosis at twice, the expected frequency. Examination of the arteries attached to the aneurysm revealed atheromatous changes in 25 of 29 specimens and atheromatous plaques in the walls of 13 of the aneurysms. Crawford (1959) compared the incidence of coronary artery disease in men (aged 45–70 years) dying from ruptured aneurysm with a control groups in which death was unrelated to vascular disease; severe coronary artery disease was nearly three times as frequent in the aneurysm groups as in the control. In his opinion there are three main factors in pathogenesis: developmental medial faults, atherosclerosis and hypertension, each of varying importance according to age. A high incidence of hypertension and of renal disease in addition to cardiovascular disease was found by Sarner and Crawford (1965). Du Boulay (1965) has studied this association of aneurysm and atherosclerosis from a different angle. Angiograms in a large series of cases of aneurysm revealed evidence of atheroma in 35% and this rose to 50% in the cases with multiple aneurysm; in a control series of angiograms of cases of tumour the incidence was 16%. Against these arguments must be set detailed observations of Hassler (1961) to which little attention has been paid. He scrutinized preparations of arteries showing atheroma and found that such changes were much less common at the sites where medial defects occur than at other sites.

An alternative view on the aetiology of disruption of the elastica is that it is the response to local stress. The work of Hassler (1961) is important in this and in other aspects. He examined the major cerebral ateries from a large number of cadavers of all ages, normal and those carrying ruptured aneurysms, scrutinizing the external and internal surfaces with a dissecting microscope and using various histological preparations. The incidence of large medial defects (up to diameters slightly over 3 mm) was higher in subjects aged over 30 years than in younger and higher in specimens bearing minute (and large) aneurysms. Minute aneurysms (of less than 2 mm diameter) were found in 17% of normal and in half the cases of ruptured aneurysms. All but 2 of 45 minute aneurysms were situated at the distal carina of arterial junctions. Hassler attaches great significance to the presence of 'intimal cushions'. These are localized thickenings of the intima, composed mainly of collagen in subjects over the age of 30 years, and of muscle and elastic tissue in the young. They were found occasionally in infants, more frequently as the age increased, in most individuals over the age of 20 years and regularly at branching points carrying medial defects and aneurysms. The situation of an intimal cushion was nearly always at the proximal angle of arterial branching, opposite the medial defect or aneurysm. In the region of the anterior communicating artery the cushions might be disposed at other points when the arterial pattern was complex; the arrangement was such that the defect or sac lay in the direct axis of the current of blood and the cushion to one side of the axis. From these studies Hassler (1961) concludes that aneurysmal sacs develop from large medial defects and that these are due to the enlargement of minute ones of congenital origin. Enlargement of the defect he suspects is connected in some way with the presence of intimal cushions, perhaps by directing the current of blood against the defect. The influence of the blood stream on the walls of the arteries and branches was examined experimentally. Models of arterial branchings made of silicone rubber within a transparent plastic case were subjected to a flow of water under varying physical conditions including pulsatile flow. Pits in the silicone rubber tubes were created at the distal carina and heaping up of the wall at proximal angles creating appearances similar to defects and cushions and at similar sites. These observations support the views of Forbus (1930) and the suggestion of Bartholow (1872) that the axial direction of the current of blood determines the distention of an inherently weak spot on an artery. Whether intimal cushions play an important role in directing this axis is arguable; it may be that they are the result of moulding by eddy currents or areas of diminished pressure. Hassler thinks that exhaustion and over-stretching may be the cause of failure of the elastic tissue supporting a medial defect but he does not discount the possibility of inflammation, because of the marked round-celled infiltration often seen in the minute aneurysms.

Neil-Dwyer et al. (1983) found that there was a deficiency of type III collagen in the skin and superficial temporal arteries in eleven of seventeen cases of cerebral aneurysm, but not in control patients with other neurosurgical conditions. As 70% of the collagen in arterial walls is of the type III variety, this group of aneurysms may result from an inherited defect of connective tissue. Ehlers–Danlos type IV is an example of a syndrome in which type III collagen is deficient and in which there is arterial fragility (Pope et al. 1981).

Much has been made by some observers of the association of aneurysm with variations in the pattern of the circle of Willis. Padget (1945) made a classical contribution to the embryology and antomy of the circle of Willis. She laid down the criteria of normality, which include symmetry either side of the median plane and relative sizes of component parts. From her own work and recorded descriptions she concluded that the 'normal' occurred in barely half the preparations. Many reports have been made since then, suggesting that a 'normal' is a minority finding; Riggs and Rupp (1963) examined 994 specimens and only 192 were 'normal'. The posterior communicating artery is subject to more variations than any other intracranial artery. In those patients in whom the luminal diameter is large, the first part of the ipsilateral posterior artery (from the basilar bifurcation to the junction with the posterior communicating artery) may be hypoplastic or absent. Hypoplasia of the stem of the anterior cerebral artery as far as its communicating branch, or of the communicating branch, is also frequent. Combinations of these variations occur in great variety and are depicted in the papers by Padget, and by Riggs and Rupp. The anterior segment of the circle is very liable to complex variations. Busse (1921) dissected 400 specimens of this portion and found a normal pattern in about 40%; in about 28% he found simple variations which comprised hypoplasia or absence of the stems of the anterior cerebral arteries; in about 20% there was a complex network of vessels and communications in the communicating artery. Almeida (1949) also depicts plexiform arrangements; aneurysmal dilatation was encountered in 10%. Padget considered variations in the circle to be twice as frequent in cases of aneurysms than those without and depicted specimens from Dandy's series. It was because he noted a high incidence of aneurysm in the region of the anterior communicating artery that Busse studied this area. Wilson et al. (1954) also found a high incidence of variation in their cases of aneurysm and that in 85% of the 40 specimens of anterior communicating aneurysm one anterior cerebral artery was hypoplastic. Similar observations have been made by others (Bassett 1949, Bassett & Lemmen 1954, Korgis et al. 1966). It is probable that variations in the pattern of the circle of Willis may influence the incidence of aneurysms in two ways. First, hypoplasia of a major element means greater calibre of other elements thus exposing sites to unusual haemodynamic stresses. Second, complex networks in the region of the anterior communicating artery result from arrest of the devolution of the primitive vascular plexus (Padget). The consequence of arrest may be an unusual number or position of sites of mural weakness. Microsurgical anatomy studies have demonstrated that in 40% there are two or even three anterior communicating arteries (Rhoton et al. 1982). Buds representing primitive arteries have been considered by some to be the origination of aneurysm at unusual sites. This is highly unlikely for the presence of buds on major arteries taken from infants would have been recorded and this is not the case, but the sites of primitive branches may remain as points of defective formation of the aterial wall and account for those few aneurysms which arise from the internal carotid, the basilar and the vertebral arteries at points where no branch is detected.

Vascular hypertension is present in perhaps 60% of patients with an aneurysm. Statistics based on clinical observations on patients admitted to hospital for rupture are unreliable, because haemorrhage of itself usually causes some and at times severe elevation of the blood pressure and patients with hemiplegic sequelae may have a reduction of previously existing hypertension. Stehbens (1954) found necropsy evidence of hypertension in 57% of cases of ruptured aneurysm and in the cases of Wilson *et al.* (1954) 67% of those under the age of 40 had cardiac hypertrophy. An unusually high incidence of ruptured aneurysm occurs in polycystic disease of the kidney and in coarctation of the aorta, both of which are characterized by hypertension. Seeing that the formation of an aneurysm and its rupture are dependent upon intra-arterial tension, it would be illogical if excessive tension did not aggravate the condition. More important perhaps is the fact that in 30–40% of cases the aneurysm develops and ruptures under the influence of a normal blood pressure.

Observations have been made on the activity of the patient at the time of rupture, to determine whether physical effort may have been a precipitating factor. Magee (1943) examined the records of 150 patients who had suffered subarachnoid haemorrhage, mostly derived from armed forces or civil defence personnel and nearly all under the age of 40 years. In 90% there was no history of physical effort, in 28% the patient was at rest, and in only 8% was an isolated incident claimed to be responsible. The Cooperative Study (V part I) examined this aspect of rupture. In 12% of cases the patient was lifting or bending, in 36% sleeping, in 32% unspecified;

emotional strain, defecation, coitus, coughing, trauma, provided small groups each of a few per cent.

## Aetiology of infarction

Arterial spasm, which is a radiographic diagnosis, is commonly invoked and accepted as a cause of ischaemia. It would indeed readily explain the distribution of infarction within the territory of parent vessels and bilateral distribution could be the result of spasm spreading to other parts of the circle of Willis. It was put forward as the result of the frequency with which narrowing of arteries in the vicinity of a ruptured aneurysm is seen in angiograms. This narrowing may be confined to a short length of the arteries proximal and distal to the sac; it often includes the internal carotid artery distal to the anterior clinoid process where the change in diameter from normal to narrow may be quite dramatic in some cases the narrowing involves vessels of the opposite side. It is thought by many that the narrowing is most likely to be seen if the angiograms have been made several days after the rupture, but as this is a common interval to elapse between rupture and angiography it is unreliable evidence. Angiography is frequently repeated for one reason or another at various intervals and these have shown that previously narrowed arteries regain a normal calibre: the duration of narrowing is generally days to weeks. That narrowing of arteries occurs and that it may endure for several weeks is indubitable but its interpretation remains controversial. Millikan (1975) in a detailed review of 198 patients concluded that there was no clinical picture consistently resulting from known vasospasm, that vasospasm had no effect on the mortality resulting from aneurysmal subarachnoid haemorrhage and that there was no relationship between the frequency of severity of the complications from therapy and the presence of absence of vasospasm. However the prevailing view is that vasospasm is one of the factors which may lead to ischaemic deficits. Fisher *et al.* (1977)

graded the degree of vasospasm according to the diameter of the angiographic column on angiograms carried out between the 4th and 13th day after the ictus. All the patients developing ischaemic deficits had grade 3 or 4 vasospasm, that is to say the diameter of the angiographic column in the proximal segment of the anterior or middle cerebral arteries of 0.5 mm or less or in the supraclinoid carotid artery was 1.5 mm or less.

Transient diminution in calibre of both small and large intracranial ateries has been observed in the exposed brain by most neurosurgeons and can be evoked by mechanical stimulation, for example rubbing the artery with an instrument. Spasm of cerebral arteries has attracted much experimentation initiated by Florey (1925) who observed the effects of mechanical and electrical stimuli. The arterial spasm observed in injured limbs when the artery is adjacent to the trauma but is not lacerated is of this nature. Florey also observed this phenomenon. A ruptured aneurysm has been thought to offer a similar stimulus; but the 2 situations are not comparable, for in one the healthy muscular wall of the artery receives a stimulus whilst in the other the rupture is of a fibrous insert sac. Byrom (1954, 1968) has made a special study of the cerebral arterial spasm seen in experimental hypertension; he regarded the contraction of the muscle of cerebral arteries as a response to its stretching by the systemic hypertension. Heifetz (1986) has suggested that the repetitive systolic thrust of a blood vessel, sensitized by irritants released from extravascular blood, against a taut pia/arachnoid fibre could produce or exacerbate arterial spasm. Denny-Brown (1956) produced spasm of small cerebral arteries by injecting saline rapidly under high pressure into a cortical vein thus abruptly raising the intraarterial pressure. Echlin (1965), Kapp et al. (1968) and others have observed the effects of fresh blood applied to the major arteries. Fresh blood is now accepted as being an initiating factor in the production of the vasospasm which develops a few days after the ictus. Evidence to support this is derived from studies (Symon et al. 1980,

Yamomoto et al. 1983) which suggest that the amount of subarachnoid blood seen on a computerized tomographic scan taken early after the haemorrhage directly correlates with the risk of developing ischaemic deficits. Fisher et al. (1980a) found that in the presence of a subarachnoid clot greater than $5 \times 3$ mm, or if the layer of blood present in the fissures of the cisterns was 1 mm or more thick, virtually all cases developed delayed ischaemic deficits. However it remains difficult to reconcile this with the fact that it is unusual at operation to see any reaction of the arteries to blood which is freshly spilled around them, even when they are denuded of arachnoid. In addition it may occur in other conditions, in only some of which is there subarachnoid blood, for example it may occur with unruptured aneurysms (Fein 1980, Peerless 1980). Various blood fractions including the breakdown products resulting from the lysis of red cells and the degradation of haemoglobin and fibrin, in addition to free radicals released during clot lysis, have been investigated to attempt to discover a spasmogenic agent. Much of the evidence, however, has been derived from basilar artery muscle strips suspended in water baths, but the contractions so produced may bear little relationship to the spasm occurring in vivo. Evidence is now accumulating to suggest that the ischaemic complications associated with angiographic vasospasm may result from a vasoproliferative disease. There is evidence that patients dying early (2–8 days) after the ictus showed damage to the endothelial surface of the arteries whereas those dying later than this had hypertrophy of the media (Kassell et al. 1980a, Peerless et al. 1980). In addition the capillaries in those dying earlier showed intimal and subintimal changes (Hughes 1980). Additional evidence of abnormalities in the vessel wall arises from the computerized tomograhic findings that abnormal contrast enhancement resulting perhaps from breakdown of the blood–brain barrier is frequently associated with a low clinical grading, angiographic vasospasm and poor outcome (Doczi et al. 1984). This raises the question of the role of the platelets; these can adhere to damaged endothelial surfaces which may be further increased by temporary clipping (Richling *et al.* 1979) and by the crunching and twisting resulting from the application of the definitive aneurysm clip. Adherence of platelets results in the release of platelet factor 4 which enters the vessel wall and can cause medial hypertophy not only at the site of adhesion of the platelet but also more remotely. The latter effect is presumably by means of a humoral agent (Stemerman 1981). In addition Grady *et al.* (1980) suggested that platelet emboli, released from platelet thrombi, might lodge more distally and result in delayed ischaemic complications.

It has been suggested that the hypothalamus might also have a role in the development of vasospasm. Wilkins (1975) has reviewed the evidence which he summarized as follows: the characteristics of vasospasm are not those associated with experimental vasospasm produced solely by exposure to blood; vasospasm occurs in some patients and not in others, but is more frequent when the aneurysm is located near to the hypothalamus, particularly if the latter is damaged. Clinically there is further evidence in the work of Neil-Dwyer *et al.* (1980) who have shown that increased sympathetic activity occurs in subarachnoid haemorrhage, frequently associated with electrocardiographic changes. Post-mortem examination revealed that 77% of the affected patients had lesions both in the hypothalamus and the myocardium whereas only 13% had hypothalamic lesions alone but neither lesion was found in control patients who had died from raised intracranial pressure from other causes (Neil-Dwyer *et al.* 1980). Adrenergic blockade resulted in less neurological deficits (Walter *et al.* 1982) particularly in women. Beta blockade was found to be better than alpha blockade.

Marion *et al.* (1986) have concluded that mortality and morbidity are related mainly to the intracranial problems. Because acute cardiac disorder does not, in their opinion, contribute significantly to the outcome, there is not an indication for administration of agents to produce prophylactic sympathetic blockade.

A large variety of ideas about how to prevent and treat vasospasm have been tried. Wilkins (1980, 1986) reviewed the drug regimes including vasodilating agents which have been used and concluded that the solution has so far escaped detection; that the most that could be done at present was to support the cerebral circulation and that detrimental factors such as the adverse autonomic ones should be avoided. The red cell mass and circulatory volume are significantly decreased in patients who have had subarachnoid haemorrhage (Maroon & Nelson 1979). The intravascular volume must therefore be expanded using both red cells and colloid in order to help maintain the cerebral circulation particularly in those patients whose autoregulation is impaired (*see* below). In the latter situation, provided the aneurysm had already been clipped, induced hypertension plus hypervolaemia has been advocated but the reported results of such treatment are conflicting (Kassell *et al.* 1980b, Ritchie *et al.* 1980, Kassell *et al* 1982). Improving the rheological characteristics of the blood, for example the use of low molecular weight dextran may also improve the circulation especially in the small vessels. More recently, following interest in evidence that vasospasm is a proliferative condition, attention is being paid to the interaction between the platelets and the vessel walls. This has lead to interest in drugs which modify these interactions for example the prostacyclins, thromboxane A2 antagonists and other drugs which modify platelet activity. In addition those advocating early surgery (see below) suggest that early removal of blood clots from the basal cisterns and fissures may reduce the incidence of vasospasm and hence the ischaemic complications (Sano & Saito 1980).

The reader interested in vasospasm should consult *Cerebral Arteriospasm* (The Proceedings of the 2nd International Workshop) which was edited by R. H. Wilkins.

However, vasospasm is not the only factor concerned in the development of delayed ischaemic deficits. Other factors include intracranial pressure, cerebral blood flow and cerebral metabolism.

## Intracranial pressure

The role of intracranial pressure measurement in subarachnoid haemorrhage is not yet clear. After describing the abrupt increases in intracranial pressure that follow rupture of an aneurysm (Nornes & Magnaes 1972), Nornes (1973) suggested that the initial elevation of pressure might reduce the risk of rehaemorrhage by tamponade. Indeed, those rehaemorrhaging tended to have a lower initial intracranial pressure. The intracranial pressure soon falls but a second slow increase occurs over the next few days (Hayashi et al. 1979). The severity of this rise correlates well with the clinical grade of the patient; the higher the mean pressure the worse the grading. Generally speaking B & C waves (see chapter 2) are of little significance in chronic intracranial hypertension but Hayashi et al. (1977) found that the worse a patient's grading the more frequently were these waves found and the greater was the amplitude of these waves. In grade 5 patients the waves were directly related to the arterial blood pressure. They therefore suggested that these waves reflected the cerebral vasomotor instability in patients graded 3 or 4 and the vasomotor paralysis in grade 5 patients. Hayashi's groups (1978) later found in patients developing angiographic vasospasm deeper initial depression in the intracranial pressure which was associated with a reduction in B & C wave activity. This was followed by the secondary increase in pressure. The onset of vasospasm coincided with the reduction in the intracranial pressure and serious neurological deficit with secondary elevation. Voldby and Enevoldsen (1982a) however found an initially higher intracranial pressure in those patients who went on to develop angiographic vasospasm and that with the onset of the latter there was a further increase in the intracranial pressure. Black (1986) concluded that vasospasm and hydrocephalus are associated because they both represent sequelae of haemorrhage into the basal cisterns.

The rise in intracranial pressure in those patients without a space occupying haematoma may result from 3 factors: the chemical meningitis which hinders the flow and reabsorption of cerebrospinal fluid; an increase in cerebral blood volume which is greater in patients with angiographic vasospasm (see below); and reduced cerebral blood flow which may lead to ischaemia and ultimately infarction, either of which will result in cerebral oedema.

Once the haemorrhage is under control, cautious reduction of the intracranial pressure to 25–30 mm mercury might have been expected to improve the clinical progress of the patient. Ventricular drainage does not always accomplish this (Voldby & Enevoldsen 1982a). However the intracranial volume pressure response shows a reduced compensatory capacity (Hamer & Kuhner 1976) which might be favourably altered, as it is in other situations, by steroids (Miller & Leech 1975).

Postoperatively, similar relationships to those found pre-operatively between intracranial pressure, including the wave forms, and the patient's clinical state have been described (Kaye & Brownbill 1981).

## Cerebral blood flow, blood volume and metabolism

Cerebral blood flow in all patients who have recently suffered a subarachnoid haemorrhage is reduced but in those who have neurological deficits or those who have vasospasm as demonstrated on angiography this reduction is significantly greater (Pitts et al. 1980). The reduction in blood flow progressively increases during the first 2 weeks and remains low for the first 3 weeks after haemorrhage. In addition the flow is also inversely related to age (Meyer et al. 1983). Cerebral oxygen utilization is also similarly reduced (Grubb 1982). The reasons for this are not clear but the rise in intracranial pressure is insufficient to account for the problem. Heilbrun et al. (1972) suggested that the reduction in cerebral blood flow is consequent upon reduced cerebral metabolism. However lactic acid concentrations in the cerebrospinal fluid are increased after subarachnoid haemorrhage. Initially this results from production by shed red blood cells. Later in those patients who have severe vasospasm, deteriorating clinical state or an increasing intracranial pressure the lactic acid level increases or is at least maintained at an abnormally high level (Voldby & Enevoldsen 1982b). This suggests that the initial event is reduced cerebral perfusion leading to hypoxia. The lactate level may then aggravate the cerebral swelling initially by causing vasomotor paralysis leading to loss of autoregulation and hyperaemia. Leakage of fluid will then occur leading to cerebral oedema. This will be compounded when depletion of adenosine triphosphate levels occurs because the maintenance of the sodium potassium ion transport mechanism is dependent upon this energy source. Thus ischaemia leads to membrane failure (Astrup 1982) which occurs in the baboon when the cortical flow drops below 8 mls/100 g/minute.

Positron emission tomography may help to improve our understanding of the relationship between local blood flow and the metabolic demands of the brain, which in turn may also allow the development of effective therapies.

How may these considerations be used to attempt to predict the outcome of aneurysm surgery pre-operatively? Dynamic isotope scanning has been suggested as a method of distinguishing those patients whose cerebral perfusion is significantly reduced and who would therefore have a high risk of developing ischaemic deficits after angiography or surgery (Kelly et al. 1979). However, a better method for predicting the outcome of surgery might be to attempt to stress the cerebral circulation for Fitch et al. (1981) showed that in baboons autologous subarachnoid haemorrhage resulted in impaired autoregulation for at least 1 week following the ictus. Some patients likewise have impaired cerebrovascular reactivity (Pickard et al. 1980). In the initial studies, carried out peroperatively, 80% of patients with impaired reactivity developed neurological deficits compared with only 7% of those with normal autoregulation. Other workers confirmed these initial findings

(Farrar et al. 1981). Initial analysis of a further 100 patients suggests comparable results (Pickard 1984). The latter's group have developed a safe pre-operative test of cerebral autoregulation using an intravenous Xenon technique and alteration in blood pressure as the challenge.

The cerebral blood volume is also increased following subarachnoid haemorrhage. However in those patients who are grade 1 or 2 (Hunt & Hess) the increase does not reach statistical significance even in those who have vasospasm demonstrated on angiography. However, the more severe the vasospasm the more marked is the increase in cerebral blood volume. This increase is most marked in patients graded 3 or 4 (Grubb 1982). Thus there must also be a significant dilatation or congestion of intraparenchymal vessels in the presence of angiographically proven spasm of the main cerebral arteries.

## Subarachnoid haemorrhage

### Symptoms and signs

The clinical manifestations of subarachnoid haemorrhage provide a diversity of patterns which can be attributed to the degree of haemorrhage, its irruption into the brain, the development of complications such as infarction and obstruction by hydrocephalus and the propensity for recurrence. Fearnsides (1916) was perhaps the first to underline recurrence of haemorrhage which he thought so characteristic as to render the diagnosis of ruptured aneurysm straightforward, a significant contrast with contemporary opinion. Collier (1933) recognized 5 syndromes:

1  *Apoplectic*: this he considered to be in no way different from severe and copious cerebral haemorrhage to which 'subarachnoid haemorrhage was a well-nigh inevitable secondary event'. [Apoplexy: a malady sudden in its attack, which

arrests the powers of sense and motion (Shorter O.E.D.).]

2 *Meningitic*: a less violent degree of haemorrhage causing the signs of 'meningeal irritation' and of raised intracranial pressure; delirium, coma and convulsions might occur.

3 *Lumbago–sciatica*: an infrequent presentation in which backache, leg pains and muscular stiffness gradually spread; it was thought that fibrin irritated the posterior spinal roots; the bleeding is probably of slight extent and the syndrome somewhat more likely to develop when the origin is in the posterior fossa or spinal canal. Such symptoms are also prominent in the stage of recovery from subarachnoid haemorrhage.

4 *Recurrent coma*: this correlates with the frequency with which intracranial aneurysms repeatedly bleed during the first few weeks after the initial ictus.

5 *Migraine*: recurrent episodes of one sided headache may precede a frank rupture. Collier considered that teichopsia and hemanopia did not occur in the migraine due to an aneurysm. He did not agree with Adie's view that ophthalmoplegic migraine was due to an aneurysm, for in his experience the patients usually made a full recovery.

Massive usually overwhelming haemorrhage is to be anticipated in patients of the first group: loss of consciousness is sudden and unannounced and if there are premonitory symptoms, the patients never lives to describe them, or cannot recall them if he recovers. Unconsiousness rapidly deepens, respirations become stertorous and airways obstructed, the blood pressure rises and the pulse rate slows at first but terminally the former fails and the latter becomes rapid. Limbs are paralysed and flaccid at the outset but later decerebrate rigidity develops. The pupils become inactive, often irregular and unequal and later usually dilate. Progressively deepening coma carries a poor prognosis and the impossibility of diagnosing the precise cause of the haemorrhage is of no practical consequence. Death is likely to occur early in this group of

patients and treatment is unavailing; Walton (1956) found that half the patients who die after a single subarachnoid haemorrhage, did so in the first 24 hours. Necropsy records of the Cooperative Study (V part 2) revealed that in half the patients dying within 72 hours of a single haemorrhage the cause was hypertensive disease, a ruptured aneurysm being present in only 36%, whereas for the complete series of the study of subarachnoid haemorrage, aneurysm was the cause in one-half and hypertensive or cerebrovascular disease in only 15%. These figures vindicate the views of Collier and accord with common clinical experience. The rapidly progressive and fatal termination in these cases is explained by the high incidence of haemorrhage into the brain; intracerebral in 80%, intracerebellar in 9% and purely subarachnoid in only 5% (Report of the Cooperative Study V part 2). Sudden loss of consciousness as the initial symptom of aneurysmal rupture is not invariably of grave significance but in these patients the coma soon lightens.

The more commonly encountered picture of subarachnoid haemorrhage corresponds to Collier's 'meningitic' syndrome, and to Symonds' second and third groups (1924). It varies from a relatively mild illness of a few days' duration in an ambulant patient to an illness of weeks, punctuated by recurrent relapses which may terminate in death or recovery. Signs indicating cranial nerve or brain damage may be absent, temporary or permanent. Conscious level may be unaffected, or depressed to the level of coma, yet recovery may occur. In the unconscious patient the potential complications of respiratory infection, difficulty in maintaining nutrition and decubitus ulceration require unceasing medical and nursing care of the highest order. Disorders of metabolism due to diencephalic damage may develop insidiously and convulsions add a risk of further brain damage as a result of hypoxia.

*Premonitory symptoms* can be elicited in a minority of patients. Vague headache, or more definite pain in the forehead on one or both sides may have occured in the previous few weeks. Unilateral ptosis particularly if associated with orbital or supraorbital pain is highly suggestive of the rapid expansion of an aneurysm sac, usually at the posterior communicating position, and rupture is likely with a few days. Pain of trigeminal distribution is an occasional and significant complaint.

Headache is a constant symptom of sub-arachnoid haemorrhage. It is usually of such sudden onset and severity that the patient can recall the time it occurred or his activity at the moment; such detail is of diagnostic value. It may be generalized or may start on one side or at the back of the head and rapidly spread all over, increasing in degree. It is persistent and only diminishes in an average case after some days but often endures to some degree in convalescence; some patients continue to suffer periodic headache when they are otherwise fully recovered. Not infrequently the initial sensation experienced by the patient is of a sudden 'snap' or 'jarring' in the head; of a blow, or of a 'bursting' feeling. These appear to be momentary and are rapidly followed by headache. There may be complaint of blurring of vision or of amaurosis perhaps due to sudden increase of pressure in the basal cisterns and subarachnoid space around the optic nerves.

*Vomiting* is common in the hours following the ictus, so common that its absence may even raise some doubt as to the diagnosis of subarachnoid haemorrhage.

*Meningism* is evident by photophobia and by the presence of neck stiffness, sometimes with head retraction and by a positive Kernig's sign. These signs develop within a few hours and the plantar responses are often extensor at this time.

*Fever* occurs in the majority of patients, usually after the first 24 hours. The degree and duration vary considerably; it is uncommon for it to exceed 39°C and to persist more than a week. Rapidly mounting and high temperatures, or a subnormal temperature occurring within the first 24 hours have a bad prognosis (as in cases of head trauma) and signify intracerebral haemorrhage with diencephalic dysfunction.

*Pulse rate* is moderately increased for a few days. Early tachycardia may be seen in intra-cerebral haemorrhage and a bradycardia suggests the development of cerebral compression.

*Blood pressure* is often considerably above the normal range when the patient is first admitted to hospital, but without knowledge of the previous level the true degree of elevation cannot at this stage be determined. Subsequent measurement often shows that the initial reading was a third or more higher than the mean arterial pressure at the time of discharge from hospital.

*Consciousness* is affected to a varying degree in the majority of cases; in only one-third of Walton's (1956) series did it remain entirely normal. Immediate and persistent loss of consciousness as noted above is typical of the 'apoplectiform' type of haemorrhage. In the meningeal group loss of consciousness is frequent shortly after the onset of headache and may return to a normal level within minutes. In its transience it resembles syncope and is not of serious import. If unconsciousness persists for several hours recovery is usually slow and is marked by stages of stupor, confusion, excitement and amnesia similar to those seen in the rising levels of consciousness which follow head injury. Intra-cerebral haemorrhage is frequent in these patients. Depression of consciousness may be delayed for hours or several days and then develops slowly. This is attributable to cerebral infarction, or to rising intracranial pressure due to intracerebral or subdural haematoma. It is in these patients that angiography is particularly liable to reveal narrowing of arteries. Fits may occasionally announce a haemorrhage, but usually they occur later and were recorded in 14% of Walton's cases. The seizure may be generalized or focal, convulsive in type or purely tonic. Tonic spasms may occur without intracerebral haemorrhage and are ascribed to massive haem-orrhage around the brain stem.

*Decerebrate rigidity* occurs in severe cases; it may be symmetrical or predominate on one side. It betokens intracerebral damage either by haem-orrhage or by infarction, but when it develops a day or so after the onset of the illness it may be due to brain stem compression from a temporal lobe or a subdural haematoma. Thus the early and the late development of decerebrate rigidity have different implications for treatment.

*Focal neurological signs.* Unilateral third nerve palsy is perhaps the commonest 'neighbourhood' sign of an aneurysm; it may occur in the prodromal period, but more commonly it develops within the first few days of rupture and takes several hours to manifest itself. The nerve may be acutely stretched by the sudden expansion of the aneurysmal sac to which it is adherent, or may be compressed by clot or may be invaded by haemorrhage. The aneurysm arises from the posterior aspect of the internal carotid artery at or near to the origin of the posterior communicating artery, or from the junction of the posterior communicating and posterior cerebral arteries. In these situations the sac lies in close contiguity with the third nerve. A complete paralysis of the oculomotor nerve in a patient with subarachnoid haemorrhage who shows no signs of intracerebral involvement is strong evidence of the location of the aneurysm. But in a drowsy or unconscious patient or in one with other abnormal neurological signs suggesting a massive bleed, the palsy may be secondary to temporal lobe herniation. This is most likely to be the cause if palsy is limited to a dilated and fixed pupil.

Defective conjugate ocular movement may be observed if the patient is sufficiently responsive to be tested, and lateral gaze is more likely to be affected. In unresponsive patients, persistent lateral conjugate deviation may be encountered; this is usually due to haemorrhage into the frontal lobe, persistent deviation being towards the side of the lesion and purposeful gaze defective away from that side; the mechanism of this has been examined by Denny-Brown (1966). A unilateral lesion in the upper brain stem may also cause unilateral deviation but, in this case, away from the side of the lesion (Denny-Brown 1960).

Hemiplegia, dysphasia and hemianopia, often identifiable only as the patient recovers from the haemorrhage, are indicative of lesions in the substance of the brain. Fortunately a considerable degree of recovery usually occurs provided no further haemorrhage or infarction takes place. Occasionally paresis is largely limited to one limb, or even to muscles of its extremity and this is usually due to the uncommon situation of an aneurysm on a peripheral branch: of the anterior cerebral artery in the case of the leg and of the middle cerebral artery in the case of the arm. Rarely premonitory symptoms of weakness, paraesthesiae or numbness may precede the rupture of such aneurysms. They have little value for diagnosis, but like other premonitory symptoms are of interest in providing clinical evidence that events take place in the sac wall, stretching or haemorrhagic infiltration, which lead to rupture.

*Grading.* A full clinical assessment of the patient is essential in determining the management and in attempting to predict the outcome. The most commonly used system is that of Hunt and Hess (1968) which is a modified version of the Botterell classification. Hunt and Hess (1968) grouped patients into five categories:

I    Asymptomatic;
II   Moderate/severe headache;
III  Drowsiness, mild focal deficit;
IV   Stupor, moderate/severe deficit;
V    Deep coma.

To these has been added a sixth grade O, to cover those who have not had a haemorrhage, for example those with a painful third nerve palsy alone.

Other systems have also been devised, for example the Nishioka (1966) system which is also an update on the Botterell system. However, Lindsay *et al.* (1983) have drawn attention to the interobserver variability which occurs when using the Hunt–Hess or the Nishioka systems and suggested that for patients at grade III or below, the Glasgow Coma Scale was a more reliable measure of the level of responsiveness. It is important to bear in mind this difficulty when assessing papers which discuss the management of patients with aneurysmal subarachnoid haemorrhage. In an attempt to reduce this difficulty the World Federation of Neurosurgical Societies Committee on Grading has proposed the following modifications to the Hunt–Hess Scale and Teasdale *et al.*'s (1984) gradings:

1  Glasgow Coma Score (GCS) 15. Neurologically intact (except for cranial nerve palsy).
2  GCS 15. Neurologically intact (except for cranial nerve palsy) with headache and/or neck stiffness.
3  GCS 13–14
3a  without focal neurological deficit
3b  with focal neurological deficit.
(3a and 3b may be combined into one group.)
4  GCS 8–12 with or without focal neurological deficit.
5  GCS 3–7 coma with or without abnormal posturing.

*Optic fundi.* Within a few hours of rupture, ophthalmoscopy may reveal numerous haemorrhages obscuring the fundus. These may be small, scattered and apparently retinal, others are large, irregular blobs of blood preretinal (subhyaloid) in situation. Although the former resolve satisfactorily the latter are more serious for they absorb slowly and may break into the vitreous leaving a permanent visual defect (Meadows 1951). Bramwell (1886) had noted at post-mortem examination extravasation of blood along the sheath of the optic nerve and into the nerve and suggested that this might be the cause of 'optic neuritis' and of optic atrophy and visual field defects in a case of haemophilia. Riddoch and Goulden (1925) obtained post-mortem information in one of 4 cases of intraocular haemorrhage. The examinations were carried out by Turnbull; the arachnoid sheath of the optic nerve was filled with blood, 'like a vein' but the nerve was not infiltrated and the pia was intact. In the excellent illustrations the optic nerve head can be seen to be swollen. They concluded that the intraocular haemorrhages were due to compression of retinal veins in the subarachnoid space surrounding the optic nerves, the mechanism invoked in papilloedema. This is generally accepted. Fundal haemorrhages are more frequently caused by aneurysms arising from the anterior part of the circle of Willis presumably because the effused blood more rapidly distends the optic nerve sheath to a high pressure.

Papilloedema of a mild degree is common within the first day or so of haemorrhage due to the immediate elevation of intracranial pressure. It may develop more slowly after a latent interval of a few days as a result of haematoma, infarction, venous congestion or of accompanying brain oedema. The latent period may be several weeks and in these the papilloedema is likely to be due to hydrocephalus, secondary to leptomeningeal obstruction.

*Metabolic disturbances.* An account of the biochemical disorders which may be encountered by the neurosurgeon in acute lesions of the brain is given in Chapter 23. In subarachnoid haemorrhage transient albuminuria and glycosuria are not infrequent. Walton (1956) recorded an incidence of 10% and of 8% respectively in which a cause other than cerebral could not be detected. He observed that the majority of such patients showed clinical evidence of hypothalamic damage and that at necropsy blood was usually found in the third ventricle. Dehydration and electrolyte imbalance of slight degree probably occur in most cases of ruptured aneurysm but in a few they provide a major therapeutic problem. Buckell *et al.* (1966) made detailed biochemical investigations in a large series of cases of subarachnoid haemorrhage and abnormality was detected in 84%. Severe muscle wasting is occasionally encountered, similar to the catabolic response to injury, but of an exaggerated and prolonged degree.

## Natural history of ruptured aneurysms

For many years information concerning the natural course of events after the rupture of an aneurysm was largely derived from series of unclassified subarachnoid haemorrhage although it was fully appreciated that while aneurysm was the commonest causative lesion, there were many other causes. In the assessment of prognosis, subarachnoid haemorrhage and ruptured aneurysm were equated for practical purposes.

This unsatisfactory and misleading practice has now been abandoned; largely owing to the activities of McKissock and his colleagues it was realized that statistical assessment of the value of surgical treatment of ruptured aneurysms was impossible without comparable precision of diagnosis in cases not subjected to operation; furthermore, that comparison demanded large numbers of unselected cases in the two groups (McKissock *et al.* 1958, 1960a).

The Cooperative Study (V part 2) isolated 830 cases of single aneurysm which had bled for the first time and for which there had been no surgical treatment. The number of deaths each successive day after the haemorrhage was the highest on the first; a progressive fall in the daily numbers was interrupted by a secondary peak around the seventh day. Over half the deaths had occurred by the end of 2 weeks and at the end of 6 weeks 55% of the patients had died. This period of time is the maximum commonly recommended by physicians for bedrest in conservative treatment. Thus we may say that about 45% of the patients survived the haemorrhage; the prognosis in these was fairly good for the figure had declined only as far as 34% in 3 years. Statistical analysis distinguished 3 groups. In one, nearly 10% of the total, the mortality was very high; three-quarters of the patients in this group died during the first 24 hours and most were dead within 5 days. In the next group comprising 47%, deaths were fewer and occurred later; the average survival was about 2 weeks but most were dead by 3 months. In the third group comprising 43%, prognosis was relatively good; they recovered from the initial ictus and during the subsequent period of follow up decline in their numbers was slow. Alvord *et al.* (1972) using data taken both from the Cooperative Study and from Pakarinen (1967) drew probability curves for survival following haemorrhage. Immediately following haemorrhage the mortality assessed at 2 months is 60% but if it is reassessed considering only those patients who survive the first 24 hours, the figure drops to 40%. Thus for a unit which admits patients directly following subarachnoid haemorrhage a management mortality of less than 60% represents an improvement upon the natural history, but if admission is delayed for only 24 hours the management mortality must be less than 40% if it is to be acceptable. Delay of one month after the ictus reduces the acceptable risk to 10% or less.

The propensity for haemorrhage to recur soon after the initial ictus was recognized by Fearnsides (1916) and is now well known. It is an important factor in the high mortality rate early in the illness and probably accounts for the secondary peak incidence of deaths around the seventh day. The Cooperative Study (V part 2) provided 1243 cases of single aneurysm arising from the anterior part of the circle of Willis, which had bled once. A second haemorrhage occurred in one-third (414) of these. Some of these patients doubtless sustained further haemorrhages but the study was not taken beyond the second. The daily incidence of the second episode was examined in the same way as for the first. The numbers of cases in which there was a second haemorrhage reached a maximum from the third to the tenth days after the initial rupture and by the end of 14 days about one-half of the recurrent haemorrhage had occurred. After this interval there was a persistent low incidence of rebleeding. The risk of rebleeding was calculated to be 10% in the first week, 12% in the second week, 7% in the third week, in the fourth week there was a slight rise in the risk, attributed to increasing activity of the patient. Kassell and Torner (1983b) in a preliminary report on the Co-operative Aneurysm Study found that in 2265 patients the maximum incidence of rehaemorrhage was on the day of the initial ictus and that there was no later peak confirming a finding in 2 previous smaller studies (Richardson *et al.* 1964, 1966). These studies differ slightly in that Richardson *et al.* found a slow decline in the incidence over days 2–14 whereas Kassell and Torner suggest that it is unchanged throughout this period. After the thirtieth day the risk drops to less than 10% in the next five months. Richardson *et al.* (1964, 1966) analysed the adverse factors which could be correlated with rehaemorrhage during the first six months. In anterior communicating aneurysms these factors were increasing age, hypertension, female gender and spherical upward pointing aneurysms but in the posterior communicating type vasospasm, haematoma, large size and female sex were the most important (Winn *et al.* 1982). After the first six months rehaemorrhage occurs at the rate of 3.5% per annum for the first 10 years and carries a mortality of 67% (Winn *et al.* 1977). Though youth was found to be no protection against rehaemorrhage in the longterm, the average time to rehaemorrhage was 9.8 years in those who were less than 40 years old and 4.4 years in those over this age at the time of the initial ictus. Longterm follow-up of the cases with ruptured intracranial aneurysms admitted to the Cooperative Study between 1958 and 1965 revealed that the rehaemorrhage rate in patients who survived a decade after the ictus was 0.86% per year for the second decade (Nishioka *et al.* 1984a). Furthermore posterior circulation aneurysms carried a more favourable prognosis after a 10 year survival than did anterior circulation aneurysms. Hypertension and female sex were associated with an increased risk of rehaemorrhage in posterior communicating aneurysms, but increased size as judged by repeat angiography at six months was not, even though an increase in size had occurred in all patients studied angiographically following a second bleed. Winn *et al.* (1977) compared this data from their study with the predicted outcome as judged by Alvord *et al.* (1972) and found that the latter's prediction of survival was over optimistic especially for ruptured posterior communicating artery aneurysms. The incidence of multiple aneurysms is about 20%; pathological studies show that the formation of aneurysms is a progressive disease. Consequently delayed recurrent haemorrhage may arise from an aneurysm which escaped detection by the first angiography, or from an aneurysm which has developed during the intervening period of time.

## Sequelae of ruptured aneurysms

*Headache* in a minority of patients fails to resolve during convalescence; in Walton's series (of undifferentiated subarachnoid haemorrhage) these comprised about one-quarter of the survivors. The headache is usually periodic like migraine and may be accompanied by malaise and vomiting though not by visual phenomena.

*Coarse neurological deficits* such as hemiparesis, dysphasia and hemianopia, the result of brain damage, usually show considerable improvement in ,the course of time. Walton found that in approximately one-half of those who showed such signs when discharged from hospital made a complete recovery. Storey (1967) gave a detailed report on a group of 209 patients who had survived the rupture of an aneurysm; one-half showed no abnormal neurological signs, one-quarter mild, and the remainder moderate to severe. The nature and degree of the defect will determine whether the patient can resume his previous employment, requires retraining, or whether as in a small proportion disablement is total and permanent. Success in rehabilitation also depends upon the extent to which mental sequelae persist.

*Psychiatric disturbance.* The gross forms seen in the acute illness usually resolve fairly rapidly. Korsakov syndrome, probably due to disturbance in the region of the anterior hypothalamus for it not infrequently follows operations on tumours in that vicinity, may take many months to clear and Walton records resolution after 11 months. Impairment of intellect was found in 40% of Storey's patients but a severe degree amounting to dementia in only 3% and in 1% of Walton's. Changes in personality are frequent and Storey records the interesting observation that the relatives of some patients considered the change to be for the better; the patient was 'easier to live with'. This he ascribed to a leucotomy effect and more frequently followed haemorrhage from anterior cerebral aneurysm. Fear of recurrent haemorrhage plays a large part in the production of anxiety symptoms and points to the need for vigorous reassurance during convalescence. It is unfortunate that some patients are warned not to undertake excessive physical exertion; not only does this invite fear, but a physical effort precipitates haemorrhage in only a very small proportion of cases.

*Epilepsy* occurs in about 10% of survivors (Storey 1967, Walton 1956). The seizures are usually infrequent and amenable to medical treatment (*see* Chapter 17).

## Differential diagnosis of subarachnoid haemorrhage

Apart from aneurysms, vascular malformations, hypertension and vascular disease, spontaneous subarachnoid bleeding can arise from any of a great variety of lesions, some very rare. The incidence in the practice of a general hospital is illustrated by the following analysis. During the years 1948–61, subarachnoid haemorrhage was diagnosed and confirmed by lumbar puncture in 452 patients admitted to the London Hospital. The causes or associated diseases, so far as could be determined, are listed below.

|  | % |
|---|---|
| Aneurysms (verified by angiography or necropsy) | 48 |
| Vascular malformation | 5 |
| Hypertension | 10 |
| Blood disease | 1.3 |
| Diabetes, endocarditis, lupus erythematosis, nephritis, pulmonary tuberculosis, coarctation of aorta, subdural haematoma, glioma | 3 |
| Undetermined | 32 |

The Cooperative Study (III) found a very similar distribution of aneurysm, malformation and other causes in 5836 cases. Necropsy in cases of the latter group showed that hypertension and vascular disease accounted for 75%, a higher proportion than Russell (1954) found for necropsies showing intracranial haemorrhage; the remaining 25% included lesions such as are listed in the table and a large number

of other unusual causes. It is notable that haemorrhage from a tumour supplied only 2%. Thus, in a patient 40–60 years of age with spontaneous subarachnoid haemorrhage, there is an even chance that the cause is an aneurysm, but if the patient's condition rapidly deteriorates the probability grows that cerebral vascular disease is responsible. A bias towards cerebrovascular disease increases with increasing age. In younger patients the pattern changes and the importance of vascular malformation emerges. In patients of the ages of 10–20 years the causes of bleeding are approximately equally divided between aneurysm, malformation and the miscellaneous group (Report on the Cooperative Study V, Fig. 44).

The history of the patient's previous health, obtained from relatives if the patient is unconscious, may give clues to the correct diagnosis. Periodic headaches or focal epilepsy for some years suggest vascular malformation; a previous stroke or heart attack makes cerebrovascular disease likely. In primary intracerebral haemorrhage unconsciousness is usually deeper and signs of paralysis immediately apparent, and in cerebral vascular occlusion the evolution of paralysis may extend over several hours, with relatively little headache and less marked impairment of consciousness than would be encountered in hemiplegia due to a ruptured aneurysm. A fall when drunk or during an epileptic seizure may suggest that the bleeding is traumatic rather than spontaneous. Chronic subdural haematoma may present acutely. Blood dyscrasias and other systemic diseases may usually be suspected from the past history or from evidence of disease elsewhere. In acute meningitis the onset of headache though it may be rapid is not abrupt as in haemorrhage, and toxic symptoms, fever, sweating, flushed face, tachycardia, are early and out of proportion to the degree of depressed consciousness. On occasions the haemorrhage has its source in the spinal canal (Chapter 21), usually from a vascular malformation, rarely from a tumour, polyarteritis nodosa or aneurysm. History of initial pain in the back later ascending to the neck and headache as a late feature suggests this possibility (Henson & Croft 1956).

Nonhypertensive patients with no other medical condition predisposing to subarachnoid haemorrhage and in whom 4 vessel cerebral angiography is normal, i.e. cases of idiopathic subarachnoid haemorrhage, have a good overall prognosis both in terms of rehaemorrhage (2.4% at mean follow-up time over 3 years) and return to work at six months, provided they survive the initial ictus (Beguelin & Seiler 1983). Nishioka et al. (1984b) in a longterm follow-up study of patients admitted to the Cooperative study found that after 6 months, the life expectancy of such patients was no difference from that of the age and sex matched United States population. The life expectancy was reduced in hypertensive patients but this may not be specific for cases who have suffered a subarachnoid haemorrhage.

## Investigations

The initial investigation of choice is computerized tomography (CT). This noninvasive study will both confirm the presence of blood in the subarachnoid space and establish whether or not a space-occupying intracranial haematoma is present. If CT fails to show intracranial subarachnoid or intracerebral blood, *lumbar puncture* should be performed in order to confirm the diagnosis. As noted earlier clear spinal fluid is occasionally though rarely encountered if an aneurysm has ruptured and bloody fluid sometimes occurs in primary intracerebral haemorrhage from atheroma. The pressure should be measured and a small sample should be collected successively into three containers, for inspection and comparison. Bleeding from the site of puncture gives diminishing degrees of colouration and mixing. Xanthochromia should be looked for in a centrifuged sample of CSF; it will be absent in cases of traumatic tap (unless there has been a previous attempt at lumbar puncture). Symonds (1924) quotes interesting examples from Froin's original thesis on the subject.

*Urine analysis* may reveal albuminuria or gly-

cosuria or both. If present, blood samples should be taken for urea and sugar estimation.

*Radiological examinations.* The skull should be X-rayed by routine projections in order to detect abnormal calcification such as may occur in athermomatous arteries, in the wall of some aneurysms, in angiomatous malformations and in tumours. A pineal opacity may be displaced by a haematoma.

*Computerized tomographic (CT) scanning* rarely shows an aneurysm. However early scanning can not only show evidence of subarachnoid blood in a high percentage of cases, but this may be predictive of the development of ischaemic complications (Fisher et al. 1980b). In addition the scan will show intracerebral haematomas and may show areas of reduced density or abnormal contrast enhancement (Doczi et al. 1984) in cases with ischaemic complications. More rarely subhyaloid haemorrhage may also be seen. The location of blood may be helpful in determining which aneurysm has bled in cases of multiple aneurysms. In patients who have been alert and then deteriorate, repeat CT scanning can be of great value in distinguishing between repeat haemorrhage and ischaemic problems. This is also the ideal method of diagnosing the communicating hydrocephalus which may complicate subarachnoid haemorrhage.

*Angiography* remains essential for the definitive diagnosis of an aneurysm and the examination may also reveal the presence of a subdural and intracerebral haemorrhage, information which will influence treatment. Concerning the aneurysm it is necessary to know its site and point of origin, size, shape, orientation and relationship to neighbouring structures, particularly major arteries: in the case of an aneurysm arising from the anterior cerebral or communicating arteries, find out whether it fills from one carotid circulation alone or freely from either (Fig. 11.6). Concerning the cerebral arteries, whether there are any of the major variations of the circle of Willis, some of which preclude certain surgical measures, and whether there is efficient or poor collateral circulation from one hemisphere to another needs to be known. Use the cross cir-

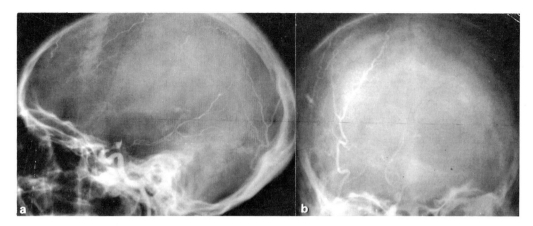

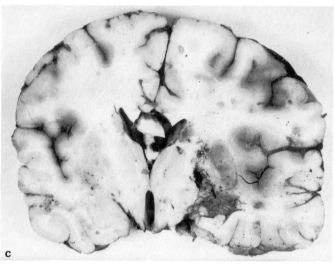

**Fig. 11.5.** Female aged 44 years: subarachnoid haemorrhage 8 days before death: comatose for last 2 days with restless movements of right limbs and none of the left except for evoked extensor movements of the arm.
(a,b) Angiography (24 hours before death) showed a probable aneurysm arising from termination of the right internal carotid: internal carotid artery at the level of the anterior clinoid process greatly narrowed and beyond this point only the posterior cerebral artery and branches are filled and are very narrow. Circulation visible in external carotid territory (superficial temporal and occipital arteries) indicating great delay or deficiency of cerebral circulation. In original film, calcified pineal displaced to the left side. The state was ascribed to cerebral ischaemia and no operation performed.
(c) Post-mortem examination revealed aneurysm of right internal carotid artery at or close to junction with posterior communicating artery, subarachnoid haemorrhage, brain swollen particularly right hemisphere, flattened convolutions and compressed sulci, poor demarcation between white and grey matter: softening and cavitation of right amygdalum, uncus and pallidum.

culation test, when one carotid is injected while the other is digitally occluded (Fig. 11.6.) The presence of narrowing of arteries, particularly if bilateral or extensive, attests to the severity of the haemorrhage and the likelihood of infarction (Fig. 11.5); displacements indicate oedema or localized collections of blood and must therefore be compared critically with the finding on computerized tomography. Not infrequently such abnormalities of the arteries are present but no aneurysm is seen; in these cases the aneurysm may be found to fill satisfactorily at a subsequent

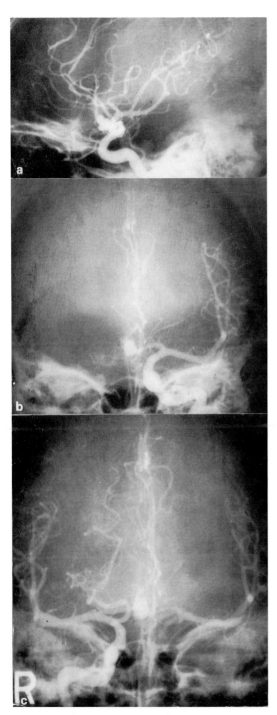

**Fig. 11.6.** Male aged 59 years: 2 attacks of subarachnoid bleeding at 2 years interval.
(a,b) Multilobulated aneurysm arising from anterior communicating artery which fills from either carotid injection.
(c) Good cross circulation with right carotid injection and left carotid occlusion.

examination, carried out 2 or more weeks later. Angiography carried out efficiently so as to give adequate information inflicts considerable stress on a cerebral circulation already impaired by the haemorrhage and its consequences; it should only be undertaken by an expert. The Cooperative Study (IV) estimated a mortality rate directly attributable to angiography of about 0.8%, but the risk of invoking further haemorrhage is negligible; approximately 1 in 300 patients died from this complication; the incidence of hemiparesis, convulsions and hyperthermia was about 3%. Complications are more frequent in patients over the age of 60 years and in those with marked atheroma and such reasons may render angiography inadvisable.

When should the examination be carried out? To some extent this will depend upon the views of the surgeon concerning operative treatment for a ruptured aneurysm. In general angiography should be performed as soon as possible in patients who are responsive, but in those who are unconscious from the outset angiography should be postponed until progressive improvement is manifest; increasing drowsiness in a patient previously alert is an indication for CT in order to detect a haematoma. How far should the examination be taken, and what degree of reliability can be achieved in revealing (or excluding) an aneurysm? The realization that 1 in 5 patients may harbour more than one aneurysm, and that aneurysms of the vertebrobasilar system can be treated surgically with increasing success have underlined the need for more thorough examination. To be set against this is the greater incidence of complications which accompanies multiple injections. In the case of the patient who is not severely ill, the minimum examination should comprise both carotid trees and cross circulation tests. In very ill patients, if the first carotid injection reveals an aneurysm, with local changes suggesting it has bled, and particularly if there is CT evidence of a haematoma at this site, the radiologist should consult with the surgeon concerned whether the opposite carotid should be injected, or whether the information available is adequate for his purpose. Full cerebral angiography can be deferred until after this aneurysm has been clipped. In these, as in all neuroradiological investigations in ill patients, close and immediate cooperation between radiologist and neurosurgeon is highly desirable and in the patients' best interests. Routine should not be blindly followed. If neither carotid examination shows an aneurysm (or other cause for bleeding) or local evidence of haemorrhage and there has been no unwanted reaction, vertebral angiography on one side should be performed. Frequently retrograde filling of the other vertebral artery occurs. If this is also negative and the haemorrhage is the patient's first attack it is wise to desist and await events. If there have been previous haemorrhages, the examination should be pursued after a few days' interval. Perrett and Bull (1959) estimated that the angiographic demonstration of a ruptured aneurysm (if present) can achieve a reliability of 96%, if the examination is thorough and the films carefully scrutinized. Sutton and Trickey (1962) analysed a series of cases of spontaneous subarachnoid haemorrhage with the following results: injection of both carotids gave positive findings in 75%, the addition of one vertebral injection improved this to 90%, and with the second vertebral injection to 96%. The value of the second vertebral injection was similar in the experience of af Bjorkesten and Halonen (1965) who found that it revealed the diagnosis in only 3 of 90 cases. The false negative rate in normal 4 vessel angiography is 1.8% (Forster et al. 1978).

Where more than one aneurysm is present it is necessary to decide which has ruptured. Local vascular abnormalities, narrowing, lack of filling and minor displacements, or the major displacements due to haematoma may clearly identify the offender. Wood (1964) found that in 87% of cases it was the largest sac which ruptured and if one of the aneurysms arose from the anterior communicating artery that was most frequently the one which had ruptured.

Funnel shaped widening of the origin of the posterior communicating artery is referred to as an infundibulum. It remains controversial as to whether this is a normal variant or represents a pre-aneurysmal state. Cases have been reported in which an aneurysm has apparently developed at the site of the infundibulum over a period of up to 9 years. After reviewing the literature, Itakura et al. (1983) identified some common features in these patients who were usually young females with multiple aneurysms. For these patients they recommended careful angiographic follow-up.

## Treatment of ruptured aneurysms

### Pre-operative management

Management of the patient is devoted to reducing the risk of a second haemorrhage and the development of other complications, for example cerebral ischaemia. The conditions most conducive to safe recovery from cerebral ischaemia should be provided. In those with a depressed consciousness it is essential to maintain the airway and adequate pulmonary function. In those who are alert it is essential to reduce anxiety and control headache, neckache and backache. Sedation may therefore be indicated in some patients but adequate analgesia is always essential. When using analgesics such as codeine phosphate it is essential that the patient not be allowed to become constipated. The risks associated with the use of a bedside commode or the toilet may be less than those resulting from the difficulties of using a bedpan. Hypertension is common in patients admitted following aneurysmal subarachnoid haemorrhage. They will divide into two groups: those with essential hypertension who will require gentle reduction and control of their blood pressure and those in whom there is a reactive hypertension, many of whom will settle with sedation and/or analgesia. Correct fluid balance is essential, and it is wise to avoid diuretics in the control of hypertension in subarachnoid haemorrhage.

Antifibrinolytic agents are capable of prolonging and consolidating experimental thrombosis. They will cross the blood–brain barrier and will result in some inhibition of fibrinolytic activity in blood and cerebrospinal fluid following subarachnoid haemorrhage (Tovi 1972). These agents have therefore been used to attempt to reduce the early rehaemorrhage risk in aneurysmal subarachnoid haemorrhage. Epsilon aminocaproic acid was used first and though there were early favourable reports, later, more critical, studies suggested that no benefit was derived from the use of this agent (Shucart et al. 1980, Ameen & Illingworth 1981). Ischaemic complications of the therapy were also reported early (Shaw & Miller 1974). Tranexamic acid has been reported as being effective in reducing the early rebleeding rate, especially in the first 10 days, but the advantage was offset by an increase in cerebral ischaemic complications (Fogstad 1982, Lindsay et al. 1984). Meyer et al. (1983) demonstrated a greater reduction in cerebral blood flow in the first 3 weeks in those patients taking tranexamic acid, as opposed to those who were not.

## Surgery

### Introduction

Fundamental to the problem are the answers to the question 'What can surgery achieve?'. Elsewhere in the body sudden haemorrhage may cause death by loss of blood and an operation can save life by controlling the haemorrhage. In intracranial haemorrhage no patient dies because of blood loss and no operation is necessary for this reason. Also, no operation can save life where haemorrhage rapidly causes lethal brain damage by its irruption into vital centres. Cessation of bleeding is entirely dependent upon natural processes; but operation may be a life-saving measure if it can prevent a recurrence of bleeding, to which aneurysms are particularly prone. In addition operation may save life and reduce morbidity by evacuating collections of blood which are producing increased intra-cranial pressure, and decompressive craniotomy may perhaps improve the cerebral circulation and diminish the degree of infarction. Finally, if hydrocephalus supervenes it can be relieved by external or internal drainage of cerebrospinal fluid.

Operations designed to prevent further rupture fall into 2 groups. In one the aneurysm is exposed by craniotomy and excluded from the circulation by closing its neck with a ligature or a clip, or the sac is obliterated by clips by intraluminal balloons or by induction of thrombosis in the sac, or if this is not possible the sac is reinforced externally. The other group is based upon the classical Hunterian operation of proximal ligation. The appropriate carotid artery is ligated in the neck, or occasionally the vertebral artery is ligated in the treatment of some aneurysms in the posterior cranial fossa; the aim is to reduce the pulse wave and blood pressure within the sac so as to lessen tension and provide time for spontaneous thrombosis. In the special case of aneurysms of the anterior cerebral and communicating arteries, an operation devised by Logue (1956) applies a similar principle but requires craniotomy; one anterior cerebral artery is occluded close to its origin from the internal carotid artery and the aneurysm is left undisturbed. The general merits of these procedures will first be considered then the timing of the operation, its modification according to site, ancillary measures to facilitate the operation, complications and results.

### Definitive operation on aneurysmal sac

*Advantages*

1   Accurate and total obliteration or exclusion of the sac prevents further rupture.
2   Efficient reinforcement offers a fair measure of protection.
3   Haematomas can be evacuated in the course of the operation.
4   Tentorial herniation can be relieved; decompression may improve the cerebral circulation and may lessen risk of further infarction.

*Disadvantages*

1   The operation is technically difficult and success demands great skill and experience, for the margin between life and death is narrow.
2   Difficulties and complications arising during the operation may cause increased morbidity.
3   The operation carries a higher mortality rate if performed soon after rupture when the risk of a second haemorrhage is greatest, than some weeks later when the risk is much less.

## Proximal ligation (extracranial)

*Advantages*

1   The operation is simple and no special skill is demanded.
2   The operation is short and puts little surgical stress upon the patient.

*Disadvantages*

1   It does not offer complete protection against further rupture.
2   Its potential effects upon the cerebral circulation are such that although a simple and short procedure, it carries a significant mortality and morbidity; as in the case of the direct operation, mortality and morbidity rates are higher when ligation is performed soon after haemorrhage, at the time when the need for protection is greatest.
3   Intracranial haematoma will still require craniotomy for evacuation of the clot.
4   The sacrifice of a major artery to the brain may have serious consequences in later years if the patient develops another aneurysm, or atheromatous stenosis in the other major arteries, a not insignificant possibility in view of the high incidence of vascular degenerative disease in these patients.

## Timing of operation

Patients who have received lethal brain damage cannot be helped; they are likely to die within 24–48 hours without regaining consciousness. That the cerebral injury is short of lethal is shown by a gradual improvement in the unconscious state and this assessment necessitates delay until a satisfactory level is attained. Operative mortality bears a close and inverse relationship to the level of consciousness immediately prior to the time of operation; this is true also for conservatively treated patients assessed at a comparable time (McKissock *et al.* 1960a).

| | Mortality (%) | |
|---|---|---|
| *Level of consciousness* | *Medical treatment (on admission)* | *Surgical treatment (before operation)* |
| Alert | 31 | 20 |
| Clouded | 56 | 40 |
| Unconscious | 31 | 81 |

Though the introduction of the microscope, advances in neuro-anaesthesia and improved aneurysm clips have greatly reduced the operative mortality to an overall level of 7% from 22% (Symon 1982, Koos & Perneczy 1982), no change has occurred in the relationship between the responsive level and the surgical outcome. Koos and Perneczy's (1982) report demonstrates this well:

| | Mortality (%) | |
|---|---|---|
| *Grade (Hunt & Hess modified)* | *Series B (premicroscope)* | *Series D (microscope)* |
| 0 | – | 0 |
| 1 | 0 | 2 |
| 2 | 17 | 4 |
| 3 | 30 | 8 |
| 4 | 50 | 20 |
| 5 | 60 | 83 |
| Overall | 22 | 7 |

In this context the level of responsiveness is the best index we possess of the integrity of the diencephalon and brain stem, whether it be assailed by direct damage, by ischaemia or by secondary intracranial hypertension. But delaying the operation strikes at its basic indication, to prevent further rupture which reaches its highest probability by the seventh to tenth day. Thereafter there is on this account a lessening indication for operation and a diminishing risk to life if it is performed. Postponement of the operation improves the 'score' as shown by mortality statistics, but does not disclose the loss of a few lives that might have been saved by earlier operation.

Adams et al. (1981) looked at the results of delayed operation with optimal medical management. At 90 days after the ictus only 46% had made a satisfactory recovery and 36% were dead. Of those admitted who were in grade 1–3 inclusive on the Hunt–Hess scale 28% were dead at 3 months and 55% were progressing well. Management mortality figures such as these have resulted in various groups moving towards early surgery (within 48–72 hours) in order to reduce the risk from early rehaemorrhage. Despite adopting a policy of early surgery, Ljunggren et al. (1985a) found that overall outcome from aneurysmal subarachnoid haemorrhage remained poor, largely because of the number of patients who are devastated by the initial haemorrhage; only 42% of their patients made a good recovery. Hunt and Hess advocated in 1968 that patients in their grades 1 and 2 should be operated upon within 24 hours if possible but that those in grade 3 or worse should be treated conservatively until they improved sufficiently to be graded 2 or better. Ljunggren et al. (1981) in a consecutive series of ruptured aneurysm of the anterior part of the circle of Willis and in which the patients graded 1–3 (Hunt–Hess) were operated upon within 48 hours were able to report an overall management mortality of 31% and good recoveries in 54%. Similar results have been reported by other workers (Hugenholtz & Elgie 1982, Bolander et al. 1984). Suzuki et al. (1979) found that closer analysis revealed that the operative mortality was lower on days 1 and 2, was at its greatest on day 3 and did not fall to the rate for the first day until day 8. Hugenholtz and Elgie (1982) not only confirmed this but also found that the morbidity was increased in those

patients coming to surgery between the third and seventh days. This is not in agreement with the findings of Yaşargil et al. (1975) that, provided the responsive level was satisfactory, there was no contraindication to operating between the third and seventh days. Morbidity is an important aspect of the outcome, but Ljunggren et al. (1981) and Bolander et al. (1984) did not find any increase in the morbidity following early surgery compared with operation undertaken after one week. Ljunggren et al. (1985a) report 76% of patients in Grades 1–3 recovering without neurological deficit following early surgery. Addition of the calcium antagonist, nimodipine, resulted in no case of fixed postoperative neurological deficit in Grade 1–3 patients with internal carotid or middle cerebral artery aneurysms despite the undoubted presence of risk factors for ischaemic deficit (Saveland et al. 1986a). However, the emotional and psychological sequelae that adversely affect outcome despite the absence of neurological deficit (Ljunggren et al. 1985b) result in only 33% of patients coming to early surgery having a fully favourable outcome.

However, it is far from universally accepted that early surgery improves the management outcome (Flamm 1982). It is possible to obtain conditions at an early operation which are slack enough to achieve the surgical objectives yet the conditions are not as good as they are later; the brain is more swollen, hyperaemic and soft. Furthermore haemorrhage into the subarachnoid space can obscure the very small vessels and hence increase the risk of damage to them.

More information is therefore required about the question of early versus late surgery before final conclusions can be drawn. Though it is not a randomized study, the International Cooperative Study on the Timing of Aneurysm Surgery should provide this. Ultimately it is likely that the view expressed by Yaşargil et al. (1975) will prove correct: that if the patient is mentally alert and in satisfactory medical condition, he is ready for operation; if he is unconscious or deeply obtunded and there is no sign of subdural or intracerebral haematoma, surgery should be delayed.

The arguments in favour of a direct attack upon a ruptured aneurysm greatly outweigh those in support of proximal ligation except in special circumstances. Craniotomy for the aneurysm will be considered first, then proximal ligation.

## Operations on the aneurysmal sac

The technical difficulties comprise access, haemorrhage from the aneurysm during its isolation and the procedure of exclusion, obliteration or reinforcement.

As in operations for tumours, the surgeon has to cope with raised intracranial pressure and brain softened by oedema; in addition brain may be swollen by haemorrhage and haemostasis may be slow and tedious. When a subdural or intracerebral haematoma is encountered, its evacuation diminishes the intracranial pressure and improves access. The presence of an intracerebral haematoma sometimes aids the surgeon for it guides him to the aneurysm and provides him with a ready-made cavity through which to work. But evacuation of haematoma leads the surgeon to approach that part of the aneurysm sac that has bled, and however gently performed, may cause the aneurysm to bleed again; the surgeon should be prepared for such trouble. Virtually all aneurysms are deeply seated and most are small and little room is available for manoeuvre unless it is provided by drainage of CSF, excision of brain, or by evacuation of a haematoma. A catheter inserted into the frontal horn of the lateral ventricle and allowed to drain during the operation is simple and effective in lowering pressure, and making space, particularly if there is hydrocephalus. The subarachnoid cisterns should be identified and opened. Continuous spinal drainage is even more effective in reducing the amount of retraction required. Some surgeons use a short course of dexamethasone pre-operatively and post-

operatively (Yaşargil *et al.* 1975). Intravenous osmotic dehydrants given shortly before the operation and the employment of controlled respiration are often of great help in diminishing brain bulk and reducing venous oozing. The rise of blood pressure which may follow dehydration as a result of increase in blood volume may cause apprehension of a further rupture of the aneurysm and may need control with a hypotensive drug. The value of induced hypotension and of hypothermia is discussed later.

The amount of retraction necessary has been greatly reduced by the introduction of microsurgical technique into aneurysm surgery. This allows stereoscopic vision despite a narrow approach with excellent lighting of the operative field and allows details of the blood vessels to be more readily recognized. With this technique the pterional approach allows access to several differently located aneurysms. Minor variations in approach allow access to aneurysms occurring at the anterior communicating, middle cerebral, internal carotid and the basilar bifurcation locations. In general, the parent artery should be dissected first, so that a temporary clip may be applied if rupture occurs which cannot be controlled by application of a cotton pledget to the aneurysm sac. Following this the opposite wall of the artery to that from which the aneurysm is arising should be exposed, before proceeding to dissect the aneurysm neck. It is wise to avoid exposing the fundus which is the thinnest and weakest part, unless this is absolutely necessary, for example if it is planned to wrap the aneurysm. It is important to check that all the small perforating arteries in addition to the major branches are dissected away from the neck before the clip is applied. A modern spring loaded clip should be used as this reduces the risk of the neck of the aneurysm being torn by muscular effort and the associated tremor. Yaşargil *et al.* (1975) recommend that before the clip is applied the neck should be lightly coagulated with bipolar diathermy in a slow intermittent regulated manner in order to toughen and elongate the neck adjacent to, but independent from the parent vessel. Once applied, it is essential to check that the clip is not partially occluding or kinking the parent vessel or a branch thereof.

The bone plate should be cut as low as possible to reduce retraction on the brain. Once it is fashioned and the dura opened, the posterior inferior part of the frontal lobe is lifted using a self retaining retractor to expose the olfactory tract which is followed posteriorly to find the optic nerve, anterior clinoid process and the carotid artery. The overlying arachnoid is opened and the internal carotid artery followed distally for aneurysms arising from this vessel. Aneurysms at the internal carotid bifurcation may require splitting of the proximal part of the Sylvian fissure to expose them. Anterior communicating artery aneurysms are exposed by carrying the dissection from the bifurcation along the first part of the anterior cerebral artery as it passes across the optic nerve and chiasm. Middle cerebral aneurysms require further opening of the Sylvian fissure. Some basilar aneurysms may also be exposed by splitting the Sylvian fissure as far as the middle cerebral bifurcation and then dissecting between the optic nerve and the carotid artery if there is sufficient space (Yaşargil *et al.* 1976), but if not, by working lateral to the carotid artery and following the inferior surface of the posterior communicating artery to the posterior cerebral and hence to the basilar bifurcartion. Great care must be taken to preserve the perforators passing to the brain stem (Sugita *et al.* 1979). Drake (1969) recommends a subtemporal approach to basilar aneurysm because it gives a better view of the brain stem perforating arteries which arise from the posterior aspect of the basilar artery. Splitting the tentorium cerebelli posterior to the sixth nerve allows access down to the level of the anterior inferior cerebellar artery. Aneurysms arising below this must be approached through a suboccipital craniectomy.

It is during the final stage, of preparing the sac and dealing with it definitively, that haemorrhage is likely to occur, at a time when a dry and clear field of vision is essential for precision. The parent vessels and fine arterial twigs must be seen so that the clip or reinforcement can be applied accurately without embarrassing the circulation in those vessels. A field flooded with blood may prove disastrous in its consequences. Ancillary methods of lowering the blood pressure within the sac are of great help, not only in lessening the risk of haemorrhage during the dissection but in diminishing the amount which must be cleared by suction, in collapsing the sac and rendering it more easily manipulated and in lessening the risk of rupture of its tenuous wall as the clip is applied. Induced hypotension is one method commonly practised; its use should be strictly limited to the time during which the sac is subjected to the stresses of manipulation, dissection, etc. Although hypotensive drugs have been widely used with impunity in other branches of surgery, for example plastic, otorhinological and orthopaedic surgery, that evidence of impunity is not valid in the surgery of the brain and particularly aneurysms. The susceptibility of the brain to structural damage by ischaemia, in terms of degree and of duration, is much greater than in other tissues, and after subarachnoid haemorrhage this susceptibility is greatly enhanced by the effects of raised intracranial pressure and by relative degrees of impaired circulation including reduced capacity for autoregulation, which may lead to swelling and patchy infarction. In addition patients subjected to operation for aneurysm are largely middle-aged or older and the cerebral vessels are frequently affected by atheroma to an extent unpredictable before operation. It is fair to regard patients with recently ruptured aneurysms as amongst the least favourable for the use of hypotensive drugs, although their value to the surgeon is undeniable.

The successful and rapid development of induced hypothermia in cardiac surgery quickly led to its application to the problems of intracranial vascular surgery. The reduction of cerebral oxygen requirements and metabolism in the hypothermic state promised an operative field rendered bloodless by the temporary occlusion of major arteries without evil consequences. Preliminary experimental work by Rosomoff and Holaday (1954) and Lougheed and Kahn (1955) indicated its practicability and Lougheed *et al.* (1955) described its use in two operations, for glioblastoma and for an extensive vascular malformation. The first series of operations for aneurysm in which temporary arterial occulusion was employed with the aid of induced hypothermia was described by Botterell *et al.* (1956). A review of hypothermia, its techniques and its effects will be found in the *British Medical Bulletin* (1961).

The oesophageal temperature was usually lowered to and maintained at 30°C at which level the oxygen requirements of the brain are reduced by about one-half; there is often a spontaneous fall of the blood pressure, to about 80–90 mmHg in a normal subject; the intracranial pressure is lessened and the operative conditions are generally improved. The technique rapidly became popular and for some years was extensively used. There has since been a retreat from it (Hamby 1963, Report of the Cooperative Study VIII past 2). It is thought by some to offer no improvement in conditions, by others that it does not protect the patient against the results of defective cerebral circulation and offer as evidence the findings at post-mortem examination of infarction and oedema which had not been anticipated. Arterial 'spasm' is thought to be aggravated by a low temperature (Allcock & Drake 1965). It is possible that hypothermia has acquired a poor reputation because too much has been expected of it. Its power to protect the brain against anoxia at the commonly used level of 30°C is but relative. At this temperature cellular activity is reduced but not abolished, as shown by a persistent oxygen requirement of about 50% of normal. The maximum safe period of total denial of cerebral circulation is probably 8 minutes at 30°C (Fairley 1961). It may be less than this if cellular vitality has been impaired by previous haemorrhage or by atheromatous narrowing of vessels. In many aneurysm operations total anaemia is not obtained by temporary arterial occlusion and this increases the margin of safety. But the exigencies of sudden operative haemorrhage may demand occlusion for longer than is safe and the technique should not be blamed

for failure in this event. Further, under hypothermia and temporary deprivation of circulation, the fine perforating vessels arising from neighbouring arteries or from the aneurysm are less easily seen and thus are likely to be damaged during the dissection more easily than in normothermic conditions. McKissock *et al.* (1960b) found that the overall operative mortality rate was unaffected by the use of hypothermia, although the conditions and ease of operation were much improved. Further analysis of these cases showed that hypothermia improved the results in those patients whose operation took place within the first 3 days of the haemorrhage. If used, hypothermia should be limited to the duration of the operation. During the period of slow rewarming the blood pressure may be labile and must be maintained at normal levels by transfusion, lowering the head of the bed and if necessary press or agents. There seems little physiological justification for prolonging the hypothermia and there are definite disadvantages in the biochemical disturbances which accompany it and in the possible damage to other organs (Fairley 1961). The figures which purport to show an increased mortality in these cases (Report of the Cooperative Study VIII part 2, table 191) may also be weighted by selection of more severely ill patients.

The introduction of profound hypothermia (below 15°C) into cardiac surgery (Drew *et al.* 1959, Drew 1961) allowing circulatory arrest for 60 minutes without brain damage, offered possibilities in aneurysm surgery. Initially thoracotomy was necessary (Uihlein *et al.* 1960, MacCarty *et al.* 1964) but the simpler method of cannulating the femoral artery and vein for the extra corporal circulation was rapidly introduced (Woodhall *et al.* 1960, Patterson & Ray (1962, 1965). Good operative conditions were obtained for operating upon the aneurysm but persistent oozing following reversal of the heparinization made haemostasis very difficult. This prevented general acceptance of the technique. An ingenious and elegant technique was evolved by Small and his colleagues (Small & Stephenson 1966, Small *et al.* 1966). Hypothermia of about 30°C was induced, an intracardiac pacemaking electrode introduced through an arm vein so as to lodge at the apex of the right ventricle, and the craniotomy is performed. During the aneurysm manoeuvres, the blood pressure could be lowered, or the circulation arrested, by 'pacing' the heart at high speeds of stimulation, which lowers cardiac output or causes ventricular fibrillation.

The prevention and control of haemorrhage and the dissection of the difficult aneurysm can be greatly assisted by the temporary occlusion of appropriate arteries. Preceding the craniotomy in patients with an aneurysm arising adjacent to the base of the skull in which difficulties in dissecting the inferior border of the neck are anticipated, tapes may be placed around the common or internal carotid arteries in the neck. At the request of the surgeon the anaesthetist can safely occlude one or both carotid arteries by traction on the tape and can release them when the danger is passed. Total ischaemia of the aneurysm is not achieved because of persistent back flow from the circle of Willis; on occasion the vertebral arteries have been temporarily occluded as well as the carotid arteries (Lougheed et al. 1955). In principle it is better to isolate as small a zone of circulation as possible; this provides more certain control of bleeding and subjects a smaller area of brain to temporary ischaemia. In middle cerebral aneurysms, the stem of the artery can be occluded by a removable spring clip; in aneurysms of the posterior aspect of the internal carotid artery occlusion of the artery intracranially by a spring clip proximal to the aneurysm is very helpful. Special clips for temporary occlusion have been designed to minimise damage to the vessel wall. Pool (1961) recommended a bifrontal exposure for anterior communicating aneurysms, with a midline approach by separating the frontal lobes; haemorrhage was controlled by temporary occlusion of both anterior cerebral arteries. In Northfield's hands this method afforded less room than a unilateral approach with resection of brain and needed more and maintained retraction of the brain to identify and occlude the anterior cer-

ebral arteries. The duration of occlusion which can be sustained without ensuring damage is indicated by the following examples: simultaneous occlusion of both internal carotid arteries up to 5 minutes and singly up to 10 minutes; the ipsilateral anterior cerebral artery for approximately 20 minutes, during which time the contralateral carotid artery was closed for 7 minutes; the stem of the middle cerebral artery for 21 minutes. Blood pressure has been maintained at about 70–80 mmHg, and oesophageal temperature at 30°C. Pool (1961) has simultaneously occluded both anterior cerebral arteries close to the anterior communicating artery for 20 minutes, the blood pressure being 'maintained'. Even under hypothermia it is unwise to use hypotensive drugs with bilateral occlusion, for they reduce collateral circulation; this is particularly important in older patients who may have atheroma to an unknown degree.

The technique of choice in direct aneurysm surgery is occlusion of the neck of the aneurysm by a modern spring loaded clip. Dandy used a clip successfully for the first time in 1937 (Dandy 1944) but the major disadvantage of the early clips was that they had to be closed actively by the surgeon. Any involuntary movement could then result in tearing of the neck of the aneurysm. Ligation was therefore introduced (Sjoquist 1954). It was less likely to tear the neck, but the anatomy could on occasion make it difficult to pass the thread around the neck. Development of spring loaded clips overcame the disadvantages of the early clips, allowing controlled application to the neck as close as possible to its origin. Furthermore if the position of the clip is not satisfactory, it can be removed and repositioned.

Reinforcement of an aneurysm is necessary when, because of size, shape, situation, fragility or because arteries are part of the sac, its total exclusion or its obliteration is not allowable. The disadvantages of the method are the need to dissect out the sac and adjacent vessels and the risk of haemorrhage during the subsequent few days until the material used and the tissues to be covered become securely bonded, though with some plastics bonding is immediate. Numerous branches arise from the anterior cerebral and the anterior communicating arteries and from the trunk and first branch of the middle cerebral artery which are perforating and nourish important areas of the diencephalon. Their presence was established last century (for example Heubner 1872) but their surgical importance is liable to be overlooked; they are well depicted in the illustrations of Lazorthes (1961), Jain (1964), Kaplan (1965). The adoption of magnification in this branch of neurosurgery renders their identification easier.

Giant aneurysms can pose special problems. In addition to the use of hypotension, hypothermia and temporary clips on the parent vessel it may be necessary to open the aneurysm and remove adherent blood clot in order to apply the clip to the neck satisfactorily. If there is a possibility that a major vessel will have to be sacrificed intracranially during the procedure an extra-cranial–intracranial arterial anastomotic bypass carried out a few weeks before the aneurysm surgery may reduce the risk of postoperative ischaemic deficits. However, in addition to the other complications described after anastomotic procedures, reflow into giant aneurysms (Robbins et al. 1984), the de novo formation of an aneurysm on the recipient cortical artery (Lantos et al. 1984), and the rupture of a previously unruptured aneurysm (Scott et al. 1972) have all been described following bypass operations.

Reinforcement was introduced by Dott (1933) who surrounded an aneurysm with muscle and McConnell (1937) obliterated an aneurysm by opening it and implanting muscle. Muscle is still popular and has the advantage that it is always readily available, is sterile, and produces no unwelcome reactions. Its disadvantage is that when the sac lies within the subarachnoid space the muscle is liable to be floated out of position by the cerebrospinal fluid. For many years Northfield used thin wisps of cotton wool which could be easily draped and interlocked around the sac and its accompanying arteries to form a cocoon (Northfield 1952). Cotton gauze is pre-ferred by other surgeons. Dutton (1956, 1959) introduced the method of investing the sac with methyl-methacrylate and Selverstone (1962) has had good results using a two-coat adherent plastic. Gelatine sponge (gelfoam) alone is sometimes used but since this useful artifical haemostatic agent is employed in neurosurgery on the grounds of its eventual absorption with little residual fibrous reaction, it is unsuitable for reinforcement. The success of reinforcement depends on the production of a brisk fibroblastic reaction in and around the wall of the sac, in the case of muscle and of cotton, or on the support given by the plastic covering.

Because of the technical difficulties and high morbidity and mortality during the early years of operating on aneursyms arising from the anterior communicating artery or its vicinity, Logue (1956) practised in these cases proximal occlusion of one anterior cerebral artery. The operation is contraindicated if angiography shows that both anterior cerebral arteries fill from only one carotid artery, which occurred in 7% of his cases (Logue 1964): the side chosen for occlusion is that which appears more responsible for filling the sac. The Sylvian fissure on that side is opened, the internal carotid artery is identified and a clip applied to the anterior cerebral artery close to its origin; the dissection is taken no further so that the adhesions and blood around the aneurysm and the perforating branches are undisturbed. Circulation through the medial (distal) portion of the artery is maintained through the median anastomotic channel and the effectiveness of preventing further rupture depends upon the lowering of the local intra-arterial pressure, upon the reduction of the pulsewave and probably also on the diversion of the axis of flow in the vicinity of the aneurysm. Improved techniques have resulted in this operation being virtually abandoned in favour of direct clipping of these aneurysms. Some aneurysms arising from a vertebral artery, because of their size, shape or situation can only be treated by proximal occlusion. The subject is dealt with later.

## Carotid ligation

In an interesting account of the history of ligation of a carotid artery, Wood (1857) considered that the pioneers in this field were Warner in 1775, Hebenstreit in 1793 and Abernethy in 1798, though there is some doubt about the dates; in all cases the indication was haemorrhage due to injury. Astley Cooper, a contemporary of Abernethy, attended Hunter's lectures and greatly respected him (Symonds 1922). From him, Cooper (Brock 1940–41) learnt of proximal ligation for popliteal aneurysm and applied this method to carotid aneurysms in the neck; the first patient died of sepsis, the second was cured (Cooper 1809). Travers (1811) ligated the common carotid artery for 'pulsating exophthalmos' presumably due to caroticocavernous fistula and Beadles (1907) stated that Horsley performed the operation in 1902 for an aneurysm in the middle cranial fossa which had been identified at an exploratory craniotomy. Carotid ligation became a relatively common operation, largely for the arrest of haemorrhage from ulcerating malignant growths of the face and the base of skull and from trauma, but also as a speculative treatment of epilepsy, neuralgia and various nervous ailments. It was gradually adopted in the treatment of saccular aneurysms following their recognition as a cause of subarachnoid haemorrhage and of paralytic neighbourhood signs. A landmark in the history of carotid ligation was the notable contribution by Schorstein (1940).

Jefferson (1938) had pointed out that new statistics were needed to assess the risk of carotid ligation for intracranial aneurysm; this led Schorstein to review the subject and he analysed 60 cases, the first large series. The mortality was 13% and neurological complications occurred in 13%; mortality and morbidity were both higher in aneurysms which had bled than in the others. From the literature he showed that the mortality of carotid ligation for traumatic haemorrhage was about 50% and for bleeding from malignant disease 35% or more. Schorstein extracted from the literature a series of 45 cases in which the operation had been performed for epilepsy and other nonhaemorrhagic lesions; these formed a control group, in which the mortality was only 2%. Schorstein arrived at important conclusions which have stood the test of time; the risks of this operation depend upon the state of the cerebral circulation at the time of the operation. It may be impaired by systemic causes, hypovolaemia from haemorrhage shock and dehydration, anaemia, debilitation and low blood pressure; it may be impaired by intracranial causes, raised intracranial pressure, local interference with blood vessels by haemorrhage or by a large aneurysm acting as a tumour and, we may add in the light of later experience, by atheromatous narrowing of cerebral arteries.

The great importance of the two factors which Schorstein emphasized, the state of the cerebral circulation and the state of the systemic circulation in determining ischaemic complications is now fully accepted and recent statistics have amply confirmed the view that hemiplegia is more likely to develop in those patients who have not recovered from the effects of the subarachnoid haemorrhage. Assuming that the systemic and cerebral circulations are healthy, ischaemia of the brain after carotid occlusion must be due either to an inadequate redistribution of blood flow in the brain due to defective collateral circulation through the circle of Willis and through the cortical anastomoses, or to obstruction of major cerebral arteries by thrombosis or by embolism, arising at the site of ligation or from the aneurysm. Failure of the collateral circulation is responsible for the hemiplegia which develops immediately or shortly after ligation; in some patients the collateral flow is marginal and proves inadequate when they first sit up, for a transient hemiparesis may develop which rapidly recovers if they promptly lie down again. This susceptibility to posture soon passes. Recognition of the overriding importance of the collateral circulation has been the stimulus for much research which is considered below. How frequently thrombosis and embolism are the cause of cerebral infarction after carotid ligation is debatable. An opinion is

often expressed that it is possible to distinguish
two groups of cases, those in which the hemiplegia develops early and those in which it is
delayed and that the latter group is determined
by organic obstruction of the cerebral arteries.
This is an erroneous opinion, for no such distinction can be made; the complications may
arise at any moment during the several days
following the act of ligation. The figures obtained
by the Cooperative Study (VIII part I) of the time
elapsing between occlusion to onset of ischaemia
describe a smooth curve which reaches a peak
by the end of 24 hours and then falls rapidly so
that approximately 84% occur within 3 days.
Post-mortem evidence of organic obstruction of
cerebral arteries is forthcoming, but it is rare.
The Co-operative Study (VIII part I) reported that
autopsy in 35 cases of fatal cerebral ischaemia
revealed thrombus extending into the circle of
Willis in only 2. Cases have been reported of
thrombosis spreading from the aneurysm into
adjacent arteries. It has been suggested that
embolism arises from fragments of clot detached
at the bifurcation of the common carotid artery
by reflux blood flow from the external to the
internal branch. The evidence for reversal of flow
in the external carotid artery in some patients is
examined later. That it may cause embolism is
unlikely since hemiplegia less frequently follows
ligation of the common than of the internal
carotid artery. Rogers (1949) believed that
emboli were thrown off from the clot above a
ligature in continuity by the transmitted impulse
of the pulse pressure; he practised division of the
artery but this does not avoid the complication.
One aspect of the problem which has received
little or no attention is the extent to which atheroma of the cerebral arteries may predispose
to postligation ischaemic damage. Battacharji
et al. (1967) have made important and detailed
observations on the incidence of atheromatous narrowing of cerebral arteries which
they consider may play an important role in
the infarction seen with stenosis of the carotid
and vertebral arteries. The middle cerebral
artery was most affected by atheromatous
narrowing, its territory the most frequent

site of infarction; postligation ischaemial lesions
seem to select this area.

An adequate blood flow in the ipsilateral hemisphere after carotid occlusion depends upon the
maintenance of a sufficient blood pressure in the
affected segment of the circle of Willis. It will be
derived 'normally' from flow through the
anterior and posterior communicating arteries
and through cortical anastomoses which link
the posterior cerebral artery and the middle and
anterior cerebral arteries. Anatomical variations
in the circle must clearly play an important part
in determining the effect of occlusion. A narrow
anterior communicating artery (its absence is
exceptionally rare), hypoplastic ipsilateral
anterior cerebral or posterior communicating
arteries and a posterior cerebral artery taking its
origin from the occluded carotid (the primitive
arrangement) will prevent a sufficient redistribution of blood flow. In addition, with the
primitive origin of the posterior cerebral artery,
the cortical anastomoses can play no part for
they are within the affected carotid field. Potter
(1959) offers convincing arguments that these
anastomoses take an important share of the load.
Diverse tests have been evolved in order to
predict whether permanent occlusion of a carotid
artery will cause ischaemic damage. They will
be described and their value assessed.

**Preligation tests**

1   Matas (1911) focused attention on the need
for a test of collateral circulation. The appropriate common carotid artery is compressed
digitally in the neck for 10 minutes, during
which time the patient is observed and tested
for signs of cerebral ischaemia which include
drowsiness, mental confusion, dysphasia and
hemiparesis. In practice the procedure is
uncomfortable for the patient, may stimulate the
carotid sinus reflex causing bradycardia and a
fall in blood pressure which invalidates the test
and it is difficult to be certain that the digital
occlusion is complete. Hamby (1952) recommended that during compression the tem-

poral artery should be palpated to confirm the absence of its pulsation. The Matas test has proved unreliable.

2   A more accurate method is to test toleration of occlusion as the first step in the definitive operation of ligation. The artery is exposed under local anaesthesia and under direct vision it is occluded by a clamp whose jaws are protected by rubber and closed only sufficiently to terminate blood flow. The temporary occlusion is maintained for 30 minutes and ligation carried out if there have been no neurological effects. It is usual to infiltrate the sheath of the artery with a local anaesthetic in order to block any carotid sinus stimuli. This test reveals only those patients whose circulation is immediately intolerant of the loss of blood flow from one carotid and these constitute about 20% (Report of the Cooperative Study VIII pat 1); the test is of no help in the other 80%. The Matas test is employed as a routine in some clinics prior to the angiographic investigation of a patient with subarachnoid haemorrhage (McKissock & Walsh 1956). It is debatable whether this is a harmless procedure in patients who may already have sustained ischaemic brain damage.

3   It was hoped that the electroencephalograph (EEG) would be helpful. Brain anaemia causes slowing of the cortical rhythms so that theta and delta activity dominate the record, and EEG monitoring has been found helpful in cardiac surgery. But as an index of toleration of carotid ligation the EEG is unreliable. Potter and Taylor (1955) used it in 34 cases and found that there was no firm correlation between the record and the clinical status and that it did not predict delayed hemiparesis. Nevertheless, the method deserves further investigation; if the EEG linked with an automatic analysis were recorded continuously for several days after occlusion a constant pattern might be found to precede the onset of delayed hemiparesis which could be used to activate an alarm system.

4   Angiography demonstrates the anatomy of the circle of Willis and thereby informs the surgeon of the presence of those important variations which militate against uneventful carotid occlusion. Cross circulation studies provide visual proof of redistribution of blood. Sedzimir (1959) applied the test as a routine on 712 patients who were investigable by angiography for various reasons. In approximately 70% the collateral circulation filled the contralateral anterior and middle cerebral arteries, in 24% it filled only the contralateral anterior cerebral, in 6% it was absent, there being no flow across the middle line. The proportions in patients with vascular lesions and in those under and those over the age of 49 years were very similar. In a number of cases in which collateral circulation was poor or absent, the test was repeated some days later; in only a few did the second test yield a different and better result. These were restricted to the group of vascular lesions and constituted 4%. Carotid ligation is clearly contraindicated when cross circulation is absent; conversely if it irrigates the contralateral middle cerebral branches ischaemic complications are less likely, though experience shows that they may still happen (Harris & Udvarhelyi 1957, Wright & Sweet 1965).

5   Measurements of the intracarotid blood pressure, introduced by Sweet and Bennett (1948) provide a more scientific method of determining the likely effects of occlusion. A catheter is passed distally into each internal carotid artery and connected with an electromanometer and a chart recorder. Sweet and Bennett noted that the blood pressure within the internal carotid artery was reduced on an average to 50% of its original value (extremes were 70% and 30%) when the artery was occluded and the pulse pressure to about 25%. By altering the sites of compression they showed that if the common carotid were closed, in some cases there might be a flow from external to internal carotid and in others from internal to external. In later papers Sweet and his colleagues (Sweet et al. 1950, Bakay & Sweet 1952, 1953) have given an account of further observations. During 30 minutes of carotid occlusion spontaneous fluctuations of pressure occurred in either direction; such fluctuations might be the clue to delayed hemiparesis and in this connection Strobos and Mount (1953) drew

attention to the fall in the systemic blood pressure which may accompany carotid ligation. Pressures were measured within branches of the major cerebral vessels down to a diameter of 0.4 mm; the percentage fall in these small vessels was of the same order as that in the internal carotid artery. As a result of the observations of Sweet and those of others, opinion formed that a fall in the carotid pressure to 50% was safe, but that pressures lower than this were potentially dangerous. Sweet has reviewed his experiences (Wright & Sweet 1965). No sequelae followed occlusion in patients with a residual intracarotid pressure of over 88 mmHg or at least 66% of the original pressure, while nearly one-half of those with residual pressures of 40 mmHg or less, or with reduction to 33% of the original pressure were intolerant of occlusion.

6   Inert tracer clearance tests for determining cerebral blood flow. Kety and Schmidt (1945) devised the nitrous oxide method of measuring cerebral blood flow; this method is accurate but time-consuming and cumbersome. The elaboration of radioactive isotopes has led to the development of more rapid methods (Lassen & Ingvar 1961) which have been adapted to the problem under discussion. Jennett et al. (1966) used [133]Xenon injected into the internal carotid artery and determined cerebral blood flow by extracranial scanning of the washout curve of radioactivity clearing from the brain. As [133] Xenon is rapidly eliminated through the lungs repeated estimations at short intervals are permissible. Miller et al. (1977) were able to outline criteria for safe carotid ligation. If the cerebral blood flow was greater than 40 ml/min/100 grams during temporary clamping, ligation was safe irrespective of the change from the control bloodflow value, but if it was less than 20 ml it was always unsafe. If the blood flow during temporary carotid occlusion lay between these two values, ligation was safe provided that the flow reduction from the control value was less than 25%. If the drop was between 25 and 35% ligation was only safe in normotensive patients in whom the back pressure in the proximally occluded internal carotid artery

exceeded 60 mmHg. The test is the most promising indication available for predicting which patient will tolerate permanent carotid ligation.

### Methods of occlusion

There is no unanimity of opinion as to whether the internal or the common carotid artery should be ligated, although the great majority of ligations are of the common (Report of the Co-operative Study VIII part 1, table 159). For the most part surgeons choose the common carotid artery because they believe that it is safer and the finding of the Cooperative Study (VIII part 1) confirm this belief; others choose this vessel so that subsequent intra-arterial pressure studies can be performed on the internal carotid artery which usually remains patent (Odom & Tindall 1968). Intra-arterial pressure readings and the use of an electromagnetic flow meter (Hardesty et al. 1961) have shown that in some patients occlusion of the common carotid artery is followed by a reversal of flow in the internal carotid artery from the brain into the external carotid artery; this can provide a 'steal' phenomenon that may account for delayed hemiparesis in some instances. The identification of a reversed flow in the internal carotid would be an indication for preferring that artery for occlusion rather than the common. Conversely in some patients there is an appreciable collateral flow into the internal carotid from the external, which diminishes the risk of ischaemia but militates against the treatment of the aneurysm; in these there is logic in ligating the internal (or internal) carotid artery as a second stage, when redistribution of blood flow has stabilized.

The artery may be occluded by a ligature and various materials have been used; the choice is unimportant provided that the ligature is not absorbable, it is coarse enough not to cut the artery and that it accepts a knot without slipping. Heavy gauge tantalum clips have been used but they have been known to open as a result of the constant thud of the pulsating artery. It is the practice of some surgeons to apply progressive closure of the lumen of the artery over the course of several days, to lessen the risk of ischaemia by encouraging the development of collateral circulation and to avoid the sudden disturbances of haemodynamics brought about by abrupt closure. Cerebral blood flow studies suggest however that there is no change in global flow until the diameter of the carotid artery has been reduced by 90%. The principle of progressive closure was put forward by Halstead (1909) who used aluminium bands around the artery applied with a special instrument. Special clamps have now been evolved, the jaws of which can be adjusted by a screw mechanism actuated by a slender handle which can protrude from the wound or is detachable. Those who take intra-carotid pressure readings determine the degree of approximation of the jaws necessary to lower the pressure by one half, then note the number of turns of the handle needed to occlude the artery completely; the jaws are readjusted to provide the 50% drop in pressure and the wound closed. If a 50% reduction of pressure is not tolerated the jaws are opened to the tolerable degree. The clamp is tightened by small increments each day until closure is complete, or until it is clear that only partial closure is possible and after several days of further observation the handle of the instrument is detached; the jaws remain *in situ*. Adjustable clamps have the advantage that they can be opened by the protruding handle immediately ischaemic symptoms appear; for this reason they are regularly used by some surgeons for abrupt closure of the artery; after an interval of observation the wound is reopened, the artery ligated proximal to the clamp which is then removed. Murphy (1965) believes that if delayed hemiparesis occurs after total occlusion and lumbar puncture shows no fresh haemorrhage, the artery should be exposed to determine whether it is thrombosed, in which case the thrombus should be removed so as to avoid the risk of embolism.

An ingenious and entirely different method of occluding the carotid artery was devised by Gibbs (1965a). The jaws of a specially constructed instrument were applied across the artery; by rotating one jaw about the other, an S-shaped loop was created in the long axis of the artery; sufficient rotation effectively blocked the artery. The handle of the instrument projected from the closed wound and adjustments could be made rapidly to open the loop in case of hemiplegia, or gradually to close it further. After several days of complete obstruction, if there were no hemological sequelae the loop was tightened then; after a further 4–6 days, the instrument was dismantled and removed. The disadvantages of this method appear to be excessive damage to the artery which can be avoided with experience, and occasional recanalization. In another paper illustrating the angiographic changes in treated aneurysms Gibbs (1965b) drew attention to the importance of the size of the posterior communicating artery; in carotid aneurysms arising at that point, a large communicating artery militates against success resulting from carotid occlusion because of the considerable blood flow from the vertebral system.

There has been some scepticism as to whether the removal of the ligature or the opening of a clamp serves any purpose once hemiparesis has developed; whether the late result would have been the same whether or not occlusion were relieved. From individual cases reported in the literature it seems that time is of paramount importance; if less than 5 minutes elapses between onset of ischaemic signs and relieving occlusion the result may be good, but when longer times elapse recovery of function follows a slow course. The Cooperative Study (VIII part 1) confirms some value; the neurological deficit persisted in 67% of patients with occluded artery and in 44% of those with release of occlusion. When considering the release of occlusion in order to favour recovery one must bear in mind the third possibility, that recovery is poor and the aneurysm still remains unprotected; there is much to recommend as a criterion for guidance, that the occlusion is not released unless it can be done within the first 5 minutes of unequivocal cerebral ischaemia.

The general advantages and disadvantages of carotid ligation which guide the choice of operation have already been given. To particularize, this operation is followed by a successful result most frequently in aneurysms arising from the internal carotid artery: successful as judged by mortality rate and by protection against recurrence of early bleeding (from the same aneurysm). The operation is less effective for anterior communicating and for middle cerebral aneurysms, for the incidence of permanent ischaemic damage is higher (Wright & Sweet 1965) and protection against further haemorrhage less effective (Odom & Tindall 1968), Report of the Cooperative Study VIII part 1).

**Other techniques**

Though direct clipping is the method of choice this is not possible with all aneurysms and in particular those arising within the cavernous sinuses, the paraclinoid aneurysms and some vertebrobasilar aneurysms. Detachable balloons both to occlude the aneurysm definitely or to temporarily occlude the carotid or vertebral artery as a test of the patient's ability to withstand ligation have been used successfully. If the patient cannot tolerate carotid ligation, an extracranial–intracranial arterial bypass between the superficial temporal artery and a suitable branch of the middle cerebral artery may be indicated prior to ligation of the internal carotid artery (Heros et al. 1983).

## Results of operation

Perusal of the literature discloses an operative mortality for the direct attack upon ruptured aneurysms ranging from 3% to 50%. The Cooperative Study (VIII part 2 1966) provided 979 patients treated in this way and 31% died; the introduction of the microscope, together with improved clips and neuroanaesthesia has resulted in a considerable improvement (Symon 1982, Koos & Perneczky 1982) in mortality figures. The more recent Cooperative figures (Adams et al. 1981) show 14% dead at 90 days

following direct surgery and 6% following carotid ligation. Similar results are reported in a large French series (Jomin et al. 1984). The surgical outcome remains dependent upon the preoperative grading (Koos & Perneczky 1982), the general medical condition of the patient and in particular, the cardiovascular state including hypertension and the patient's age (Fortuny et al. 1980). Martindale and Garfield (1978) found that very few patients aged 60 years or over had a favourable outcome, though this has been vigorously disputed by others.

It is not possible to ascertain accurately the degree of protection provided by the various methods of dealing directly with the aneurysm, but it is probably very high. Crompton (1966a) reported on a number of specimens obtained at necropsy and was impressed by the degree of fibrosis induced in the wall of the aneurysm by reinforcement with cotton. Moreover, recurrence of subarachnoid haemorrhage may not necessarily be from the same aneurysm; indeed the accumulating observations on aetiology suggest that haemorrhage recurring several years after a technically successful operation is at least as likely to be due to a fresh aneurysm as to the former one.

Logue (1959) reported an operative mortality of 20% following proximal clipping of the anterior cerebral artery in 87 patients. As with other operations for recently ruptured aneurysms, the fatalities are more frequent in ill patients than in those clinically recovered from the effects of haemorrhage. Amongst the 18 deaths, recurrent haemorrhage was the cause in 6, but in 2 of these the operation was incomplete; there were no late recurrences of haemorrhage.

Relatively few series have been reported devoted solely to the results of surgery for aneurysms occurring in the vertebrobasilar territory. It is only in recent years that the full possibilities of surgery have been explored. The list opposite summarizes some of these results.

Those arising from the basilar artery and particularly from its rostral end are the most difficult. The results of direct attack on these aneurysms have improved with the development of the sub-

| Reference | Number of patients | Number of deaths |
|---|---|---|
| Co-operative Study III part 2 | 31 | 13 |
| Höök et al. (1963) | 12 | 0 |
| Logue (1964) | 12 | 2 |
| Drake (1961, 1965, 1968) | 31 | 7 |
| Jamieson (1964, 1968) | 28 | 12 |
| Yasargil et al. (1976) | 38 | 3 |
| Sugita et al. (1979) | 32 | 2 |

temporal (Drake 1968) the pterional (Yasargil et al. 1976) and the transsylvian (Sugita et al. 1979) microsurgical approaches. The latter two groups of authors reported mortality rates of 6–7%, poor results in a further 7 and 3% respectively and good results in 65% and 88% respectively.

### Vertebrobasilar and carotid occlusion

The risk of proximal vertebral artery occlusion in cases of aneurysm is still undetermined and the situation now may be compared with that of carotid occlusion in 1938 when Jefferson pointed out the need for fresh statistics. There is information concerning ligation of the vertebral artery in the neck for traumatic aneurysms and for arteriovenous fistulae in its extracranial course (Elkin & Harris 1946, Killian 1950, Jefferson et al. 1956). Occasional reports in the literature concern the imperative need to clip the artery in the course of the removal of a posterior fossa neoplasm on account of haemorrhage or because the tumour involved the artery, usually with fatal brain stem ischaemia. Alexander is said to have 'tied the vertebral arteries, sometimes both at one sitting, thirty six times with no more than three deaths' in a mistaken notion that it would cure epilepsy (Jefferson et al. 1956). In arteriovenous fistulae and angiomatous malformations there is a dilatation of the blood vessels in the territories of the vessels concerned and of their collaterals, anatomical and haemo-

dynamic changes which reduce the risks of ischaemia below that to be expected in the normal. In the presence of tumours, including large aneurysms, whether they have ruptured or not, and particularly when these are situated in the posterior fossa which is such a small compartment, the situation is reversed, for the blood supply to the brain stem is already embarrassed by compression and its further impairment by occluding a major artery is more than likely to lead to ischaemia. Details have been found of 24 examples of vertebral occlusion for aneurysm, fatal in 7 cases (Dandy 1944, Hamilton & Falconer 1959, Paulson et al. 1959, Poppen 1959, Logue 1964, Report of the Cooperative Study VIII part 2). In one patient death was due to recurrent haemorrhage, in the others it appears to have been the direct result of occlusion. In the survivors the records reveal little or no evidence of ischaemia sequelae. If vertebral artery occlusion is under consideration, it is imperative to determine that the opposite artery is of normal size. Krayenbühl and Yaṣargil (1957) state that in 11% per cent of their angiographic studies one vertebral artery was markedly hypoplastic and slightly so in a much higher proportion. In the course of their studies of intravascular pressures, Wright and Sweet (1963) found that the pressure in the vertebral artery was usually unaffected by proximal occlusion, but partial occlusion of its fellow at the same time caused an appreciable drop. It should be mentioned here that this operation was performed for an angiomatous malformation in the posterior fossa which had bled repeatedly; the operation proved successful in preventing further haemorrhage during a follow-up of 6 years.

In the case of inoperable vertebrobasilar aneurysms and in particular the giant ones, occlusion of both vertebral arteries or the basilar artery has been advocated to promote thrombosis with the lumen of the aneurysm. Pelz et al. (1984) reviewed 71 cases and found that the angiographic morphology of the posterior communicating arteries was the most important predictive indicator as to whether the patient would tolerate occlusion of the vertebrobasilar system.

Overall the procedure resulted in an excellent or good outcome in 66% of cases. Drake (1975) also reported favourable results from both unilateral and bilateral vertebral occlusion for large vertebrobasilar aneurysms but found that occlusion of the basilar artery was dangerous even though it was effective in producing thrombosis within the aneurysm. He felt that basilar occlusion should only be carried out after testing under local anaesthetic. However if the basilar artery filled spontaneously from the carotid tree the use of a general anaesthetic could be considered. When ligating the vertebral artery, the site of occlusion should ideally be distal to the origin of the posterior inferior cerebellar artery. Ligation proximal to this artery can lead to unacceptably high morbidity.

Setting aside the ischaemic complications of carotid ligation which have already been considered, what degree of protection can be achieved by this method of treating aneurysms? Jefferson (1952) had a large experience; in 142 cases there was a mortality of 8% within the first 6 weeks and 6% in the survivors after this time (a total of 20 patients); in 8 patients the same aneurysm bled again, but in only 2 did this occur after the first month. Johnson (1952) analysed the cases further and pointed out that 12 deaths occurred in 29 patients whose carotid was ligated a few hours after haemorrhage, underlining the greater risk of operating shortly after haemorrhage and common to all methods. Jefferson's summing up is fully justified: 'the method is one that has, to put it soberly, considerable merit'. The Cooperative Study (VIII part 1) makes the valuable distinction between carotid ligation for ruptured and for unruptured aneurysms. In the former group of 667 cases the mortality was 23%, ranging from 6% to 90% according to the clinical state of the patient. In the group of unruptured aneurysms (125) mortality was only 6%. Winn et al. (1977) following up patients 8 years after carotid ligation found that once 6 months had elapsed the late rehaemorrhage rate was no different from patients who had been treated conservatively, i.e. non surgically.

**Functional outcome after surgery**

What is the functional capacity of those patients who survive haemorrhage from an aneurysm? Fortuny and Prieto-Valiente (1981) in a detailed study of patients who were graded I to III pre-operatively found that overall 62% were neurologically intact, 83% were totally independent, 64% returned to their social activities but only 51% returned to the same work. However though 64% had no psychiatric disability only 40% subjectively felt as well as they had prior to the onset of the illness. The factors which lead to morbidity were vasospasm, increasing age, hypertension and a less good clinical pre-operative grade. The higher percentage of residual neurological deficits in patients with left sided aneurysms was due to a high incidence of dysphasic disorders in this group. The Report of the Co-operative Study (1974) showed the highest incidence of hemiparesis and dysphasia follows surgery for internal carotid aneurysms with a lower incidence for middle cerebral and anterior cerebral group ones. Confusion and dementia however were much more common in the anterior cerebral group and very unusual in the middle cerebral aneurysm. Sengupta et al. (1975) analysing the results of direct anterior communicating artery aneurysm surgery using psychometric measures found that though there were no deficits in intellectual ability, there were personality changes which manifested themselves as loss of interest, initiative and drive. They found that these difficulties were worse in those with a low pre-operative grade and deduced therefore that in the majority of cases these problems were the result of the initial damage inflicted by the haemorrhage. In contrast Ljunggren et al. (1983) considering patients in grades I–III (Hunt–Hess) could not attribute more than 17% of all unfavourable results including death to the initial haemorrhage. The latter authors agreed with Fortuny and Prieto-Valiente (1981) that the timing of surgery did not influence the outcome. After carotid ligation in addition to the continuing low risk of late rehaemorrhage Winn et al. (1977) found that, compared with a conservatively treated group of patients, there was an increased incidence of hypertension. Rossi *et al.* (1981) reported that, over an average follow up period of over 8 years, 10% of patients undergoing a common carotid ligation suffered transient ischaemic attacks and 10% developed monocular blindness. In those patients undergoing internal carotid artery ligation one sixth developed transient ischaemic attacks, two thirds of whom later experienced completed strokes, over an average follow up period of 12 years. A further 5% of those undergoing internal carotid artery ligation had a stroke in the contralateral cerebral hemisphere.

### Hydrocephalus

In the chapter on hydrocephalus attention is drawn to leptomeningeal obstruction, by exudate at first and by fibrosis later, which follows subarachnoid diffusion of blood. A mild degree of hydrocephalus is commonplace after subarachnoid haemorrhage from an aneurysm and usually causes little or no clinical disturbance. Occasionally the degree of obstruction is severe, persistent and demands investigation and treatment. It is particularly prone to complicate the recovery from otherwise successful operations on aneurysms in the posterior fossa. The reason may be that the operative manoeuvres increase the degree of meningeal adhesions in an area where the pathways for cerebrospinal fluid are normally relatively restricted. Acute hydrocephalus is associated with increased mortality from cerebral infarction. This can often be explained by hyponatraemia and hypovolaemia, but not by failure to institute surgical drainage of the ventricular system (Van Gijn *et al.* 1985).

## Incidental aneurysms

Since the time of Bramwell (1866) it has been usual and useful to separate aneurysms into two clinical groups, those that cause symptoms by bleeding and those whose symptoms arise from pressure upon neighbouring structures, the 'paralytic' group. As a result of angiography, a third group has emerged, small but important; it comprises those aneurysms which are detected by angiography undertaken for some other reason and which are clearly not the source of the patient's illness. They are important because, in view of their potential gravity, the question will arise whether an 'insurance' operation should be recommended. In the Cooperative Study (V part 2) 2.6% of all the aneurysms were incidental findings and it is argued that the figure is probably nearer 8%. About two thirds were disclosed by angiography, the rest by autopsy; multiple aneurysms one of which had ruptured were excluded. The site, age and sex distribution are similar to those which rupture, but the majority of these sacs are smaller being less than 6 mm in diameter. Little information is available as to prognosis but deductions may be justifiably drawn from the natural history of 165 aneurysms which had not ruptured but which gave rise to symptoms; few of these sacs were less than 7 mm in diameter. In this group 34 were not treated and of these 9 (26%) died of haemorrhage. Presented with the case of an aneurysm found incidentally and aside from such factors as its site, the age and fitness of the patient, the decision will rest largely upon size. Kassell and Torner (1983a) analysed more recent Cooperative data and suggested that aneurysms of under 1 cm in diameter are hazardous, particularly if over 5 mm. They suggest that all aneurysms over this size should be clipped even if a second craniotomy at a later date is required to gain access to the unruptured aneurysm. If less than 5 mm they recommend repeat angiography at one or two year intervals. Mount and Brisman (1974) found that 10% of unruptured aneurysms haemorrhage within an average follow-up period of 5 years. Heiskanen (1981) found a lower risk of haemorrhage; 11.5% during 10 years follow-up with the fatal risk being almost 7% but 6 further patients suffered recurrent haemorrhage more than 10 years after diagnosis and half of them died. This brought the risk of death from haemorrhage over an average follow-up period of 16 years to over 11%. He therefore advocates surgery for unruptured aneurysms. Winn *et al.* (1983) found a similar rate (1% per annum) of rupture in incidental aneurysms but that hypertension increased the risk. Wirth *et al.* (1983) reported 107 patients with incidental aneurysms operated upon with no mortality and 6.5% morbidity. Further information is required concerning the risks of haemorrhage from an unruptured aneurysm, paticularly as the introduction of digital subtraction angiography may increase the frequency with which the problem is encountered.

## Aneurysms causing symptoms by local compression

Like tumours, aneurysms of the paralytic group cause well defined syndromes determined by their anatomical situation. The most important are those arising from the internal carotid artery within the cavernous sinus (infraclinoid), those above this level (supraclinoid) which commonly implicate the optic pathway in the vicinity of the chiasm and those from its posterior aspect which may compress the third cranial nerve. Aneurysms from the anterior cerebral artery may also affect vision, while others from this artery and from the middle cerebral artery if large enough may cause epilepsy or mental symptoms. Large basilar aneurysms cause brain stem symptoms. Saccular aneurysms which had not ruptured but were causing symptoms comprised 7% of the total examined by the Cooperative Study (V part 2).

### Intracavernous aneurysms

Intracavernous aneurysms (nonfistulous) formed only about 1% of the Cooperative Study, although Jefferson (1960) had a personal experience of 35 cases, which is likely to remain unrivalled. Our knowledge of the clinical evolution and the correlation between the morbid and the normal anatomy is largely due to his

acute observations (1938), though he names and gives credit to those who preceded him and in particular to Bartholow (1872). These aneurysms are characterized by the symptoms produced by pressure upon the structures within the cavernous sinus, facial pain at times of excruciating degree, and ocular palsy; this syndrome of the cavernous sinus produced also by other lesions is frequently named eponymously 'of Foix' (Foix 1922) but Jefferson points out that this commemoration is undeserved for earlier observers had fully described the clinical picture. Infraclinoid aneurysms which have not reached a size sufficient to cause pressure symptoms are occasionally encountered as incidental findings. At this stage they may rupture within the cavernous sinus, creating an arteriovenous fistula (*see* below). As the sac enlarges it obtains the support of the walls of the sinus and then rupture is very rare. In the Cooperative Study (V parts 1 and 2) 2 ruptured and caused subarachnoid haemorrhage as against 44 unruptured, of which 16 were incidental findings. An unexplained feature of these aneurysms commented on by all with experience is their curious predilection for females; in Jefferson's series of 36 patients 33 were females (Fig. 11.7).

The evolution of symptoms may be abrupt or spread over several weeks; the initial symptom is generally pain or at least discomfort in the trigeminal field, but sooner or later it is almost invariable and usually severe. It is distinguished from paroxysmal trigeminal neuralgia by its continuity and the objective evidence of impaired cutaneous sensibility. Ptosis and paralysis of the muscles of the eye accompany or soon follow the trigeminal symptoms. Often a total internal and external ophthalmoplegia develops, rarely the oculomotor, trochlear and abducens nerves are involved in isolation. The pupil may not be fully dilated although nonreactive and this is ascribed to the interruption of its sympathetic nerve supply. Jefferson distinguished three groups according to the situation of the aneurysm in the posterior, in the middle and in the anterior part of the sinus, the latter being the most usual. The distinction depends upon the extent of the

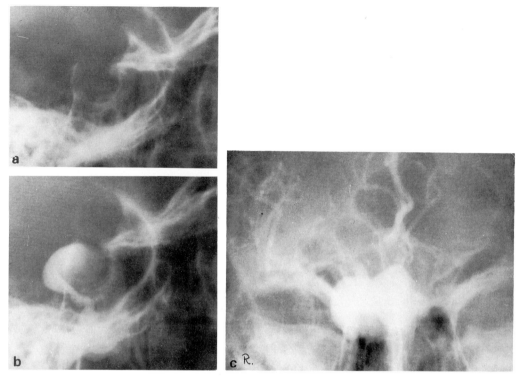

**Fig. 11.7.** Female aged 35 years: sudden left-sided frontoparietal headache and blurring of vision, followed by third left nerve palsy: no blood in CSF: visual fields full.
(a) Slight ballooning of sella turcica, anterior and posterior clinoid processes eroded.
(b,c) Right carotid subclinoid aneurysm within cavernous sinus, extending into the sella tutcica. Carotid ligation, recovery of palsy.

trigeminal sensory loss; the posterior situation will affect all divisions of the fifth nerve, the intermediate, the maxillary and ophthalmic, whilst the aneurysm placed well forward in the sinus will only compress the ophthalmic division. 'It is this anaesthetic accompaniment of an ocular muscle palsy which makes the diagnosis of an infraclinoid aneurysm a matter of the utmost nicety and precision.' This distinctive picture is occasionally lacking; Rischbieth and Bull (1958) found that in 4 of 23 cases pain was absent and the chief features were loss of vision, palsy of third and of sixth nerves respectively. Although the walls of the cavernous sinus protect the sac from rupture, they gradually give to the relentless impulse within it and thus the aneurysm may assume a large size. Pain may eventually be abolished by the overstretching and atrophy of nerve fibres, the sphenoid is partially eroded in a characteristic pattern (*see* below) and upward expansion may compress the optic nerve, causing atrophy and blindness (Meadows 1951). Deafness and tinnitus have been recorded, thought to be due to pressure upon the eustachian tube and Meadows noted a bruit in one patient. A slight degree of non-pulsatile proptosis is frequent but not the orbital congestion and protrusion seen in caroticocavernous fistula and thrombosis of the cavernous sinus. Encroachment medially into the pituitary fossa may give rise to depression of endocrine functions (*see* below). Infraclinoid aneurysms may undergo spontaneous thrombosis and cure, may become quiescent with persistent ophthalmoplegia but relatively little pain, or may rupture into the paranasal air sinuses and exceptionally into the subarachnoid space.

The differential diagnosis is mainly from malignant tumours invading this area, in particular those originating in the nasopharyngeal tissues and in the paranasal sinuses; pituitary adenoma (Jefferson's case 12 was later shown to be a pituitary adenoma: Jefferson 1955), meningioma, chordoma, schwannoma of the fifth and of the eighth nerves may at time cause uncertainty in clinical diagnosis. Inflammatory lesions of the orbital tissues by causing ocular paresis and local pain (the superior orbital fissure syndrome) may come to mind but the trigeminal pain is not severe, nor is there sensory loss.

Radiological investigation establishes the diagnosis with certainty. In a number of cases curvilinear calcification on plain X-ray of the skull is strong presumptive evidence of aneurysm, though the size and the situation of the arc may not precisely define the sac. The pattern of bone destruction was the most reliable evidence prior to angiography. Forward pulsation of the aneurysm or a displaced carotid siphon erodes the medial part of the great wing of the sphenoid; in particular it enlarges the superior orbital fissure and may destroy the slender strut of bone which supports the lesser wing and forms the inferolateral boundary of the optic foramen. Jefferson and Twining (Jefferson 1936) considered this to be pathognomonic of aneurysm. Rischbieth and Bull made a critical comparison of the radiological changes produced by infraclinoid aneurysms with those due to pituitary tumours, meningiomas, orbital tumours and chordoma and confirmed the value of this sign, though it is not peculiar to aneurysms. It is usually accompanied by asymmetrical erosion of the sella turcica and Rischbieth and Bull found the ipsilateral anterior clinoid process to be elevated and eroded in 20 of their 23 cases of infraclinoid aneurysm. The enlargement of the sella may mimic faithfully that due to a pituitary adenoma causing diagnostic difficulty. Computerized tomographic scanning may not resolve this problem. Angiography is the final step in diagnosis: unless there is some compelling contra-

indication it should be carried out on both sides, not only for preligation tests but to detect a similar lesion on the other side, which is not an infrequent occurrence. The sac may appear smaller than expected and present a bizarre shape due to mural clot.

The treatment is carotid ligation or intraluminal balloon occlusion. However, surgery may not be required or may be deferred in those patients in whom spontaneous cure or quiescence appears to have taken place. The chief indication is pain, which responds satisfactorily to operation; ptosis may improve but ophthalmoplegia to some extent persists. The incidence of postligation morbidity is low compared with that in supraclinoid aneurysms which have ruptured. In Jefferson's series 21 ligations were performed; there were no deaths and only 3 showed passing signs of ischaemia. In the Cooperative Study (VIII part 1) there was a mortality of 2.7% following carotid occlusion for unruptured aneurysm of the internal carotid artery in 111 patients; the site of the aneurysm is not defined in this group, nor the incidence of complications.

**Aneurysms compressing the optic pathways**

The close proximity of the anterior part of the circle of Willis to the optic nerves, chiasm and tracts renders their compression by an aneurysm arising from the component arteries almost inevitable if the sac instead of rupturing gradually enlarges. Those from the carotid artery impinge upon the lateral angle of the chiasm, or upon the optic nerve or commonly on both by the time help is sought. Their precise point of origin is rarely identifiable except at post-mortem and then rarely sought or recorded: it is notable that the smaller aneurysms arising at the origin of the ophthalmic artery, which usually manifest themselves by haemorrhage, rarely cause visual symptoms; only 1 in the series of 14 reported by Drake et al. (1968). In addition, the optic pathways are also at risk from those infraclinoid aneurysms which insinuate themselves medially into the sella turcica, whence they may expand upwards and mimic a pituitary adenoma. Aneurysms derived from the anterior cerebral artery usually compress the optic nerve and the chiasma from above, but may insinuate themselves under these structures and elevate them. Jefferson (1937, 1955) made 2 impressive contributions to the subject of aneurysmal compression of the optic pathways based on a personal experience of 30 examples and of 66 published records. Excluding those in which the precise origin of the aneurysm could not be determined or was not stated, there were 52 from the internal carotid artery and 20 from the anterior cerebral or communicating artery. An unusual cause for chiasmal compression is an aneurysm arising from the termination of the basilar artery. The optic tract or radiation may very rarely be compressed by an aneurysm from the middle cerebral, the posterior communicating and the posterior cerebral arteries.

The syndrome of chiasmal and optic nerve compression is fully described in Chapter 9 and careful analysis of the changes in the visual fields (provided they are not very advanced) will usually indicate the site of the compressing lesion. The features which may help to distinguish an aneurysm are the bizarre patterns of visual field loss which often develop, their fluctuation from time to time, the tempo of which may be quite abrupt in either direction; the frequent association with facial pain, usually ocular or periorbital. The differential diagnosis is from: anterior basal meningioma, usually slowly and relentlessly progressive, sometimes associated with anosmia, but rarely painful; pituitary adenoma, which because it is occasionally accompanied by ocular pain and trigeminal pain and because an aneurysm may cause endocrine failure, often provides the most difficult clinical problem; retrobulbar optic neuritis (Meadows 1951). It is the aneurysm arising from the anterior cerebral artery which is liable to evade detection, for visual failure may be very slow and other signs entirely absent; X-ray examination of the skull will show no abnormality but computerized tomographic scanning may show a mass which enhances if there is any residual patent lumen. Progressive visual failure 'of unknown cause' always requires the fullest radiological examination and is not complete without angiography. The problem of diagnosis is further aggravated by the fact that angiography is ocasionally negative, presumably as a result of partial thrombosis of the aneurysm (Klingler 1951) and that the aneurysm may fill by carotid injection on the side with better vision. Dementia has been reported in a sufficient proportion of large supraclinoid aneurysms to suggest that it is more than a coincidental finding. It is unlikely that size alone is responsible, and it may be that the sac interferes with the circulation through its parent vessels and thereby with the nourishment of extensive areas of the brain.

The treatment of the supraclinoid aneurysms compressing the optic pathways may present a major problem. Carotid ligation in the neck is likely to be the preference for those arising from the internal carotid artery provided collateral circulation is adequate and this may be imperilled by the very size of the sac if supraclinoid. Those from the anterior cerebral artery require a direct approach. Angiography may show that circulation across the midline would allow excision of the sac by clipping the parent artery either side, close to the sac so as not to sacrifice perforating branches.

### Compression of the oculomotor nerve

The morbid anatomy of paralysis of the third cranial nerve has been described earlier. Not only may it occur as a result of haemorrhage from an aneurysm, but it may be the only evidence of aneurysm. It is so well recognized as to be almost banal, but Jefferson (1947) found the subject of sufficient interest to warrant a contribution, which concerned 55 cases of isolated oculomotor palsy, in 15 of which there was no rupture. In 52 the aneurysm arose from the posterior aspect of the carotid artery, at or about the origin of the posterior communicating artery; in the others it sprang from the posterior end of the communicating artery. Aneurysms of the basilar artery may compress the third nerve, but not in isolation. The palsy takes several hours to a day or so to develop fully and consequently the patient may awaken with it. Although the ptosis is the obvious feature for the patient, Jefferson stated that in all his cases it was preceded by a brief period of diplopia or confused vision. Supraorbital pain is a frequent accompaniment, probably due to the pressure of the aneurysm on the tentorium, to the free edge or undersurface of which it is often adherent. Although spontaneous recovery is frequent, it is rarely complete for all the muscles concerned; elevation of the lid is usually adequate if not complete, but this may be a nuisance because of the diplopia from imperfect muscle balance. Botterell et al. (1962) made a useful study of the recovery from oculomotor palsy in 40 patients, of whom 4 received no surgical treatment, in 8 the carotid artery was ligated and in 28 the aneurysm was obliterated. The cases did not correspond precisely with Jefferson's because there were other cranial nerve palsies due to aneurysmal pressure, namely of the second, the fourth and the fifth. In each of the 8 patients treated by carotid occlusion recovery was incomplete. In the 22 patients surviving craniotomy for obliteration of the sac, recovery was partial in 14 and complete in 8; 6 of the latter operations took place within 10 days of the onset. Duration of recovery was usually 3 months, but it might continue for upwards of a year.

### Hypopituitarism

Pituitary failure may occasionally follow subarachnoid haemorrhage and the cause is probably hypothalamic damage from minute infarctions and haemorrhage (Tomlinson 1959, Crompton 1963). Similar lesions might affect the stalk of the gland. The manner in which large aneurysms may compress the optic nerves and chiasma was dealt with in an earlier paragraph. In a few of these cases compression affects the pituitary gland. Rarely the aneurysm arises from

the anterior cerebral artery and compresses the infundibulum; more commonly it arises from the intracavernous part of the internal carotid artery and expanding medially compresses the gland within the sella turcica. White (1964) reported 3 cases of his own and 33 from other sources, in which an aneurysm simulated a pituitary adenoma, on account of the visual field defects and the enlargement of the sella turcica. In approximately half of these cases there was clinical evidence of endocrine failure, but in only 5 was it of a pronounced degree. Van T'Hoff et al. (1961) described 3 examples of severe hypopituitarism due to aneurysm in which endocrine status was fully investigated. They draw attention to recorded examples not of impairment but of abnormal pituitary function, namely acromegaly and Cushing syndrome in association with aneurysm (see also Chapter 9). Seeing that either aneurysm or adenoma can at times give rise to visual field defects, ocular palsy, ophthalmic division pain and sensory loss, endocrine failure, enlargement of the sella, and subarachnoid haemorrhage (in the case of adenoma from spontaneous bleeding in its substance), it is not surprising that differential diagnosis may occasion great difficulty and can only be solved by angiography. Mistakes will be made and the lesson to be learnt is always to aspirate before incising a mass causing chiasmal compression.

### Optic nerve compression by the carotid artery

A rare cause of visual failure is compression of the optic nerve by an enlarged or diseased carotid artery. Bernheimer (1891) reported the autopsy findings on 2 patients who had not complained of disturbance of vision: the undersurface of the optic nerves was deeply notched by the ophthalmic arteries and the carotid arteries showed calcification and dilatation. Smith (1909) and Stopford (1917) described similar pressure effects which they had observed in anatomical specimens. Considering the close apposition of these structures, clinical records of visual disturbance are surprisingly few. Arteriosclerotic fusiform dilatation of the carotid artery has been reported and in some cases the compression may be exerted by a normal terminal portion of the artery which is hoisted up by the more proximally situation dilatation (Dandy 1944, Fig. 41). Meadows (1951) records compression of the optic tract causing an incongruous homonymous hemianopia. Ley (1950) and Mitts and McQueen (1965) have described in detail personal cases and have reviewed the literature. The duration of the history varies between months and many years and symptoms commence after the age of 30 years. Both eyes are usually affected, to an unequal degree and the visual field defects are irregular and asymmetrical although there is often a discernible pattern of altitudinal hemianopia; the loss of vision may be in the upper or the lower halves. Papilloedema has frequently been observed in the eye more recently affected, the other showing optic atrophy; this combination comprising a Foster Kennedy syndrome could give grounds for suspecting a meningioma. McLean and Ray (1947) report a case of optic atrophy in which operative exploration revealed rigid atheromatous carotid arteries, similar in description to that of Bernheimer, alluded to above. Periarteritis of the carotid artery was the cause of a cavernous sinus syndrome in a case described by Tolosa (1954), but the optic nerve was unaffected. The correct diagnosis will be clear if the angiogram reveals dilatation of the carotid artery, or irregularity of the lumen suggesting thickening of its walls; often only exploratory craniotomy will disclose the presence of optic nerve compression although the combination of optic atrophy without other evident cause and calcification of the carotid arteries should arouse suspicions. The only treatment which may improve or preserve vision is removal of the roof of the optic canal, with the object of allowing the optic nerve to drift away from the artery, but the results are disappointing. It is likely that in many cases the nerve has suffered irretrievable damage, by pressure atrophy (Bernheimer's histological preparations show severe attenuation of the nerve) or by involvement of the optic nerve arteries in scler-otic degeneration or periarteritis. Further information is given by Duke-Elder (1949).

## Caroticocavernous fistula

A fistulous communication between the internal carotid artery in its intracavernous course and the surrounding sinus may arise as a result of trauma or spontaneously, in the ratio of 3 to 1. Males predominate in the former group, attributable to their greater exposure to accidents and in particular to the incidence of war injuries; in the latter group females predominate. Injury may be penetrating or closed and the latter are usually of a severe nature, associated with prolonged unconsciousness and with clinical if not radiological evidence of fracture of the base of the skull. The fixity imposed upon the artery in its course through the base of the skull and the cavernous sinus renders it susceptible to the same severe shearing stresses which give rise to fractures across the body of the sphenoid and the petrous bone, frequently seen in autopsies following fatal head injury. Small tears of the wall of the artery in its intraosseous course may not be infrequent and are compatible with survival unless they give rise to thrombosis. Those within the cavernous sinus will cause a fistula, immediately or later. The latency, which may be weeks or months, suggests that in these the injury caused an incomplete tear of the vessel wall which gradually forms a traumatic aneurysm and then ruptures. Proof that an aneurysm in the cavernous sinus can arise as a result of trauma is provided by the case reported by Araki et al. (1965) although a fistula did not develop. In the spontaneous variety, the cause is with fair certainty rupture of a saccular aneurysm; their incidental occurrence on this portion of the carotid artery is well established and the high proportion amongst females is in accord with that of massive aneurysms within the sinus. In his classical monograph Sattler (1920) reviewed 352 cases of 'pulsating exophthalmos' which included 30 due to a vascular tumour or orbital meningocoele, 246 to traumatic, and 76 to spontaneous fistulae. He appended a valuable account of autopsy findings, describing the tears in the artery following trauma; in some of the spontaneous examples aneurysms were detected, in others they were not apparent and the force of the rupture may have destroyed the sac, as happens sometimes in cerebral aneurysms. The excellent account by Dandy (1937) reviews the writings of Sattler and others and describes 8 cases in detail; it is beautifully illustrated. A later review is that of Hamby and Dohn (1964).

As a result of the fistula arterial blood is injected into the cavernous sinus, causing great distension of all the venous channels which communicate with the sinus and in the course of time the sinus itself enlarges (Fig. 11.8). The orbital veins are the most important because of the immediate and obvious clinical effects of their distention; the superior ophthalmic vein forms an enormous serpentine sac continuous with enlarged supraorbital and angular veins; communication with the opposite cavernous sinus by way of the circular sinus and dural channels on the clivus gives rise to bilateral signs. These channels are well illustrated in Dandy's article. A large fistulous opening leads to a redistribution of blood flow in the circle of Willis so that the ipsilateral hemisphere depends for some of its supply on the opposite carotid and on the vertebral arteries. Cervical ligation of the ipsilateral carotid artery may be followed by ischaemia owing to the retrograde escape of blood from the circle of Willis through the fistula. This event may be anticipated if at angiography the cerebral arteries fail to fill with medium during ipsilateral carotid injection.

The onset of symptoms in both spontaneous and delayed traumatic varieties is abrupt. It is usually painless though the patient is aware that something has happened, but pain, often severe,

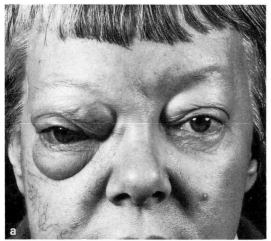

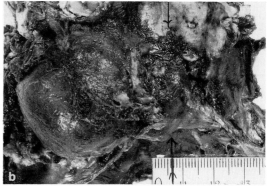

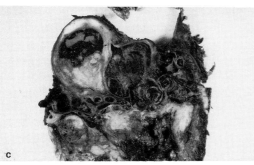

Fig. 11.8. Left caroticocavernous fistula: female aged 45 years. Fell and struck left side of head: no immediate sequelae: 6 weeks later sudden onset of pain, redness and swelling of left 'eye': left eye blind, total internal and external ophthalmoplegia, slight pulsating proptosis, bruit. Multiple intra- and extracranial carotid ligations; in time complained of left trigeminal pain and numbness and right eye became markedly prominent. Died of intracranial haemorrhage 6 years after onset of symptoms.
(a) Five years after onset when pulsating exophthalmos, venous congestion and bruit worse on right side.
(b) The specimen comprises body of sphenoid with cavernous sinuses and aneurysmal swelling: arrows indicate median plane.
(c) Coronal section through approximately its middle revealing many vascular channels, some containing organized clot.

soon develops in the forehead and around and in the eye. The pain tends gradually to subside though it may persist as an important symptom. A noise in the head synchronous with the pulse is usually immediately perceived by the patient, persists with variable intensity and for some patients it is a constant source of disturbance and annoyance. A bruit is audible on auscultation, loudest in the region of the orbit but often widely transmitted and reduced or abolished by carotid compression in the neck. It may be so loud as to be noticeable to a bystander. It is regarded as the most reliable sign of the side on which the fistula has developed and its permanent cessation indicates closure whether by natural causes or by operation.

Pulsating exophthalmos is the most obvious and constant sign, taking several days to become evident and many weeks or months to reach its maximum extent. When well developed the protrusion of the eyeball is considerable and there is much oedema and vascular congestion of the conjunctiva, so that the lids cannot be closed. The pulsating movement of the globe is best perceived by looking at it from the side. In longstanding cases veins of the face and forehead become distended and thickened and a thrill may be palpable if the finger partially occludes one. In addition to protrusion the globe is usually displaced outwards and downwards by the distended superior ophthalmic vein which lies in the upper medial part of the orbit. Severe prolonged congestion may lead to impaired vision from papilloedema and optic atrophy, haemorrhages on the retina and opacity of the media, lens and cornea. Vision is also at risk from dehydration of the cornea and superimposed infection as a result of inability to close the lids. Sattler found that about a quarter of the patients became blind: this would be a pessimistic view of the results of modern treatment unless the condition had been neglected. Jefferson (1952) reported defective vision in only 2 of 26 patients and the incidence was low in Hamby's series. Congestion of the nasal mucosa may give rise to epistaxis. Ophthalmoplegia is variable in degree, usually in accordance with the severity of the lesion; in the

traumatic cases it may have been caused at the time of injury by damage to the nerves in the cavernous sinus or in the superior orbital fissure; in both groups the nerves may be stretched with the distension of the sinus, or by compression and displacement within the orbit by the enlarged and thickened veins. Considerable variation occurs in the extent to which both eyes are affected. Unilateral signs are more common and the contralateral eye is affected to a lesser degree in perhaps one-fifth of the cases. Exceptionally, the signs are more marked in, or are entirely restricted to, the contralateral eye. These variations depend upon the freedom of intersinus communications and upon anatomical differences in the venous drainage in the orbit. Dandy pointed out that signs are usually restricted to the ipsilateral side probably because 'in most instances the path of least resistance is into the ophthalmic vein'. Ramos and Mount (1953) described a case with entirely contralateral signs in which angiography revealed the fistula draining by a large anterior segment of the circular sinus into the opposite cavernous sinus and thence into the distended ophthalmic vein. In traumatic fistulae, an alternative to anatomical variation is thrombosis of venous channels as a result of the injury.

Provided the three cardinal signs are present, exophthalmos, pulsation and bruit, there is little doubt about the diagnosis. The abruptness of onset distinguishes a caroticocavernous fistula from other vascular lesions such as angiomatous malformation and tumour. Arteriovenous fistula in the neck produce a cervical swelling and thrill and bruit are maximal over it. Cavernous sinus thrombosis has an abrupt origin and presents the orbital signs, but there is no pulsation or bruit and systemic disturbances are severe. Congenital defects of the orbit may cause pulsating exophthalmos but the other characteristic features of a fistula are absent. If the volume of shunted blood is sufficient, arteriovenous fistulae give rise to cardiovascular changes. Such observations are rare in caroticocavernous fistulae although Keegan (1933) showed in two cases a much higher oxygen saturation in the internal jugular venous blood than in arm venous blood.

The indications for treatment are the danger of blindness, noise, pain and disfigurement. Spontaneous cure occurs in an appreciable number and provides encouragement for the patient if for any reason operation is not undertaken. In Sattler's series the fistula closed spontaneously in 5.6% of cases and Potter (1954) reported this in no fewer than 5 of 15 patients; in 2 it followed hypotensive episodes (syncope in one and haemorrhagic shock at amputation in the other) and in 2 it followed angiography. Because spontaneous cure may occur and because in the past the results of operation have often been disappointing, an expectant attitude is commonly adopted for months and even years. It is likely that postponement of surgical treatment militates against success, by allowing the orifice of the fistula and the collateral arteries to enlarge. Brooks (1930a) gave a succinct account of the altered haemodynamics in traumatic arteriorvenous fistulae of the limbs and recommended delaying operation for no longer than was necessary for the (accidental) wound to heal. His arguments might well be applied to caroticocavernous examples in the light of accumulated experience.

*Operative treatment.* Operations fall into two groups: arterial ligations aimed at isolation of the fistula, and direct closure or obturation of its lumen. In contradistinction to the successful results of carotid ligation in the neck for simple intracavernous aneurysms, the same operation for fistulae has proved much less effective. Various combinations of occlusion of the cervical carotid arteries have resulted in permanent cure in some 30% to 50% of cases. In the others there has been improvement, but commonly the condition fully reasserts itself. Proximal ligation alone is an insufficient procedure because it only partially reduces the amount of blood flowing through the fistula. As Dandy emphasized, it succeeds at times, only because a temporarily reduced circulation through the fistula allows thrombosis to gain a foothold; success may depend upon a small opening. The fistula creates

a point of low pressure in the local circulation comparable with the electrical 'sink' of neurophysiology. Closure of one artery increases the reflux flow through collaterals, which consequently enlarge. The most important fraction of this flow comes through the carotid above the fistula and next in importance is the ophthalmic artery which freely communicates with the external carotid system. The contribution which the ophthalmic system can make to the circle of Willis has been well recognized clinically and identified angiographically in cases of atheromatous thrombosis of the internal carotid artery. Falconer and Hoare (1951) have demonstrated this circulation by angiography in a case of caroticocavernous fistula. Minute branches between the two internal carotid arteries in their intracavernous course also enlarge and provide collateral flow; they have been displayed by the dissections of Parkinson (1964) and Ramos and Mount (1953) have demonstrated hypertrophy of the posterior communicating artery. The presence of the congenital anomaly carotid–basilar anastomosis, will also provide an additional and large blood flow to the fistula.

In a review of the various ligations undertaken in a series of 36 cases, Hamby (1964, 1966) condemned fractional and staged procedure; for the reasons given above 'each fractional attack induces more widespread anastomoses that bypass the occluded artery'. He recommended closure of the intracranial end of the carotid segment by ligation proximal to the posterior communicating artery, occlusion of the ophthalmic artery (which may be technically difficult or impossible if there is much distension of the cavernous sinus) and finally ligation of the internal carotid artery in the neck, in one stage. This programme, with minor modifications in some cases, achieved a cure in 11 of 12 patients. Ligation of the ophthalmic artery does not always cause blindness because of collateral circulation from the external carotid artery, but the effect of this operation upon vision in the ipsilateral eye is unpredictable.

Obliteration or obturation of the fistula may be achieved by the ingenious and elegant operation of Brooks (1930b). This depends upon the principle of embolization; a piece of muscle is inserted into the lumen of the internal carotid artery and is driven into its cavernous section by the blood flow. Hamby and Gardner (1933) found that 6 days after a muscle embolus 'the size of a pea' the bruit returned; it was abolished permanently by carotid ligation. Röttgen (1948) found the method effective in 2 cases but he combined it with cervical ligation of the internal carotid artery as have other surgeons. Lang and Bucy (1965) cured a patient by muscle embolization without arterial ligation. This operation, or more recent modifications employing a detachable balloon as an embolus, (De Brun & Fox 1982) has now become the method of first choice (Black *et al.* 1973). Mullen (1979) described thrombogenic techniques which preserved the integrity of the carotid artery. If the fistulous connection can be identified, copperclad steel thrombogenic wires are inserted into the fistula via the lateral wall of the cavernous sinus. If the neck of the fistula cannot be identified but the flow is predominantly into one group of distended draining veins, the latter are packed with thrombogenic material, for example oxidized cellulose. In the event of failure, as a last resort, direct exposure of the intracavernous segment of the carotid artery may be considered. Parkinson (1973) has described a microsurgical technique for directly ligating the fistulous connection under hypothermia (8–10°C) and complete femoral circulatory bypass. He emphasized that operation within the cavernous sinus but outside the venous and arterial components was possible. Browder (1937) cured a case by packing muscle into a bulging cavernous sinus, but whether this entered the fistulous part of the artery or the surrounding sinus is not clear in the description. In longstanding cases, exophthalmos may persist to a disfiguring degree even when the fistula has been successfully closed. This is due to the mass of thick walled veins within the orbit; excision of the largest may be advisable.

## Brain stem compression by aneurysm

Large aneurysms arising from the vertebrovasilar system may indent the pons, medulla or upper segments of the spinal cord, giving rise to a clinical picture which simulates a tumour. They may be saccular or fusiform in type and because they are so obvious a lesion at autopsy they form a large proportion of the earlier statistics on aneurysms. Although Gull (1959) was well acquainted with aneurysmal rupture and emphasized the need to search thoroughly at post-mortem examination for this origin of an intracranial haemorrhage, he wrote that the basilar artery must be 'the most frequent seat' for an aneurysm (a third of his specimens were so situated) and that they form a 'natural group'. In present day experience they are relatively rare and Meadows (1951) emphasized the varied clinical picture which 'explains why most basilar aneurysms are suprise post-mortem findings'. The history usually extends for a year or so and in the early stage may be characterized by the involvement of a single cranial nerve. Depending upon the site of origin, the third, fifth, seventh or the eighth cranial nerve may be picked out. In the case of the fifth cranial nerve the initial symptom will be trigeminal pain; in the case of the seventh, hemifacial spasm (2 good examples were described by Campbell & Keedy 1947) and the eighth, vertigo resembling Meniere disease. These features establish a similarity with cerebellopontine angle tumours. Progress in the size of the aneurysm leads to the involvement of other cranial nerves and because fusiform aneurysms are often serpentine in shape and cause much distortion of the pons and medulla (Fig. 11.9) asymmetrical bilateral cranial nerve palsies may develop. Compression of the brain stem gives rise to pyramidal signs and disturbance of equilibrium, nystagmus, palatal palsy, dysarthria and dysphagia. Alajouanine *et al.* (1948) stated that though pyramidal signs are practically constant, the sensory tracts remain unaffected and ataxia of the limbs does not develop. These points are useful in distinguishing aneurysmal compression from an intra-

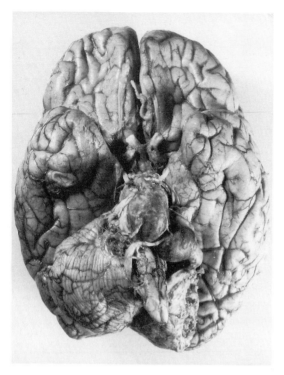

**Fig. 11.9.** Fusiform vertebrobasilar aneurysm. Male aged 60 years: progressive symptoms and signs for 6 years of a left cerebellopontine angle lesion, with episodes of painful stiffness of neck: no radiological abnormalities: lumbar CSF contained 110 mg protein/100 ml. Presumptive diagnosis acoustic schwannoma: operative exploration revealed aneurysm, death from bulbar palsy 2 weeks later. The caudal portion of the aneurysm is in the course of the left vertebral artery: the right vertebral artery enters close to the junction with the rostral portion: the terminal portion of the basilar artery is seen emerging from the rostral pole of the aneurysm. Severe atheroma of cerebral arteries.

medullary neoplasm. Meadows mentions that alternating hemiparesis has been described and that remission of symptoms simulates multiple sclerosis. An aneurysm from the vertebral artery may lie astride the foramen magnum and will then compress the uppermost segments of the cervical spinal cord (Symonds & Meadows 1937). Occipital pain radiating into the shoulder and arm was found by Alajouanine *et al.* (1948) to be the commonest first symptom; its presence suggests that the aneurysm is low in the posterior fossa, or even at the foramen magnum. They found vomiting was frequent, but papilloedema

did not develop; in the later stages the patients were wasted and weak.

Fluctuation and alteration of signs mimics vertebrobasilar ischaemia from atheroma. Indeed it is probable that in aneurysms this is an important factor in the course of the disease. Multiple sclerosis, syringobulbia, glioma and polioencephalomyelitis, also enter into the differential diagnosis, but the commonest difficulty is distinction from extramedullary tumours, in particular schwannomas of the trigeminal and acoustic nerves, meningioma, chordoma and a malignant tumour invading the base of the skull. X-ray examination of the base of the skull may show bone destruction typical of these various tumours; fractional air encephalography may reveal a mass without providing information sufficient for its identification. Vertebral angiography often supplies valuable evidence in cases of tumour and will immediately identify an aneurysm, provided both vertebral arteries are displayed.

Although the surgical treatment of giant aneurysms has made some strides in recent years, these massive aneurysms remain a difficult problem in the posterior fossa. The saccular examples are so intimately applied and adherent to important penetrating arterial twigs that even if dissection from adjacent cranial nerves and brain stem were successfully achieved and the sac amputated after closure of its base, total ischaemic infarction seems inevitable. Perhaps a combination of hypothermia, circulatory arrest, and microsurgery might allow a successful form of endo-aneurysmorrhaphy, with reconstruction of the parent artery, as evolved by Matas. One can see no radical way of treating a fusiform aneurysm, though Dandy (1944, Case 11) ligated one vertebral artery for such a condition, and the patient was 'well' 2 years later. If a significant reduction of intrabasilar pressure followed vertebral or basilar occlusion one would then be fearful of pontine ischaemia because of the failure of circulation through fine penetrating arteries whose mouths were partially occluded by the atheroma.

# References

ADAMS H.P., KASSELL N.F., TORNER J.C., NIBBELINK D.W. & SAHS A.L. (1981) *J. Neurosurg.*, **54**, 141.

AF BJORKESTEN G. & HALONEN V. (1965) *J. Neurosurg.*, **23**, 29.

ALAJOUANINE T., LE BEAU J. & HOUDART R. (1948) *Rev. Neurol.*, **80**, 321.

ALLCOCK J.M. & DRAKE C.G. (1965) *J. Neurosurg.*, **22**, 21.

ALMEIDA F. DE (1949) In *Cerebral Angiography* (Ed. Lima, P.A.) Oxford University Press, London.

ARAKI C., HANDA H., HANDA J. & JOSHIDA K. (1965) *J. Neurosurg.*, **23**, 64.

ALVORD E.C., LOESER J.D., BAILEY W.L. & COPASS M.K. (1972) *Arch. Neurol.*, **27**, 273.

AMEEN A.A. & ILLINGWORTH R. (1981) *J. Neurol. Neurosurg. Psychiat.*, **44**, 220.

ASTRUP J. (1982) *J. Neurosurg.*, **56**, 482.

ATKINSON W.J. (1949) *J. Neurol. Neurosurg. Psychiat.*, **12**, 137.

ATKINSON W.J. (1950) *Ann. roy. Coll. Surg. Eng.*, **7**, 38.

BAKAY L. & SWEET W.H. (1952) *Surg. Gynaec. Obstet.*, **95**, 67.

BAKAY L. & SWEET W.H. (1953) *J. Neurosurg.*, **10**, 353.

BARTHOLOW R. (1872) *Amer. J. Med. Sci.*, **64**, 373.

BASSETT R.C. (1949) *J. Neurosurg.*, **6**, 216.

BASSETT R.C. & LEMMEN C.J. (1954) *J. Neurosurg.*, **11**, 135.

BATTACHARJI S.K., HUTCHINSON E.C. & McCALL A.J. (1967) *Brit. med. J.*, **2**, 270.

BEADLES C.F. (1907) *Brain*, **30**, 331.

BEGUELIN C. & SEILER R. (1983) *Neurosurgery*, **13**, 409.

BERNHEIMER S. (1891) *Von Graefe's Arch. Ophth.*, **37(2)**, 37.

BIERSE S.H. & TOM M.I. (1960) *Neurology*, **10**, 101.

BLACK P.M. (1986) *Neurosurgery*, **18**, 12.

BLACK P., SUMIOVEMATSU C.M., PEROVIC M. & WALKER A.E. (1973) *J. Neurosurg.*, **38**, 113.

BOLANDER H.G., KOURTOPOULOS H. & WEST K.A. (1984) *Acta. Neurochir.*, **70**, 31.

BOTTERELL E.H., LLOYD C.A. & HOFFMAN H.J. (1962) *Amer. J. Ophth.*, **54**, 609.

BOTTERELL E.H., LOUGHEED W.M., SCOTT J.W. & VANDEWATER S.L. (1956) *J. Neurosurg.*, **13**, 1.

BRAMWELL B. (1886) *Ed. med. J.*, **87**, 32.

BRINTON W. (1852) *Trans. Path. Soc. London*, **3**, 49.

BRITISH MEDICAL BULLETIN (1961) Vol. 17, No. 1, *Hypothermia and the Effects of Cold*. Medical Dept. Brit. Council, London.

BROCK R.C. (1940–41) *Guy's Hosp. Reps.*, **90**, 104.

BROOKS B. (1930a) *South. med. J.*, **23**, 100.

BROOKS B. (1930b) *Trans. South. Surg. Ass.*, **43**, 176.

BROWDER J. (1937) *Arch. Ophth.*, **18**, 95.

BRUCE A., PIRIE J.H.H. & MacDONALD W.K. (1908) *Rev. Neurol. Psychiat.*, **6**, 449.

BUCKELL M. (1966) *J. Neurol. Neurosurg. Psychiat.*, **29**, 291.

BUCKELL M., RICHARDSON A. & SARNER M. (1966) *J. Neurol. Neurosurg. Psychiat.*, **29**, 293.

BULL J.W.D. (1962a) *The London Clinic med. J.*, **3**, 47.

BULL J.W.D. (1962b) *Brit. Med. J.*, **2**, 1701.

BULL J.W.D. (1969) *Brain*, **92**, 535.

BUSSE O. (1921) *Virchow's Arch. Path. Anat. Physiol.*, **229**, 178.

BYROM F.B. (1954) *Lancet*, **2**, 201.

BYROM F.B. (1968) *Proc. roy. Soc. Med.*, **61**, 605.

CAMPBELL E. & KEEDY C. (1947) *J. Neurosurg.*, **4**, 342.

CARMICHAEL R. (1945) *J. Path. Bact.*, **57**, 345.

CARMICHAEL R. (1950) *J. Path. Bact.*, **62**, 1.

CLARKE E. & WALTON J.N. (1953) *Brain*, **76**, 378.

COLLIER J. (1933) In *Text Book of the Practice of Medicine*, 4th edn. (Ed. Price F.W.) p. 1538. Oxford University Press, London.

COOPER A.P. (1809) *Med. Chirurg. Trans.*, **1**, (reprinted in Guy's Hosp. Reps. 1940–41, **90**, 123).

COURVILLE C.B. (1965) *Bull. Los. Angel. Neurol. Soc.*, **30**, 1.

CRAWFORD M.D. & SARNER M. (1965) *Lancet*, **2**, 1254.

CRAWFORD T. (1959) *J. Neurol. Neurosurg. Psychiat.*, **22**, 259.

CROMPTON M.R. (1962) *Lancet*, **2**, 421.

CROMPTON M.R. (1963) *Brain*, **86**, 301.

CROMPTON M.R. (1964) *Brain*, **87**, 263.

CROMPTON M.R. (1966a) *J. Neurol. Neurosurg. Psychiat.*, **29**, 164.

CROMPTON M.R. (1966b) *Brit. med. J.*, **1**, 1138.

CROMPTON M.R. (1967) *Lancet*, **1**, 48.

DANDY W.E. (1937) *Zbl. Neurochirurg.*, **2**, 77 and 165.

DANDY W.E. (1944) *Intracranial Arterial Aneurysms*. Comstock, New York.

DE BRUN G. & FOX A.J. (1982) In *Clinical Management of Intracranial Aneurysms*. (Ed. Hopkins L.N. & Long D.M.) Raven Press, New York.

DENNY-BROWN D. (1956) *J. Neuropath. Exp. Neurol.*, **15**, 146.

DENNY-BROWN D. (1960) In *Handbook of Physiology*, Section 1. Neurophysiology. (Ed. Field J., Magoun H.W. & Hall V.E.) Vol. 2, p. 781. Williams and Wilkins, Baltimore.

DENNY-BROWN D. (1966) *The Cerebral Control of Movement*. Liverpool University Press, Liverpool.

DINNING T.A.R. & FALCONER M.A. (1953) *Lancet*, **2**, 799.

DOCZI T., AMBROSE J. & O'LAOIRE S. (1984) *J. Neurosurg.*, **60**, 335.

DOTT N.M. (1933) *Trans. Med. Chirurg. Soc. Ed.*, **47**, 219.

DRAKE C.G. (1961) *J. Neurosurg.*, **18**, 230.

DRAKE C.G. (1965) *J. Neurosurg.*, **23**, 457.

DRAKE C.G. (1968) *J. Neurosurg.*, **29**, 372 and 436.

DRAKE C.G. (1969) *J. Neurosurg.*, **29**, 436.

DRAKE C.G. (1975) *J. Neurosurg.*, **43**, 255.

DRAKE C.G., VANDERLINDEN R.G. & AMACHER A.L. (1968) *J. Neurosurg.*, **29**, 24.

DREW C.E., KEEN G. & BENAZON D.B. (1959) *Lancet*, **1**, 745.

DREW C.E. (1961) *Brit. med. Bull.*, **17**, 30.

DU BOULAY G.H. (1963) *Acta Radiol. N.S.*, **1**, 257.

DU BOULAY G.H. (1965) *Brit. J. Radiol.*, **38**, 721.

DUKE–ELDER W.S. (1949) *Text Book of Ophthalmology*, Vol. 4. p. 3534 and 3535. Kimpton, London.

DUTTON J.E.M. (1956) *Brit. med. J.*, **2**, 585.

DUTTON J.E.M. (1959) *Brit. med. J.*, **2**, 597.

ECHLIN F.A. (1965) *J. Neurosurg.*, **23**, 1.

ELKIN D.C. & HARRIS M.H. (1946) *Ann. Surg.*, **124**, 934.

EPPINGER H. (1887) *Arch. klin. Chirurg.*, **35**, Suppl.

FAIRLEY H.B. (1961) *Brit. med. Bull.*, **17**, 52.

FALCONER M.A. & HOARE R.D. (1951) *Proc. roy. Soc. Med.*, **45**, 225.

FARRAR J.K., GAMACHE F.W., FERGUSON G.G., BARKER J., VARKEY G.P. & DRAKE C.G. (1981) *J. Neurosurg.*, **55**, 857.

FEARNSIDES E.G. (1916) *Brain*, **39**, 224.

FEIN J.M. (1980) In *Cerebral Arterial Spasm*. (Ed. Wilkins R.H.) Chapt. 80. Williams & Wilkins, Baltimore.

FISHER C.M., ROBERTSON G.H. & OJEMANN R.S. (1977) *Neurosurgery*, **1**, 245.

FISHER C.M., KISTLER J.P. & DAVIS J.M. (1980a) In *Cerebral*

*Arterial Spasm.* (Ed. Wilkins R.H.) Chapt. 60. Williams & Wilkins, Baltimore.

FISHER C.M., KRISTLER J.P. & DAVIS J.M. (1980b) *Neurosurgery*, **6**, 1.

FITCH W., PICKARD J.D. & GRAHAM D.I. (1981) *J. Cerebral Blood Flow & Metabol.*, **1**, suppl. 1, 5556.

FLAMM E.S. (1982) In *Clinical Management of Intracranial Aneurysms.* (Ed. Hopkins L.N. & Long D.M.) Raven Press, New York.

FLOREY H. (1925) *Brain*, **48**, 43.

FODSTEAD H. (1982) *Acta Neurochir.*, **63**, 233.

FOIX C. (1922) *Rev. Neurol.*, **29**, 827.

FORBUS W.D. (1930) *Bull. Johns. Hopk. Hosp.*, **47**, 239.

FORSTER D.M.C., STEINER L., HAKANSON S. & BERGVALL U. (1978) *J. Neurosurg.*, **48**, 712.

FORTUNY L.A., ADAMS C.B.T. & BRIGGS M. (1980) *J. Neurol. Neurosurg. Psychiat.*, **43**, 879.

FORTUNY L.A. & PRIETO-VALIENTE L. (1981) *J. Neurosurg.*, **54**, 35.

GIBBS J.R. (1965a) *Brit. J. Surg.*, **52**, 947.

GIBBS J.R. (1965b) *J. Neurol. Neurosurg. Psychiat.*, **28**, 383.

GILLINGHAM F.J. (1958) *Ann. roy. Coll. Surg.Eng.*, **23**, 89.

GLYNN L.E. (1940) *J. Path. Bact.*, **51**, 213.

GRADY P.A., BLAUMANIS O.R. & NELSON E.R. (1980) In *Cerebral Arterial Spasm.* (Ed. Wilkins R.H.) Chapt 15. Williams & Wilkins, Baltimore.

GRUBB R.L. (1982) In *Clinical Management of Intracranial Aneurysms.* (Ed. Hopkins L.N. & Long D.M.) Raven Press, New York.

GULL W. (1959) *Guy's Hosp. Reps.*, **5**, 281.

HALSTED W.S. (1909) *J. Exp. Med.*, **11**, 373.

HAMBY W.B. (1952) *Intracranial Aneurysms.* Thomas, Springfield, Illinois.

HAMBY W.B. (1963) *J. Neurosurg.*, **20**, 4.

HAMBY W.B. (1964) *J. Neurosurg.*, **21**, 859.

HAMBY W.B. (1966) *Proc. Third Int. Cong. Neurol. Surg. Int. Congress Series.*, No. 110, p.667. Exc. Med. Foundation, Amsterdam.

HAMBY W.B. & DOHN D.F. (1964) *Clin. Neurosurg.*, **11**, 150.

HAMBY W.B. & GARDNER W.J. (1933) *Arch. Surg.*, **27**, 676.

HAMER J. & KUHNER A. (1976) In *Intracranial Pressure III*, (Ed. Beks J.W.F., Bosch D.A. & Brock M.) p. 157. Springer-Verlag, Berlin.

HARRIS P. & UDVARHELYI G.B. (1957) *J. Neurosurg.*, **14**, 180.

HAMILTON J.G. & FALCONER M.A. (1959) *J. Neurosurg.*, **16**, 514.

HARDESTY W.H., ROBERTS B., TOOLE J.F. & ROYSTON H.P. (1961) *Surgery*, **49**, 251.

HASSLER O. (1961) *Acta Psychiat. Neurol. Scand. Suppl.*, 154.

HAYASHI M., MARUKAWA S., FUJII H., KITANO T., KOBAYASHI H., & YAMAMOTO S. (1977) *J. Neurosurg.*, **46**, 584.

HAYASHI M., MARUKAWA S., FUJII H., KITANO T., KOBAYASHI H., MUNEMOTO S. & YAMAMOTO S. (1978) *Acta Neurochir.*, **44**, 81.

HEIFETZ M.D. (1986) *Neurosurgery*, **19**, 665.

HEILBRUN M.P., OLSEN J. & LASSEN N.A. (1972) *J. Neurosurg.*, **37**, 36.

HEISKANEN O. (1981) *J. Neurosurg.*, **55**, 524.

HENSON R.A. & CROFT P.B. (1956) *Quart. J. Med.*, **25**, 53.

HEROS R.C., NELSON P.B., OJEMANN R.G., CROWELL R.M. & DEBRUN G. (1983) *Neurosurgery*, **12**, 153.

HEUBNER O. (1872) *Abl. Med. Wiss.*, **10**, 817.

HIDJRA A., VAN GIJN J., STEFANKOS S., VAN DONGEN K.J., VERMEULEN M. & VAN CREVEL H. (1986) *Neurology*, **36**, 329.

HOOK O. & NORLEN G. (1964) *Acta Neurol. Scand.*, **40**, 200 and 219.

HUGENHOLTZ H. & ELGIE R.G. (1982) *J. Neurosurg.*, **56**, 180.

HUGHES J.T. (1980) In *Cerebral Arterial Spasm.* (Ed. Wilkins R.H.) Chapt. 77. Williams & Wilkins, Baltimore.

HUNT W.E. & HESS R.M. (1968) *J. Neurosurg.*, **28**, 14.

HYLAND H.H. & BARNETT H.J.M. (1953) *Proc. roy. Soc. Med.*, **47**, 141.

HYPOTHERMIA IN NEUROL. SURG. (1964) *Second European Congress Neurol. Surg. Acta Neurochirur.*, Suppl. 13.

ITAKURA T., OZAKI F., NAKAI E., FUJII T., HAYASHI S. & KOMAL N. (1983) *J. Neurosurg.*, **58**, 117.

JAIN K.K. (1963) *Surgery*, **54**, 347.

JAIN K.K. (1964) *Canad. J. Surg.*, **7**, 134.

JAMIESON K.G. (1964) *J. Neurosurg.*, **21**, 781.

JAMIESON K.G. (1968) *J. Neurosurg.*, **28**, 544.

JEFFERSON G. (1936) *Proc. roy. Soc. Med.*, **29**, 1169.

JEFFERSON G.J. (1937) *Brain*, **40**, 444.

JEFFERSON G.J. (1938) *Brit. J. Surg.*, **26**, 267.

JEFFERSON G. (1947) *Proc. roy. Soc. Med.*, **40**, 419.

JEFFERSON G. (1952) *Proc. roy. Soc. Med.*, **45**, 300.

JEFFERSON G. (1955) The Third Sherrington Lecture 'The Invasive Adenomas of the Anterior Pituitary'. Liverpool University Press, Liverpool.

JEFFERSON G. (1960) *Selected Papers.* Pitman Med. Publ. Co. Ltd., London (p. 301, a postscript to *Brit. J. Surg.*, **26**, 267).

JEFFERSON G., BAILEY R.A. & KERR A.S. (1956) *J. Bone Jt. Surg.*, **38B**, 114.

JENNETT W.B., HARPER A.M. & GILLESPIE F.C. (1966) *Lancet*, **2**, 1162.

JOHNSON R. (1952) *Proc. roy. Soc. Med.*, **45**, 301.

JOMIN M., LESOIN F. & LOZES G. (1984) *Surg. Neurol.*, **21**, 13.

KAPLAN H.A. (1965) *J. Neurosurg.*, **23**, 305.

KAPP J., MAHALEY M.S. & ODOM G.L. (1968) *J. Neurosurg.*, **29**, 331, 339 and 350.

KASSELL N.F., PEERLESS S.J., DURWARD Q.J., BECK D.W., DRAKE C.G. & ADAMS H.P. (1980a) In *Cerebral Arterial Spasm.* (Ed. Wilkins R.H.) Chapt. 111. Williams & Wilkins, Baltimore.

KASSELL N.F., PEERLESS S.J. & DRAKE C.G. (1980b) In *Cerebral Arterial Spasm.* (Ed. Wilkins R.H.) Chapt. 12. Williams & Wilkins, Baltimore.

KASSELL N.F., PEERLESS S.J., DURWARD Q.J., BECK D.W., DRAKE C.G. & ADAMS H.P. (1982) *Neurosurgery*, **11**, 337.

KASSELL N.F. & TORNER J.C. (1983a) *Neurosurgery*, **23**, 291.

KASSELL N.F. & TORNER J.C. (1983b) *Neurosurgery*, **13**, 479.

KAYE A.H. & BROWNBILL D. (1981) *J. Neurosurg.*, **54**, 726.

KEEGAN J.G. (1933) *Surg. Gynae. Obstet.*, **57**, 368.

KELLY P.J., GORTEN R.J., ROSE J.E., GROSSMAN R.G. & EISENBERG H.M. (1979) *Neurosurgery*, **5**, 202.

KETY S.S. & SCHMIDT C.F. (1945) *Amer. J. Physiol.*, **143**, 53.

KILLIAN H. (1950) *Langenbeck's Arch. Klin. Chirurg.*, **263**, 437.

KLINGLER M. (1951) *Confin. Neurol.*, **11**, 261.

KOOS W. TH. & PERNECZKY A. (1982) *Acta. Neurochir.*, **63**, 125.

KORGIS H., FISHER W.L., LLEWELLYN R.C. & PEEBLES E.M.C. (1966) *J. Neurosurg.*, **25**, 73.

KRAYENBUHL H. & YASARGIL M.G. (1957) *Die Vascularen Erkrankungen im Gebiet der Arteria Vertebralis und Arteria Basilaris.* Thieme, Stuttgart.

KRAYENBUHL H. & YASARGIL M. G. (1958) *Das Hirnaneurysma*. Geigy S. A., Basle.

LANG E. R. & BUCY P. C. (1965) *J. Neurosurg.*, **22**, 387.

LANTOS G., FEIN J. M. & KNEP S. (1984) *J. Neurosurg.*, **60**, 636.

LASSEN N. A. & INGVAR D. H. (1961) *Lancet*, **2**, 806.

LAZORTHES G. (1961) *Vascularisation et Circulation cerebrales*, Masson, Paris.

LEY A. (1950) *J. Neurol. Neurosurg. Psychiat.*, **13**, 75.

LINDSAY K. W., TEASDALE G. M. & KNILL-JONES R. P. (1983) *J. Neurosurg.*, **58**, 57.

LINDSAY K. W., VERMEULEN M., MURRAY G., CHEAH F., HIJDRA A., MUIZELAAR J. P., SCHANNONG M., TEASDALE G. M., VAN CREVEL H. & VAN GIJN J. (1984) S.B.N.S. report. J. Neurol. Neurosurg. Psychiat. In press. Full report: Vermeulen M., Lindsay K. W., Murray G., Cheah F., Hijdra A., Muizelaar J. P., Schannong M., Teasdale G. M., van Crevel H. & van Gijn J. (1984) *New Engl. J. Med.*, **311**, 432.

LJUNGGREN B., BRANDT L., KAGSTROM E. & SUNBARG G. (1981) *J. Neurosurg.*, **54**, 473.

LJUNGGREN B., SAVELAND H. & BRANDT L. (1983) *Neurosurgery*, **13**, 629.

LJUNGGREN B., SAVELAND H., BRANDT L. & ZYGMUNT S. (1985a) *J. Nurosurg.*, **62**, 547.

LJUNGGREN B., SONESSON B., SAVELAND H. & BRANDT L. (1985b) *J. Neurosurg.*, **62**, 673.

LOGUE V. (1956) *Brit. med. J.*, **1**, 473.

LOGUE V. (1959) In *L'Aneurusme de l'Artere Communicante Anterieure* (Ed. Krayenbuhl H.) p. 113. Masson, Paris.

LOGUE V. (1964) *Clin. Neurosurg.*, **11**, 183 and 218.

LOGUE V., DURWARD M., PRATT R. T. C., PIERCY M. & NIXON W. L. B. (1968) *Brit. J. Psychiat.*, **114**, 137.

LOUGHEED W. M. & KAHN D. S. (1955) *J. Neurosurg.*, **12**, 226.

LOUGHEED W. M., SWEET W. M., WHITE J. C. & BREWSTER W. R. (1955) *J. Neurosurg.*, **12**, 240.

MACCARTY C. S., MICHENFELDER J. D. & UIHLEIN H. (1964) *J. Neurosurg.*, **21**, 372.

MAGEE C. G. (1943) *Lancet*, **2**, 497.

MARION D. W., SEGAL R. & THOMPSON M. E. (1986) *Neurosurgery*, **18**, 101.

MARTINDALE B. V. & GARFIELD J. (1978) *Brit. med. J.*, **1**, 465.

MAROON J. C. & NELSON P. B. (1979) *Neurosurgery*, **4**, 223.

MATAS R. (1911) *Ann. Surg.*, **53**, 1.

MATSON D. D. (1965) *J. Neurosurg.*, **23**, 579.

MCCONNELL A. A. (1937) *Zbl. Neurochirurg.*, **2**, 269.

MCDONALD C. A. & KORB M. (1939) *Arch. Neurol. Psychiat.*, **42**, 298.

MCKISSOCK W., PAINE K. W. E. & WALSH L. S. (1958) *J. Neurol. Neurosurg. Psychiat.*, **21**, 239.

MCKISSOCK W., PAINE K. W. E. & WALSH L. S. (1960a) *J. Neurosurg.*, **17**, 762.

MCKISSOCK W., PAINE K. W. E. & WALSH L. S. (1960b) *J. Neurosurg.*, **17**, 700.

MCKISSOCK W., RICHARDSON A., WALSH L. & OWEN E. (1964) *Lancet*, **1**, 623.

MCKISSOCK W. & WALSH L. S. (1956) *Brit. med. J.*, **2**, 559.

MCLEAN J. M. & RAY A. S. (1947) *Arch. Ophth.*, **38**, 154.

MEADOWS S. P. (1951) In *Modern Trends in Neurology*. (Ed. Feiling A.) p. 391. Butterworth, London.

MEYER C. H. A., LOWE D., MEYER M., RICHARDSON P. L. & NEIL-DWYER G. (1983) *Neurosurgery*, **12**, 58.

MILLER J. D., JAWAD K. & JENNETT W. B. (1977) *J. Neurol. Neurosurg. Psychiat.*, **40**, 64.

MILLER J. D. & LEECH P. (1975) *J. Neurosurg.*, **423**, 274.

MILLIKAN C. H. (1975) *Arch. Neurol.*, **32**, 433.

MITTS M. G. & MCQUEEN J. D. (1965) *J. Neurosurg.*, **23**, 33.

MONIZ E. (1927) *Rev. Neurol.*, **2**, 72.

MONIZ E. (1934) *L'Angiographie Cerebrale*. Masson, Paris.

MOUNT L. A. & BRISMAN R. (1974) *Clin. Neurosurg.*, **21**, 166.

MULLEN S. (1979) *J. Neurosurg.*, **50**, 131.

MURPHEY F. (1965) In *Intracranial Aneurysms and Subarachnoid Haemorrhage*. (Ed. Fields W. S. & Sahs A. L.) p. 315. Thomas, Springfield, Illinois.

NEIL-DWYER G., BARTLETT J. R., NICHOLLS A. C., NARCISI P. & POPE F. M. (1983) *J. Neurosurg.*, **59**, 16.

NEIL-DWYER G., CRUICKSHANK J., DOSHI A. & WALTER P. (1980) In *Cerebral Arterial Spasm*. (Ed. Wilkins R. H.) Chapt. 35. Williams & Wilkins, Baltimore.

NISHIOKA H. (1966) *J. Neurosurg.*, **25**, 574.

NISHIOKA H., TORNER J. C., GRAF C. J., KASSELL N. F., SAHS A. L. & GOETTLER L. C. (1984a) *Arch. Neurol.*, **41**, 1142.

NISHIOKA H., TORNER J. C., GRAF C. J., KASSELL N. F., SAHS A. L. & GOETTLER L. C. (1984b) *Arch. Neurol.*, **41**, 1147.

NORNES H. (1973) *J. Neurosurg.*, **39**, 226.

NORNES H. & MAGNAES B. (1972) *J. Neurosurg.*, **36**, 537.

NORTHFIELD D. W. C. (1952) *Proc. roy. Soc. Med.*, **45**, 302.

ODOM G. L. & TINDALL G. T. (1968) *Clin. Neurosurg.*, **15**, 101.

PADGET D. H. (1945) In *Intracranial Arterial Aneurysms*. (Ed. Dandy W. E.) . 67., Comstock, New York.

PAKARINEN S. (1967) *Acta Neurol. Scand.*, **43**, Suppl. 29.

PARKINSON D. (1964) *Canad. J. Surg.*, **7**, 251.

PARKINSON D. (1973) *J. Neurosurg.*, **38**, 99.

PATTERSON R. H. & RAY B. S. (1962) *Ann. Surg.*, **156**, 377.

PATTERSON R. H. & RAY B. S. (1965) *J. Neurosurg.*, **23**, 184.

PAULSON G., NASHOLD B. S. & MARGOLIS G. (1959) *Neurology*, **9**, 590.

PEERLESS S. J. (1980) In *Cerebral Arterial Spasm*. (Ed. Wilkins R. H.) Chapt. 79. Williams & Wilkins, Baltimore.

PEERLESS S. J., KASSELL N. F., KOMATSU K. & HUNTER I. G. (1980) In *Cerebral Arterial Spasm*. (Ed. Wilkins R. H.) Chapt. 13. Williams & Wilkins, Baltimore.

PELZ D. M., VINUELA F., FOX A. J. & DRAKE C. G. (1984) *J. Neurosurg.*, **60**, 560.

PERRETT L. V. & BULL J. W. D. (1959) *Brit. J. Radiol.*, **32**, 85.

PICKARD J. D. (1984) Personal communication.

PICKARD J. D., MATHESON M., PATTERSON J. & WYPER D. (1980) *J. Neurosurg.*, **53**, 305.

POOL J. L. (1961) *J. Neurosurg.*, **18**, 98.

PITTS L. H., MACPHERSON P., WYPER D. J., JENNETT B., BLAIR I. & COOKE M. B. D. (1980) In *Cerebral Arterial Spasm*. (Ed. Wilkins R. H.) Chapt 49. Williams & Wilkins, Baltimore.

POPE F. M., NICHOLLS A. C., NARCISI P., BARTLETT J., NEIL-DWYER G. & DOSHI B. (1981) *Lancet*, **1**, 973.

POPPEN J. L. (1959) *Clin. Neurosurg.*, **6**, 198.

POTTER J. M. (1954) *Brit. med. J.*, **2**, 786.

POTTER J. M. & TAYLOR F. M. (1955) *Arch. Neurol. Psychiat.*, **74**, 414.

POTTER J. M. (1959) *Brain*, **82**, 367.

RAMOS M. & MOUNT L. A. (1953) *J. Neurosurg.*, **10**, 178.

Report of the Cooperative Study of Intracranial Aneurysm and Subarachnoid Haemorrhage (1966) *J. Neurosurg.*

| Sect. I | vol. 24 | p. 782 |
| Sect. II | vol. 24 | p. 922 |
| Sect. III | vol. 24 | p. 1034 |
| Sect. IV | vol. 25 | p. 98 |

Sect. V     part 1, vol. 25   p. 219
Sect. V     part 2, vol. 25   p. 311
Sect. VI    vol. 25           p. 467
Sect. VII   part 1, vol. 25   p. 574
Sect. VII   part 2, vol. 25   p. 593
Sect. VIII  part 1, vol. 25   p. 660
Sect. VIII  part 2, vol. 25   p. 683
Report on Randomized Treatment Study (1974) *Stroke*, Sect III, **Vol. 5**, p. 557.
RHOTON A. Z., FUJII K., SAEKI N., PERLMUTTER D. & ZEAL A. (1982) In *Clinical Management of Intracranial Aneurysms*. (Eds. Hopkins L. N. & Long D. M.) Raven Press, New York.
RICHARDSON A. E., JANE J. A. & PAYNE P. M. (1964) *J. Neurosurg.*, **21**, 266.
RICHARDSON A. E., JANE J. A. & YASHON D. (1966) *Arch. Neurol.*, **14**, 172.
RICHLING B., GRIESMAYR G., LAMETSCHWANDTNER A. & SCHEIBLBRANDNER (1979) *J. Neurosurg.*, **51**, 654.
RIDDOCH G. & GOULDEN C. (1925) *Brit. J. Ophth.*, **9**, 209.
RIGGS H. E. & RUPP C. (1963) *Arch. Neurol.*, **8**, 8.
RISCHBIETH R. H. C. & BULL J. W. D. (1958) *Brit. J. Radiol.*, **31**, 125.
RITCHIE W. L., OVERTON T. R. & WEIR B. K. A. (1980) In *Cerebral Arterial Spasm*. (Ed. Wilkins R. H.) Chapt 112. Williams & Wilkins, Baltimore.
ROBBINS J., FEIN J. M., LANTOS G. & HOOSHANGI N. (1984) *Neurosurgery*, **15**, 121.
ROBERTSON E. G. (1949) *Brain*, **72**, 150.
ROGERS L. (1949) *Lancet*, **1**, 949.
ROSKI R. N., SPETZLER R. F., NULSEN F. E. (1981) *J. Neurosurg.*, **54**, 583.
ROSOMOFF H. L. & HOLADAY D. A. (1954) *Amer. J. Physiol.*, **179**, 85.
RÖTTGEN P. (1948) *Langenbeck's Arch. Klin. Chirurg.*, **260**, 613.
RUSSELL D. S. (1954) *Proc. roy. Soc. Med.*, **47**, 689.
SANO K. & SAITO I. (1980) In *Cerebral Arterial Spasm*. (Ed. Wilkins R. H.) Chapt. 82. Williams & Wilkins, Baltimore.
SARNER M. & CRAWFORD M. D. (1965) *Lancet*, **2**, 1251.
SATTLER C. H. (1920) *Graefe-Saemisch Handbuch der ges. Augenheilk*, **9**, part 2, 1.
SAVELAND H., LJUNGGREN B., BRANDT B. & MESSETER K. (1986a) *Neurosurgery*, **18**, 146.
SAVELAND H., SONESSON B., LJUNGGREN B., BRANDT L., USKI T., ZYGMUNT S. & HINDFELDT B. (1986b) *J. Neurosurg.*, **64**, 191.
SCHNECK S. A. (1964) *Neurology*, **14**, 691.
SCHORSTEIN J. (1940) *Brit. J. Surg.*, **28**, 50.
SCOTT R. M., LIU H. S., YUAN R. & ADELMAN L. (1982) *Neurosurgery*, **37**, 361.
SEDZIMIR C. B. (1959) *J. Neurosurg. Psychiat.*, **22**, 64.
SENGUPTA R. P., CHIU J. S. P. & BRIERLEY H. (1975) *J. Neurosurg.*, **43**, 58.
SELVERSTONE B. (1962) *J. Neurosurg.*, **29**, 884.
SHAW M. D. M. & MILLER J. D. (1974) *Lancet*, **11**, 847.
SHUCART W. A., HUSSAIN S. K. & COOPER P. R. (1980) *J. Neurosurg.*, **53**, 28.
SJOQUIST O. (1954) *Cinque Congres Neurol. Int. Lisbonne. Comptes Rendus III*, p. 108.
SMALL J. M. & STEPHENSON, S. C. F. (1966) *Lancet*, **1**, 569.
SMALL J. M., STEPHENSON S. C. F., CAMPKIN T. V., DAVISON P. H. & MCILVEEN, D. J. S. (1966) *Lancet*, **1**, 570.
SMITH B. (1963) *J. Neurol. Neurosurg. Psychiat.*, **26**, 535.

SMITH G. E. (1909) *J. Anat. Physiol.*, **43**, 410.
STEHBENS W. E. (1954) *Aust. Ann. Med.*, **3**, 214.
STEMERMAN M. B. (1981) In *Interactions Between Platelets & Vessel Walls*. (Eds. Born G. V. R. & Vane J. R.) The Royal Society, London.
STOPFORD J. B. S. (1917) *J. Anat. Physiol.*, **51**, 250.
STOREY P. B. (1967) *Brit. med. J.*, **3**, 261.
STROBOS R. R. J. & MOUNT L. A. (1953) *Arch. Neurol. Psychiat.*, **69**, 118.
SUGITA K., KOBAYASHI S., SHINTANI A. & MUTSUGA N. (1979) *J. Neurosurg.*, **51**, 615.
SUTTON D. & TRICKEY S. E. (1962) *Clin. Radiol.*, **13**, 297.
SUZUKI J., ONUMA T., YOSHIMOTO T. (1979) *Surg. Neurol.*, **11**, 407.
SWEET W. H. & BENNETT H. S. (1948) *J. Neurosurg.*, **5**, 178.
SWEET W. H., SARNOFF, S. J. & BAKAY, L. (1950) *Surg. Gynaec. Obstet.*, **90**, 327.
SYMON L. (1967) *J. Neurol. Neurosurg. Psychiat.*, **30**, 497.
SYMON L. (1982) *Acta Neurochir.*, **63**, 5.
SYMON L., BELL B. A. & KENDALL B. (1980) In *Cerebral Arterial Spasm*. (Ed. Wilkins R. H.) Chapt. 61. Williams & Wilkins, Baltimore.
SYMONDS C. P. (1922) *Guy's Hosp. Reps.*, **71**, 129 (reprinted 1940–41, **90**, 73).
SYMONDS C. P. (1923) *Guy's Hosp. Reps.*, **73**, 139.
SYMONDS C. P. (1924) *Quart. J. Med.*, **18**, 93.
SYMONDS C. P. & MEADOWS S. P. (1937) *Brain*, **60**, 52.
TEASDALE G. M., LINDSAY K. W., DHARKER S. & MILLS G. (1985) *J. Neurol. Neurosurg. Psychiat.*, **148**, 597.
TOLOSA E. (1954) *J. Neurol. Neurosurg. Psychiat.*, **17**, 300.
TOMLINSON B. E. (1959) *J. Clin. Path.*, **12**, 391.
TOVI D. (1972) In *The Central Nervous System with Special Reference to Intracranial Haemorrhage and to the Effect of Anti-fibrinolytic Drugs*. Umea University Medical Dissertations No. 8.
TRAVERS (1811) *Med. Chirurg. Trans.*, **2**, 1.
TURNBULL H. M. (1915) *Quart. J. Med.*, **8**, 201.
TURNBULL H. M. (1918) *Brain*, **41**, 50.
UIHLEIN A., THEYE R. A., DAWSON B., TERRY H. H., MCGOON D. C., DAW E. F. & KIRKLIN J. W. (1960) *Proc. Staff. Mtgs. Mayo Clinic*, **35**, 567.
VAN GIJN J., HIJDRA A., WIJDICKS E. F. M. VERMEULEN M. & VAN CREVEL H. (1985) *J. Neurosurg.*, **63**, 355.
VAN T'HOFF W., HORNABROOK R. W. & MARKS V. (1961) *Brit. med. J.*, **2**, 1190.
VOLDBY B. & ENEVOLDSEN E. M. (1982a) *J. Neurosurg.*, **56**, 186.
VOLDBY B. & ENEVOLDSEN E. M. (1982b) *J. Neurosurg.*, **56**, 197.
WALKER A. E. & ALLEGRE G. (1954) *J. Neuropath. exp. Neurol.*, **13**, 248.
WALTER P., NEIL-DWYER G. & CRUICKSHANK J. M. (1982) *Brit. med. J.*, **1**, 1661.
WALTON J. N. (1956) *Subarachnoid Haemorrhage*. Livingstone, Edinburgh.
WHITE J. C. (1964) *Clin. Neurosurg.*, **10**, 224.
WILKINS R. H. (1975) *Surg. Neurol.*, **4**, 472.
WILKINS R. H. (1980) *Neurosurgery*, **6**, 198.
WILKINS R. H. (1980) (Ed.) *Cerebral Arterial Spasm*. Williams & Wilkins, Baltimore.
WILKINS R. H. (1986) *Neurosurgery*, **18**, 808.
WILSON G., RIGGS H. E. & RUPP C. (1954) *J. Neurosurg.*, **11**, 128.

WINN H. R., RICHARDSON A. E. & JANE J. A. (1977) *J. Neurosurg.*, **47**, 727.

WINN H. R., RICHARDSON A. E. & JANE J. A. (1978) *Ann. Neurol.*, **4**, 418.

WINN H. R., RICHARDSON A. E. & JANE J. A. (1982) In *Clinical Management of Intracranial Aneurysms.* (Eds Hopkins L. N. & Long D. M.) Raven Press, New York.

WINN H. R., ALMAANI W. S., BERGA S. L., JANE J. A. & RICHARDSON A. E. (1983) *J. Neurosurg.*, **59**, 642.

WIRTH F. P., LAWS E. R., PIEPGRAS D., SCOTT R. M. (1983) *Neurosurgery*, **12**, 507.

WOOD E. H. (1964) *J. Neurosurg.*, **21**, 182.

WOOD J. R. (1857) *New York J. Med.*, **3**, 9.

WOODHALL B., SEALY W. C., HALL K. D. & FLOYD W. L. (1960) *Ann. Surg.*, **152**, 37.

WOODHALL B., SEALY W. C., HALL K. D. & FLOYD E. H. (1964) *J. Neurosurg.*, **21**.

WRIGHT R. D. & SWEET W. H. (1963) *Clin. Neurosurg.*, **9**, 163.

WRIGHT R. L. & SWEET W. H. (1965) In *Intracranial Aneurysms and Subarachnoid Haemorrhage.* (Eds. Fields W. S. & Sahs A. L.) p. 324. Thomas, Springfield, Illinois.

YAMOMOTO I, HARA M., OGURA K., SUZUKI Y, NAKANE T. & KAGEYAMA N. (1983) *Neurosurgery*, **12**, 169.

YASARGIL M. G., ANTIE J., LACIGA R., JAIN K. K., HODOSH R. M. & SMITH R. D. (1976) *Surg. Neurol.*, **6**, 83.

YASARGIL M. G., FOX J. L. & RAY M. W. (1975) In *Advances and Technical Standards in Neurosurgery*, Vol. 2. (Ed. Krayenbuhl H.) Springer-Verlag, Wein.

# Chapter 12
# Vascular Malformations of the Brain

## M. D. M. SHAW

Congenital malformations of the blood vessels of the brain are of importance to the neurosurgeon because they may bleed, may cause ischaemic damage to the brain and may give rise to epilepsy (probably the result of focal gliosis due to haemorrhage or ischaemia). The conveniently brief term angioma is commonly used, but they are not neoplastic, although in the cerebellum and in the spinal cord they may occasionally be associated with haemangioblastoma. They are vascular hamartomas, the result of aberrant development in the primitive vascular network and may be of microscopic size (then not infrequently multiple) or may be so extensive as to occupy much of a cerebral hemisphere. The formation of the skull and cerebral membranes splits the vascular mesenchyme into layers; as a consequence the same malformation may in continuity occasionally affect the brain, its membranous coverings, the skull and the scalp. Occasionally arteries may communicate directly with dural sinuses (Kunc & Bret 1969). Vascular malformations may give rise to progressive neurological deficit mimicking a tumour even to the extent of causing papilloedema. As will be seen later, these effects are due to minor haemorrhages, to thrombosis and in some to the presence of arteriovenous communications or shunts, which may increase in number or degree with the passage of time.

The literature has become voluminous since the application of computerized tomography and angiography have rendered accurate diagnosis possible and more frequent. Among the older contributions on morbid anatomy must be mentioned those of Cushing and Bailey (1928), Bergstrand et al. (1936), Pluvinage (1954), Russell and Rubinstein (1971) and the succinct account by McCormick (1966). The vascular malformations can be divided into the following simple groups: (1) capillary (telangiectasis), (2) cavernous, (3) venous, (4) arteriovenous, (5) Sturge–Weber disease.

## 1. Capillary telangiectasis

As the name implies, this is a focus of dilated capillaries, often so small as to be missed by casual inspection; to the naked eye it may resemble a petechial haemorrhage. The pons is the commonest site. Microscopical examination reveals aneurysmal and irregular dilatation of the abnormal capillaries. Adjacent arteries are normal, but Blackwood (1941) described enlargement of the relevant veins. Angiography is unlikely to display a telangiectasis because of its small size, but conceivably its venous drainage might be demonstrated. Interstitial calcareous deposits are not described by Russell and Rubinstein (1971), a point of radiological distinction from other forms of vascular hamartoma. The potential capacity to bleed is the only feature which may bring it into the neurosurgeon's field of work, but since these rare lesions are usually in the pons haemorrhage is commonly fatal.

## 2. Cavernous malformation (syn: cavernoma, cavernous angioma, angioma calcificans)

These vascular anomalies are probably more common than the above type, cover a wider range of sizes up to several centimetres in diameter and are more frequent in the cerebral hemispheres than elsewhere. They form discrete plum-coloured masses which comprise a sponge-like collection of irregular blood filled spaces and the surrounding tissue may be stained brown from old haemorrhage. They are firm to touch as a result of the organization of thrombus and often gritty. Microscopic examination shows intervening fibrous tissue, calcification (occasionally ossification), blood pigment and surrounding gliosis. The blood spaces of irregular shape and size have collagenous walls lined with endothelium. There is no enlargement of afferent or of efferent vessels. It is generally accepted that no brain parenchyma can be found separating the individual vascular elements, which distinguishes them from other vascular hamartomas. For Cushing and Bailey (1928) the absence of intervening cerebral tissue indicated their neoplastic nature, but this is not the present opinion. Their association with similar lesions elsewhere in the body and their relationship to telangiectasis and to haemangioblastoma were reviewed by Russell and Rubenstein (1971). In the cerebral hemisphere they may be subcortical with a particular frequency in the region of the central fissure, in the basal ganglia and may cause hydrocephalus by third ventricular obstruction; they may also be found on cranial nerves. Although the pathological findings show that minor local extravasations of blood are frequent, massive haemorrhage is an uncommon presentation. The neurosurgeon is more likely to encounter them as the focal cause of epilepsy, as a mass lesion mimicking a brain tumour or on account of hydrocephalus. Krayenbühl (1957) reported on 5 cases, occurring in a series of 77 supratentorial vascular malformations, which ran a short course with epilepsy and manifestations of an expanding lesion simulating a glioblastoma. Angiography revealed small spotty areas of contrast medium in the capillary phase. Finkemeyer and Kautsky (1968) described 3 cases involving the cavernous sinus. The angiograms showed irregular blotchy collections of contrast medium in the arterial phase and displacement of neighbouring arteries, an unusual appearance. Cavernomas can be seen on com-

puterized tomographic scans. Vaquero *et al.* (1983) report the appearances as showing a nodule which is slightly hyperdense, which does not enhance, but may contain areas of calcification. There is a hypodense area surrounding the lesion and there may be displacement suggesting a mass effect. Removal if situated in an accessible site has been advocated because of the small risk of haemorrhage (Vaquero *et al.* 1983) but care must be exercised when advocating an essentially prophylactic operation in a condition which is otherwise benign.

## 3. Venous malformations

These are uncommon and one may feel uncertain whether an abnormal leash of cortical veins or a large solitary vein merits the term malformation. In the older writings, some of the illustrations of lesions disclosed at craniotomy appear to be identical with arteriovenous lesions with which neurosurgeons are now very familiar. Papilloedema was present in 2 of the 5 cases recorded by Cushing and Bailey and it is difficult to reconcile this with a purely venous anomaly which is not situated so as to cause obstructive hydrocephalus. Russell (1954) questions 'as to whether pure venous malformations do in fact exist' because in her experience microscopic examination has constantly shown an arterial element, abnormal in size and structure. Angiography provides a method which demonstrates reliably in life an arterial component if present, either by showing abnormal arteries, or by the early filling of the relevant veins; a purely venous anomaly will appear synchronous with other cortical veins (Moniz & Guerra 1953). Pluvinage (1954) recorded 2 cases in which weakness of the leg appeared to be caused by an abnormal congeries of veins in the superior Rolandic region; weakness improved after their excision. An interesting case was reported by Robertson (1938) of an adult who since infancy had suffered from left sided fits and a mild left spastic hemiparesis with underdevelopment.

Ventriculography revealed a parietal diverticulum. Craniotomy over this area disclosed a mass of pial vessels, and this portion of the brain was resected down to the ventricle. Histological examination showed that the vascular anomaly consisted of veins and no abnormal vessels penetrated the cortex; the neurons were abnormal in number and their architecture was abnormal. This case underlines the observations of Bailey (1961) that vascular malformations may be accompanied by a maldevelopment of the adjacent brain tissue; this, as apparently in Robertson's case, may be the cause of neurological deficit rather than the vascular anomaly. Moniz considered that venous malformations were probably always associated with cerebral malformation. Other examples have been described by Wolfe and Brock (1935). When deeply situated they may be the cause of sudden intracerebral haemorrhage (Crawford & Russell 1956).

## 4. Arteriovenous malformations (syn: arterio-venous aneurysm)

These are the most common, and to the neurosurgeon, the most important of the vascular hamartomas. Their frequency relative to the other varieties cannot be accurately estimated because the latter are usually necropsy findings whereas the former are now diagnosed by computerized tomography and angiography and less frequently enter the records of a department of morbid anatomy. Berry *et al.* (1966) reported that during a period of 21 years there were 22 examples of telangiectasis (all by autopsy), 12 of cavernous (7 autopsy, 5 biopsy) and 58 of arteriovenous malformation (12 autopsy, 12 biopsy, 34 diagnosed by angiography). This probably represents too low a proportion of arteriovenous lesions; in large series of brain tumours they comprise between 2% and 7% (Zülch 1965). A preponderance amongst males is commonly reported (Krenchel 1961) but in the series analysed by the Cooperative Study (VI) the sexes were nearly equally represented.

Although they may occur in any part of the brain, about one-half arise in the territory of the middle cerebral artery and only about 5% lie in the posterior cranial fossa. The majority of those in the cerebral hemispheres occupy the surface of the brain forming a wedge-shaped mass with its apex reaching the wall of the ventricle, but the smallest lesions (to which further reference will be made) lie buried in a sulcus with little or no surface evidence of their presence or lie deep in the brain. The basal ganglia and brain stem are involved in about 10% and these form a small but clinically important group. Wyburn-Mason (1943) drew attention to certain brain stem vascular anomalies which can be traced forwards in the optic pathways to the retina and are accompanied by a cutaneous naevus of trigeminal distribution, a pattern determined embryologically.

The superficial aspect of an arteriovenous malformation presents a most impressive and unmistakable appearance when exposed at operation. A tangled mass of vessels of varying calibre; from its periphery greatly enlarged veins (a diameter of 1–2 cm is not uncommon) diverge to join the sagittal and lateral sinuses; the central portion pulsates vigorously. Careful inspection usually reveals that some of the thin walled apparent veins contain bright red blood; in some instances streams of arterial and of venous blood can be seen swirling unmixed in a vessel. In the central area the cortex may be covered by a felt-work of bright red vessels. Occasionally the loop of an important feeding artery may be detected, identified by its smooth rounded calibre and vigorous pulsation; more commonly they lie hidden in the sulci. The arachnoid is patchily thickened to form a white fibrous membrane which may be adherent to the overlying dura mater and may be directly involved in the vascular anomaly. For these reasons reflection of the dura mater demands great care in order to avoid the rupture of a vessel. At post-mortem examination the absence of distension and of pulsation renders the surface appearances relatively unimpressive. Section of the brain exposes the full extent of the lesion which often attains the wall of the ventricle. It

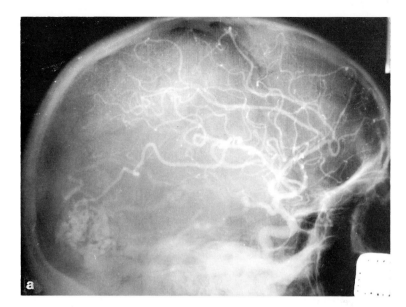

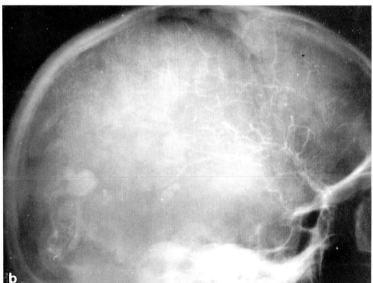

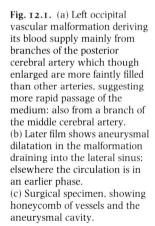

**Fig. 12.1.** (a) Left occipital vascular malformation deriving its blood supply mainly from branches of the posterior cerebral artery which though enlarged are more faintly filled than other arteries, suggesting more rapid passage of the medium: also from a branch of the middle cerebral artery.
(b) Later film shows aneurysmal dilatation in the malformation draining into the lateral sinus; elsewhere the circulation is in an earlier phase.
(c) Surgical specimen, showing honeycomb of vessels and the aneurysmal cavity.

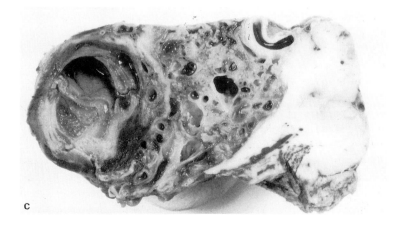

comprises a mass of closely packed vessels of irregular shape and size some of which are clearly arterial; their walls are firm and thick and retain a circular lumen. Aneurysmal cavities may be encountered (Fig. 12.1). The mass is generally firmer in consistency than the surrounding brain as a result of fibrosis; calcareous nodules may be palpable. Discoloration due to the altered blood of past haemorrhages permeates and surrounds the lesion and alongside there may be a haematoma or blood in the ventricles. The surrounding brain may be softened and contain small necrotic cavities; the involved cortex may be atrophied. Histological examination confirms the great variety of shape, size and structure of the vessels. Their walls show much distortion in the distribution and quantity of the various elements of muscle, elastic and fibrous tissue. The same vessel may in one area show all layers and in another little but endothelium and connective tissue. There may be large intraluminal projections of muscle or of endothelium; aneurysms develop; fibrosis, atheroma, thrombosis and mural calcification occur. Between the vessels and around the lesion there is evidence of old haemorrhage, fibrosis, gliosis and breakdown of myelin and of neuron.

Cushing and Bailey (1928) suggested that an arteriovenous hamartoma is determined in the second stage of development of the vascular system, when the primitive network of blood vessels begins to differentiate into arteries, capillaries and veins. A failure to form capillaries would leave arteries and veins in direct communication. As Kaplan *et al.* (1961) put it, the anomaly represents 'a perpetuation of a primitive arteriovenous communication, a shunt which normally would be replaced by an intervening capillary network'. The view frequently put forward, that absence of a capillary bed is primarily responsible for the complicated arteriovenous network as a result of the lack of capillary 'resistance' to blood flow is a misleading simplification. It ignores the all important physiological role played by the arterioles and precapillaries in providing the peripheral resistance. These must be involved in the mal-

development if a shunt is to form and the histological picture certainly supports the view that in addition to the absence of capillaries all vessels are structurally defective. The arteriovenous fistulous communication is proven by observations at operation, by the high oxygen content of the venous blood leaving the brain (Horton & Zeigler 1930), by the two- or threefold increase of total cerebral blood flow (Shenkin *et al.* 1948), by the increased regional blood flow (Häggendal *et al.* 1965, Feindel *et al.* 1965) and by angiography which reveals morphology and provides a means of measuring the speed of transit through the anomaly (Tönnis 1957). The fistulous nature of the lesion has important consequences. It is responsible for the frequency with which they bleed, for the development of aneurysms within the lesion, for the enlargement of the arteries which irrigate it and in consequence for the secondary development of saccular aneurysms not infrequently seen on those arteries, probably the results of increased and abnormal stress (Moniz and Guerra 1953, Anderson and Blackwood 1959). Saccular aneurysms are also seen on arteries not supplying the malformation but these may be no more than chance association (Boyd-Wilson 1959). The papilloedema which occasionally develops in the absence of bleeding or of obstructive hydrocephalus can be explained by a raised intracranial venous pressure and by increase in the size of the malformation as a result of the fistulae. Olivecrona and Riives (1948) and Potter (1955) have shown by angiography that expansion may occur over a period of time; Potter suggested that rupture of a vessel may aggravate the fistula. The arteriovenous shunt is also generally considered to be the cause of progressive intellectual deterioration which may manifest in some patients with very large lesions and also partly the cause of focal disturbances such as epilepsy and paresis. Using high speed serial angiography (4–6 exposures per second) Greitz (1956) found that although circulation time through the malformation was much reduced, in the rest of the brain it was within the upper limit of normal except in one patient who had recently suffered a haemorrhage. Computerized tomographic scanning may show ventricular dilatation, local under the lesion and sometimes general; the latter may be the result of longstanding elevated venous pressure, or of haemorrhage. There is certainly cortical atrophy, loss of neurons and gliosis in and adherent to the lesion. But to what extent this is due to anoxia from the shunt, to local pressure, repeated small haemorrhage (these lesions are rarely if ever free from such traces) and thrombosis is hardly susceptible of proof. It is likely that all factors play a part in producing brain damage in the region of the malformation; whether the fistulous lesion can cause a generalized deficiency of cerebral circulation leading to dementia is as yet unproven; such dementia as occurs can often be explained by the effect of local damage, which in large malformations covers a wide area, to which must be added the results of hydrocephalus, due to meningeal fibrosis from recurrent haemorrhage and to enlargement of the vein of Galen.

Kaplan et al. (1961) stressed the importance of the two venous systems, the superficial and the central or Galenical, in arteriovenous malformations. Where these are large and extend deeply, or are situated centrally, their drainage will largely flow along the transcerebral veins which are orientated towards the walls of the ventricles and along the basal veins, to the veins of Galen. These deep dilated veins, easily detectable by angiography, are significant for the assessment of the depth of the lesion, particularly if operation is contemplated and the fistulous portion is so small as to be dubious in the angiogram. Hydrocephalus due to distension of the great vein of Galen secondary to arteriovenous fistulae was mentioned in a case record by Jaeger et al. (1937) but to which attention was drawn by the important paper of Russel and Nevin (1940). A considerable number of cases has since been reported (Nayrac et al. 1956, Hirano & Terry 1958, Litvak et al. 1960). Aneurysm formation may be part of a general dilatation of the internal cerebral veins due to a distant but deeply extending malformation or it may be the more localized effect of an adjacent lesion (Fig. 12.2).

In a number of cases there has been no angiomatous malformation, but a congenital arteriovenous fistula between an anomalous branch usually of the posterior cerebral artery and the internal cerebral veins or the great vein itself; bilateral fistulae may be present (see also Padget 1956).

In common with arteriovenous fistulae elsewhere in the body (including caroticocavernous), an arteriovenous malformation in the brain may affect the cardiovascular system. In 1920, Schmitt remarked upon cardiac enlargement and hypertrophy of the left ventricle, a paper which Brock and Duke (1932) considered to be the first on the subject. Lewis and Drury (1923) investigated the physiological disturbances in 2 cases of limb arteriovenous fistulae consequent upon battle injury sustained in the war of 1914–19. Detailed investigations in 8 cases of cerebral arteriovenous malformation have been described by Kauntze and McGill (1962). The shunt lowers the peripheral resistance and to compensate for the consequent fall in blood pressure there is an increase in the cardiac output and in the blood volume and an arteriolar constriction. In the 8 cases, low blood pressure was recorded in 3, high cardiac output in 4, left ventricular hypertrophy in 7, tachycardia in 1, collapsing pulse in 3 and a raised jugular venous pressure in 2. Intellectual deterioration had occurred in 3 of these patients, and the authors discuss the part played by impairment of the cerebral circulation, to which an earlier reference was made. It is possible that the cardiovascular effects are as important as the local shunt in impoverishing the cerebral circulation.

### Cerebral blood flow

Arteriovenous malformations have a low vascular resistance, resulting in high flow through the malformation and stealing the blood from the higher resistance capillary bed in the adjacent brain. Häggendal et al. (1965) using intraarterial Xenon found a large peak of activity in the primary curve representing the rapid passage

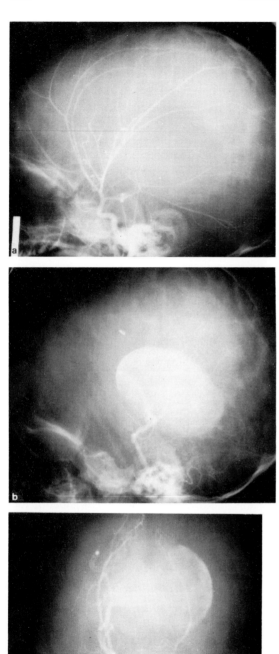

**Fig. 12.2.** Aneurysms of vein of Galen. Female aged 4 months: enlargement of the head noticed for 3 weeks: routine AEG indicated a centrally placed lesion causing obstructive hydrocephalus.

(a) Carotid angiogram reveals typical pattern of arteries in hydrocephalus. (b) Vertebral angiograms show large centrally placed aneurysm fed by (c) an enlarged branch of the posterior cerebral artery which is much larger than the left. The artery appears to be in direct fistulous communication with the aneurysm, the medium dispersing fanwise within it. The two posterior cerebral arteries are widely separated by the sac. Operative treatment: (1) ventriculocaval shunt (2) occlusion of fistula. (By courtesy of Mr T. T. King.)

of blood through the shunt. Assessment of the blood flow deep to the malformation suggested that it came from the contralateral carotid artery which therefore supports the underlying brain. Abolition of the initial peak per- or postoperatively suggests that the fistula has been controlled (Häggendal *et al.* 1965, Feindel *et al.* 1971).

More recently assessment of local cerebral blood flow has become more accurate using Xenon-enhanced computerized tomographic scanning (Okabe *et al.* 1983). This reveals low flow adjacent to the arteriovenous malformation which correlates well with progressive or fluctuating neurophysiological deficits. After removal of the malformation the local flows both in grey and white matter return to normal levels.

Defective autoregulation in the area around a malformation can result in a swollen haemorrhagic brain at operation when the lesion is removed and blood flow to the surrounding brain is increased. This has been termed 'normal perfusion breakthrough' (Spetzler *et al.* 1978) and is discussed below in the section on treatment.

## Clinical manifestations

### Haemorrhage

Haemorrhage is the commonest first symptom of an arteriovenous malformation, the incidence varying between 40% (Krenchel 1961) to 60% (Report of Cooperative Study VI). Bleeding is not invariable in the course of the disease, but occurs in upwards of 80%. In sharp contrast to the haemorrhage due to the rupture of an aneurysm, the peak incidence occurs in youth. The Co-operative Study (VI) found it to be between the ages of 15 and 20 years, though the first haemorrhage may happen throughout the full range of life; 72% of all first haemorrhage had occurred by the age of 40 years. That intracranial haemorrhage in a young person is most likely to be due to an angiomatous malformation has of course been recognized and emphasized for many years (Jefferson 1948) although only recently

have large numbers proved the point. As in aneurysmal disease, bleeding is likely to recur, but unlike it the mortality is much lower, for the primary and for subsequent haemorrhages and the recurrences are widely spaced in time. Svien and McRae (1965) found the mortality of the first haemorrhage to be only 6% and the figure was the same for subsequent haemorrhages; somewhat similar figures were reported by Henderson and Gomez (1967) and in the 2 series the ultimate mortality from haemorrhage was 12% and 19% respectively. The Cooperative Study (VI) showed that the mortality from the haemorrhage for which the patient was admitted was 10%. Henderson and Gomez noted that the interval between recurrent haemorrhages was less than 6 weeks in only 13% and from 5 to 26 years in 30%.

Haemorrhage may occur into and remain restricted within the white matter to form an intracerebral haematoma; it may leak into the ventricle, or it may be primarily intraventricular and blood appears in the subarachnoid spaces. Unlike a ruptured aneurysm, primary subarachnoid haemorrhage and subdural haematoma are rare. The latter occurred in 3 of the 110 cases of Paterson and McKissock (1956). Head injury or physical effort may both precipitate haemorrhage; these factors were present in 6% and 16% respectively in Krenchel's series. The recognition of a vascular malformation causing intracranial haemorrhage after a head injury has forensic importance. Focal signs, for example motor or sensory paresis, dysphasia, hemianopia, are more common when haemorrhage results from a vascular malformation than when it is due to an aneurysm, probably because of the frequent location of the lesion in the territory of the middle cerebral artery. About 50% of the patients in the Cooperative Study (VI) sustained neurological deficits as a result of the first haemorrhage. Infarction, adjacent and remote and narrowing of arteries in the angiograms, so characteristic of aneurysmal rupture, are rare. This, the absence of damage to central and basal parts of the brain, except where tentorial herniation occurs, and the usually less severe degree of bleeding, account for the lower mortality. The prognosis for recovery from neurological deficits is relatively good.

*Epilepsy*

Epilepsy is next in frequency as a first symptom (incidence 36% Krenchel, 23% Cooperative Study VI) and develops sooner or later in about half the patients. When it is the first symptom it usually occurs at a somewhat earlier age than does bleeding as a first symptom. As might be anticipated, the incidence of epilepsy is much higher in malformations involving the cortex than in the deeply situated ones and is highest in those situated in the centroparietal region, reaching 86% in the experience of Tönnis (1957). The seizures may be focal or generalized or both; McKenzie (1953) found that at some time or other focal seizures nearly always occurred.

*Headache*

Headache of a migrainous type occurs in perhaps a fifth of the patients and for many years may prove to be the only complaint. The pain is of a severe throbbing nature, commonly affecting only one side of the head, usually that on which the lesion is situated and lasting many hours. Visual hallucinations and transient paresis of visual function are common. In a case recorded by Northfield (1940) a man aged 52 years had experienced severe migraine for 37 years. The headache was usually heralded by a scotoma scintillans and in later years was sometimes accompanied by dysphasia, loss of power in the right arm, and loss of consciousness; the patient finally developed a partial right homonymous hemianopia. Angiography revealed a vascular malformation in the territory of the left middle cerebral artery. McKenzie, amongst whose patients there were several with a similarly long history of migraine, considered that a distinction could be made from 'idiopathic' migraine by the

constancy with which the headache and its accompaniments affected the one side and by the longer duration of the accompaniments. It is said that migrainous headache is more common with occipital lesions and that the 'flashing lights' of a visual hallucination are synchronous with the heart beat (Dimsdale 1957). Headache of a more generalized and banal character is a frequent complaint and may be related to increased venous pressure. When haemorrhage occurs the headache is sudden and violent and has been fully described in the section on ruptured aneurysm. Raised intracranial pressure from obstructive hydrocephalus may also be a cause of headache.

*Hemiparesis*

Hemiparesis of a slowly progressive nature, developing over a course of a number of years is a not infrequent symptom. It is rarely accompanied by sensory disturbance and is generally found in large malformations about the centroparietal region and in those involving basal ganglia or brain stem. There may be hypoplasia of the affected side, indicating that the hemiparesis originated in childhood. The absence of episodic worsening of the paresis shows that in these patients recurrent haemorrhage is not the cause; it is attributed to the local ischaemia induced by the shunt and to increase in the size of the lesion. Hemianopia may develop in a similar manner and the patient may be quite unaware of the defect. Recurrent transient hemiparesis which does not fully recover also occurs, the result of small haemorrhages and of thrombosis and softening.

*Psychosis*

Impairment of mental function, in the form of intellectual deterioration or disorders of a neurotic or psychotic nature, is encountered to a slight degree fairly frequently, to a severe degree uncommonly and in these the lesion is usually large. Krenchel found mental changes more frequent when the dominant hemisphere was affected, in the proportion of 17–10 in 150 patients. The reported incidence of mental changes varies between 7% (Potter 1955) and 50% (Tönnis 1961). Discrepancies must be due to the adoption of different criteria for assessment.

Frank psychosis may occur in cases with frontal malformations. Parkinson and Bachers (1980) reported a 14% incidence in these cases.

*Bruit and other vascular signs*

The presence of a bruit in the head, occasionally audible to the patient, is a useful sign in the small number of cases in which it is present. Taken with the history and any other physical signs it provides an immediate clue to the diagnosis. It is usually most audible when auscultation is made over the eye, the temple, or directly over the lesion; it is rarely loud and not comparable in that respect with a caroticocavernous fistula. It may be heard only with the patient in a particular position (for example sitting up or recumbent) and only after exertion. Although a cranial bruit may be heard in other conditions (for example raised intracranial pressure in children, highly vascular tumours situated close to or in the skull, severe anaemia) these are on other counts usually distinctive. The absence of a bruit is not significant.

Physical examination may reveal signs of which the patient is unaware. In children the head may be enlarged. There may be abnormal vascularity of the scalp and face sometimes amounting to a 'cirsoid aneurysm'; excessive pulsation, enlargement and even tortuosity of the carotid arteries in the neck may be detected. Wadia (1960) described rapid filling of the external jugular vein, when emptied by expressing its contents. A port-wine naevus may be found on the face. Papilloedema may be present; in some patients this may be obviously the result of recent haemorrhage, or may prove explicable on the basis of an obstructive site of the lesion. Occasion-

ally no such explanation is admissable and the fundal changes must be attributed to the malformation, the effect of its bulk or of raised intracranial venous pressure secondary to the vascular shunt. In these the swelling of the disc is rarely severe, the veins are enlarged and tortuous and may be seen to pulsate and visual acuity is unaffected. A retinal vascular malformation may be seen. Optic atrophy has been described, due to pressure on the nerve and chiasma by abnormal vascular tissue (Hobbs 1957). There may be proptosis, nonpulsatile, on one or both sides. Signs of focal damage to the affected cerebral hemisphere are frequent and were present in 70% of the series recorded by Paterson and McKissock (1956). The syndromes produced by vascular malformations in the brain stem and cerebellum and by those involving the great vein of Galen will be given consideration later. The remote cardiovascular effects have been described.

In a small group of cases Northfield (1940) noted that those which presented with headache and epilepsy and those presenting with haemorrhage appeared to form distinct groups. This has been confirmed in that haemorrhage is more frequently an initial symptom in small angiomatous malformations, which are less likely by reason of size or situation to give rise to headache or to epilepsy. Krenchel divided his cases into those in which the lesion was small (less than 3 cm in diameter), intermediate and large (greater than 6 cm in diameter). There were 70 small lesions and of these 55 (80%) had bled and 14 (20%) had caused epilepsy; there were 27 large, of which 7 (26%) had bled and 18 (67%) had caused epilepsy. This aspect of the natural history of angiomatous malformations has been illuminated by the increasing recognition of the frequency with which intracerebral haemorrhage, in particular in young people, is caused by one of these small lesions. Special attention was drawn to this subject by Margolis *et al.* (1951) and by Crawford and Russell (1956). The latter reported 20 cases, in 15 of which the age was below 20 years; in 10 the hamartoma was in the cerebral hemisphere, in 4 in the basal ganglia and in 6 in the cerebellum (a much higher incidence than of vascular hamartomas in general). The clinical picture was one either of sudden apoplexy which was often rapidly fatal within hours, or with a slower time course so that the possibility of brain abscess or rapidly growing tumour entered the differential diagnosis. Crawford and Russell emphasized again the point made by others (Hawkins & Rewell 1946) that in these cases the vascular anomaly may well be so small as to escape detection, in the angiogram, at operation and post-mortem; for this reason they designated them 'cryptic'. The walls of the cavity created by the haematoma need careful scrutiny and the blood clot should be searched, for the force of the bleeding may detach the lesion and often destroys it. The majority are arteriovenous; examples of the other varieties of vascular hamartoma have been reported but histological diagnosis may be uncertain when the available fragment of tissue is very small. (*See also* Gerlach & Jensen 1961, Courville 1963, Krayenbühl & Seibenmann 1965).

*Brain stem involvement*

Vascular malformations of the brain stem deserve special mention because they present a clinical pattern different from those in the cerebral hemispheres. Their age incidence and liablity to haemorrhage is not peculiar but they rarely cause epilepsy; their chief feature is the production of motor and sensory long tract signs, in conjunction with irregular cranial nerve palsies, nystagmus, ataxia and tremor. Trigeminal neuralgia is an unexpected and interesting feature in a small proportion of cases. The disease follows a fluctuating course, rapid exacerbation being followed by slow partial recovery. Unlike a malformation in the basal ganglia the hemiparesis may alternate from side to side and exacerbation may be accompanied by vertigo and vomiting and additional cranial nerve involvement. Headache and neck stiffness in an acute attack signifies subarachnoid haemor-

rhage, but often these symptoms are absent and the episode is attributable, as in lesions elsewhere, to small haemorrhages confined within the parenchyma or to infarction. The progressive nature of the illness, the absence of rasied intracranial pressure and the pattern of the physical signs usually suggest a glioma of the brain stem, but an episodic course with relative recovery often leads to a diagnosis of multiple sclerosis, while the initial attack may resemble a mesencephalic encephalitis. The condition might be mistaken for atheroma of the basilar artery but the age groups are dissimilar. An important diagnostic point is made by Logue and Monckton (1954) that in some patients the history of the disorder may be of many years' duration, without any attack of subarachnoid haemorrhage. This was so in 2 of their cases, the history dating back 15 years; in both the diagnosis was confirmed by angiography. Walter and Bischoff (1966) have analysed a large series. Reference has been made to the rare subgroup described by Wyburn-Mason (1943), distinguished by the combination of brain stem signs with a vascular anomaly within the eye, exophthalmos and facial naevus. There may be highly organized dream-like hallucinations such as Lhermitte (1932) described from lesions in the vicinity of the peduncles.

*Cerebellum*

In the series of 'cryptic hamartomas' described by Crawford and Russell 6 of the 20 cases were situated in the cerebellum, a high proportion compared with the distribution in the brain of vascular malformations as a whole. Three of these patients died very rapidly from sudden haemorrhage. In the others the illness evolved relatively slowly, lasting 4 months in one patient and presenting the typical features of obstructive hydrocephalus with signs of cerebellar disorder. This epitomizes the clinical picture which may result from involvement of the cerebellum. Infarction of the cerebellum may produce a similar clinical picture (Norris *et al.* 1969).

In a review by Walter *et al.* (1967) of posterior fossa vascular malformations (including those in the brain stem) the high incidence of papilloedema (in two-thirds of the cases) and of obstructive hydrocephalus is underlined. Trigeminal neuralgia occurred in 11%, presumably attributable to a brain stem location.

## Diagnosis

The ease and accuracy of clinical diagnosis will depend upon whether the patient presents with the picture of intracranial haemorrhage or not. The diagnosis of this condition has already been discussed in the section on aneurysms. The Cooperative Study (V part I) found that vascular malformations were the cause of 6% of their cases of subarachnoid haemorrhage. This is probably an underestimate of the percentage of intracranial haemorrhage, because about 10% of haemorrhages from malformations do not reach the spinal fluid (Paterson & McKissock 1956). The distinctive feature of this cause of spontaneous intracranial haemorrhage is its frequency in young people, threequarters of the first attacks taking place before the age of 40 years. Although malformations are commoner in patients presenting aged 25 years or less, aneurysms remain the commonest cause even in this age group. A haemorrhage which has produced crisp focal signs of cerebral damage with little or no general cerebral disturbance, for instance brief unconsciousness, little or no obfuscation, is likely to be due to malformation. A past history of previous haemorrhage, which sometimes masquerades under the diagnosis of 'meningitis' of epilepsy and of hemicranial pain and the external stigmata of vascular malformation will be of great value. Sudden massive intracerebral haemorrhage, apoplexy, in a child or young person is very likely to be due to a vascular anomaly provided there is no history suggestive of blood dyscrasia. Evolution in some cases has a more subacute character and must be distinguished from brain abscess and cystic tumour. Where haemorrhage is not the presenting illness, a careful enquiry may elicit a history of past symptoms, sometimes many years earlier, suggestive of haemorrhage or meningitis. Since bleeding occurs at some time or another in some 80% of cases, this item in the history is of great diagnostic importance. Fits and headaches are banal symptoms of tumour, the usual alternative diagnosis, but the headaches of raised intracranial pressure due to a tumour are rarely consistently unilateral and rarely persist for years without papilloedema. The differential diagnosis of central and of brainstem angiomatous malformations has already been considered. To entertain the diagnosis leads to a search for confirmatory signs, however insignificant they may seem; facial naevus, enlarged scalp vessels, slight proptosis and bruit are those which are frequently overlooked.

## Investigations

Radiological examination of the skull reveals abnormality in about a quarter of the cases. There may be greatly increased diploic channels and enlarged or newly formed emissary foramina, excessive grooving by sphenoparietal, superior sagittal sinuses and by meningeal vessels. In the base of the skull there may be enlargement of the foramina spinosa, the carotid canals and the jugular foramina. Hoare (1953) drew attention to the importance in posterior fossa malformations of enlargement of the jugular foramina and of grooving of the arch of the atlas and enlargement of the foramina of the cervical vertebral transverse processes by hypertrophied vertebral arteries. Pathological deposits of calcification are visible in about a quarter of the cases (Paterson & McKissock). This is rarely marked, as may be the case in some gliomas and usually consists of fairly dense, homogenous irregular spotty deposits, perhaps only one; occasionally it may have a sinuous shape suggesting the course of a vessel, but this should not be confused with the opacities seen in Sturge–Weber disease. Occasionally the calcification is curvilinear and lies within the wall of an aneurysm in the lesion or of the great vein of Galen.

Static or dynamic isotope scanning reveals an area of high activity but is not diagnostic. The first line investigation of choice is now computerized tomographic scanning, which can detect smaller amounts of pathological calcification than are visible on plain skull radiographs. In addition there may be evidence of haemorrhage, hydrocephalus and areas of altered density which may be either hypo- or hyperdense. Contrast enhancement may show serpiginous vessels supplying or draining the fistula. Because of the varied appearances care must always be taken in the interpretation of the computerized tomographic scan (Foy et al. 1981). Air encephalography has no place now, though prior to computerized scanning it was used in the search for causes of epilepsy. However it was often normal, it being rare that an arteriovenous malformation causes irregularity or displacement of the ventricular wall. In cases where hydrocephalus was suspected clinically, ventriculography was to be preferred particularly as it was potentially less risky.

Angiography is an essential investigation and if excision of the malformation is under consideration it should be pursued thoroughly until full information is obtained of the situation and extent and of feeding and draining vessels (Fig. 12.1). This may be achieved by injecting separately both external and internal carotids, and frequently requires bilateral vertebral examination in addition. Small frontal lesions may be in the territory of a single enlarged branch of one anterior cerebral artery; large posteriorly placed examples may receive blood from the major branches of both cerebral hemispheres and from the vertebral arteries. Where there are signs of abnormal vascularity of the scalp or skull it is a wise precaution separately to examine the external carotid system. If the arteriovenous shunt is copious, the draining veins may be so large and may fill so early that they obscure the malformation and in these rapid serial angiography is necessary; also in showing the minute malformations which may be missed by ordinary

techniques in which the timing of the exposures may happen not to synchronize with the passage of contrast through the abnormal vessels. Stereo-angiograms may be of help in planning treatment in that it may allow easier identification of the feeding vessels (Parkinson & Bachers 1980). Driesen (1968) re-examined the films of 50 cases of spontaneous cerebral haemorrhage in young persons, in which originally no causative lesion had been detected; careful scrutiny revealed a minute vascular anomaly in 5; the abnormality only comprised a small abnormal artery and 'early filling' vein.

Vessel displacements will reveal a haematoma and a saccular aneurysm may be present, which may be the cause of haemorrhage rather than the malformation. It is interesting in this context to note that the narrowing of vessels often seen in aneurysmal rupture usually called spasm and attributed by some to a spasmogenic substance in effused blood, is rarely seen in the angiograms of recently ruptured angiomatous lesions and then at the periphery of a haematoma where it is accepted as the effect of compression.

Occasionally it may be difficult to distinguish a vascular anomaly from the abnormal vascularity of tumours, usually the glioblastoma multiforme and the meningioma. Points to look for are: hypertrophy of a feeding artery, unusual except in malformation; great irregularity in calibre and in course in glioblastoma, while in malformation the vessels run a smoothly sinuous irregularity; the diffuse capillary shadow (blush) characteristic of a meningioma is rarely seen. Tumours displace major vessels in the vicinity but this only occurs with malformation if a haematoma is present.

## Natural history

As in the case of saccular aneurysms, surgical treatment should be viewed against the background of the natural history of the disease. The formation of a haematoma within the brain which endangers life demands operative relief, though when massive the situation may be irretrievable and death occurs within 24 hours. But this happens in relatively few cases for as noted earlier the mortality from the first haemorrhage is about 6% and from recurrence up to twice that figure.

Svien and McRae (1965) and Henderson and Gomez (1967) have made valuable studies of the natural history of angiomatous malformations, patients having been observed over periods of up to 46 years after the onset of symptoms. In these two surveys 16% and 22% respectively died from causes directly related to the lesion, usually haemorrhage. In many of these the malformation was in a situation or of a size judged at that time to be unsuitable for excision; Svien and McRae considered that polar lesions were suitable for excision but these constituted only 18% of their series. In the series of Henderson and Gomez 13 of the 15 malformations which ultimately caused the death of the patient were judged then to be unsuitable for removal. Svien and McRae present an analysis in epochs of five years of the quality of survival; the category 'good' comprised patients who were working and had but minor symptoms and in the first 5 years of follow-up they included 75%; in the epoch 15–19 years the proportion had only fallen to 68%. The corresponding proportions of invalids were 1% and 7% respectively. The authors of both these series consider that in about 80% of cases, nonoperative treatment is appropriate but that prompt evacuation of a haematoma is necessary and the excision of the vascular malformation should be undertaken at the same time if practical. Graf et al. (1983) analysed the risks in 2 groups of patients with arteriovenous malformations; 57 presenting with an unruptured lesion and 134 following rupture. In those with an unruptured malformation, 74% of whom presented with epilepsy, the average yearly risk of rupture was 2.3%. In males there was a higher risk during the first year but the females were at greater risk by 10 years. This difference had averaged out by 20 years. In the few presenting without epilepsy the risk of haemorrhage was higher; 17% by 5 years and 45% by 10 years. Small malformations (3 cm or less) were more

likely to rupture than large ones both at one year (0% v. 10%) and at 5 years (10% v. 52%). Though caution must be exercised in interpreting such small numbers, these figures do give some valuable help in assessing the risk in a patient presenting with an unruptured malformation. In those who present after rupture and haemorrhage from the lesion, the risk of further haemorrhage overall in the first year is 6% and thereafter 2% per annum. Factors occurring at the time of the first haemorrhage which were likely to indicate a higher risk were the presence of an intracerebral haematoma and the neurological grade of the patient; grade II had the earliest rebleeds whilst in grade III the risk was less than 1% over the first 15 years. The other risk factor was advancing age, irrespective of the actual age at presentation. There was no correlation between the size of the malformation and its propensity to rehaemorrhage.

In reviewing the natural history, Wilkins (1985) reported a risk of bleeding of 2–3% per annum with 1% mortality in previously ruptured malformations. After haemorrhage had occured, however, there was a 6% risk of recurrent bleeding in the survivors during the first years, dropping to 2–3% in subsequent years. The mortality for the second haemorrhage was 13%. Initial life survival analysis of 217 patients with arteriovenous malformations presenting to the Mersey Regional Unit over a 30 year period and managed nonsurgically reveals a similar risk of haemorrhage or rehaemorrhage: 42% during the 20 years after diagnosis (Crawford et al. 1986). This risk was increased in those presenting with haemorrhage and in the elderly and was reduced in the young and in those with a nonhaemorrhagic presentation or a malformation involving the parietal lobe. The initial mortality at diagnosis was 4% but though 29% were dead at 20 years only two-thirds of the deaths were related to the malformation. Haemorrhage from the malformation did not increase the risk of death but arteriovenous malformations in the parietal lobe were less likely to be fatal than those at other sites. Six per cent had a major neurological disability at the time of diagnosis but though over 20 years 27% developed a neurological deficit only one sixth of these new deficits rendered the patient dependent. The risks of developing *de novo* epilepsy after diagnosis was 18% over 20 years. There is the occasional report of an arteriovenous malformation which has undergone spontaneous regression (Nehls & Pittman 1982).

## Treatment

The objective is to prevent further haemorrhage, to eliminate further damage to the brain from ischaemia and compression, to relieve raised intracranial pressure and to cure epilepsy. Migrainous headache is often abolished by excision of the lesion, though this symptom rarely if ever qualifies as an indication for treatment.

The danger to life from haemorrhage, taking all cases into consideration, is not nearly so great as in aneurysms; the indication for excision is less compelling nor is it so urgent (except in massive haematoma) because recurrence of bleeding takes place at much longer intervals. That haemorrhage occurs more frequently from the smaller lesions and in the young, in whom the cerebral vessels are likely to be healthy, makes excision generally less hazardous than occluding an aneurysm. Unfortunately these hopeful generalizations are modified by the preponderant localization of malformations in the territory of the middle cerebral artery. 'The principal problem is not the technique of excision but whether it can be done without important neurological sequelae' (Jefferson 1948). When excision is deemed necessary because of the risk to life from bleeding, then even a severe neurological deficit may be justified. Excision in order to insure the patient against a future hemiparesis or against the worsening of an existing one is a failure if it leaves the patient hemiparetic. The indications for the surgical treatment of epilepsy are discussed in Chapter 17. The seizures due to a vascular malformation are usually sufficiently controlled by medication as to render operation unnecessary. It is an axiom in the surgery of

epilepsy that operation should not inflict a physical disability. This principle excludes many cases of malformation (if epilepsy is the sole or major reason for excision) because seizures have a high incidence in the centroparietal lesions; polar lesions are suitable and in particular those which occur in the temporal lobe. Paterson and McKissock (1956) found that about 44% of those patients who had suffered from epilepsy before excision, were improved or relieved of this symptom.

In which vascular malformations is excision likely to prove feasible? Those affecting the poles of the cerebral hemispheres can usually be extirpated by modified lobectomy. Those up to 3–4 cm in diameter on the convexity, the medial and the inferior surfaces of the hemispheres, can usually be excised without great difficulty, except those which impinge upon or involve the pre- and postcentral gyri and the 'speech areas'. Small deeply placed lesions and those in the cerebellum, in which the indication for operation is usually a lifethreatening haematoma, should be excised; fortunately the haematoma has often carried out part of the dissection for the surgeon.

Excision of large malformations (5 cm and over) is rarely practical if they involve middle cerebral territory, the basal ganglia and if they communicate with several major arteries. Although it has been suggested that the brain closely applied to such malformations is not functional, thus allowing excision provided that the operator stays very close to the malformation, only recurrent massive bleeding is likely to force the decision and this event is uncommon. Extension of anomalous vessels into the ventricle, the choroid plexus and the brain stem is a contraindication to excision in any case; the angiographic examination should make this clear. In judging the size of the malformation, attention should be paid to the tangle of vessels which constitutes the arteriovenous core and not to the superficial draining veins which though possibly enormous are relatively unimportant. Specially timed films may be necessary in order to distinguish the essential part of the lesion. Great distension of deep veins, particularly the internal cerebral, is important in suggesting a deeper extension than might have been thought likely and which may render total excision dangerous or impossible. However, others (Kunc 1974) argue that arteriovenous malformations situated in the centre of the speech and sensorimotor cortex are resectable because these functions do not reside in the malformation and the vessels supplying it do not supply the functional cortex. Size is not a contraindication provided there is good demarcation of the edges of the malformation. Luessenhop and Rosa (1984) feel that overall the surgical risk is now less than that of the natural history in 65–75% of all patients with an arteriovenous malformation. In their view, only in those patients who are past their fourth decade, who are grade III or worse and have an extensive malformation are the risks of surgery unacceptable. Spetzler and Martin (1986) have proposed a six-point grading system for arteriovenous malformations, based upon size, venous drainage pattern, and the identifiable neurological function in adjacent brain. This has been used to predict the operative mortality for a particular malformation. Shi and Chen (1986) have used a four-point grading system, based upon size, location and depth, arterial supply and venous drainage.

As in the case of aneurysms, judicious use of induced arterial hypotension, preoperative steroids, hypothermia and shrinkage of the brain by intravenous osmotic agents have greatly assisted the surgeon in this field of surgery. The youth of the patient and of the arteries, the absence in most cases of basal brain damage by bleeding and by infarction, renders him a much better subject for these helpful ancillary techniques and they are in general use. The steps in the operation are, first, to identify the hypertrophied feeding artery and to follow it without damaging its normal branches until, by the sudden local increase in vascularity of the brain and by guidance from the angiograms, the point of junction with the abnormal core of vessels has been reached. The feeding artery, now usually an abormal branch of the enlarged parent trunk, is divided between clips or silk ligatures. Other feeding arteries are similarly dealt with. At this stage, if all important arteries have been divided there will be a notable shrinkage in the mass and in the surface veins in which the colour of the blood will have changed from red to dark purple. The largest arterial stump is now used as a pedicle and the arteriovenous mass is gently dissected from its bed. Great care is necessary to maintain close contact with the plane around the malformation; if abnormal vessels are left behind they are likely to cause a subsequent and frequently fatal haemorrhage. The final step is the division of the large veins, superficial and deep; if these are occluded too soon there will be great engorgement and a high risk of rupture. The degree to which encroachment upon functionally eloquent areas of cortex will result in important neurological deficits is to some extent unpredictable. On the whole, more liberties can be taken in these dissections than in those for glioma and a greater recovery of function can be anticipated. It may be due to the presence of healthy brain in the immediate vicinity, to which there is improvement in the circulation as a result of the abolition of the shunt. Immediately adjacent brain damaged by ischaemia and by minor haemorrhage is functionless and dissection through this zone need not inflict further damage (Kunc 1974). Meticulous attention to the dissection and the use of considerable hypotension has in recent years led to a more radical surgical approach to these cases; experience has shown that it is sometimes possible to remove lesions from eloquent areas of cortex with little or no disability (Kunc 1965, Walter & Brock 1966). Deep malformations may be more easily located at surgery using a pulsed Doppler echo technique (Nornes et al. 1979), thus facilitating the planning of the cortical incision and identification of the vessels involved.

In only about half the cases diagnosed is excision of the lesion carried out; the proportion is higher in those malformations that have bled than in the others. In the Cooperative Study VI, operation was performed for 20% of the non-bleeding malformations and for nearly 60% of those that had bled; the majority of these operations were excisions. The mortality rate for excision varies from series to series, lying between 4% (McKissock & Hankinson 1957) and 11% (Cooperative Study VI). It is somewhat higher than the average if an intracerebral haematoma is present; not because this makes excision technically more difficult, indeed often the reverse is true, but because of the disturbances secondary to the haematoma, which may render the patient unfit for an operation; this was so in 10% of the patients of Krenchel, admitted with an intracerebral haematoma. They died within 24 hours. The late results of excision are good. A few patients died later; some from further haemorrhage presumably due to incomplete excision, others from intercurrent infection consequent upon invalidism and from unrelated causes. In the series of 68 patients of McKissock and Hankinson treated by excision, 3 died shortly after the operation; 6 died later and 56 were leading normal working lives (86% of those surviving the operation). Vasospasm is very rare but recently defective autoregulation has been recognized as being the cause of swollen haemorrhagic brain (termed normal perfusion pressure breakthrough by Spetzler *et al.* 1978) which may occur (Mullen 1983) when the haemodynamic state is converted from a high flow low resistance situation in the presence of the malformation to a lower flow high resistance state following its removal. This inability of the feeding vessels to adjust their calibre rapidly following the haemodynamic change is more common with increasing age and the larger the diameter of the vessel (Garretson 1979). It has been suggested that the phenomenon of normal perfusion pressure breakthrough can be controlled by high dose barbiturate anaesthesia, controlled ventilation, blood pressure control, steroids, osmotic diuretics and late removal of any haematomas (Day *et al.* 1982). An alternative approach might be to remove arteriovenous malformations, particularly large ones, in multiple stages using both embolization (*see* below) and resection. This might allow some degree of autoregulation to return to surrounding vasculature (Solomon & Michelsen 1984).

What alternatives are available for cases unsuitable for excision? Any technique which is to be successful in the long term must result in filling up or removing the low resistance sink at the heart of the malformation, for failure to achieve this will just result in other feeding vessels opening up to supply the sink. Carotid ligation has been tried in a number of cases. Owing to the unpredictable course of the disease particularly with regard to the long interval that may occur before recurrence of haemorrhage, its value on this score is difficult to assess. Its success in diminishing the arteriovenous shunt is as poor as for caroticocavernous fistula, and for similar reasons; there are disadvantages, for permanent hemiplegia may follow ligations (Olivecrona 1950). Occlusion of the individual feeding arteries, close to the malformation is favoured by some surgeons. On theoretical grounds, judging by the model of the caroticocavernous fistula, this is likely to be permanently successful only if the malformation can be entirely excluded from the arterial side of the circulation. In practice, this operation is desirable for the large or deeply placed lesions unsuitable for excision, yet in these the feeding arteries are usually multiple and sometimes inaccessible. Although angiography performed immediately after occlusion of some of these vessels may show the lesion to be smaller or less dense, when this is repeated years later the shunt may be as copious as ever, in keeping with the known malign influences of arteriovenous communications. This form of treatment does not insure against recurrent bleeding; Paterson and McKissock (1956) found that carotid ligation had some success in reducing the frequency of fits, and that it abolished the migraine in 2 patients, the only patients of those treated in this way who had suffered migrainous headaches, an observation of considerable interest. They had not known the operation to be followed by any adverse effects. In recent years highly ingenious techniques of artifical embolization have been evolved in an attempt to occlude the arteriovenous communications and the feeding vessels (Luessenhop & Spence 1960, Luessenhop *et al.* 1965). Initally plastic or silicone rubber spheres enclosing a metal ball for radiological identification, in a range of diameters of from 1.0 mm to 6.0 mm were used. The appropriate size was chosen in accordance with the size of the enlarged feeding vessels and was introduced into the internal carotid artery; their progress and lodgement were observed radiologically. Postoperative major intracerebral haemorrhage, however, has been described following embolization using silastic spheres (Kvam et al. 1980). More recently other materials have been used to embolize including muscle, polyvicryl alcohol foam and oxidized cellulose. With the advent of improved flexible balloon catheters which can be 'floated' into distal cerebral arterial branches (Vinuela et al. 1983) the possibility now exists of allowing the relatively safe injection of a polymerising substance such as isobutyl-2-cyanoacrylate directly into the malformation (Samson et al. 1981, Debrun et al. 1982). In addition, this technique can be used at open operation, when it may be combined with surgical excision. Satisfactory results have been reported even in the absence of complete obliteration of the malformation (Kusse & Kelly 1974, Debrun et al. 1982) though others (Wolpert 1982) found no effect upon seizures or the progression or incidence of focal neurological signs. Only longterm follow up will resolve this. Neurological deficits may result from direct injection of the polymerizing agent into normal cerebral vessels or leakage away from the malformation into normal vessels. There is as yet no information concerning the longterm risks of these materials in man (Debrun et al. 1982). Isobutyl-2-cyanoacrylate, injected into the peritoneal cavity of the rodent, results in neoplastic change (Samson 1986). At the present time, in the UK, this agent can be used for injection into a cerebral AVM only on a named patient basis.

Radiotherapy has been employed in the past from time to time by most surgeons in cases unsuitable for operation. The decision has often been made on the grounds that nothing else was available. The only therapeutic effect that might be expected from irradiation is an endothelial reaction leading to obliteration of the smallest vessels. If it is these minute vessels that bleed, benefit might result. But there is little evidence that these are the prime or the major source. It is more probable that it occurs from rupture of vessels with malformed and thin walls, from aneurysmal dilatations, directly communicating with the arterial inflow. The closure of arteriovenous fistulae by fibrosis can hardly be expected. Standard radiotherapeutic treatment has for the most part been discontinued as beneficial effects have not been generally experienced. Stereotactic radiotherapy (Backlund 1979, Leksell 1983), on the other hand, has a valuable contribution to make in treating inaccessible arteriovenous malformations provided that their diameter does not exceed 30–35 mm. Leksell found that in 83% of patients followed for 2 years there was obliteration of the abnormal vessels but that there was a long latency (6–18 months) before any change occurred. Stereotactic Bragg–peak proton-beam therapy induces subendothelial deposition of collagen and hyaline substance which narrows the lumen by thickening the wall in small bore blood vessels during the first 2 years after irradiation. Kjellberg et al. (1983) reported 74 cases with follow-ups of 2–16 years. Two fatal haemorrhages occurred within the first year after therapy. Thereafter no fatal or disabling bleed occurred. If the threshold dose (which varies depending upon the beam diameter) for cerebral necrosis is exceeded, neurological damage can occur but in this report no patient died from causes directly related to the therapy. Preliminary reports of photocoagulation using argon or neodymium:yttrium–aluminium–garnet (YAG) lasers have suggested satisfactory results can be obtained in obliterating arteriovenous malformations (and possibly aneurysms) whilst maintaining the patency of normal cerebral arteries. The numbers of patients treated are as yet small and follow-up short (Fasano et al. 1982).

Subtemporal decompression has a small part to play in arteriovenous malformations, which by reason of their size cause raised intracranial pressure and which cannot be excised or dealt with by arterial ligation. A decompression will have no beneficial effect upon the lesion, nor upon the complications of bleeding, epilepsy or paresis. But by providing an elastic vent to the rigid skull it has been known to relieve headache and papilloedema.

Obstructive hydrocephalus, consequent upon meningeal fibrosis from haemorrhage or due to the situation of the lesion should be treated by one of the methods outlined in Chapter 15.

## Dural arteriovenous malformations

Dural arteriovenous malformations are rare. The majority of those occurring are congenital, but occasionally they result from trauma (Feldman *et al.* 1980). The symptoms are similar to those resulting from cerebral malformations, i.e. sub-arachnoid haemorrhage, headache, hydro-cephalus, neurological deficits and bruits. The blood supply is primarily from the external carotid circulation and only secondarily from the internal carotid and vertebral systems. The flow difficulties arise not from steal but from the ele-vated venous pressure (Kosnik *et al.* 1974).

At operation the fistula must be excised *in toto* even if it includes part of one of the venous sinuses. In the latter instance the collateral venous drainage seems to be sufficient to cope satisfactorily (Kosnik *et al.* 1974). Incomplete excision is followed inevitably by enlargement of the remnant.

## Aneurysmal dilatation of the great vein of Galen

Aneurysms of the vein of Galen are rare, present in infants and children, and have been associated with a poor prognosis. The intracranial space is not only compromised by the mass of the large lesion but also by the concomitant hydro-cephalus. The latter is usually obvious in infants and it is usually on this account that they are brought to medical notice. Lorber (1967) stated that in the 50 or so cases which had been recorded, males predominated. Features which distinguished these infants from those with more

banal forms of hydrocephalus included dilated facial veins (usually in the scalp in common hydrocephalus), proptosis and blindness, con-vulsions and cranial bruit often with high output heart failure. Occasional cases have been reported in which the aneurysm had undergone spontaneous thrombosis (Olin *et al.* 1982).

Computerized tomographic scanning reveals a large midline globular mass which enhances strongly upon injection of contrast intrav-enously. Four vessel cerebral angiography is necessary to define the feeding vessels, which are multiple, both from the anterior and posterior circulations.

Surgical management is difficult. The best results occur in those patients presenting in later infancy with a large head and a bruit but no heart failure and conversely the worst results in the larger group of neonates who are in heart failure. Surgical removal is the treatment of choice (Long *et al.* 1974, Yaşargil *et al.* 1976, Smith and Donat 1981) if this can be achieved without causing irreparable damage to the corpus callosum and the posterior part of the thalamus. It is possible in this type of mal-formation to clip all the feeding vessels, thus isolating the arteriovenous fistula from the intra-cranial circulation. It is essential to check that this has been achieved by aspirating the aneur-ysm until it has collapsed (Amacher & Shillito 1973). With improvements in the technique it may become possible to use embolization tech-niques to reduce the flow through the aneurysm, thus allowing the definitive surgery to be delayed until the child is out of the neonatal period. Ultimately the technique may be so improved that the fistula can be closed entirely by embol-ization, obviating the need for surgery.

The hydrocephalus usually requires treat-ment. Lazar (1980) suggested that drainage should be undertaken before the definitive direct surgery in order to be certain of pre- and post-operative control of the intracranial pressure. In addition CSF shunting reduces the risk of haem-orrhage from the subependymal veins, which become markedly dilated following the removal of the aneurysm (Yaşargil *et al.* 1976).

## Intracerebral haematoma

Haemorrhage into the brain, often termed spontaneous to distinguish it from a traumatic aetiology, provides a diversity of clinical patterns ranging from the apoplectic to the simulation of a tumour. In appropriate cases timely operation is lifesaving and the ultimate functional recovery rewarding; in others the damage to the brain is lethal and operation an error of judgement. One aspect of this subject has been examined in the context of aneurysmal rupture. The other varieties of intracerebral haemorrhage will now be considered.

In the series of 461 autopsy records analysed by Russell (1954) the important causes of fatal brain haemorrhage were vascular hypertension in 50%, saccular aneurysm in 20%, blood diseases in 8%, mycotic aneurysm in 6% and vascular hamartoma in 5%. Odom et al. (1966) found in a clinical series of 151 cases that the haemorrhage was due to hypertension in 33%, to a saccular aneurysm in 33% and to a vascular hamartoma in 11%; other or unknown causes were responsible in the remainder. In the patients with hypertensive haemorrhage, the blood pressure at the time of admission averaged 214 mmHg systolic and 126 mmHg diastolic; in patients with a ruptured aneurysm the figures were 160 mm and 90 mm respectively; in the cases of bleeding vascular hamartoma they were not reported. That intracranial haemorrhage may temporarily raise the blood pressure has already been noted in regard to aneurysmal rupture. Beck (1954) reported that a high blood pressure initially present in 8 cases of intracerebral haemorrhage persisted after operation in only 3. The pattern of distribution of hypertensive haemorrhage is fundamental in determining the outcome, as regards both life and function. The majority involve the basal ganglia or brain stem; in the cases of Odom et al. (1966) 60% affected the basal ganglia and a further 14% the midbrain and pons. Thus in perhaps three-quarters of the cases of fatal cerebral haemorrhage due to hypertension it is the situation of the lesion which renders it lethal. The rapidity with which patients succumb to a haemorrhage involving vital areas is illustrated by Rose's enquiry (1948) which was based on autopsies. The average survival following basal ganglia haemorrhage was 21 hours and following brain stem haemorrhage 14 hours. On the other hand, in a small proportion of cases bleeding occurs remote from vital centres and more accessible to the surgeon; some 10% of the hypertensive haemorrhages in Russell's series were in the cerebral white matter. It is of considerable interest that the micro-aneurysms on small cerebral arteries demonstrated by Ross Russell (1963) appear to have a similar general distribution between the white matter and basal ganglia. The death rate from 'cerebral haemorrhage' varies with different authorities. Kinnier Wilson quotes estimates up to 85%; in 1000 cases of 'apoplexia cerebri' (which also included thrombosis and embolism) Dalsgaard-Nielsen (1955) found it to be 62%. Such assessments are based on clinical diagnoses and in survivors there is no proof of accuracy. In a series (McKissock et al. 1961) in which diagnosis was supported by radiological investigation the illness ended fatally in 51%. An important observation of Dalsgaard-Nielsen concerned the state of the survivors; only 12% were left with negligible or slight disability; in the others disability was moderate to severe and 19% were totally dependent. Nor is the longterm natural history favourable. In reviewing the management of intracranial haematoma, Tsementzis (1985) quoted a 5-year survival of 10% or less in medically managed cases.

Reference has already been made to the importance of tiny 'cryptic' (Crawford & Russell 1956) vascular malformations or 'micro-angiomas' (Gerlach & Jensen 1961) as sources of haemorrhage. They may be in the depths of a fissure, in the white matter, rarely in the deep grey masses of cerebrum and in the cerebellum. They betray their presence by haemorrhage, rarely by any of the other symptoms of an angiomatous malformation; in some there may have been a previous episode of bleeding. Intracerebral haemorrhage due to these lesions occurs predominantly in the young, the ages averaging about 30 years; a sharp contrast to haemorrhage from aneurysm and hypertension which is more commonly seen in patients some 20 years or more older. In the great majority the lesion and consequently the haemorrhage is favourably placed for surgical relief although in a few bleeding is so copious that the patient is rapidly overwhelmed. Careful scrutiny of the angiograms is necessary in order to detect the minute abnormality which may comprise only an unduly early filling of a vein; and similar scrutiny of the walls of the haematoma and of its contents are essential if the lesion is not to be overlooked. In spite of this care, the origin of the bleeding may not be discovered and the probability is supported only by the age of the patient and the absence of other predisposing cause. In the series of Krayenbühl and Siebenmann (1965) confirmation of the lesion was lacking in 9 of 24 cases. Gerlach and Jensen demonstrated it by angiography in 18 of 20.

Some confusion arises in the use of the terms haemorrhage and haematoma. Haemorrhage describes the process of bleeding; it comprises extravasations of blood into tissues with and without their destruction and, in the case of the brain, into the ventricles and into the subarachnoid spaces; at post-mortem examination it provides a convenient label for all collections of blood external to its normal anatomical boundaries. Haematoma implies a localized discrete collection of blood resulting from haemorrhage; it may be solid, semisolid or liquid and is contained within a cavity in the brain created by disruption or necrosis of the tissue, or in a pre-existing space, for example subdural. It does not cover the process of bleeding although this may occasionally continue in small quantities, for example recent haemorrhage into a chronic subdural haematoma, and perhaps in some intracerebral haematomas which only slowly manifest themselves. In neurological parlance, haemorrhage and haematoma are often used synonymously; the process of bleeding and the formation of a haematoma merge insensibly but all haemorrhages do not become haematomas: death may occur in the stage of diffuse infil-

tration, or small quantities of blood may be absorbed without significant cavitation. It is essential that the neurosurgeon should envisage as clearly as possible the morbid anatomy of the lesion for which he proposes to operate. His aim is to evacuate an abnormal collection of blood which by compression and by chemically induced vasoconstriction is causing further ischaemic damage to adjacent brain and by virtue of its occupation of space is elevating intracranial pressure; his interference must cause the minimum of damage. A freshly formed haematoma is usually of tar-like consistency and its margins ragged and ill defined; the surrounding brain is soft and hyperaemic. After some days the contents become firmer and, later still, liquid; the walls of the cavity become smoother and better defined and the adjacent brain is firmer and less hyperaemic. Thus early operation is desirable in order to relieve or forestall the effects of rising intracranial pressure and to prevent further local damage to brain tissue by blood; but evacuation of a haematoma is technically easier at a later stage when the acute reactive changes in its walls have somewhat subsided. The statement is sometimes made that an intracerebral haematoma becomes 'encapsulated'; this is rare; usually a reactive gliosis slowly occurs around a haematoma, embodied in the walls of its cavity rendering them smooth and firm and fading peripherally into the surrounding healthy brain. Jewesbury (1947) mentions a case of encapsulated haematoma which was enucleated and Greenfield reported that it had a fibrous capsule.

Intracerebral haematomas may take the form of an acute or of a subacute illness. In the former group are those in which the haemorrhage, by reason of depth or of speed, overwhelms the patient in a few hours. This is the picture presented by many cases of hypertensive haemorrhage and by a few originating from a cryptic angiomatous malformation. As Kinnier Wilson dramatically describes it, 'a brief second of bewilderment, a cry of pain, a vague momentary alarm, a tragic ejaculation—'Oh, my head!'— heralds immediate and profound insensibility'.

The rapid development of hemiplegia or of decerebrate rigidity, abnormal size and responses of the pupils, conjugate ocular deviation and disturbances of vital signs indicate the depth and the severity of the lesion. In other cases which run an acute course, headache and vomiting precede a gradual failure of consciousness and coarse neurological abnormalities become evident more slowly; the accompaniments of rising intracranial pressure and of consequent temporal lobe herniation are manifest within 24–48 hours. In the subacute form of the illness, the initial symptoms of headache, vomiting, confusion, drowsiness, may be transient, the patient after several days appearing to recover, but only to develop symptoms and signs of focal brain damage and of slowly increasing intracranial pressure in the course of the succeeding days or weeks. This pattern of presentation of an intracerebral haematoma may be mistaken for an abscess or a tumour. A variety of atypical cases was recorded by Jewesbury.

Whatever may have been the cause, if intracerebral haemorrhage has a catastrophic onset, causing immediate and rapidly increasing coma and other signs indicating massive and deep damage, operation has no part to play unless and until there is evidence that the patient is rallying. This is likely to be at least 2 days. In other cases in which the fall in the level of consciousness and the emergence of signs of focal brain damage run a measurably slower time course, investigation with a view to operation should be undertaken as soon as possible, particularly in young subjects in whom there may be an angiomatous malformation, with the proviso that there is no reason to suspect a blood disease. In the subacute presentation, the decision will present no difficulties unless an abscess is mistakenly suspected, in which case the desire to await the response to antibiotics may endanger life. The value of a lumbar puncture is dubious. The presence of blood in the cerebrospinal fluid confirms a haemorrhagic aetiology, but its absence in no way excludes it: xanthochromia is a sequel of recent bleeding: pleiocytosis may be found in cases of intracerebral haematoma as in abscess though a count of over 100 cells per cubic millimetre would strongly favour abscess. The overriding need to relieve increasing intracranial pressure and consequent brain herniation is a general principle which should guide judgement in these problems, and computerized tomography should always take precedence over lumbar puncture.

Computerized tomographic scanning will confirm the presence of an intracerebral haematoma, but will usually not exclude the possibility of an underlying vascular lesion such as an aneurysm, an arteriovenous malformation or occlusion of a major vessel. Angiography is therefore essential for that purpose. As a localizing investigation it is less effective. McKissock et al. (1959) found that angiography was successful in localizing a haematoma in only 70%; they found that an increased interval between the stems of the middle and the anterior cerebral arteries in the anteroposterior film, separation of the limbs of the U, was a useful sign of basal ganglia haemorrhage. Other signs are displacement of deep veins, whilst stretching and elevation of the pericallosal arteries suggest hydrocephalus, Ventriculography is indicated only if angiography provides inadequate information and computerized tomographic scanning is not available.

Aspiration through a burr hole rarely if ever achieves success because the contents are too thick; adequate evacuation of the haematoma requires an osteoplastic flap. The cortex is incised over the most accessible portion, the blood is removed by gentle suction, with as little disturbance to the walls of the cavity as possible, unless there is evidence of an angiomatous malformation, which should be removed if the exigencies of the situation allow. In acute haematoma a too thorough cleaning of its walls causes small vessel bleeding which may be difficult to arrest and in the attempt to do so unnecessary damage may be inflicted. However if possible the walls of the haematoma cavity should be examined to try to exclude the possibility of an angiographically cryptic malformation or that the haemorrhage has occurred within a primary or metastatic brain tumour (Shuey *et al.* 1979, Cohen *et al.* 1982). If the latter possibility seems likely a biopsy of the cavity wall should be taken. The operating microscope is an important aid in this operation. The general mortality rate following the evacuation of spontaneous intracerebral haematomas is indicated by the published reports of 602 cases collected by Weber (1963). Death occurred in 172 (29%). In his own series of 37 operations, death followed in 2 of 3 acute cases, in 7 of 28 subacute cases and no deaths occurred in 8 chronic cases. In the series of Odom *et al.* (1966) the operative mortality for haematomas of hypertensive origin was 50%, approximately the same for those due to aneurysmal rupture, but only 14.3% for those of angiomatous origin. In the small consecutive series of 11 cases of mixed aetiology reported by Beck (1954) there were no deaths. All the 24 cases of Krayenbühl and Siebermann were believed to be due to small vascular malformations: 2 patients died without operation: only 1 death followed operation in the other 22. The degree of recovery of function may be surprisingly good: in 21 survivors 'full recovery' was recorded in 10; a spastic hemiparesis persisted in 2 and the others exhibited lesser degrees of neurological deficit. The results of operation in patients who have sustained a cerebral haemorrhage of hypertensive or of unidentified origin are in general disappointing in terms of saving life and of recovery of function, but they should be viewed realistically against the background of aetiology and of localization. Elkington (1958) and Kelly (1958) had no doubt of the value of operation in selected cases. A large number have been reported by McKissock *et al.* (1959, 1961). In the 1959 series of 244 consecutive cases, of which 152 patients were hypertensive, the overall mortality rate was 51%, varying between 35% for frontal and 93% for capsular haematomas. With a hypertensive aetiology the death rate was 58%, in others 35%. In the 1961 series comprising 180 cases (hypertension in 151) a controlled trial of conservative and surgical treatment was carried out, comparable with that undertaken in the treatment

of ruptured aneurysms. Death occurred in 51% of the patients treated conservatively and 65% of those treated surgically. One-third of the survivors of operation returned to full work and one-quarter of the others. These figures support no advantage of surgical over conservative treatment so far as saving life is concerned (in fact somewhat the reverse), but it is likely that certain criteria for including a patient in the series would have led many surgeons to delay operation. Volpin *et al.* (1984) analysed the volume of the intracerebral haematoma as judged on computerized tomographic scanning in 132 patients of whom 50 came to surgery. They concluded that in comatose patients evacuation of the haematoma increased the survival rate if the volume of the clot was between 26 and 85 ml but that such a survival was associated with a high probability of serious neurological deficit, particularly if the haematoma was situated in the basal ganglia. They felt that surgery should be carried out in these cases soon after the ictus in contradistinction to the 4–5 days that many surgeons wait before taking out more superficial haematomas. Kanno *et al.* (1984) reviewing an uncontrolled retrospective series of 459 cases of hypertensive intracerebral haematoma found no significant improvements in the overall outcome between the surgically and nonsurgically treated groups. However, in putaminal haemorrhage as opposed to haemorrhage in other sites there were some differences in outcome between the 2 treatment groups. Putaminal haemorrhage was divided into 4 groups: mild, involving the external capsule; moderate, in which mainly the external capsule was involved but there was encroachment upon the internal capsule which typically extended into the corona radiata; severe subtype 1, in which the haematoma extended downwards in the internal capsule but stopped short of the midbrain, and subtype 2, in which it extended to the midbrain, compressing the latter; very severe, in which the haematoma extended into the midbrain. Those with either moderate or severe subtype 1 putaminal haemorrhage did better with surgery provided that it was carried out within 6 hours of the ictus.

According to Kinnier Wilson cerebellar haemorrhage is 'extremely uncommon'. But Russell (1954) found 18 examples amongst 232 hypertensive haemorrhages, and in their series of cryptic hamartomas Crawford and Russell showed 6 out of 20 were in the cerebellum. McKissock *et al.* (1960) did not regard cerebellar haemorrhages as so rare; in their experience they supplied 8% of all primary brain haemorrhages. Of 34 cases, hypertension was the presumed cause in 22, angiomatous malformation in 6 and aneurysm in 2. In half the cases the haemorrhage remained confined to the cerebellum, important for survival; in the other cases it spread into the brain stem or ruptured into the fourth ventricle. In children there are numerous causes including vascular malformations, aneurysms, neoplasms, infection, blood dyscrasias and the occasional idiopathic case (Kazimiroff *et al.* 1980). As in cerebral haemorrhage the illness may take an acute catastrophic course, or evolve subacutely over the course of a week or so. Although onset may be sudden (in 28 of their cases) consciousness is frequently at first unaffected (in 18) nevertheless deterioration may be very rapid and small fixed pupils, periodic respirations, conjugate ocular deviation away from the side of the lesion (towards a hemiparesis if present) were ominous developments. Only one-quarter presented signs of cerebellar disorder and consequently in the majority there were no distinguishing features. Some help in the selection of cases is provided by an interesting analysis of primary pontine haemorrhages made by Silverstein (1967). Outstanding points were the rarity of spasticity and decerebrate rigidity, the frequency of pupillary abnormalities, of a marked degree of slowing of the respirations (which reached 3 to 5 per minute in some cases) and of hyperthermia.

Computerized tomographic scanning is the initial investigation of choice. It will allow localization of the haematoma within the posterior fossa and in particular will allow differentiation between pontine and intracerebral haemorrhage. Angiography is essential to exclude an underlying vascular cause. It will also show more major degrees of hydrocephalus but if computerized tomographic scanning is not available, ventriculography can be of value in confirming the hydrocephalus and may give information as to the localization of the lesion within the posterior fossa. A stronger case has been made for surgical evacuation of cerebellar haemotomas. In patients subjected to a posterior fossa craniectomy the mortality was 36%; those treated by ventricular tapping or drainage all died. Therefore, unlike those patients with a supratentorial haematoma, patients with a cerebellar haematoma should undergo urgent removal of the clot. However, Kanno *et al.* (1984) have recently cast some doubt upon the role of surgery, particularly when performed early. They found that conservatively managed cases could have a good outcome even when the lesion was large. Further assessment of this problem is required.

**Sturge–Weber disease**

Historical accounts of this disorder are numerous; those by Bergstrand *et al.* (1936), Wohlwill and Yakovlef (1957) and Alexander and Norman (1960) give full details and extensive bibliographies. Other names are sometimes added to the eponyms for their owner's share and priority in describing important features, but that of Sturge (1879) is outstanding. By recognizing that epilepsy arising at the age of 6 months and hemiparesis in a patient with a facial naevus and buphthalmos were not fortuitous associations but might have a common aetiology in angiomatosis, he showed clinical acumen and imagination of a high order. Kalischer (1897, 1901) reported post-mortem confirmations of meningeal angiomatosis in a similar case. Radiological opacity within the skull of a patient presenting the syndrome was described by Weber in 1922; curiously in that paper he made no suggestion that the opacity was due to calcium deposits, but stated that the left half of the brain 'appears to be sclerosed'. The quality of the reproduction (or of the original films) is so poor that

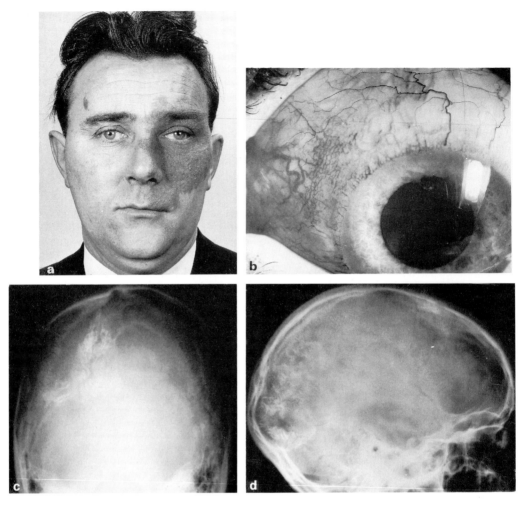

**Fig. 12.3.** Sturge–Weber disease: male aged 33 years with recurrent episodes all his life of blurred vision right eye (left behind), malaise and violent headache: occasional epilepsy.

(a) Facial naevus.

(b) Naevoid sclera of left eye: raised introccular tension, primary atrophy with deep cup. Calcification was present in left occipital pole.

(c, d) Typical calcification in right occipital lobe: the right hemicranium is smaller than the left. (By courtesy of Dr K. G. Heathfield.)

the texture and pattern of the opacity cannot be determined (in 1928 the case was again reported with films showing the typical appearance). Credit for drawing attention to the curious pattern of calcification should really go to Dimitri (1923) who described a case accompanied by an excellent reproduction of a good X-ray. Krabbe (1932) described the first autopsy findings in a case with radiological evidence of calcification;

histological preparations revealed heavy calcareous deposits in the cerebral cortex. In 1934 he published 6 cases; further X-ray examination of one patient showed no increase in the calcification after an interval of 8 years.

The essential feature of the syndrome is the angiomatosis: cutaneous affecting the face (port-wine stain, capillary naevus, naevus flammeus) and leptomeningeal affecting the cerebrum, usually its posterior half (Fig. 12.3). Epilepsy and cerebral calcification appear sooner or later in practically every case and ocular abnormalities in a large number. The extent to which some of the features may be absent and the diagnosis still acceptable or the case regarded as an atypical example is a matter of opinion. Angiomatosis of the skin and of the pia is generally regarded as the minimum requirement although Lichtenstein (1953) and Huber and Zweigmuller (1954) described cases in which the cerebral lesion was typical but there was no abnormality of the skin or of the mucosa of the mouth and pharynx. In that reported by Norlen (1959) calcification was present in both occipital lobes which were amputated; microscopy revealed abnormal vessels in one specimen but not in the other; it is not recorded whether a facial naevus was present. Typical calcification alone is probably an insufficient qualification for the diagnosis, for Alexander and Woodhall (1943) have drawn attention to the deposition of calcium salts in this pattern in other lesions. Terminological exactitude is perhaps satisfied if 'syndrome' is applied to those cases conforming precisely with Sturge's description, and 'disease' to those with strong similarities but lacking some of the features.

## Cutaneous naevus

Arteriovenous malformations of the brain may occasionally be accompanied by a vascular naevus of the face, and of the spinal cord by a naevus on the trunk in corresponding metameres. In the Sturge–Weber syndrome the face is always affected, though the naevus may cover only part of it and may extend elsewhere for considerable distances; the distinctive feature is its occupation, at least to some extent, of the forehead and upper lid. Alexander and Norman (1960) traced in the literature 257 cases satisfying their criteria and in every case part of the facial naevus involved this area of skin. They have found no authentic case in which forehead and eyelid were entirely free. Kautsky (1949)

analysed a large number of cases and suggested that a relationship existed between cutaneous involvement of the first, second and third trigeminal divisions and occipital parietal and frontal distribution of the cerebral lesion. He makes an unconvincing case, and Alexander and Norman offer an alternative embryological explanation; they agree that an extensive cerebral lesion often goes with an extensive facial naevus.

## Cerebral lesions

*Vascular malformation.* Ipsilateral to the facial naevus (so far as it involved the specific area) the leptomeninges, most commonly over the posterior part of the cerebrum, are thickened and contain a felt-work of abnormal vessels. These are mainly fine in calibre and include arteries and veins. Various degrees of thickening and of abnormal structure are seen; calcification is found in the walls of smaller arteries. Vessels in the grey matter take but little part in the angiomatosis.

*Calcification* in the grey matter and to a slight degree in the subjacent white matter occurs in all cases and is restricted to the superficial extent of the meningeal angiomatosis. It is slight in infancy, gradually becoming denser until the maximum degree is attained probably by the age of 20 years. Although in Case 5 of Alexander and Norman, calcification was not detected radiologically at the age of 1 year, it was very marked in the histological preparations. Some of the calcium is deposited around the capillaries, large irregular masses accumulate, disposed so that the largest lie nearest the surface; on the cut section they are visible to the naked eye. Degenerative changes are severe in the cortex and white matter subjacent to the vascular anomaly: shrinkage of gyri, loss of nerve cells and fibres and gliosis. Atrophy and gliosis are also found in other areas (Lichtenstein), and the entire hemisphere is reduced in size. Wohlwill and Yakovlev (1957) found errors of development beyond the confines of the angiomatosis.

The cerebral calcification and focal degeneration are generally ascribed to the stasis and anoxia induced by the abnormal leptomeningeal vessels; in several of the cases described by Alexander and Norman, the angiomatous area presented a cyanotic hue at operation. Hypoxia during repeated convulsions also aggravates local damage and may be responsible for degeneration elsewhere in the brain. But the considerable discrepancy in size of the two hemispheres of patients who have died in infancy leads some authorities to believe than an error of development must play an important part. Alexander and Norman 'favour the view that the stunted size of the hemisphere is secondary to the vascular anomaly'.

### Ocular manifestations

Alexander and Norman estimated that buphthalmos was reported in about one-fifth of the cases and glaucoma in a proportion of these. Angiomatosis of the choroid is found in some, congenital abnormalities in others, but the cause of the intra-ocular hypertension is often unexplained. Intra-ocular calcification has been reported.

### Epilepsy

Epilepsy 'has occurred in nearly every published case where the essential lesions of the Sturge–Weber anomaly have been present. This fact is noteworthy and unique among potentially epileptogenic lesions' (Alexander and Norman). The fits usually commence in infancy and increase in frequency and in severity in spite of medical treatment. Spontaneous remissions of several years may occur; Norlen records a continuing absence of fits for 7 years in a patient who had suffered from them for 30 years. Focal and generalized patterns occur but a visual aura is apparently unusual although the occipital lobe is so commonly affected. Following a severe bout, postepileptic contralateral hemiparesis may

make imperfect recovery, so that in time there is a permanent spastic hemiparesis and the affected limbs are stunted. In other cases the hemiparesis may precede the development of fits.

### Mental symptoms

These take the form of behaviour disorders and of progressive mental retardation, which may reach the degree of idiocy. Intellectual deterioration, or failure to develop, often dates from childhood. All except one of the patients described by Alexander and Norman were retarded. In the series of 23 cases reported by Tönnis and Friedmann (1964) mental disturbances were noted in 6; one-third of the 15 patients of Norlen (1959) were severely affected and 5 of the 8 of Krayenbühl et al. (1957). Alexander and Norman consider that admission to an institution in late childhood and death in status epilepticus is the usual fate of these patients.

Physical examination should take note of the extent of the cutaneous naevus and in particular whether the forehead and upper lid are affected, the condition of the eyes (expert ophthalmological advice should be sought) and evidence of hemiatrophy of the skull, which was clearly described by Kalischer. No cranial bruit is found in these patients. If cooperation is sufficient, a hemianopia can be detected. Spastic hemiparesis to some degree, often with underdevelopment of the affected limbs is frequent and there may be impairment of discriminative sensory function. Plantar responses may be extensor on both sides. Psychometric testing should be performed. X-rays of the skull may reveal that its capacity is diminished on one side and here the vault may be thickened. In children below the age of 2 years calcification is rarely detectable, but with increasing age virtually always present. It takes the form of wavy, sinuous shadows, often of delicate gradation, which have a double contour, the 'tramlines' appearance. The double lines were formerly attributed to deposits depicting the contours of cortical vessels, but Krabbe (1932) showed that the density of the linear shadow is due to the calcerous deposit in sulcal cortex projected perpendicular to the film, the contiguous surfaces of the sulcus providing the double line. There is no correspondence between the X-ray appearances and that of the angiomatous malformation. The radiological appearances of resected specimens are beautifully reproduced in the monograph of Bergstrand *et al.* (1936, Figs. 27 and 28). Calcification is most common in the occipital lobe and it may clearly outline the pole; it may be so extensive as to involve most of the hemisphere; occasionally it is found in the frontal lobe. When well developed the opacity is unmistakable; when ill defined it could be confused with calcification in an oligodendroglioma. Computerized tomographic scanning may not resolve this difficulty without serial scanning over a considerable period. In Sturge–Weber syndrome it is unlikely that there will be any displacement of structures, whereas in the case of a slow growing neoplasm space occupation will eventually occur. There may even be enlargement of the ipsilateral ventricle, or part of it, and of the overlying subarachnoid spaces. (In the absence of computerized tomographic scanning the latter can be demonstrated by air encephalography.) Angiography frequently shows no abnormality and this has been attributed to a slow circulation in the angiomatous area; a diffuse shadow due to the filling of fine vessels is illustrated by Krayenbühl and Yaşargil (1965, Fig. 312b).

## Treatment

Resection of the affected area of brain has been carried out in a relatively small number of patients in an attempt to cure the epilepsy, to arrest the progress of intellectual deterioration and to improve behaviour. These indications for operation are similar to those for hemispherectomy in certain cases of infantile hemiplegia (Chapter 17). Although the pathological changes in the brain in the two conditions are different the clinical effects are somewhat similar, except that the mental changes in Sturge–Weber disease are often more severe. The macroscopic lesion is commonly smaller and consequently hemispherectomy in these patients is too mutilating. If the calcification and the angiomatous meninges are restricted to the occipital pole (or rarely the frontal) a lobectomy can be performed; a hemianiopia is often already present, or is likely to develop as the disease matures. Where the lesion is placed further forward a local resection is performed, and should extend sufficiently deeply into the white matter to extirpate all seemingly abnormal tissue. If a considerable degree of hemiparesis has developed a hemispherectomy should be seriously considered. Where calcification is very extensive, includes the temporoparietal region and a considerable hemiparesis is present, it is likely that the healthy hemisphere is dominant and extensive resection will have no deleterious effect upon speech. Guttman (1942) in a study of aphasia in children quotes a statement attributed to Cotard: 'whichever the side of the lesion, individuals hemiplegic since infancy never present aphasia'. When the lesion is distant from such important cortical areas resection should not cause any disturbance. In Case 2 (age 8 years) of Alexander and Norman, a left occipital lobectomy was performed without dysphasic sequelae; there was no familial left-handedness but she was partially left-handed and significantly speech was late in developing. Case 5 was a rightsided occipito-oparietal resection at the age of 1 year. An episode of aphasia occurred 6 months after the operation and a history of familial left-handedness was traced. The disease extended and the result 2 years later was poor. It is probable that up to the age of about 3 years operation on either hemisphere can be tolerated and the development of speech and other functions predominantly unilateral will prove satisfactory (*see also* Basser 1962). In older patients the problem is more difficult though when the patient is old enough (and intelligent enough) to cooperate, the 'localization' of speech for the purposes in question can be determined by an intracarotid injection of sodium amytal (*see* Chapter 17).

Resection of the brain to an extent corresponding with that of the visible lesion is an oversimplification of the surgical problem, so far as it concerns the epilepsy (*see* Chapter 17). Although removal of abnormal tissue from the brain is a *sine qua non*, because it may be the ultimate 'exciting' cause and of the angiomatous meninges because they may cause further damage to underlying cortex, nevertheless electroencephalography (EEG) has shown that apparently healthy brain remote from a coarse lesion may be partly or totally responsible for epileptic discharges. Consequently the decision to operate and the extent of resection should be judged in relation to the scalp EEG findings and may be aided by electrocorticography. These may show abnormality characteristic of epilepsy not only in the vicinity of the lesion but remote from it (Radermacker 1951). In infancy and childhood the EEG records may be difficult to interpret and older patients may be unsatisfactory subjects for the repeated and prolonged examination necessary for reliable information. There are few records of surgeons seeking EEG guidance; Alexander and Norman discuss the EEG findings but largely those related to the depressed electrical activity in the area of the lesion; less attention seems to have been paid to the examination of adjacent cortex for outlying epileptic activity. Broager and Hertz (1949) reported the excision of an area of frontal cortex which exhibited EEG manifestations of epilepsy, while ignoring the occipital lesion; improvement was noted for 1 year.

In Table 12.1 are listed the results of operation derived from a brief search of the literature.

Thus in 64% of these patients the epilepsy was 'improved'; this expression is used for brevity's sake and in many instances there were no further fits after operation. But as Norlen points out the duration of postoperative observation is often too limited for a reliable judgement of the value of the operation, particularly as spontaneous remission of fits for a number of years is not uncommon. The series may also be misleading because isolated cases in which operation has been of no benefit are unlikely to be published. Alexander and Norman believe that better results might be achieved if the vascular anomaly were removed before it induced severe changes in the underlying brain and consequential epilepsy and mental retardation; they make a plea for operation within a few months of birth.

The Sturge–Weber syndrome is rare and few neurosurgeons will encounter more than several examples during their professional career. This in itself is a hindrance to the assembling of information suitable for the development of the best line of treatment. A greater emphasis upon EEG investigations and control during operation may

**Table 12.1.**   Results of operation for Sturge–Weber disease.

| References | Number of cases | Nature of operation | Effect on epilepsy | Duration of follow-up |
|---|---|---|---|---|
| Bentzen (1947) | 2 | resection | 2 improved | 6 months |
| Lund (1949) | 6 | resection or coagulation | 3 improved | 1–4 years |
| Green *et al.* (1950) | 1 | resection | 1 improved | 6 months |
| Cairns & Davidson (1951) | 1 | hemispherectomy | 1 improved | 1 year |
| Polani (1952) | 3 | hemispherectomy | 3 improved | 6 wks–1 yr |
| Obrador-Alcade (1954) | 1 | resection | 1 improved | 2 years |
| French *et al.* (1955) | 1 | hemispherectomy | 1 improved | 2 years |
| Goodall (1957) | 1 | hemispherectomy | 1 improved | over 6 months |
| Norlen (1959) | 10 | resection | 2 improved | 14–26 years |
| Alexander & Norman (1960) | 5 | resection | 3 improved | 4–8 years |
| Falconer & Rushworth (1960) | 5 | hemispherectomy | all fit free | 3–8 years |
| Totals | 36 | | 23 | |

prove helpful. At present the evidence suggests that extensive brain resections are more likely to be successful than limited resections, in keeping with the experience gained from the surgical treatment of epilepsy due to other causes; that improvement in behaviour depends upon the degree to which the epilepsy improves but severe intellectual failure is unlikely to be repaired though the result may prove sufficient to ease the burden of caring for such patients.

# References

ALEXANDER G. L. & NORMAN R. M. (1960) *The Sturge–Weber Syndrome*. Wright, Bristol.

ALEXANDER L. & WOODHALL B. (1943) *J. Neuropath. Exp. Neurol.*, **2**, 1.

AMACHER A. L. & SHILLITO J. (1973) *J. Neurosurg.*, **39**, 89.

ANDERSON R. McD. & BLACKWOOD W. (1959) *J. Path. Bact.*, **77**, 101.

BACKLUND E. O. (1979) *Advances and Technical Standards in Neurosurgery*, Vol. 6 (Ed. Krayenbühl H.) Springer-Verlag, Wien.

BAILEY O. T. (1961) *J. Neuropath. Exp. Neurol.*, **20**, 170.

BASSER L. S. (1962) *Brain*, **85**, 427.

BECK D. J. K. (1954) *Proc. roy. Soc. Med.*, **47**, 700.

BENTZEN O. (1947) *Nord. Medicin.*, **33**, 465.

BERGSTRAND H., OLIVECRONA H. & TONNIS W. (1936) *Gefassmissbildungen und Gefassgeschwulste des Gehirns*. Thieme, Leipzig.

BERRY R. G., ALPERS B. J. & WHITE J. C. (1966) *Res. Pub. Ass. Ner. Ment. Dis.*, **41**, 61.

BLACKWOOD W. (1941) *J. Path. Bact.*, **52**, 209.

BOYD-WILSON J. S. (1959) *J. Neurol. Neurosurg. Psychiat.*, **22**, 218.

BROAGER B. & HERTZ H. (1949) *Acta Psychiat. Neurol. Kbh.*, **24**, 1.

BROCK S. & DYKE G. (1932) *Arch. Neurol. Psychiat.*, **2**, 247.

CAIRNS H. & DAVIDSON M. A. (1951) *Lancet*, **2**, 411.

COHEN H. C. M., TUCKER W. S., HUMPHREYS R. P. & PERRIN R. J. (1982) *Neurosurg.*, **10**, 704.

COURVILLE C. B. (1963) *J. Neuropath Exp. Neurol.*, **22**, 274.

CRAWFORD J. V. & RUSSELL D. S. (1956) *J. Neurol. Neurosurg. Psychiat.*, **19**, 1.

CRAWFORD P., CHADWICK D. W., WEST C. & SHAW M. D. M. (1986) *J. Neurol. Neurosurg. Psychiat.*, **49**, 1.

CUSHING H. & BAILEY P. (1928) *Tumours Arising from the Blood Vessels of the Brain*. Baillière, Tindall & Cox, London.

DAALSGAARD-NIELSEN T. (1955) *Acta Psychiat. Neurol. Scand.*, **30**, 169.

DAY A. V., FRIEDMAN W. A., SYPERT G. W. & MICKLE J. P. (1982) *Neurosurgery*, **11**, 625.

DEBRUN G., VINUELA F., FOX A. & DRAKE C. G. (1982) *J. Neurosurg.*, **56**, 615.

DIMITRI V. (1923) *Rev. Ass. Med. Argent.*, **26**, 1029.

DIMSDALE H. (1957) *Proc. roy. Soc. Med.*, **50**, 85.

DRIESEN W. (1968) *Zbl. Neurochirurg.*, **29**, 17.

ELKINGTON J. ST. C. (1958) *Lancet*, **2**, 327.

FALCONER M. A. & RUSHWORTH R. G. (1960) *Arch. Dis. Childh.*, **35**, 433.

FASANO V. A., URCIVOLI R. & PONZIO R. A. (1982) *Neurosurg.*, **11**, 754.

FEINDEL W., GARRETSON H., YAMAMATO Y. L., PEROT P. & RUMIN N. (1965) *J. Neurosurg.*, **23**, 12.

FEINDEL W., YAMAMOTO Y. L. & HODGE C. P. (1971) *J. Neurosurg.*, **35**, 167.

FELDMAN R. A., HIESHIMA G., GIANNOTTA S. L. & GADE G. F. (1980) *Neurosurg.*, **6**, 670.

FINKEMEYER H. & KAUTSKY R. (1968) *Zbl. Neurochirurg.*, **29**, 23.

FOY P. M., LOZADA L., SHAW M. D. (1981) *J. Neurosurg.*, **54**, 125.

FRENCH L. A., JOHNSON J. R., BROWN I. A. & VAN BURGEN F. B. (1955) *J. Neurosurg.*, **12**, 154.

GARRETSON H. D. (1979) *Neurosurg.*, **4**, 544.

GERLACH J. & JENSEN H. P. (1961) *Acta Neurochirurg. Suppl.*, **71**, 367.

GOODALL R. J. (1957) *Neurology*, **7**, 151.

GRAF C. J., PERRET G. E. & TORNER J. C. (1983) *J. Neurosurg.*, **58**, 331.

GREEN J. R., FOSTER J. & BERENS D. L. (1950) *Amer. J. Roentgenol.*, **64**, 391.

GREENFIELD (1963) *Neuropathology* 2nd Ed. Arnold, London.

GREITZ T. (1956) *Acta Radiol. Suppl.*, **140**, 70.

GUTTMAN E. (1942) *Brain*, **65**, 205.

HÄGGENDAL E., INGVAR D. H., LASSEN N. A., NILLSON N. J., NORLEN G., WICKBOM I. & ZWETNOW N. (1965) *J. Neurosurg.*, **22**, 1.

HAWKINS C. F. & REWELL R. E. (1946) *Guy's Hosp. Reps.*, **95**, 88.

HENDERSON W. R. & GOMEZ R. DE R. L. (1967) *Brit. med. J.*, **2**, 571.

HIRANO A. & TERRY R. D. (1958) *J. Neuropath. Exp. Neurol.*, **17**, 424.

HOARE R. D. (1953) *Acta Radiol.*, **40**, 96.

HOBBS H. E. (1957) *Proc. roy. Soc. Med.*, **50**, 89.

HORTON B. T. & ZEIGLER L. H. (1930) *Proc. Staff Mtgs. Mayo Clinic.*, **5**, 178.

HUBER K. & ZWEIGMULLER E. (1954) *Wien Zsch. Nervenheilk.*, **9**, 459.

JAEGER J. R., FORBES R. P. & DANDY W. E. (1937) *Trans. Amer. Neurol. Ass.*, 173.

JEFFERSON G. J. (1948) *Rev. Neurol.*, **80**, 413.

JEWESBURY E.C.O. (1947) *Brain*, **70**, 275.

KALISCHER S. (1897) *Berlin Klin. Wochenschr.*, **34**, 1057.

KALISCHER S. (1901) *Arch. Psychiat. Nervenheilk*, **34**, 171.

KANNO T., SANO H., SHINOMIYA Y., KATADA K., NAGATA J., HOSHINO M. & MITSUYAMA F. (1984) *J. Neurosurg.*, **61**, 1091.

KAPLAN H. A., ARONSON S. M. & BROWDER E. J. (1961) *J. Neurosurg.*, **18**, 630.

KAUNTZE R. & McGILL D. (1962) *Guy's Hosp. Reps.*, **111**, 235.

KAUTSKY R. (1949) *D. Zscht. Nervenheilk*, **161**, 506.

KAZIMIROFF P. B., WEICHSEL M. E., GRINNELL V. & YOUNG R. F. (1980) *Neurosurg.*, **6**, 524.

KELLY R. (1958) *Proc. roy. Soc. Med.*, **51**, 213.

KJELLBERG R. N., HANAMURA T., DAVIS K. R., LYONS S. L. & ADAMS R. D. (1983) *New Engl. J. Med.*, **309**, 269.

KOSNIK E. J., HUNT W. E. & MILLER C. A. (1974) *J. Neurosurg.*, **40**, 322.

KRABBE K. (1932) *Rev. Neurol.*, **39(i)**, 1394.

KRAYENBÜHL H. (1957) *Premier Congres Int. Neurochirurgie Rapports et Discussions.* p. 263. Acta Med. Belg., Bruxelles.

KRAYENBÜHL H. & SIEBERMANN R. (1965) *J. Neurosurg.*, **22**, 7.

KRAYENBÜHL H. & YAŞARGIL M. G. (1965) *Die Zerebrale Angiographie.* Thieme, Stuttgart.

KRAYENBÜHL H., YAŞARGIL M. G. & UEHLINGER E. (1957) *Dermatologica*, **115**, 555.

KRENCHEL N. J. (1961) *Intracranial Racemose Angiomas.* Universitets Forlagert, Aarhus.

KUNC Z. (1965) *J. Neurol. Neurosurg. Psychiat.*, **28**, 183.

KUNC Z. (1974) *J. Neurosurg.*, **40**, 293.

KUNC Z. & BRET J. (1969) *Acta Neurochirung.*, **20**, 85.

KUSSE J. A. & KELLY W. A. (1974) *J. Neurosurg.*, **40**, 313.

KVAM D. A., MICHELSON W. J. & QUEST D. O. (1980) *Neurosurgery*, **7**, 491.

LAZAR M. L. (1980) *Neurosurgery*, **7**, 278.

LEKSELL L. (1983) *J. Neurol. Neurosurg. Psychiat.*, **46**, 797.

LEWIS T. & DRURY A. N. (1923) *Heart*, **10**, 301.

LHERMITTE J. (1932) *Encephale*, **27**, 422.

LICHTENSTEIN B. W. (1953) *Fifth Int. Cong. Neurol. (Lisbon) Comptes-rendus.*, **vol. 3**, p. 242.

LITVAK J., YAHR M. D. & RANSOHOFF J. (1960) *J. Neurosurg.*, **17**, 945.

LOGUE V. & MONCKTON G. (1954) *Brain*, **77**, 252.

LONG D. M., SELJESKOG E. L., CHOU S. N. & FRENCH L. A. (1974) *J. Neurosurg.*, **40**, 304.

LORBER J. (1967) *Proc. roy. Soc. Med.*, **60**, 20.

LUESSENHOP A. J., KACHMANN R., SHELVIN W. & FERRERO A. A. (1965) *J. Neurosurg.*, **23**, 400.

LUESSENHOP A. J. & SPENCE W. T. (1960) *J. Amer. med. Ass.*, **172**, 1153.

LUESSENHOP A. J. & ROSA L. (1984) *J. Neurosurg.*, **60**, 14.

LUND (1949) *Acta Psychiat.*, **24**, 569.

MCCORMICK W. F. (1966) *J. Neurosurg.*, **24**, 807.

MCKENZIE J. (1953) *Brain*, **76**, 184.

MCKISSOCK W. & HANKINSON J. (1957) *Premier Cong. Int. Neurochirurgie. Rapports et Discussions*, p. 263. Acta Med. Belg., Bruxelles.

MCKISSOCK W., RICHARDSON A. & WALSH L. (1959) *Lancet*, **2**, 683.

MCKISSOCK W., RICHARDSON A. & WALSH L. (1960) *Brain*, **83**, 1.

MCKISSOCK W., RICHARDSON A. & TAYLOR J. (1961) *Lancet*, **2**, 221.

MARGOLIS G., ODOM G. L., WOODHALL B. & BLOOR B. M. (1951) *J. Neurosurg.*, **8**, 564.

MONIZ E. & GUERRA M. (1953) *Fifth Int. Cong. Neurol.*, vol. 1, p. 79. Serevo-Freitas-Mega, Lisboa.

MULLEN S. (1983) In *Controversies in Neurology* (Eds. Thompaon R. A. & Green J. R.) Raven Press, New York.

NAYRAC P., LAINE E., FORTAN J., DELANDTSHEER J. M. & GALIBERT )P. (1956) *Neurochirurgie*, **2**, 85.

NEHLS D. G. & PITTMAN H. W. (1982) *Neurosurgery*, **11**, 776.

NORLEN G. (1959) *Neurochirurgica*, **1**, 242.

NORNES H., GRIP A. & WIKEBY P. (1979) *J. Neurosurg.*, **50**, 145.

NORRIS J. W., EISEN A. A. & BRANCH C. L. (1969) *Neurology*, **19**, 1043.

NORTHFIELD D. W. C. (1940) *Guy's Hosp. Reps.*, **90**, 149.

OBRADOR-ALCADE S. (1954) *Arch. Neurobiol.*, **17**, 75.

ODOM G. L., TINDALL G. T., CUPP H. & WOODHALL B. (1966) *Res. Pub. Ass. Nerv. Ment. Dis.*, **41**, 145.

OKABE T., MEYR J. S., OKAYASU H., HARPER R., ROSE J., GROSSMAN R. G., CENTENO R., TACHYBANA H. & LEE Y. Y. (1983) *J. Neurosurg.*, **59**, 21.

OLIN M. S., ELTOMEY A. A., DUNSMORE R. H. & ROBERTS M. P. (1982) *Neurosurgery*, **10**, 258.

OLIVECRONA H. (1950) *Dtsch. Med. Wschrift.*, **75**, 1169.

OLIVECRONA H. & RIIVES J. (1948) *Arch. Neurol. Psychiat.*, **59**, 567.

PADGET D. H. (1956) *Amer. J. Anat.*, **98**, 307.

PARKINSON D. & BACKERS E. (1980) *J. Neurosurg.*, **53**, 285.

PATERSON J. H. & MCKISSOCK W. (1956) *Brain*, **79**, 233.

PLUVINAGE R. (1954) *Malformations et Tumeurs Vasculaires du Cerveau.* Masson, Paris.

POLANI P. E. (1952) *Proc. roy. Soc. Med.*, **45**, 860.

POTTER J. M. (1955) *Ann. roy. Coll. Surg. Eng.*, **16**, 227.

RADERMACKER J. (1951) *Acta Neurol. Psychiat. Belge*, **51**, 427. Report of Cooperative Study of Intracranial Aneurysm and Subarachnoid Haemorrhage, Section VI (1966) *J. Neurosurg.*, **25**, 467.

ROBERTSON E. G. (1938) *Med. J. Aust.*, **2**, 245.

ROSE W. McI. (1948) *Lancet*, **2**, 561.

ROSS RUSSELL R. W. (1963) *Brain*, **86**, 425.

RUSSELL D. S. (1954) *Proc. roy. Soc. Med.*, **47**, 689.

RUSSELL D. S. & NEVIN S. (1940) *J. Path. Bact.*, **51**, 375.

RUSSELL D. S. & RUBINSTEIN L. J. (1971) *Pathology of Tumours of the Central Nervous System*, 3rd ed. p. 93. Arnold, London.

SAMSON D. (1986) *Neurosurgery*, **19**, 885.

SAMSON D., DITMORE M. & BEYER C. W. (1981) *Neurosurgery*, **8**, 43.

SCHMITT O. (1920) *Beitrage Klin. Chirurg.*, **118**, 178.

SHENKIN H. A., SPITZ E. B., GRANT F. C. & KETY S. S. (1948) *J. Neurosurgery*, **5**, 164.

SHI Y. Q. & CHEN X. C. (1986) *J. Neurosurg.*, **65**, 484.

SHUEY H. M., DAY A. L., QUISLING R. G., SYPERT G. W. (1979) *Neurosurgery*, **5**, 476.

SILVERSTEIN A. (1967) *Confin. Neurol.*, **29**, 33.

SMITH D. R. & DONAT J. F. (1981) *Neurosurgery*, **8**, 378.

SOLOMON R. A. & MICHELSEN W. J. (1984) *Neurosurgery*, **14**, 78.

SPETZLER R. F. & MARTIN N. A. (1986) *J. Neurosurgery*, **65**, 476.

SPETZLER R. F., WILSON C. B., WEINSTEIN P., MEHDORN M., TOWNSEND J. & TELLES D. (1978) *Clin. Neurosurg.*, **25**, 651.

STURGE W. A. (1879) *Trans. Clin. Soc. London*, **12**, 162.

SVIEN H. J. & McRAE J. A. (1965) *J. Neurosurg.*, **23**, 23.

TÖNNIS W. (1957) *Premier Congres Int. Neurochirurgie. Rapports et Discussions*, p. 205. Acta Med. Belg., Bruxelles.

TÖNNIS W. & FRIEDMANN G. (1964) *Zbl. Neuroshirur.*, **25**, 1.

TSEMENTZIS S. A. (1985) *Neurosurgery*, **16**, 562.

VAQUERO J., LEUNDA G., MARTINEZ R. & BRAVO G. (1983) *Neurosurgery*, **12**, 208.

VINUELA F. V., DEBRUN G. M., FOX A. J. & KAN S. (1983) *J. Neurosurg.*, **58**, 817.

VOLPIN L., CERVELLINI P., COLOMBO F., ZANUSSO M. & BENEDETTI A. (1984) *Neurosurgery*, **15**, 663.

WADIA N. A. (1960) *Brain*, **83**, 425.

WALTER W. & BISCHOFF W. (1966) *Acta Neurochirurg.*, **9**, 150.

WALTER W. & BROCK M. 1966) *Proc. Third. Int. Cong. Neurol. Surg. Int. Cong. Series no. 110*, p. 686. Exc. Med. Foundation, Amsterdam.

WALTER W., SCHETTLER G. & BISCHOFF W. (1967) *Dtsch. Zsch. Nervenheilk.*, **191**, 39.

WEBER F. P. (1922) *J. Neurol. Psychopath.*, **3**, 134.

WEBER F. P. (1928) *Proc. roy. Soc. Med.* **22**, 431.

WEBER J. (1963) *Schweiz, Arch. Neurol. Neurochirurg. Psychiat.*, **91**, 510.

WILKINS R. H. (1985) *Neurosurg.*, **16**, 421.

WOHLWILL F. J. & YAKOVLEV P. I. (1957) *J. Neuropath. Exp. Neurol.*, **6**, 341.

WOLF A. & BROCK S. (1935) *Bull. Neurol. Inst. New York*, **4**, 144.

WOLPERT S. M., BARNETT F. J. & PRAGER R. J. (1982) *Amer. J. Roentgenol.*, **138**, 99.

WYBURN-MASON R. (1943) *Brain*, **66**, 163.

YASARGIL M. G., ANTIC J., LACIGA R., JAIN K. K. & BOONE S. C. (1976) *Surg. Neurol.*, **6**, 195.

ZÜLCH K. J. (1965) *Brain Tumours*. Heinemann, London.

# Chapter 13
# Other Cerebrovascular Diseases

P. R. D. HUMPHREY

Cerebrovascular disease is one of the commonest causes of death and prolonged disability in the United Kingdom. A cerebrovascular accident or stroke is defined by WHO as rapidly developing clinical signs of focal or at times global (applied to patients in deep coma and to those with sub-arachnoid haemorrhage) loss of function with symptoms lasting more than 24 hours or leading to death, with no apparent cause other than that of vascular origin. If the event is shortlived and full recovery occurs in less than 24 hours, the episode is termed a transient ischaemic attack (TIA). These may also involve the ophthalmic arteries and therefore episodes of transient uni-lateral visual loss (amaurosis fugax) with or without focal neurological deficit are included in the definition of TIAs. A further term, reversible ischaemic neurological deficit (RIND) is some-times used and refers to events lasting between 24 hours and three weeks with full functional recovery.

## Incidence

The Framingham Study in the United States has shown that stroke is the third commonest cause of death, accounting for 11% of all deaths. The incidence has been estimated to be approxi-mately 200 per 100,000 population (Kannel & Wolf 1983). In this country, the Oxford Com-munity Stroke Study has shown an incidence of 195 per 100,000 per annum (Oxfordshire Com-munity Stroke Project 1983). Thus 95,000 patients will suffer a stroke in England and Wales each year. Mortality figures vary but ap-proximately 30% will die in the acute phase; of

the survivors 70% will be left with some perma-nent disability.

In the last 20 years, the incidence of stroke has fallen (Nicholls & Johansen 1983). Whisnant (1984) in the Rochester Study has shown a 76% fall in mortality rates from stroke since 1950. The incidence of both cerebral infarction and of haemorrhage has fallen. There has been much debate about the cause of this decline (Whisnant 1984, Hachinski 1984). It seems unlikely that it can be explained entirely on the basis of reclassi-fication of disease although the realization that atherosclerotic dementia is uncommon may be partly responsible. Furthermore the reduction has not been seen in subarachnoid haemorrhage. Whilst Whisnant (1984) argues that the active treatment of hypertension is the most relevant factor, this is unlikely to explain the whole picture. Whisnant's figures suggest that the inci-dence of stroke was falling even over the period 1950–60, before the treatment of hypertension became widely practised and there were effective acceptable hypotensive drugs. Hachinski (1984) argues that the reduction in rheumatic heart disease, the reclassification of cerebrovascular disease and the recognition and treatment of TIAs may also be important. Data for England and Wales has also shown a fall, although the magnitude of the reduction (approximately 20–30%) is not so great (Haberman et al. 1982).

The percentage of strokes which are haem-orrhagic, embolic or thrombotic is also con-troversial. Much of the early data relates to post-mortem studies which clearly cannot be extrapo-lated to the community at large. The clinical differentiation of cerebral haemorrhage and thromboembolic disease is notoriously inaccurate. Allen (1983) has recently introduced a scoring system to try and improve this clinical differentiation; there remains, however, considerable clinical overlap between these two groups. Examination of the CSF to look for haemorrhage is also unreliable as some infarcts become haemorrhagic and some haemorrhages remain entirely intracerebral and do not communicate with the CSF. It is clear with the advent of CT scanning that many small haemorrhages which did not rupture into the subarachnoid space were previously incorrectly characterized as thrombotic. The Oxford Community Stroke Study has obtained CT scans or post-mortems on 89% of all strokes occurring over a one year period. This suggests that 8% are due to primary intracerebral haemorrhage, 5% to subarachnoid haemorrhage and 75% to cerebral infarction secondary to thromboembolic disease (Sandercock *et al.* 1985).

What percentage of cerebral infarction is secondary to emboli and what to thrombosis is even less clear. Post-mortem data (Torvik & Jorgensen 1964, Blackwood *et al.* 1969) suggests that as many as 50% of cerebral infarcts are secondary to cardiac emboli. However, most clinical data suggests that only 5–20% of strokes arise from cardiac emboli (Carter 1957, Kurtzke 1976, Groch *et al.* 1961); only Gautier and Morelot (1975) have found clinical evidence to suggest that cardiac emboli account for approximately half of all strokes. The percentage of artery to artery emboli (for example from internal carotid stenosis) is even more difficult to define. It seems likely that the percentage of cerebral infarcts secondary to emboli has been severely underestimated in the past. Carotid angiography and more intensive cardiac investigations suggest that emboli from the heart and proximal arteries are a common cause of cerebral infarction. However, there are limitations with techniques such as echocardiography and cerebral angiography and it is likely that a significant number of embolic strokes are still being missed (Ports *et al.* 1978, Asinger *et al.* 1983, Humphrey & Harrison 1985). Unfortunately the detection of a cardiac source for emboli does not necessarily mean that embolization has occurred; this is especially so in the elderly where vascular lesions at multiple sites are common.

## Pathogenesis

### Stroke

*Cerebral thrombosis*

Thrombosis usually occurs on an atheromatous plaque. It can occur in any of the major cerebral arteries but is particularly common in the internal carotid and basilar vessels. Hypertension is the major risk factor for cerebral artery thrombosis. In hypertensive patients the extent of the atheroma is increased in all vessels (Robertson & Strong 1968). In addition, however, lipohyaline changes in the vessel wall with microaneurysm formation tend to occur in the deep penetrating arteries of the internal capsule, thalamus and pons (Ross Russell 1963).

Thrombosis in the larger arteries tends to produce larger peripheral wedge shaped cortical infarcts (Fig. 13.1). Those that occur in the small penetrating arteries result in smaller lacunar shaped infarcts (Fig. 13.2) which are associated

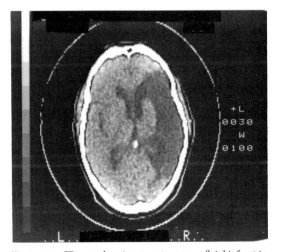

**Fig. 13.1** CT scan showing a mature superficial infarct in the middle cerebral artery territory.

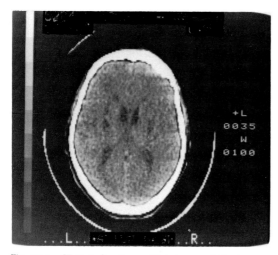

Fig. 13.2   CT scan showing multiple lacunar infarcts.

with an ever increasing number of different clinical syndromes which Miller Fisher has so carefully described (Fisher 1982). However, with increasing use of CT scanning, it has become apparent that the clinical features of the lacunar syndromes may be seen in superficial cortical infarcts so that the clinical differentiation between superficial cortical infarcts and deep lacunar infarcts is less clear cut (Nelson *et al.* 1980).

Damaged cerebral tissue tends to swell from accumulation of water in glial cells (cytotoxic oedema). In addition with the breakdown of the blood brain barrier, extracellular (vasogenic) oedema occurs (O'Brien 1979, Harrison & Ross Russell 1983). Ischaemic oedema is a mixture of cytotoxic oedema which occurs within hours of the event and vasogenic oedema which reaches a peak after 3–4 days. The combined effect is to cause extensive cerebral oedema sometimes with herniation and compression of adjacent structures leading to the clinical deterioration and drowsiness seen in the first few days after a cerebral thrombosis.

### Cerebral emboli

Cerebral emboli also cause cerebral infarction. The emboli usually come from either the heart (Table 13.1) or the great vessels in the neck (de Bono 1983, Harrison & Marshall 1976). The resultant infarcts, which may be multiple and sometimes occur in different vascular territories, often become haemorrhagic. The ophthalmic and middle cerebral arteries are common sites for emboli to lodge. As more noninvasive methods for looking at the heart and extracranial arteries become available, it is likely that the clinical incidence of embolic disease will rise.

It is well established that congenital and rheumatic heart disease, bacterial endocarditis, mural thrombi following recent myocardial infarction, and arrhythmias, particularly atrial fibrillation, are common sources of emboli (de Bono 1983). These are largely composed of fibrin, red cells and platelets. In recent years minor cardiac valvular abnormalities such as mitral annulus calcification and mitral valve prolapse have been recognized as possible sources of emboli. The latter is common to the general population and

Table 13.1   Cardiac sources of emboli.

*Left atrium*
   thrombus (usually secondary to atrial fibrillation)
   myxoma
   paradoxical embolism

*Mitral valve*
   rheumatic endocarditis
   infective endocarditis
   marantic endocarditis
   prosthetic valve
   mitral valve prolapse
   mitral annulus calcification

*Left ventricle*
   thrombus—myocardial infarction, cardiomyopathy

*Aortic valve*
   rheumatic endocarditis
   infective endocarditis
   marantic endocarditis
   bicuspid valve
   aortic sclerosis and calcification
   prosthetic valve
   syphilitic aortitis

*Congenital cardiac disorders*

*Cardiac Surgery*
   air embolism
   platelet/fibrin embolism

there has been much debate about the significance of this lesion (Oakley 1984).

Emboli from proximal atheromatous plaques are also common. These particularly occur at the origin of the internal carotid artery where atheromatous narrowing is common. These plaques tend to ulcerate. This may be due to rupture of lipid-laden plaques into the lumen or result from haemorrhage into the plaque with the formation of either cholesterol emboli or fibrin–platelet emboli. As these friable atherosclerotic plaques become re-endothelialized the emboli cease and the lesion becomes incorporated into the intima of the artery.

Emboli may sometimes be observed on fundoscopy (Fisher 1959). Platelet emboli are only seen transiently before breaking up and moving on whilst cholesterol emboli often remain in the retinal arteries and are sometimes visible for months after the clinical attack. Sometimes emboli from the great vessels or heart valves are calcific. Rarely fibrin – platelet emboli occur on the heart valves in patients with carcinoma, particularly carcinoma of the pancreas, or come from the leg veins having passed through an atrial septal defect to enter the cerebral circulation, the so-called paradoxical embolus.

### Spontaneous cerebral haemorrhage

Spontaneous intracerebral haemorrhage originates from small intracerebral arteries affected by lipohyaline degeneration. This occurs in certain well defined sites: basal ganglia, cerebellum, pons and subcortical white matter (Ross Russell 1963). Lipohyaline change is caused by plasma permeating into the walls of arterioles which have become weakened through loss of elastic and smooth muscle tissue as a result of chronic hypertension. Small microaneurysms (Charcot–Bouchard aneurysms) form, which tend to rupture, producing small lacunar haemorrhages. Sometimes these are larger and may rupture into the subarachnoid space; brain swelling, herniation and brain stem compression may

Table 13.2 Causes of cerebral haemorrhage.

| | |
|---|---|
| 1 | Hypertension |
| 2 | Aneurysm |
| 3 | Arteriovenous malformation |
| 4 | Anticoagulant treatment |
| 5 | Primary or secondary tumour |
| 6 | Clotting abnormalities/thrombocytopenia |
| 7 | Leukaemia |
| 8 | Amyloid angiopathy |
| 9 | Venous infarction |

follow. If the patient survives, the haemorrhage usually absorbs leaving a cystic cavity.

The major causes of cerebral haemorrhage are detailed in Table 13.2.

### Transient ischaemic attacks (TIAs)

#### Carotid

*Embolic*   The vast majority of carotid TIAs are due to emboli. These may be seen passing through the retinal circulation particularly during an attack of amaurosis fugax (Ross Russell 1968). Cholesterol emboli have also been seen in the brain at autopsy (McDonald 1967). Angiography and subsequent endarterectomy often show a loose thrombus at the origin of the internal carotid artery in patients having TIAs (Harrison & Marshall 1977). These lesions may be ulcerated, with haemorrhage into the plaque: this finding is more common in patients with TIAs compared to asymptomatic patients with only atheroma.

Endarterectomy is often successful in stopping TIAs. Attacks also tend to cease when the carotid artery occludes spontaneously. Symptoms in successive attacks may either be similar or may involve different arterial territories; thus a patient may have episodes of amaurosis fugax alternating with weakness of the contralateral limbs.

It would be difficult to explain these observations on a haemodynamic basis but relatively easy on the basis of emboli. Furthermore, Brice *et al.* (1964) showed that blood flow does not fall until the lumen of a vessel is narrowed by at least

75%; TIAs, however, may occur when there is only mild atheroma. There is thus a host of evidence supporting the embolic aetiology of TIAs.

*Haeomodynamic*   A minority of TIAs may have a haemodynamic basis. Eastcott *et al.* (1954) described a patient with tight internal carotid stenosis who had frequent simultaneous attacks of amaurosis in one eye with contralateral limb symptoms which occurred at the time of a cardiac tachyarrhythmia. Surgical repair of the carotid artery prevented the neurological attacks although the episodes of cardiac arrhythmia continued. It is unlikely that arrhythmias alone are a common cause of TIAs in patients with normal vascular trees. The majority of patients with arrhythmias complain of syncopal symptoms such as dizziness, light-headedness and loss of consciousness due to diffuse lowering of cerebral blood flow without any focal symptoms. Kendall and Marshall (1963) studied 37 patients with TIAs on a tilt table and lowered their blood pressure with ganglion blocking agents. Diffuse symptoms were common, including loss of consciousness, but only one patient had a focal attack of the sort described previous to the experiment.

Fisher (1976) has described a patient whose frequent TIAs stopped when hypotensive drugs were withdrawn. Furthermore Ross Russell and Page (1983) described four patients with extensive occlusive disease who suffered attacks of visual loss due to transient retinal ischaemia; these attacks were usually provoked by standing or exercise. The attacks in these patients occurred many times a day and were often precipitated by these specific manœuvres unlike embolic TIAs. Ophthalmodynamometry, which measures the perfusion pressure in the ophthalmic artery, was low and fell during an attack. Surgical reconstruction to improve blood flow resulted in relief of symptoms. These factors suggest that these attacks were occurring on a haemodynamic rather than embolic basis.

Stark and Wodak (1983) have recently described four patients who developed cerebral symptoms on standing some of which resembled focal TIAs; these were often accompanied by dizziness and faintness. All had severe vascular disease. Others have described similar groups of patients (Caplan & Sergay 1976). There thus seems little doubt that a small percentage of carotid TIAs do occur as a result of generalized hypoperfusion. These are usually patients with severe occlusive vascular disease often with occlusion or stenosis of at least three of the major cerebral arteries. There are often clear provocative factors, such as standing, exercising, straining or even eating (Pantin & Young 1980), prior to the development of focal symptoms which may be associated with dizziness and faintness. Haemodynamic TIAs frequently occur many times a day. Whilst haemodynamic TIAs are rare compared to embolic TIAs, it is important to differentiate these two types as different therapeutic measures are often necessary to control the symptoms.

*Vertebrobasilar TIAs*

TIAs in the vertebrobasilar territory also usually occur secondary to emboli. However some are undoubtedly haemodynamic. It is well known that extension of the neck is a cause of vertebrobasilar TIAs. These presumably occur on a haemodynamic basis with kinking of the arterial supply (Payne & Spillane 1957). Sheehan *et al.* (1960) demonstrated that one could find compression of the vertebral artery by osteophytes in the cervical region when the neck was turned and extended. It is doubtful however if this is a common cause of vertebrobasilar TIAs. It is probably only significant where there is coexistent narrowing or occlusion of the carotid arteries in which case the circulation is dependent on its vertebral arteries for cerebral perfusion.

The subclavian steal syndrome is a characteristic cause of haemodynamic vertebrobasilar TIAs. Here there is a stenosis or occlusion of the subclavian artery, usually on the left. As a result, the vertebral artery on this side fails to fill in the normal direction but fills retrogradely from the other vertebral artery or from the carotid arteries via the circle of Willis. Because of the blocked subclavian artery, the blood supply to that arm is dependent on flow in the vertebral artery being retrograde and these patients develop symptoms of vertebrobasilar insufficiency when the arm is exercised; these occur because of the haemodynamic stealing of blood away from the brain stem towards the arm. It is rarely a cause of brain stem infarction and is surprisingly often asymptomatic (Hennerici *et al.* 1981). Fields and Lemak (1972) described a group of 168 cases; they emphasized that the risk of a major brain stem infarct was small.

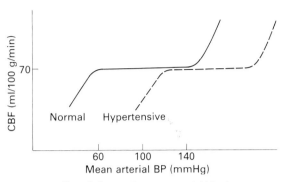

**Fig. 13.3** Effect of changes in mean arterial blood pressure on CBF in normal and hypertensive subjects. (Courtesy of the *British Journal of Hospital Medicine*.)

## Pathophysiology

### Metabolic control of cerebral blood flow (CBF)

An understanding of the major factors controlling CBF is important in the rational management of cerebrovascular disease. In normal controls, there is a close correlation between CBF and $pCO_2$ as well as an inverse correlation between CBF and the oxygen saturation of blood (Kety & Schmidt 1948). There is also a close link between CBF and metabolic demand so that CBF rises as the metabolic rate increases and vice versa.

### Blood pressure, hypertension and cerebral blood flow

CBF remains constant throughout the normal range of blood pressure by autoregulation (Fig. 13.3). It remains constant over a mean arterial blood pressure range of around 60–140 mmHg, that is approximately 80–170 mmHg systolic (Lassen 1959). Below this range, CBF falls and above it the CBF rises.

In hypertension, autoregulation is still present but the whole curve is shifted to the right (Strandgaard *et al.* 1973). As blood pressure is reduced CBF begins to fall at a higher level of mean arterial blood pressure in patients who have been suffering from arterial hypertension compared with controls. This is important in the management of chronically elevated blood pressure. Sudden reduction of blood pressure may be sufficient to cause a fall in CBF even though the absolute level to which the blood pressure has fallen may not normally be regarded in the hypotensive range.

There is good evidence that vascular complications can follow rapid reduction in blood pressure (Kumar *et al.* 1976, Cove *et al.* 1979). Ledingham and Rajagopalan (1979) described 10 patients who developed CNS deficits after such an event. One of their patients developed left hemisphere signs and symptoms after the blood pressure was rapidly reduced from 240/155 to 140/80. The latter blood pressure would normally be regarded as satisfactory but in that previously hypertensive subject, a blood pressure of 140/80 could well have been below the lower limit of autoregulation.

Unless the patient has eclampsia, hypertensive encephalopathy, left ventricular failure secondary to hypertension or aortic dissection, it would seem prudent to lower the blood pressure gradually over a period of days. This is not an argument against treating hypertension; mortality studies show this is the major risk factor in vascular disease. It merely supports gentle reduction of blood pressure. In hypertension, there is evidence that the autoregulatory curve shifts back towards normal after treatment (Vorstrup *et al.* 1984).

*Ischaemia*

Infarction follows thrombosis if the collateral circulation is inadequate. A central zone of necrosis develops. Animal experiments suggest that around this there is an ischaemic penumbra which is viable but functionless (Branston *et al.* 1977). Necrosis of neurons occurs with cerebral blood flow below 10 ml/100 g/min; below 20 ml/100 g/min electrical function ceases, so that between 10 and 20 ml/100 g/min, it is possible to restore electrical function by increasing CBF (normal CBF 50–60 ml/100 g/min).

Following an occlusive episode, CBF tends to be low (Fieschi *et al.* 1966). However there are occasions when the flow is high compared with the metabolic rate, so called luxury perfusion (Lassen 1966). Recent studies with positron emission scans in which both CBF and metabolic rate are measured have confirmed that ischaemia is usually only seen early after a stroke and that luxury perfusion is common (Wise *et al.* 1983). In ischaemia there are two compensatory mechanisms which attempt to maintain metabolic supply. Firstly there is an increase in the extraction of oxygen from blood. Secondly the cerebral blood volume rises again to maximize the delivery of oxygen and other nutrients to the ischaemic area (Gibbs *et al.* 1984). It is only when these compensatory mechanisms are exhausted that ischaemia occurs.

The finding of low flow after an occlusive episode led for a while to the use of carbon dioxide as a vasodilator to increase CBF. However, when CBF to the ischaemic region was measured after carbon dioxide administration, there was evidence to suggest that it had fallen. It appears that the blood vessels in an ischaemic area lose their ability to respond normally to carbon dioxide, being in a state of vasoparalysis (Paulson 1970). Vasodilation to carbon dioxide occurs in the normal parts of the brain with the result that blood is directed away from the ischaemic area towards the rest of the brain, this phenomenon being called intracerebral steal.

Vasoparalysis also affects the response to vasodilator drugs which may, like carbon dioxide, provoke an intracerebral steal rather than the desired increase in flow to the ischaemic area. Measures directed at improving the viscosity of blood do not suffer from this drawback because a reduction in blood viscosity should improve flow to both the normal and ischaemic regions.

Following an occlusive episode, there is also loss of the autoregulatory response to changes in blood pressure (Paulson 1970). Experimental work suggests that CBF is then directly proportional to mean arterial blood pressure (Symon *et al.* 1976). Thus any reduction in blood pressure will be followed by a fall in CBF. The rationale, therefore, for lowering blood pressure in acute strokes is questionable. Indeed by raising blood pressure it is possible to raise CBF (Merory *et al.* 1980). Unfortunately elevating the blood flow after ischaemia may also increase the rate of formation of oedema which will have a deleterious effect (Hossmann 1976).

Most would not now lower the blood pressure in acute stroke patients unless there was evidence of hypertensive encephalopathy or cerebral haemorrhage. It is often difficult to differentiate cerebral haemorrhage and thrombosis without CT scanning. However, clinically, the incidence of cerebral haemorrhage and hypertensive encephalopathy is much greater if the diastolic exceeds 130 mmHg. It seems reasonable to lower the blood pressure in the acute situation if it is greater than 130 mmHg, to diastolic values of about 100–110 mmHg.

It is important to appreciate, however, that the long term situation is different. Patients who recover from an acute stroke and are found to have raised blood pressure (diastolic greater than 100 mmHg) have a better prognosis if treated with hypotensive agents. There is evidence to suggest that autoregulation may partially return after a stroke although it may still be impaired three years after an infarct (Waltz 1970, Symon *et al.* 1975). Although exact guidelines cannot be given, if the blood pressure remains elevated (greater than 100 mmHg diastolic) a month after the acute ischaemic episode, it is reasonable to institute hypotensive therapy. It is then safe to lower blood pressure, although prudent to lower it gradually for the reasons outlined above.

### Transient ischaemic attacks (TIAs)

Regional changes in CBF may long outlive the duration of the TIA (Rees *et al.* 1970). In one recorded case, the regional CBF was found still to be low 90 days after the last attack. It is important to emphasize that these changes were regional; the overall CBF remained normal. Van der Drift and Kok (1973) demonstrated small infarcts at post-mortem in patients who had only had a TIA clinically. These findings emphasize that the differentiation of thromboembolic cerebrovascular disease into strokes and TIAs is somewhat artificial. The idea that TIAs are not associated with any structural damage or permanent change is probably naïve. The evidence suggests that fundamentally there is little difference between strokes and TIAs and that TIAs and strokes with recovery should be investigated in the same way to prevent a further attack.

## Risk factors

### Age

Needless to say, age is one of the important predictive factors in cerebrovascular disease. The incidence of stroke is low before the age of 40 when the annual incidence is considerably less than one per 1,000 per year and rises to approximately 20 per 1,000 per year by the age of 75 (Kannel & Wolf 1983).

### Hypertension

After the age of the patient, arterial hypertension is the next most powerful risk factor for both haemorrhagic and atherosclerotic cerebrovascular disease. Whilst most physicians use the diastolic blood pressure for long term follow-up, it is the systolic blood pressure which reflects most closely the risk of future stroke. The Framingham Study suggests there is no clear cut-off in blood pressure levels at which the risk begins to rise; it increases progressively with increasing . systolic blood pressure even from within the normotensive range (Kannel & Wolf 1983).

Ross Russell (1963), reaffirming Charcot and Bouchard's findings, found that hypertensive patients were more likely to have small microaneurysms which particularly occur in the basal ganglia, cerebellum, pons and subcortical white matter. These may rupture causing 'lacunar haemorrhages' or thrombose resulting in 'lacunar infarcts'. In addition, atherosclerosis is more advanced in hypertension (Robertson & Strong 1968).

In the past it has been suggested that hypotension, with a resultant fall in cerebral blood flow is also a risk factor for stroke. Epidemiological data suggests that this is rare. It is seen usually following a cardiac arrest where diffuse damage occurs particularly in the watershed areas. Very rarely a stroke seems to follow hypotensive treatment in patients with severe widespread occlusive cerebrovascular disease. However, there is no doubt that it is the preceding hypertension which is the most important risk factor in cerebrovascular disease.

### Transient ischaemic attacks

After a TIA there is an undoubted increased risk of stroke. It is difficult to put a definite figure on this because different studies have shown the risk of stroke after a TIA varies between zero and 50% (Brust 1977). This is largely due to differing methods of data collection. Most would accept that the risk of stroke is approximately 10% per annum, the greatest risk being in the first year (Mohr 1978, Kannel & Wolf 1983). The Framingham data suggests that the risk of stroke is increased by at least 10 times in the first year after a TIA (Kannel & Wolf 1983).

*Coronary artery disease*

Atherosclerosis is a widespread disease; it is not surprising therefore that patients with coronary artery disease are at an increased risk of stroke. Cardiac enlargement on chest X-ray, congestive cardiac failure and ECG abnormalities such as left ventricular enlargement, intraventricular conduction disturbances and ST/T wave changes, are all associated with an increased risk of cerebrovascular disease (Kannel & Wolf 1983). This association is further emphasized by mortality data which shows that coronary artery disease and not a further stroke is the chief cause of death following a stroke (Sacco *et al.* 1982).

*Diabetes mellitus*

An elevated blood sugar appears to be an independent risk factor according to the Framingham data (Kannel & Wolf 1983).

*Haematocrit*

Whilst there is no doubt that polycythaemia rubra vera is associated with cerebrovascular disease, it has only recently become apparent that haematocrit values in the high normal range may also represent an independent risk factor (Kannel & Wolf 1983).

*Other risk factors*

A variety of other parameters such as cholesterol, smoking, lack of exercise and obesity have all been suggested as independent risk factors (Kannel & Wolf 1983). Whilst elevated lipid levels and smoking are definite independent risk factors in the aetiology of coronary artery disease, their role in cerebrovascular disease is less clear. As a practical policy, it is best to take account of the latter risk factors because several of them are amenable to treatment; furthermore to divorce coronary and cerebrovascular risk

**Table 13.3**   Other causes of cerebral infarction.

| | |
|---|---|
| 1 | Migraine |
| 2 | Haematological disorders (*see* Table 13.4) |
| 3 | Inflammatory arterial disease (*see* Table 13.5) |
| 4 | Fibromuscular hyperplasia |
| 5 | Venous thrombosis |
| 6 | Moya-Moya disease |
| 7 | Trauma to neck |
| 8 | Pregnancy |
| 9 | Metabolic disorders, for example homocysteinuria |
| 10 | Fat embolism |
| 11 | Infection |
| 12 | Malignancy—neoplastic angioendotheliosis |
| 13 | Fabry pseudoxanthoma elasticum |
| 14 | Hypertensive encephalopathy |
| 15 | Cerebral arteriography |
| 16 | Subarachnoid haemorrhage |
| 17 | Post therapeutic irradiation |
| 18 | Oral contraceptives |

**Table 13.4**   Haematological disorders causing stroke.

| | |
|---|---|
| 1 | Polycythaemia rubra vera |
| 2 | Sickle cell disease |
| 3 | Essential thrombocythaemia |
| 4 | Leukaemia |
| 5 | Thrombocytopenia |
| 6 | Thrombotic thrombocytopenia purpura |
| 7 | Hyperviscosity multiple myeloma Waldenstrom macroglobulinaemia |
| 8 | Paroxysmal nocturnal haemoglobinuria |
| 9 | Lupus anticoagulant |

**Table 13.5**   Inflammatory arterial disease.

| | |
|---|---|
| 1 | Systemic lupus erythematosis |
| 2 | Giant cell arteritis |
| 3 | Polyarteritis nodosa |
| 4 | Granulomatous angiitis |
| 5 | Wegener granulomatosis |
| 6 | Behcet disease |
| 7 | Sarcoid angiitis |
| 8 | Scleroderma |
| 9 | Rheumatoid arthritis |
| 10 | Rheumatic fever |
| 11 | Aortic arch syndrome Takayasu arteritis syphilis transient emboligenic aortoarteritis |
| 12 | Necrotizing angiitis with drug abuse |

factors into separate groups for management purposes is naïve because most stroke patients die of coronary artery disease.

This section has largely dealt with the risk factors responsible for cerebral atherosclerosis. Independent of this, there are a variety of other conditions which may present with ischaemic cerebrovascular episodes unrelated to atherosclerosis (Tables 13.3, 13.4 and 13.5).

## Clinical diagnosis

### Carotid territory

*Anterior cerebral artery*

The anterior cerebral artery passes forwards and over the corpus callosum supplying the medial part of the cerebral hemisphere including the entire motor and sensory cortex controlling the leg area. Urgency or incontinence of micturition may occur because the area concerned with the voluntary control of bladder function lies just anterior to the leg area. Because this artery also supplies the frontal pole, there may be disturbances of intellect, judgement and emotional control. Branches of the anterior cerebral artery also supply the anterior limb of the internal capsule, ischaemia of which results in hemiplegia.

*Middle cerebral artery*

The middle cerebral artery supplies most of the lateral surface of the cerebral hemisphere. It also gives off small penetrating branches (lenticulostriate arteries) which pass deep into the cerebral hemispheres and supply part of the basal ganglia and internal capsule.

Ischaemia produces a hemiparesis with hemisensory loss affecting mainly the face and arm. There may be a homonymous hemianopia. This pattern of neurological dysfunction may be due to superficial cortical infarcts or deep lacunar infarcts.

If the dominant hemisphere is affected, then dysphasia is common. Nondominant hemisphere lesions produce topographical disorientation

with inattention and neglect of the left side: there may be difficulty with dressing.

The symptomatology of TIAs is similar. Sometimes symptoms may be confined to the arm or hand only, and it is important not to confuse this with a more peripheral lesion.

*Internal carotid artery*

This produces a syndrome resembling combined anterior and middle cerebral artery occlusion. Furthermore, the first branch of the internal carotid artery is the ophthalmic artery; loss of vision to one eye may accompany carotid artery occlusion, particularly if both the internal and external arteries are involved. More frequently, episodes of fleeting visual loss (amaurosis fugax) occur. These are usually embolic and produce either transient complete unilateral loss of vision or altitudinal field loss if only the upper or lower half of the retina is involved. Rarely these attacks are haemodynamic in which case there is a clear provocative feature before each attack such as standing, exercise or straining at stool, all of which tend to reduce retinal perfusion (Ross Russell & Page 1983).

In addition an ipsilateral Horner syndrome may be present following damage to the sympathetic fibres in the carotid sheath. Because of the increased collateral blood flow, the external carotid branches such as the superficial temporal artery, may be more prominent and sometimes even painful on the side of an internal carotid artery occlusion.

*Posterior cerebral artery*

These paired vessels are formed by the bifurcation of the basilar trunk. They supply the occipital lobes, the upper part of the brain stem and the medial surface of the temporal lobe. Homonymous visual field defects, usually unilateral, are the principal result of ischaemia in the posterior cerebral territory. Lesions on both sides may result in cortical blindness. Pupillary responses are spared as the pupillary fibres travelling to the midbrain are not involved. The patient often confabulates, has hallucinations, little insight and may even deny his blindness (Anton syndrome).

Transient amnesia is common because of ischaemia to the medial aspect of the temporal lobes. The posterior cerebral artery also supplies part of the thalamus. Infarction produces sensory impairment over the contralateral side of the body sometimes accompanied by a very unpleasant pain which may be spontaneous or induced by light contact with the skin (thalamic syndrome).

*Vertebrobasilar ischaemia*

The symptoms and signs following vertebrobasilar ischaemia depend on the level of the lesion in the brain stem (Caplan 1981). Occlusion of the terminal basilar artery may produce signs of posterior cerebral artery occlusion.

In midbrain lesions pupillary changes with impaired vertical gaze or oculomotor nerve dysfunction are seen. Fixed constricted pupils and horizontal gaze palsy with facial weakness and sensory loss follow damage to the pons. In either case a hemiparesis or quadriparesis may also occur.

A wide range of other syndromes, many of which Fisher (1982) classifies as lacunar infarcts, are reported to follow ischaemia to localized regions of the brain stem. The basic pattern is similar. They consist of ipsilateral cranial nerve palsies with contralateral paresis or sensory loss which affects either the arm and leg or arm, leg and face depending on the level in the brain stem; this may be combined with ipsilateral cerebellar signs. Thrombosis of the posterior inferior cerebellar artery serves as a useful example. This produces ischaemia of the dorsolateral medulla with cranial nerve palsies V, VI, VII, IX and X, cerebellar ataxia and a Horner syndrome on the same side of the lesion with contralateral spinothalamic loss in the arm and leg. Pain

and temperature loss may occur over the ipsilateral face due to damage to the descending tract and nucleus of V. Hemiplegia is rare because the pyramidal tracts lying ventrally are spared.

Occlusion of the basilar artery itself often results in fatal coma with flaccid tetraplegia and loss of brain stem reflexes. It is important to distinguish this from the rare 'locked-in' syndrome in which there is ventral ischaemia of the midbrain (Hawkes 1974). The clinical picture appears similar; the patient is immobile and superficially appears unconscious but may be fully alert. The only voluntary movement consists of vertical movements of the eyes and occasionally the eye lids. Thus it is important to check these eye movements before accepting that any patient is truly unconscious.

Postural vertigo is often thought to be synonymous with vertebrobasilar ischaemia; this is rarely so. It is much more likely to be due to inner ear disease. It is better not to label such cases as vertebrobasilar ischaemia, unless there is other good evidence for cerebrovascular disease.

*Subclavian steal syndrome*

Typically the patient develops symptoms of vertebrobasilar ischaemia after exercising the arm. Although this is the classical presentation, the TIAs may be unrelated to arm exercise; it is only with the advent of noninvasive Doppler studies that the relatively common occurrence of this vascular pattern of disease has been appreciated.

*Lacunes*

Lacunar states overlap with some of the previous clinical groups described. These small microinfarcts, are common, mostly occur in hypertensive patients, and give rise to many clinical syndromes described (Fisher 1982). The four most widely described and the site of the lesion in each type are shown in Table 13.6.

Sometimes multiple lacunar infarcts (l'état

**Table 13.6** Common lacunar infarcts.

| Clinical type | Site of lesion |
| --- | --- |
| Pure hemisensory loss | Thalamus |
| Pure motor hemiplegia | Internal capsule, pons, cerebral peduncle |
| Ataxic hemiparesis | Pons, internal capsule |
| Dysarthria/clumsy hand syndrome | Pons, internal capsule |

lacunaire) occur; the clinical syndrome then consists of a pseudobulbar palsy, dementia, dysarthria, small-stepping gait (marche à petit pas), imbalance and incontinence. The history is usually progressive with additional episodes of focal neurological loss, particularly hemiplegia.

*Boundary zone infarcts*

The clinical patterns so far described follow occlusion of individual arteries. Sometimes, however, there is a generalized reduction in cerebral blood flow (Torvik 1984). This particularly follows a cardiac arrest or hypoxic damage during cardiac surgery. Ischaemia is then most marked in the boundary zone between the territories of the individual distributing cerebral arteries, because it is here that cerebral perfusion pressure is lowest. Most commonly, this occurs in the parieto-occipital zone, where infarcts produce visual field defects (often only partial), reading difficulties, visual disorientation and constructional apraxia (Ross Russell & Bharucha 1978). In the frontal border zone mental slowing, grasp reflexes, gait disturbance and incontinence may occur.

*Spinal cord*

*See* spinal cord disease (Chapter 21 and 22).

## Clinical examination

In the assessment of cerebrovascular disease it is particularly important to include a full general and cardiovascular examination, paying particular attention to heart sounds and murmurs and checking the peripheral pulses. Asymmetry of the blood pressure in each arm (more than 15 mmHg systolic) with or without a supraclavicular bruit suggests subclavian occlusion or stenosis. Even though a carotid bruit at the angle of the jaw is the best clinical guide to an internal carotid stenosis, there are many false positives and negatives (Humphrey & Bradbury 1984). Bruits are thought to arise from arterial wall vibration due to turbulence in the arterial flow. This is most commonly seen with an internal carotid stenosis. However, they sometimes occur if there is a contralateral or ipsilateral internal carotid occlusion, if there is just atheroma in the

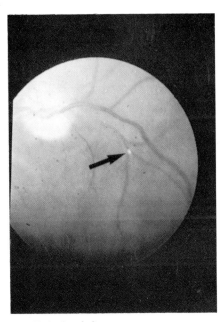

**Fig. 13.4** Retinal emboli.

internal carotid artery or rarely if there is an external carotid stenosis. Furthermore the bruit disappears as an internal carotid stenosis exceeds 90%. Whilst a bruit is the best clinical guide to an internal carotid stenosis, attacks of amaurosis fugax combined with contralateral hemiparesis, coexistent intermittent claudication, age over 50 years and hypertension, all increase the chance of finding a stenosis at angiography (Harrison & Marshall 1975, Wilson & Ross Russell 1977).

Examination of the ocular fundus may show emboli which usually lodge in the major retinal arteries or at their bifurcations (Fig. 13.4). Sometimes in patients with haemodynamic TIAs evidence of slow flow retinopathy may be visible (Ross Russell & Page 1983).

**Differential diagnosis**

*Transient ischaemic attacks (TIAs)*

Attacks similar to TIAs may occur in migraine (Bartleson 1984); it is important to ask about the presence of other migrainous symptoms in the attack such as headache, nausea, vomiting and photophobia as well as a past history of more typical migrainous episodes with or without a visual aura.

Rarely symptoms of TIAs may occur in hypoglycaemia (Meyer & Portnoy 1958). Hyperviscosity states and hepatic and renal failure may occasionally produce unilateral disturbances as can hyponatraemia (Faris & Poser 1964) and hypercalcaemia (Longo & Witherspoon 1980).

Tumours often present with focal epilepsy; sometimes however they present as transient episodes of focal neurological disturbance without epileptic features (Ross 1983, Loeb 1979). Giant aneurysms which are often filled with thrombotic material occasionally give rise to embolic TIAs (Steel *et al.* 1982). Finally chronic subdural haematomas may present with attacks identical to TIAs (Luxom & Harrison, 1979).

*Stroke*

Like TIA, stroke is merely a descriptive term for a set of clinical symptoms and signs. Rarely a cerebral tumour, subdural haematoma, encephalitis, abscess or episode of demyelination may all present with an acute onset of focal neurological deficit, particularly if it occurs in a stepwise manner or evolves over a period of hours or days (Luxom & Harrison 1979). Unfortunately, however, vascular disease can also present subacutely. This is especially likely if there is further propagation of the original thrombus, additional emboli, secondary oedema or haemorrhage.

One may also use clinical criteria to try and distinguish cerebral haemorrhage from infarction (Allen 1983); as already mentioned this is unreliable. A history of previous TIAs, presence of emboli in the retina or clear cardiac source of emboli, strongly suggest embolism. Early headache and loss of consciousness, drowsiness, vomiting, meningism, bilateral extensor plantar responses and elevated diastolic blood pressure point towards a haemorrhagic episode.

**Investigations**

Investigation involves confirming the diagnosis and identifying any risk factors. All patients with strokes or TIAs should have the tests shown in Table 13.7.

Any abnormality needs appropriate further investigation. In young patients it is particularly important to consider the more unusual causes of strokes mentioned in Tables 13.3, 13.4 and

Table 13.7   Routine tests on all strokes or TIAs.

Full blood count, platelet count, ESR
Urea and electrolytes, biochemistry profile
Blood sugar and fasting lipids
Serology for syphilis
Test for sickling in black patients, haemoglobin,
   electrophoresis
Chest X-ray, Skull X-ray
ECG
MSU

13.5. All young patients (less than 55 years) should have an echocardiogram to look for sub-clinical heart disease; M-mode provides good information on the heart valves but fails often to demonstrate mural thrombi for which two dimensional echocardiography (2DE) is more useful (Ports *et al.* 1978, Asinger *et al.* 1983).

If there is doubt about the diagnosis, then CT scanning is indicated; ideally it should be performed on all stroke patients especially on those in whom angiography is planned. However, whilst the CT scan may provide helpful information and will undoubtedly differentiate haemorrhage and infarction, it may not be able to differentiate a tumour from an infarct. In fact Norris and Hachinski (1982) showed that it was not a substitute for careful clinical assessment.

Angiography of the cerebral vessels is usually reserved for those with carotid TIAs or stroke who have made a good recovery and thus have a lot to lose from a further attack; it is sometimes performed in vertebrobasilar TIAs uncontrolled by medical means or if signs of subclavian stenosis are present. It is only indicated in those who are otherwise fit for surgery. It is virtually never indicated for acute stroke unless there is evidence of trauma to the neck vessels, subarachnoid haemorrhage or cerebellar haemorrhage.

Angiography may provide information on unusual causes of stroke such as fibromuscular dysplasia. More frequently it is used to look for an operable stenosis at the origin of the internal carotid artery. Unfortunately only approximately 30% of all patients referred to a neurological centre with carotid TIAs have an operable lesion (Humphrey & Marshall 1981). This has led to the assessment of noninvasive methods for detecting carotid bifurcation disease. These are based on two distinct mechanisms (Woodcock 1981). The first uses Doppler ultrasonography which is particularly useful in detecting carotid stenosis greater than 50% and carotid occlusions (Hennerici *et al.* 1981). The second uses B-mode ultrasonic imaging to create anatomical pictures of the vessel wall and is useful in all degrees of atheroma especially those with mild to moderate atheroma (Ginsberg & Cebul 1983). These two

methods have been combined in the so-called Duplex scanners which give good correlation with angiography throughout all grades of atheromatous disease. These techniques are particularly operator dependent and need considerable practice and time to master the technique and interpret the results.

Angiography remains the standard method for visualizing the vascular tree. Until recently, this has either been by catheter studies or by direct puncture, and requires good biplanar views of both carotid artery bifurcation and the intra-cerebral circulation. Although arch angiograms are often taken prior to catheter studies of the carotid arteries, these are rarely necessary as they infrequently contribute to the surgical management of the individual patient (Goldstein *et al.* 1981). One policy is first to obtain views of the symptomatic carotid bifurcation; if this is normal then no further X-rays are necessary. If there is an internal carotid stenosis or occlusion, then views of the contralateral carotid artery must be taken as a prelude to possible surgery. With a very tight stenosis, it is important to take delayed films with subtraction to look for the thin trickle of contrast media signifying that the stenosis has not completely occluded, the so-called pseudo-occlusion. If a complete occlusion of the internal carotid artery is demonstrated then it is important to look for a persistent internal carotid stump (Fig. 13.5) which can be a source of continuing emboli (Bogousslavsky *et al.* 1981).

Internal carotid artery occlusion is usually accompanied by reversed flow in the ophthalmic artery which is now supplied through the orbit (Fig. 13.6) by branches of the external carotid artery; this is most easily demonstrated by Doppler ultrasound (Trockel *et al.* 1984). It is therefore possible for embolic TIAs to continue after an internal carotid occlusion if there is a coexistent external carotid artery stenosis or persistent internal carotid artery stump with emboli reaching the cerebral circulation through the external carotid artery via the ophthalmic artery.

Angiography, however, still carries a small risk of stroke. Whilst most would put this at

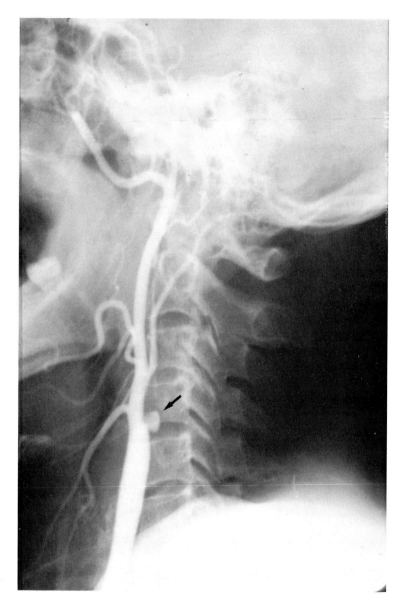

**Fig. 13.5** Internal carotid artery occlusion with a persistent patent stump at the origin of the internal carotid.

about 1% a recent prospective survey has suggested that when looked for carefully, the risks may be higher (Steiner *et al.* 1983). This combined with the risks of surgery, accounts for the marked variation in the use of angiography in different centres in the United Kingdom (United Kingdom TIA Study Group 1983).

Recently, digital subtraction angiography with computerized imaging of the cerebral vessels after either intravenous or small intra-arterial injections of contrast media has become available. This may be less hazardous than conventional angiography and provides good quality pictures in approximately 80% of cases (Little *et al.* 1982). It is likely that this will replace conventional angiography in most patients with cerebrovascular disease although even digital venous angiography has a definite morbidity and mortality (Aaron *et al.* 1984).

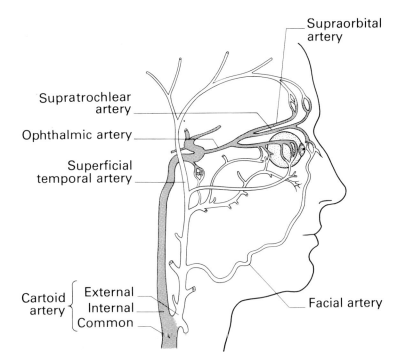

Supraorbital artery

Supratrochlear artery

Ophthalmic artery

Superficial temporal artery

Cartoid artery
- External
- Internal
- Common

Facial artery

**Fig. 13.6** Anatomy of the anastomoses linking the internal and external carotid arteries.

## Management

### Acute stroke

Preservation of the airway, maintaining fluid balance and nursing in the semiprone position are important if the patient is drowsy. Cerebral oedema is a significant factor in large infarcts and may be associated with a deteriorating level of consciousness. Steroids have not been shown to be of any consistent use and there is no justification for their routine use (Mulley *et al.* 1978). Hyperosmolar agents, such as mannitol and glycerol, may reduce the degree of cerebral oedema although as yet the clinical value of this is unclear (Frithz & Werner 1975).

Low molecular weight dextran reduces haematocrit and improves cerebral blood flow. However, controlled clinical studies have shown no worthwhile benefit in acute stroke (Matthews *et al.* 1976).

There is much debate about the treatment of hypertension in acute stroke. If there is no evidence of aortic dissection, cerebral haemorrhage or hypertensive encephalopathy, (Dimsdale 1982), then it is prudent not to lower blood pressure. Unfortunately it is difficult clinically to differentiate cerebral haemorrhage and thrombosis without CT scanning. The incidence of haemorrhage or hypertensive encephalopathy is much greater if the diastolic exceeds 130 mmHg. Thus if the diastolic blood pressure exceeds this, gentle lowering is probably indicated; because this will be associated with a fall in cerebral blood flow, it is wise not to lower the blood pressure below 100–110 mmHg diastolic.

Anticoagulants have no part to play in thrombotic strokes. However, where there is a clear source of emboli, then anticoagulants need to be considered. Secondary bleeding into an infarct is the major risk of anticoagulants and needs to be balanced against the risk of further emboli. In rheumatic heart disease with or without atrial fibrillation, anticoagulants are usually given early although some authors delay for 2–3 weeks to minimize the risks of bleeding into the infarct. Although not conclusive, evidence suggests that the risks of secondary haemorrhage due to anticoagulant treatment are less than the risks of further emboli (Koller 1982, Furlan *et al.* 1982). All patients should have a CT scan prior to anticoagulation to exclude an intracerebral haemorrhage or haemorrhagic infarct.

The risks of further emboli in lone atrial fibrillation are also substantial (Wolf *et al.* 1983); whether long term anticoagulation improves the prognosis is unclear but most physicians would anticoagulate for at least six months when the risk of further emboli is greatest. Mural thrombi are a rare cause of cerebral emboli and usually occur in the first four weeks after a myocardial infarct (Bean 1938); short term anticoagulation for 3–6 months is necessary. Where a left ventricular aneurysm is present, then anticoagulation should be long term if surgical correction is not deemed possible.

**Stroke in evolution**

Anticoagulation should be considered with stuttering or progressive stroke in evolution to prevent further deterioration even if there is no embolic source. If there is no sign of haemorrhage on CT or on examination of the cerebrospinal fluid then short term anticoagulation is given in the hope of preventing further propagation of the thrombus (Millikan & McDowell 1981).

Surgery has no part to play in the management of acute stroke unless there is cerebellar haemorrhage or infarction in which case there is good evidence that urgent evacuation of the haemorrhage or decompression may be followed by dramatic recovery (Heros 1982). In the unoperated cases, if there is a progressive deterioration in the level of consciousness, the prognosis is invariably poor. The role of surgery in the management of intracerebral haemorrhage remains controversial.

# Long term management, rehabilitation and prognosis

Prognosis in patients who have suffered a stroke depends largely on the level of consciousness of the patient when first seen. Eighty-ninety per cent of those in coma die within a few weeks of admission compared with 30% mortality in patients who are alert. In survivors, the prognosis is worst in those with urinary incontinence, complete hemiplegia with severe joint position loss, and those who have a gaze palsy and difficulty sitting unaided (Oxbury *et al.* 1975, Prescott *et al.* 1982). Most improvement occurs within the first three months although recovery can continue for up to 6–12 months (Wade *et al.* 1983). Approximately 60% of those who recover become functionally independent.

Physiotherapy, occupational therapy and attention to speech disorders help to encourage maximum utilization of the neurological function that slowly returns. The role of specialized stroke units and highly trained speech therapists remains uncertain. It is clear that the motivation of the patients, combined with simple practical advice and the attitude of the clinical team and family, are important in coming to terms with the disability and making the most of the recovery that does occur (Howell 1984).

Aids to daily living with home assessment can make it possible to get many people back to the community. Spasticity may be helped by physiotherapy, physical methods of treatment such as ice packs and antispastic drugs namely, baclofen, dantrolene sodium or diazepam. In some cases, however, usually where the leg is very weak, the spasticity may help the patient to use the leg as a prop. In this case, antispastic drugs may remove the spasticity and unmask severe weakness, rendering the limb less useful.

Advice for the future and treatment concerning any risk factors is required. There is often a fear that treating hypertension in this situation may be dangerous as it will tend to lower CBF. Experimental evidence suggests that autoregulation partially returns after a stroke. Clinical trials suggest that the prognosis is better in hypertensive patients with a stroke if the blood pressure is treated (Johnston *et al.* 1981). However, it is wise to lower blood pressure slowly and to aim for a diastolic blood pressure of around 100 mmHg. In spite of this, there do seem to be a small number of stable patients with a stroke who become worse after hypotensive treatment; it is not yet possible to predict clinically who these patients are. It seems likely that either their blood pressure falls precipitously without anyone realizing it or that their compensatory cerebral vasodilatory mechanisms were already maximally operative so that any fall in blood pressure was followed by a fall in CBF. Thus in the rare clinical case where deterioration occurs immediately following hypotensive treatment, it is probably wise to cease hypotensive therapy and leave the arterial pressure at the untreated level.

The long term prognosis of the patient who has suffered a stroke suggests that the risk of a further major stroke is small. The majority die from a myocardial infarct (Sacco *et al.* 1982), emphasizing that this is a diffuse disease and one cannot consider cerebrovascular disease in isolation from the other manifestations of arteriosclerotic disease.

## Transient ischaemic attacks and strokes with recovery

### Medical treatment

Patients who have made a full recovery, whether it be from a TIA or stroke, should be considered for full investigation. The risk of a further permanent stroke in these patients is approximately 5–10% per annum (Brust 1977). The risk of further stroke is probably greater if the initial episode occurred in the carotid artery territory.

Advice and treatment to deal with any risk factors described earlier is necessary. Hypertension is far and away the most important risk factor for both cerebral haemorrhage and infarction. Routine blood pressure in excess of 100

mmHg diastolic should be lowered to 90–95 mmHg. The systolic pressure is a better prognostic guide, but is more liable to fluctuate and therefore more difficult to control. It is important to lower blood pressure gradually as the autoregulatory range is higher in hypertension (Fig. 13.3). There is now good evidence that the autoregulation threshold may revert back towards normal after prolonged treatment (Vorstrup *et al.* 1984). This is not an argument against treating hypertension but merely a word of caution regarding the rate at which arterial pressure is lowered.

Dietary advice in hyperlipidaemia should also be given even though it is, as yet, of unproven value in cerebrovascular disease. However there is good evidence that cholesterol is a risk factor for cardiac disease, and the majority of patients with cerebrovascular disease die of myocardial disease. For the same reasons, patients should be urged to refrain from smoking.

In the majority of patients, there is no operable lesion (*see* next section). The choice of therapy for embolic or thrombotic events lies between antiplatelet and anticoagulant drugs. Antiplatelet drugs are used extensively in the prevention of stroke. Three large trials, from the United States, Canada and France, all have suggested that aspirin is useful in the prevention of stroke after an initial stroke (Fields *et al.* 1977, Canadian Cooperative Study Group 1978, Bousser *et al.* 1983). All three studies used approximately 1,300 mg of aspirin per day. The ideal dose is unclear. There is some laboratory evidence that low dose aspirin (about 60 mg) is better (Masotti *et al.* 1979). Much has been made of the effect of aspirin on prostaglandin synthesis. In platelets, there is thromboxane $A_2$ ($TXA_2$ which causes vasoconstriction and platelet aggregation and is blocked by low dose aspirin. In the vessel wall, prostacyclin (epoprostenol, $PGI_2$) is produced; this causes vasodilation and platelet disaggregation. 1,300 mg of aspirin blocks both $TXA_2$ and $PGI_2$ production whereas low dose only inhibits $TXA_2$. Ideally therefore low dose aspirin to block $TXA_2$ and leave $PGI_2$ production intact is indicated. As yet there is no clinical trial evidence to support this pattern of dosage. The UK TIA Study Group (1987) has shown no significant difference between doses of 1200 mg and 300 mg per day, so that 300 mg now appears to be the dose recommended on the basis of data from clinical trials.

The role of two other antiplatelet agents, dipyridamole and sulphinpyrazone, is also unclear. There is a great deal of experimental evidence to support their antiplatelet effects. However there is no good clinical evidence that sulphinpyrazone is of any use (Canadian Cooperative Study 1978). This also applies to dipyridamole (Bousser et al. 1983) apart from one study in which it was useful in preventing emboli from prosthetic heart valves when combined with anticoagulants (Sullivan et al. 1968). One practice is to reserve dipyridamole for those patients in whom aspirin is medically contraindicated or fails to control TIAs.

The place of anticoagulants in the management of TIAs without any clear source of cardiac emboli is controversial (Brust 1977). Most of the trials are open to considerable criticism. Anticoagulants are usually reserved for those cases in which antiplatelet drugs fail to control TIAs. As the risk of stroke after a TIA is highest in the first six months, anticoagulants are rarely given for a longer period except in those with cardiac emboli. Anticoagulants are clearly not without risks and much more difficult to manage than antiplatelet therapy.

Long term anticoagulation is mainly reserved for cardiac emboli due to rheumatic heart disease with or without atrial fibrillation (Easton & Sherman 1980). Occasionally heart valve replacement may be necessary where there is a persistent source of emboli which cannot be controlled by anticoagulant and antiplatelet drugs. The place of long term anticoagulants in those with lone atrial fibrillation is unclear. With mild valvular abnormalities such as mitral valve prolapse, there is insufficient information and anticoagulants are not usually given.

**Surgical treatment**

*Internal carotid endarterectomy*

About 25% of TIAs in the carotid territory arise from an operable stenosis at the origin of the internal carotid artery (Harrison & Marshall 1975, Humphrey & Marshall 1981). The five year risk of a completed stroke after carotid TIAs is approximately 35%. Ever since the first carotid reconstruction by Eastcott et al. (1954), it has been largely accepted that surgery was the procedure of choice to prevent total occlusion and remove an ulcerated atheromatous plaque or stenosis which acts as a source of emboli. Those with a particular interest in carotid endarterectomy quote operative morbidity and mortality figures below 1% (Thompson & Talkington 1976). No randomized trial has shown a clear benefit from surgical treatment (Warlow 1984). It was only when the results of a study from a general surgical vascular unit in the Midwest of the United States were bravely published showing an operative morbidity and mortality in excess of 20% that grave doubts about the risks of carotid endarterectomy arose (Easton & Sherman 1977). That same group has since reported more recent figures concerning mortality and morbidity which have considerably improved. In the United Kingdom, however, the doubt about endarterectomy persists; this led to the setting up of the European Endarterectomy Study which is based in the United Kingdom and is currently comparing medical treatment and endarterectomy in carotid stenosis. Operative mortality and morbidity figures of close to 1% have been reported by those with a particular interest in vascular surgery in the United Kingdom (Browse & Ross Russell, 1984). Carotid endarterectomy should probably only be performed by those who do the operation frequently and have an overall mortality and morbidity of less than 5% for angiography and surgery combined.

The risks of endarterectomy are greater after a preoperative stroke, even if there has been full recovery, than after a TIA (Harrison 1982). The risks are also greater if there is contralateral carotid occlusion or stenosis. The place of surgery in the management of nonstenotic ulcerated plaques is unclear; most physicians would treat these medically and consider surgery only if the attacks continued despite medical treatment.

The complications of endarterectomy either follow local vascular problems such as mural thrombosis, cessation of blood flow during the operation or embolization at the time of surgery or damage to local nonvascular structures. There has been much debate about the place of intravascular shunts to enable blood to bypass the endarterectomy site whilst the operation is in progress (Ferguson 1982, Sundt 1983). The risks of causing local damage or emboli seem to balance the benefits of preserving flow in the carotid artery. If there is low stump pressure (less than 50 mmHg) in the distal part of the clamped internal carotid artery, then it would seem prudent to use a shunt to maintain distal carotid artery perfusion. Intraoperative monitoring of the EEG may also help in making this decision.

The local complications of carotid surgery include damage to the hypoglossal nerve, recurrent laryngeal nerve, sympathetic fibres in the carotid sheath, glossopharyngeal and facial nerves as well as sensory loss to the skin of the neck and around the ear (Dehn & Taylor 1983). The majority of deficits are transient and recover in less than 12 months. There is one practical point if bilateral carotid endarterectomy is planned: after the first operation it is important to check that there is no paralysis of the vocal cord on that side. If the nerve supply of the other vocal cord is damaged at the second endarterectomy, it is vital to know that the vocal cord was functioning normally after the first operation or extubation will be exceedingly hazardous.

*Internal carotid occlusion: extracranial to intracranial vascular anastomosis*

Over the last decade much interest has been focused on surgical methods of improving blood flow after a stroke. The majority involve anastomosing branches of the extracranial arteries to the intracranial arteries (EC–IC anastomosis). The most widely used method anastomoses a branch of the superficial temporal artery to a convenient superficial branch of the middle cerebral artery through a small craniectomy (STA–MCA anastomosis). With standard microsurgical techniques it is a straightforward operation and this partly accounts for how widespread the procedure has become before being fully assessed. The value of STA–MCA anastomosis has been investigated by Barnett *et al.* (EC–IC Bypass Study Group 1985). No clear benefit was found, for any group of patients.

A variety of factors needs to be considered if complete occlusion of the carotid artery is demonstrated. There is no value in trying to remove the occlusion in patients with acute infarction; this is likely to aggravate the situation by turning a pale infarct into a haemorrhagic lesion with a greater space-occupying effect.

After a complete internal carotid occlusion, flow in the supraorbital and supratrochlear arteries, which are branches of the superficial temporal artery, is usually reversed (Trockel *et al.* 1984) so that the external carotid artery is now supplying the cerebral hemisphere through the ophthalmic artery partly compensating for the loss of flow in the internal carotid artery. Thus the majority of patients have already achieved their own EC–IC anastomosis. This is sometimes demonstrable at angiography but is more easily demonstrated by Doppler ultrasonography. It is unlikely further benefit can be gained by performing EC–IC anastomosis surgically, if the patient is stable or recovering, once the acute stroke period has passed.

If, however, TIAs continue after a known internal carotid occlusion, it is important to note that emboli can now reach the cerebral circulation via the external carotid artery. In this situation, the proximal stump of the internal carotid artery may persist, acting as a potential source of emboli (Fig. 13.5) (Bogousslavsky *et al.* 1981); alternatively there may be an external carotid stenosis (Fig. 13.7). Either of these can be

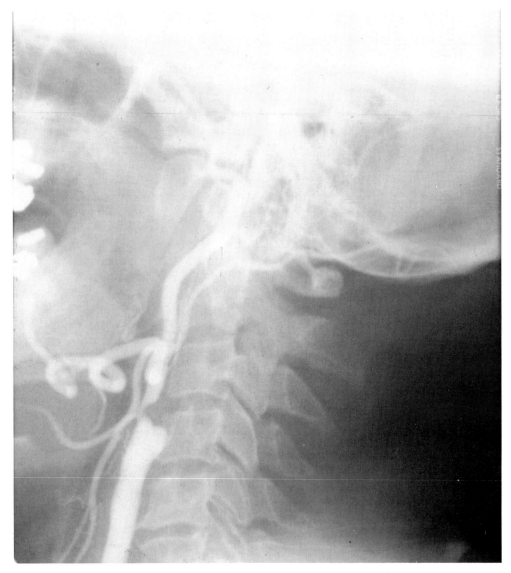

**Fig. 13.7**   Angiogram showing an internal carotid occlusion with an external carotid stenosis.

a potential source of cerebral emboli and should be considered for surgical correction, by either excising the internal carotid stump or performing an endarterectomy on the external carotid stenosis, whichever is appropriate.

Several groups of patients have been considered for EC–IC bypass surgery (Marshall 1982). The first comprises those who continue to have ipsilateral TIAs in spite of medical treatment in the presence of either unilateral or bilat-

eral carotid occlusion and not associated with a proximal internal carotid stump or external carotid stenosis. EC–IC anastomosis may be indicated if the TIAs are thought to be occurring on a haemodynamic basis as judged by the clinical and angiographic data. The second group comprised those with an intracranial carotid stenosis in the carotid siphon. A direct surgical approach is impossible. If the TIAs are thought to be embolic, antiplatelet or anticoagulant therapy is initially indicated; however if this fails, or there is evidence that the TIAs are haemodynamic in origin, then EC–IC anastomosis was proposed.

The third indication for EC–IC anastomosis was proximal middle cerebral artery stenosis or occlusion if symptons were not controlled by medical treatment. This condition is rare and again is not readily amenable to direct surgery. STA–MCA may improve flow in the territory of the middle cerebral artery. The prognosis in untreated middle cerebral artery occlusive disease is as yet unclear; most suggest the prognosis is good (Sacquegna *et al.* 1984), although Corston *et al.* (1984) found a 24% risk of stroke over a seven year follow up.

There has been much debate about the role of EC–IC anastomosis in multi-infarct dementia. Without doubt this condition has been greatly overdiagnosed in the past prior to computerized tomography. Most patients have had a progressive Alzheimer type of dementia (Brust 1983). There is, however, a small group who suffer multiple infarcts on the basis of both the clinical picture and CT scan and who have widespread vascular occlusive disease in whom there may improvement after EC–IC anastomosis. As yet, it is difficult to define this group clinically. The mere presence of a low cerebral blood flow does not warrant bypass surgery as the low CBF is usually secondary to the reduced metabolic demand of the already damaged ischaemic brain. Whether tests of CBF reserve by measuring the response of flow to carbon dioxide or positron emission tomographic (PET) scanning will allow one to delineate the group in whom low CBF is the limiting factor is too early to say (Gibbs *et al.* 1984).

Finally EC–IC anastomosis may be performed as a prelude to endarterectomy for internal carotid stenosis if there is a contralateral internal carotid occlusion. This is usually done on the contralateral side to help maintain blood flow to the brain during the endarterectomy.

A wide range of other EC–IC anastomoses have been postulated. The rationale for all of these is to improve flow to an ischaemic area in the brain. It may be of little use if the increase in flow that results from the operation is superfluous to the needs of the tissue supplied unless it protects against the effects of further ischaemic or embolic events. How often continuing ischaemia is truly the limiting factor is difficult to know on present data. PET scanning suggests it may not be as common as was once thought (Wise *et al.* 1983). The EC–IC Bypass Study Group (1985) showed that superficial temporal to middle cerebral artery anastomosis is of no proven benefit in the groups studied. This includes stroke and TIA patients with either internal carotid occlusion, middle cerebral artery stenosis or intracranial carotid stenosis. It emphasizes the importance of subjecting these surgical techniques to controlled studies before accepting that they are 'intrinsically' beneficial.

## Asymptomatic bruits

There has been a vogue in recent years mainly in the United States for prophylactic endarterectomy for asymptomatic internal carotid stenosis. Asymptomatic bruits occur in 3–4% of patients aged 45–65 years and in 7% over the age of 65 years. However, longterm studies suggest that the risk of stroke is relatively small in these patients at about 4% per annum. Furthermore, less than 50% of these strokes occur in the vascular territory of the vessel with the bruit. There seems little indication for operating on patients with an asymptomatic bruit which is merely an indicator of generalized disease rather than a specific risk factor in a specified arterial territory (Wolf *et al.* 1981). Only surgical centres with combined morbidity and mortality figures for surgery and angiography of under 1–2% could begin to justify such action.

The prognosis of asymptomatic bruits in those about to undergo general or cardiac surgery has also been studied. There is a slightly increased risk of stroke in these patients, perhaps because of intraoperative episodes of arterial hypotension. Again, of the few strokes that did occur, several were not in the territory of the bruit. There thus seems little evidence to justify routine endarterectomy prior to either coronary or peripheral vascular or general surgery in patients with asymptomatic carotid stenosis (Yatsu & Hart 1983).

## Fibromuscular dysplasia

Fibromuscular dysplasia most commonly affects the mid cervical part of the internal carotid artery. There is alternate thickening, due to excess fibrosis, and thinning, due to loss of elastic tissue and muscle fibre, of the medial coat of the arterial. This produces a characteristic angiographic picture usually described as a string of beads (Fig. 13.8).

It is frequently bilateral and may affect other vessels such as the renal arteries. It is associated with an increased incidence of intracranial aneurysms and approximately one fifth of patients present with subarachnoid haemorrhage (So et al. 1981). Other common presentations include TIAs and completed stroke although in about a third it is an incidental finding at angiography.

The longterm risks of further thromboembolic events is unclear. Most reports suggest the lesion is benign (Corrin et al. 1981, Wells & Smith 1982). Wells and Smith (1982) followed up 16 patients for an average of 3.8 years; two developed a hemiplegia although both were noted to have severe concurrent arteriosclerosis.

A direct surgical approach is often not possible as the lesion is too distal to be easily accessible; some have attempted graduated internal dilatation (Starr et al. 1981). Initially, symptoms should be managed medically with antiplatelet agents, or anticoagulants if these fail.

## Cerebral venous thrombosis

Cerebral venous thrombosis can be conveniently considered as two separate entities; the symptoms and signs may follow either dural sinus thrombosis or cortical vein thrombosis (Humphrey et al. 1983). Dural sinus thrombosis usually produces the symptoms and signs of raised intracranial pressure. Frequently, however, the cortical veins are also involved and

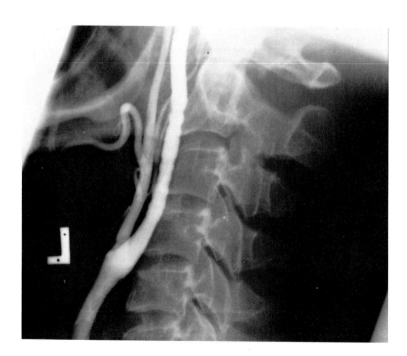

Fig. 13.8 Fibromuscular dysplasia showing the alternate constriction and dilatation of the internal carotid artery.

the clinical features which follow largely result from venous infarction which often produces intracerebral or subarachnoid haemorrhage.

Headache is common and may be associated with nausea, vomiting and neck stiffness. Epilepsy, which may be generalized or focal, is frequent and follows intracerebral haemorrhage. This is often followed by prolonged ischaemic focal neurological deficit and it may be difficult to distinguish the clinical picture from cerebral arterial disease, subarachnoid haemorrhage or meningoencephalitis.

It is especially common in systemic disease such as malignancy, in many haematological disorders, such as thrombocythaemia, polycythaemia rubra vera and leukaemia, or after local sepsis, for example sinusitis and trauma. It also tends to occur in the puerperium or on the contraceptive pill.

Diagnosis is difficult as angiography with delayed and oblique views is the only reliable investigation. Fever, leucocytosis and a raised ESR are frequently present. The cerebrospinal fluid varies from being normal to showing changes suggestive of subarachnoid bleeding or meningoencephalitis. The computerized tomographic scan is sometimes useful and may show multiple haemorrhagic infarcts (Fig. 13.9). Usually however it is normal or just shows multiple low attenuation areas. Patronas *et al.* (1981) suggested that a triangular area of increased density, before contrast, along the course of the superior sagittal sinus was a useful finding. This is thought to be due to unorganized thrombus. It lasts only a few days and is then replaced by a low or normal attenuation area as the clot becomes organized. This low attenuation may be highlighted by giving contrast, following which a triangular area of enhancement appears around the sinus.

Therapy is directed at any predisposing cause. Symptomatic treatment to deal with the epilepsy or raised intracranial pressure is important. The management of the thrombosis itself is unsatisfactory because of the high incidence of haemorrhagic venous infarction. If the thrombosis is confined to the dural sinuses then it is reasonable to consider anticoagulants or perhaps fibrinolytic agents. If there is any evidence of focal signs or epilepsy suggesting cortical vein thrombosis, and thus haemorrhagic infarction, their use is clearly hazardous.

## Traumatic dissections of the carotid artery

These usually occur in young people and either cause complete or partial occlusion of the internal carotid artery. The dissection begins just above the carotid bifurcation (Fig. 13.10) and often tracts up as far as the base of the skull.

It may follow local trauma including angiography, but sometimes occurs in fibromuscular dysplasia, Marfan syndrome, Ehlers–Danlos syndrome or pseudoxanthoma elasticum. The majority are associated with pain in either the face, eye or neck (Fisher 1982) and symptoms of thrombo-embolic disease; Horner syndrome may be present.

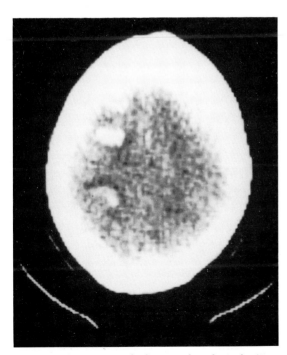

**Fig. 13.9** CT scan in cerebral venous thrombosis showing multiple small haemorrhagic infarcts.

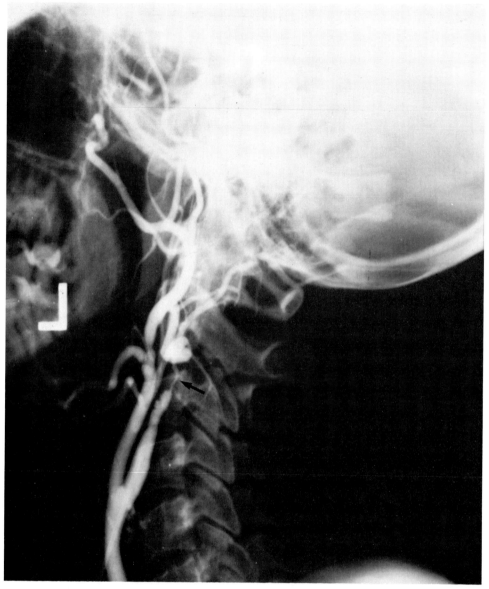

**Fig. 13.10**   Angiogram showing a traumatic dissection of the internal carotid artery with a progressive narrowing leading to string sign.

Often surgical reconstruction is not feasible because of the length of the dissection. The overall prognosis is good; if emboli occur, then anticoagulation is indicated (Stringer & Kelly 1980, Friedman *et al.* 1980). Rarely local surgery or EC–IC anastomosis may be considered if medical treatment fails to control the symptoms.

## Takayasu disease (aortic arch syndrome or pulseless disease)

This syndrome follows occlusion of the major arteries to the head and arms (Fig. 13.11). This is often asymptomatic in the early stages and symptoms only begin to appear when there is a significant reduction in cerebral blood flow

**Fig. 13.11** Takayasu disease. Only a single (right) vertebral artery remains supplying the head with many prominent small collateral vessels. (Courtesy of Dr B. Kendall).

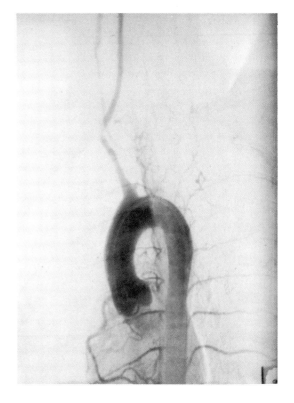

which cannot be met by collateral supply. Most patients present with symptoms of generalized cerebral ischaemia, such as vertigo, light-headedness, confusion, syncope or occasional fits. Focal deficits such as hemipareses or episodes of visual loss occur late in the disease; these are haemodynamic in origin and often tend to be precipitated by standing, exercise or straining, sometimes occurring many times a day (Ross Russell & Page 1983). Other symptoms may include claudication of the jaw, ischaemic pain in the arms after exercise and progressive dementia (Ross Russell 1983).

The characteristic findings on examination are reduced pulses in the neck and arms sometimes with unrecordable blood pressure. Many cases occur in Oriental women in whom pathological studies show a low grade arteritis; there is fibrous proliferation of the arterial wall, mononuclear infiltration and occasional giant cells. It is important to exclude syphilitic aortitis and giant cell arteritis.

If there is evidence of a systemic disorder with fever, anaemia, arthralgia and erythema nodosum, along with a raised erythrocyte sedimentation rate, then steroid therapy is indicated (Ross Russell 1983). For most, however, there is no specific treatment; reconstructive surgical procedures to improve cerebral flow may ameliorate some symptoms (Ross Russell & Page 1983).

## Moya-Moya disease

This is a radiological description, first described in Japan, which refers to the network of small collateral vessels seen around a terminal carotid occlusion (Fig. 13.12). It occurs mainly in children and young adults and presents with recurrent episodes of cerebral ischaemia such as hemiparesis, with or without mental deterioration. These abnormal vessels may rupture and there is an increased incidence of cerebral and subarachnoid haemorrhage especially in adults (Suzuki & Kodama 1983).

Yamashita *et al.* (1983) have demonstrated microaneurysm formation, focal fibrin deposits and marked attenuation of the wall with diminution of the elastic lamina. At times, there is also fibrous intimal thickening with collapse of the vascular lumen and thrombosis.

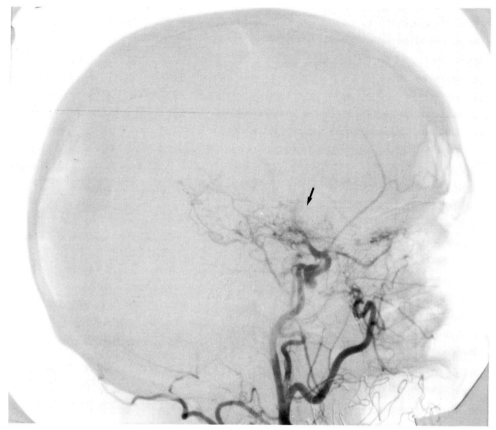

**Fig. 13.12**   Moya-Moya disease showing the network of small blood vessels at the terminal internal carotid artery.

Similar radiological appearances are sometimes seen in neurofibromatosis, thromboembolic occlusive disease, X-ray therapy, basal meningitis and basal tumours. Suzuki and Kodama (1983) emphasize the frequency of a past history of chronic inflammation in the cervical region in patients with Moya-Moya.

Treatment is unsatisfactory; bypass procedures to improve cerebral blood flow have not been shown to be of any consistent benefit, because of the small calibre of the intracranial vessels.

## Arteritis

This may follow acute inflammation of the tonsils or retropharyngeal tissues with resultant throm-

bosis in the carotid artery (Ross Russell 1983). Sometimes it follows cavernous sinus thrombosis (Clifford-Jones *et al.* 1982) or local herpes zoster (MacKenzie *et al.* 1981). Meningitis, either acute or chronic, may be followed by inflammation and thrombosis of the circle of Willis and its branches. This may occur with bacterial infections such as pneumococcal, meningococcal, tuberculous or syphilitic meningitis and fungal infections like mucor mycosis, aspergillosis or candidiasis.

Other inflammatory diseases such as polyarteritis nodosa, systemic lupus erythematosis, giant cell arteritis, Behcet disease, Wegener's granulomatosis and isolated granulomatous angiitis of the central nervous system may all present with cerebral vascular occlusive disease (Moore & Cupps 1983, Haas 1982, Ross Russell 1983, Howard *et al.* 1984).

Drug abuse is likely to become an increasing cause of cerebrovascular disease in the young (Caplan *et al.* 1982). There is also good evidence that the early high dose contraceptive pill was associated with an increased risk of thromboembolic disease. Whether the risks remain with the low dose oestrogen pill is as yet unclear (Meade *et al.* 1980, Beral & Kay 1977).

# References

AARON J. O., HESSELINK J. R., OOT R., JONES R. L., DARIS K. R. & TAVERAS J. M. (1984) *Radiology*, **153**, 675.

ALLEN C. M. C. (1983) *Quart. J.*, **52**, 515.

ASINGER R. W., MIKELL F. L., SHARMA B. & HODGES M. (1983) *Amer. J. Cardiol.*, **47**, 145.

BARTLESON J. D. (1984) *Stroke*, **15**, 383.

BEAN W. B. (1938) *Ann. Intern. Med.*, **12**, 71.

BERAL V. & KAY C. R. (1977) Royal College of General Practitioners Contraception Study, *Lancet*, **ii**, 727.

BLACKWOOD W., HALLPIKE J. F., KOCEN R. S. AND MAIR W. G. P. (1969) *Brain*, **92**, 897.

BOGOUSSLAVSKY J., REGLI F., HUNGERBÜHLER J P & CIMANOWSKI R. (1981) *Stroke*, **5**, 627.

BOUSSER M. G., ESCHWEGE E., HAGUENAU M., LEFAUCCONNIER J. M., THIBOULT N., TOUBOUL D. & TOUBOUL P. J. (1983) *Stroke*, **14**, 5.

BRANSTON N. M., STRONG A. J. & SYMON L. (1977) *Neurol. Sci.*, **32**, 305.

BRICE J. G., DOWSETT D. J. & LOWE R. D. (1964) *Brit. Med. J.*, **ii**, 1363.

BROWSE N. L. & ROSS RUSSELL R. (1984) *Brit. J. Surg.*, **71**, 53.

BRUST J. C. M. (1977) *Neurology*, **27**, 701.

BRUST J. C. M. (1983) *Stroke*, **14**, 298.

CANADIAN COOPERATIVE STUDY GROUP (1978) *New Eng. J. Med.*, **299**, 53.

CAPLAN L. R. (1981) *Stroke*, **12**, 111.

CAPLAN L. R. & SERGAY S. (1976) *J. Neurol. Neurosurg. Psychiat.*, **39**, 385.

CAPLAN L. R., HIER D. B. & BANKS G. (1982) *Stroke*, **13**, 869.

CARTER A. B. (1957) *Quart. J. Med.*, **50**, 335.

CLIFFORD-JONES R. E., ELLIS C. J. K., STEVENS J. M. & TURNER A. (1982) *J. Neurol. Neurosurg. Psychiat.*, **45**, 1092.

CORRIN L. S., SANDOK, B. A. & HOUSER O. W. (1981) *Arch. Neurol.*, **38**, 616.

CORSTON R. N., KENDALL B. E. & MARSHALL J. (1984) *Stroke*, **15**, 237.

COVE D. H., SEDDON M., FLETCHER R. F. & DUKES D. C. (1979) *Brit. med. J.*, **ii**, 245.

DE BONO D. P. (1983) In *Cerebral Arterial Disease*, (Ed. Ross Russell R. W.) 324–336.

DEHN T. C. B. & TAYLOR G. W. (1983) In *Progress in Stroke Research 2*. (Eds Greenhalgh R. M. & Clifford-Rose F.) pp. 484–491. Pitman, London.

DIMSDALE H. B. (1982) *Stroke*, **13**, 717.

EASTCOTT H. H. G., PICKERING G. W. AND ROB C. (1954) *Lancet*, **ii**, 994–996.

EASTON J. D. & SHERMAN D. G. (1977) *Stroke*, **8**, 565.

EASTON J. D. & SHERMAN D. G. (1980) *Stroke*, **11**, 433.

EC–IC BYPASS STUDY GROUP (1985) *New Engl. J. Med.*, **313**, 1191.

FARIS A. A. & POSER C. M. (1964) *Neurology (Minneap.)*, **14**, 206.

FERGUSON G. C. (1982) *Stroke*, **13**, 287.

FIELDS W. S. & LEMAK N. A. (1972) *J. Amer. Med. Assoc.*, **222**, 1139.

FIELDS W. S., LEMAK N. A., FRANKOWSKI R. F. & HARDY R. J. (1977) *Stroke*, **8**, 301.

FIESCHI C., AGNOLI A., BATTISTINI N. & BOZZAO L. (1966) *Arch. Neurol.*, **15**, 653.

FISHER C. M. (1959) *Neurology (Minneap.)*, **9**, 333.

FISHER C. M. (1976) *Cerebrovascular Diseases – 10th Princeton Conference*, (Ed. SCHEINBERG P.) pp. 50–53. Raven Press, New York.

FISHER C. M. (1982a) *Headache*, **22**, 60.

FISHER C. M. (1982b) *Neurology*, **32**, 871.

FRIEDMAN W. A., DAY A. L., QUISLING R. G., SYPERT G. W. & RHOTON A. L. (1980) *Neurosurgery*, **7**, 207.

FRITHZ G. & WERNER I. (1975) *Acta. Med. Scand.*, **198**, 287.

FURLAN A. J., CAVALIER S. J., HOBBS R. E., WEINSTEIN M. A. & MODIC M. T. (1982) *Neurology*, **32**, 280.

GAUTIER J. C. & MORELOT D. (1975) *Nouv. Presse Med.*, **4**, 2575.

GIBBS J. M., WISE R. J. S., LEENDERS K. L. & JONES T. (1984) *Lancet*, **i**, 182.

GINSBERG M. D. & CEBUL R. D. (1983) In *Cerebral Vascular Disease*, (Eds HARRISON M. J. G. & DYKEN M. L.) **3**, 215–253. Butterworths International Medical Reviews, London.

GOLDSTEIN S. J., FRIED A. M., YOUNG B. & TIBBS P. A. (1981) *Amer. J. Neuroradiol.*, **2**, 559.

GROCH S., McDEVITT E. & WRIGHT I. S. (1961) *Ann. Intern. Med.*, **55**, 358.

HAAS L. F. (1982) *J. Neurol. Neurosurg. Psychiat.*, **45**, 554.

HABERMAN S., CAPILDEO R. & CLIFFORD-ROSE F. (1982) *Stroke*, **13**, 582.

HACHINSKI V. (1984) *Stroke*, **15**, 376.

HARRISON M. J. G. (1982) In *Topical Reviews in Neurosurgery*, Vol. 1, (Ed. RICE EDWARDS J. M.) pp. 57–80. John Wright and Sons, Bristol; and PSG, Baltimore.

HARRISON M. J. G. & MARSHALL J. (1975) *Brit. med. J.*, **i**, 616.

HARRISON M. J. G. & MARSHALL J. (1976) *Brit. med. J.*, **i**, 205.

HARRISON M. J. G. & MARSHALL J. (1977) *Brit. J. Surg.*, **64**, 511.

HARRISON M. J. G. & ROSS RUSSELL R. W. (1983) In *Cerebral Vascular Disease*. (Eds HARRISON M. J. G. & DYKEN M. L.) **3**, 258. Butterworths, London.

HAWKES C. H. (1974) *Brit. Med. J.*, **iv**, 379.

HENNERICI M., AULICH A., SANDMANN W. & FREUND H. J. (1981) *Stroke*, **12**, 750.

HEROS R. C. (1982) *Stroke*, **13**, 106.

HOSSMANN K. A. (1976) In *Dynamics in Brain Oedema* (Eds PAPPIUS H. M. & FEINDEL W.) p. 219. Springer-Verlag, New York.

HOWARD G. F., HO S. U., KIM K. S. & WALLACH J. (1984) *Ann. Neurol.*, **15**, 204.

HOWELL T. H. (1984) *Brit. med. J.*, **ii**, 35.

HUMPHREY P. R. D. & BRADBURY P. G. (1984) *J. Neurol. Neurosurg. Psychiat.*, **47**, 1128.

HUMPHREY P. R. D. & HARRISON M. J. G. (1985) *Postgrad. Med. J.*, **61**, 1039.

HUMPHREY P. R. D. & MARSHALL J. (1981) *Stroke*, **12**, 765.

HUMPHREY P. R. D., CLARKE C. R. A. & GREENWOOD R. J. (1983) In *Cerebral Vascular Disease* (Eds HARRISON M. J. G. & DYKEN M. L.) pp. 309–319. Butterworths, London.

JOHNSTON J. H., BEEVERS D. G., DUNN F. G., LARKIN H. & TITTERINGTON D. M. (1981) *Postgrad. Med. J.*, **57**, 690.

KANNEL W. B. & WOLF P. A. (1983) In *Vascular disease of the Central Nervous System* (Ed. ROSS RUSSELL R. W.) pp. 1–24. Churchill Livingstone, Edinburgh.

KENDALL B. E. & MARSHALL J. (1963) *Brit. med. J.*, **ii**, 344.

KETY S. S. & SCHMIDT C. F. (1948) *J. clin. Invest.*, **27**, 484.

KOLLER R. L. (1982) *Neurology*, **32**, 283.

KUMAR G. K., DASTOOR F. C., ROBAGO J. R. & RASSAQUE M. A. (1976) *J. Amer. med. Ass.*, **235**, 275.

KURTZE J. F. (1976) In *Cerebrovascular Diseases – Tenth Princeton Conference* (Ed. SCHEINBERG P.) Raven Press, New York.

LASSEN N. A. (1959) *Physiol. Rev.*, **36**, 183.

LASSEN N. A. (1966) *Lancet*, **ii**, 1113.

LEDINGHAM J. G. G. & RAJAGOPALAN B. (1979) *Quart J. Med.*, **48**, 25.

LITTLE J. R., FURLAN A. J., MODIC M. T. & WEINSTEIN M. A. (1982) *Stroke*, **13**, 557.

LOEB C. (1979) In *Advances in Neurology*, Vol. 25 (Eds GOLDSTEIN M. L., BOLIS L., FIESCHI C., GORINI S. & MILLIKAN C. H. pp. 141–148. Raven Press, New York.

LONGO D. L. & WITHERSPOON J. M. (1980) *Neurology (Minneap.)*, **30**, 200.

LUXON L. M. & HARRISON M. J. G. (1979) *Quart. J. Med.*, **48**, 43.

MacDONALD W. I. (1967) *J. Neurol. Neurosurg. Psychiat.*, **30**, 489.

MacKENZIE R. A., FORBES G. S. & KARNES W. E. (1981) *Ann. Neurol.*, **10**, 458.

MARSHALL J. (1982) In *Tropical Reviews in Neurosurgery*, Vol. 1. (Ed. RICE EDWARDS J. M.) pp. 57–80. John Wright and Sons, Bristol; and PSG, Baltimore.

MASOTTI G., GALANTI G., POGGESI L., ABBATE R. & NERI SERNERI C. G. (1979) *Lancet*, **ii**, 1213.

MATTHEWS W. B., OXBURY J. M. & GRAINER K. M. R. (1976) *Brain*, **99**, 193.

MEADE T. W., GREENBERG G., THOMPSON S. G. (1980) *Brit. med. J.*, **i**, 1157.

MERORY J., THOMAS D. J., HUMPHREY P. R. D., du BOULAY G. H., MARSHALL J., ROSS RUSSELL R. W. & SYMON L. (1980) *J. Neurol. Neurosurg. Psychiat.*, **43**, 214.

MEYER J. S. & PORTNOY H. S. (1958) *Neurology (Minneap.)*, **8**, 601.

MILLIKAN C. H. & McDOWELL F. H. (1981) *Stroke*, **12**, 397.

MOHR J. P. (1978) *New Eng. J. Med.*, **299**, 93.

MOORE P. M. & CUPPS T. R. (1983) *Ann. Neurol.*, **14**, 155.

MULLEY G., WILCOX R. G. & MITCHELL J. R. A. (1978) *Brit. med. J.*, **ii**, 994.

NELSON R. F., PULLICINO P., KENDALL B. E. & MARSHALL J. (1980) *Stroke*, **11**, 256.

NICHOLLS E. & JOHANSEN H. (1983) *Stroke*, **14**, 153.

NORRIS J. W. & HACHINSKI V. C. (1982) *Lancet*, **1**, 328.

OAKLEY C. M. (1984) *Brit. med. J.*, **i**, 1853.

O'BRIEN M. D. (1979) *Stroke*, **10**, 623.

OXBURY J. M., GREENHALL R. C. D. & GRAINGER K. M. R. (1975) *Brit. med. J.*, **ii**, 125.

OXFORDSHIRE COMMUNITY STROKE PROJECT (1983) *Brit. med. J.*, **ii**, 713.

PANTIN C. F. A. & YOUNG R. A. L. (1980) *Brit. med. J.*, **ii**, 1686.

PATRONAS N. J., DUDA E. E., MIRFAKHRAEE M. & WOLLMANN R. L. (1981) *Surg. Neurol.*, **15**, 11.

PAULSON O. B. (1970) *Neurology*, **20**, 63.

PAYNE E. E. & SPILLANE J. D. (1957) *Brain*, **80**, 571.

PORTS T. A., COGAN J., SCHILLER N. B. & RAPAPORT E. (1978) *Circulation*, **58**, 528.

PRESCOTT R. J., GARRAWAY W. M., AKHTAR A. J. (1982) *Stroke*, **13**, 641.

REES J. E., du BOULAY G. H., BULL J. W. D., MARSHALL J., ROSS RUSSELL R. W. & SYMON L. (1970) *Lancet*, **ii**, 1210.

ROBERTSON W. B. & STRONG J. P. (1968) *Lab. Invest.*, **18**, 538.

ROSS R. T. (1983) *Arch. Neurol.*, **40**, 633.

ROSS RUSSELL R. W. (1963) *Brain*, **86**, 425.

ROSS RUSSELL R. W. (1968) *Lancet*, **ii**, 789.

ROSS RUSSELL R. W. (1983) *Vascular Disease of the Central Nervous System*, pp. 368–404. Churchill Livingstone, Edinburgh.

ROSS RUSSELL R. W. & BHARUCHA N. (1978) *Quart. J. Med.*, **47**, 303.

ROSS RUSSELL R. W. & PAGE N. G. R. (1983) *Brain*, **106**, 419.

SACCO R. L., WOLF P. A., KANNEL W. B. & McNAMARA P. (1982) *Stroke*, **13**, 290.

SACQUEGNA T., de CAROLIS P., ANDREOLI A., FERRARA R., LIMONI P., TESTA C. & LUGARESSI E. (1984) *Brit. med. J.*, **288**, 1490.

SANDERCOCK P., MOLYNEUX A. & WARLOW C. (1985) *Brit. med. J.*, **290**, 193.

SHEEHAN S., BAUER R. B. & MEYER J. S. (1960) *Neurology (Minneap.)*, **10**, 968.

SO E. L., TOOLE J. F., DALAL P. & MOODY D. M. (1981) *Arch. Neurol.*, **38**, 619.

STARK R. J. & WODAK J. (1983) *J. Neurol. Neurosurg. Psychiat.*, **46**, 883.

STARR D. S., LAWRIE G. M. & MORRIS G. C. (1981) *Stroke*, **12**, 196.

STEEL J. G., THOMAS H. A. & STROLLO P. J. (1982) *Stroke*, **13**, 712.

STEINER T. J., McIVOR J., PERKIN G. D., GREENHALGH R. M. & ROSE F. C. (1983) In *Progress in Stroke Research*, 2, 136–153 (Eds GREENHALGH R. M. & ROSE F. C.). Pitman, London.

STRANDGAARD S., OLESEN J., SKINHØJ E. & LASSEN N. A. (1973) *Brit. med. J.*, **i**, 507.

STRINGER L. S. & KELLY D. L. (1980) *Neurosurgery*, **6**, 123.

SULLIVAN J. M., HARKEN O. E. & GORLIN R. (1968) *New Eng. J. Med.*, **279**, 576.

SUNDT T. M. (1983) *Stroke*, **14**, 93.

SUZUKI J. & KODAMA N. (1983) *Stroke*, **14**, 104.

SYMON L. BRANSTON N. M. & STRONG A. J. (1976) *Stroke*, **7**, 547.

SYMON L., CROCKARD H. A., DORSCH N. W. C., BRANSTON N. M. & JUHASZ J. (1975) *Stroke*, **6**, 482.

THOMPSON J. E. & TALKINGTON C. M. (1976) *Ann. Surg.*, **184**, 1.

TORVIK A. (1984) *Stroke*, **15**, 221.

TORVIK A. & JORGENSEN L. (1964) *J. Neurol. Sci.*, **1**, 24.

TROCKEL U., HENNERICI M., AULICH A. & SANDMANN W, (1984) *J. Neurol. Neurosurg. Psychiat.*, **47**, 43.

UNITED KINGDOM TIA STUDY GROUP (1983) *Brit. med. J.*, **i**, 514.

UNITED KINGDOM TIA STUDY GROUP (1987) *Brit. med. J.*, in press.

VAN DER DRIFT J. H. A. & KOK N. K. D. (1973) In *Cerebrovascular Disease, Sixth International Conference, Salzburg.* (Eds MEYER J. S., LECHNER H., REIVICH M. & EICHORN O.) (1973) Thieme, Stuttgart.

VORSTRUP S., BARRY D. I., JARDEN J. O., SVENDSEN U. G., BRAENDSTRUP O., GRAHAM D. I. & STRANDGAARD S. (1984) *Stroke,* **15,** 312.

WADE D. T., LANGTON–HEWER R., WOOD V. A., SKILBECK C. E. & ISMAIL H. M. (1983) *J. Neurol. Neurosurg Psychiat.,* **46,** 521.

WALTZ A. G. (1970) *Stroke,* **1,** 27.

WARLOW C. P. (1984) *Stroke,* **15,** 1068.

WELLS R. P. & SMITH R. R. (1982) *Neurosurgery,* **10,** 39.

WHISNANT J. P. (1984) *Stroke,* **15,** 160.

WILSON L. A. & ROSS RUSSELL R. W. (1977) *Brit. med. J.,* **ii,** 435.

WISE R. J. S., BERNARDI S., FRACKWIAK R. S. J., LEGG N. J. & JONES T. (1983) *Brain,* **106,** 197.

WOLF P. A., KANNEL W. B., McGEE D. L., MEEKS S. L., BHARUCHA N. E. & McNAMARA P. M. (1983) *Stroke,* **14,** 664.

WOLF P. A., KANNEL W. B., SORLIE P. & McNAMARA P. (1981) *J. Amer. med. Ass.,* **245,** 1442.

WOODCOCK J. P. (1981) *Brit. J. Anaesth.,* **53,** 719.

YAMASHITA M., OKA K. & TANAKA K. (1983) *Stroke,* **14,** 50.

YATSU F. M. & HART R. G. (1983) *Stroke,* **14,** 301.

# Chapter 14
# Brain Abscess and Other Inflammatory Conditions

## M. D. M. SHAW

## Brain abscess

### Introduction

Abscess of the brain may arise by the direct spread of microorganisms from an adjacent focus of infection, often in the cranium but occasionally in the surrounding soft tissues, for example a boil on the face; by their implantation as in penetrating wounds of the head; or by their deposition in the brain by the blood stream, having been derived from a remote septic focus. The causative focus may still be active at the time the abscess manifests itself, thus facilitating diagnosis; on the other hand not infrequently the focus of infection may have completely resolved, naturally or as a result of treatment. Dependent upon the numbers of organisms gaining entrance to the brain and upon their virulence, the speed

of evolution varies considerably: in haematogenous infection there may be more than one abscess. These general factors play an important part in rendering diagnosis a matter of great difficulty in some cases.

### Aetiology

An analysis of the common routes of infection of the brain is set out in Table 14.1, the figures being derived from various sources. The cases of Evans (1931) were from necropsy material based upon post-mortem examinations performed in the London Hospital between 1908 and 1925. Careful search failed to reveal the source of infection in 9%. The other figures come from neurosurgical centres. Those of Pennybacker (1951) and of Krayenbühl (1967b) include a con-

Table 14.1. Common routes of infection of the brain.

| Source | Number of cases | Direct spread (%) | | | Haematogenous (%) | | Uncertain |
|---|---|---|---|---|---|---|---|
| | | Ear | Para-nasal | Others | Lung | Others | |
| Evans (1931) | 194 | 56 | 6 | 5 | 11 | 11 | 9 |
| Pennybacker (1951) | 110 | 42 | 10 | 16 | 20 | 14 | — |
| Tutton (1953) | 68 | 37 | 16 | 13 | 24 | 10 | — |
| Bonnal et al. (1960) | 545 | 24 | 5 | 23 | 12 | 15 | 21 |
| Krayenbühl (1967b) | 130 | 12 | 15 | 5 | 21 | 26 | 20 |
| Sampson & Clarke (1973) | 42 | 19 | | 24 | 17 | 28 | 12 |
| Beller et al. (1973) | 89 | 30 | 8 | 19 | 6 | 18 | 19 |
| Jefferson & Keogh (1977) | 49 | 65 | 16 | 12 | — | 6 | — |
| McClelland et al. (1978) | 172 | 26 | 8 | 14 | 17 | 20 | 15 |
| Weisberg (1981) | 14 | — | — | 7 | 22 | 71 | — |
| Yang (1981) | 400 | 65.75 | 0.5 | 6.75 | — | 17 | 10 |
| Bradley & Shaw (1983) | 325 | 41 | 17 | 5 | 16 | 7 | 14 |

siderable number of cases from the pre-antibiotic era in contrast to those of Tutton and of Bonnal *et al.* (1960) which include only cases since the introduction of antibiotics. In Krayenbühl's series the proportion of otitic abscesses is remarkably low. Possibly some of the abscesses of unknown aetiology (of which there were 20%) were due to ear disease which had resolved; in favour of this is the fact that of 32 temporal lobe abscesses, only 7 were deemed to be otogenic, whereas there were 9 otogenic cerebellar abscesses. It is more common for ear disease to infect the temporal lobe than the cerebellum, in the ratio of about 2:1. Krayenbühl points out that in his experience the commonest cause of a brain abscess is chest infection. This is not the experience in other countries; Bonnal *et al.* give the combined figures of several widely separated European centres; of 928 cases, 30% were 'metastatic' and in probably one-half of these the primary infection was pulmonary. Recent evidence suggests that the incidence of brain abscess in the United Kingdom is falling (Bradley & Shaw 1983) but that otogenic and sinus disease remains the commonest cause, as was found by other UK workers (Jefferson & Keogh 1977, McClelland *et al.* 1978). However both causes were found to be on the decline and this was more marked for otogenic than for sinus disease. Bradley and Shaw also found that pulmonary infection as a cause of brain abscess had declined markedly over the last 20 years. In some parts of the world metastatic infections are now the commonest cause of nontraumatic cerebral abscesses (Carey *et al.* 1972, Sampson & Clarke 1973, Weisberg 1981) but not in others (Beller *et al.* 1975, Yang 1981). This change may well reflect improved surgical and antibiotic management of both acute and chronic infections of the ears and nasal air sinuses.

The table needs further explanatory comment. 'Other' causes of abscess as a result of direct spread (the 'adjacent' abscess of some writers) include osteomyelitis of the skull (secondary to scalp wounds), facial and scalp sepsis and head injury. The latter formed a high proportion of the 23% of Bonnal *et al.* Bradley and Shaw

(1983) found an increasing proportion of brain abscesses as the result of trauma over a 30 year period in Merseyside. Although it is well known that brain abscess may follow a penetrating injury of the skull, it may occasionally follow a closed injury, without scalp abrasion or underlying osteomyelitis. The reason is obscure; whether a focal cerebral contusion provides a *locus resistentiae minoris* is unproven, but further consideration is given later to this and to other allied problems in the section on pathogenesis. 'Other' causes of haematogenous brain abscess include infective endocarditis, pyaemia, and distant foci of suppuration which can be virtually in any part of the body. A small, important and apparently increasing proportion of cases arise in patients with cyanotic congenital heart disease and with angiomatous malformations in the lungs. The factors operating in these, in thoracogenic, in paranasal and in otitic abscesses are treated in detail below.

### Bacteriology

It would be of little value to list all the microorganisms which have been recovered from brain abscesses, for most of those which may invade the body have on occasion been reported. In general the aetiology of the brain abscess may give a clue as to the infecting organisms. However confirmation of the type and its sensitivities has greatly improved following the development of more discriminating microbiological techniques, for example streptococci have been frequently described but until the anaerobic culture techniques were improved there was a high incidence in the reported series of 'sterile cultures'. That these 'sterile' abscesses might be caused by anaerobes including anaerobic streptococci and bacteroides was suggested by Heinemann and Brande (1963). Meticulous techniques including prompt inoculation of cultures (de Louvois *et al.* 1977a) confirmed streptococci to be the commonest organism isolated from brain abscesses no matter what the primary source; most were streptococcus milleri, Lancefield Group F or

Ottens & Winkler Type O III. Staphylococci predominated in cases complicating head injury or surgery. The importance of both aerobic (including proteus, enterobacteriaceae and haemophilus) and anaerobic (most frequently bacteroides) Gram-negative bacteria was emphasized by the same workers. Bacteroides was found almost invariably, though often in combination with other organisms from otogenic abscesses (de Louvois *et al.* 1977a, Ingram *et al.* 1977) but rarely in abscesses resulting from other primary foci of infection (de Louvois *et al.* 1977a).

### Fungal infections

Invasion of the central nervous system by other microorganisms occurs less frequently. The main group are the fungi which may be divided into two groups: the pathogenic and the opportunistic. The former following implantation or inhalation by the host may overcome the defence mechanisms and lead to disease. These fungi include histoplasma, coccidioides and blastomyces.

The second group, the opportunistic infections, include candida, aspergillus, nocardia and cryptococcus. They are unable to cause disease in the healthy host, but if the defence mechanisms are impaired as the result of either a disease process or treatment leading to immunosuppression (for example the therapy required to prevent rejection of transplanted organs or the chemotherapy used in the treatment of malignant disease) they may act as pathogens and cause disease. Schober and Herman (1973) found that 16% of patients who had undergone cardiac transplant and came to post-mortem had fungal infections of the brain. Similarly, patients who develop T-cell deficiency (the acquired immune deficiency syndrome) are very likely to develop a wide spectrum of opportunistic infections including cerebral toxoplasmosis (Handler *et al.* 1983).

Each of the fungal and parasitic infections of the nervous system is discussed in detail in Volume 35 of the *Handbook of Clinical Neurology*

(Eds. Winken & Bruyn). Amphotericin B is the most effective antifungal agent available for central nervous system fungal infections (Bell 1981) but it may have to be used in combination with other agents, for example 5-fluorocytosine, miconazole or ketoconazole. These drugs are rather toxic and may have to be given intrathecally because of the poor cerebrospinal fluid penetration.

### Location

The relative frequency with which abscesses are encountered in the various regions of the brain is largely determined by aetiology. The frontal lobe is a common site on account of the adjacent paranasal sinuses, the incidence of injuries to the fore part of the head and of facial sepsis. The temporal lobe is frequently affected, largely due to infection arising in the ear. The parietal lobe is next in sequence and most of these abscesses are haematogenous; cerebellar abscesses are nearly as numerous, ear disease being responsible for practically all. The occipital pole is an uncommon site for an abscess (5% in Tutton's and 12% in Krayenbuhl's series) and it is usually metastatic. Although blood borne organisms may be deposited anywhere in the brain, abscesses from this or any other cause are rare in the brain stem.

### Pathology

By whatever route the brain becomes infected the structural changes leading to the fully developed abscess are similar. The changes are often referred to as 'stages'; this is a word of convenience for descriptive purposes only, for the process is smoothly continuous, one 'stage' merging imperceptibly with the next. The abscess develops in the white matter, rarely in the grey matter which apparently offers considerable resistance probably due to its greater vascularity. The initial change is that of a steadily expanding area of septic encephalitis, showing the characteristic accompaniments of acute inflammation. The white matter is swollen with oedema and there is dilatation of vessels, diapedesis, rupture and thrombosis of small vessels and petechial haemorrhages. The centre, where the changes are more advanced, becomes softened, partly as a result of intense oedema and partly from necrosis of tissue, then liquefies. Extension of the necrotic area is accelerated by further vascular occlusion around its periphery (Putnam & Alexander 1938, fig. 238). The total extent of oedema may now occupy much of a lobe, though its purulent core may measure only a centimetre or so (Fig. 14.1). The cavity walls are poorly defined and irregular and there may be several areas of necrosis which subsequently coalesce. Histological examination reveals necrosis bordered by hyperaemic tissue infiltrated with polymorphonuclear cells and veins heavily cuffed; beyond this there is a zone of microglial activity and oedema in diminishing intensity. The abscess cavity expands, its wall becomes smoother, can be identified by sight and it is palpably firmer than the surrounding brain. This stage of the abscess can be correlated histologically with the development of a lining of granulation tissue, the fibroblasts being derived from the proliferating capillaries bordering the necrotic zone, or by migration from nearby meninges. There is vigorous scavenging activity by microglia and beyond this, proliferation of atrocytes. The granulation tissue matures to form an inner fibrous wall to the abscess cavity several millimetres thick which can become so tough as to require a sharp instrument to penetrate it and it is surrounded by an ensheathing astrogliosis which fades into the surrounding brain; this gliosis is frequently irregular in deposition, so that the surgeon, when excising the abscess, may be led astray in his dissection by irregular trabeculae of firm tissue. The oedema of the surrounding brain steadily diminishes during the maturation of the abscess wall; the optimum moment for excision occurs when the wall is sufficiently firm to withstand surgical manoeuvres without rupturing, whilst the

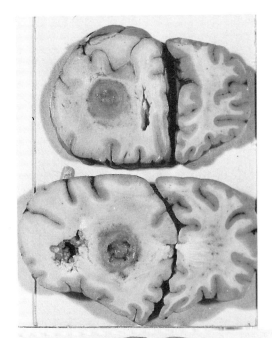

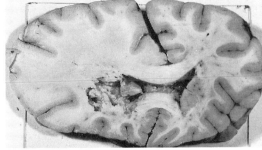

Fig. 14.1. Left frontal lobe abscess: the cavity of the abscess is small but oedema is extensive and the white matter so softened that ragged cavities have appeared. Posteriorly such a cavity communicates with the lateral ventricle. One month's history of headache following a 'cold': patient died suddenly with respiratory arrest following a series of attacks of decerebrate rigidity.

immediate surrounding brain is still slightly soft from oedema. Earlier than this the abscess wall easily breaks up if handled surgically, which not only contaminates the field but introduces the risk of leaving a fragment of granulation tissue in the brain; later than this the surrounding brain becomes tough from gliosis. The fibroblastic response which creates the abscess wall and which seals off the suppurative process, is not of uniform vigour around all aspects of the cavity. It is more advanced, and therefore the wall is thicker and firmer, on its cortical aspect, the least brisk and the wall thinnest on its deepest aspect. This variation of fibroblastic response is probably related to the richer vascular hyperplasia available from the cortical vessels. It has important consequences; as the pus increases in amount the cavity will more easily distend in a deep direction, towards the ventricle and as the wall is thin the abscess may rupture into the ventricle. This complication will be discussed later.

In its simplest form, a fully developed brain abscess is round or pear shaped. Frequently, however, it is multilocular or several separate cavities may be grouped together. These variants may arise as a result of areas of multicentric necrosis, fusing or remaining separate, or as a result of deeper spread of infection at an early stage. In the series of Bonnal et al. (1960) about one-third of the abscesses were multilocular.

The mobilization of natural defences is clearly of vital importance in limiting the spread of infection within the brain and the fibroblastic reaction around the centre of necrosis a matter of great interest to the surgeon. In a study of experimentally produced abscesses various 'stages' seen in the human brain were reproduced (Russell et al. 1941, Falconer et al. 1943). The authors paid particular attention to the development of the fibrous wall of the abscess cavity (the so-called 'capsule') to determine whether, as has been suggested, the fibrous reaction is hindered if the organisms are anaerobic or Gram-negative cocci. They found no evidence for this. They also observed that the incorporation of thorotrast with the inoculum of bacteria hastened the formation of fibrous tissue. The experiments reproduced the observations in man, described earlier, that the fibroblastic response is much slower in the depths of the white matter than in the subcortical zone; they also demonstrated formation of a deep loculus and the thinness of the wall adjacent to the ventricle (Falconer et al. 1943).

Abscess of the brain is commonly associated with pronounced oedema; only around multiple small abscesses, such as arise in pyaemia, may there be little oedema, and in these cases it is probable that death supervenes before the process has had time to develop. Oedema causes enlargement of the relevant portion of the brain and the development of internal herniations dealt with in detail in the section on intracranial pressure (Chapter 2). Intracranial pressure is elevated in most patients suffering from brain abscess (88% of the large series collected by Bonnal et al.) and its relief is the immediate problem to be treated because it is the commonest cause of death as revealed by the post-mortem demonstration of brain herniation and shift (Northfield 1942, Tutton 1953).

Purulent meningitis is the next most common cause of death. The leptomeninges may be directly infected by the adjacent septic focus which causes the abscess; this is more likely to happen in chronic ear disease owing to the proximity of the basal cisterns to the lateral sinus and the posterior surface of the petrous bone. The interactions which occur between the meninges and the organisms and which lead to meningitis are not clear. However, evidence suggests that cerebrospinal fluid is an immunological vacuum, in that there is marked deficiency or absence of complement and opsonic proteins. This allows bacteria the freedom to divide at least initially during which time there is slow targeting of polymorphs into the cerebrospinal fluid and a lack of specific antibody. These factors increase the risk of the infection becoming established (Garvey 1983). Meningitis arising as the result of direct extension, though creating a diagnostic problem, is usually susceptible to antibiotics but leptomeningitis can occur secondary to the spread of infection from the abscess to the lateral ventricle. As described above, increase in the size of an abscess occurs mainly on its deep aspect, towards the ventricle. Its superficial aspect may extensively undermine the cortex but rarely breaks through it or infects the subarachnoid space over it, because the space is largely obliterated by local pressure and because the superficial part of the wall is the thickest. Since the deep position of the wall is the least mature it provides less physical resistance to the tension of the pus within its cavity. Oedema tends to be more severe around the deep pole of the abscess and the white matter may soften to the extent that the ependyma lining the adjacent ventricle gives way; cerebrospinal fluid seeps into and breaks up the softened white matter (Fig. 14.1). The physical barriers separating the cavity of the abscess from that of the ventricle are weakened, so that microorganisms can readily reach the ventricle by direct extension or as a result of rupture of the abscess. Pyocephalus occurs, usually signified by an abrupt and rapid deterioration in the state of the patient and the infection quickly spreads through to the leptomeninges. Purulent meningitis secondary to pyocephalus is more difficult to treat than the primary variety because of persistent contamination of the ventricle from the abscess and because the patient often dies from the ventriculitis before appropriate treatment has had time to take effect. Absorption of abnormal constituents from within the ventricles is rapid and many substances, even blood, have profound nocuous effects; intraventricular injection of purified penicillin in doses exceeding 20,000 units may cause loss of consciousness and a state of shock. The experiments of Feldberg and Sherwood (1953) and coworkers (Feldberg 1965) show that certain drugs introduced into the ventricles have a selective action on cell masses bordering the ventricles; these observations were foreshadowed by those of Cushing (1931) who found that the intraventricular injection of pituitrin had an effect different from that following its subcutaneous injection.

## Pathogenesis

Although the process of invasion of the intracranial cavity by microorganisms from a focus of suppuration, say in the ear, is well understood and documented by post-mortem examinations, the method of invasion of the brain which leads to an abscess is still somewhat conjectural. Our knowledge and opinions are largely based on the observations made in the first quarter of this century. Present techniques of treatment and the lowering of mortality progressively diminish opportunities for direct observations which might extend our knowledge of pathogenesis. The first defence to be breached is the skull. Infection may transverse naturally occurring portals of entry, such as the olfactory foraminae, the occipital emissary vein foraminae, the labyrinth and thence the internal auditory meatus and the aqueductus vestibuli, congenital deficiencies, fissured fractures and suture lines, for example petrosquamoid (Turner & Reynolds 1931, figs. 2–5). Infection spreading along the sheaths of the olfactory nerves (Turner & Reynolds 1931, figs. 68–70) and of the auditory nerve pours directly into capacious leptomeningeal spaces and causes acute meningitis but rarely abscess.

Bone infection, of the walls of the paranasal sinuses or of the middle and inner ears, is the usual precursor of brain abscess which in consequence is a complication of chronic (or an acute exacerbation of chronic) rather than of acute disease. Analysing the records of 1225 cases, Courville and Nielsen (1934) found that in 80% of otitic abscesses the ear disease was chronic. The bone is infected through a necrotic area of mucosa, or by spread through lymphatics and veins penetrating the bone and an osteomyelitis develops (Turner and Reynolds 1931, figs. 24–27, 35–36 and 58). In longstanding cases caries of the bone leads to dehiscence; the common sites are the posterior wall of the frontal sinus, the tegmen tympani, the lateral part of the posterior surface of the petrous bone (Trautmann's triangle).

The second line of defence is the dura mater which offers considerable protection against infection on account of its close and tough texture and its good blood supply; although to the naked eye it has an avascular appearance, it can rapidly become visibly hyperaemic, a response with which the surgeon is familiar, for when an extradural haemorrhage is evacuated the membrane then weeps from fine blood vessels which may be troublesome to control. The obser-

vations of Rowbotham and Little (1965) emphasize this vascularity. The dura mater may
completely resist infection so that an extradural
abscess is formed and in the process its outer
surface becomes covered with granulation tissue.
Penetration of the dura mater probably takes
place along the course of the small vessels which
transverse its thickness; they may thrombose and
provide convenient pathways (Turner & Reynolds 1931, fig. 19, Brunner 1946, figs. 29b and
41). The membrane swells as a result of the
inflammatory reaction and granulation tissue
replaces its normal sheen and silvery appearance. This state is called pachymeningitis and if
the wall of a venous sinus is involved, thrombosis
ensues. This may remain restricted to part of the
circumference of the sinus (mural) or the whole
wall may be involved and the sinus thereby
becomes occluded. Purulent exudate may form
on the inner surface of the infected dura mater
occupying the subdural space (Fig. 14.2); if it
accumulates rapidly it spreads widely and is
termed a subdural empyema.

Little is known of the degree of resistance of
the arachnoid to infection; that it is appreciable
is proven by the fact that in subdural empyema
there is often no leptomeningeal infection. That it
can be breached is proven by the acute meningitis
which may complicate an extradural abscess
and particularly dural sinus thrombophlebitis.
It is likely that the membrane is directly invaded
from the pachymeningitis or by thrombosis of
the small veins which transverse it from the subarachnoid space to the dura mater. The account
given of the stages leading to the establishment
of a focus of pachymeningitis can be sub-
stantiated by macroscopic and microscopic
records, to which references have been given.
But from here onwards the mechanism of brain
infection becomes progressively more speculative. In the majority of specimens of brain
abscesses secondary to adjacent bone disease, the
brain is adherent to the patch of inflamed dura
mater. It is at this point that the abscess cavity
usually most nearly approaches the surface and
indeed in the junction zone there may be no
cortex (Brunner 1946, Fig. 78). This point of

attachment is often described as the stalk of the
abscess and cases have been described in which
the abscess has discharged its contents through
the 'stalk', through a hole in the dura mater and
in the carious bone, to the exterior. Macewen
(1893) considered that spread of inflammation
to the inner aspect of the dura mater 'may result
in a "soldering" of the inner membranes, the
subjacent arachnoid and even the pia becoming
adherent by the fibrinous meshes of the
exudation. Once this occurs general leptomeningitis is guarded against'. The causes which
determine the occurrence of a diffuse purulent
leptomeningitis, localized adhesive meningitis
(soldering) or subdural empyema remain
obscure; they are probably related to the speed
with which the infection spreads, a function of
the virulence of the microorganism and the reaction of the host. Occasionally at the site of localized adhesion of the brain to its coverings, an
abscess develops which involves the membranes
and the cortex of the brain. Macewen described
this as ulceration of the brain (case 10). It can be
adequately explained by direct spread of infection
across the pia causing a localized and entirely
superficial necrosis of the cortex, as a result of
thrombosis. To account for the formation of the
common type of abscess, Macewen (p. 81) considered that infection spread 'along the paths of
the cerebral vessels which penetrate the white
substance of the brain'; this hypothesis has been
generally accepted. The anatomy of the mic-
rocirculation of the brain provides plausibility.
Small arteries from the pial network enter the
cortex perpendicularly and break up into a rich
capillary bed to supply the various layers; the
deepest reach the subcortical white matter. The
vessels terminate in a T-shaped branch, or a
sprouting of branches (the 'candelabra' of Rowbotham & Little 1963) before entering the capillary bed. There appears to be little or no
anastomosis between small arteries beyond the
pial network. Other arteries, of larger diameter
than the cortical ones, traverse the cortex and
penetrate the white matter to varying distances,
some reaching the walls of the ventricles, and
some to the periphery of the basal ganglia which

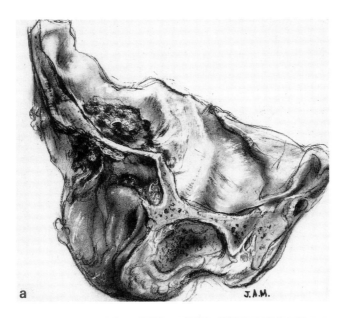

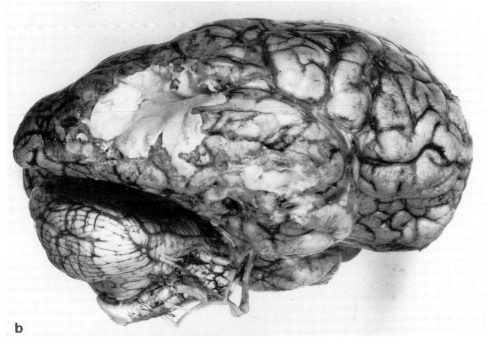

**Fig. 14.2.** Male aged 47: discharging right ear for many years, sudden onset of acute suppurative meningitis and slight left hemiparesis: symptoms and signs subsided with antibiotics, angiography showed evidence of a temporal lobe abscess: radical mastoidectomy; subsequently his condition rapidly worsened and he died 1 week later after operation.

(a) Right petrous bone seen from in front and above, showing deficit of bone and dura mater in region of tegmen tympani which exuded pus.

(b) Subdural purulent exudate covering temporal lobe: some of the smaller veins showed thrombophlebitis. Cortex of lateral and inferior surfaces of pole was soft and pus exuded from small superficial cavity within the brain. A zone of haemorrhage softening without pus formation was found anterior to this superficial abscess.

are supplied by central arteries entering the base of the brain (Lazorthes 1961, Rowbotham & Little 1965). These arteries of the white matter have collateral branches but do not anastomose with one another, nor with the central arteries. The veins of the cortex empty into the surface cortical system (Campbell 1938, p. 83); those of the white matter return blood to the surface system and also to the ventricular and basal systems (Lazorthes 1961). It is therefore anatomically feasible for purulent exudate to extend into the white matter along the perivascular sheath of a penetrating artery; purulent thromboangiitis will create an area of infarction and the depth of this nidus will depend upon the distribution of the vessel. Whether infection along the course of a penetrating vein will have similar consequences is uncertain but the different drainage of the white matter veins may make this less likely. Proof that this is the pathogenesis of brain abscess is hard to come by because it is destroyed as the abscess gets larger. Preysing (1901) described and illustrated a frontal abscess which had an attachment to the dura mater covering an ethmoid air cell. Crossing this attachment, which contained an opening into the abscess, was a cortical vein obliterated at this point; he considered that the vein might have provided the pathway of infection into the brain. Atkinson (1934, Fig. 13) depicts a small subcortical abscess; overlying it is a pial vein containing pus; small areas of subcortical necrosis of white matter adjacent to sulci filled with purulent exudate are also illustrated (Figs. 10 and 11).

The pathogenesis of metastatic abscess at first sight seems simple; the occurrence of septic embolization. Alexander and Putnam (1938) described and illustrated a brain with multiple abscesses (Fig. 204). One area of white matter free of any visible abscess appeared hyperaemic to the naked eye (Fig. 205) and microscopic examination of this area revealed purulent thromboangiitis, perivascular haemorrhages and early necrosis (Fig. 706). They considered that these were the changes preceding the formation of an abscess. Macewen describes a case and quotes another, in which erosion of bone had

extended from the middle ear to the carotid canal and thrombus was found within the internal carotid artery, partially occluding its lumen. A metastatic abscess might well arise from such a source; this may be the explanation of those abscesses which are occasionally encountered in the brain remote from an infected ear. Embolization however does not explain why metastatic abscesses rarely occur in the cortex, unless the emboli are of a size too large to enter the cortical arteries but not too large to enter those which traverse the cortex and enter the white matter. It may be that the greater vascularity of the grey matter, though it renders the cortex more liable to receive the embolus, enhances its resistance to the infection. Rowbotham and Little (1963) consider that the capillary distributions of individual cortical arteries overlap to some extent; if this be so then infarction of grey matter will be less readily produced. Another problem is whether the bolus must be of minimum size in order to pass the pulmonary filter (in the absence of a congenital alternative pathway) and if the minute bolus comprising a few microorganisms such as occurs in bacteraemia is adequate to infect the brain. If this be so, then it is difficult to account for the infrequence of brain abscess, when transient bacteraemia is relatively common in illness, during operations on infected tissues and the occurrence in apparently healthy persons (Butler 1937). A further anomaly is the relative infrequence of brain abscess in subacute bacterial endocarditis. Sperling (quoted by Collis 1944) found that in 76 cases of endocarditis involving the left side of the heart and causing multiple emboli, abscesses were present in the kidney in 57, in the spleen in 39, but in the brain is only 15. Commenting on the difficulty of producing experimental brain abscess by injecting bacteria into the blood stream, Gates et al. (1950) estimated that the incidence of metastatic brain abscess is about 0.4% of necropsies; they point out that on this basis only one positive result would occur in 250 animals and that no experiments had been carried out on such a large scale. Molinari et al. (1973) in an experimental model found that there had to be pre-existing or concurrent brain damage, for example as the result of trauma or vascular occlusion, before bacteria could invade the parenchyma.

The commonest cause of haematogenous brain abscess was chronic suppurative pulmonary disease and according to Schorstein the first case was recorded by Powell in 1815. Schorstein (1909) found records of 19 in 3700 necropsies at the Brompton Hospital for Diseases of the Chest; the most frequent cause was bronchiectasis, present in 14. Gates et al. combining figures from the literature found the following incidence: bronchiectasis 39%, empyema 23%, lung abscess 19%, the remainder showing mixed lesions. Schorstein comments that infarcts and abscesses elsewhere were unusual and that although it was generally assumed that tiny infected thrombi were discharged into the circulation from the pulmonary veins, 'there was very little proof; no thrombi were found in arteries of the brain' Collis (1944) reviewed the theories and found them wanting. He considered that the infected material was carried by veins from the chest wall to the rich paravertebral plexus of veins, which communicate freely with the cerebral veins. These lines of venous communication, and the direction of blood flow in them, have been examined by Batson (1940) and Anderson (1951) in the context of cerebral metastases of cancer, particularly common from carcinoma of the lung and of the breast, both of which may invade the chest wall. But evidence against this route of infection is well nigh overwhelming. Abscesses along the course of these veins practically never occur; in 42 necropsies on cases of thoracogenic brain abscess Gates et al. found only 1 case of spinal cord abscess and 1 of vertebral osteomyelitis and the latter was the result of direct spread from an empyema; there were no instances of venous thrombosis.

In a small but important group of brain abscesses the patients have cyanotic congenital heart disease. Campbell (1957) states that the first example was recorded in 1814 by Farre and that Ballet in 1884 thought the association to be significant. Campbell found 14 metastatic abscesses in 800 such patients. None had endo-carditis and all had central cyanosis due to congenital abnormalities which created a shunt of blood from the right to the left side. Newton (1956) found 72 cases in the literature and added 7. In a few the congenital defect was limited to the septum and in these it is suggested that an intermittent shunt occurs. Closely similar to these are the cases of metastatic brain abscess in association with a pulmonary angiomatous malformation (Stern & Naffziger 1953) and in hereditary haemorrhagic telangiectasia (Dyer 1967). Although thoracogenic brain abscesses are multiple in about 40% of cases, in cases of congenital heart disease, abscesses are multiple in only about 10% of cases. These patients are usually young; in Newton's series the ages fell between 5 and 20 years. Although the shunt explains the pathway taken by the infective material, the susceptibility of the brain is not explained, for it is rare to find a primary thrombus or to find emboli elsewhere in the body. Newton states that a primary focus of infection was found in only 8%. Thus transient bacteraemia which escapes the pulmonary filter remains a convenient but unproven assumption. Campbell comments on the unexplained problems of pathogenesis and draws attention to three phenomena which characterize patients with cyanotic heart disease. They are prone to cerebral thrombosis because of the associated polycythaemia and in which a retardation of the cerebral circulation may play a part; they are cyanosed and areas of hypoxic cerebral damage may occur which could act as permissive loci at which infection could become established and lead to the development of an abscess. In this respect it is of interest to recall that a brain abscess may arise in a patient who has sustained a closed head injury with no scalp or bone infection; it has been suggested that in these rare cases, a local nidus for infection would be provided by a focal contusion. In this context the observations of Falconer et al. (1943) may be of significance. When they inoculated the brains (of rabbits) with a broth culture of organisms, the incidence of a well formed abscess was much lower than when the inoculation consisted of agar, yet containing only one tenth the number of organisms. 'The use of agar in the inoculum appears to favour the establishment of an infection. When one correlates the various difficulties encountered in attempting an explanation of the pathogenesis of brain abscess, it seems necessary to implicate a local factor in the brain, such as a nidus of tissue whose vitality is impaired, in order to 'establish infection'. This is valid both for abscesses due to the spread of a nearby septic focus and for haematogenous abscesses. The nature and the cause of the 'nidus' in many cases remains conjectural.

### Symptoms and signs

It is usual to divide these into three groups; those of toxic or infective origin, those due to raised intracranial tension and those indicating neurological disturbance.

An uncomplicated brain abscess gives rise to little or no evidence of its inflammatory nature and as Kinnier Wilson wrote 'the symptoms due to intracranial pus are often confused with those due to the process'. Marked toxic symptoms are usually attributable to the lesion causing the abscess, or to complicating ventriculitis or meningitis. Emaciation described in the older writings is now rarely seen. Although the temperature is usually subnormal in an established abscess, slight and transient episodes of fever often occur for a few days during the initial stages. In the large series of Bonnal et al. 30% of the cases evolved without a rise of temperature but in 60% there was a transitory slight rise. In patients with outspoken toxic symptoms of an adjacent suppurative process, the evidence that an intracranial lesion may be inflammatory is obvious. By contrast, in patients lacking any overt primary focus of infection, the possibility that a suspected intracranial lesion may be an abscess can easily be overlooked; in these the detection of slight fever is significant. Leucocytosis and elevation of the erythrocyte sedimentation rate may occur but may be due to the primary focus, or to an associated respiratory

tract infection which so often develops in a drowsy patient; commonly the blood examination is normal. Meningitis and the changes which may occur in the cerebrospinal fluid will be considered later.

Recognition of the symptoms of raised intracranial pressure is of the greatest importance in diagnosis for they, rather than the neurological disturbances, often dominate the clinical picture. The subject has been considered in detail in Chapter 2 and only a few comments need be added here. Headache is the commonest and the most significant; initially it may be unilateral, or occipital in cerebellar abscess, but it later becomes generalized and progressively more severe. Disease of the frontal sinus or of the ear may cause considerable local pain but if a brain abscess develops the headache involves a much greater area even if it is at first unilateral and takes on a throbbing intensity which may respond to change in posture. On occasion progress is so rapid that confusion and drowsiness overtake the patient before there has been much complaint of headache. Vomiting is more common in cerebellar than in cerebral abscess. Slowing of the mental processes, confusion, drowsiness and coma are late symptoms of raised pressure, due to the development of internal brain herniations causing embarrassment of the circulation in the brain stem; they signify the urgency of the condition. At this time the temperature is usually subnormal, the pulse rate is slow and the respiratory rhythm and rate may be affected; respirations may suddenly cease without warning or in an attack of coughing or vomiting, or when the patient is turned. Papilloedema is an inconstant finding and is often absent in acute or fulminating cases. It is more frequent in those which develop slowly and in which the abscess has acquired a wall; Bonnal et al. reported papilloedema in 70% of 301 cases of formed abscess.

The focal neurological disturbances occasioned by an abscess are essentially similar to those due to a tumour or other space occupying lesion and will depend upon the locality of the abscess. Only the more common and important ones will be recounted here. Physical signs referable to internal herniation and in particular those due to temporal lobe herniation and brain stem compression may rapidly dominate the clinical picture and conceal the localizing signs of the abscess. Epilepsy occurs in about one-quarter of the cases (Jooma *et al.* 1951, Bonnal *et al.* 1960) usually early in the course of the disease. The attacks are infrequent and may be generalized or focal; only the latter provide help in localization.

Frontal lobe abscesses may give rise to apathy, defective memory and personality and marked slowing of mental processes. Such symptoms also arise as a result of increased intracranial pressure from abscesses elsewhere; only when they seem disproportionately prominent with a well retained level of consciousness are they reliable evidence of a frontal abscess. Hemiparesis is caused by an abscess in the postfrontal region, but may also be due to herniation.

Temporal lobe abscess is characterized by a contralateral homonymous upper quadrantanopia, an almost constant feature if the abscess is otogenic. The upper quadrant is always lost first; the lower quadrant will also be affected if the abscess or surrounding oedema has extended further back or more deeply. If the abscess is in the anterior third of the temporal lobe 'Meyer's loop' of the optic radiation may escape and the visual fields will be unaffected, but an otogenic abscess so far forward is unusual. A partial hemiparesis may be detected, the mildest and most common degree being a contralateral facial weakness affecting the lower part of the musculature. If the abscess is on the dominant side, it may cause dysphasia; the disorder most commonly encountered is for the naming of objects (nominal dysphasia). Quadrantic hemianopia and nominal dysphasia are the two most valuable signs of a temporal lobe abscess; they may be overlooked in examination, or the patient's condition may render their detection impossible.

Cerebellar abscess nearly always causes nystagmus, the slower and coarser component being evoked when gaze is directed to the side of the lesion. There may be defective conjugate movement of the eyes towards the side affected; it signifies a rapidly progressing or large abscess and consequently that the condition is urgent. Ataxia and hypotonia of the ipsilateral limbs are usually present though tests may be difficult to apply and the results to evaluate in an ill patient.

Brain stem abscess presents with nystagmus, hemiparesis, dysphasia, dysarthria and ocular, facial and hypoglossal palsies.

The clinical evolution of an abscess is frequently described as occurring in three stages; the initial characterized by transitory malaise, fever, headache, seizure, limb weakness etc.; the latent, when such symptoms having largely disappeared the patient seems relatively well; the terminal in which the full clinical picture develops. It is true that in some cases a critical examination of the history may reveal minor events pointing to the initiation stage. Such observations are more likely to be available if the patient is under medical care at that time, for example when an abscess develops after a mastoid operation, or after a head injury. Occasionally a metastatic abscess may start abruptly as a mild stroke. But early manifestations of this kind are rare in current practice, perhaps as a result of the use of antibiotics in the treatment of the primary infection. The 'second' stage is hardly latent, but rather one of insidious development of the symptoms of raised intracranial pressure which merge with the more florid manifestations of a focal brain lesion or of brain herniation. Macewen regarded 'latent' as a misnomer if applied to an acute abscess for this 'second stage ... abounds in symptoms of cerebral disturbance ... though it is true that in many cases the symptoms may be so unobtrusive that they may be overlooked unless specially sought for'. Kinnier Wilson considered the defining of clinical stages to be misleading.

The speed with which brain abscesses develop is subject to great variation and the course which an individual case takes is unpredictable, in that the deterioration which heralds herniation or infection of the ventricle may occur abruptly with little or no premonitory warning. In the case of Bonnal *et al.* about one-quarter had symptoms for 2 weeks or less and nearly one-half of these for only a week; in 40% the duration was from 2 to 4 weeks; in the remainder the history was spread over several months, and in a few there was a latent period of years. Chronic abscesses giving rise to symptoms up to 24 years after a penetrating brain injury have been reported (Cairns & Donald 1934, Arseni & Ghilescu 1967). It is noteworthy that even after such long periods of quiescence, organisms can be cultured from the inspissated contents.

### Differential diagnosis

In a case of suspected abscess secondary to an adjacent focus of suppuration, of which paranasal sinusitis and mastoid disease are the commonest examples, it may be difficult to determine whether extradural or subdural abscess or dural sinus thrombophlebitis adequately explains the condition. Pain is often severe but usually localized to the diseased area and accompanied by local tenderness and swelling if there is superficial osteomyelitis, particularly in children, in whom the bone is thinner and softer. Lateral sinus thrombosis frequently causes local tenderness, swelling and stiffness of the neck and enlargement of lymph nodes; as well as papilloedema; extensive sagittal sinus thrombosis is manifest by obstruction to venous drainage from the cerebrum with symptoms of intracranial hypertension; thrombophlebitis extending into the cortical veins causes fits and paresis. Purulent sinus thrombosis may give rise to rigors. Extradural abscess is rarely of such a size as to cause intracranial hypertension and focal brain damage. On the other hand subdural pus (empyema) may collect in large quantities and rapidly produce hemiplegia, signs of compression of the brain and seizures. A subdural empyema in the posterior fossa is usually too diffuse to cause signs of cerebellar disturbance. A subdural empyema may elude clinical localization or distinction from intracerebral suppuration, but the possibility of its presence, like that of an abscess,

requires only to be recognized for appropriate diagnostic measures to be undertaken. When local suppurative processes are solely the cause of symptoms, they will usually be accompanied by the systemic disturbances of loculated pus. The problem of diagnosis is most difficult in patients in whom a brain abscess is developing in addition to extensive local suppuration. The two most important symptoms are headache, as distinct from local pain, and progressive mental dulling and drowsiness; if these are present, a tentative diagnosis of abscess should be maintained until it has been excluded by radiological methods.

In acute meningitis the general clinical picture is usually one of a vigorous systemic reaction to the infection, in contrast to that seen in abscess; the temperature and the pulse rate are markedly elevated, the respiration rate may be raised, the face flushed and the body sweating. The mental state may be that of confusion or drowsiness; coma is likely only in the terminal stages either as a result of brain damage from associated encephalitis or vascular lesions (Cairns & Russell 1946) or of hydrocephalus from leptomeningeal adhesions. If an abscess is also present, the meningeal infection having arisen concurrently, its effect is generally to dominate the picture; headache and drowsiness and the elevation of temperature and of pulse rate are less marked than would be anticipated in meningitis alone. The finding of abnormal neurological signs indicating a focal lesion is of great help, with the proviso that in severe meningitis there may be scattered cranial nerve palsies and extensor plantar responses and in tuberculous meningitis focal signs may be due to arteritis (Smith & Daniel 1947).

Meningitis may be a later complication of an abscess as a result of ventricular spread and this is the more common experience. A critical reappraisal of the history will often reveal the true course of events and is time well spent. Such patients are usually desperately ill, deterioration having been catastrophic in speed and in degree; examination reveals coma, severe neck rigidity and marked Kernig's sign, hemiplegia or decerebrate rigidity, dilated and poorly reacting pupils, high fever, a rapid pulse rate and irregular respirations and often a low blood pressure. The picture is one of terminal brain herniation, meningitis and a state of shock.

Reference has already been made to dural sinus thrombosis in the context of local suppurative disease. Benign forms occur in which the local inflammatory condition is mild and transient; they have been called 'toxic' (McAlpine 1952) and 'otitic' (Symonds 1931) hydrocephalus. They are characterized by mild symptoms of raised intracranial pressure, papilloedema which may be pronounced, frequently an abducens weakness, but no signs of a focal brain lesion. If the picture does not conform to this benign pattern, abscess should be suspected. Thrombosis may also affect the cortical veins; if many are involved and if there is associated thrombosis of dural sinuses, venous drainage is severely obstructed, leading in some cases to infarction and necrosis of the relevant area of brain. Epilepsy is the common first symptom, often focal and frequently repeated. This may be followed by hemiparesis or other evidence of disturbed brain function appropriate to the region concerned. In restricted cortical venous thrombosis there are no signs of raised intracranial pressure and the patient remains alert between the fits, which are usually more frequent than is the case in an abscess. But if the thrombosis is widespread, the patient's condition may deteriorate and the level of consciousness fall; it may then be impossible to exclude an abscess without other investigations. The subject is dealt with more fully later.

Occasionally it may be difficult to distinguish between abscess and tumour. Chronic abscess may be encountered in an exploratory craniotomy for tumour; conversely a stuporose patient with a discharging ear, or with a history of ear disease may be suffering from a tumour. This is a particular difficulty in cases of brain stem abscesses which may present as chronic problems and in whom no primary infective source may be discovered (Russell & Shaw 1977). Exploration and aspiration may be the only way of distinguishing between abscess and glioma at this site.

Encephalitis and in particular that caused by herpes simplex virus may be difficult to differentiate from an area of bacterial cerebritis. The diagnosis of herpes simplex encephalitis is considered later.

### Investigations

Examination of the blood is rarely of diagnostic value. In an uncomplicated case of brain abscess leucocytosis rarely reaches a level seen in pus concealed elsewhere in the body. Krayenbühl (1967b) found the erythrocyte sedimentation rate raised in a large proportion of his cases and considered it useful.

Analysis of cerebrospinal fluid can be of value in diagnosis, for it is rarely normal with an abscess in the cerebrum and virtually never normal in a case of cerebellar abscess. But, as in cases of brain tumour, there is considerable risk in performing a lumbar puncture if an abscess (or subdural empyema) is present, because brain herniation may be aggravated. It should be avoided if the information can be dispensed with; but if the information is essential, as it may be if there is accompanying meningitis, the risk can be diminished by the preliminary tapping of a lateral ventricle to lower the pressure immediately prior to lumbar puncture, at which not more than 2 mls should be removed. A constant abnormality in a case of abscess is elevation of the protein; 1g/l is a common figure. The cells are usually increased in number, in uncomplicated cases up to $200/mm^3$; whether polymorphonuclear cells predominate or not depends upon the acuteness of the lesion. A common problem is that of a visibly purulent fluid, containing several thousand cells, but in which no organisms can be seen in the direct film, the culture remains sterile and the sugar content is slightly below normal. Such a fluid is typical of an abscess associated with extensive oedema, or if the abscess is adjacent to the ventricles; unfortunately this is frequently not recognized and a diagnosis of 'meningitis' is made, its treatment instituted, but further investigation for an abscess is postponed. Tutton (1953) reported that in 68 cases of abscess, more than a third presented with meningitis, the criterion being a CSF containing over 2,000 white cells/mm³; three-quarters of these fluids were sterile on culture.

Electro-encephalography (EEG) has, in the past, been found helpful; Tutton (1952) found it a reliable method of localization. Recording causes little or no disturbance to the patient, and serial observations provide evidence as to the progress of events within the skull. In the early years of the clinical application of EEG, Williams and Gibbs (1938) and Walter (1940) first drew attention to its potential value in the diagnosis of brain abscess. Courjon and Corriol (1949) emphasized the localized abnormalities which may be recorded over an abscess of the cerebral hemisphere. Haas and Laubichler (1967) analysed the records of 33 cases, and attempted to correlate them with the pathological states. Diffuse and bilateral abnormality characterized by the presence of irregular (theta and delta) slow waves, diminution or loss of background frequencies and of alpha rhythm, worse on the affected side, is seen in spreading purulent encephalitis and widespread oedema. The slower the activity the worse the clinical state. Diffuse irregular slow activity may also occur in purulent meningitis and in extensive thrombophlebitis. A well localized abscess with mature wall and restricted oedema is recognized by an overlying focus of high voltage slow (0.5–2Hz) waves with phase reversal. On occasion, if the abscess is large and superficial it may be marked by an area of electrical silence. The record may show little or no abnormality elsewhere, except for a reduction in amplitude of the ipsilateral alpha. Between the two extremes, of diffuse bilateral gross abnormality and of well defined focus of slow waves, combinations occur according to the pathological state. Hasaerts et al. (1960) draw attention to the influence of impaired consciousness in masking localization; abnormality was localized in each of 10 alert patients, but in

17 stuporose or comatose patients a focus could be detected in only 4. It is a disadvantage that in such patients, in whom the difficulties of clinical localization are greatest, the EEG may also provide the least help. The intravenous administration of a dehydrating agent may sometimes reduce the diffuse and uncover the sought-for local abnormality (Radermecker 1956). Tutton (1953) underlined the assistance afforded by serial records during treatment; shrinkage of the abscess as a result of aspiration was reflected in the lessening of diffuse disorganisation and better definition of the focal abnormality, while the reverse changes indicate the need for reaspiration. It should be noted that in posterior fossa abscess the EEG gives no localizing signs, though the record is generally abnormal.

Ultrasound (echo-encephalography) and isotope scanning (gamma-encephalography) were useful diagnostic methods which have been applied to the detection of abscesses, in common with other space occupying lesions. The former would indicate whether or not there is displacement of midline structures, information sometimes supplied by X-ray if the pineal body is calcified and is seen to be displaced to one side. The special value of scanning was in the detection of multiple abscesses.

Radiological examination provides the most reliable information and should be undertaken without delay when an abscess is suspected. X-rays of the skull may reveal unsuspected areas of bone infection; in-driven fragments of bone or opaque foreign bodies, relics of a head injury, may be disclosed or the line of an old fracture through the frontal sinus may suggest the possibility of a frontal abscess. Very occasionally a bubble of gas may be seen, produced by a gas forming organism.

Isotope brain scanning will often reveal an area of increased radioactivity corresponding to the localization of a brain abscess, but the test is not specific for an inflammatory process. Radio-labelled leucocytes have been used to enhance the specifity of the test, however, and computerized tomography is now the diagnostic method of choice. Formerly, ventriculography was employed in diagnosis, but it has serious limitations. There is frequently such extensive oedema of the affected cerebral hemisphere that the lateral ventricle on that side is too compressed to contain air; films reveal air only on the opposite side, much displaced to that side. In cerebellar abscess, air ventriculography reveals dilated lateral and third ventricles; it is rare to obtain filling of the aqueduct and fourth ventricle so that localization within the cerebellum, often achieved in a tumour, is not possible. But the clinical findings taken in conjunction with the proof of hydrocephalus are usually sufficient for surgical purposes. Ventriculography carries a considerable risk to life in cases of abscess, because it may aggravate cerebral herniations and may precipitate rupture into the ventricle. The accuracy of the method in excluding an abscess, even if the examination satisfactorily explores all portions of the ventricular system is discussed later.

Angiography largely superseded ventriculography in the investigation of a patient with a suspected abscess. It carries little risk in the hands of an expert and provides information which may lead to the diagnosis of other inflammatory conditions which mimic abscess, for instance subdural empyema. Clinical and other methods may make it clear that carotid puncture on one side only is necessary, though if a haematogenous aetiology is suspected, both sides should be examined. If the anterior cerebral artery is in the middle line and is stretched and swept upwards, hydrocephalus is present, which may be caused either by a posterior fossa abscess or by the obstructive effects of meningitis. Computerized tomography or ventriculography is necessary to make the distinction. When a cerebral abscess is present, displacements of vessels occur. An important finding is an area of relative lack of vascularity. The avascular area corresponds to the zone of oedema, not to the abscess cavity. When an abscess has developed a well formed wall, this may sometimes be depicted in the angiograms. Lima (1950) drew attention to this and Heep (1949) described a capillary 'blush' outlining an abscess, appearing early in the venous phase. Weber (1960) detected pathological vessels in 13 of 61 cases. Although of infrequent occurrence, the recognition of these appearances is important because of their correlation with the maturation of the wall. During treatment, failure to improve may be due to the multilocular character of the abscess and angiography may demonstrate clearly that the lesion is much larger than that indicated by the pyogram (see below). It may also reveal abscesses elsewhere and evidence of cortical venous or sinus thrombosis.

Computerized tomographic scanning has now virtually replaced angiography in the investigation of brain abscess. It is essential that good scans without movement artefact are obtained. If there is ventricular distortion, enlargement or an area of reduced density in the parenchyma, contrast enhancement is necessary. A 'halo' appearance, which is thought to be due to the area of hyperaemia around the abscess

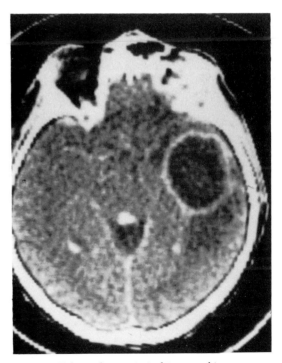

Fig. 14.3. Enhanced computerized tomographic scan showing an abscess in the right temporal lobe.

(Huckman 1975), even though it has been described prior to contrast enhancement (Keogh 1976) is accepted as one of the major features of an abscess. (Fig. 14.3). The degree of enhancement may be reduced if steroids are being used (Black & Farhat 1984). This appearance is not specific for the condition as it also occurs in other lesions with a necrotic centre (Fig. 14.3). If this appearance is found no further investigation is necessary but if there is no enhancement it may be necessary, particularly if there is fourth ventricular displacement or absence, to proceed to ventriculography to be certain that there is no infratentorial lesion. In the case of supratentorial ventricular displacement it will be necessary to proceed to exclude the possibility of subdural pus (see below). Computerized tomography also allows detection of multiple abscesses including daughter abscesses. This is of particular value during the initial follow up of treated abscess.

The computerized tomographic scan is very accurate in the diagnosis and localization of intracranial abscess, the false negative and positive rates being of the order of 1% each (Shaw & Russell 1977). This contrasts with the reported accuracy of angiography; temporal 100%, frontal 65%, parietal 67% and subdural 68% (Garfield 1969): and that for ventriculography; temporal 71%, frontal 81%, parietal 96%, subdural 83% (Garfield 1969) and cerebellar 97% (Shaw & Russell 1975). However it will always be difficult to distinguish on the computerized scan the intermediate zones between cerebritis and frank pus formation. Recently Britt and Enzmann (1983) have described criteria which help to distinguish cerebritis from an encapsulated abscess. These depend upon the time-density curves and patterns of enhancements judged from sequential computerized tomographic scans following intravenous infusion of contrast medium.

Computerized tomography does not always distinguish with certainty between an abscess and tumour. Brain scintigraphy using [111]Indium-labelled leucocytes improves diagnostic accuracy but does not absolutely confirm or exclude the diagnosis of brain abscess (Rehncrona et al. 1985).

The position of nuclear magnetic resonance in the diagnosis of brain abscess is not yet clear. Experimental work suggests that spin echo nuclear magnetic resonance images are more sensitive to the extent, particularly of the surrounding oedema, than is computerized tomographic scanning but that the latter is better at predicting the periphery of the inflammatory focus, i.e. the capsule. Inversion recovery nuclear magnetic resonance imaging more closely approximates to the findings on computerized tomographic scanning, though it may be better at assessing the oedema (Brant-Zawadzki et al. 1983).

**Treatment**

Amongst the earliest accounts of brain abscess must be those of Fabricius Hildanus (1560–1634) who recommended trephining, and of Morgagni (1682–1771) who recognized their otogenic nature in certain cases (Ballance 1922). Dupuytren (1839) vividly describes the events in a soldier who had sustained a compound fracture of the skull several years previously and who developed a hemiplegia; the wound was opened, the dura mater incised and a bistoury 'plunged' into the brain, evacuating pus; the man recovered. In 1876, Macewen made his first definite localizing diagnosis of brain abscess; the lesion was thought to be in Broca's area and operation was recommended but permission was refused; the patient died shortly afterwards and post-mortem examination confirmed the diagnosis. In 1881 he carried out his first operation, and in 1893 described his experiences of 25 cases in a publication which remains a milestone in neurosurgery. Operation was performed in 19 patients and 18 recovered, an operation mortality of 5.5% and a total case mortality of 24%. These results at a time when recovery was a rarity are astonishing and have remained so. His success was in part due to the type of abscess; many had a long history and appear to have acquired a well formed wall, but the case records reveal that in many patients there was clinical evidence of brain stem compression. It was also in part due to the meticulous care with which he cleansed the abscess cavity of pus and of sloughs, inserted and secured the drainage tube and to the avoidance of frequent change of dressing. Macewen was also aware of the danger of general anaesthesia in these patients, particularly in abscess of the cerebellum, by causing sudden arrest of respiration. Treatment by external drainage remained the method of choice for many years, though the techniques for securing drainage were modified from time to time; a historical review is given by King and Turney (1954). One method which gained favour was marsupialization; through a small craniectomy over the abscess, the overlying brain was excised and the abscess wall stitched to the dura mater; or the cavity was packed with gauze, the latter being gradually extruded by the intracranial pressure. Using this method King (1942) reported a mortality of 9%; the total number of patients observed was 79 of whom 42 died. Aspiration of the abscess was recommended by Spasokukolsky in 1916, according to King and Turney and again later by Dandy (1926), who appreciated that the problem of abscess in the brain was very different from that elsewhere, on account of the delicacy of the tissue and the slowness of reaction to infection except for the oedema which favours its spread. Sargent (1928) appears to have been the first to regard enucleation as the proper treatment of a thick-walled abscess. This he performed in 6 patients, all of whom recovered, in spite of rupture of the abscess in one. Some years were to elapse before the experience of Vincent led to the first major change in treatment. In 1934 in the course of a frontal craniotomy, aspiration revealed that the suspected tumour was an abscess; the patient's condition thereafter improved and 17 days later the abscess was again aspirated; a month later it was excised. Vincent perceived that decompression could control the distension of the abscess; time thus gained permitted the natural processes to wall off the infection rendering

enucleation feasible. He also showed that wound infection need not occur (Vincent et al. 1937). Vincent did not open the dura mater in the area of the decompression but this can be done safely if no pus is 'spilt' and provides a greater degree of relief of pressure. The method is applicable to both cerebral and cerebellar abscesses. The avoidance of open drainage considerably reduced mortality; at the London Hospital during the years 1936–41, 31 patients were treated. In each of 12 the abscess was drained and 9 patients died (75%); in some of these decompression and aspiration were also employed. In 19 patients no drainage was employed, only combinations of aspiration, decompression and enucleation; 42% died (Northfield 1942). But a radical reduction of mortality rates was not achieved until the introduction of antibiotics; the first case of brain abscess treated by the instillation of penicillin occurred early in 1942 (Pennybacker 1951). Part of the improvement should perhaps be attributed to the general adoption of angiography in preference to ventriculography (for reasons given above) which was taking place at about the same time.

Success demands early and accurate localizing diagnosis, energetic treatment with the appropriate intravenous antibiotic in large doses which both limits the spread of encephalitis and controls meningitis, accurate and repeated aspiration and intracavitary instillation of antibiotic and in many cases enucleation at the appropriate time. Decompressive craniotomy has become less frequently necessary since the use of antibiotics; intravenous dehydrating injections help to tide some patients over an episode of intracranial hypertension, but decompression can still be a life-saving measure though some surgeons prefer excision of the purulent area in such an extremity. Alderson et al. (1981) were unable to find any evidence for or against the use of steroids.

Early and accurate diagnosis is a primary requirement because of the unpredictable course in any case of abscess, emphasized long ago by Cairns (1930). As mentioned above, the clinical picture may change abruptly within a few hours with little or no warning, the result of brain stem compression or of ventriculitis. Tutton (1953) drew attention to the difference in mortality between a series which includes all cases, whether diagnosed in life or not and a series in which the abscess was diagnosed and was found at operation. In the former category mortality was 30%, in the latter it was 13%; the difference is due to 14 fatal cases, in 5 of which an abscess was not suspected, in 5 it was not found at operation and in the remainder the patients were moribund or operation was refused.

Diagnosis should be immediately followed by aspiration. In a cooperative patient the operation can be performed under a local anaesthetic; in the unconscious patient endotracheal intubation is advisable so that ventilation can be easily maintained if respiration suddenly fails and it provides an opportunity for tracheobronchial toilet. The burr hole should be made through intact skin at a point which appears to be closest to the abscess. Its likely point of origin is important; the frontal abscess secondary to frontal sinusitis is usually low down and far forward and the incision should be made just above the eyebrow; the temporal otogenic abscess is best approached by an incision just above and behind the external auditory meatus; the cerebellar abscess requires a posterior fossa incision as it is important to obtain a wide bony decompression including removal of the arch of the atlas, even in cases in which an aspiration alone as opposed to excision is to be carried out (Griffith 1969). It is generally agreed that aspiration through the wound of operation for frontal sinusitis or mastoiditis is inadvisable for fear of introducing infection into the brain; further aspirations in any case demand a separate and cleanly healed incision. Aspiration is performed with a large bore brain cannula, introduced slowly in the appropriate direction, as judged from the investigations and aetiology and guided by CT-stereotactic methods, by scanning ultrasound or by hand, as local facilities permit. The abscess may be entered without the surgeon recognizing it and for this reason the stylet of the cannula should be removed every few millimetres of advance, to

allow pus to escape; the stylet should be reinserted after each pause, so that softened brain does not enter and plug the lumen of the cannula. In some cases the resistance of the abscess wall will be encountered as the cavity is entered; this observation of depth is of importance and should be recorded. When the abscess has been located, the cannula should be kept still, as it is easily displaced from the cavity which may not readily be found again; the pus is allowed to escape and when it ceases to flow, a few millilitres of antibiotic solution (and if computerized scanning is not available, a sterile radio-opaque particulate medium, for example a suspension of finely ground barium sulphate) may be instilled. A specimen of the pus is immediately sent for bacteriological examination. If the abscess is not located, up to a depth of about 5 cm in the cerebrum, and about 4 cm in the cerebellum, as measured from the dura mater, the cannula is withdrawn and inserted in a different direction. It is inadvisable to explore by hand-guided needle in more than three directions; if localization has been accurate it is unlikely that a large abscess will be missed, and if the abscess is small the danger to life resides in the oedema and herniation; excessive needling of softened brain may spread infection or may precipitate haemorrhage. The evacuation of a large quantity of pus, 30 ml or more from the cerebrum, 10 ml or more from the cerebellum, provides a considerable reduction of intracranial pressure and consequently some improvement in the patient's condition may be anticipated forthwith. The computerized tomographic scan should be repeated at a suitable time interval (*see* section above on radiographic investigation) or in the absence of this, plain radiographs of the skull in 2 planes are carried out, which will reveal the abscess cavity as outlined by the opaque medium, the pyogram, a technique introduced by Kahn (1939). According to the progress of the patient and the appearances on the serial computerized tomographic scans (or changes in the pyogram), further aspirations are performed; on each occasion antibiotic may be installed (and further opaque medium if the pyogram is of poor quality); the pus should be cultivated. Aspiration may be needed every few days, or at weekly intervals, until the abscess steadily shrinks and the cannula penetrates the abscess with difficulty owing to the firmness of its wall. At this stage the decision must be made whether to enucleate the abscess or not; this is discussed later.

If aspiration has been unsuccessful all the relevant data in the case, history, physical signs and investigations should be carefully reviewed in order to confirm the diagnosis, to consider the state of the intracranial pressure and the amount of temporal lobe (or tonsilar) herniation. High intracranial pressure may be temporarily reduced by intravenous dehydration; tapping a lateral ventricle will relieve the acute hydrocephalus due to a cerebellar abscess, but in the case of an abscess in the cerebral hemisphere lowering the ventricular pressure may precipitate rupture into the ventricle of an adjacent abscess. If such measures in conjunction with systemic antibiotics and the maintenance of an unobstructed airway in the unconscious patient do not lead to an unequivocal improvement in the clinical state, or if the review of the case made it clear that internal herniation was present, decompressive craniotomy should be performed (Fig. 14.4). Some surgeons would widely excise the infected area of brain at this early stage. The flap should be fashioned over the site of the abscess; for example based on the temporal fossa where a large craniectomy can provide the

necessary decompression; in the case of a cerebellar abscess a suboccipital craniectomy is performed; in either event the dura mater must be opened. To relieve tentorial herniation, theoretically the temporal lobe should be elevated and its hippocampal border disimpacted but this is often impractical because the brain is too soft and too swollen; some surgeons resect the inferior portion of the lobe in such circumstances thus gaining access to the edge of the tentorium. To liberate herniated cerebellar tonsils it is frequently necessary to remove the posterior arch of the atlas in order to divide the dura mater adequately. A further attempt at aspiration of the abscess should be made a day or so later, when the abscess cavity may have enlarged sufficiently to be encountered.

When the initial aspiration reveals that the abscess has already acquired a firm wall, and this may have been deduced from the computerized tomographic scan, the decision must be made whether further treatment should be by repeated aspiration or by enucleation.

*Choice of antibiotics.* The primary procedure in the treatment of abscess should be surgical drainage of the pus not only in order to confirm the diagnosis and to give immediate relief, but also to obtain a specimen so that the organisms can be identified and their sensitivity to antibiotics determined. At the first aspiration these are unknown and the choice of antibiotic depends

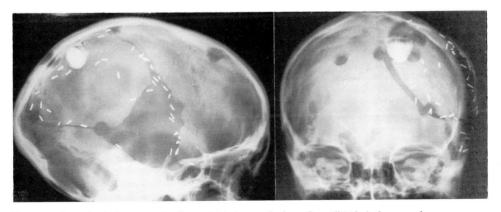

**Fig. 14.4.** Osteoplastic decompression for parietal abscess: the bone flap still 'rides' after 4 weeks.

upon the probability of various organisms being present. In abscesses resulting from sinus disease streptococci are the most likely organisms and hence penicillin would be the antibiotic of choice, whereas in those arising from an otogenic source the flora is mixed and a wide spectrum antibiotic (for example chloramphenicol, aminoglycosides) is required, perhaps in combination (de Louvois *et al.* 1977b). Ingram *et al.* (1977) suggested that metronidazole should be added to control the anaerobes which are very commonly present in otogenic abscesses. Multiple therapy is also recommended for metastatic abscesses (de Louvois *et al.* 1977b). It is essential that metronidazole be given in all cases in which anaerobes are suspected. Later the antibiotic should be changed to a more appropriate one if indicated by sensitivity tests. Systemic administration should also be given in high doses because of their value in controlling the advancing cerebritis until the acute stage has subsided: there is clinical evidence that antibiotics pass the blood–brain barrier in areas of acute inflammation and the blood–CSF barrier in acute meningitis, provided the dose is sufficiently high. Penicillin in doses of 1 million units or more every hour or chloramphenicol up to 6 grams daily are suitable. Bonnal *et al.* (1960) quote the case of a proteus infection, of poor sensitivity to penicillin *in vitro*, in which 20 million units of penicillin daily intravenously proved successful. Chloramphenicol carries a small risk of aplastic anaemia, but has the advantage of a broad 'spectrum' and of penetrating into brain and CSF better than most. Exceptionally, intrathecal administration is necessary for purulent meningitis due to organisms sensitive only to unusual antibiotics; ventricular instillation at doses of 1% or less of the systemic dose should be vigorously employed if there is ventriculitis.

Penetration of abscesses by systemically administered antibiotics varies considerably when judged by the antibiotic activity found in the pus removed during surgical drainage. This may be due to failure to penetrate the abscess or to tissue products in the blood which are capable of degrading the antibiotic. Nor does it give information about the concentration in the wall of the abscess. De Louvois *et al.* (1977b) found that penicillin penetrated well but that this was not the case for other betalactam antibiotics; that chloramphenicol may penetrate well but was erratic in its behaviour and that aminoglycosides had poor penetrating properties. Black *et al.* (1973) felt that chloramphenicol penetrated satisfactorily if the blood levels were adequate and therefore felt that local instillation of this or penicillin was not justified. De Louvois *et al.* (1977b) found that sulphonamides and cotrimoxazole could not be reliably estimated but Ingram *et al.* (1977) found metronidazole penetrated satisfactorily. These considerations are of great importance in the choice of antibiotics in those cases in which there are small metastatic abscesses deeply placed in the brain, which are often multiple and hence are unsuitable for surgical drainage (Rosenblum *et al.* 1980).

The follow-up of a treated abscess is best conducted using serial computerized tomographic scans. However, Moseley and Zilkha (1984) suggested that with large numbers of repeat computerized tomographic scans in patients with abscesses a radiation dose might be reached that poses a threat to vision. This must be balanced against the undoubted threat that these lesions pose to life. They have therefore suggested that routine postoperative scanning should not be undertaken, but be repeated only if further surgical intervention is contemplated for any reason including clinical deterioration or failure to improve over a reasonable period; that repeat scans should be done with contrast enhancement unless postoperative haemorrhage is suspected; that fine detail scans are not required; and finally that other radiological procedures such as angiography and sinus views can largely be dispensed with as they do not add significantly to the information gained from computerized tomography in the majority of cases. If computerized tomographic scanning is not available pyograms provide a useful method of following the course of the abscess. Thorotrast was the first medium used (Kahn 1939) but is no longer used because reported cases of malignancy particularly in the liver followed its use. Now a suspension of finely divided barium sulphate would be used (Micropaque). Both are taken up by the wall of the abscess and can provide visual evidence on skull radiographs that the wall is contracting. If micropaque comes in contact with the meninges a marked fibrous reaction occurs. Unlike computerized tomographic scan, the pyogram will give no evidence about any daughter loci or other abscesses which may be developing.

*Enucleation.* Whether an abscess should be treated by repeated aspiration until it is sterilized and shrivels up, or whether at an appropriate moment it should be excised is still largely a matter of opinion. The arguments against enucleation are as follows:

1  that it is unnecessary if cure is taking place;
2  that it is an additional risk to the patient's life;
3  that the dissection may cause, increase, or may make permanent a neurological deficit;
4  that the removal of the abscess scar is only achieved by replacing it with a surgical one.

The answers to these objections and further indications for enucleation are as follows:

1  Recrudescence of an abscess treated by aspiration may occur; in one series 8% recurred at the same site, from 3 months to 13 years later and all ended fatally (Jooma *et al.* 1951). Only enucleation prevents this.
2  The added risk to life of enucleation under antibiotic cover is very small, certainly less than that of recurrence quoted in (1).
3  That neurological deficit may be made permanent is admitted; this aspect is elaborated later.
4  The surgical scar resulting from a skilfully performed excision is less epileptogenic than the mixed glial and fibroblastic one of an abscess. The risk of subsequent epilepsy is not abolished and there is little evidence that it is lessened (*see* below).
5  In multilocular abscesses, aspiration fre-

quently fails to reach and to sterilize all loculi and enucleation is obligatory.
6  Chronic thick walled abscesses and post-traumatic abscesses containing fragments of bone or foreign bodies.
7  Thoracogenic and other abscesses in the acute stage which are not responding to aspiration (*see* below).

Although the two schools of thought lead to different actions in many cases, there is a considerable measure of agreement. All surgeons excise multilocular abscesses that are not showing satisfactory progress (5), thick walled or post-traumatic abscesses (6), those of (7) and as the primary treatment for the majority of cerebellar abscesses; enucleation would not be undertaken by its proponents if a resolving abscess is situated very deeply or in an 'eloquent' are of the brain, where the inevitable neurological deficit would be incapacitating. This would be the case for instance in abscesses under the central fissure, in the internal capsule, brain stem, basal ganglia or in the 'speech' areas.

With the advent of antibiotics of great variety, more radical initial surgery has been advocated. Le Beau (1946) recorded the recovery of cases in which abscesses which had not acquired a wall were enucleated by suction together with surrounding softened brain, thus rapidly relieving herniation. The heavy contamination of the cavity in the brain which inevitably accompanies such a fragmentary manner of removal of infected tissue was controlled by leaving penicillin in the cavity and in the ventricles and by systemic penicillin postoperatively.

Alderson *et al.* (1981) found that primary excision of abscesses produced as good results as did aspiration but they employed this method only in those patients whose responsive level was no worse than drowsy and disorientated. Choudhury *et al.* (1977) felt that their experience supported the contention that primary excision was the method of choice in the majority of cases and that such treatment did not increase the postoperative morbidity indeed in only two of their fifteen survivors was there any residual neurological deficit. Van Alphen and Dreissen (1976) present evidence to support the view that primary excision may result in increased damage to the swollen, friable and haemorrhagic brain and hence in more severe neurological deficit in this group than in those treated by aspiration with or without secondary excision. More recently Maurice-Williams (1983) has reported favourable results from widely incising abscesses at open operation and removing the pus thoroughly under direct vision. The value of radical surgery in the early stages of an abscess which is not responding favourably to less drastic methods is now established and if ventricular infection has occurred, is the only method likely to prove successful. To quote Ballantyne and White (1953) a brain abscess can be operated upon at any time that evidence of increasing intracranial pressure or threatened rupture makes intervention imperative.

What criteria guide one in choosing the appropriate moment for elective enucleation? Ideal conditions for dissection are an abscess wall sufficiently firm and surrounding brain still soft so that they separate easily. Earlier than this the wall too readily ruptures and though this is no longer a disaster it should be strenuously avoided: an intact abscess is more easily manoeuvred and there is no risk of leaving fragments. If too long delayed, surrounding gliosis may be so dense as to lead the dissector astray. The rate at which fibrosis develops varies considerably from case to case, so that determining maturity by the assumed 'age' of the process may be misleading, particularly as the dating of brain infection may be unreliable. Experience before antibiotic therapy suggested an 'age' of 8–12 weeks (Northfield) but with the acceleration of the natural processes as a result of antibiotics the period is nearer 4–8 weeks. Computerized tomographic scanning and the lessening of neurological deficits provide evidence of shrinkage of the abscess and the resistance to the aspirating needle is palpable proof of the firmness of its wall. Enucleation is carried out through an osteoplastic craniotomy for a cerebral abscess and through a unilateral suboccipital craniectomy

for a cerebellar abscess. The abscess is exposed by excising sufficient overlying portion of brain (uncapping) and partially emptied by aspiration; dissection is performed with moistened pledgets of wool and the greatest care must be exercised as the deep aspect is approached: here the wall is thinnest and ramifying loculi may be encountered. If the abscess arises from adjacent bone disease, the surgeon must anticipate the presence of a 'stalk'. This should be removed with the abscess, together with any diseased dura mater; a deficit in the dura mater should be closed with a free graft of temporal fascia, pericranium, or fascia lata, thus sealing the route of infection and avoiding a cerebrospinal fluid fistula if a track exists through the bone. Appropriate antibiotics may be instilled into the operative cavity. Not infrequently the ventricle is opened during the deeper part of the dissection; an abscess in the temporal lobe is often adherent to the choroid plexus and brisk haemorrhage may be evoked during the division of these adhesions. It is advisable to inject antibiotic into the lateral ventricle at the end of the operation if it has been opened, and if pus has been spilt instillation may be repeated for several days.

The question will arise as to when a patient may be considered cured. An affirmative answer may be more confidently given if the abscess has been excised than if aspiration only has been employed. In both, particularly if the aetiology has been uncertain or haematogenous, another quiescent abscess must be excluded; an aspirated abscess may have unsuspected loculi. Smooth clinical improvement and improving appearances on computerized tomographic scanning are encouraging.

*Treatment of the primary focus.* When an abscess arises from a known source of infection, this must also be treated. If it involves surgery, the question of priority arises. In general there is little doubt that the intracranial abscess constitutes the immediate threat to life and its treatment must be instituted forthwith. Where suppuration exists in the paranasal sinuses or in the ear, operation should be carried out immediately the patient's condition allows and should never be postponed indefinitely. Only eradication of the local bone disease will avoid the possibility of a recurrence of the abscess (Wright & Grimaldi 1973). Pennybacker and Sellors (1948) drew attention to the prime importance of this principle in thoracogenic brain abscess. They point out that the high mortality in these cases is due partly to the exhausted state of the patient as a result of the thoracic infection and partly to the interference with pulmonary ventilation and coughing consequent upon the impaired state of consciousness. The second factor is the more important because it may be fatal. They recommend early excision of the brain abscess and vigorous treatment of the pulmonary lesion including its excision if this is appropriate. Further abscesses are likely if the chronic chest infection cannot be controlled or eradicated.

## Prognosis

With the use of antibiotics, the mortality of treated abscesses has been approximately halved. Detailed analyses are to be found in the papers of Jooma et al. (1951), Tutton (1953) and Bonnal et al. (1960). In the last named the total mortality for 967 cases was 32%; this is broken down to reveal the death rates according to procedure, to anatomy of the abscess (single, multiple and multilocular) and to its morbid anatomy at the time treatment was started. In all series aspiration is linked with a higher mortality than enucleation, but the two groups are not comparable, because those of aspiration are weighted by the very ill or moribund who succumb shortly after the institution of treatment. In Tutton's series of 54 patients operated upon the mortality was 13%, the majority being treated by aspiration. Krayenbuhl reports a reduction of mortality in cases treated by excision from 47% (period 1937–44) to 7.6% (period 1960–65). Pennybacker (1961) achieved a mortality rate in all otogenic abscesses of 5.7% for the years 1950–60; it was higher for cerebellar than for temporal lobe abscesses. Thoracogenic abscess

still carried a very high mortality rate, between 30% (Tutton) and 47% (Bonnal et al. 1960). Pennybacker and Sellors reported recovery in 5 of 6 patients.

In more recent papers covering large series of abscesses over many years the mortality has remained high. However in each successive 5–10 year period there has been a continuous decline in the mortality rate. Alderson et al. (1981) reviewing a fifteen year period found that, when split into consecutive 5 year periods, the mortality fell from 42 to 21 to 9.7%. The cause of this improvement is far from certain. Effective antibiotics and more accurate localization by computerized tomographic scanning may have helped, but an increasing awareness of the potential diagnosis and hence early surgery not only for the abscess but also for the primary source must be one of the most important factors and is likely to be the factor which could lead to further improvement.

Sequelae may constitute a serious, even total disablement and comprise neurological deficits, psychiatric disturbances and epilepsy; all are attributable to brain damage and depend upon its extent, intensity and localization. In many cases of uncomplicated abscess, the final result is excellent and the patient returns to his original work with no residual neurological abnormality apart from his scars. In others, a small neurological deficit may occasion no disability; for instance, in temporal lobe abscess an upper quadrantic field defect is commonly permanent but the patient may hardly be aware of it, and in cerebellar abscess ataxia or disequilibrium is usually well compensated in due course. But the sequel to an abscess in the vicinity of the Rolandic fissure or in the dominant parietal lobe is very different; hemiplegia or dysphasia may be totally incapacitating. In abscesses complicated by meningitis, high intracranial pressure and temporal lobe herniation, not only is there the local necrosis of the brain due to the abscess, but there is in addition widespread diffuse neuronal damage, both cortical and central, in part due to the effect of oedema and of ischaemia and in part due to hypoxia from the impaired pulmonary ventilation during coma and during fits which may have occurred. Convalescence in these patients is prolonged and it is these which are likely to be left with psychiatric disturbance. They include personality changes, lack of concentration and of initiative, general invalidism, impaired memory and intellectual deterioration. Similar sequelae are seen in another group of patients in which diffuse as well as focal damage may occur, namely severe brain trauma. In the large series of Bonnal *et al.* approximately one-third of the patients had neurological or psychiatric sequelae; in this group of 121 patients the abnormalities were hemiplegia 58, psychiatric trouble 54, dysphasia 15 and visual disturbance 40. Matthijs (1963) examined 103 who had survived an abscess for up to 39 years. Neurological deficit was detected in 40%; pyramidal damage was the most frequent and 18 of 42 so affected were in consequence unemployable. Psychic disturbance occurred in 17%. A return to full work was achieved by 60% of the patients.

The incidence of epilepsy following supratentorial abscess is very high and the effectiveness of prophylactic anticonvulsants is not certain (*see* Chapter 17). It has been suggested that in early excision of supratentorial abscesses the incidence of epilepsy may be lower than following burr hole aspiration (Choudhury *et al.* 1977). However the statistical evidence and the duration of follow-up in these cases is not sufficient to be certain of this.

## Extradural abscess

Extradural pus is difficult to diagnose on angiography or ventriculography, but computerized tomographic scanning is very accurate. The neurosurgeon may encounter an extradural collection of pus in the course of an exploration for brain abscess; it originates from the primary adjacent lesion. The collection should be thoroughly evacuated by suction, the cavity irrigated with antibiotic and the original aim of the operation pursued. The definitive treatment of the extradural abscess depends upon eradication of the local bone disease, usually a matter for the appropriate specialist surgeon. Extradural abscess may be consequent upon osteomyelitis of the vault. Formerly this was treated by extensive resection of all infected bone, sometimes a formidable procedure, but with the advent of antibiotics this is no longer necessary; an intensive and prolonged systemic course often preserves much bone that would otherwise have been sacrificed. Sequestrectomy may be necessary at a later stage when radiological examination reveals the need. In the early stages a small incision in the centre of a subgaleal collection of pus will provide for bacteriological examination and at the same time a burr hole will reveal an extradural collection, which should be evacuated and antibiotic instilled.

Infection of a craniotomy wound may lead to osteomyelitis of the bone flap and an underlying collection of pus. If infection is severe, prompt removal of the bone flap is preferable. This saves time and is in the patient's best interest for it avoids sinus formation and frequent minor operations for the evacuation of small abscesses along the imperfectly healed wound.

## Subdural empyema

The subdural space normally contains but the thinnest film of fluid and is bounded on the one hand by the endothelium lining the inner surface of the dura mater and on the other hand by the arachnoid mater. Apart from arachnoidal granulations embedded in the dura, blood vessels and nerves passing to and fro, the space is in continuity over the brain on each side of the falx and the tentorium and through the foramen magnum over the spinal cord. Consequently there is free communication within this space from one end of the neuraxis to the other so that pus from a lesion in the frontal region may be encountered in the spinal subdural space in the course of a lumbar puncture (Case 3, Schiller *et al.* 1948). Although communication is free within the intact skull, immediately a burr hole is created brain bulges into and plugs the opening obstructing further drainage. The untrammelled rapid spread of pus, the vulnerability to thrombophlebitis of the veins traversing the subdural space and the swift increase of intracranial pressure due to the accumulation of fluid and to the venous engorgement of the brain are responsible for the neurological pattern and the grave nature of the disease; the difficulty of draining the subdural space constitutes the problem of surgical treatment. Subdural empyema, by analogy with pleural empyema, is an appropriate and now the generally accepted term for the disease. In the course of time the dura and to a lesser extent the arachnoid react to the presence of pus; where endothelial surfaces are still in contact they adhere by plastic exudate and the membranes enclosing the pus produce granulation tissue. These reactions are similar to, but faster and more severe than, those seen in chronic subdural haematoma. Loculation of pus is often termed subdural abscess. 'Purulent pachymeningitis' has been used synonymously, but this term should be reserved for the local area of dura mater adjacent to osteomyelitis, where the full thickness of the membrane becomes swollen, inflamed and may be infiltrated with minute abscesses. In the early stages the leptomeningeal space is preserved and the cerebrospinal fluid contains only a mild excess of cells and of protein; purulent meningitis may however also be present as a result of direct infection of the leptomeninges by the causative suppurative lesion. Organization around a loculus incorporates the adjacent pia-arachnoid and the encapsulated subdural abscess becomes firmly bonded to the brain. Cortical thrombophlebitis is almost universally present and the clots may become purulent. When severe it leads to extensive cortical damage, even infarction, and paves the way for secondary intracerebral abscess. The dural sinuses may be involved by extension of the venous thrombosis and by direct spread of infection from the primary lesion. The morbid anatomy of subdural empyema is fully surveyed in the papers by Courville (1944) and Schiller et al. (1948).

Paranasal sinusitis is by far the commonest precursor of subdural empyema and spreading osteomyelitis of the skull is nearly always the immediate cause. The 33 cases comprising the basis of the paper by Schiller et al. were due to sinusitis in 23, to mastoiditis in 6 and to a distant focus of suppuration in 4. Osteomyelitis was present in three-quarters of each group, totalling 26 cases in all. Other lesions were extradural abscess in 16, thrombophlebitis or sinus thromboses in 8, cerebral abscess in 8, suppurative meningitis in 7 and pulmonary abscess in 2. In approximately half the patients the empyema was loculated. Bannister et al. (1981) found a similar distribution of causative infections. Such analyses underline the widely ranging nature of the infection.

**Clinical features**

The clinical picture of subdural empyema differs in many respects from that of brain abscess. The high incidence of acute osteomyelitis means that in many patients the overlying scalp is swollen and tender (Pott's puffy tumour) and systemic disturbance is pronounced; the patient looks toxic and may have rigors. The neurological disturbance consists of a rapidly progressive flaccid hemiplegia usually starting in the face or arm and involving sensory function and a homonymous hemianopia. Schiller et al. drew attention to the frequency of paralysis of ocular conjugate movement towards the paralysed side and of the consequent persistent deviation of the eyes to the opposite side, a feature of acute destructive (or compressive) lesions of the frontal lobe and not peculiar to this disease. Paralysis of the cortical functions of one hemisphere may be total in 24 hours and if it be the dominant one the patient is speechless. Focal epileptic seizures may occur in the early stages but usually do not persist. The local pain of osteomyelitis is replaced by headache of rising intracranial tension. Although a subdural empyema gives rise to tentorial herniation, this may be difficult to detect because the empyema has already caused hemiplegia. Neck rigidity may be present, though this may be due to an associated meningitis; only pupillary changes may give the hint of brain stem compression. Pus spreading from mastoid disease may extend under the hemisphere on the tentorium to the occipital pole so that hemianopia may precede hemiparesis. In this situation it is clinically frequently mistaken for a deep intracerebral abscess; the anatomy is made clear by computerized tomography. If pus flows between the hemispheres under the falx the first 'eloquent' area of cortex to be affected is often the opposite paracentral lobule. This is revealed clinically as an extension of the hemiplegia to the opposite lower limb. Keith (1949) drew attention to the frequency with which the leg is paralysed before the arm during the initial hemiparesis, an important clinical detail because it indicates that the pus envelopes the hemisphere via the median fissure and this should receive special attention during operation.

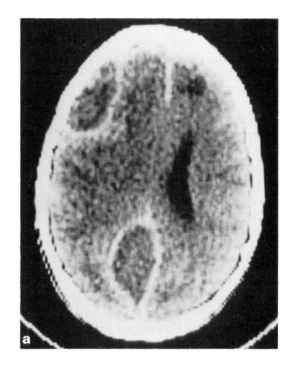

### Investigation

In contrast to brain abscess, a high leucocytosis is usual and blood culture may be positive. Ultrasonic examination reveals a midline shift unless the empyema is bilateral. The EEG is grossly disorganized, slow waves predominating, and without localizing feature unless the amplitude is greatly reduced ('flat') over the affected side, as is sometimes seen in subdural haematoma. Radiological examination of the skull may confirm the presence of osteomyelitis if it has been present for several weeks.

Computerized tomographic scanning is the diagnostic method of choice (Danziger *et al.* 1980). Though subdural empyemas can spread freely, often loculation occurs resulting in crescentic areas of low density occurring with compression or displacement of the ipsilateral ventricle. Following administration of intravenous contrast, enhancement occurs at the interface between the cortex and the pus (Fig. 14.5). Parafalcine collections may occur (Joubert & Stephano 1977). A few cases have been

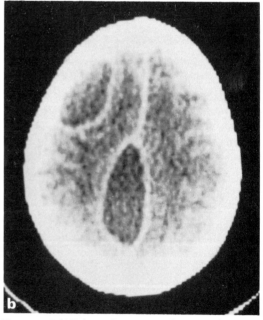

**Fig. 14.5.** (a,b) Enhanced computerized tomographic scan showing collections of loculated subdural pus both over the convexity on the left and parafalcine.

reported (Shaw & Russell 1977) in which ven-tricular displacement with or without low density changes and no enhancement on con-trast administration occurs.

Angiography is a most useful diagnostic inves-tigation. The exposure of the films must be timed so that the terminal cortical arteries are clearly shown; because of the high intracranial tension, circulation is often considerably delayed. The cortical vessels do not reach the calvarial shadow and this clear space is best seen in the AP pro-jection when effusion is over the convexity. This film may also reveal a collection alongside the falx, when the pericallosal artery and its bran-ches will be displaced from the midline; the opposite carotid injection will confirm this and comparison of the two films may reveal a bicon-vex clear area. Collections of pus around the occipital lobe may require vertebral angio-graphy.

Ventriculography (like angiography) may reveal an appearance similar to subdural hae-matoma but often the diagnosis will be made when the dura mater is incised, by the escape of subdural pus; in that event the ventricles should not be tapped.

If, following investigation, there is still doubt as to the presence of subdural pus, or if the patient is deemed too ill for angiography or ven-triculography the diagnosis must be made by multiple burr holes, through which treatment can be commenced. Negative burr hole explo-ration cannot reliably exclude collections of pus under the inferior surface of the hemispheres, nor in the median fissure; intensive antibiotic treatment should be commenced, and angio-graphy resorted to as soon as possible.

**Treatment**

Drainage of the subdural space is unsat-isfactory because burr holes are blocked by brain. Formerly mortality was virtually 100% because of the limitations of the diagnostic pro-cedures, inadequate evacuation of pus and over-whelming bacterial invasion; if the acute stage was safely passed an undiscovered loculation proved fatal later. Computerized tomographic scanning, angiography and antibiotics have greatly improved the results of treatment, although evacuation of the pus through multiple burr holes has remained the operation of choice for many surgeons. In cases arising from paran-asal sinusitis, a burr hole is made low in the forehead near the midline, or over the site of maximal scalp swelling if this is present. Sub-periosteal pus is evacuated and the skull drilled; if the bone is infected it bleeds readily and beads of pus may be seen in the diploe; any extradural pus is evacuated, enlarging the hole if necessary. On opening the dura mater subdural pus will well out, but the flow ceases as the depressed brain rises and blocks the opening. The brain should be gently depressed with a smooth instru-ment in several directions to facilitate further flow and this will be aided by an earlier admin-istration of urea or mannitol to reduce brain bulk. Further burr holes should be made: at the midline to give access to the space either side of the falx, over the frontal pole, in both parietal regions, and elsewhere as seems advisable in order to reach the limits of the empyema. Pus under and medial to the occipital pole requires burr holes close to the lateral and to the sagittal sinuses. Narrow-bore catheters are inserted into several of the burr holes so that they reach the limits of the empyema which is gently irrigated to evacuate further pus, its egress being aided by depression of the brain. The wounds are closed around the catheters into which low dose anti-biotic solution can be injected.

McKenzie (Keith 1949) recommended the removal of a midline gutter of bone in the frontal region in order to ensure adequate examination of the median fissure. Glass (1947) and Le Beau (1949) considered that only by an osteoplastic flap can the subdural space be completely emptied of pus. Bannister et al. (1981) also recommend that subdural empyema should be treated primarily by craniotomy. In this series they achieved much better results (see below) than they did with burr hole aspiration. Intensive systemic antibiotic treatment must be continued for many weeks in cases of acute osteomyelitis; Cairns (Schiller *et al.* 1948) recommended 8 weeks systemic administration. Epilepsy complicates recovery in a third of cases and requires prophylactic anticonvulsants. General measures for combating severe toxaemia and septicaemia must be applied vigorously.

If diagnosis has been early, before the cortex has sustained structural damage, a favourable response to treatment should be reflected in a rapid and progressive lessening of the signs of cortical paralysis. If this fails to take place, if improvements ceases, or further signs accrue, the cause is likely to be a loculated subdural abscess or an abscess in the brain. Computerized tomography should be undertaken forthwith and a fresh burr hole made at a site which will provide the most direct route to the abscess.

Treatment for the primary adjacent focus must be undertaken at the earliest possible moment in order to reduce the risk of reinfection.


**Results**

Prior to the discovery of the sulphonamides and penicillin, acute subdural empyema was almost without exception fatal. Keith (1949) described a series of 6 cases all of which recovered; all received chemotherapy and the last 2 penicillin in addition. In the important contribution by Schiller *et al.* (1948) 33 cases are reviewed; 18 patients treated before the introduction of penicillin died; 5 were encountered when the supplies of penicillin were inadequate and all died; 10 were treated with 'adequate' doses of penicillin and 7 recovered. Cairns (1930) restricted his operations to multiple burr holes. The more drastic method of an osteoplastic craniotomy was used by Le Beau (1949) and his colleagues in 8 patients and 7 recovered. Bannister *et al.* (1981) report a 92% survival rate following primary craniotomy compared with a 48% mortality in those treated by burr hole aspiration alone. Initial burr holes were instrumental in saving life in 19% but if this failed and repeat aspiration was required the mortality increased steeply to

58%. In those in whom the repeat procedure was a craniotomy 81% survived. However, early recognition which allows early decisive surgery is the most important factor in determining a favourable outcome. Prompt diagnosis remains the real challenge in the management (Renaudin & Frazee 1980).


## Sinus thrombosis and thrombophlebitis

Thrombosis of dural sinuses and cerebral veins provides a diversity of clinical syndromes according to the speed, the extent and the situation of the obstructive process. Such cases usually come to the neurosurgeon for the clarification of diagnosis; surgical treatment is restricted to that of a primary septic focus if present and occasionally to the relief of persistent intracranial hypertension. Thrombosis of the transverse (lateral and sigmoid) sinus was probably the first to be recognized. Macewen gives priority to Abercrombie who described an example in 1816. Ribes in 1825 recorded a case of thrombosis of the superior sagittal and transverse sinuses (Kalbag & Wolff 1967). Thereafter the condition was recognized with increasing frequency, and Gowers (1888 p. 416) devoted 6 pages to the condition. He divides the cases into two groups according to aetiology: (1) primary 'due to the state of the blood and circulation generally' (2) secondary due to 'disease adjacent to the sinuses'. Such a division is still adopted for descriptive purposes although in many cases in which the diagnosis can be confirmed by modern radiological methods a distinction between the two aetiological origins cannot be drawn. It is noteworthy that Gowers entertained the possibility of thrombosis within the cerebral veins not having spread from the sinuses. The concept of thrombophlebitis restricted to cortical veins owes much to the studies of Symonds (1937) and Martin and Sheehan (1941). In some of the latter's cases verification was provided by autopsy or by the appearances at craniotomy.

Dural sinus thrombosis secondary to an adjacent septic focus is becoming less frequent as a result of the earlier eradication of such foci by operations and by antibiotics. The incidence of transverse sinus thrombosis encountered in the course of mastoid operations was found by Archer (1952) to be 3.5% for the period 1921–36 and 1% for the period 1946–51. Surprisingly there was no similar fall in the incidence of brain abscess which was 2.6% and 3.0% respectively. Thrombosis of the cavernous sinus is usually secondary to septic infection of the face and nose and is now rare. Thrombosis occurring in the superior sagittal sinus is commonly of the primary variety, though it may be secondary to paranasal sinusitis as noted in the description of subdural empyema, to osteomyelitis of the calvarium and to open and closed head injury. In the absence of congenital abnormality there is free communication between the dural sinuses and the clotting process readily spreads, so that for example thrombosis commencing in the middle one-third of the superior sagittal sinus, a common site, may eventually occlude the torcular Herophili, the internal cerebral veins (the Galenic system), a transverse sinus and jugular bulb. Conversely a relatively silent thrombosis of a transverse sinus may spread via the superior petrosal sinus to the cavernous sinus causing florid signs.

Although the pathological changes leading to thrombosis of a sinus secondary to inflammation of its wall are well understood, those inducing primary thrombosis remain obscure. The following associated conditions have been recorded and are considered to play an important role in aetiology: wasting, dehydration, hypernatraemia, oligaemia, anaemia, pregnancy and puerperium, thrombophlebitis elsewhere, operation, trauma, heart disease and cerebral artery occlusion, blood diseases, fever, insulin and steroid therapy. Some of these conditions share common factors: diminished blood volume and pressure, abnormalities of blood clotting mechanism, local changes in the cerebral circulation. The 73 cases reported by Krayenbühl (1967a) included 30 associated with infections (11 adjacent), 16 with pregnancy or puerperium and 15 without detectable aetiological factor. That the

thrombus most frequently starts in the superior sagittal sinus has been ascribed to its anatomy. Its walls are relatively rigid, as is the case with the straight and transverse sinuses; consequently any diminution in the quantity of blood transmitted in unit time (blood flow) must be accompanied by a diminution in velocity which facilitates thrombus formation. Its lumen is traversed by trabeculae and the current of blood issuing from its tributary veins is directed anteriorly, contrary to the direction of flow in the sinus. Against these local factors which might appear to favour thrombosis must be set the difficulty of inducing a spreading thrombosis in experiments on animals. Beck and Russell (1946) used various methods including obstruction by a clip, by a plug of muscle and of cotton wool and by introducing into the sinus thrombin and a chemical irritant ethamolin used to obliterate varicose veins; thrombosis beyond the site of operative obstruction was not achieved. Similar resistance to thrombosis occurred in the experiments of Owens et al. (1957) which were undertaken as a consequence of the experience of Meirowsky (1953) in dealing with battle injuries of the superior sagittal sinus. These injuries might be regarded as the human prototype of the experimental injuries in animals. Meirowsky dealt with 112 cases of injury involving sinuses; in many there was severe brain damage. In 15 lacerations of the superior sagittal sinus, which were repaired by a muscle graft, the sinus subsequently thrombosed in only 1.

Sinus thrombosis obstructs the venous drainage of the brain and the rapidity with which it occurs and the extent of the thrombosis determines the degree of damage sustained by the brain. Gradual occlusion allows time for the opening up of collateral pathways of which the network of cortical veins is the most important; well developed anastomic veins of Trolard and Labbé and the Sylvian veins provide large communicating channels between the midline single and the paired lateral sinuses. Emissary and diploic veins serve a similar purpose though their capacity to enlarge is limited by the surrounding bone; extensive thrombosis closes them. If collateral drainage is adequate there may be no more than a rise of intracranial pressure which subsides as the clot is recanalized, a matter of several weeks. Venous return may prove to be inadequate because of anatomical variations in the richness or size of collaterals, or because they in turn become permeated by thrombosis. Brain damage is then swift, severe, irrevocable and often lethal. Intense congestion leads to widespread oedema of the brain, capillary damage and transudation, subpial and subarachnoid haemorrhage, infarction and intracerebral haemorrhage. The fulminating course in some cases is illustrated by No. 17 of Kalbag and Woolf; a young woman whose first sympton of sinus thrombosis appeared 16 days after parturition died 39 hours later; thrombosis involved not only the superior sagittal but also the straight and both transverse sinus, some cortical veins and the Galenic venous system. The experimental occlusion of the veins of Galen in animals has little or no ill effect (Bedford 1934, Schlesinger 1939) and it does not cause spreading thrombosis. Their partial compression by tumours of the pineal body gives rise to no damage attributable to venous obstruction, presumably because alternative pathways are adequate; the hydrocephalus in these cases is due to obstruction of the outlet of the third ventricle by the tumour. But unlike simple occlusion by a 'clip' thrombophlebitis of the veins of Galen and their tributaries blocks collaterals and gives rise to total haemorrhagic infarction of the basal ganglia. This has been encountered as a complication of the removal of a colloid cyst in a young woman who was thought to be 2 months pregnant but whose uterus was found at necropsy to contain a hydatiform mole. Thrombosis of dural sinuses is also an occasional complication of craniotomy. If sinus thrombosis is not immediately fatal, the late results are seen as areas of cortical scarring, porencephaly and in infants widespread dissolution of white matter which at this stage of immaturity appears to be particularly susceptible to damage. The early and late pathological changes are described in detail and beautifully illustrated in the excellent mono-

graph of Kalbag and Woolf (1967). Enlargement of the ventricles may be found in some patients who survive for long periods (Bailey & Hass 1937, Holub 1953) and Kinal (1962) has described hydrocephalus in cases of stenosis of the transverse sinus and of the jugular bulb. The cause of the hydrocephalus is disputed, whether it is the result of the excessive secretion or of the defective absorption of cerebrospinal fluid or whether it is *ex vacuo*, from hypoxic damage to white matter revealed as oedema subsides. The cerebrospinal fluid usually contains an excess of white cells and of protein attributable to intense brain oedema; in severe cases it may be xanthochromic and contain red blood cells. Occasionally subdural effusions of yellow or blood stained fluid occur, probably due to the rupture of small veins where they traverse the space to gain the superior sagittal sinus.

**Clinical features**

The chief symptoms are headache (usually the first), drowsiness and vomiting bespeaking intracranial hypertension; in favourable cases without extensive spread no abnormal neurological signs may develop, apart from retinal congestion or papilloedema, and an abducens paresis. Occasionally there is neck stiffness and in children oedema of the scalp, enlargement of the scalp veins and increase in the size of the head. In the majority of cases however, paralytic signs give evidence of focal brain lesions. The commonest is hemiparesis which was seen in 64% of Krayenbühl's cases; its development is slower than that due to an arterial cause, taking several hours or a day or so to become maximal. It may be preceded or accompanied by convulsions, general or focal; in some patients the epileptic seizures may be very frequent and Holub (1953) mentions a case in which status epilepticus was the reason for admission to hospital. Less frequent are sensory hemiparesis, hemianopia and dysphasia. Both paresis and epilepsy may spread to both sides indicating progressive involvement of the tributaries of the superior sagittal sinus.

It is generally assumed that the syndrome of recurrent seizures and paralysis which is such a characteristic feature of intracranial thrombophlebitis always betokens spread of the process into the cortical veins. There is good clinical evidence in support of this view, for benign cases occur in which a diagnosis of cortical thrombophlebitis seems justified by focal fits and paresis affecting one limb only, without evidence of sinus thrombosis, in a setting of infection or thrombosis elsewhere (Symonds 1940, Kendall 1948). But in some cases, defective communications in the cortical venous network may well be sufficient to cause an intense focal congestion, if the mouth of a vein is obstructed by thrombus in the sagittal sinus, though not invaded. It is interesting to compare the paresis described by Holmes and Sargent in their paper on *Injuries of the Superior Longitudinal Sinus* (1915) with that seen in primary superior sagittal sinus thrombosis. Holmes and Sargent were much impressed to find that the lower limbs were more frequently and more severely affected than the upper limbs, the distribution being such that the distal part of the upper limbs was most likely to escape and the distal part of the lower limb most likely to be severely affected, the reverse of that seen in capsular lesions. The authors ascribed this to venous thrombosis and obstruction affecting most severely that portion of the cortical territory nearest the sinus, which includes the paracentral lobule. Another feature which attracted their attention was the intense rigidity which accompanied and ran parallel to the paresis. By contrast the paresis accompanying non traumatic sinus thrombosis commonly affects the upper limbs before and more than than the lower; the affected muscles are often hypotonic, or only slightly spastic. In the 5 cases described in detail by Symonds (1940) the leg was affected first in only 2. Initial and more severe weakness of the leg is ascribed to thrombosis of the veins draining the medial surface of the hemisphere which may enter the sagittal sinus separate from the convexity veins (Martin & Sheehan 1941). In describing their 70 cases, Holmes and Sargent state that in many there was 'no direct damage

to brain either by projectile or by depressed fragment of bone'. The injuries were commonly gutter or tangential wounds in the midline of the head. Post-mortem specimens revealed thrombosed veins and swollen brain and 'minute haemorrhages which were grouped more closely in the neighbourhood of the wound'. Such a description fits more accurately contusion of brain by the projectile, and it is now well recognized that a glancing (tangential) trajectory causes severe and widespread damage to underlying brain, even in the absence of a fracture. It is more likely that the particular pattern of paresis so carefully observed by Holmes and Sargent was the result of direct cerebral damage and in favour of this interpretation is their comment that the associated intense muscular rigidity was immediately noticed by the soldier at the time of wounding, if he was not rendered unconscious. The immediacy and intensity of muscular rigidity and the posture adopted by the limbs is very similar to that which Denny-Brown (1966) called 'dystonia' and which followed the bilateral removal of cortical extrapyramidal areas.

Constitutional disturbance varies with aetiology and with the extent of the thrombosis. Infective cases commonly show some elevation of temperature and of pulse rate, but when intracranial pressure is markedly raised these may become depressed.

The differential diagnosis includes abscess and meningitis (both of which may be present) in addition to thrombophlebitis, subdural empyema, subdural haematoma, intracerebral and spontaneous subarachnoid haemorrhage and encephalitis. The history of a recent infective illness, the presence of sepsis or of venous thrombosis elsewhere, the use of oral contraceptives (Atkinson *et al.* 1970) and pregnancy or recent confinement should bring the possibility to mind.

### Investigations

Phillips (1948) considered that an increase in the plasma fibrinogen-B was a useful test, and

Kendall (1948) drew attention to the high plate-let count, their increased stickiness and the shortening of the coagulation time. Krayenbühl (1967a) reported an increase of the erythrocyte sedimentation rate in three-quarters of his cases and a leucocytosis in one-third. A lumbar punc-ture reveals an increase in the pressure of the spinal fluid which may contain an excess of cells and of protein; in severe cases the fluid is xan-thochromic and blood-stained.

Christophe (1951) drew attention to the changes which are to be found in the EEG namely a generalized irregular slowing. Burkhardt and Regli (1964) have analysed the records of 27 cases. No normal record was encountered. The mortality rate was 50% in those patients whose records early in the ill-ness revealed moderate to severe diffuse abnormal-ity, whereas none died whose records were only slightly or moderately abnormal.

The abnormality comprised depressed back-ground activity, loss of alpha, irregular slow waves and in about one-half a delta focus was detected. Intermittent rhythmic frontal delta was sometimes seen which they ascribed to upper brain stem disturbance (probably related to inter-nal herniation). Although epileptic attacks occur-red in 19 patients, in only 7 were epileptiform types of discharge seen in the EEG. Post-mortem examination showed that a persistent delta focus was likely to indicate an intracerebral collection; where there was little or no lateral pre-ponderance of abnormality, the superior sagittal sinus was usually affected. Clinical improvement was reflected in an improvement in the EEG; this may help to distinguish between thrombosis and abscess, though not between abscess and hae-matoma. In both these conditions a focus of delta activity may be uncovered as a record improves generally.

Computerized tomographic scanning is the radiographic investigation of first choice. In the case of sinus thrombosis bilateral low density lesions are seen, often with areas of secondary haemorrhage. Following the administration intravenously of contrast the walls of the sinus involved may enhance, but the lumen at the site of the thrombosis does not enhance. In cases of cortical venous thrombosis wedge shaped areas of low density develop.

Confirmation of the diagnosis can be obtained by angiography or by sinography. Krayenbühl prefers the former method, believing that the latter may spread thrombosis to the veins. He emphasizes the necessity to expose more films than usual so as to cover a longer postinjection period, 12 seconds, because of the great slowing of the venous circulation. This slowing is one feature to be sought; others are the lack of filling of groups of veins or isolated veins, the dilatation and tortuosity of veins and the lack of filling of dural sinuses. If a subdural effusion is present it will be clearly demonstrated. Sinography (by direct cannulation of the sagittal sinus through a midline burr hole in line with the coronal suture) introduced by Frenckner (1934 & 1937) may give more definite information about the superior sagittal sinus if carotid angiograms prove unsatisfactory, but if the total flow from this sinus passes into one lateral sinus, com-monly the right, thrombosis of the other lateral sinus cannot be assumed because occasionally there is no torcular communication between the paired lateral sinuses; retrograde jugulography (Ray et al. 1951, Gejrot & Lauren 1964) may then be advisable. Ventriculography provides little help; the lateral ventricles are small so that it may be difficult to engage them with the brain cannula and haemorrhage can easily be pro-voked in the softened and engorged brain. Uni-lateral extension to cortical veins may cause a slight deviation from the middle line. A large displacement of the ventricle to one side suggests an intracerebral haematoma or abscess.

**Treatment**

Antibiotics are essential if there is an evident infective aetiology but since this is not always overt, antibiotics should be given in all cases. Epilepsy requires anticonvulsant therapy; dosage must be sufficient to bring the attacks fully under control because of the danger of additional hypoxic brain damage. Kalbag and Woolf suggest the use of low molecular weight dextran, which might improve the cerebral circulation by diminishing the viscosity of the blood. Anti-coagulant therapy seems first to have been employed in this country by Stansfield (1942) and later by Kendall (1948) but the fear of precipitating intracranial haemorrhage has inhibited its general adoption. Some restrict anti-coagulants to those patients in whom paresis or fits have not occurred, reasoning that in these thrombosis has not spread to the veins and there-fore there are no infarcts. Krayenbuhl (1967a) strongly favours anticoagulant treatment and states that he has encountered no intracerebral haemorrhage attributable to such treatment when properly controlled. Steroids and dehy-dration by hypertonic solutions may also help in the less severe cases, by reducing oedema and diminishing intracranial pressure.

Surgery has only a limited scope. Clot has been removed from the sagittal sinus but thrombosis slowly recurred in spite of anticoagulant therapy (Ray & Dunbar 1951). Nevertheless it is likely that the operation opened up alternative venous pathways, because papilloedema subsided, having been unrelieved by bitemporal decom-pressions performed 8 months earlier. To be useful such a measure must be undertaken before thrombosis extends to the veins. Occasionally an intracerebral haematoma may be sufficiently large to warrant evacuation (Paillas & Sedan 1960, Krayenbühl 1967a) and the possibility of abscess should always be borne in mind. Sub-dural effusions need aspiration. The value of decompression for the relief of intracranial pres-sure is debatable and there is considerable risk that the swollen and softened brain will rupture when exposed.

### Prognosis

The reported mortality from sinus and venous thrombosis varies between 30 and 50%, though Kalbag and Woolf consider that the overall figure is lower than this. It is probable that lesser degrees of cortical thrombophlebitis com-plicating ear disease are more common than appears from the literature and this usually resolves satisfactorily. At the other extreme are the cases of spreading superior sagittal sinus thrombosis which usually end fatally. The sur-vivors are frequently left with severe disabilities including spastic diplegia, bilateral hemiplegia or in the young, mental retardation. In Krayenbühl's series, which covers a wide variety of cases, 34% died. In 20 patients no treatment was given and 70% died; this group included the very ill, some dying within a few hours of admission to hospi-tal. In 33 patients treated with antibiotics the mortality rate was 31% and in 17 treated with anticoagulants it was 5%; a few craniotomies were performed in both groups. Of the 48 sur-vivors, 3 were left with a residual disabling hem-iparesis and 3 with mild epilepsy.

## Pituitary abscess

Abscesses within the pituitary gland are rare. Domingue and Wilson (1977) found only 50 cases in the literature and all had been diagnosed at operation or post-mortem examination. They added a further 7 cases. In most of the cases in which sufficient detail had been recorded for analysis (29 in all) they found pre-existing disease in the pituitary gland including aden-omas and craniopharyngiomas. A primary focus for the infection is by no means always evident, but meningitis in known or suspected pituitary disease, or a patient with visual field defects should lead to a presumptive diagnosis of pitu-itary abscess. An enlarged pituitary fossa on skull radiographs or computerized tomographic scan-ning would virtually confirm the diagnosis. In the latter investigation the appearances of an abscess may be present. Dominque and Wilson (1977) recommend prompt treatment with appropriate antibiotics and replacement steroids. If improvement is not rapid, the abscess should be drained preferably by the transphenoidal route. They reported a mortality rate of 28%.

## Tuberculoma

Tuberculoma was formerly one of the commonest space-occupying lesions of the brain. In their analysis of a large series of autopsy records in Leeds, covering the years 1910–1931, Garland and Armitage (1933) found that approximately one-third of the brain tumours were tuberculomas, and gliomas provided a similar proportion. Van Wagenen (1927) examined the records of the Boston Children's and Infants Hospitals; during the 10 year period commencing 1915 there were 98 necropsies for tuberculosis of the central nervous system and in 9% the lesion was a tuberculoma. The incidence has steadily fallen to the extent that in 1963 Olivecrona was reported by Higazi not to have seen one in the last 20 years; that would be the experience of most neurosurgeons in Western Europe and North America, but in countries where malnutrition and tuberculosis are rife, tuberculoma still provides a considerable proportion of brain tumours, for example India 20% (Ramamurthi & Varadaraan 1961), Chile 16% (Asenjo *et al.* 1951), Rumania 9% (Arseni 1957). The increasing ease of movement of individuals from one country to another enhances the possibility of sporadic encounters with such rare tumours, yet the speedy recognition of its nature when revealed at operation is essential for its cure.

Tuberculoma may occur at any age but about one-half of the patients are less than 20 years of age. The cerebellum is frequently affected, particularly in the young. In his series of 201 cases Arseni (1958) reported an incidence of 62% in the cerebellum; in adults the incidence above and below the tentorium was about equal but in the young, cerebellar lesions predominated. Other large series are in rough agreement with this. Multiple foci may be present; in 15% of Arseni's cases and in 33% of those of Asenjo *et al.* Dastur and Desai (1965) point out that these may give rise to misleading signs. An associated tuberculous meningitis is rare, but tuberculous disease elsewhere in the body, usually in the lungs, is detectable in about one-half. In a population in which this disease is common, it will also be found in patients with intracranial neoplasms but Dastur and Desai encountered extracranial tuberculous disease in only 4 of 107 patients with a verified glioma, and in 47 of 108 patients with a tuberculoma.

### Morbid anatomy

A subcortical tuberculoma is usually yellowish white, avascular, hard, sharply demarcated and of rounded shape; the majority are caseous, a few sclerotic and occasionally they may contain pus or cystic fluid. A few are of irregular shape suggesting the confluence of multiple small foci (Dastur & Desai). They are generally surrounded by considerable oedema which Descuns *et al.* (1954) ascribe to a tuberculous encephalitis. Higazi states that the hard mass lying in jelly-like softened brain renders the naked eye appearances characteristic. In about half the cases (Dastur & Desai) tuberculomas involve the cortex, leptomeninges and dura mater. These are usually more vascular than the deep ones and may be mistaken for meningioma; often they are studded with tubercles by which they may be immediately recognized. If a tuberculoma is situated in the ventrolateral part of the cerebellum, involvement of the meninges and adjacent cranial nerves gives rise to a cerebellopontine angle syndrome; these accounted for one-fifth of Ramamurthi's cases (1957). In a small proportion of superficial tuberculomas the lesions are of considerable extent but of little depth and have been called 'meningo-encephalite *en plaque*'. They may cause considerable neurological deficit with relatively little rise of intracranial tension.

### Diagnosis

The symptoms and signs of a tuberculoma are those of an expanding lesion, in accordance with its anatomical situation and in some cases rendered complex by the multiplicity of lesions. The great majority of patients develop severe papil-loedema and in about one-half consecutive optic atrophy causes permanent blindness or severe loss of vision (Descuns *et al.* 1954, Dastur & Desai 1965). In those countries in which tuberculosis is common, tuberculoma of the brain appears to run a more virulent course, with a greater degree of systemic disturbance than in those in which the cases are of sporadic incidence. This in itself aids a correct pre-operative pathological diag-nosis in the first instance but renders it less likely in the second. The duration of symptoms may be as brief as 10 days, or as long as 9 years (Asenjo *et al.* 1951) but it is commonly between 3 months and a year. The importance of associated tuberculous disease elsewhere and of contact with diseased relatives has been pointed out, but their absence in no way excludes the diagnosis. Examination of the lumbar cerebrospinal fluid will often be impracticable because of increased intracranial pressure; the fluid may be normal or may contain a moderate increase of cells (lym-phocytes) and of protein. Arseni reported an increase of ESR in only 15% of cases. Many papers emphasize that the symptoms are often precipitated by some other illness, by trauma and by pregnancy.

Radiological investigations are important. In children there is usually radiographic evidence of raised intracranial pressure. Occasionally focal disease of cranial bones is revealed; this indicates involvement of the dura mater and epidural spread. Higazi describes a case in which proptosis and changes in the sphenoidal ridge simulated a meningioma. Calcium deposits are rare, occur-ring in about 6% of cases. Radiological exam-ination of the lungs for pulmonary and lymph node disease and of the skeletal bones to which attention may be drawn by reason of pain, swell-ing or chronic sinus is an obvious necessity. Computerized tomographic scanning is the radiological investigation of choice. The appear-ances change over time, because the tuber-culoma is an evolving granulomatous lesion (Vengsarkar *et al.* 1986). Initially the appearance of a tuberculoma is an isodense mass which enhances markedly with contrast. The edges are irregular but well defined and there is a sur-rounding low density reaction. Later the inflammatory reaction disappears and the centre undergoes caseation. At this stage the appear-ances are of a mass lesion with peripheral ring enhancement and a necrotic centre (Rovira *et al.* 1980). If this investigation is not available angiography and ventriculography are both useful but as with other tumours causing severe intracranial hypertension, angiography is pref-erable as it is tolerated better; it has the added advantage that multiple lesions are more likely to be disclosed. The vessel displacements are often considerable on account of the severe oedema. Higazi (1963) and Ramamurthi and Vara-darajan (1961) have noted that pathological vessels may be present forming a homogeneous opacity similar to the so called 'blush' of a men-ingioma and appearing in the arterial phase.

## Treatment

As penicillin opened a new era in the treatment of brain abscess, so the introduction of strep-tomycin and the more recent antituberculous agents (such as rifampicin) has radically changed the outlook in the treatment of tuber-culoma. In 1927 Van Wagenen reviewed the past results of operative removal and stated that in the literature there were records of about 50 cases of attempted removal and that permanent recovery was very rare. The common cause of death was tuberculous meningitis, signs of which developed a few weeks after the operation. Tuberculous disease elsewhere in the body proved fatal in some patients who recovered from operation. In 17 cases from the Peter Bent Brigham Hospital treated surgically, only one patient survived any length of time, a child who was alive and well 6 years after a decompression. Arseni (1958) reported a mortality of 45% in 60 cases, reaching 85% following radical excision; mortality ascribable to meningitis was 40%, being 100% in excision of cerebellar tuber-culomas. Dott and Levin (1939) examined the records of 94 cases provided by members of the

Society of British Neurological Surgeons and these showed 'comparatively favourable results'. All had been treated surgically and 43 survived; tuberculous meningitis occurred in 16 (17%). In an instructive paper on tuberculous disease of the central nervous system, Smith and Daniel (1947) expressed the hope that streptomycin might prove to be an effective therapeutic agent and in 1950 Obrador and Urquiza were able to give a preliminary report confirming its value. When first used, streptomycin was instilled at operation into the cavity created by removal of the tuberculoma and was given systemically and intrathecally for several weeks after the return of the lumbar spinal fluid to normal. In 1959 Obrador gave a further account of his experiences and stated that he had discontinued the practice of postoperative intrathecal injections, but was giving isoniazid in addition to systemic streptomycin. This is now the common practice in those clinics dealing with many cases and paraaminosalicylic acid (PAS) is also frequently administered. Prophylaxis against meningitis is not the only determinant of the duration of treatment; it must be continued until tuberculous disease elsewhere in the body is extinguished for this is an important factor in the mortality rate. Details of dosage are given by Arseni (1957) and Obrador (1959).

The indications for and the nature of the operation will depend upon the situation of the tuberculoma, whether there are multiple lesions and the degree of intracranial hypertension. If intracranial pressure is but little raised and in cases where the lesion is meningocortical, systemic treatment alone is often successful; the response is judged by symptomatic improvement, confirmed if necessary by computerized tomography it should be evident in a week or so. Inaccessible lesions causing severe intracranial hypertension require a decompression: in the case of brain stem tuberculoma a CSF shunting procedure will relieve hydrocephalus. Excision of the tuberculoma is possible and is necessary in the majority. Although the ideal is enucleation in one mass and formerly was obligatory for success, the use of antibiotics and chemotherapy makes piecemeal removal permissible, as in the case of pyogenic abscess. This is a valuable advance in treatment because tuberculomas in the cerebellum are often firmly adherent to the tentorium or to the ventrolateral walls of the posterior fossa, rendering their removal difficult, dangerous and at times impossible without fragmentation (Tolosa 1955). It should be noted that if there is any doubt as to the nature of the lesion, a rapid histological examination should be carried out so that specific therapy can be commenced without delay.

### Prognosis

Arseni, whose earlier results have been quoted above, had a total mortality of 12% in 141 cases using streptomycin; of the last 71 patients only 2 died and there was no case of meningitis. Palliative decompression was performed in only 6 cases, all tuberculomas of the brain stem; in the other 135 cases the operation was radical excision. Similar results were reported by Obrador (1959) and by Dastur and Desai (1965). The latter article contains much useful information and compares the authors' experience of tuberculomas with that of gliomas; they make the interesting observation that of 114 patients with verified tuberculomas, 89 were known to be alive at the time of writing, whereas of 107 with verified gliomas only 29 were alive. The postoperative mortality in the two groups was 7 and 30% respectively.

## Viral infections

In relationship to the frequency of viral infections in the population at large, viral infection of the central nervous system is relatively infrequent. This is not because the pathogens capable of invading the nervous system are rare, for example enteroviruses and herpes simplex, but perhaps because of the relative rarity of flaws in the defence mechanism which normally prevents the viruses from entering and infecting susceptible cells within the central nervous system (Johnson & Griffin 1978). Normally the body has several barriers against the entry of viruses. The most extensive is the skin but the other portals of entry through the mucous membranes are protected by immunoglobulins if the host has been exposed to the virus before. In addition the mucus in the respiratory tract has non specific inhibitors and the cilia eject the film of mucus including incorporated particles. Acidity and enzymatic activity help to protect the gastrointestinal tract. Once established in the body, however, nearly all viruses have the facility to invade the central nervous system. Entry to the central nervous system may be as the result of centrifugal spread along the peripheral nerves or the olfactory nerve or by the blood stream (Johnson 1982). The latter is the most important method of infection in man. Normally replication occurs at the site of inoculation, followed by a viraemia. The reticuloendothelial system attempts to clear the virus particles from the blood and its success is an important determinant as to whether infection of the central nervous system occurs. The viruses can pass into the brain or cerebrospinal fluid by several mechanisms: by infecting the vascular endothelial cells and thence to the glial cells and the neurons; by pinocytic transport across the vascular endothelium; or infrequently in leucocytes crossing the endothelial cells. Once within the central nervous system disease will occur only if the viruses attach themselves to and penetrate susceptible cells. The various cells show different susceptibilities to the range of infecting viruses (Johnson 1982) which may explain why some viruses produce only meningitic signs in man whilst others produce gross effects from damage to the cerebral parenchyma.

Since the survey in 1968 by Miller and Ross of 68 patients with encephalitis presenting to a neurosurgical unit, herpes simplex has been recognized as the single most common cause in the United Kingdom of severe encephalitis. By 1973 Adams and Miller were able to report 22 cases.

# Herpes simplex encephalitis

Herpes simplex virus causes an acute necrotizing encephalitis involving both neurons and glial cells. Though petechial haemorrhages commonly occur the endothelial cells themselves do not seem to be infected (Baringer 1978). Though a generalized infection the characteristic sites are the medial parts of the temporal lobe, the cingulate gyri and the subfrontal regions.

**Clinical features**

Herpes simplex encephalitis is primarily a disease of adults with no sex preference and the majority have been in good health previously. There is no increased incidence in the past history of cold sores as compared with the general population (Whitley et al. 1977). The onset may be insidious or fulminant. Commonly personality and behavioural changes occur followed by fever and headache. Some 40% experience seizures (Olson et al. 1967). Hemiparesis, aphasia and upper quadrantic visual deficits may occur, whilst some patients progress rapidly into coma without the development of obvious localizing signs.

**Investigation**

The cerebrospinal fluid is often under pressure and, except for very early in the disease, a lymphocytic pleocytosis with a raised protein and possibly mildly decreased sugar content is found. Red cells are often found in the cerebrospinal fluid. The electroencephalogram may show diffuse slowing and often periodic slow wave complexes occurring at regular intervals of 2–3/s from one or both temporal leads. An isotope brain scan may reveal increased activity in the temporal regions whilst computerized tomographic scanning may be normal initially. Later low density space-occupying changes may occur in one or both temporal regions. Parts of these areas may enhance with intravenous contrast. Angiography may show evidence of temporal masses, slow circulation time and local increased vascularity (Pexman 1974).

Early definitive diagnosis is dependant upon cerebral biopsy specimens which are subjected to light and electron microscopy/fluorescent antibody staining and inoculation into cell culture or animals. The latter gives the most reliable results. Serological studies involve too great a delay to be of value in helping to decide about antiviral therapy. Possibly methods of detecting specific virus protein or enzymes in cerebrospinal fluid may provide a reliable non-invasive diagnostic test in the future (Johnson 1982).

**Treatment**

There are 2 components to treatment: the control of the mass effect and hence the intracranial pressure with steroids; and the use of antiviral agents. Whitley *et al* (1981) reported a study using vidarabine in which the mortality of the treated group was 32%. However age and responsive level at the onset of treatment were major determinants in this study. Those under 30 years of age had a mortality of 24% compared with 52% for over this age. If the younger patients were only lethargic the mortality dropped to 9% but if the patients were in coma the mortality was nearly 60% irrespective of age. Cytosine arabinoside did not improve the mortality (over 70% in both treated and untreated patients Johnson 1982). Acyclovir is theoretically the most ideal antiviral agent as it is phosphorylated to the active substance in infected cells only. Assessment in human herpes encephalitis is in progress. If successful the final outcome for the patient will depend upon early diagnosis, at a stage before irreparable damage (in particular to the temporal lobes) has been done. At present 50% of those who survive are severely disabled often by an amnesic syndrome and by major focal deficits.

# References

ADAMS H. & MILLER J. D. (1973) *Postgrad. med. J.*, **49**, 393.

ALDERSON D., STRONG A. J., INGRAM H. R. & SELTON J. B. (1981) *Neurosurg.*, **8**, 1.

ALEXANDER L. & PUTNAM T. J. (1938) *Res. Pub. Ass. Res. Nerv. Ment. Dis.*, **18**, 471.

ANDERSON R. (1951) *J. Neurosurg.*, **8**, 411.

ARCHER G. E. (1952) *Proc. roy. Soc. Med.*, **45**, 121.

ARSENI C. (1957) *J. Neurol. Neurosurg. Psychiat.*, **21**, 308.

ARSENI C. (1958) *Confin. Neurol.*, **17**, 258.

ARSENI C. & GHILESCU M. (1967) *Acta Neurochirurg.*, **16**, 201.

ASENJO A., VALLADARES H. & FIERRO J. (1951) *Arch. Neurol. Neurosurg. Psychiat.*, **65**, 146.

ATKINSON E. A., FAIRBURN B. & HEATHFIELD K. W. G. (1970) *Lancet.*, **1**, 914.

ATKINSON E. M. (1934) *Abscess of the Brain*. London Medical Publications, London.

BAILEY O. T. & HAAS G. M. (1937) *Brain.*, **60**, 293.

BALLANCE C. A. (1922) *A Glimpse into the History of the Surgery of the Brain*. (The Thomas Vicary Lecture). Macmillan, London.

BALLANTYNE H. T. & WHITE J. C. (1953) *New Engl. J. Med.*, **24**, 8.

BANNISTER G., WILLIAMS B. & SMITH S. (1981) *J. Neurosurg.*, **55**, 82.

BARINGER J. R. (1978) In *Handbook of Clinical Neurology*, vol. 34 (Eds. Vinken P. J. & Bruyn G. W.) Chapter 8. North-Holland Publishing Co., Amsterdam.

BATSON O. V. (1940) *Ann. Surg.*, **112**, 138.

BECK D. J. K. & RUSSELL D. S. (1946) *J. Neurosurg.*, **3**, 337.

BEDFORD T. H. B. (1934) *Brain*, **57**, 1 and 255.

BELL W. E. (1981) *Ann. Neurol.*, **9**, 417.

BELLER A. J., SAHAR A. & PRAISS I. (1973) *J. Neurol. Neurosurg. Psychiat.*, **36**, 757.

BLACK K. L. & FARHAT S. M. (1984) *Neurosurgery*, **14**, 215.

BLACK P. GRAYBILL J. R. & CHARACHE P. (1973) *J. Neurosurg.*, **38**, 705.

BONNAL J., DESCUNS P. & DUPLAY J. (1960) *Les Abces Encephaliques a l'Ere des Antibiotiques*. Masson, Paris.

BRADLEY P. J. & SHAW M. D. M. (1983) *J. roy. Coll. Surg. Edin.*, **28**, 223.

BRANT-ZAWADZKI M., ENZMANN D. R., BRITT R. H. & SHELDON P. (1983) *Amer. J. Neuroradiol.*, **4**, 250.

BRITT R. H. & ENZMANN D. R. (1983) *J. Neurosurg.*, **59**, 972.

BRUNNER H. (1946) *Intracranial Complications of Ear, Nose and Throat Infections*. The Year Book Publishers, Chicago.

BURKHARDT S. & REGLI F. (1964) *Schweiz. Arch. Neurol.*, **94**, 1.

BUTLER H. M. (1937) *Blood Cultures and their Significance*. Churchill, London.

CAIRNS H. (1930) *Proc. roy. Soc. Med.*, **23**, 1049.

CAIRNS H. & DONALD C. (1934) *Proc. roy. Soc. Med.*, **27**, 111.

CAIRNS H. & RUSSELL D. S. (1946) *J. Path. Bact.*, **58**, 649.

CAMPBELL A. C. P. (1938) *Res. Pub. Ass. Res. Nerv. Ment. Dis.*, **18**, 83.

CAMPBELL M. (1957) *Lancet*, **1**, 111.

CAREY M. E., CHOU S. N. & FRENCH L. A. (1972) *J. Neurosurg.*, **36**, 1.

CHOUDHURY A. R., TAYLOR J. C. & WHITTAKER R. (1977) *Brit. med. J.*, **2**, 1119.

CHRISTOPHE L. (1951) *Presse Med.*, **59**, 1194.

CLARKE P.R.R., LANGMAID C. & WRAY S. (1961) Neur-ochirurgia 4, 211.

COLLIS J.L. (1944) *J. Thor. Surg.*, **13**, 445.

COURJON J. & CORRIOL J. (1949) *Rev. Neurol.*, **81**, 542.

COURVILLE C.B. (1944) *Arch. Otolaryng.*, **39**, 211.

COURVILLE C.B. & NIELSEN J.M. (1934) *Acta Otolaryngol.*, **21**, 19.

CUSHING H. (1931) *Proc. nat. Acad. Sci.* **17**, 163 and 239.

DANDY W.E. (1926) *J. Amer. med. Ass.*, **87**, 1477.

DANZIGER A., PRICE H., SCHECHTER M.M. (1980) *Neuroradiol.*, **19**, 31.

DASTUR H.M. & DESAI A.D. (1965) *Brain*, **88**, 375.

DE LOUVOIS J., GORTVAI P. & HURLEY R. (1977a) *Brit. med. J.*, **2**, 981.

DE LOUVOIS J., GORTVAI P. & HURLEY R. (1977b) *Brit. med. J.*, **2**, 985.

DENNY-BROWN D. (1966) *The Cerebral Control of Movement.* Liverpool University Press, Liverpool.

DESCUNS P., GARRE H. & PHELINE C. (1954) *J. Neurosurg.*, **11**, 243.

DOMINGUE J.N. & WILSON C.B. (1977) *J. Neurosurg.*, **46**, 601.

DOTT N.M. & LEVIN E. (1939) *Edin. med. J.*, **46**, 36.

DUPUYTREN G. (1839) *Lecons Orales de Clinique Chirurgicale*, 2nd edn., vol. 6, p. 146. Ballière, Paris.

DYER N.H. (1967) *J. Neurol. Neurosurg. Psychiat.*, **30**, 563.

EVANS W. (1931) *Lancet*, **1**, 1231.

FALCONER M.A., McFARLANE A.M. & RUSSELL D.S. (1943) *Brit. J. Surg.*, **30**, 245.

FELDBERG W. (1965) *Proc. roy. Soc. Med.*, **58**, 395.

FELDBERG W. & SHERWOOD S.L. (1953) *J. Physiol.*, **120**, 3P.

FRENCKNER P. (1934) *Acta Otolaryngol.*, **20**, 477.

FRENCKNER P. (1937) *Acta Otolaryngol.*, **25**, 441.

GARFIELD J. (1969) *Brit. med. J.*, **2**, 7.

GARLAND H.G. & ARMITAGE G. (1933) *J. Path. Bact.*, **37**, 461.

GARVEY G. (1983) *J. Neurosurg.*, **59**, 735.

GATES E., KERNOHAN J.W. & CRAIG W.McK. (1950) *Medicine.*, **29**, 71.

GEJROT T. & LAUREN T. (1964) *Acta Otolaryngol.*, **58**, 191.

GLASS R.L. (1947) *J. Neurosurg.*, **4**, 391.

GOWERS W.R. (1888) *A Manual of Diseases of the Nervous System*, vol. 2. Churchill, London.

GRIFFITH H. (1968) *J. Neurol. Neurosurg. Psychiat.*, **31**, 89.

HAAS R. & LAUBICHLER W. (1967) *Acta Neurochirur.*, **16**, 79.

HANDLER M., HO V., WHELAN M. & BUDZILOVICH G. (1983) *J. Neurosurg.*, **59**, 1001.

HASAERTS R., RETIF J. & GRAFF G. (1960) *Neurochirurgie.*, **6**, 382.

HEEP W. (1949) *Zbl. Neurochirurg.*, **1**, 2.

HEINEMANN H.S. & BRANDE, A.I. (1963) *Amer. J. Med.* **35**, 682.

HIGAZI I. (1963) *J. Neurosurg.*, **20**, 378.

HOLMES G. & SARGENT P. (1915) *Brit. med. J.*, **2**, 493.

HOLUB K. (1953) *Wien. klin. Wochenscht.*, **65**, 540.

HUCKMAN M.S. (1975) *Surg. Neurol.*, **3**, 297.

INGRAM H.R., SELKON J.B. & ROXBY C.D. (1977), *Brit. med. J.*, **2**, 991.

JEFFERSON A.A. & KEOGH A.J. (1977) *Quart. J. Med.*, **183**, 389.

JOHNSON R.T. (1982) *Virus Infections of the Nervous System.* Raven Press, New York.

JOHNSON R.T. & GRIFFIN D.E. (1978) In *Handbook of Clinical Neurology*, vol. 34 (Eds Vinken P.J. & Bruyn G.W.) Chapt. 2 North-Holland Publishing Co., Amsterdam.

JOOMA O.V., PENNYBACKER J.B. & TUTTON G.K. (1951) *J. Neurol. Neurosurg. Psychiat.*, **14**, 308.

JOUBERT M.J. & STEPHANO V.S. (1977) *J. Neurosurg.*, **47**, 73.

KAHN E.A. (1939) *Arch. Neurol. Psychiat.*, **41**, 158.

KALBAG R.M. & WOLFF A.L. (1967) *Cerebral Venous Thrombosis.* Oxford University Press, London.

KEITH W.S. (1949) *J. Neurosurg.*, **6**, 127.

KENDALL D. (1948) *Brain*, **71**, 386.

KEOGH A.J. (1976) *J. Neurol. Neurosurg. Psychiat.*, **39**, 920.

KINAL M.E. (1962) *J. Neurosurg.*, **19**, 195.

KING J.E.J. (1942) *Bull. N.Y. Acad. Med.*, **18**, 813.

KING J.E.J. & TURNEY F. (1954) *Ann. Surg.*, **139**, 587.

KRAYENBÜHL H. (1967a) *Clin. Neurosurg.*, **14**, 1.

KRAYENBÜHL H. (1967b) *Clin. Neurosurg.*, **14**, 25.

LAZORTHES G. (1961) *Vascularisation et Circulation Cerebrales.* Masson, Paris.

LE BEAU J. (1946) *J. Neurosurg.*, **3**, 359.

LE BEAU J. (1949) *Acta Psychiat. Neurol. Scand.*, **24**, 547.

LIMA P.A. (1950) *Cerebral Angiography.* Oxford University Press, London.

McALPINE D. (1952) *Arch. Middlesex Hosp.*, **2**, 149.

McCLELLAND C.J., CRAIG B.F. & CROCKARD H.A. (1978) *J. Neurol. Neurosurg. Psychiat.*, **41**, 1043.

MACEWEN W. (1893) *Pyogenic Infective Diseases of the Brain and Spinal Cord.* Maclehose, Glasgow.

MARTIN J.P. & SHEEHAN H.L. (1941) *Brit. med. J.*, **1**, 349.

MATTHIJS R. (1963) *Acta Neurol. Psychiat. Belg.*, **63**, 583.

MAURICE-WILLIAMS (1983) *J. Neurol. Neurosurg. Psychiat.*, **46**, 697.

MEIROWSKY A.M. (1953) *J. Neurosurg.*, **10**, 496.

MILLER J.D. & ROSS C.A.C. (1968) *Lancet*, **i**, 1121.

MOLINARI G.F., SMITH L., GOLDSTEIN M.N. & SATRAN R. (1973) *Neurology.*, **23**, 1205.

MOSELEY I.F. & ZILKHA E. (1984) *Brit. J. Radiol.*, **57**, 303.

NEWTON E.J. (1956) *Quart. J. Med.*, **25**, 201.

NORTHCROFT G.B. & WYKE B.D. (1957) *J. Neurosurg.* **14**, 249

NORTHFIELD D.W.C. (1942) *J. Neurol. Neurosurg. Psychiat.*, **5**, 1.

OBRADOR S. (1959) *Neurochirurgia.*, **1**, 150.

OBRADOR S. & URQUIZA P. (1950) *J. Neurol. Neurosurg. Psychiat.*, **13**, 66.

OLSON L.C., BUESCHER E.L., ARTENSTEIN M.S. & PARKMAN P.D. (1967) *N. Engl. J. Med.*, **277**, 1271.

OWENS G., STAHLMAN G., CAPPS J. & MEIROWSKY A.M. (1957) *J. Neurosurg.*, **47**, 640.

PAILLAS J.E. & SEDAN R. (1960) *Neurochirurgie.*, **6**, 268.

PENNYBACKER J. (1951) In *Modern Trends in Neurology* (Ed. Feiling A.) p. 257. Butterworth, London.

PENNYBACKER J. (1961) *Proc. roy. Soc. Med.*, **54**, 309.

PENNYBACKER J.B. & SELLORS T.H. (1948) *Lancet*, **1**, 90.

PEXMAN J.H.W. (1974) *Brit. J. Radiol.*, **74**, 179.

PHILLIPS G. (1948) *J. Neurol. Neurosurg. Psychiat.*, **11**, 263.

PREYSING H. (1901) *Arch. Ohrenheilk.*, **51**, 262.

PUTNAM T.J. & ALEXANDER L. (1938) *Res. Pub. Ass. Res. Nerv. Ment. Dis.*, **18**, 556.

RADERMACKER J. (1956) *EEG Clin. Neurophysiol.*, Suppl. **5**.

RAMARMURTHI B. (1957) *First Int. Cong. Neurol. Surg. Abstracts* 93. Exc. Med. Foundation, Amsterdam.

RAMARMURTHI B. & VARADARAJAN M.G. (1961) *J. Neurosurg.*, **18**, 1.

Ray B. S. & Dunbar H. S. (1951) *Ann. Surg.*, **134**, 376.

Ray B. S., Dunbar H. S. & Dotter C. T. (1951) *J. Neurosurg.*, **8**, 23.

Rehncrona S., Brisma J. & Holtas S. (1985) *Neurosurg.*, **16**, 23.

Renaudin J. W. & Frazee J. (1980) *Neurosurgery* **7**, 477.

Rosenblum M. L., Hoff J. T., Norman D., Edwards M. S. & Berg B. O. (1980) *J. Neurosurg.*, **52**, 217.

Rovira M., Romero F., Torrent O. & Ibarra B. (1980) *Neuroradiol.*, **19**, 137.

Rowbotham G. F. & Little E. (1963) *Brit. J. Surg.*, **50**, 694.

Rowbotham G. F. & Little E. (1965) *Brit. J. Surg.*, **52**, 8.

Russell D. S., Falconer M. A. & McFarlan A. M. (1941) *J. Neurol. Neurosurg. Psychiat.*, **4**, 273.

Russell J. A. & Shaw M. D. M. (1977) *J. Neurol. Neurosurg. Psychiat.*, **40**, 625.

Sampson D. S. & Clark K. (1973) *Amer. J. Med.*, **54**, 201.

Sargent P. (1928) *Brit. med. J.*, **2**, 971.

Schiller F., Cairns H. & Russell D. S. (1948) *J. Neurosurg. Neurol Psychiat.*, **11**, 143.

Schlesinger B. (1939) *Brain*, **62**, 274.

Schober R. & Herman M. M. (1973) *Lancet*, **1**, 962.

Schorstein G. I. (1909) *Lancet*, **2**, 843.

Shaw M. D. M. & Russell J. A. (1975) *J. Neurol. Neurosurg. Psychiat.*, **38**, 429.

Shaw M. D. M. & Russell J. A. (1977) *J. Neurol. Neurosurg. Psychiat.*, **40**, 214.

Smith H. V. & Daniel P. (1947) *Tubercle*, **28**, 64.

Stansfield F. R. (1942) *Brit. Med. J.*, **1**, 436.

Stern W. E. & Naffziger H. C. (1953) *Ann. Surg.*, **138**, 521.

Symonds C. P. (1931) *Brain*, **54**, 55.

Symonds C. P. (1937) *Brain*, **60**, 531.

Symonds C. P. (1940) *Brit. med. J.*, **2**, 348.

Tolosa M. E. (1955) *Neurochirurgie*, **1**, 211.

Turner A. L. & Reynolds F. E. (1931) *Intracranial Pyogenic Diseases*. Oliver & Boyd, Edinburgh.

Tutton G. K. (1952) *Brain Abscess*. Thesis, Manchester University.

Tutton G. K. (1953) *Ann. roy. Coll. Surg. Eng.*, **13**, 281.

van Alphen H. A. M. & Dreissen J. J. R. (1976) *J. Neurol. Neurosurg. Psychiat.*, **39**, 481.

van Wagenen W. P. (1927) *Arch. Neurol. Psychiat.*, **17**, 57.

Vengsarkar V. S., Pisipaty R. P., Parekh B., Panchal V. G. & Shetty M. N. (1986) *J. Neurosurg.*, **64**, 568.

Vincent C., David M. & Askenasy H. (1937) *J. Chirurgie*, **49**, 1.

Walter W. G. (1940) *Pract. Otorhinolaryngol.*, **3**, 17.

Weber G. (1960) *Neurochirurgie*, **6**, 317.

Weisberg L. A. (1981) *Neurology*, **31**, 575.

Whitley R. J., Soong S. J., Dolin R., Galasso G. J., Ch'ien L. T. & Alford C. A. (1977) *N. Engl. J. Med.*, **297**, 289.

Whitley R. J., Soong S. J., Hirsch M. S., Karohmer A. W., Dolin R., Gallaso G. J., Dunnick J. K. & Alford C. A. (1981) *N. Engl. J. Med.*, **304**, 313.

Williams D. & Gibbs F. A. (1938) *New Engl. J. Med.*, **218**, 998.

Winken P. J. & Bruyn G. W. (1978) (Eds.) *Handbook of Clinical Neurology*, vol. 35. North-Holland Publishing Co., Amsterdam.

Wright J. L. W. & Grimaldi P. M. G. B. (1973) *J. Laryngology & Otology*, **87**, 1085.

Yang S. (1981) *J. Neurosurg.*, **55**, 794.

# Chapter 15
# Hydrocephalus

## R. V. JEFFREYS

Although it is usual to define hydrocephalus as 'an increase in the volume of the cerebrospinal fluid within the skull' (Brain 1962) such a definition embraces conditions which are not normally considered in clinical differential diagnosis. Should we include the enlargement of the ventricles and the capacious subarachnoid spaces which accompany certain diffuse brain diseases? In these the passive accumulation of fluid merely compensates for the shrinkage of brain tissue; findings which can be demonstrated on computerized tomography or at autopsy and for which the term 'hydrocephalus ex vacuo' has been used (Fig. 15.1). Such cases come under the remit of cerebral atrophy and should be excluded. In so far as hydrocephalus results from an imbalance of CSF formation and absorption the term should be reserved for these cases.

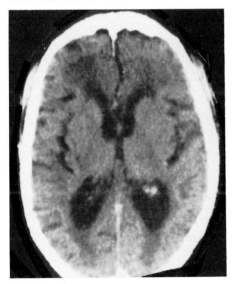

**Fig. 15.1** CT scan of 55-year-old man with dementia, showing widespread atrophy as well as ventricular enlargement.

Hydrocephalus will therefore be defined as 'an excessive accumulation of CSF within the head due to a disturbance of formation, flow or absorption'.

The advanced clinical condition was doubtless known in ancient medicine if only because of the great size of the head that might result. Russell (1949) quotes a passage from Vesalius in which it is clear that the feature which attracted attention was the enlarged head 'bigger than two men's heads', and he proceeds, 'this disease was that the ancients called hydrocephalus from the water which is stored in the head and gradually collects'.

The various classifications of hydrocephalus are based on clinical features, morbid anatomy or time of onset. Each has its own merits, but in a condition as broad as hydrocephalus no single classification will be perfect. Dandy and Blackfan (1913, 1914) subdivided hydrocephalus into two major groups: communicating and noncommunicating. In the former there is full communication between the ventricular system and the subarachnoid space; in the latter CSF cannot escape from the ventricular system. This classification has found most favour, since it can be modified by aetiological description (Milhorat 1972).

The causes of hydrocephalus will be considered under the following headings: tumours, congenital malformations, inflammation and absorption blockages. Presentation on a pathological basis is clearer than one based on anatomy, though the site of a lesion determines its effect. This follows the example set by the outstanding monographs of Russell (1949, 1966) and Milhorat (1972).

# Causes of hydrocephalus

## Tumours

These are the commonest cause of hydro-cephalus in adults, though in infants congenital malformations and postinflammatory scarring are more usual. The manner in which tumours may displace and compress the brain and according to the situation may obstruct the flow of CSF has been described in the various chapters on tumours and radiological techniques; only a brief summary is necessary here.

Tumours within or compressing one cerebral hemisphere may cause dilatation of the opposite lateral ventricle by compressing the foramen of Monro, the third ventricle or the aqueduct, thereby impeding the caudal passage of CSF. Compression may be due to the mass itself, to oedema increasing the bulk of the hemisphere, or to herniation of the temporal lobe through the tentorial hiatus. The ipsilateral ventricle cannot dilate because of its compression by tumour or oedema. Tumours of the basal ganglia and hypothalamic region also compress the third ventricle and cause dilatation of both lateral ventricles. All tumours lying within the third ventricle, the aqueduct of Sylvius and the fourth ventricle, or bulging into them from without, thereby compressing these anatomically strategic channels, give rise to hydrocephalus affecting all ventricular cavities proximal to the lesion. It follows that most tumours lying in the posterior fossa cause hydrocephalus (Fig. 15.2). Those arising extrinsically (for example schwannoma, meningioma, chordoma) may reach a considerable size without so doing, by reason of their slow growth and their distance from the fourth ventricle. Tumours which lie within the basal cisterns may obstruct the flow of CSF within the leptomeningeal spaces and thereby cause hydrocephalus; a meningioma in the posterior fossa is more likely to do this than a schwannoma because bulk for bulk it usually has a more widespread attachment to the dura mater and consequently affects a greater extent of the subarachnoid space. Tumours in the vicinity of

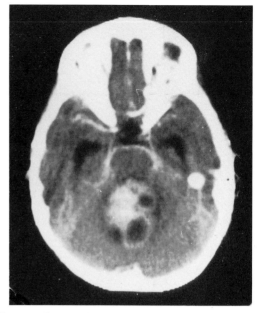

Fig. 15.2 CT scan of 8-year-old boy showing a solid and cystic turnover of the cerebellar vermis with hydrocephalus (the dilated temporal horns can be seen).

the tentorial hiatus may embarrass the upward flow of CSF, by obstructing the cisterna ambiens around the midbrain. The hiatus may be partially occupied by tumour or by herniated brain tissue, the medial margins of the temporal lobes from above downwards, or the superior cerebellum from below upwards.

The single possible case of hydrocephalus caused by over-secretion of CSF is with choroid plexus papillomas (Fig. 15.3). Milhorat (1972) felt that although these tumours might over-secrete CSF there was no convincing evidence for this, and, citing the fact that these tumours always occur within the ventricles and shed debris, he considered that they cause hydrocephalus by obstruction. However Eisenberg et al. (1974) have convincingly demonstrated that CSF production was increased by four times the normal in a neonate with a choroid plexus papilloma of the lateral ventricle.

Tumours can give rise to hydrocephalus in a more insidious manner, which at times eludes diagnosis. Neoplastic cells may spread through the CSF pathways and obstruct the flow of CSF;

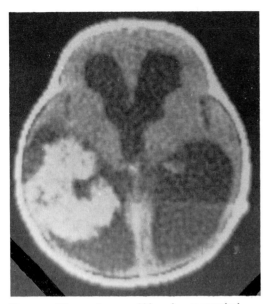

Fig. 15.3 CT scan of 1-year-old boy showing marked hydrocephalus due to a large choroid plexus papilloma of the left lateral ventricle.

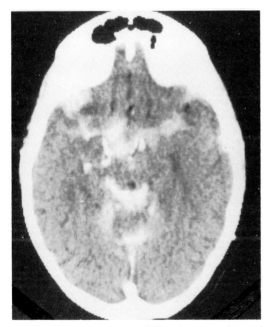

Fig. 15.4 CT scan of 12-year-old boy showing widespread leptomeningeal infiltration from a cerebellar ependymoma excised 2 years previously.

this is seen in gliomatosis of the meninges, a common occurrence in medulloblastoma but may occur with any glioma (Fig. 15.4). This event can also occur with metastatic tumours in the CNS, producing carcinomatosis of the meninges.

## Malformations

### Aqueductal obstruction

Congenital narrowing of the aqueduct of Sylvius is a frequent cause of hydrocephalus, usually giving rise to symptoms in infancy or childhood; on occasions the onset is deferred to adult years. Milhorat (1972) states that in approximately 2 out of 3 patients with congenital hydrocephalus a lesion obstructing the aqueduct of Sylvius can be demonstrated. The normal anatomical configuration of this channel has been studied by Woollam and Millen (1953) and MacFarlane and Maloney (1957). There is general agreement that the channel is not of uniform calibre, but presents two zones of narrowing and that the shape of the lumen changes as it is traced distally. Woollam and Millen arbitrarily defined the aqueduct as extending from a plane caudal to the posterior commissure, to that immediately caudal to the inferior colliculus, the plane lying perpendicular to the long axis of the brain stem. The length varied from 7 mm to 12 mm, the average being 11 mm. The upper constriction was situated at the level of the superior colliculus and the lower at the level of the intercollicular sulcus. The two constrictions divide the aqueduct into three portions, and the following are the more important of the cross-sectional measurements of Woollam and Millen (1953):

Average of cross sectional areas
1.3 mm$^2$ (range 0.6–2.0)
Average at upper constriction
0.9 mm$^2$ (range 0.2–1.8)
Average at lower constriction
0.8 mm$^2$ (range 0.4–1.5)

These authors also noted an inverse relation-ship between length of aqueduct and size of lumen; a long aqueduct tended to have a small lumen and vice versa.

It is of importance to identify the smallest dimension which can occur without hydro-cephalus. From the studies of Woollam and Millen (1953) it appears that a cross sectional area of 0.2 mm–0.3 mm$^2$ probably represents the minimum calibre of the aqueduct which is com-patible with a normal flow of CSF. But this is not the only parameter which influences the rate at which fluid passes through a tube. Length is also a determining factor. Impedence to flow is a function of cross sectional area and length; a narrow aperture of very short length offers less obstruction than a somewhat less narrow aper-ture extending for some distance. Measurements of the size of an allegedly narrowed aqueduct are incomplete if the longitudinal extent of the narrowing is not stated. There are three main types of aqueductal obstruction (stenosis):

### Forking, septum and gliosis

*Forking.* This term was introduced by Russell (1949) in preference to 'atresia' which was for-merly applied to the condition and which implies absence of the aqueduct. Forking is a common cause of hydrocephalus and in contrast to aque-ductal gliosis does not develop as an acquired lesion (Fig. 15.5), and is often associated with other congenital anomalies such as spina bifida, meningomyelocele and Arnold–Chiari mal-formation (Milhorat 1972). In forking, the aque-duct is represented by two channels lying one above the other separated by normal nervous tissue; one channel usually terminates blindly, or both may fuse to form a single channel. The channels are lined by ependymal epithelium; the dorsal one often has a complex infolded shape surrounded by secondary tubules, the ventral is usually a simple slit. A clear distinction between aqueductal gliosis and forking is occasionally difficult to make, since superimposed ventriculitis can obscure the histological findings (Alvord 1961).

*Septum* of the aqueduct occasionally occurs. Russell (1949) described two specimens and found three other reported cases. The septum is usually situated at the inferior end of the aque-duct and may be paper thin or may exhibit tiny perforations. Russell regarded this condition as congenital, though Milhorat feels that the overall evidence points to acquired reactive gliosis.

*Gliosis.* Aqueductal gliosis causes obstruction to the aqueduct by an overgrowth of glia. It is necessary at this point to underline the need for clarity in nomenclature. As is often the case in medicine, morbid anatomy leads the way in the accurate definement and classification of lesions. The distinction between gliosis and stenosis is an important one, which the pathologist may have no difficulty in drawing: in the latter the aque-duct is too narrow by normal anatomical criteria;

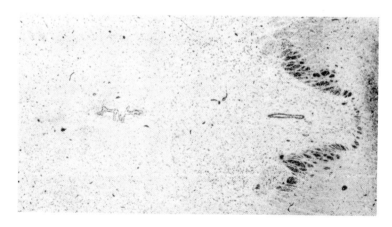

**Fig. 15.5** Section of midbrain. Forking of aqueduct; the aqueduct consists of two narrow channels separated by normal brain tissue.

in the former there are well marked histological changes in addition to the diminished size of the lumen. But the clinicians can rarely diagnose accurately the pathological nature of a benign (i.e. nontumourous) obstruction of the aqueduct. Considerations of age, associated malformations, past history of inflammatory disease may enable them to make a guess though how far from the truth only autopsy will reveal. It follows that neurosurgeons need a term denoting non-neoplastic obstruction and for this they often uses the word 'stenosis' or 'stricture', but it should be clearly recognized that this clinical diagnosis does not equate with the neuro-pathological one.

The two criteria necessary for a histological diagnosis of gliosis are narrowing of the lumen with loss of ependymal lining, and an over-growth of fibrillary glia. The lumen may be reduced to a minute canal, bare of ependyma and surrounded by glial fibres, and beyond this the ghost of the original canal may be provided by a more dense layer of glial cells interspersed with scattered ependymal cells (Russell 1949). In other cases the ependymal cells are arranged to form minute canals and tubules and in some specimens the appearances are a combination of both forking and gliosis.

The aetiology of aqueductal gliosis is obscure. Spiller (1916), who was the first to describe the lesion, considered it to be of developmental origin, a distortion of the normal closure of the aqueduct, the calibre of which is larger in the fetus than in the adult. Russell (1949) main-tained that the histological findings were incon-sistent with a maldevelopment, and suggested that they were an expression of a more wide-spread ependymitis. Milhorat (1972) points out that aqueductal stenosis is a regular finding in experimental animals innoculated either intra-cerebrally or intranasally with common viruses; the lesion is not only strikingly similar to that occurring in mankind, but evolves in the same pathological sequence as described by Russell.

*Arnold–Chiari malformation*

This remarkable deformity of the hindbrain was described at the end of the last century (Cleland 1883, Chiari 1891, 1896, Arnold 1894). Papers dealing with the Arnold–Chiari malformation often quote the categories into which Chiari divided his 24 specimens. *Type I* comprised those in which only the cerebellar tonsils protruded through the foramen magnum and which were due to long-standing hydrocephalus. In *Type III* the brain stem showed the characteristic elonga-tion but the ectopic cerebellar tissue lay within a cervical meningocele. *Type IV* comprised 2 cases of hypoplastic cerebellum. *Type II* com-prised the abnormality as it is generally under-stood and which will now be discussed. Since the paper by two of Arnold's pupils (Schwalbe & Gredig 1907) the term Arnold–Chiari has been used. The subject attracted little attention until Russell and Donald (1935) reported the presence of the malformation in each of 10 consecutive cases of meningomyelocele. Their interest in the subject was prompted by a desire to determine the cause of the 'frequent association of hydro-cephalus with spina bifida'. The important role played by this malformation in the production of hydrocephalus and of rather more obscure neurological syndromes is now well appreciated, though the mechanism may be less well under-stood.

The essential features of the Type II Arnold–Chiari malformation concern the cerebellum and the medulla, which are found to lie partly within the cervical portion of the spinal canal. They are often described as being 'displaced' into the spinal canal, but the use of this word carries the aeti-ological assumption that they have moved caud-ally during fetal development; this may or may not be true. When the specimen is examined from its dorsal aspect, a tongue of cerebellar tissue is seen protruding through the foramen magnum; its length varies, usually it is several centimetres but its tip has been known to extend as low as the second thoracic vertebra. The tongue of tissue is flattened, somewhat firm and fibrous, and is applied and adherent to the medulla and spinal cord. It is generally regarded as being derived from the inferior vermis (Cameron 1957a, Daniel & Strich 1958). Russell and Donald pointed out that the cerebellum is usually hypoplastic, lacking differentiation into vermis and lateral lobes and that tonsils and flocculi can seldom be identified. The junction of cerebellum and tongue is grooved by the margin of the foramen magnum. The pons and medulla are long, narrow and thin, occupying a more distal position than normal, so that the medulla lies to a variable extent within the upper spinal canal (Figs. 15.6 and 15.7). Cameron (1957a) has seen the pons level with the foramen magnum. As a corollary, part of the fourth ventricle, the foramen of Magendie and in severe examples the foramina of Luschka, are intraspinal. A characteristic abnormality of the medulla is a curious hump or lip which projects from its dorsal surface at its junction with the spinal cord; on sagittal section this is found to be just distal to the gracile and cuneate nuclei and is associated with a kink in the posterior columns (Peach 1965b). Abnormalities of the tectal plate have been noted in which there is a beaking deformity (mesencephalic spur) and these indicate that the Arnold–Chiari malformation involves the midbrain as well as the hindbrain (Adeloye 1976). In consequence of the occupation of the upper spinal canal by the medulla, the upper cervical spinal segments of the spinal cord lie at a lower level than normal and their nerve roots travel obliquely upwards to enter their respective intervertebral foramina. In a similar fashion the low position of the pons and medulla impose a longer course for the relevant cranial nerves to reach their respective cranial foramina.

The anatomy of the region of the foramen of Magendie may be complex. The tip of the cerebellar tongue may terminate rostral to the obex, leaving the inferior end of the fourth ventricle exposed, or it may extend caudal to the obex to overlap the cervical cord. Choroid plexus may lie within the ventricle, or it may be extraventricular, lying over and bound to the dorsal surface of the tongue. The opening of the central canal of the spinal cord lies in the distal part of the floor of the fourth ventricle. The site of the foramen of Magendie may be occupied by a pouch-like extension of the ventricle (Peach 1964b). The leptomeninges enveloping the hindbrain in the vicinity of the foramen magnum are usually thickened and fibrous, contain haemosiderin, and there is much congestion of blood vessels.

Other abnormalities of the brain frequently accompany the Arnold–Chiari malformation. They include hydrocephalus in most cases, stenosis and forking of the aqueduct, fusion of the thalami, microgyria, obliteration of the interhemispheric fissure and hypoplasia of the falx and of the tentorium. In consequence of the caudal situation of the hindbrain, the attachment of the tentorium to the parietal dura mater and consequently the transverse sinuses are unusually low, so that the posterior fossa is small.

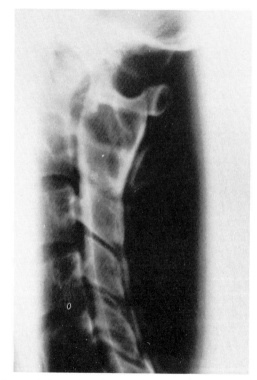

**Fig. 15.6** Cervical myelogram of 25-year-old woman with ataxia showing Arnold–Chiari malformation as filling defect in the column of contrast material as far down as C2.

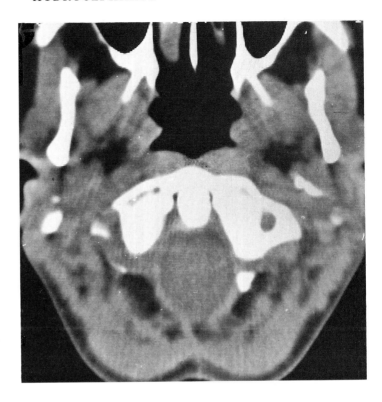

**Fig. 15.7** Same case as Fig. 15.6. Postoperative CT scan after decompressive surgery. CT at junction of C1 and C2 showing medulla within cervical canal.

The Arnold–Chiari malformation is associated with congenital anomalies of the spinal cord, meningomyelocele being the most common, though hydromyelia, syringomyelia and diastomatomyelia are also found. Milhorat (1972) found that 97% of cases with meningomyelocele had ventricular enlargement almost certainly consequent upon Arnold–Chiari malformations. Occasionally the Arnold–Chiari malformation may occur in the adult with or without accompanying spinal abnormalities. Recently Paul *et al.* (1983) have reported their findings in adults with type I Arnold–Chiari malformation; they regard cerebellar descent as the essential part of the anomaly in their patients and have paid no attention to the situation of the medulla. In this series there was a 32% association with syringomyelia.

The hydrocephalus which accompanies the malformation in 65% of cases (Milhorat 1972) is due to obstruction of the aqueduct of Sylvius. In cases of the malformation without aqueductal obstruction, hydrocephalus can be brought about in several ways, and probably more than one operates in an individual case. The abnormalities around the foramen of Magendie, described above, impede egress of CSF from the fourth ventricle. The crowding of the hindbrain in the small posterior fossa and in the spinal canal may also impede the flow of CSF even if the foramen of Magendie is patent. Marked leptomeningeal fibrosis around the malformation, particularly at the site of grooving by the foramen magnum, accentuates the problem. Finally Russell and Donald (1935) noted in some cases the hydrocephalus was of the communicating variety. From their observations on the spread of indian ink injected into the lateral ventricles and on the distribution of purulent exidate in cases dying with meningitis, they concluded that CSF might readily attain the spinal subarachnoid space, but its flow into the head was obstructed within the leptomeningeal spaces at the level of the foramen magnum.

A number of theories have been advanced, and hotly debated, to explain the morphogenesis of the Arnold–Chiari malformation. There are three leading theories: *hydrocephalic, traction* and *maldevelopment*. The hydrocephalic theory was first propounded by Chiari (1891) but remained in abeyance until taken up with enthusiasm by Gardner (1959), who added that hydrocephalus was responsible for other associated anomalies of syringomyelia and hydromyelia. Strong support has come from Margolis and Kilham (1969) with their work on hydrocephalus produced in suckling hamsters by retroviruses. The most telling objection to this theory lies in the fact that it does not explain the absence of the Arnold–Chiari malformation in most cases of hydrocephalus, nor does it explain the absence of hydrocephalus in some cases of the malformation.

The great frequency with which the Arnold–Chiari malformation and myelocele are associated has led to the notion that the myelocele is the prime cause, because it tethers the lower spinal cord and causes a relative downward displacement of the cerebellum and brainstem. However this theory fails to explain why and how in some cases the malformation occurs in the absence of a spina bifida defect. Neither does it explain the dorsal buckling of the medulla. Finally the nerves of the thoracic area run a normal course, so that any traction applied to the cord must be dissipated below this level. (Barry *et al.* 1957, Milhorat 1972).

Daniel and Strich (1958) link the Arnold–Chiari malformation and the myelocele only for the purposes of dating their onset in embryogenesis, which they suggest is about the fourth or fifth week of intrauterine life. Peach (1965a) supported the maldevelopment theory since most of the anomalies of the Arnold–Chiari malformation can be explained on the basis of an arrest in development of the neuraxis, particularly at the level of the pontine flexure. As Milhorat (1972) points out this theory explains the frequent association of the Arnold–Chiari malformation with other anomalies, it accounts for the appearance of the malformation without spinal cord anomalies, and it explains why the malformation can be experimentally induced by a variety of agents such as X-irradiation, drugs and vitamin deficiencies.

*Atresia of foramina of Magendie and Luschka*

Congenital absence of the foraminal exits from the fourth ventricle is rare and must be distinguished from inflammatory obliteration which is more frequent and in which there are adhesions and fibrosis of the overlying leptomeninges. In a monograph on hydrocephalus Russell (1949) could only find reference to 12 cases and added one from her experience, though by 1962 Portugal and Brock were able to review 45 cases in the literature. Interest in the malformation lies not only in the hydrocephalus, but in the accompanying deformity of the cerebellum, and the overall condition is now commonly known as the Dandy–Walker syndrome. Taggart and Walker (1942) drew attention to a case recorded by Blackfan and Dandy in 1914 which was similar to their own and gave a detailed description of the findings.

There is severe dilatation of the whole of the ventricular system and the aqueduct of Sylvius. The lateral lobes of the cerebellum are widely separated and at first glance the vermis appears to be absent. The broad interval between the cerebellar lobes is bridged by a tenuous membrane, usually transparent, which in the intact state bulges outwards like a cyst and through which can be seen the greatly dilated fourth ventricle. This membrane is the roof of the fourth ventricle. The arachnoid mater invests it as a separate layer, at its margins continuing over the cerebellum and medulla. When the greatly thinned membrane is incised and scrutinized, its periphery is seen to be attached to, and to fuse with the cerebellar cortex except caudally where its attachment passes onto the medulla (Fig. 15.8). Histological examination of the membrane identifies its nervous origin; on its inner surface it is lined with ependyma and Russell found fragments of cerebellar cortex in one part of the membrane. The vermis can be

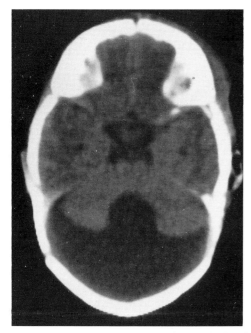

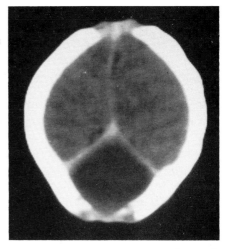

Fig. 15.9 Same case as Fig. 15.8. CT scan showing high attachment of tentorium.

Fig. 15.8 Dandy–Walker syndrome: 3-month-old girl with enlarging head. CT scan showing huge dilatation of the fourth ventricle and hypoplastic cerebellum.

identified when the fourth ventricle is opened or the specimen divided in the sagittal plane, as a small rounded mass of cerebellar tissue, bulging into the mouth of the dilated aqueduct. These features are clearly illustrated in the paper by Brodal and Haughlie-Hanssen (1959). Scrutiny for the foramina often reveals their absence, though in some cases the foramen of Magendie is absent and those of Luschka present. It seems fairly certain that closure of all three foramina is not an essential accompaniment and this may account for the delay, for many years in some cases, of symptoms attributable to the hydrocephalus. The choroid plexus may be absent, rudimentary or displaced caudally within the ventricle (Milhorat 1972). In a number of cases agenesis of the corpus callosum occurs (Raimondi *et al.* 1969).

A noteworthy feature of this malformation is its influence on the posterior cranial fossa which is larger than normal due to a high attach-ment of the tentorium in contradistinction to the low position in the Arnold–Chiari malformation (Fig. 15.9). Taggart and Walker (1942) pointed out that radiological examination of the skull may reveal this by the presence of high lateral sinus grooves. Not only is this sign pathognomonic (though not always present) but it clearly proves that the obstructive process in the posterior fossa dates from early fetal life. In the young embryo the lateral sinuses are situated far forward in the head and with the development of the cerebrum gradually migrate caudally, reaching the lambdoid region between the third and fourth month of intrauterine life; there they remain in the Dandy–Walker syndrome. There are two main schools of thought regarding the aetiology of this condition. On the one hand there are those (Taggart & Walker 1942, Gardner 1959) who feel that the primary disorder is a failure of the foraminal outlets to develop thereby leading to the train of events described above; and on the other are those (Brodal & Haughlie-Hanssen 1959, Benda 1954) who feel the condition represents something akin to cerebellar dysraphism.

*Benign intracranial cysts*

The most common cysts that need to be discussed are arachnoid cysts and ependymal cysts.

Although arachnoid cysts may occur anywhere within the skull, those arising within the posterior fossa are likely to produce hydrocephalus by obstructing the egress of CSF from the fourth ventricle. The most common sites are overlying the posterior-inferior surface of the cerebellum, in the cerebellopontine angle and overlying the superior surface of the cerebellum close to the tentorium (Milhorat 1972). Histologically the walls of a cyst are very similar to normal arachnoid. The majority connect with the CSF pathways.

Ependymal cysts are most commonly found in the third ventricle, in the region of the quadrigeminal plate and the cerebellopontine angle (Zülch 1965). Those in the third ventricle are also called colloid cysts and lie beneath the columns of the fornices caudal to the foramina of Monro (Little & MacCarty 1974) (Fig. 15.10). The centre of the cyst contains an amorphous proteinaceous substance (colloid) which stains with the periodic acid-Schiff reagent, and the wall is lined with low columnar ciliated epithelium. Their origin remains a mystery; they may arise from the ependymal epithelium (Kappers 1956, Zülch 1965) or from the paraphysis which is a vestigial organ that is present in embryos of 17–100 mm (Poppen *et al* 1953). However, as Milhorat points out, they rarely produce symptoms until adult life, and examples exist of their being found as an incidental finding at autopsy.

*Vascular malformations*

Vascular malformations occurring in the midline of the brain are a rare cause of congenital hydrocephalus, the most common of which is the so called 'aneurysm of the vein of Galen'. In reality this is an arteriovenous fistula which leads to

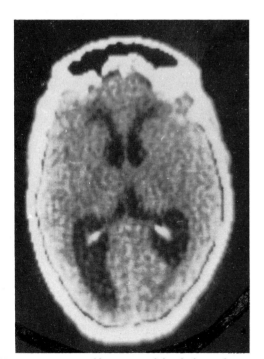

Fig. 15.10 40-year-old woman with headaches and dementia. CT scan showing hydrocephalus with nonfilling of third ventricle due to a colloid cyst (some colloid cysts show up as enhancing lesions on CT).

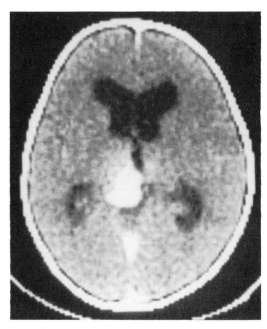

Fig. 15.11 Aneurysm of Vein of Galen: 1-year-old boy with heart failure and an audible cranial bruit. CT scan showing enhancing lesion behind and to the left of the third ventricle.

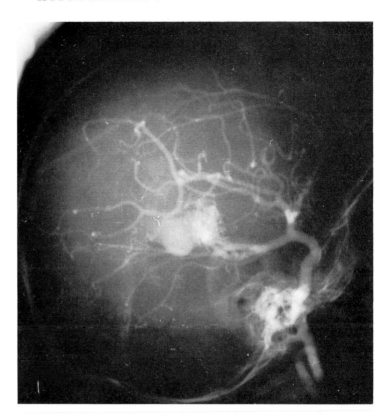

**Fig. 15.12** Same case as Fig. 15.11. Left carotid angiogram aneurysm of the vein of Galen due to arteriovenous fistulae.

enlargement of the vein of Galen which may distort the aqueduct of Sylvius thereby leading to hydrocephalus (Figs. 15.11 and 15.12). However any hydrocephalus is of more minor import when compared to the severe heart failure that infants exhibit as a consequence of the large arteriovenous shunt. In addition to the heart failure the tremendous flow of blood through the fistula deprives the cerebrum of blood and may lead to gross parenchymal brain damage (Norman & Becker 1974). Between 1937 and 1982 128 such cases had been reported in the literature (Hoffman *et al.* 1982).

## Inflammation

The plastic and fibrous reactions aroused by inflammation within the ventricles and leptomeninges are a potent and frequent cause of hydrocephalus. Acute inflammation leads to a cellular exudate which may later progress to chronic fibrosis and obstruction of the CSF pathways. The two most common leptomeningeal inflammations are those due to infection and haemorrhage, and there is also a miscellaneous collection of causes to which brief mention will be made.

In acute purulent meningitis the viscid exudate delays the passage of CSF through the foramina of the fourth ventricle and through the cisterns. Subsequent organization may partially or totally occlude these pathways. A common site for obstructive leptomeningeal fibrosis is the collar of arachnoid ensheathing the midbrain in the tentorial hiatus, a strategically placed channel through which the CSF must pass to gain the supratentorial pathways.

Bacterial infections are the commonest cause of purulent meningitis, the organism to some extent varying with age. Milhorat (1972) has categorized these as follows:

1  Birth to 3 months: *Escherichia coli, staphylococcus aureus,* and a variety of Gram-negative enteric bacilli.

2  3 months to 3 years: *Haemophilus influenzae,* pneumococcus, meningococcus and *Staphylococcus aureus.*

3  3 years and older: meningococcus, pneumococcus, streptococcus, gonococcus and *Haemophilus influenzae.*

Although, due to improved immunization programmes, tuberculosis is now rare in the United Kingdom, cases do occur and the neurosurgeon should be aware of the problems that tuberculous meningitis can cause (Kocen 1977, Parsons 1982), not the least being a severe hydrocephalus. Fungal infections of the leptomeninges occur and lead to hydrocephalus, and often they are exceedingly difficult to diagnose.

The relationship between haemorrhage and hydrocephalus was first delineated by Foltz and Ward (1956), who pointed out that subarachnoid haemorrhage can incite a basal arachnoiditis which in turn can lead to a communicating hydrocephalus. The most common causes of the haemorrhage are from ruptured intracranial aneurysms, head injury and intracranial operations. Hydrocephalus is a common complication following ruptured intracranial aneurysm, occurring in 63% of patients when assessment was carried out by CT scanning (Wening *et al.* 1979); however in the large majority of cases the hydrocephalus resolves spontaneously and surgical drainage procedures are only necessary in a small proportion (7% in the series of Vassilouthis & Richardson 1979; 13% in the series of Jeffreys 1981). Hydrocephalus consequent upon head injury was reported by Lewin (1968) when he described 20 such cases, all with communicating hydrocephalus due to a block to the passage of CSF through the basal cisterns, presumably as a result of traumatic subarachnoid haemorrhage. Hydrocephalus, usually communicating, is an occasional postoperative complication; it is more likely to follow intraventricular and posterior fossa procedures. Frequently repeated examinations of the CSF show a cellular response but no bacteria are found on either cytology or culture, and the possibility must be accepted that blood and necrotic tissue are the responsible irritants.

Foreign particulate material introduced into the subarachnoid spaces evokes an acute inflammatory response that may lead to chronic fibrous arachnoiditis, and this has been exploited in the experimental production of hydrocephalus. Substances that have been used include lampblack (Weed 1920), trypan blue (Wislocki & Putnam 1921), kaolin (McLaurin *et al.* 1954) and silicone oils (Wisniewski *et al.* 1969). In humans similar findings were encountered with some of the original contrast materials used in radiology such as Thorotrast (Russel 1949) and microfilmed barium sulphate. Endogenous material may also produce the same result; dissemination of the contents of an epidermoid cyst or craniopharyngioma can result in hydrocephalus. In the rare condition of 'gargoylism' (Type I mucopolysaccharidosis) the leptomeninges contain lipid deposits, chronic inflammatory cells and fibrosis (Russell 1949) resulting in hydrocephalus.

*Normal pressure hydrocephalus*

This syndrome is probably better called intermittent raised pressure hydrocephalus or adult nontumourous hydrocephalus (Jeffreys & Wood 1978) for reasons that will be apparent later. Hakim (1964) first drew attention to normal pressure hydrocephalus and this was followed by later collaborative work (Adams *et al.* 1965). In this condition there is a progressive hydrocephalus due to a block to the passage of CSF over the cerebral hemispheres. Usually there is no history of antecedent intracranial disease, though it does occur in a few cases of head injury and cases with leptomeningeal inflammation (Jeffreys & Wood 1978, Pickard 1982). Originally measurement of the lumbar CSF pressure revealed normal pressure, but with the introduction of the technique of continuous intracranial pressure monitoring (Lundberg 1972) it quickly became apparent that at times, and particularly during sleep, the intracranial pressure is quite severely raised (Symon *et al.* 1972, Jeffreys & Wood 1978). The cerebral blood flow is diminished (Greitz *et al.* 1969). Histological examination reveals leptomeningeal fibrosis with or without changes in the arachnoid granulations (Di Rocco *et al.* 1977).

## Anatomical consequences of hydrocephalus

The naked-eye effects of hydrocephalus are its most obvious features: the expansion of the ventricles and, according to the site of the obstructive lesion, of the communicating passages, foramina and leptomeningeal spaces. The ventricles are not affected to an equal degree, nor uniformly within the same cavity. The frontal and temporal horns of the lateral ventricles are usually the first to suffer and to a greater extent; in infants the convexity brain tissue ultimately becomes the thinnest. The corpus callosum is elevated and tenuous and the septum pellucidum so stretched that it may be fenestrated. In children these changes are much more severe than in adults partly because expansion of the skull, consequent upon diastasis of the sutures, allows the cerebral tissue to be stretched; partly because of the susceptibility to damage of the immature brain. In congenital hydrocephalus the ventricles may achieve enormous size, for example Milhorat (1972) quotes Vesalius who in 1725 described a 2–year-old girl whose head at death contained '9 pounds of water, or 3 Augsburg wine measures (so help me God!)'. The lateral walls of the third ventricle are supported by the basal ganglia which limit the expansion in the transverse plane; but the thin floor becomes greatly distended and may extend down into the pituitary fossa. As a result hypothalamic–hypophyseal connections may be disturbed. The normal suprapineal recess of the third ventricle may be distended to form a considerable pouch. The degree of dilatation of the aqueduct of

Sylvius varies considerably. Although the fourth ventricle takes part in the hydrocephalus when the obstruction is at or distal to its exit foramina, the enlargement is rarely severe except in foraminal occlusions.

The histological changes which take place were studied by Penfield and Elvidge (1932), Russell (1949) and Blackwood *et al* (1963). The grey matter is much more resistant to the disintegrating effects of stretching and compression than the white matter, partly because of its richer blood supply; the white matter suffers more perhaps because its basal and central blood supply is more likely to be impaired by compression and stretching from within outwards and because of changes in the ependyma to be described. The relative preservation of the grey matter is doubtless a factor to be taken into account in the unexpected intellectual development which occurs in some children in whom hydrocephalus has been successfully relieved. Penfield and Elvidge (1932) pointed out that if neurons are spared then their main axons must also to some extent be preserved, and the major atrophic process in hydrocephalus probably involves the neuroglia and axonal collaterals, at least in the earlier phases (Milhorat 1972). Yakovlev (1947) has offered an interesting explanation of the spastic weakness of the legs which accompanies severe hydrocephalus; the long and unprotected course of the capsular fibres from the upper part of the motor cortex subjects them to a greater degree of pressure and of stretching than those from the lower part, passing to arm and face, which are protected by the caudate nucleus.

Hydrocephalus has adverse effects upon the ependyma. The stretching of the walls of the ventricles leads to gaps in the continuity of the ependymal lining, for the ependymal cells have little or no regenerative capacity (Russell 1949), and there is no evidence that the ependyma proliferates in an attempt to cover these bare areas (Greenfield 1976). These denuded areas are not visible macroscopically, but the exposed subependymal glia reacts by proliferation, often in the form of minute polypoid masses. These are visible to the naked eye, giving a faint roughness or granular appearance to what is normally a smooth and shining surface; hence the term granular ependymitis which is a regular feature of noninflammatory hydrocephalus. The breaches that occur in the continuity of the ependymal lining may account for the periventricular oedema that is seen on CT scans in patients with hydrocephalus (Granholm 1976).

## Hydrodynamics of hydrocephalus

Although the identification of lesions which lead to hydrocephalus is successful during life in perhaps 90% of cases and at post-mortem examination in virtually every case, this does not dispose of all the problems. A simple example is hydrocephalus which occurs with benign forms of obstruction of the aqueduct of Sylvius. In such cases the lateral ventricles may be dilated to a capacity of several hundred mls. The normal production of CSF in humans has been estimated to be 0.35–0.40 ml/min or about 500 ml/24 hours (Davson & Segal 1971). Assuming the capacity of the normal human lateral and third ventricles to be about 20 ml (Last & Tompsett 1953 give 22.4 ml, Bull 1961 gives 20 ml for all ventricles) and assuming that three-quarters of CSF production is formed within the lateral and third ventricles, i.e. 0.30 ml/min, then the contents of these ventricles will be replaced in just over one hour. If an obstruction of the aqueduct causes hydrocephalus of the order of 300 ml then normal production of CSF can replace this in 36 hours. From the experiments of Bering and Sato (1963) it can be calculated that in the normal dog the contents of the lateral and third ventricles would be replaced every 2 hours; in the hydrocephalic dog, in which the aqueduct was blocked, replacement takes just over 7 hours. These figures can only be approximate but they clearly pose the question: what happens to the CSF which is apparently being produced in chronic hydrocephalus and which cannot drain through the aqueduct? The problem in chronic hydrocephalus is probably quite different from

that which obtains in acute hydrocephalus. Clinical experience shows that if an acute obstruction is not rapidly relieved death occurs quickly; for example when a blockage develops in a shunt system, which has until then been successfully treating a chronic hydrocephalus, symptoms occur more rapidly and the need for relief is more urgent than was the case prior to the insertion of the shunt. It has been assumed by clinicians that secretion of CSF diminishes in chronic hydrocephalus, because of failure to secrete against a high intracranial pressure. While there is some experimental evidence to support this hypothesis (Sahar *et al.* 1971), the reduction in CSF production observed in the hydrocephalic cat with raised intracranial pressure was only of the order of 30%. Only when intracranial pressure is so high that cerebral blood flow is reduced does the CSF production rate fall off considerably. Other possible compensatory mechanisms have to be considered; all these might serve to dissipate the pressure gradient between the ventricles and the brain, and might, if the CSF obstruction is incomplete (as it usually is in humans) reduce the pathological process (Milhorat 1972). These mechanisms include expansion of the skull volume (in the child before the sutures have fused), reduction in the cerebrovascular volume and enlargement of the ventricular system. All of these may serve to slow down the evolution of hydrocephalus. Later, cerebral atrophy may also serve to slow the process. Hakim (1964) introduced the principles of mechanics into the subject to explain enlargement of the ventricular system in the absence of severely raised intracranial pressure. He pointed out that:

$$Pressure = \frac{Force}{Area}$$

What this means is that a normal CSF pressure will apply greater total force upon an expanded ventricular system than upon a normal one, and that although the intraventricular pressure may be only slightly raised the ventricles will continue to expand. It is likely, however, that the major compensatory mechanism in chronic hydro-cephalus is transventricular absorption of CSF; this suggestion was made by Bering and Sato (1963) and has been supported by other workers (Sahar *et al.* 1971). The sites of transventricular absorption have not been fully identified, though the two most likely are transchoroidal and trans-ependymal, and there is some experimental evidence to support both of these hypotheses (Milhorat 1972). Periventricular lucency on the CT scan has been cited as evidence of trans-ventricular CSF passage but this remains an area of controversy since similar appearances can occur in the absence of CSF pathway obstructions.

## Clinical features of hydrocephalus

### Infants

The symptoms of increasing intracranial pressure are not as easily recognized in the infant as in older patients, because individually they may be caused by other diseases and because of the inability of the infant to communicate symptoms. These include lack of activity, drowsiness, fretfulness, failure to thrive, vomiting, unexplained fever, attacks of crying, stiffening of the limbs, opisthotonus, convulsions and finally coma. Examination is all important, and the enlargement of the head is often obvious but not always so; the circumference of the head should be measured and compared on a standard chart of head circumference with the norm for the appropriate age. The tape measure is applied in the plane of the maximum girth; an inaccurate record is avoided by moving the tape measure up and down until the largest reading is obtained, and this should be entered on the head circumference chart. In doubtful cases a record of repeated measurements will demonstrate graphically an abnormally rapid expansion of the skull. The fontanelles are larger than normal; they bulge and do not pulsate, though crying vitiates this test. It is often possible to palpate suture separation. The head is of globular shape and the temporal fossae are convex, in contrast to the normal slight concavity. The scalp veins are frequently distended. If there is much enlargement of the head, by contrast the face appears small and the eyeballs sunken as a result of protrusion of the forehead. This tends to elevate the upper eyelids so that an excessive amount of sclera is exposed. this is aggravated by a downward deviation of the ocular axes, to an extent that sometimes the pupils are hidden by the lower eyelids (the so called *sunset* appearance). This downward deviation is probably due to disturbance of the midbrain, and quickly disappears upon relief of the hydrocephalus. Ocular muscle palsies may be seen, abducent most commonly; the pupils are commonly dilated and react sluggishly to light, but failure to react is rare. The optic discs are usually pale; papilloedema is rarely encountered unless the hydrocephalus is due to a tumour. The neck muscles may feel rigid, spontaneous limb movements often appear unusually jerky and in advanced cases may be spastic. Examination should include a careful inspection for spina bifida and for other malformations.

### Children

The development of speech, vocabulary and intelligence enables the child to describe the various symptoms of raised intracranial pressure. The rapidity with which the lesion causes obstruction dictates the speed of evolution of the symptoms and their severity. Compared with obstruction due to a tumour, the hydrocephalus from benign causes is manifest more slowly. Dulling of mental faculties and a slowing of scholastic ability may be apparent to parents and teachers. The head is often enlarged and globular, the fontanelles are closed and a 'cracked pot sound' may be evoked on percussing the skull (Macewen sign). Papilloedema may be present. Squint, usually due to an abducens paresis, often fluctuates; defects of ocular deviation occur in the later stages. There may be attacks of vertigo, of sudden loss of consciousness and convulsions. Although weakness of the limbs is uncommon, there is often a tremulousness and clumsiness of the upper limbs, and the gait may be ataxic or the child may suffer from frequent falls. There may be evidence of long tract signs in the limbs, though sensory functions are preserved. When hydrocephalus is severe and has been present for some years a diversity of endocrine disturbances may occur: stunting of skeletal growth, delayed sexual development, obesity, diabetes insipidus, pubertas praecox have all been recorded (Guillaume & Rogé 1950).

**Adults**

The symptoms that occur in adults may be due to hydrocephalus or a tumour, or to combinations of these. Since the nature and site of origin of tumours that cause hydrocephalus are varied, it will perhaps be of more benefit in this section to concentrate on the symptomatology of non-neoplastic hydrocephalus though at the same time realizing that cases with tumour may well develop some or all of the symptoms described. The clinical features of hydrocephalus in the adult fall roughly into two groups, though they merge and features from both may be encountered in the same patient.

The first group comprises many of those features which have already been described in children. They are recognizable as symptoms of raised intracranial pressure and headache is often conspicuous and intermittent; when they have been present for some years they are liable to be discounted. Enlargement of the head is occasionally encountered, though not a cracked pot note, for the sutures close with the cessation of growth. A large head, unless a family trait, indicates that the responsible lesion was present in early life. Convulsions are rare in adults compared to infants and children. Papilloedema is often found, as are disorders of eye movements. There may be incoordination of the limbs as well as trunkal ataxia, and long tract signs may be found particularly in the lower limbs. Character

changes or behavioural disorders may be reported by relatives or friends. Occasionally, with inconspicuous or no previous symptoms, patients may present in an acute confusional state which may be brief and may be misdiagnosed as hysteria; from which state they may rapidly pass into coma. Minor degrees of head trauma may lead to signs out of all proportion to the severity of the blow. This may be the mode of onset of symptomatic acqueduct stenosis in the adult.

The second group is characterized by the predominance of those symptoms and signs which indicate diffuse organic brain damage and by a relative or complete absence of symptoms of raised intracranial pressure. Since the processes of hydrocephalus so far as we know are identical in both groups, it is pertinent to enquire why such a difference can occur. It seems probable that the explanation lies in the slightness or absence of those symptoms of raised intracranial pressure which demand relief, namely headache, vomiting and papilloedema. In their absence, damage to the brain by hydrocephalus advances insidiously to a more overt degree and is liable to be attributed to a degenerative disease of the brain. Alternatively, the exact opposite may pertain, that is to say some hydrocephalic causes may develop so slowly that at no stage does overt and continuous raised intracranial pressure appear and yet there is slow expansion of the ventricular system that leads to parenchymal brain damage. For the present there is no definitive answer to this problem. Continuous monitoring of intracranial pressure usually reveals a pattern of intermittent elevations of pressure of moderate severity from a background of a normal resting pressure.

The earliest and the most prominent disturbance in these patients is progressive deterioration of mental faculties. Slowing of performance both mental and physical, failing memory, lack of initiative and attention, poverty of thought, speech and activity, pass gradually into a frank dementia with incontinence and neglect of personal appearance. Episodes of akinetic mutism and of lack of spontaneous movement ultimately merge with stupor and coma. On the physical side, the disorders of the motor system present as unsteadiness of gait which may progress to an inability to walk unaided or at all. Incoordination of the upper limbs is less obvious. There is rarely evidence of limb weakness, though the reflexes are often exaggerated.

## Differential diagnosis

At all ages the possibility that hydrocephalus is due to tumour must be considered and excluded. In infants it is least likely to be the case; at all other ages a tumour is more likely. In many cases local symptoms and signs due to the tumour make it clear that hydrocephalus alone cannot explain the clinical picture, even though a correct interpretation for localizing purposes may not be possible. On the other hand symptoms and signs of cerebellar disturbance may be pronounced in cases of hydrocephalus from benign non-neoplastic lesions (Bramwell 1899). Pronounced mental deterioration in late adult life may well be due to an invasive glioma, a chronic subdural haematoma or degenerative brain disease. Papilloedema in infants is rarely due to hydrocephalus of benign origin; MacNab (1955) never observed it in a series of 160 cases. The commonest lesion simulating infantile hydrocephalus is a subdural haematoma or effusion; it may be excluded by computerized tomography, or if this is not available, by performing bilateral subdural taps. Diagnostic investigations in which radiology plays a dominant role are necessary to exclude tumour and other lesions and to identify the anatomical situation of the obstruction to the flow of CSF.

## Investigations

### Radiology

*X-ray examination of the skull* should not be omitted, even in infants. It affords confirmation of raised intracranial pressure in many cases and a record for later comparison. Important items to be noted are pathological calcification; asymmetry due to a localized collection of fluid or to a slow growing neoplasm; the situation of the transverse sinus grooves, suggesting the large posterior fossa of the Dandy–Walker syndrome and a small posterior fossa of the Arnold–Chiari malformation; and abnormalities in the craniovertebral junction.

*CT scanning* has revolutionized the further investigation, particularly so since in the vast majority of cases it is sufficiently diagnostically accurate to avoid invasion of the CSF pathways with contrast material. Although for many patients CT scanning can be a simple and non-invasive test, it is important to realize that for children under five years of age and for confused and noncooperative adults general anaesthesia may be necessary. The unenhanced CT scan will reveal the shape and size of the CSF pathways, together with any localized distortion; in addition to assessing ventricular size it is also important to look at the basal cisterns and the subarachnoid spaces over the cerebral hemispheres, since the absence of these will suggest a degree of 'tightness' within the skull and their presence conversely a lack of fullness implying absence of space occupation. It is essential in every case to perform an intravenous contrast enhanced scan, particularly looking for a tumour. If no tumour is seen then one needs to return to the unenhanced scan and study the CSF pathways more carefully. A discrepancy in size between enlarged supratentorial ventricles and a smaller fourth ventricle will suggest a stenosis of the aqueduct of Sylvius, in which case contrast ventriculography may be necessary (*see* below). Large lateral ventricles with a poorly demonstrated third ventricle may indicate a tumour within its lumen, since it should be understood that colloid cysts do not always enhance with contrast materials, and here again contrast ventriculography or magnetic resonance imaging will be required.

CT scanning is essentially a radiological test to produce anatomical information of the intracranial contents, and is very good at so doing

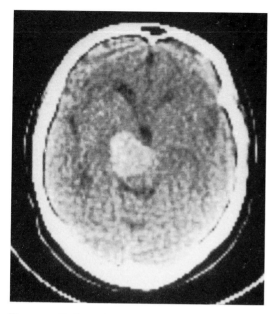

**Fig. 15.13** Basilar artery aneumysm: 58-year-old woman with headaches and ataxia. CT scan showing enhancing lesion to the left of the third ventricle.

with reference to the CSF pathways. However CT scanning cannot produce physiological data, particularly with regard to flow and absorption of CSF and other techniques are required. If a cystic lesion is found which does not enhance, it will be necessary to demonstrate whether or not it communicates with the CSF pathways; water-soluble iodine compounds may be installed into the CSF (usually by lumbar or cisternal puncture) and the passage of the contrast material can then be followed on CT scanning. In an adult the presence of uniformly dilated ventricles with prominent cisterns may suggest a non-tumourous communicating hydrocephalus, though this will need to be distinguished from cerebral atrophy; in such a case continuous intracranial pressure monitoring, together with some form of volume challenge test, will be necessary prior to a decision being taken on whether to drain the CSF pathways (*see* below).

*Contrast ventriculography*, since the intro-

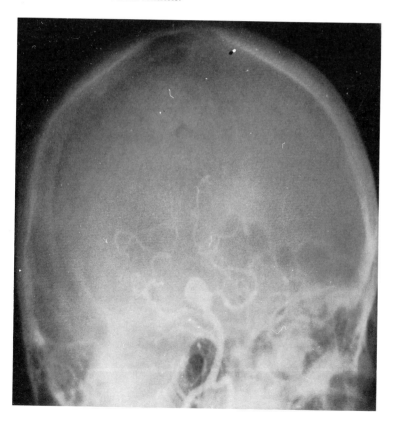

**Fig. 15.14** Same case as Fig. 15.13. Vertebral angiogram showing aneurysm of the bifurcation of the basilar artery.

duction of CT scanning, has a much more limited place than hitherto. Some of the indications have been discussed above. In the case of a suspected aqueduct stenosis or a third ventricular tumour it should be performed by instilling contrast material through a catheter inserted into the lateral ventricle through a right frontal burr hole. The contrast agent, being somewhat more dense than CSF, can be manoeuvred from the frontal horn through the foramen of Monro by tilting the head. This technique also is of value in assessing whether or not a mass is within a lateral ventricle or outside it and merely bulging inwards. Examination of the posterior fossa may be carried out by installing contrast material from below, provided there is no evidence of raised intracranial pressure and provided there is no evidence of distortion of the fourth ventricle; if these are present then it is wiser to insert a frontal burr hole, as a readily available safety valve, before proceeding.

In infants with an open fontanelle, *ultrasound scanning* can be used to demonstrate enlargement of the ventricular system.

*Spinal myelography* has a very limited place; it can be useful in the demonstration of Arnold–Chiari malformation and of a possible associated syringomyelia. *Magnetic resonance imaging* is now the method of choice in this situation. Although angiography may demonstrate hydrocephalus and tonsillar herniation it is rarely used as a primary investigation. However if an aneurysm is suspected then it is mandatory; such suspicions would arise if an enhancing lesion on CT scanning were seen in the third ventricle that might be due to a large anterior communicating artery or basilar artery neurysm (Figs. 5.13 and 5.14); in the case of enhancement in the pineal region in a child that might suggest an arteriovenous fistula of the vein of Galen.

**Cerebrospinal fluid**

Examination of the CSF should be performed only after CT scanning. If a tumour is demonstrated on CT scanning then it is wiser to leave the CSF pathways intact until operation; however if the patient is deteriorating rapidly then external ventricular drainage may reduce raised intracranial pressure prior to more definitive treatment. In the case of hydrocephalus without any space-occupying cause or aqueduct stenosis, examination of the CSF is required, in particular looking for any possible infective cause from either bacteria or fungi. Before the insertion of a ventricular shunt it is mandatory to exclude infection in those cases that have either suffered from meningitis or who have undergone intracranial or spinal surgery that may have contaminated the CSF pathways.

*Intracranial pressure monitoring* can be of value in distinguishing which cases with non-tumourous hydrocephalus will respond to ventribular drainage operations; it is unnecessary in cases with aqueduct stenosis since the presence of ventricular enlargement is by itself sufficient proof that there is both an anatomical and physiological blockage that requires shunting. The technique requires a frontal burr hole and some form of pressure monitoring system which can be an internal transducer or a ventricular catheter filled with saline connected to an external transducer (Pickard 1982). Monitoring is carried out for at least 24 hours; those most likely to respond to shunting will exhibit raised intracranial pressure either continuously or paroxysmally (B waves), particularly during sleep (Symon *et al.* 1972, Chawla *et al.* 1974, Jeffreys & Wood 1978). If after monitoring for 24 hours doubt still remains then the CSF pathways may be challenged either by a bolus injection of saline into the ventricles (Jeffreys & Wood 1978) or by a CSF infusion test (Lorenzo *et al.* 1974, Katzmann 1977).

## Treatment

The basic anatomical problems of hydrocephalus were defined by Dandy and Blackfan (1914), and a few years later Dandy devised two operations for its relief. In the 60 years which have elapsed many ingenious operations have been invented but only a few have stood the test of time, notably the development of mechanical CSF bypass shunts. But in 1972 Milhorat pointed out that 'unfortunately all methods of current therapy have certain disadvantages and it is widely acknowledged that the ideal treatment of hydrocephalus is not yet at hand'. There are no effective medical treatments for hydrocephalus; therefore, when indicated, treatment is surgical. Before describing the various surgical techniques currently available it is pertinent to discuss the indications for both operating and not operating.

## Indications for surgery

The indications for surgical treatment in children and adolescents are not quite as clear-cut as they are in adults, mainly for the reason that many of these young patients are suffering from co-existing abnormalities that may have a major bearing on the ultimate outcome and prognosis. Matson (1969) suggested subdividing children into three groups for the purposes of treatment:

1   Patients with progressive hydrocephalus and no evidence of irreversible brain damage.
2   Patients with progressive hydrocephalus and evidence of irreversible brain damage and/or associated major congenital abnormalities.
3   Patients with arrested hydrocephalus.

Group 1 patients require operation, the nature of which will depend on the anatomical and pathological problem. It is Group 2 patients who pose the greatest problem. The evidence for irreversible brain damage is often difficult to obtain (Milhorat 1972). Many workers have attested to the fact that there is no correlation between ventricular size and outcome, though others have demonstrated correlation between the thickness of the cortical mantle and the development of mental and motor skills (Foltz & Shurtleff 1963, Laurence & Coates 1962, Scarff 1959). As a rough guide a cerebral mantle of 1 cm or less indicates a poor prognosis, and one of 2 cm or more a good prognosis (Matson 1969) but

most neurosurgeons will know of individual exceptions to this rule. A full neuropsychological assessment of the patient should be carried out, and the expert advice of a paediatric neurologist should be sought. In the end the whole patient with his/her family must be considered, together with the particular ethical and philosophical views of the surgeon and paediatric neurologist before a decision is taken whether or not to treat; no clear guide-lines can be laid down on these issues. However it is worth pointing out that if in young children hydrocephalus is untreated the head may enlarge to grotesque proportions, presenting major aesthetic and nursing problems, and it may be wiser to prevent this by shunting. Group 3 patients require very careful observation, since the diagnosis of arrested hydrocephalus should not be made unless there is evidence of satisfactory continuing neuropsychological development (Milhorat 1972). Sequential follow-up CT scans must be laid alongside the clinical evidence (in particular school reports) each time the child is reviewed. It would be true to state that many neurosurgeons feel that this condition does not exist, and that what one sees is a hydrocephalic process which is evolving more slowly than is normally the case (see below).

Adults present fewer problems, mainly because the majority of patients with major congenital disorders have already been assessed as children or adolescents. The two congenital disorders that may present for the first time in adulthood are aqueduct stenosis and the Arnold–Chiari malformation; in the former, hydrocephalus will invariably require treatment though the latter may present with problems around the foramen magnum without hydrocephalus, but when hydrocephalus is present it will usually require treatment. In every case, with one exception, when true chronic hydrocephalus is found in an adult it will require treatment either by removal of the causative lesion and/or by a shunting procedure. The exception is nontumourous hydrocephalus which must first be distinguished from cerebral atrophy; while patients with true chronic hydrocephalus can be dramatically improved by shunting, patients with cerebral atrophy can be made worse (Jeffreys & Wood 1978). As discussed above, continuous intracranial pressure monitoring can provide valuable additional information which will help in reaching a decision on whether or not to treat.

## Operations

Contemporary operations for the relief of hydrocephalus fall into three main groups: *direct, intracranial shunting* and *extracranial shunting*. For an individual patient these are not exclusive, for example, although it is correct to remove a tumour of the posterior fossa first, it may also be necessary later to perform a CSF shunting procedure.

### Direct

Whenever possible it is best to remove a mass lesion that is causing hydrocephalus. If circumstances allow it is wiser to leave the CSF pathways intact prior to surgery. In the case of supratentorial mass lesions within the ventricles the presence of expanded ventricles allows the surgeon safer access to the ventricle and thence to the lesion itself; in the case of posterior fossa mass lesions, drainage of the lateral ventricles prior to, or at the start of the operation will aid both the anaesthetist and the surgeon in providing better operating conditions in the posterior fossa. At the end of the operation it is wise to leave an in-dwelling ventricular catheter in place; so that it is available should postoperative drainage of CSF be required. Otherwise it is probably better to keep the drain closed as ventricular drainage may increase the development of subarachnoid space blockage in the posterior fossa and the need for permanent postoperative CSF shunting.

### Intracranial shunting

*Third ventriculostomy.* In 1922 Dandy described an operation for the relief of non-communicating hydrocephalus. A hole was made in the greatly thinned floor of the third ventricle; through this fistula CSF could pass into the chiasmatic cistern, thus bypassing the obstruction. In his early operations he sacrificed an optic nerve in order to obtain access, but later he described a lateral approach beneath the temporal lobe, the hole being made in the floor of the third ventricle (1933). His results depended on the age of the patient; there were good results in patients over one year of age but poor results in infants. He attributed the poor results in infants to the lack of development of the subarachnoid spaces (1945). Stookey and Scarff (1936) improved upon this operation; they pointed out that the greatly thinned lamina terminalis can easily be exposed if the frontal pole be elevated, for it then baloons out like a bluish cyst above (dorsal to) the optic chiasm. The membrane is opened, a blunt instrument passed into the distended third ventricle and a hole made in the posterior part of its floor; the position of the hole can be determined by feeling for the dorsum sellae with the instrument, and making a rent immediately behind it (Scarff 1951). This fistula makes communication between the third ventricle and the interpeduncular cistern; the advantage of this method is that the arachnoid overlying the fistula is undamaged avoiding the risk of closure of the fistula by reactive adhesions, and drainage is into a cistern whose walls do not collapse when the intracranial pressure is lowered during the operation. This procedure will be successful only if the cerebrospinal fluid can be freely transported upward through the cisterna ambiens and absorbed at the superior sagittal sinus.

*Ventriculocisternostomy* was devised by Torkildsen (1939). One end of a thin silastic tube is inserted into a lateral ventricle through an occipital burr hole: the foramen magnum is exposed, its posterior border removed, the dura mater opened and the cisterna magna identified.

The silastic tube is passed through a subgaleal tunnel and its lower end inserted into the cisterna magna. In cases of a third ventricle tumour which isolate the lateral ventricles by obstructing both foramina of Monro it will be necessary to perform a bilateral operation. Attention to certain details is essential for success; the length of the tube must be such that the intraventricular portion is not so long that the end engages the choroid plexus or the anterior wall of the frontal or temporal horns; nor so short that with increase in the thickness of the brain contact with the ventricle is lost; the cisternal end must be within the cisterna magna and if its arachnoid roof is carelessly torn during the manoeuvre it is difficult to be certain of correct placement; closure of the wound over the foramen magnum must be watertight. If a leak of CSF develops in this wound, meningitis is a frequent sequel. In infants, due to the fact that there are often large dural venous sinuses in the posterior fossa, Matson (1969) suggested avoiding the posterior fossa and instead performed a hemilaminectomy of C1–C3 and inserted the lower end of the tube in the spinal subarachnoid space anterior to the dentate ligaments.

The operation is appropriate only for patients with CSF obstruction along the 'central narrows' and yet with CSF patency along the basal cisterns and over the cerebral hemispheres; in particular for tumours obstructing the third ventricle, aqueduct of Sylvius and fourth ventricle and for congenital stenosis of the aqueduct. Since the effectiveness of the operation is entirely dependent upon a free flow of CSF from the cisterna magna upwards through the tentorial hiatus, it is unfortunate that the operation has been employed in cases of posterior fossa tumour, in which, sooner or later, the ambient and basal cisterns become obstructed by tumour or tentorial herniation; such misapplications may have contributed towards bringing this operation into ill repute. The major reported shortcoming of this procedure is the high failure rate of 42% (Milhorat 1972). However frequency and severity of late complications are less than in ventriculoatrial shunting.

*Extracranial shunting*

Although the operations of third ventriculostomy and ventriculocisternostomy were major advances at the time of their introduction, they have only a limited place today. Neurosurgeons continued to seek better methods and their attention turned to the drainage of CSF without the skull. Two early operations, quickly abandoned, were ventriculomastoidotomy (Nosik 1950) and arachnoidureterostomy (Matson 1949). Diversion of CSF into the peritoneal cavity was first described in 1908 by Kausch, though not until 1949 were successful results first reported (Cone et al. 1949). The ventriculopleural shunt was introduced in 1954 by Ransohoff for palliative treatment of unresectable third ventricular tumours, though later he employed this operation for the treatment of infantile hydrocephalus (Ransohoff et al. 1960). The real turning point came in 1952 with the introduction, by Nulsen and Spitz, of the ventriculoatrial shunt designed by Holter; thereafter called the Spitz–Holter valve. In 1957 came the second ventriculoatrial shunt designed by Pudenz et al. These two systems were a great step forward and were cornerstones of the treatment of hydrocephalus until 1970, when there was a swing back to ventriculoperitoneal shunting. All shunt systems have their complications and the ideal treatment of hydrocephalus has not yet arrived. That such a number of shunt systems is presently available is both a reflection of the imperfections that exist in all such systems as well as a tribute to the enthusiasm of some neurosurgeons to place their names on the patent roll of honour!

This plethora of shunt systems will be confusing to neurosurgeons in training, and they will have difficulty in deciding which system to use; they can only be guided by teachers when in training, and thereafter by commonsense and developing experience in assessing the rival claims of both neurosurgeons and manufacturers alike.

## Ventriculoatrial shunting

All ventriculoatrial shunts (VA shunts) have three major component parts that may come separate and require joining together at the time of operation or may come already joined together: a ventricular catheter, a one-way valve working at a preset opening pressure and an atrial catheter. Only the two most widely used shunts are discussed, the Spitz–Holter and Pudenz systems: in the Spitz–Holter system the valve lies buried on the surface of the skull and has a roughly cylindrical shape whereas in the Pudenz system the valve comprises 4 slits at the end of the atrial catheter; the Pudenz system has a reservoir, roughly hemispheric in shape, which lies over the burr hole and which can serve as a method of assessing shunt patency; shunt patency is assessed in the Spitz–Holter system by palpating the middle of the valve which is compressible.

The operation is performed under general endotracheal anaesthesia; the patient is supine with the head rotated to the left, since it is usually the neck veins on the right which pass more vertically into the heart and consequently it is easier to pass the atrial catheter downwards from the neck veins into the right atrium. A transverse incision in Lange's lines is made two finger breadths below the angle of the jaw to expose the medial border of the sternocleidomastoid muscle; the deep cervical fascia is divided. Whenever possible, the common facial vein is used for cannulation; this is easier in the neonate when the vein is disproportionately larger; in adults it may become so small that cannulation is impossible. In that event the internal jugular vein must be used. It is essential to check the opening pressure of the valve against a column of saline before introduction. Once introduced into the venous system the catheter is advanced down the internal jugular vein towards the right atrium. Accurate placement of the lower end is essential; this may be effected either by radiographic control or by the electrocardiographic method introduced by Robertson *et al.* (1961). In this latter method the catheter is filled with saline and connected

to an electrocardiogram by one of the bipolar leads, and as the catheter is advanced it acts as a probing cardiac electrode; the P-wave becomes bifid as the tip is advanced into the right atrium. This method has the advantage over the radiographic method in not disturbing the drapes and thereby decreasing the risks of infection. The catheter is positioned at the level of the sixth thoracic vertebra in the radiographic method.

The route by which the lateral ventricle is cannulated is a matter for debate and it is probably true to state that there are no absolute rules. For the first operation in a patient with enlarged ventricles the parieto-occipital approach, above and behind the right ear, is perfectly satisfactory; if the ventricular catheter repeatedly blocks or if the ventricles are small then the frontal route is better. At either site a curvilinear incision is made and a small scalp flap raised, followed by a semicircular pericranial flap which is used to cover the valve or reservoir. After drilling a burr hole the dura is opened and the ventricle cannulated without releasing more than a few drops of CSF. The ventricular catheter is inserted to lie 1–2 cm within the lateral ventricle, and is connected either to the valve in the case of the Holter system or the reservoir in the Pudenz system. The upper end of the atrial catheter is brought up subcutaneously to the scalp wound and connected to the rest of the system. Shunt systems are manufactured with a variety of opening pressures ranging from 10 mm to 100 mm $H_2O$. These variations stem from differing opinions as to the optimum pressure at which to drain the ventricles. There is no simple answer, though the inexperienced surgeon will not go very far wrong if he uses shunt systems with opening pressures between 50–70 mm $H_2O$. Finally it is essential to stress that these shunt systems are self regulating and do not require pumping, a fact that must be emphasized to both patient and relatives.

## Ventriculo- and lumboperitoneal shunts

The peritoneum may be used to absorb CSF that is brought thither either from the ventricles or from the lumbar subarachnoid space. Ventriculoperitoneal shunts (VP shunts) have the same indications as have VA shunts, whereas lumboperitoneal shunts can only be used in communicating hydrocephalus. Most neurosurgeons now favour VP shunts as a first choice; the reasons depending in the main on the complication rate, particularly the occurrence of 'shunt nephritis' after VA shunting. VP shunts have the theoretical advantage that if there is doubt on the bacteriological sterility of the CSF (as for example after meningitis or in a child with an open meningomyelocoele) or if the CSF contains malignant cells (for example medulloblastoma) it may be safer to run such impurities into the peritoneal cavity rather than into the blood stream. If in a patient VA shunts have already been inserted and both internal jugular veins occluded then a VP shunt clearly is indicated. The upper end of the operation is the same as for VA shunting, and the lower end of the catheter is taken subcutaneously along the chest wall to a small laparatomy which can either be placed subcostally or at MacBurney's point. The catheter is placed in the peritoneal cavity, usually into the right paracolic gutter or over the dome of the liver.

Lumboperitoneal shunts are inserted by performing a small laminectomy of one or two segments in the mid-lumbar region and inserting a catheter into the subarachnoid space for 2–3 mm and then dealing with the peritoneal end in the same way as for a VP shunt. Recently a system has been introduced in which a shunt system can be inserted transcutaneously, the only shunt system which can be so inserted.

## Complications of ventricular shunts

These fall into four main categories: obstruction, infection, intracranial haematoma and thromboembolism.

### Obstruction

Obstruction of an external ventricular shunt may be insidious, intermittent or sudden in onset and the clinical effect corresponds. Where the hydrocephalus is of the noncommunicating type failure of the shunt produces severe and rapidly progressive symptoms of raised intracranial pressure, often worse than those preceding the operation. If the hydrocephalus was communicating in type the relapse evolves more slowly, probably because the basal cisterns and spinal theca can accommodate some of the CSF which is not passing through the shunt. However caution must be exercised since cases have been reported in which shunting has converted a communicating into a noncommunicating hydrocephalus (Foltz & Shurtleff 1966). Obstructions that are slow in evolution may be suspected by the development of headaches, strabismus and intellectual arrest or decline.

Palpation of either the valve (in the Holter system) or the reservoir (in the Pudenz system) may make it clear that (a) the ventricular catheter is blocked, for the contents can be compressed but the valve/reservoir refills very slowly or not at all; (b) the block lies in the valve or distal catheter, because the valve/reservoir is incompressible; (c) the shunt is apparently working normally.

A normally working shunt should empty easily without resistance and refill within a short time that ranges from 5 to 30 seconds. The refilling rate will lengthen as the ventricles become smaller and some allowance must be made for this phenomenon.

The clinical examination is important and should override any conclusions reached on shunt patency from palpation of the valve or reservoir. If there is any suspicion of a shunt obstruction then it is wiser to evaluate the shunt by a repeat CT scan (looking at the size of the CSF pathways) and measurement of the intracranial pressure either through the valve or reservoir or by ventricular tap in the case of noncommunicating hydrocephalus or by lumbar puncture for communicating hydrocephalus. In this assessment it is wise to monitor intracranial pressure for at least one overnight period. The patency of the shunt system can be tested by injecting water-soluble iodine contrast materials into the valve or reservoir (shuntogram); this technique not only outlines the shunt (which also can be seen on plain x-ray since most shunt tubing is impregnated with radio-opaque barium) but, by taking serial x-rays over 30 minutes, also gives an indication of the rate at which the dye is cleared through the system. Recently Graham *et al.* (1982) have advocated using $Tc^{99}$ DTPA as a method of performing a shuntogram.

The ventricular catheter may be obstructed by debris or coagulum, by contact with the choroid plexus, or by brain as a result of diminution of the size of the ventricle. Obstruction may be due to disconnection of items of assembly, sometimes by ligatures cutting through the tubing and sometimes following a head injury when a blow in the vicinity of the valve or reservoir may rupture the silastic tubing. The distal catheter may, in the case of a VA shunt, be obstructed within the right atrium by thrombus, but the more usual cause is the position of the tip. It is generally agreed (Nulsen 1961, Milhorat 1972) that the catheter will become obstructed if its distal end recedes as high as the superior vena cava or T4. It is rare for the distal catheter to block in adults once it has been accurately placed (Jeffreys 1978); however in neonates and children natural growth will inevitably lead to proximal migration of the distal catheter. Some surgeons favour elective lengthening of the catheter (Becker & Nulsen 1968). In the case of VP shunts the distal catheter may become occluded by omentum or peritoneal adhesions.

The management of a shunt blockage is clear; it must be explored and all aspects of the shunt rechecked at surgery. In the case of recurrent blockages to the ventricular catheter it is often wiser to reposition it in the frontal horn, in the hope that in this position it will be less likely to come into contact with choroid plexus. If the current shunt system cannot be made to work then it will be necessary to change the system, i.e. VA to VP or vice versa.

The frequency of shunt blockage seems to depend on the age at which the first shunt was inserted; in neonates and children the incidence is 25–40% within two years of operation, and 40–100% at five years or longer (Milhorat 1972); in adults the rate is lower ranging from 7% (Jeffreys 1978) to 21% (Illingworth *et al.* 1971).

## Infection

This is the second most common complication of ventricular shunting and occurs in 10–20% of children (Matson 1969), though the rate in adults is less being 8–9% (Illingworth *et al.* 1971, Jeffreys 1978). The reasons for this are twofold; firstly more shunt revisions are necessary in children due to growth, and secondly series of children contain within their midst those with open myelomeningocoele. The effects of infection tend to be more numerous and more serious in patients with VA shunts than those with VP shunts; the reason being that infection of a VA shunt may lead to bacteraemia with all its attendant problems.

Shunt infection is encountered in three main forms:

1 *Wound infection* from imperfect healing or from faulty technique. The skin over the valve/reservoir may necrose, and this complication can be minimized by ensuring pericranial cover in addition to skin cover.
2 *Ventriculitis* and *meningitis* may occur from spread of skin infection, from an open myelomeningocele or from contamination of the shunt system during operation.
3 *Infection of the shunt system* may lead to infection within the blood system in the case of VA shunts; bacterial endocarditis, infected pulmonary embolism, bacteraemia and septicaemia, and proliferating glomerulonephritis have all been described (Milhorat 1972). In the case of VP shunts peritoneal infections occur, though

usually these are not as devastating as is the case for VA shunts.

The majority of shunt infections occur immediately or within a few months of insertion; in which case it is difficult to refute the opinion that bacterial contamination occurred during operation. However in some patients a VA shunt can work well for many months or even years, seemingly without any evidence of infection, only for a shunt infection to become apparent a short while after a systemic infection such as pneumonia or urinary tract infection; in such cases it is less easy to incriminate intraoperative contamination.

The most common bacillus is *Staphylococcus epidermis* (*S. albus*) which is coagulase-negative and is a common skin contaminant. Less commonly *S. aureus*, *Pseudomonas aeruginosa* and *Escherichia coli* are found.

The treatment of shunt infections must be aggressive so that the coincidental effects mentioned above are prevented or eliminated. Initially a course of intravenous antibiotic can be tried, but if the infection has not been eliminated within 7–10 days the shunt system must be removed in its entirety, the hydrocephalus controlled by continuous external ventricular drainage and again the appropriate antibiotic administered intravenously. A new shunt system can only be inserted after all infection has been eliminated, particularly judged by a normal cell count in the CSF.

### Intracranial haematoma

After a hydrocephalus has been drained by the insertion of a shunt system a variable period of time will elapse before the brain can expand and occupy the skull fully. During this period there exists a considerable potential for the formation of subdural haematoma from a ruptured cortical vein leaking into the potential space that exists; this possibility is enhanced by trauma to the head, albeit of a minor nature. Furthermore shunts produce a siphon effect when the patient

is in the erect or sitting position, whereby the intracranial pressure may be subatmospheric (McCullough & Fox 1974), and for this reason some shunt systems incorporate an antisyphon device. The incidence of intracranial haematoma was 4% in the series of Ilingworth *et al.* (1971) and 2% in Jeffreys' series (1978), who felt that the incidence might be lessened by avoiding excessive drainage of CSF during the insertion of the shunt, and by keeping the patient supine for the first 3–4 postoperative days.

Once the complication occurs it can be very difficult to treat. Burr hole drainage of the haematoma should be attempted first and this may be all that is required. Unfortunately in some patients the haematoma may recur and in this event it may be necessary to temporarily clamp off the shunt system for a few days in order to allow the brain to expand and occlude the subdural space.

### Thromboembolism

In the earlier days of VA shunting thromboembolism was a common complication such that Anderson (1959) mentioned the presence of pulmonary embolism in 2 of 12 post-mortem examinations in a series of 36 operations and Freidman *et al.* (1964) found pulmonary vascular lesions in 57% of cases reaching autopsy. Since the introduction of modern plastics (silastic) the incidence of this complication appears to have fallen since little mention is made in more recent series. This may, however, be related more to the fact that fewer VA shunts are now performed as most neurosurgeons favour ventriculoperitoneal shunts.

## Results and prognosis

The outcome for a patient with hydrocephalus will depend on various factors which include the age at diagnosis and initial treatment, the degree of cerebral function before treatment and the underlying cause of the hydrocephalus. The first two factors will be discussed separately. The last factor involves many differing factors, for example the outcome for a patient in whom a medulloblastoma has been removed, the neur-axis X-irradiated and the hydrocephalus shunted will depend more on the prognosis for the medulloblastoma than for the hydrocephalus and shunting. For this reason outcome for many of the pathological causes of hydrocephalus will be found elsewhere in the appropriate sections. However the peri-operative mortality rate for shunting hydrocephalus can be reasonably assessed irrespective of the pathological processes Guthkelch (1967a), operating mainly on children, had 5 postoperative deaths in 166 consecutive cases and Jeffreys (1978), operating mainly on adults, had no postoperative deaths in 56 consecutive cases.

## Children

It is clear that when considering treatment for hydrocephalus this must be better than the natural history. Laurence (1958) examined the outcome in 182 children in whom no operation was performed and the major findings were as follows: 49% died during follow-up, 45% were alive and were classified as having arrested hydrocephalus, 5% had progressive hydrocephalus and 1% were lost to follow-up. Although these findings have been quoted as representative of untreated congenital hydrocephalus Milhorat (1972) points out that of the 182 cases only 27% were the result of malformations and the rest were examples of acquired hydrocephalus such as infection and birth trauma. Even though the strictures of Milhorat should be taken seriously Laurence's series still provides a useful yardstick against which to compare contemporary treatment.

Laurence stated that the criteria for spontaneous arrest were cessation of skull enlargement, loss of tension in the fontanelle, return of the ocular axes to normal and a 'striking improvement in physical and mental development'. Judged by these criteria arrest took place usually between the ages of 9 months and 2 years. It is pertinent, though largely conjectural, to enquire what may be the anatomical and pathological changes which could lead to a spontaneous cessation of hydrocephalus? Whether the choroid plexuses atrophy (Laurence & Coates 1962), or secrete less against longstanding obstruction is undetermined; the experimental evidence is unfavourable, though clinical experience suggests the possibility. The histological appearances of forking and of gliosis of the aqueduct of Sylvius do not favour a spontaneous dilatation under the influence of high intraventricular pressure; but this might well happen in stenosis in which no pathological process surrounds the canal, since the aqueduct regularly dilates in posterior fossa obstruction. The obstruction offered by the Arnold–Chiari malformation may lessen in some cases as a result of growth of the posterior fossa; congenital atresia of the foramina of Luschka and Magendie may be incomplete and very thin septa might give way in some cases. There are even authenticated records of the spontaneous formation of fistulas between ventricles and subarachnoid cisterns (Sweet 1940, Tandon & Harkmark 1959, Leslie & Alker 1964). Spontaneous resolution of obstruction is most credible in communicating hydrocephalus due to leptomeningeal occlusion, in which adhesions might gradually resolve and complex subarachnoid pathways open up under the persistent and pulsatile prying of CSF.

Are the criteria described by Laurence adequate to ascertain arrest? A 'striking' improvement occurring over a short period of time is persuasive; but cessation of enlargement of the head after the age of 2 years may be attributable in part to the natural increase of resistance of sutures to distraction. Schick and Matson (1961) are probably correct in demanding a stricter criterion related to head size. Not only must the head cease to enlarge but it should start to grow again only when it is near to or within the curve of the 90th percentile and it should maintain that relationship. The studies of Lorber (1961) have shown that ventricular enlargement is in advance of head enlargement, proving that brain tissue offers less resistance than the cranial envelope. Can a 'striking improvement in physical and mental development' be accepted as reliable evidence of arrest? Examination of the intelligence quotient (I.Q.) of the 40% survivors in Laurence's series revealed that in 27% it was 50 or below, in 32% it was 50–84, in 41% it was in excess of 85 (in the United Kingdom, for a child to attend a normal state school, the I.Q. must be above 70; any child with an I.Q. below 70 is deemed educationally subnormal and will attend a special school; a child with an I.Q. below 50 does not attend any school).

To what extent were Laurence's results the effect of brain damage before arrest and to what extent were they due to unrecognized persistent hydrocephalus? Experience of adult hydrocephalus shows that in some cases of benign aqueduct obstruction causes gradual distension of the ventricles for many years before the occult becomes overt. Previously serial estimations of ventricular size and the width of the cortical mantle were dependent on ventriculography or encephalography, and it was clear that these procedures could not easily be repeated. However the introduction of CT scanning has added a new dimension and serial examinations of these parameters can easily be effected. Unfortunately nearly every child with evidence of obstructive hydrocephalus undergoes a shunting procedure and up-to-date series of nonoperated children do not exist. Some of the arguments will persist.

Milhorat (1972) has assembled the results from various series of children who have undergone surgical treatment and these are tabulated in his monograph. The best results would appear to be those of Lorber and Zachary (1968) who studied 30 children and showed that of the 25 survivors 8% had I.Q. of 120–129, 48% were between 90 and 119, 28% were between 70 and 89, 8% were between 50 and 69 and 8% were below 50; moreover 52% had no physical defects. More recently Shurtleff et al. (1975) have been more sanguine; they reviewed 454 hydrocephalic children with and without myelo-

meningocele, of whom 115 patients were not shunted for reasons which included a frontal cortical mantle less than 1 cm, other major congenital abnormalities and systemic causes of hydrocephalus such as mucopolysaccharidoses; all these required custodial care. Of the 91 patients with hydrocephalus alone who underwent VA shunting, by 14 years of age 48% were dead, 26% were alive but mentally retarded and 26% were alive and with a 'normal' I.Q.

These results underline the complexity of evaluating the prognosis for such patients. The two most important factors seem to be the initial brain function and the occurrence or otherwise of shunt complications. In an attempt to assess the occurrence of complications a collaborative West German series was evaluated (Leem & Miltz 1978). The series involved a retrospective study of 1,612 patients with hydrocephalus who underwent VA or VP shunting, and of whom 83% were less than one year of age at the time of their first operation. It was found that 40% of patients required a shunt revision; these revisions in all necessitated 1,019 operations of which 37% were for blocked ventricular catheters, 11% for malfunctions of the reservoir or valve, 42% for blocked atrial catheters and 10% for blocked peritoneal catheters; the overall infection rate was 3%.

A critical study of the 'prognostic significance of the cerebral mantle' was carried out by Yashon et al. (1965) on untreated cases and they reviewed the observations of others. They concluded that the head circumference and the thickness of the mantle could not be correlated with the ultimate neurological status. Foltz and Shurtleff (1963) held a contrary view; their measurements led them to conclude that a 'width of the cerebral mantle less than 1.2 cm is associated with low I.Q.'. It would of course be contrary to common experience and commonsense to assume from the data available that the anatomical effects of hydrocephalus upon the cerebral hemispheres exert no deleterious influence over intellectual development. What emerges is the encouraging evidence that severe hydrocephalus is not always a bar to a considerable

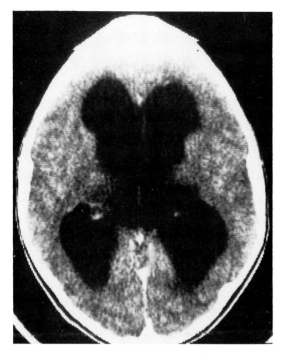

**Fig. 15.15** 12-year-old boy with gross truncal ataxia and poor scholastic development. CT scan showing huge hydrocephalus, which was found on ventriculography to be due to aqueductal stenosis.

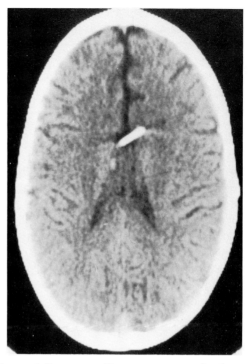

**Fig. 15.16** Same case as Fig. 15.15, one year after the insertion of a ventriculo-atrial shunt. CT scan showing small ventricles. The boy was now playing sport and was performing well scholastically.

degree of development of the intellectual faculties, provided that the hydrocephalus is relieved by natural process or by operation (Figs. 15.15 and 15.16). Conversely anatomical relief of hydrocephalus, even at a very early age, may be followed by a disappointing degree of mental retardation. Multiple pathological factors are operating, all of which have not been fully elucidated, and until that happens their individual influences cannot be assessed. The child with an originally thin pallium and which observation proves can develop considerably after operation and who attains a 'normal' I.Q. on entry to school, is only on the threshold of intellectual activity and of environmental problems demanding abstract thought. It is the absence of the latter which characterizes and handicaps the 'leucotomized' patient, who may otherwise perform quite well in formal intelligence tests. The total effects of hydrocephalus cannot be fully assessed until the child has reached adult years and has attempted to grapple with adult problems. Even when performance is satisfactory, the superimposition of a head injury of even moderate severity can produce devastating disability, suggesting that such patients are functioning at the limit of capacity.

**Adults**

The assessment of the results of treatment and prognosis is easier for adults than for children; the majority of patients have an acquired hydrocephalus, and even if they develop late problems from a congenital hydrocephalus a baseline of intelligence and behaviour exists prior to diagnosis and any possible treatment. In many cases hydrocephalus is caused by a space-occupying lesion, and it is likely that it is this primary pathological process which will determine the result of treatment rather than the treatment of the hydrocephalus *per se*. The condition which best lends itself as a model for assessing the results of treatment is nontumourous (normal) pressure hydrocephalus. In this condition each patient can act as his own scientific control both with respect to any physical change and with respect to pre- and postoperative psychometry (Jeffreys & Wood 1978). In patients with the triad of dementia, gait disturbance and incontinence there is a growing consensus that useful improvement occurs in up to 65% with complete recovery in 35% (Pickard 1982), though the prognosis for gait and incontinence is better than for intellectual function. Age, duration of symptoms and degree of disability do not appear to affect the outcome.

# References

ADAMS R. D., FISHER C. M., HAKIM S., OJEMANN R. G. & SWEET W. H. (1965) *New Eng. J. Med.*, 273, 117.

ADELOYE A. (1976) *J. Neurosurg.*, 45, 415.

ALVORD E. C. (1961) In *Disorders of the developing Nervous System.* (Eds. Fields W. S. & Desmond M. M.) Thomas, Springfield, Illinois.

ANDERSON F. M. (1959) *J. Neurosurg*, 16, 551.

ARNOLD J. (1894) *Beitrag. Anat. Allg. Path.*, 16, 1.

BARRY A., PATTEN B. M. & STEWART B. H. (1957) *J. Neurosurg.*, 14, 285.

BECKER D. P. & NULSEN F. E. (1968) *J. Neurosurg.*, 28, 215.

BENDA C. E. (1954) *J. Neuropath. Exp. Neurol.*, 13, 14.

BERING E. A. & SATO O. (1963) *J. Neurosurg.*, 20, 1050.

BLACKWOOD W., MCMENEMEY W. H., MEYER A., NORMAN R. M. & RUSSELLS D. S. (1963) In *Greenfield's Pathology.* Arnold, London.

BRAIN, LORD (1962) *Diseases of the Nervous System,* 6th edition. Oxford University Press, London.

BRAMWELL B. (1899) *Brain*, 22, 66.

BRODAL A. & HAUGLIE-HANSSEN E. (1959) *J. Neurol. Neurosurg. Psychiat.*, 22, 99.

BULL J. W. D. (1961) *Neurology*, 11, 1.

CAMERON A. H. (1957a) *J. Path. Bact.*, 73, 195.

CAMERON A. H. (1957b)) *J. Path Bact.*, 73, 213.

CHAWLA J. C., HULME A. & COOPER R. (1974) *J. Neurosurg.*, 40, 376.

CHIARI H. (1891) *Dtsch. Med. Wschr.*, 17, 1172.

CHIARI H. (1896) *Dtsch. Akad. Wiss. Wien.*, 63, 71.

CLELAND G. (1883) *J. Anat. Physiol.*, 17, 257.

CONE W. V., LEWIS R. D. & JACKSON I. J. (1949) *Shunting of cerebrospinal fluid into the peritoneal cavity.* Presented at the Meeting of American College of Physicians, Montreal.

DANDY W. E. (1922) *Johns. Hopk. Hosp. Bull.*, 33, 189.

DANDY W. E. (1933) In *Lewis's Practice of Surgery.*, 12, 247. Prior Co. Inc, Hagerstown.

DANDY W. E. (1945) *Arch. Surg.*,, 51, 1.

DANDY W. E. & BLACKFAN K. D. (1913) *J. Amer. med. Ass.*, 61, 2216.

DANDY W. E. & BLACKFAN K. D. (1914) *Amer. J. Dis. Child.*, 8, 406.

DANIEL P. M. & STRICH S. J. (1958) *J. Neuropath. Exp. Neurol.*, 17, 255.

DAVSON H. & SEGAL M. B. (1971) *Acta. Neurol. Lat. Amer.*, (suppl 1). 17, 99.

DI ROCCO C., DI TRAPANI G., MAIRA G., MACCHI G. & ROSSI G. F. (1977) *J. Neurol. Sci.*, 33, 437.

EISENBERG H. M., MCCOMB J. G. & LORENZO A. V. (1974) *J. Neurosurg.*, 40, 381.

FOLTZ E. L. & SHURTLEFF D. B. (1963) *J. Neurosurg.*, 20, 1064.

FOLTZ E. L. & SHURTLEFF D. D. (1966) *J. Neurosurg.*, 24, 520.

FOTLZ E. L. & WARD A. A. (1956) *J. Neurosurg.*, 13, 546.

FRIEDMAN S., ZITA-GOZUM C & CHATTEN J. (1964) *J. Paediat.*, 64, 305.

GARDNER W. J. (1959) *Cleveland. Clin. Quart.*, 26, 206.

GARDNER W. J. & ANGEL J. V. (1959) *Clin. Neurosurg.*, 6, 131.

GRAHAM P., HOWMAN-GILES R., JOHNSTON I. & BESSER M. (1982) *J. Neursurg.*, 57, 262.

GRANHOLM L. (1976) In *Intracranial Pressure III.* (Eds Beks J. W. F. & Al.), 173. Springer, Berlin.

GREITZ T. (1969) *Acta. Radiol.*, 8, 376.

GUILLAUME J. & ROGÉ R. (1950) *Rev. Neurol.*, 82, 424.

GUTHKELCH A. N. (1967a) *Brit. J. Surg.*, 54, 665.

GUTHKELCH A. N. (1967b) *Proc. roy. Soc. Med.*, 60, 1263.

HAKIM S. (1964) MD Thesis No. 957, Javeriana University School of Medicine, Bogota.

HOFFMAN H. J., CHUANG S., HENDRICK E. B. & HUMPHREYS R. P. (1982) *J. Neurosurg.*, 57, 316.

ILLINGWORTH R. D., LOGUE V., SYMON L. & UEMURA K. (1971) *J. Neurosurg.*, 35, 681.

JEFFREYS R. V. (1978) In *Advances in Neurosurgery, no 6.* (Eds. Wüllenweber R., Weker H., Brock M. & Klinger M.) Springer, Berlin.

JEFFREYS R. V. & WOOD M. M. (1978) *Acta. Neurochir.*, 45, 103.

JEFFREYS R. V. (1981) *Acta. Neurochir*, 56, 39.

KAPPERS J. A. (1955) *J. Comp. Neurol.*, 102, 425.

KATZMANN R. (1977) *Contemp. Neurol.*, 15, 69.

KOCEN R. S. (1977) *Brit. J. Hosp. Med.*, 18, 436.

LAST R. J. & TOMPSETT D. H. (1953) *Brit. J. Surg.*, 40, 425.

LAURENCE K. M. (1958) *Lancet*, 2, 1152.

LAURENCE K. M. & COATES S. (1962) *Arch. Dis. Child.*, 37, 345.

LEEM W. & MILTZ H. (1978) In *Recent Advances in Neurosurgery, no 6* (Eds Wüllenweber R., Wenker H., Brock M. & Klinger M.) Springer, Berlin.

LESLIE E. V. & ALKER G. J. (1964) *Radiol.*, 83, 683.

LEWIN W. S. (1968) *Brit. J. Surg.*, 55, 747.

LITTLE J. R. & MacCARTY C. S. (1974) *J. Neurosurg.*, 40, 320.

LORBER J. (1961) *Arch. Dis. Child.*, 36, 381.

LORBER J. & ZACHARY R. B. (1968) *Arch. Dis. Child.*, 43, 516.

LORENZO A. V., BRESNAN M. J. & BARLOW C. F. (1974) *Arch. Neurol.*, 30, 387.

LUNDBERG N. (1972) In *Scientific Foundations of Neurology* (Eds. Critchley M., O'Leary J. & Jennett W. B. Heinemann, London.

MACFARLANE A. & MALONEY A. F. J. (1957) *Brain*, 80, 479.

McCULLOUGH D. C. & FOX J. F. (1974) *J. Neurosurg.*, 40, 372.

MACNAB G. H. (1955) *Proc. roy. Soc. Med.*, **48**, 846.
MARGOLIS G. & KILHAM L. (1969) *Lab. Invest.*, **21**, 189.
MATSON D. D. (1949) *J. Neurosurg.*, **6**, 238.
MATSON D. D. (1969) *Neurosurgery of Infancy and Childhood.* 2nd edition. Thomas, Springfield, Illinois.
MCLAURIN R. L., BAILEY O. T., SCHURR P. A. & INGRAHAM F. D. (1954) *Arch. Path.*, **57**, 138.
MILHORAT T. H. (1972) *Hydrocephalus and The Cerebrospinal Fluid.* Williams & Wilkins, Baltimore.
NORMAN M. G. & BECKER L. E. (1974) *J. Neurol. Neurosurg. Psychiat.*, **37**, 252.
NOSIK W. A. (1950) *J. Neurosurg.*, **7**, 236.
NULSEN F. E. & SPITZ E. B. (1952) *Surg. Forum.*, **2**, 399.
NULSEN F. E. (1961) *Excerpta Medica*, **36**, 40.
PARSONS M. (1982) *Brit. J. Hosp. Med.*, **27**, 682.
PAUL K. S., LYE R. H., STRANG A. & DUTTON J. (1983) *J. Neurosurg.*, **58**, 183.
PEACH B. (1964a) *Arch. Neurol.*, **10**, 497.
PEACH B. (1964b) *Arch. Neurol.*, **11**, 609.
PEACH B. (1965a)) *Arch. Neurol.*, **12**, 527.
PEACH B. (1965b) *Arch. Neurol.*, **12**, 613.
PENFIELD W. & ELVIDGE A. R. (1932) In *Cytology and Cellular Pathology of the Nervous System* (Ed. Penfield), **3**, 1203. Hoeber, New York.
PICKARD J. D. (1982) *Brit. J. Hosp. Med.*, **27**, 35.
POPPEN J. L., REYES V. & HORRAX G. (1953) *J. Neurosurg.*, **10**, 242.
PORTUGAL VON J. R. & BROCK M. (1962) *Zblt. Neurochir.*, **23**, 80.
PUDENZ R. H., RUSSELL F. E., HURD A. H. & SHELDON C. H. (1957) *J. Neurosurg.*, **14**, 171.
RAIMONDI A. J., SAMUELSON G., YARZAGARAY L. & NORTON T. (1969) *J. Neurosurg.*, **31**, 202.
RANSOHOFF J. (1954) *J. Neursurg.*, **11**, 295.
RANSOHOFF J., SHULMAN K. & FISHMAN R. (1960) *J. Paed.* **56**, 399.
ROBERTSON J. T., SCHICK R. W., MORGAN F. & MATSON D. D. (1961) *J. Neurosurg.*, **18**, 255.
RUSSELL D. S. (1949) *Observations on the Pathology of Hydrocephalus.* MRC Sp Rep Series 265. HMSO, London.
RUSSELL, D. S. (1966) *Observations on the Pathology of Hydrocephalus. Med. Res. Coun. Sp. Rep. Series* No. 265. Third imp. with Appendix. H.M.S.O., London.
RUSSELL D. S. & DONALD C. (1935) *Brain*, **58**, 203.
SAHAR A., HOCHWALD G. M. & RANSOHOFF J. (1971) *Neurol.*, **21**, 218.
SCARFF J. E. (1951) *J. Neurosurg.*, **8**, 204.
SCARFF J. E. (1959) *Acta. Psychiat. Neurol. Scand.*, **34**, 354.
SCHWALBE E. & GREDIG M. (1907) *Beitrag. Path. Anat. Allg. Pathol.*, **40**, 132.
SCHICK R. W. & MATSON D. W. (1961) *J. Paed.*, **58**, 791.
SHURTLEFF D. B., KRONMAL R. & FOLTZ E. L. (1975) *J. Neurosurg.*, **42**, 61.
SPILLER W. G. (1916) *J. nerv. Ment. Dis.*, **44**, 395.
STOOKEY B. & SCARFF J. (1936) *Bull. Neurol. Inst. New York*, **5**, 348.
SWEET W. H. (1940) *Arch. Neurol. Psychiat.*, **44**, 532.
SYMON L., DORSCH N. W. C. & STEPHENS R. J. (1972) *Lancet*, **2**, 1291.
TAGGART J. K. & WALKER A. E. (1942) *Arch. Neurol. Psychiat.*, **48**, 583.
TANDON P. N. & HARKMARK W. (1959) *Neurol.*, **9**, 699.
TORKILDSEN A. (1939) *Acta. Chirug. Scand.*, **82**, 117.
VASSILOUTHIS J. & RICHARDSON A. E. (1979) *J. Neurosurg.*, **51**, 341.
WEED L. H. (1920) *Contributions to Embryology*, **9**, 425. Carnegie Inst, Washington.
WENIG C., HUBER G. & EMDE H. (1979) *Eur. Neurol.*, **18**, 1.
WISLOCKI G. B. & PUTNAM T. J. (1921) *Amer. J. Anat.*, **29**, 313.
WISNIEWSKI H., WELLER R. O. & TERRY R. D. (1969) *J. Neurosurg.*, **31**, 10.
WOOLLAM D. H. M. & MILLEN J. W. (1953) *Brain*, **76**, 104.
YAKOVLEV P. I. (1947) *Amer. J. Ment. Defic.*, **51**, 561.
YASHON D., JANE J. A. & SUGAR O. (1965) *J. Neurosurg.*, **23**, 509.
ZÜLCH K. J. (1965) *Brain Tumors, Their Biology and Pathology.* 2nd ed. Springer, New York.

# Chapter 16
# Common malformations of the nervous system

## G. F. G. FINDLAY

## Introduction

Although the nervous system is subject to a diversity of malformations, relatively few require or are amenable to surgical treatment. Only those malformations for which some sort of corrective therapy exists will be considered, including some skeletal malformations which affect neural function such as craniostenosis. Vascular malformations affecting the brain are considered in Chapter 12 and those which affect the spine are discussed in Chapter 21.

The formation and closure of the neural tube and its isolation by mesoderm are highly complex processes and failure to follow the normal pattern is the origin of most of the developmental abnormalities which confront the neurosurgeon. The term 'dysraphic state' was introduced by Fuchs in 1909 to embrace all lesions attributable to embryological errors of this nature. Bremer (1927) noted that other anomalies of skin, bone and nervous tissue were frequently present and that there could be a high genetic influence. The aetiological mechanisms involved in the generation of neurological developmental abnormalities are often unclear in the individual case. Many have a genetic basis; either as a random mutation or as an inherited syndrome such as Apert syndrome. The majority, however, seem to have a multifactorial basis. Here also genetic factors play an important role as in spina bifida but many other factors may be at work. Viral influences are not uncommon, the most commonly implicated being rubella and cytomegalovirus. Ionizing radiation is recognized as being a rare factor. More common agents include: drugs (for example thalidomide); alcohol (fetal alcohol syndrome); dietary and vitamin

deficiency (possibly implicated in spina bifida); and maternal disease (such as insulin dependent diabetes). The exact role of any factor in the production of abnormality is unclear but the subject has been extensively reviewed by Melnick (1977).

Probably the most intensively investigated neurological abnormality is spina bifida and associated hydrocephalus. The general incidence of spina bifida was quoted by McKeown & Record (1960) as about 2–3 per 1000 births. The modern figure appears to be gradually diminishing due to greater use of prenatal screening for raised alpha fetoprotein levels which allow detection of potentially affected fetuses at a stage where termination on medical grounds is feasible. Laurence *et al.* (1968) identified a marked local geographic variation of incidence and, although several factors were suggested as being culpable, no generally accepted reason for this has become apparent. The undoubted genetic influence was emphasized by Lorber (1965) who found that 8% of siblings born to parents with one affected child was affected by either spina bifida, anencephalus or hydrocephalus. Carter and Roberts (1967) estimated the risk of a third infant being affected to be 10%.

## Cranial encephalocele

Defective closure of the skull and consequent protrusion of its contents is less common than spinal defects in a proportion of about 1:8 (Ingraham & Matson 1954). Although these defects are usually described as encephaloceles, some contain no neural tissue and are truly meningoceles. The majority are completely covered with epithelium, often with full thickness skin, but occasionally epithelium is absent and brain tissue exposed. There is great variation in size and in the occipital region they may even attain the dimensions of the head. The orifice by which the contents of the hernia communicate with those of the cranium, the neck of the sac, may be quite small compared with the dimensions of the sac, consequently these cranial swellings may be sessile or pedunculated. Encephaloceles occur in the median plane, although those through the anterior cranial fossa may deviate to one side as they expand; three-quarters arise in the occipital region.

### Frontal encephalocele

Although these malformations are seemingly rare in this country and in North America, elsewhere they are more frequent. Nearly one-third of the craniovertebral malformations in a Moroccan centre were encephaloceles (Aquaviva *et al.* 1966) and in Thailand the incidence of frontal encephaloceles is put at 1 in 5000 live births (Suwanwela & Hongsaprobbas 1966). There may be a swelling at the root of the nose with broadening of the bridge and it may extend to one or both sides of the nose below the orbits; it may be within the orbit causing proptosis and lateral displacement of the eyeball or there may be no external disfigurement, the hernia bulging into the nasal cavity causing airway obstruction. In this situation it may be mistaken for a simple inflammatory polyp. The defect in the cranium is usually at the junction of the frontal and ethmoidal bones, forming a central circular opening; occasionally the opening is on one or both sides as a result of defective development of the anterior extremity of the cribriform plate. The sac usually contains a plug of brain tissue. Operation is necessary for aesthetic reasons, for the correction of displacement of the eyeball, or to relieve nasal obstruction and to prevent ulceration and infection.

In the past surgical correction of such abnormalities was often deferred until long beyond the neonatal stage due to the high risks of infant surgery. However, the adverse effect which an anterior fossa encephalocele exerts on the development of the facial skeleton is severe. With improvements in neonatal care, it is now accepted that the initial and main surgical correction should be performed during the first six months of life with many surgical teams opting for the early part of this period. The surgery is primarily transcranial but this can allow radical skull base surgery at the same time to correct any degree of facial deformity, the commonest type of which is hypertelorism. This, along with the peroperative management of such a young child, provides the main surgical difficulties. The isolation, reduction and ligation of the dural sac does not usually pose major problems, in fact Dandy introduced such a procedure in 1929.

### Occipital encephalocele

The position of the bony opening varies so that the sac may contain either part of the occipital lobe or of the cerebellum; in which case there may be associated hindbrain abnormalities. Occasionally the swelling proves to be a simple meningocele. It is advisable to determine the nature of the contents of the sac and the presence or otherwise of associated abnormalities. This usually can be determined by CT scanning, though on occasions ventriculography may be necessary. It is of interest to recall that the first attempt made by Horsley (1884) to stimulate the human brain electrically was on such a case: he wished to know whether the swelling contained brain. The decision to operate will depend upon the extent of brain herniation and the nature of other malformations, but hydrocephalus is not a bar. In cases of doubt it is wise to postpone the decision but if there is no contraindication excision should be performed early in order to solve nursing problems. An elliptical incision through healthy skin near the base of the sac is employed; it can be extended in a vertical direction if the sac communicates with the posterior fossa, so that the anatomical structures involved can be identified. In meningocele, it is only necessary to excise the sac and to make a watertight closure of the dura mater and the skin. Small bone defects will gradually fill with a firm plug of scar tissue. Large ones may require reinforcement with a bone graft or other firm material at a later date. The treatment of herniated brain will depend on its amount and identity; although sacrifice of a portion of cerebellum may be of little importance, loss of part of the occipital pole might result in hemianopia. If hydrocephalus is present, whether due to aqueduct obstruction, hindbrain malformation or of communicating type, it should be treated by a diversionary or shunting procedure at the same time as closure of the encephalocele as this will reduce the risk of leakage of cerebrospinal fluid through the site of dural repair. Encephaloceles arising in the parietal area are usually small and present no technical difficulties in their removal. They may be mistaken for dermoid cysts; both form sessile midline lumps and a dermoid may be anchored in a bony depression.

The prognosis of infants with encephaloceles varies markedly. Those with simple meningoceles fare best; whilst those with large encephaloceles and microcephaly do worst. Guthkelch (1970) found that 86% of patients with a meningocele fared well with normal or better intelligence. However, of those with an encephalocele, only 40% achieved such survival. The presence of hydrocephalus served to reduce both these figures further. It is to be hoped that with more effective management of the hydrocephalus this can be improved but no figures are actually available to support this contention.

## Spina bifida and other dysraphic states

Two groups of cases can be distinguished, on the basis of anatomy and of clinical presentation. Spina bifida cystica comprises those in which herniation of part or of all the spinal contents forms an obvious protrusion; it includes meningocele, myelocele, and rachischisis. In spina bifida occulta, mesodermal differentiation has progressed sufficiently to prevent herniation so that there is little or no external bulge; if a local swelling is present it is due to a lipomatous mass and by contrast in some cases a depression or dimple in the skin overlies the hidden malformation. Spina bifida may be accompanied by other dysraphic errors; myelodysplasia, syringomyelia, hydromyelia and partial or total axial division of the spinal cord with or without partial division of the spinal canal, diastematomyelia. These may be at a higher segmental level and occasionally at a considerable distance. Their association is important for they may be responsible for neurological deficits in cases of spina bifida occulta and of meningocele which cannot be explained by the more ovbious malformation. Congenital obstruction of the aqueduct of Sylvius and Arnold–Chiari malformation are frequent causes of hydrocephalus in the more severe degrees of spina bifida. Figures derived from the records of the Children's Medical Centre, Boston (Ingraham & Matson 1954) during a period of 20 years, give the incidence of spina bifida occulta as 8%; these were patients admitted to hospital. The incidence of malformation of a neural arch has been as high as 17% of all spines X-rayed (Curtius & Lorenz 1934) but such accidental findings have no clinical relevance. Approximately one-half of the Boston examples of spina bifida cystica were meningoceles but in MacNab's (1957) series of 200 cases the proportion was much lower, 20% and similar to that reported by Doran and Guthkelch (1961). The occult malformation is nearly always in the lumbar region; the cystic variety may occur in any part of the spine but over two-thirds of the Boston cases were lumbar or lumbosacral, the remaining one-third being spread fairly evenly throughout the rest of the spine and included the rare thoracic and pelvic anterior (or anterolateral) herniation.

### Meningocele

This benign and simple cystic herniation may be sessile or pedunculated; it is covered with healthy skin (unless ulcerated by pressure) and by defin-ition contains no nervous structures. Depending upon the size and the patency of its neck, its volume and tension increases with straining and also in the erect posture if it is lumbar (conversely this may then diminish if it is cervical). Its con-tents can be partially expressed into the spinal canal by gentle compression. The internal layer of the sac comprises dura mater with an endo-thelial lining which represents the arachnoid mater; the latter can be identified as a separate membrane only near the neck, or within the spinal canal. Skin covering the fundus may be thin and fused with the dural wall, or irregular masses of adipose tissue sometimes forming a fibrolipoma may intervene; similar tissue sur-rounds the base of the new sac. The extent to which the malformation affects the roof of the spinal canal is variable; from a narrow dehi-scence of one lamina on one side or an absence of a spinous process, to absence of several neural arches, widening of the transverse diameter of the canal which is shallow and bordered either side by peg-like process of bone attached to the pedicles and representing vestigial laminae. Extensive bone deformity is uncommon in men-ingocele but usual in myelocele. The dural sac narrows to form the neck where it traverses the roof of the spinal canal, to become smoothly continuous with the theca. Occasionally the lumen of a narrow neck becomes obliterated by adhesions; the sac is often traversed by filmy adhesions which may cause loculation of cere-brospinal fluid. Not uncommonly adhesions may take the form of fibrous cords which simulate nerve roots; nerve roots may herniate into the sac and be anchored to its wall by adhesions, but careful dissection will trace the root back into the spinal theca before it enters its exit sheath.

General examination of the infant should include a careful search for other malformations and for evidence of neurological abnormality, for example hydrocephalus, lack of spontaneous movements in a limb, patulous anus and club foot. Neurological abnormality, or deformity resulting therefrom, suggests that the spinal lesion is not a simple meningocele or that there is associated malformation such as myelodysplasia. Transillumination of the swelling may exclude any solid structure within it.

Excision of a meningocele can be deferred until the infant is from 3 to 6 months of age unless the fundus of the sac is so thin that it may give way or unless the swelling is inconveniently large. A transverse elliptical incision is made near its base, preserving sufficient skin to provide apposition without tension and deepened until the dural sac wall is encountered. It is opened and the interior examined to confirm the simple nature of the lesion. The fundus is excised and the neck traced to the theca; the interior of the spinal canal is examined for any further abnor-mality though it is inadvisable to enlarge the deficiency in its roof for this purpose, the neck is cut short and the stump securely closed.

The results of the excision of a spinal men-ingocele are highly satisfactory. In a series of 61 children in whom a meningocele was removed Doran and Guthkelch (1961) reported no mor-tality: 9 had slight lower limb weakness (due to diastematomyelia in 3), delayed or impaired control of sphincters occurred in 4 and in 6 there was postoperative increased intracranial pressure which subsided after 2 months.

### Myelocele (myelomeningocele)

In this form of spina bifida cystica, by far the commonest and the most serious, mesoderm fails to separate the relevant portion of the spinal cord from the ectoderm; in consequence it remains attached to the skin of the fundus of the sac or itself forms the fundus. In the latter event the cord is then usually malformed, with evidence of varying degrees of failure of fusion of the lips of the neural tube. In the worst cases (rachischisis) there is little or no bulging or cyst formation owing to the escape of cerebrospinal fluid and the spinal cord presents as an oval flat plaque of soft reddish tissue merging with thin epithel-ialized fibrous tissue at its margins. At times a midline groove can be discerned terminating at either end in a hole, representing the original neural groove and its continuation with the central canal of the rest of the cord. Stimulation of the plaque may elicit motor responses and these excitable points lie close to the midline (Brocklehurst *et al.* 1967) and on the deep aspect. The 'anterior' roots are attached to the deformed tissue either side of the midline, and the posterior roots lateral to these, near the margin. Malformations of this degree and affecting a considerable extent of the spinal cord are rare and commonly cause death soon after birth, but involvement of one or two segments is a common form of spina bifida cystica; indeed in necropsy specimens (Cameron 1956) it is the commonest, and it is questionable whether the retention of the term meningomyelocele (or myelomeningocele) serves any useful purpose; the important feature of these cases is the presence of spinal cord in the sac. In all there is a diversity of dysplasia of the ectopic nervous tissue. Whether it is covered by a thin layer of skin or whether it is exposed and whether it bulges or not are clinical aspects which may influence treatment. Lichtenstein (1940) showed that a severe degree of myelodysplasia may accompany little external abnormality and that even if the cord is covered with skin (the commonly termed myelomeningocele) there may be an intimate mixture of skin, connective tissue, neural elements and ectopic ependymal canals. MacNab (1957) stated that in 50% of post-mortem specimens there were pathological changes in the spinal cord above the sac. In addition to the macroscopic dysplasias he reported that Cameron had noted retardation of myelinization, and Lendon (1968) found a reduction in the neuron population of apparently normal segments.

In the newly born a fully developed myelocele presents as a cystic spina bifida the centre of which is occupied by moist greyish-pink tissue, the *area medullovasculosa* of von Recklinghausen, which is friable and readily bleeds. At its periphery it blends with parchment-like epithelialized membrane which merges with normal skin. The degree of bulging varies considerably and probably depends upon the extent

to which cerebrospinal fluid has leaked, from an open central canal or through rents in the membrane. The neural plaque can rapidly become infected and within a few days may be covered by granulation tissue and purulent exudate. If death does not supervene the raw surface gradually epithelializes and in the course of several months the plaque is incorporated in a puckered leathery scar; according to the degree of inflammatory reaction the previous cystic swelling may virtually subside. In the lesser degrees of malformation, the displaced portion of spinal cord is covered with thin skin (which may rapidly ulcerate) and the swelling may resemble a meningocele, though the fundus may feel firmer than normal. Transillumination and X-ray examination after insufflation of air or CT scanning will reveal the presence of solid tissue at the fundus and often the shadows of the nerve roots traversing the sac. Palpation of the spine around the base of the sac will give some indication of the extent of the bony malformation; a row of bony spurs can be felt either side, representing the stubs of laminae and pedicles, the two rows being separated by a wide and shallow gutter, the roofless spinal canal. Radiographs will confirm the increased width of the spinal canal and may reveal anomalies of the vertebral bodies. In older children the midline spur of a diastematomyelia may be revealed but in infants ossification is seldom sufficiently advanced for it to be seen.

In marked contrast to meningoceles, greater or lesser degrees of paralysis distinguish the myelocele. Doran and Guthkelch (1963) reported that in approximately one-half of their cases of closed myeloceles there was no paralysis; paralysis was present in all the open cases and it was complete in 86%. Identification of muscle weakness in the infant depends as much upon the eye as upon the hand; careful scrutiny of the limbs when the child is crying or restless will disclose which segments of a limb are not being moved or in which direction there is no movement and palpation will confirm this excluding other causes such as joint deformity. If present, the latter may have a paralytic origin. Reflex movements of limbs in response to stimulation must be discounted. The absence of tendon reflexes should be noted. Examination of the anus will reveal a patulous sphincter and continuous dribbling of urine indicates bladder involvement. Both sphincters may be defective when there are no other signs of paralysis. Sensory response to gentle pin-prick can be roughly estimated when the child is quiet and the test is of particular value in determining the upper limit of cord damage in thoracic lesions, when the lower limbs are totally paralysed.

The most frequent and the most serious complication of myelocele is hydrocephalus and its incidence may be as high as 75% (Laurence 1957). Since some infants may die of meningitis or from other causes before hydrocephalus becomes clinically manifest and may die at home without necropsy, this estimate is probably conservative. In the experience of MacNab (1954) when hydrocephalus complicates spina bifida cystica, in 90% of cases this is evident by the fourth month. Enlargement of the ventricles precedes unequivocal increase in the circumference of the head. Lorber (1961) carried out systematic ventriculography in a series of infants with myeloceles and the ventricles were demonstrably larger than normal in 83%; in one-third of these the size of the head was within normal range. The aetiology of hydrocephalus has been discussed fully at an earlier stage but, in the context of spina bifida, it is usually a hindbrain deformity of the Arnold–Chiari type which is responsible, often with associated aqueduct obstruction. Gardner (1968) suggested that maldevelopment in the rhomboencephalic roof led to diversion of cerebrospinal flow into the central canal with the resulting build-up of pressure being sufficient to rupture the caudal end of the neural tube thus producing the myelomeningocele.

Purulent meningitis is not as frequent a sequel of myelocele as might be anticipated, occurring in 18% of MacNab's cases (Jolly 1957) and causing death in 13% of those of Doran and Guthkelch (1961). Meningeal fibrosis consequent upon infection is probably an important factor in precipitating hydrocephalus in those cases in which brain malformation alone narrows but does not completely block the natural pathways of the cerebrospinal fluid.

## Treatment

In few branches of neurosurgery, indeed of surgery in general and of paediatrics, has there been such a change of attitude as there has towards the treatment of the more severe forms of spina bifida. The natural history of the lesion has been established for many years; many of the infants have severely paralysed lower limbs; hydrocephalus is common; and the natural death rate is high. To attempt to close an open myelocele, even with the introduction of antibiotics making this feasible, may seem unrewarding and, in the opinion of many, meddlesome surgery. On the one hand, prolonging a miserable existence for both child and family because of cerebral damage, paraplegia and incontinence of urine and of faeces may make it seem that early death by natural causes would prove the kindlier solution in most cases and so surgical interference may be withheld except for the more benign malformations. However, statistical evidence to support this attitude was not available for a long time and among paediatricians there was a growing body of opinion that a considerable number of children with hydrocephalus and with paralytic deformities from healed myeloceles survived for many years (Jolly 1955). This view led to a sense of dissatisfaction with the laissez-faire attitude of many, though not of all, neurosurgeons. Laurence (1958, Laurence & Coates 1962) made an outstanding contribution to the study of hydrocephalus, by his analysis of its consequences if no operation were attempted. He showed that approximately one-half of affected patients died; the other half survived for a sufficient length of time for the hydrocephalus to be considered as arrested and 75% of these children were educable. A study of spina bifida (Laurence 1964) revealed that a similar proportion of children with a myelocele lived for some years, although only 29% were expected to reach the age of 12 years. These figures added momentum to the change which was taking place in the case of these infants, a change which was largely brought about by the development of the treatment of hydrocephalus by shunting procedures. Impetus to this revolution was also provided by the public interest in the eduction and training of children suffering from spastic diplegia and in the successful rehabilitation of paraplegics. Experience in the latter group of patients not only showed how diverse paralytic deformities might be alleviated, but stimulated interest in management of the urinary and bowel complications. In more recent years this enthusiastic approach has diminished somewhat and greater emphasis has been placed on prevention and in attempts to assess the severity of the lesion at birth with the resultant prognosis of neurological damage (Lorber 1971). Such assessment is extremely difficult to make in the neonate but in general it is possible to estimate the approximate upper level of the lesion and thus gain some guide as to the likely deficit. Using this and taking into consideration the parental circumstances and reactions, a sensible decision can be reached as to whether or not to operate. If the decision is made not to operate, the problem of the medical, nutritional and social management of the child poses enormous difficulties demanding careful assessment. Fortunately, the more widespread use of prenatal screening as mentioned earlier has led to a reduction of the number of occasions on which such distressing situations arise.

If an operative course is elected, surgery is usually performed in the first 24 hours of life. Sharrard (1967) felt that early closure resulted in some improvement of final neurological status. It is, however, likely that any such improvement stems from the protection of the exposed cord tissues to further damage rather than to any real increase in function and Brocklehurst *et al.* (1967) felt that early closure made no difference to the final result, save in the protection which it conferred against meningitis. Operative repair of the myelomeningocele is governed by the same principles which apply to a meningocele: isolation and removal of the sac with watertight closure of the dural elements and skin. It is technically much more demanding due to the need to free and preserve neural structures and the difficulties of achieving skin closure. The details were fully described by Ingraham and Matson (1954). The skin incision is usually placed transversely and is sited as close to the neural plaque as is consistent with skin viability. It is deepened to expose the sac which is then opened. The cord and its roots are gently mobilized and adhesions freed sufficiently to allow it to sink into the spinal canal, though frequently the 'canal' is so malformed that it is merely a shallow groove. It has been recommended that the cord and canal should be explored to determine the presence of a diastematous spur; whether to do this will depend upon the exigencies of the situation, and in any event such a spur is often at a higher level. The membranes of the sac are mobilized and trimmed so that they can be brought together and closed over the cord. In some cases there is insufficient tissue to do this without subjecting the cord to compression; it may be necessary to use lumbar fascia to close the defect. Sufficient skin may be available for apposition without tension, but mobilization by undercutting is usually necessary and in some cases needs rotation flaps and remote tension-relieving incisions. Bare areas are covered by skin grafts. Appropriate antibiotics must be given and to diminish the risk of cerebrospinal fluid leak the infant should be nursed prone with the buttocks raised until the wound appears firmly healed. Intracranial tension may be raised after the operation and whether this is due to meningeal reaction, meningitis, or to exacerbation of hydrocephalus, it should be relieved by periodically puncturing the lateral ventricle or by inserting an indwelling catheter. Loss of cerebrospinal fluid during the operation or subsequently by drainage requires the correction of water and electrolyte deficiency. The appearance of clinically obvious raised intracranial pressure due to hydrocephalus can be confirmed by CT scanning and a shunting procedure then undertaken.

The management of a child with a myelomeningocele only begins with the operations to close the lesion and treat any hydrocephalus. A multidisciplinary team approach is necessary to treat or prevent the associated problems of bladder and bowel function, orthopaedic deformity of spine and lower limbs and the educational and social problems. With regard to associated spinal deformity, this may appear as a scoliosis, kyphoscoliosis or isolated kyphus. The mechanisms of such deformities are complex. They are related to the effect upon spinal growth of paravertebral muscular paralysis and the not infrequent finding of associated bony abnormalities such as diastomatomyelia, block or hemivertebra, or areas of failure of vertebral segmentation. Correction of paediatric spinal deformity is usually undertaken by specially organized orthopaedic teams; however, neurological compromise, due to diastomatomyelia or bony kyphus, often involves neurosurgical involvement to perform decompression. Such procedures should never be performed in isolation and should always be combined with corrective spinal surgery either at the same time or at a staged second procedure.

## Spina bifida occulta

Although radiological evidence of defective fusion of the neural arch is common in otherwise normal people, associated neurological dysfunction is rare. The site of such malformations may be marked by an overlying patch of hairy skin, by a cutaneous vascular naevus, by a mass of fatty tissue sometimes very bulky, or by a depression in the skin. The latter may constitute the superficial extremity of a dermal sinus or tract. The neurological abnormalities and deformations of the lower limbs are similar to those described in cases of myelocele though of a much less severe degree and there may be an associated scoliosis. Unlike cases of myelocele these disturbances are usually not perceived by the parents until the child starts to walk; in some not for several years, in others minor disturbance of function passes without complaint for several years and then appears to get worse. The parents' complaint may be of faulty posture, limp or stumbling because of a clumsy foot. Pain is an unusual feature. Callosities and pressure sores on the feet may be noticed and significantly, may be painless. Faulty control of micturition, manifest as delay in acquiring normal habits or subsequent loss of them, may be the only evidence of spina bifida occulta and its associated intraspinal lesions.

It is unusual for neurological deficit to be due directly to some neural maldevelopment. Rather it is likely to be due to some associated problem such as: diastematomelia; tethered cord; intradural lipoma; or dermoid cyst. Radiological examination should include the skull and whole spine to detect malformation at other levels and myelography is also essential to show the nonbony associated conditions mentioned above. Surgical intervention solely to attempt repair of the occult spina bifida is unnecessary but is indicated if neurological deficit develops due to associated hamartomatous conditions such as lipoma or dermoid (Chapter 21) or to abnormal cord fixation by diastematomyelia or cord tethering (see below).

## Other meningoceles

Diverticula of the spinal theca, probably of developmental origin, occur at sites other than posterior spina bifida. Anterior meningocele which passes through a divided vertebral body resembles the problems of a neurenteric cyst. Below, out-pouching of the theca in the thoracic and in the sacral regions are considered.

### Lateral intrathoracic meningocele

A symptomless diverticulum of the dura mater, lined by arachnoid, may pass through an intervertebral foramen and form a rounded sac within the thoracic cavity, displacing the pleura and lung and lying in the paravertebral gutter if of sufficient size. It may be discovered during radio-

logical examination of the lungs for other
purposes, throwing a soft-tissue shadow. Meningoceles, single or multiple, are prone to occur
in cases of von Recklinghausen neurofibromatosis, often in association with kyphoscoliosis.
They may cause intercostal pain and backache
but do not give signs of spinal cord implication
though these may be present if there are intrathecal neurofibromata. A large meningocele may
cause dyspnoea on exertion, particularly if pulmonary function is impaired by a severe kyphoscoliosis. X-ray examination of the spine shows
changes compatible with a dumb-bell tumour:
great enlargement of an intervertebral
foramen, increase in the interpedicular distance,
hollowing of the sides and of the posterior
aspects of the vertebral borders (scalloping)
and separation and erosion of adjacent ribs. If a
spinal curvature is present, its level coincides
with the changes due to the meningocele, and
there may be severe deformities of the vertebral
bodies.

Skeletal dysplasia is a frequent accompaniment of von Recklinghausen neurofibromatosis
and Heard (quoted by Heard & Payne 1962)
found changes in the bones of nearly one-half of
a series of 79 cases and the vertebrae were
affected in one-half of these. Apart from kyphoscoliosis the vertebral abnormalities include scalloping, widening of the interpedicular distance
and enlargement of the intervertebral foramina;
the spinal canal is enlarged but the intervertebral
discs are unaffected (except for irrelevant
degenerative changes). These abnormalities may
be present at the level of the spinal curvature
and they may be found in the lumbosacral region
identical with those reported by Jefferson (1955)
and considered congenital.

The correct diagnosis of the nature of a paravertebral soft tissue shadow in a patient with
neurofibromatosis, particularly if there is kyphoscoliosis, will rarely be in doubt. A meningocele
is much the more likely cause; a spinal neurofibroma large enough to cause the changes of a
dumb-bell tumour is not usually in keeping with
the character of von Recklinghausen disease.
Greater difficulty may arise in patients without
the stigmata of that disease; the distinction may
be made on the extent of the radiological abnormalities. In dumb-bell tumour only one foramen
is enlarged and expansion of the spinal canal is
likely to be limited to the immediately adjacent
vertebrae. In meningocele these changes are
usually seen in several vertebrae and may also
be present elsewhere in the canal. Myelography
will be conclusive.

The prime indication for surgery is that of
disturbance of pulmonary function. The
approach is by thoracotomy to allow excision of
the sac. The main difficulty is of dural closure
and, to achieve this, it may be necessary to
expose an area of dura by cautious enlargement
of the affected intervertebral foramen. Failure to
achieve watertight closure can lead to massive
pleural effusion with further respiratory embarrassment.

*Sacral meningocele*

Sacral meningoceles may present as a painless,
ill-defined sessile swelling in the buttock or perineum, this being distinguished from the midline
swelling of the much more common spina bifida.
Attention may have been drawn to the swelling
by its inconvenience or discomfort when seated.
Occasionally it causes mild pain in the buttock
and leg by its pressure on local nerves. Anterior
meningocele forms a soft swelling in the sacral
hollow, palpable by vaginal or rectal examination. It may be discovered in the course of pelvic
examination for other reasons, or as a result of
vague symptoms of pelvic fullness or ache, or of
disturbance of bladder and rectum. The anterior
meningocele is said to be more common in
women than in men but as Sutton (1963) has
suggested it may be more frequently discovered
in women because of the more frequent pelvic
examinations in that sex. The swelling of a meningocele may sometimes be clearly distinguished
from that of a true cyst by increase in its tension
and size as a result of changes in position affecting the pressure of the spinal fluid. Elevation of
the buttocks usually reduces tension and size,

but this will depend upon the diameter of its neck, commonly large.

Radiological examination reveals the bony defect which may be of varying size ranging from foraminal enlargement to sacral agenesis. The usual finding is of a bony defect lying laterally which leaves a characteristic shape to the remainder of the sacrum often referred to as 'scimitar-shaped'. There is often an associated defect in the posterior part of the sacrum.

There is a definite tendency for these lesions to gradually enlarge and so cause increasing sacral neurological deficit which demands surgical intervention. It is evident that transrectal aspiration carries a high risk of meningitis but, if the nature of the lesion is not recognized, such a manoeuvre may have been performed. Laminectomy of the remaining sacral laminae will allow safer aspiration but the dura in this area is extremely difficult to close in a watertight manner. Should such a procedure fail, the sac may be approached by either an abdominal or perineal route which is technically more difficult but can make closure of the neck easier as more tissue is available with which to reinforce the repair.

## Problems of abnormal cord fixation

Many differing abnormalities of mesoblastic differentiation may result in lesions which fixate the cord in an abnormal way such as the development of a conus lipoma or dermoid. In such cases, attention is naturally drawn to the hamartomatous lesion. Neurological disturbance more closely related to the actual abnormal fixation of the cord occurs primarily in two ways: by cord tethering; or by diastematomyelia.

### The tethered cord

Until the third month of fetal life the spinal cord and the spinal canal are of equal length. Thereafter the more rapid longitudinal growth of the vertebral column is such that at birth the tip of the conus usually lies opposite L3. If growth continues unimpeded until maturity, the conus 'ascends' further to lie opposite L1 in the adult. Abnormal fixation of the conus either directly or via the cauda equina may result in tethering of the cord such that its 'ascent' is impeded and so remains at a lower vertebral level and may be under tension.

The majority of patients with a tethered cord also have abnormalities of the lumbar spine ranging from a single level spina bifida occulta to much more widespread neural arch abnormality. The commonest agent which seems to be responsible for the tethering seems to be an abnormally thickened filum terminale with anything over 2 mm in width on myelogram being considered abnormal (James & Lassman 1972). More rarely, the conus itself is seen to be adherent to the dorsal dura. This occurrence has been related to a previously closed myelomeningocoele (Heinz et al. 1979) but is more usually seen without obvious cause, though a dermal sinus tract has also been implicated (Anderson 1975). The most likely explanation of this disorder is based on intradural adhesions (Yashon & Bealty 1966), though again the reason for such adhesions is not clear. Tethering of any nature is often associated with other abnormalities; notably, diastematomyelia and intradural lipoma.

The clinical presentation of a tethered filum is closely similar to that of diastematomyelia and is discussed later. However, it should be observed that, whereas presentation of a diastematomyelia in adult life is rare, the presentation of a tethered filum alone is much more common in adults than is usually accepted (Pang & Wilberger 1982) though approximately one-half of these adult patients had a pre-existing but static skeletal or neurological deficit. The presentation in adult life differed from that of childhood by having a much higher incidence of pain as a feature and a lower incidence of both cutaneous abnormalities and progressive kyphoscoliosis.

The same problems with regard to prophylactic surgery apply to tethered filum as do to diastematomyelia but a progressing neurological deficit is an absolute indication for early surgery.

Recovery of established deficit is rare, therefore diagnosis and treatment must take place at an early stage to prevent severe motor, sensory and sphincteric disturbance. Surgery is directed simply towards release of the tethering agent; all that is usually required is division of the filum. Associated hamartomatous lesions also require attention if present. Great care is necessary to ensure that only the filum is divided as there are often adherent neural filaments. Lindsay *et al.* (1980) have described a technique of intra-operative stimulation which greatly aids this process. Watertight dural closure can be difficult to achieve because the dura is often abnormally thin.

### Diastematomyelia

Diastematomyelia is a term which signifies pathological splitting of the spinal cord; it is usually associated with varying degrees of apparent reduplication of the cord, or diplomyelia. Indeed, such authorities as Cameron (1957) felt that the associated midline bony or cartilaginous septum represented an abortive attempt at spinal reduplication, but most agree with Lichtenstein (1940) who considered the anomaly to be primarily a split in the developing cord or 'pseudo-duplication' which may be related to the temporary presence of a neuroenteric canal *in utero* (Bremer 1952). Each half of the split cord is ensheathed with pia mater and frequently with a duplicated dural sheath. Lying in the split is found a midline septum arising from the posterior aspect of the vertebral body and passing posteriorly to a varying degree, sometimes reaching the neural arch. This septum may be bony and as such visible on plain radiology or tomography but, equally, it can be formed only of fibrous or cartilaginous material. The split may occur at any level of the cord but is usually found in the thoracolumbar area. Spurs usually occupy less than one vertebral level though on occasions they may be longer. Due to the effect of traction produced on the 'ascending' cord the split in the cord can extend over several levels usually starting closely applied to the lower end of the spur. Distal abnormalities such as tethered filum terminale are also commonly found.

Clinically, neurological deficit may be present at birth but more commonly presents with skeletal growth during early childhood. Presentation *de novo* in the adult is rare and may be associated with other factors as in a case of the author's where one of the hemichord channels had undergone spondylotic changes. Cutaneous stigmata over the back such as hairy patches are common and an associated progressive kyphoscoliosis or scoliosis is common in the growing child. Indeed, scoliosis is often the actual symptom leading to presentation. Inequality in lower limb growth and, especially in foot size, is common. Pain is unusual in children and if the presentation is not due to spinal deformity, it is usually due to progressing lower limb neurological disturbance or sphincteric abnormality. Plain radiology will reveal neural arch abnormality of greater or lesser degree and may show the midline spur if it is sufficiently ossified. In any event, myelography and CT scanning is necessary to exactly delineate the split and to show any associated abnormality such as a tethered filum or lipoma.

In cases where undoubted neurological deterioration is in progress at the time of presentation, surgery is indicated at that stage to prevent further deterioration. When diastematomyelia is diagnosed at a stage prior to the development of neurological deficit, the situation is less clear. The majority of North American authorities (for example Sheptak & Susen 1967) advocate prophylactic surgery but in this country a more conservative approach is often adopted with regular follow-up of the patient, surgery being performed at the earliest evidence of neurological change. The commonest situation where diastematomyelia is discovered prior to development of neurological deficit is in the investigation of scoliosis. In such an instance, it is customary to excise the spur prior to, or at the same time as, spinal correction to avoid the risk of increasing the traction on the cord during the distraction of the spinal column required for correction of the scoliosis.

The surgical technique for treatment of diastematomyelia involves an approach by laminectomy which can be very difficult due to the anomalous and often thickened neural arches. Having completed this, the dura above and below the split should be opened, followed by dural opening over each of the split cord segments. This is easiest to achieve starting at the rostral end of the split as the cord is less applied to the spur at this point. This manoeuvre results in the spur being left with a dural collar; all of these structures are then removed by a combination of rongeurs and air drill used under the operating microscope until the clearance is flush with the vertebral body. The posterior dura is then closed as a single tube. If a thickened filum terminale is present, this is often divided at the same procedure, though this manoeuvre often requires a further laminectomy at a lower level. Several authorities, however, feel that such a manoeuvre as a routine is unnecessary (Matson et al. 1950, James & Lassman 1972). Finally, comment has to be made on the occurrence of diastematomyelia with a single dural tube as described by Herren and Edwards (1940). In their series, James and Lassman also encountered this entity and felt that the agent responsible for the split was a fibrous band running from the dorsal rather than the ventral structures. The key to diagnosis is the finding of a low lying conus with no abnormal filum. Management is as for the more usual types of diastematomyelia.

**Lipomyelomeningocele.**

Lipomyelomeningoceles present a complex problem associated with the dysraphic process producing, not only the bony canal deformities of spina bifida, but also a subcutaneous lumbosacral lipoma which communicates through a dural defect with an abnormal and tethered spinal cord. The lipoma is often intimately related to the abnormally low conus. Chapman (1982) separated these lesions into three types, namely, dorsal, transitional and caudal. It is generally accepted that the dorsal type often present lesions which are relatively amenable to surgical excision whilst the other types present surgical difficulties of increasing proportions which make excision difficult but not impossible (Hoffman et al. 1985). In that paper, Hoffman and his colleagues stressed that the older the child was at presentation the more likely was it that neurological deficit would have appeared and, therefore, made a strong plea for investigation and surgery at a very early stage in these infants. They justify this by showing an extremely low morbidity from surgery even when performed at less than six months of age.

## Syringomyelia and hydromyelia

Syringomyelia and hydromyelia are not synonymous. Hydromyelia is, strictly speaking, the dilatation of the central canal of the cord. The size and extent of such dilatation may vary but the cavity must run through most of the cord and its wall must be lined with ependyma for the cavity to be ascribed to hydromyelia. The ependymal lining, however, may be patchily incomplete and in such areas there is glial overgrowth of the lining. Occasionally, in such an area denuded of ependyma, there may be an extension of the cavity into the cord tissue, thus forming an associated syringomyelia. Peach (1965) observed that the embryonic central canal is relatively large in diameter and that the normal narrowing of the lumen was due to development and proliferation of glia and neural tissue. He regarded hydromyelia as a persistence of this normal embryonic state due to arrest in the development of the subependymal glia.

Syringomyelia constitutes the formation of cavities within the actual parenchyma of the spinal cord (or brainstem in the case of syringobulbia). The consequent destruction of neural elements and their replacement by gliosis and cavitation leads to the associated neurological disturbance.

The walls of a syringomyelic cavity, or syrinx, include degenerate and oedematous tissue with overgrowth of glia and obliteration of some blood vessels. Such changes may be present with little or no cavitation and can extend into the cord at either end of the cavity. The disease usually affects the cervical part of the cord most severely, though extension into the first cervical segment and brainstem does occur. The cavity lies mainly in the grey matter dorsal to the central canal extending posteriorly into the dorsal columns and ventrally into the area of the anterior commisure. A syrinx may extend over much or all of the cord even reaching the filum terminale (Schlesinger *et al.* 1981 Williams & Fahy 1983), though its width typically varies at differing levels and it may even appear segmented rather akin to a string of sausages. It may either obliterate the central canal or take it up into its wall, thus explaining the occasional area of ependymal lining.

With regard to the aetiology of syringomyelia, many differing mechanisms and pathologies have been implicated. In 1969, Williams introduced the concept of communicating and non-communicating syringomyelia, referring to any existing connection between syrinx cavity and the fourth ventricle. The majority of patients with a communicating syrinx also have some form of hindbrain abnormality such as Arnold–Chiari malformation or Dandy–Walker cyst with resulting obstruction to the normal outlets of the fourth ventricle. Earlier feeling that the aetiological nature of syringomyelia was primarily a developmental fault in the spinal central canal has largely been replaced by the development of the theories of Gardner (Gardner *et al.* 1957). He suggested that the obstructed fourth ventricle could not dissipate the surges of CSF pressure related to the normal intracranial pulse wave. The only remaining outlet to the fourth ventricle lies in the opening of the central canal and the repetitive 'water-hammer' effect of the pulsation results in progressive hydromyelia with its consequent rupture into the cord substance forming a syrinx. Gardner (1968) even proposed that such a process in the fetal neural tube could lead to a caudal rupture of the tube causing myelomeningocele. Although lateral ventricular dilatation occurs in one-third of

patients with syringomyelia (West & Williams 1980) frank raised intracranial pressure is rare. Ball and Dayan (1972) further felt that the normal intracranial pulse pressure was insufficient to produce the progressive dilatation of the syrinx. Williams felt the explanation to be based upon repetitive but short-lasting pressure changes. He felt that actions such as coughing or straining resulted in an increased intraspinal pressure leading to CSF being forced upwards past the hindbrain hernia at the foramen magnum but unable to descend again due to recurrence of the tonsillar herniation on relaxation. The fluid trapped in the posterior fossa then forces CSF down the central canal. In an earlier communication, Williams (1969) had speculated that such pressure changes could also be applied to the intracranial veins which, coupled with partial blockage of the subarachnoid space at the foramen magnum, could produce a pressure greater in the spinal central canal than that of the spinal subarachnoid space which could encourage distension of the cord. Williams (1981) has produced *in vivo* evidence that such craniospinal pressure dissociation can exist. Other mechanisms of syrinx production have been suggested. Ball and Dayan (1972) suggested that fluid could reach the cord cavity by passing along abnormally large Virchow–Robin perivascular spaces as there would be an abnormally high intraspinal subarachnoid pressure due to hindbrain herniation. Others have suggested that the fluid within the syrinx is actively secreted either by glia (Barnett 1973) or by areas of ependyma. More recently, Williams and Fahy (1983) have tentatively suggested a scenario where several of these mechanisms could be active at different stages of the development of a syrinx linking it to the factor of birth trauma which is a common feature of patients with syringomyelia.

The noncommunicating type of syringomyelia is less common and relates primarily to the extension of cystic cavities within the cord or to blockage of the central canal within the cord. As is discussed in Chapter 21 intramedullary neoplasms may be associated with cystic components which may extend over many segments. Indeed, Epstein and Epstein (1982) have even suggested the possibility of syringomyelia being due to a neoplasm with a major cystic component in which the tumour involutes: a possibility discussed by Simon in 1895.

A syrinx may develop as a late event in a severe traumatic spinal cord lesion (Barnett & Jousse 1973). The development of such a complication is indicated by a late upward extension of the neurological level often many years after the injury. For an account of the possible mechanisms involved, the reader is referred to the reviews of Barnett (1973) and Schleip (1978). Some aspects of treatment have been discussed by Shannon et al. (1981) with particular emphasis on indwelling extraspinal catheter drainage. It has been claimed that arachnoiditis may be responsible at least as part of the aetiological basis for post-traumatic syringomyelia and Barnett (1973) also reviewed the rare occurrence of a syrinx in pure arachnoiditis.

The clinical features of syringomyelia are, like so many cord diseases, protean and depend to a large extent on the distribution of the lesion. The so-called classical picture is that of a stepwise though persistent deterioration culminating in a picture of dissociated sensory loss, lower motor neuron damage in the upper limbs, upper motor neuron changes affecting the lower limbs and trophic skin changes. Episodes of deterioration are often heralded by incidents of minor trauma. The early extension of the syrinx cavity into the area of the anterior commisure explains the dissociation of the sensory changes; pain and temperature sensation, the pathways for which largely cross the midline at this point, are severely affected over several segments, while other modalities which ascend in the posterior columns, though often affected to some extent, are relatively spared. Other clinical features which may be present are scoliosis, neurogenic arthropathy and, if syringobulbia is present, cranial nerve involvement. Plain radiology of the spine will show the scoliosis if present but otherwise will merely show canal expansion or be normal. Myelography may show an expanded

cord; if it also shows a hindbrain deformity on supine screening, this is very suggestive of syrinx. In the absence of hindbrain deformity the differentiation from an intramedullary tumour may be very difficult and even demonstration of a cavity by CT or endomyelography does not exclude a cystic neoplasm. The use of air or gas myelography to show 'collapse' of the cord seems to be losing popularity. CT cranial scanning should also be performed to identify any posterior fossa anomaly and to check the size of the ventricles. Magnetic resonance imaging is now the preferred method for demonstrating most clearly both the syrinx and any craniospinal junction abnormality.

The ideal management of syringomyelia is not yet clear. No method of treatment frequently results in objective improvement, though a subjective feeling of improvement by the patient is more commonly reported. It is important to be aware that any improvement may be due to the rest, increased care and physiotherapy which accompanies the surgical procedure. Surgery, especially at the cranial base, has a significant morbidity and mortality. Varying series report arrest of a previous deterioration in between one-half and three-quarters of cases but a considerable majority of those go on to later relapse.

It was Gardner who, in 1965, proposed the concept of posterior fossa decompression which has become a mainstay of treatment. As a consequence of his ideas of aetiology he advocated decompressive posterior fossa craniotomy combined with upper cervical laminectomy. He suggested that the dura should be opened and the tonsils separated or amputated, with an attempt being made to open the foramen of Magendie. The exit of the fourth ventricular floor was then explored at the obex and, if this was patent, the opening should be plugged with muscle. Whilst most agree with the posterior fossa decompression, many authors (for example Van der Zwan 1963) feel that it is the decompression which is effective and that plugging the obex or indeed separating the tonsils is unnecessary, and may be damaging. Further differences of opinion exist as to whether the syrinx cavity should be aspirated, drained by myelotomy or diverted by a tube into the subarachnoid space or to an extraspinal site. In addition, it does seem advisable to sample the cyst fluid in case it could be neoplastic in origin.

Certain factors in some of the aetiological arguments, especially the production of syringomyelia in experimental kaolin-induced hydrocephalus (Williams 1980), would favour the treatment of any associated hydrocephalus. Whilst this is not infrequently performed, it should be appreciated that the presence of ventricular enlargement does not necessarily imply an active hydrocephalus and intracranial pressure monitoring prior to CSF shunting would seem desirable. Myelotomy alone, with or without a drainage procedure but without a posterior fossa decompression, has been advocated but the difficulties of maintaining drainage long enough to allow collapse and 'fusion' of the cavity are major problems. Extending this approach and based on further suggestions by Gardner *et al.* (1957), Williams and Fahy (1983) have reported the results of what they term 'terminal ventriculostomy'. On the basis that in certain cases the syrinx cavity may extend in the filum terminale, they excised the filum and terminal conus in 34 patients, only 17 of whom had had previous surgical procedures. Although in 20 of the cases no fluid was seen escaping from the cut cord, 19 of the 34 patients reported improvement though they note that this was usually only of a subjective type. Williams and Fahy have suggested that craniovertebral decompression should remain the initial treatment of choice; if marked hydrocephalus is present, it should be treated by shunting; myelotomy, if performed, should be made where the syrinx is widest and is more likely to succeed if the fluid is drained to a low-pressure area such as the peritoneum; terminal ventriculostomy has only a restricted place in the overall management.

## Craniovertebral malformations

Abnormalities of the cranial base and the upper two cervical vertebrae, usually of congenital origin, are considered together because they may give rise to, or be associated with, somewhat similar neurological disturbances, attributable to interference with the hindbrain and the upper segments of the spinal cord. One or more of the malformations may be present in the same patient who may have other congenital stigmata; the craniovertebral abnormalities may cause no disability in one patient while in another they may lead to total disablement and death. The onset of symptoms may be precipitated by trauma of almost insignificant degree and run a rapid course; on the other hand symptoms may develop slowly and insidiously over many years and their relationship to the abnormal configuration of bone and of joint may not be apparent, particularly if these are not of a severe degree. The malformations comprise primarily: basilar impression, synostosis of the atlas and occiput (assimilation); and atlanto-axial dislocation. Their occurrence without other features of skeletal dysplasia is unusual and the whole spine should be examined. In particular, anomalous lower cervical vertebral fusions are common. Schmidt *et al.* (1978) have published a detailed review of this topic.

### Basilar impression

Bull *et al.* (1955) computed the frequency of basilar impression to be at least 1 in 3000. The essential feature is a deformation of the basi-occiput, in which the rim of the foramen magnum, the condyles and the neighbouring bone are invaginated upwards into the posterior fossa (Fig. 16.1). When severe, the intracranial surface of the basi-occiput may be as high as the level of the posterior clinoid processes. The clivus is shortened; the invagination of the margins of the foramen magnum diminishes its diameters; and the ascent of the occipital condyles carries with it the atlas so that the odontoid process

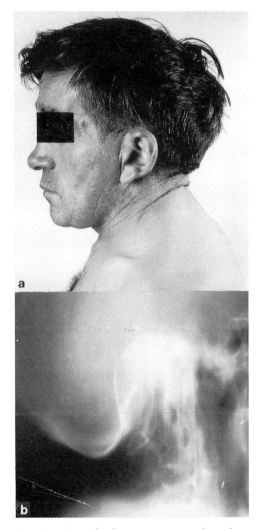

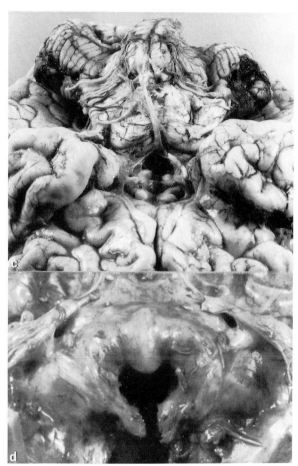

**Fig. 16.1**  Severe basilar impression in male aged 45.
(a) The short neck and overhanging occiput.
(b) Ascent of basi-occiput into cranial cavity.
(c) Deeply grooved cerebellum and deformed brain-stem.
(d) Stenosis of foramen magnum with encroachment by dens: the posterior deficiency is operative.

projects into the anterior part of the foramen magnum whose lumen is thus further reduced in its anteroposterior diameter. The arch of the atlas may be partly or wholly fused with the occipital bone, the condyles of which are often deformed asymmetrically with corresponding deformation of the articular masses of the atlas. The anterior part of the occiput is usually deformed to a greater extent than the posterior,

tilting the skull downwards and forwards and producing a compensatory cervical lordosis which may be so pronounced that it can cause difficulty in endotracheal intubation.

Basilar impression may occur with a familial incidence; Bull *et al.* found a high incidence of radiological abnormalities in relatives of clinically affected patients. It may be associated, particularly in children, with posterior fossa

abnormalities such as Arnold–Chiari malformation or Dandy–Walker cyst but it is debated
whether the much commoner finding of a degree
of cerebellar tonsillar herniation is a primary
feature or due to the upward migration of the
skull base. There is also an association with syringomyelia but to a lesser extent than with
Arnold–Chiari malformations. Basilar
impression may occur secondary to diseases
which lead to softening of bone texture such
as Paget disease, osteomalacia and osteogenesis
imperfecta.

The terms platybasia and basilar impression
are often erroneously used synonymously. Platybasia is merely a flattening of the cranial base
and, in isolation, is of no clinical significance.
The radiological criteria of true basilar impression have been widely studied and several
arbitrary lines have been proposed on which to
base measurements relating the tip of the dens
to the plane of the foramen magnum. Those most
commonly still in use are:

1  Chamberlain's (1939) line which is drawn
from the posterior margin of the hard palate to
the posterior lip of the foramen magnum: the tip
of the dens is normally below this line;
2  McGregor's (1948) line which is drawn from
the posterior margin of the hard palate to
subtend the lowest part of the occipital curve,
and below which line the tip of the dens again
should lie.

### Assimilation of the atlas

Fusion of the atlas to the occipital bone is a
developmental error; the most caudal portion of
the occiput and the most cranial portion of the
atlas having a common segmental origin. The
entire atlas may be incorporated in the occiput
with the tip of the odontoid process fused with
the lip of the foramen magnum. Incomplete
assimilation is more usual and is often associated
with a degree of occipital dysplasia. Uncomplicated assimilation is probably of no clinical
significance but it is often complicated with

abnormalities of the odontoid and/or atlanto-
axial ligaments resulting in instability. Because
of this it is important to complement plain radiology with flexion and extension views;

### Congenital atlanto-axial dislocation

This serious abnormality may arise as a complication of assimilation of the atlas due to undue
laxity of the alar ligaments of the odontoid
process and of the transverse ligaments of the
atlas. It should be distinguished from the more
common form associated with rheumatoid
arthritis. Whether the laxity in this case is a
congenital weakness or whether it is due to the
added strain imposed on them by the lack of
movement between atlas and occiput is not
known. Comparison of lateral X-ray films taken
with the head in flexion and with it in extension
reveals an increased separation of the anterior
arch of the atlas from the dens. McRae (1955)
considered that an increase greater than 3 mm
was abnormal and if the interval between the
posterior surface of the dens and the anterior
surface of the posterior arch of the atlas was

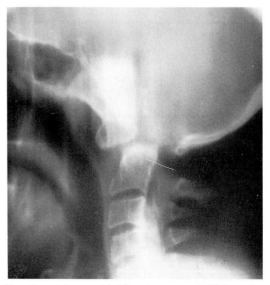

**Fig. 16.2** Atlanto-axial dislocation: congenital failure of
odontoid fusion. Also shows assimilation of the axis.

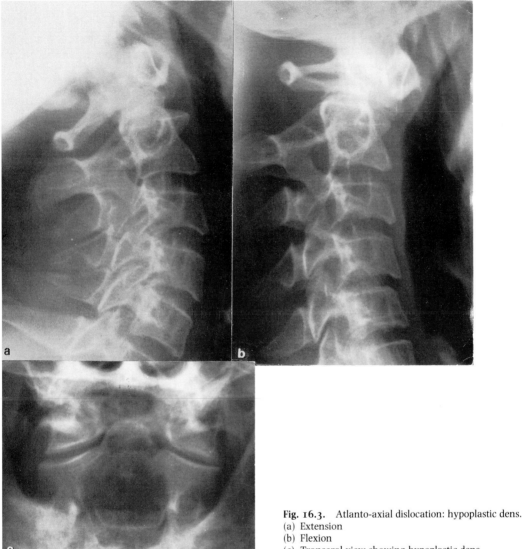

**Fig. 16.3.**  Atlanto-axial dislocation: hypoplastic dens.
(a) Extension
(b) Flexion
(c) Transoral view showing hypoplastic dens.

less than 19 mm neurological disturbance was always present. Dislocation may also arise as a result of the failure of the odontoid process to fuse with the body of the axis vertebra (Fig. 16.2) or of its aplasia (Fig. 16.3). In the former case, radiological examination demonstrates that in flexion the detached dens glides forwards with the atlas and the spinal canal becomes narrowed by the approximation of the posterior arch of the atlas to the posterosuperior margin of the body of the axis.

**Intracranial findings**

The displacement of normal structures due to these craniovertebral anomalies often causes abnormality in the posterior fossa. Basilar impression causes the brain stem to be forced upwards and compressed by the odontoid. Fibrosis and adhesions combined with the displacement may so disturb CSF circulation that hydrocephalus develops and the apparent downward dislocation of the tonsils may mimic an

Arnold–Chiari malformation. As a consequence of the deformation of the floor of the posterior fossa, the lower cranial nerves may be distorted resulting in paresis. Driesen (1961) commented on the frequency of vascular abnormalities. These comprise irregularity of calibre, hypoplasia, angiomatous malformation and irregularity of course. The vessels observed were the vertebral, posterior inferior cerebellar and posterior spinal arteries.

Sections of the deformed brain stem show nuclear degeneration, loss of myelin and gliosis. Purkinje cell loss and gliosis may be found in the cerebellum. Atlanto-axial dislocation may produce extreme flattening of the cervicomedullary junction with degeneration of the pyramidal tracts and posterior columns. Anterior horn cell loss at lower levels may also be seen. Occasionally, cavitation resulting in hydromyelia, syringomyelia or syringobulbia may be found.

### Clinical features

The external appearance of a patient with craniovertebral abnormality may be striking. A short neck, low hair-line and limitation of neck movements, features of Klippel–Feil syndrome, are frequently seen, and in some patients there may also be torticollis. In basilar impression the skull may be broader than normal and the occiput approaches the upper cervical spinous processes.

All patients with radiological evidence of craniovertebral abnormality do not have neurological sequelae; in McRae's series (1953) about one-third were asymptomatic. Symptoms may commence in childhood or may not appear until after the age of 60 years, but in about three-quarters the onset is between the ages of 10 and 40 years. The duration of symptoms varies considerably; more than half of the patients reported by Spillane et al. (1957) had had symptoms for more than 6 years. Trauma is an important precipitating factor in about a quarter of cases, but more particularly in assimilation of

the atlas. Apart from the effects of trauma, the progression of symptoms and disability is usually slow with episodes of remission in the early stages. Occasionally the onset of signs may be dramatic suggesting a vascular occlusion (Taylor & Chakravorty 1964).

In general, the function of pons, medulla and cerebellum are more frequently disturbed by basilar impression, and of the medulla and cervical cord by the anomalies of the atlas and odontoid process. But there is much overlap and blurring of syndromes produced by associated ischaemic damage, by herniation and malformation and by cavitation. Painful restriction of neck movement is usual and forceful passive movement of the head is liable to evoke faintness and a sense of weakness of the limbs. The following are also frequent complaints: diplopia, vertigo, episodes of faintness or of loss of consciousness; tinnitus; hoarseness and nasal twang of voice, dysarthria, dysphagia, vomiting and nasal regurgitation of food; respiratory embarrassment; weakness of the lower limbs aggravated by forced movements of the head and neck; ataxia of limbs and of gait; sphincter disturbance. Occasionally symptoms of raised intracranial pressure develop and papilloedema is detected.

Movement of the head and neck is generally restricted and painful and may evoke giddiness, limb paraesthesiae and even syncope. Evidence of cranial nerve paresis, especially the accessory nerve, may be present. Pyramidal signs are present in most cases sometimes amounting to severe quadriparesis. The musculature of the upper limb may show pronounced wasting; this may be symmetrical or unilateral and may affect the whole limb or only the hand. Ataxia of the limbs is more common in basilar impression, while ataxia of gait is common to all disorders. Sensory impairment may present a variety of patterns. Again it may be either symmetrical or asymmetrical involving an upper limb perhaps with spread to the trunk. Dissociated sensory loss is often associated with upper limb wasting, thus suggesting syringomyelia. Loss of proprioceptive sensation is, however, the commonest sensory disturbance, primarily of the upper limbs but also often affecting the legs.

Spillane *et al.* (1957) underlined two unusual physical signs. Mirror movements of the hands were first described by Bauman (1932) in the Klippel–Feil syndrome. Purposeful movements of the digits, hand or arm of one side are accompanied by precisely similar movements in the other limb. Nystagmus and other abnormalities of eye movements including oscillopsia are not uncommon in patients with craniovertebral abnormality.

Differential diagnosis includes many diseases which may affect the cervicomedullary junction. Important amongst these are: Arnold–Chiari malformation; tumours of the foramen magnum area such as meningioma or chordoma; syringobulbia and syringomyelia; disseminated sclerosis; and amyotrophic lateral sclerosis. Correct diagnosis depends largely on precise radiographic examination of the cranial base, utilizing plain and motion radiography, tomography myelography and CT scanning.

## Treatment

The indications for treatment are primarily those of progressive or recurrent neurological complications and occasionally hydrocephalus. Conservative measures, such as immobilization in an occipitomental collar or case, may be effective especially in cases with intermittent disability (Phillips 1955) but the majority of patients require surgical intervention. The aim of the operation is to reduce tension within the posterior fossa and on the upper cervical cord. The usual procedure is to combine posterior fossa decompression with upper cervical laminectomy. This is applicable to patients with neurological compression particularly in basilar impression but patients with pain and evident instability (particularly in atlanto-axial dislocation) also require a fusion procedure.

Particular care during intubation and patient positioning is necessary; indeed, in severe basilar impression intubation may be so difficult that tracheostomy is necessary. Postoperatively, great care is also necessary as respiratory depression and failure is not uncommon and largely accounts for the mortality of operation, which can be considerable. In 1957, Gatai found a mortality of 33% in 98 recorded cases, though by 1966 Driesen *et al.* were able to report on 75 patients only four of whom died. The posterior fossa craniectomy may be extremely difficult due to the invagination of the posterior lip of the foramen magnum, aggravated by the accompanying cervical lordosis. The dura bulges over this receding lip and its division is difficult due to its thickness, vascularity and the often close proximity of the medulla. Theoretically, it is probably advisable to divide arachnoidal adhesions which often bind down the cerebellar tonsils to the brain stem but this manoeuvre may be extremely hazardous and is often avoided, treating any hydrocephalus by a shunting procedure. Where there is major compression on either the upper cervical cord or medulla by the displaced odontoid, decompression can only be achieved satisfactorily by excision of the odontoid by a transoral route (Fang & Ong 1962).

In cases of atlanto-axial dislocation, preoperative reduction of deformity may be necessary by the use of skull traction. When reduction is complete, posterior atlanto-axial fusion is undertaken. Several methods exist but usually a combined wire and bony fusion is used. If the arch of the atlas is hypoplastic, absent or assimilated, then an occipitocervical fusion is necessary. If pre-operative reduction does not relieve the neurological deficit, a posterior decompressive procedure is hazardous as it increases the instability and there is a strong case for a transoral decompression either combined with simultaneous fusion of the atlanto-axial joints or with a standard posterior fusion.

## Craniostenosis

At birth, the bones of the skull are connected by fibrous tissue (continuous with pericranium and with the dura mater) which allows for the normal growth of the brain and for an abnormal rate of increase in the size of the head in states of raised intracranial pressure. By the age of 6 months, during which time the brain has nearly doubled its weight, the intervening bridge of fibrous tissue between neighbouring bones of the vault is narrow and the serrated junction characteristic of a suture is recognizable radiologically. The suture has considerable strength but it is still susceptible to stretching by intracranial hypertension; radiological examination of the skull of a five-year-old child with a slowly progressive hydrocephalus may reveal sutures which form a band, a centimeter wide, of interdigitating spike-like processes derived from the contiguous bones. Separation (diastasis) of sutures is negligible after 10 years of age and the sutures become obliterated by fusion (synostosis) in late adult life, commencing at the inner surface of the skull after the third decade. Craniosynostosis is therefore a normal ageing process but the term, referred to commonly as craniostenosis, is restricted to abnormalities in which premature and abnormal suture closure results in cranial and facial deformity.

The exact cause of craniostenosis is not clear other than in instances of so-called 'secondary craniostenosis'. This refers to the occasional fusion of a suture resulting from overlap of adjacent bones consequent on using a ventricular shunt with an excessively low valve pressure in the treatment of a child with marked hydrocephalus. In primary craniostenosis, however, current theory (Moss 1975) places greater stress on the role which skull base development plays in creating deformity, with most authorities agreeing that it is abnormal dural tension arising from the skull base which in some way promotes the premature closure of the calvarial suture lines. However, others feel that the prime event is sutural closure itself (Albright & Byrd 1981). Premature craniostenosis is often considered in three main categories: cranial synostosis alone; craniofacial dysostosis (Crouzon disease); and acrocephalosyndactyly (Apert syndrome). It is likely, however, that similar aetiological processes are active in each category.

The abnormalities active in the skull base are also felt to be important in preventing proper development of the midfacial skeleton resulting in the typical deformities found in the Crouzon and Apert cases of maxillary hypoplasia and the shortening of the orbits leading to severe exophthalmos. The skull deformity resulting from sutural closure depends on the number and site of the affected sutures. The various types and their associated syndromes were reviewed by Cohen (1975).

As the name implies, craniostenosis is characterized by a skull with too small a capacity. It must be distinguished from the small skull of microcephaly, in which the reduced size of the brain determines the size of the skull. In craniostenosis the skull develops in an asymmetrical manner towards unfused sutures and affected sutures are often easily palpable. The commonest isolated suture to close is the sagittal, leading to scaphocephaly. This usually causes only cosmetic problems but other sutural closure syndromes can be associated with major clinical problems such as raised intracranial pressure, hydrocephalus and papilloedema. Associated midfacial problems can cause exophthalmos, proptosis and ocular damage along with upper airway obstruction. Although the most common indication for surgical correction is a cosmetic one, the presence or potential development of any of these associated features can make surgery essential.

The therapy of craniostenosis has made great developments following the lead of the treatment of other forms of craniofacial deformity such as hypertelorism. Methods of releasing, and attempting to prevent regrowth of, prematurely closed sutures by means of linear craniectomy, calvarial morcellement or silastic covering of sutures have been widely advocated in the past, but now should probably be reserved for the treatment of solitary sagittal synostosis. More complicated forms of craniosynostosis are now treated in a more radical manner. Gillies and Harrison (1959) reported the first high Le Fort III osteotomy performed in a patient with craniostenosis. This work was greatly extended by Tessier (1967), forming the foundation for today's practice. This practice involves a multidisciplinary team of plastic, faciomaxillary and neurosurgeons, who, in addition to performing linear craniectomy, proceed to perform an anterior fossa advancement by means of a skull base osteotomy and bone grafting. This has the combined benefits of orbital enlargement and at least partial release of the skull base sutures allowing improved facial development. This procedure can be combined with definitive surgery to the facial deformity at the same time or this may be done or refined at a later stage. Such midfacial surgery is easier to perform in an older child but modern practice is to perform the calvarial and anterior fossa advancement surgery as early as possible, ideally at about six weeks of life, to allow less neurological and ocular damage and to promote facial development, thus reducing the degree of correction required in later years (Tessier 1971).

# References

ALBRIGHT A. L. & BYRD R. P. (1981) *J. Neurosurg.*, **54**, 384.
ANDERSON F. M. (1975) *Paediatrics*, **55**, 826.
AQUAVIVA R., TAMIC P. M., BRU P., TEBASCLE J. & KENDONDI H. (1966) *Proc. Third Int. Cong. Neurol. Surg.*, p. 839. Exc. Med. Foundation, Amsterdam.
BALL M. J. & DAYAN A. D. (1972) *Lancet*, **2**, 799.
BARNETT H. J. (1973) In *Syringomyelia*, p. 174. (Ed Barnett H. J. *et al.*). Saunders, London.
BARNETT H. J. & JOUSSE A. T. (1973) In *Syringomyelia*, p. 129. (Eds. Barnett H. J. *et al*). Saunders, London.
BAUMAN G. I. (1932) *J. Amer. med. Ass.*, **98**, 129.
BREMER F. W. (1927) *Dtsch. Z. Nervenheilk.*, **99**, 104.
BREMER F. W. (1952) *Arch. Path.*, **54**, 132.
BROCKLEHURST G., GLEAVE J. R. & LEWIN W. (1967) *Brit. med. J.*, **1**, 666.
BULL J. W., NIXON W. L. & PRATT R. T. (1955) *Brain*, **78**, 229.
CAMERON A. H. (1956) *Lancet*, **2**, 171.
CAMERON A. H. (1957) *J. Path. Bact.*, **73**, 213.
CARTER C. O. & ROBERTS J. A. (1967) *Lancet*, **1**, 306.
CHAMBERLAIN W. E. (1939) *Yale J. Biol. Med.*, **11**, 487.
CHAPMAN P. H. (1982) *Child's Brain*, **9**, 37.
COHEN M. M. (1975) In *Malformation Syndromes*, p. 137. (Ed. Bergsma D.). Excerpta Medica, Amsterdam.
CURTIUS F. & LORENZ I. (1934) *Zbl. ges. Neurol. Psychiat.*, **149**, 1.
DORAN P. A. & GUTHKELCH A. N. (1961) *J. Neurol. Neurosurg. Psychiat.*, **24**, 331.
DORAN P. A. & GUTHKELCH A. N. (1963) *J. Neurol. Neurosurg. Psychiat.*, **26**, 545.

DRIESEN W. (1961) *Acta Neurochirurg.*, **9**, 19.
DRIESEN W., OLDENKOTT P. & ROSSI K. (1966) *Acta Neurochirurg.*, **15**, 83.
EPSTEIN F. & EPSTEIN N. (1982) *J. Neurosurg.*, **57**, 685.
FANG H. S. & ONG G. B. (1962) *J. Bone Jt. Surg.*, **44A**, 1588.
FUCHS A. (1909) *Wien. Med. Wschr.*, **59**, 2142.
GARDNER W. J. (1965) *J. Neurol. Neurosurg. Psychiat.*, **28**, 247.
GARDNER W. J. (1968) *Clin. Neurosurg.*, **15**, 57.
GARDNER W. J., ABDULLAH A. F. & McCORMACK L. J. (1957) *J. Neurosurg.*, **14**, 591.
GARDNER W. J., BELL H. S., POOLOS P. N. *et al.* (1977) *J. Neurosurg.*, **46**, 609.
GATAI G. (1957) *Zbl. Neurochir.*, **17**, 264.
GILLIES H. & HARRISON S. H. (1951) *Brit. J. Plast. Surg.*, **3**, 123.
GUTHKELCH A. N. (1970) *Arch. Dis. Child*, **45**, 104.
HEARD G. & PAYNE E. E. (1962) *J. Neurol. Neurosurg. Psychiat.*, **25**, 345.
HEINZ E. R., ROSENBAUM A. E., SCARFF T. B., *et al.* (1979) *Radiology*, **131**, 153.
HERREN R. Y. & EDWARDS J. E. (1940) *Arch. Path.*, **30**, 1203.
HOFFMAN H. J., TAECHOLARN C., HENDRICK E. B., *et al.* (1985) *J. Neurosurg.*, **62**, 1.
HORSLEY V. (1884) *Brain*, **7**, 228.
INGRAHAM F. D. & MATSON D. D. (1954) *Neurosurgery of Infancy and Childhood*, Thomas, Springfield, Illinois.
JAMES C. C. & LASSMAN L. P. (1972) In *Spinal Dysraphism*, Butterworth, London.
JEFFERSON A. (1955) *J. Neurol. Neurosurg. Psychiat.*, **18**, 305.
JOLLY H. (1955) *Proc. roy. Soc. Med.*, **48**, 843.
JOLLY H. (1957) *Proc. roy. Soc. Med.*, **50**, 746.
LAURENCE K. M. (1957) *Proc. roy. Soc. Med.*, **50**, 745
LAURENCE K. M. (1958) *Lancet*, **2**, 1152.
LAURENCE K. M. (1964) *Arch. Dis. Childh.*, **39**, 41.
LAURENCE K. M. & COATES S. (1962) *Arch. Dis. Childh.*, **37**, 345.
LAURENCE K. M., CARTER C. O. & DAVID P. A. (1968) *Brit. J. Proc. Soc. Med.*, **22**, 146.
LENDON R. C. (1968) *Dev. Med. Child. Neurol.*, Suppl. **15**, 50.
LICHTENSTEIN B. W. (1940) *Arch. Neurol. Psychiat.*, **44**, 792.
LINDSAY K. W. & TEASDALE G. M. (1980) *Surg. Neurol.*, **14**, 49.
LORBER J. (1961) *Arch. Dis. Childh.*, **36**, 381.
LORBER J. (1965) *Paediatrics*, **35**, 589.
LORBER J. (1971) *Dev. Med. Child. Neurol.*, **13**, 279.
MacNAB G. H. (1954) *Ann. roy. Coll. Surg. Eng.*, **14**, 124.
MacNAB G. H. (1957) *Proc. roy. Soc. Med.*, **50**, 738.
MATSON D. D., WOODS R. F., CAMPBELL J. B. *et al* (1950) *Paediatrics*, **6**, 98.
McGREGOR M (1948) *Brit. J. Radiol.*, **21**, 171.
McKEOWN T. & RECORD R. G. (1960) In *Ciba Foundation Symposium on Congenital malformations*, p. 2, Churchill, London.
McRAE D. L. (1953) *Acta Radiol.*, **40**, 335.
MELNICK M. (1977) In *Handbook of Clinical Neurology*, Vol. 30, Chapter 4 (Eds. Vinken P. S. & Bruavyn G. W.), Elsevier, Amsterdam.
MOSS M. L. (1975) *Child's Brain*, **1**, 22.
PANG D. & WILBERGER J. E. (1982) *J. Neurosurg.*, **57**, 32.
PEACH B. (1965) *Arch. Neurol.*, **12**, 527.
PHILLIPS D. G. (1955) *J. Neurol. Neurosurg. Psychiat*, **18**, 58.
SCHMIDT H., SARTOR K. & HECKL R. W. (1978) In *Handbook of*

*Clinical Neurology, Vol. 32, Chap 1,* (Eds. Vinken P. S. & Bruyn G. W.) Elsevier, Amsterdam.

SCHLEIP G. (1978) In *Handbook of Clinical Neurology,* Vol. 32, Chap 10 (Eds. Vinkwen P. J. & Bruyn G. W.) Elsevier, Amsterdam.

SCHLESINGER E. B., ANTUNES J. L., MICHELSON W, J,. *et al.* (1981) *Neurosurgery,* **9**, 356.

SHANNON N., SYMON L., LOGUE V. *et al.* (1981) *J. Neurol. Neurosurg. Psychiat.,* **44**, 35.

SHARRARD W. J. W. (1967) *Proc. roy. Soc. Med.,* **60**, 676.

SHARRARD W. J., ZACHARY R. S., LORBER J. *et al.* (1963) Arch. Dis. Childh. **38**, 18.

SHEPTAK P. E. & SUSEN A. F. (1967) *Amer. J. Dis. Child,* **113**, 210.

SPILLANE J. D., PALLIS C. & JONES A, M. (1957) *Brain,* **80**, 11.

SUTTON D. (1963) *Acta Radiol.,* **1**, 787.

SUWANWELA C. & HONGSAPROBHAS D. (1966) *Proc. Third Int. Cong. Neurol. Surg.,* p. 835. Exc. Med. Foundation, Amsterdam.

TAYLOR A. R. & CHAKRAVORTY B. C. (1964) *Arch. Neurol.,* **10**, 475.

TESSIER P. (1967) *Ann. Chir. Plast,* **12**, 273.

TESSIER P. (1971) *Plast. Reconstr. Surg.,* **48**, 224.

VAN DER ZWAN, A. (1963) *J. Neurol. Neurosurg. Psychiat.,* **26**, 97.

WEST R. J. & WILLIAMS B. (1980) *Neuroradiology,* **20**, 5.

WILLIAMS B (1969) *Lancet,* **2**, 189.

WILLIAMS B. (1980) *J. Neurol. Sci.,* **48**, 109.

WILLIAMS B. (1981) *Acta Neurochir.,* **59**; 123.

WILLIAMS B. & FAHY G. (1983) *J. Neurosorg.,* **58**, 188.

YASHON D. & BEALTY R. A. (1966) *J. Neurol. Neurosurg. Psychiat.,* **29**, 244.

# Chapter 17
# Epilepsy and neurosurgery

M. D. M. SHAW, D. W. CHADWICK

## Introduction

Epilepsy is a common symptom of a wide variety
of cerebral disorders, and in one form or another
affects 0.5–1.0% of the population at some time
during their lives. Epilepsy caused by neurosurgical conditions or their treatment, or indeed
treatable by neurosurgical procedures, makes up
only a small part of the total spectrum of the
disorder. This chapter aims to discuss the neurosurgical management of epilepsy in relation to
the condition as a whole.

Evidence of craniotomy is to be found among
skulls surviving from neolithic and later periods,
and it is surmised that some of these primitive
operations may have been performed to relieve
convulsions. Hippocrates recognized that paralysis or convulsion on one side of the body might
be due to a disorder of the brain on the opposite
side and believed that it might be relieved by an
opening in the skull. The relationship between
injury to the convexity of the skull and the subsequent development of epilepsy was noted
during the eighteenth century; Percival Pott is
said to have appreciated that the important link
was brain damage. Sporadic reports of successful
operation began to appear, but progress in this,
as in other branches of surgery, awaited the
development of anaesthetics, of anti- and aseptic
techniques and of sufficient knowledge of physiology. Horsley was working at a time when the
first of these two requirements had been achieved
and when investigation into brain function was
expanding rapidly; he played an important part
in that expansion by his experimental observations on animals and on humans (Northfield
1968). His first operation after appointment as
surgeon to the National Hospital for the Para-

lysed and Epileptic (as it was then called) in
Queen Square was for the relief of epilepsy resulting from the effects of a compound fracture of
the skull which the patient had sustained 15
years previously. Similar operations and experiments related to cortical localization of function
formed a considerable proportion of his work. At
the same time physicians (in particular Hughlings Jackson and William Gowers) were paying
critical attention to the subject of epilepsy,
making major contributions by clinical study
and classification. Medical and physiological
activities continued steadily, but surgical interest
flagged. It is likely that two factors were responsible. The development of improved craftmanship
revealed the possibilities of the surgical treatment
of brain tumours; as a result more tumours and
other expanding lesions were referred to surgeons for treatment. The results were increasingly gratifying and such patients were more
urgently in need of attention than 'epileptics'; as
a consequence those surgeons interested in brain
operations found their time fully occupied to the
exclusion of epilepsy. The other factor leading to
the decline of a surgical interest in epilepsy was
the low success rate of rendering the patient free
of attacks. Improvement in the results depended
upon greater understanding of the mechanisms
involved, improved classifications and selection
and the use of technical investigations during
procedures.

Penfield was the first of the modern neurosurgeons to resurrect interest in epilepsy and he
was largely responsible for establishing the value
of operative treatment in the relief of this particularly unpleasant disorder of central nervous
function. Study of his work reveals the requirements necessary for success in this field of

597

surgery; special interest in the disorder and its consequences for the sufferer, a penetrating knowledge of the physiology and anatomy of the organ concerned, a high order of technical skill of a particularly deliberate character. These qualities are of course valid for all branches of modern surgery; they are essential for those who intend to involve themselves in the treatment of epilepsy.

## Neurophysiology

In the words of Hughlings Jackson, 'Epilepsy is the name for occasional, sudden, excessive, rapid and local discharge of grey matter'. Although stated a century ago (1873, see *Selected Writings*) at a time when precise information on the localization of function and on the physiology of the nervous system was scanty, this definition is still a satisfactorily concise generalization of a complex disorder.

Epilepsy is a phenomenon inherent in nerve cells, an abnormal manner of reaction to normal stimuli which can be brought about by a great variety of influences. It comprises two fundamental and essential processes; that a group of neurons discharge in unison and continue to do so; that this synchronous discharge is communicated to adjacent nerve cells and to those at a distance by spread through neuronal pathways. The surgery of epilepsy is for the most part based upon the conception of a locus of abnormality from which the phenomenon is initiated.

### The control of cellular excitability

There is now greater insight into the phenomena which control seizure threshold at a cellular level in epileptogenic foci. This has resulted from study of both acute (local application of penicillin) and chronic (sub-pial alumina gel) models of focal seizures as well as study of human material obtained during neurosurgical procedures.

Normal cells have both inhibitory and excitory

influences causing excitory and inhibitory post-synaptic potentials (EPSPs and IPSPs). Once a critical membrane depolarization occurs an action potential is propagated. This leads to firing of individual neurons in a repetitive fashion, with quiescence, usually for more than 5ms between successive action potentials (Evarts 1964).

Neurons in epileptogenic foci (experimentally produced by penicillin or alumina gel, or in human foci), exhibit a different pattern of firing. The prime characteristic of epileptic neurons is the paroxysmal depolarization shift (PDS) which is more prolonged than the EPSP (Prince 1968). It results in burst firing of neurons with interspike intervals of less than 5ms, instead of isolated spike firing (Wyler *et al.* 1982). Bursts of action potentials from epileptic neurons terminate spontaneously and the cell then remains refractory for a prolonged period of time until the next burst of action potentials.

Such 'Group 1' epileptic neurons are found at the centre of an epileptic focus and fire spontaneously, usually uninfluenced by afferent inputs. (They may rarely fire in response to afferent stimuli, but when they do so, they again respond with a burst rather than a single spike.) They thus act as an epileptic 'pacemaker'. Immediately surrounding a population of such neurons 'Group II' neurons are found. These neurons can fire in normal patterns, and can be influenced by afferent inputs, but they can also exhibit PDS, and burst firing. They may be recruited by primary neurons at the centre of a focus. It appears that burst firing by neurons at the centre of a focus may be the basis of the cortical spike, the electroencephalographic (EEG) interictal discharge characteristic of an epileptic focus (Prince 1968). This is true in acute focal epilepsy induced by the topical application of penicillin (Wyler *et al.* 1982), although a less direct relationship between these two phenomena may exist in chronic models of focal epilepsy and human epilepsy. When a critical mass of surrounding Group II neurons is recruited this may then result in a focal seizure and corresponding EEG discharge.

The fundamental question that must be

addressed concerns the changes within a focus that result in this altered functional activity. A number of possibilities have been suggested, and it may be that a combination of these is necessary to explain why widely differing phenomena such as acute application of penicillin, or the development of gliosis following alumina gel or naturally occurring human pathology, can ultimately result in similar neurophysiological abnormalities.

The first question to be resolved is whether PDS is a result of abnormal afferent input to normal neurons, or a primary abnormality of neurons within a focus. Whilst normal pyramidal tract neurons (particularly in prefrontal and hippocampal regions) can, under some circumstances, exhibit burst firing, the structure of such bursts and those evoked by orthodromic stimulation of thalamic neurons differs from those seen in neurons within epileptic foci (Wyler et al. 1973). It therefore seems unlikely that burst firing is evoked by a hypersynchronous afferent input.

Given the assumption that PDS and burst firing are intrinsic functions of epileptic cortical neurons, a number of factors might be implicated in such an abnormality. All must have a final common pathway either by altering ionic conductances of membranes, or by modifying responses to neurotransmitter release. The pathological changes capable of giving rise to focal epilepsies are diverse, and include tumours, arteriovenous malformation and cortical scarring. All may be associated with one or more of three histopathological changes: neuronal cell loss, neuronal degeneration and morphological change, and gliosis.

There is mounting evidence of selective loss of inhibitory interneurons within epileptic foci. It has been demonstrated that loss of aspinous and sparsely spinous stellate neurons occurs within alumina gel foci. Axon terminals of such neurons contain the enzyme glutamic acid decarboxylase (GAD), suggesting that their synapses onto pyramidal neurons release gamma-amino butyric acid (GABA), a major inhibitory CNS transmitter (Ribak et al. 1981). Similar loss of GABA-

ergic inhibitory terminals is seen in infant monkeys following hypoxia (Sloper et al. 1980), and decreased GAD activity (Lloyd et al. 1981) and in some instances decreased GABA content may be found within human epileptic foci removed at operation (Van Gelder et al. 1972). As penicillin probably owes its convulsant properties to its GABA receptor antagonist action (Woodbury 1980), a crucial role for the selective loss of GABAergic function within foci is attractive, although a causal relationship has yet to be proved.

Pyramidal cells receive excitatory synaptic inputs mainly from dendritic spines and fine dendritic terminations. Pyramidal neurons from alumina gel foci show loss of dendritic spines and terminal branches (Ward 1969) as do hippocampal pyramidal cells from temporal lobectomy specimens (Scheibel & Scheibel 1973). This phenomenon might give rise to hyperexcitability and paroxysmal discharge either due to cortical deafferentation and resultant receptor supersensitivity (Sharpless 1969), or to displacement of synaptic EPSPs closer to the action potential initiation zone of the initial segment of pyramidal neurons, where they might possess a greater potency in triggering burst firing (Schwartzkroin & Wyler 1980).

Reactive gliosis is a prominent feature in and around many epileptogenic foci. It has been suggested that as glial cells are important in controlling extracellular concentrations of $K^+$ and excitatory neurotransmitters, that increased numbers of fibrous or reactive glial cells might impair these processes contributing to membrane instability (Ward 1978). This hypothesis lacks firm experimental support.

## The spread of epileptic activity

Whatever the mechanisms of focal discharge, the pathways by which such activity spreads to influence activity in other cortical areas are of fundamental importance to the surgical treatment of epilepsy. Of prime importance are those mechanisms by which focal seizures become generalized, with synchronized EEG activity over both hemispheres and impaired consciousness.

Normal consciousness is maintained by the interaction of cortical structures with brainstem reticular formation, the latter influencing cortical activity via nonspecific thalamocortical pathways. These pathways offer a route by which cortical activity might become synchronized, either when a discharge arises in a primary fashion at a reticular or thalamic level, or if such a pathway is activated secondarily to a focal cortical discharge.

That such a discharge might arise centrally has classically been accepted to explain primary generalized tonic–clonic seizures and absences (petit mal) as 'centrencephalic epilepsies' (Penfield & Jasper 1954). This was based on the classical observations of Jasper and Droogleever-Fortuyn (1946) that stimulation of the thalamic nuclei at low frequency could evoke generalized cortical spike and wave disturbance, similar to that seen in patients with petit mal epilepsy. This phenomenon was dependent on the degree of arousal of the experimental animal, suggesting that changes in the reticular activity were also important. Indeed stimulation of the midbrain reticular formation at the same rate as thalamic stimulation augmented the response (Perot 1963). However, the role of a reticular or thalamic pacemaker in the generation of generalized epileptiform discharge has become increasingly questioned for a number of reasons.

Bennet (1953) demonstrated that whilst intracarotid injection of metrazol in the cat produced spike and wave discharge, intravertebral arterial injection (affecting the thalamus and reticular formation) did not. Further evidence supporting the primary importance of the cortex in generation of generalized discharges has come from the animal model of epilepsy produced by the systemic injection of penicillin (Prince & Farrell 1969). This produces both absence seizures and generalized spike and wave, the latter appearing first in the cortex, and only subsequently spreading to subcortical structures (Fisher & Prince 1977). Furthermore, both metrazol and conjugated oestrogen can evoke spike and wave discharge, and apparent absence seizures, when applied bilaterally to the frontal cortex of cat and monkey (Marcus & Watson 1966 and 1968). The synchrony of this discharge was disrupted by corpus callosum section, but not by isolation of the two homologous areas of frontal cortex from other structures as long as the corpus callosum connection between the two areas was maintained. This illustrated that at least in this model bilateral synchrony was achieved by callosal rather than thalamic pathways.

The relationship between one area of cortex and its homologous area in the contralateral hemisphere is of particular importance to the surgical treatment of temporal lobe epilepsies. An experimentally induced lesion in one hemisphere, may after a latent period lead to the development of spike discharge from the contralateral homologous cortex. Initially, spiking in the two areas is time linked, but eventually the 'mirror focus' may become independent, and abnormal activity may continue after the removal of the originally injured cortex (Morrell 1960). The development of a mirror image focus may be prevented by commisure section (Lowrie et al. 1978). This has important clinical implications as temporal spikes are frequently seen to be bilateral and apparently independent in human epilepsies. Fortunately it may still be possible to demonstrate that activity on one side is primary, by showing that unilateral carotid injections of amylobarbitone abolishes spikes bilaterally. In any event, temporal lobectomy appears as beneficial in patients with bilateral spiking, as in those with unilateral spikes (Engel et al. 1975).

## Classification

Hughlings Jackson was able to provide an adequate physiological definition of epilepsy as 'a recurrent abnormal discharge of neural tissue'. No such easy clinical definition can be proposed because of the infinite variety of clinical manifestations of such a discharge. It is necessary to describe and classify both seizures themselves, as well as the way in which recurrent and various seizure types combine in an individual patient's epilepsy.

## Seizures

Table 17.1 summarizes a 1981 international classification of seizures. The major division in this classification is between partial and generalized seizures; the former begin locally at the cortex, in which there is an aura which reflects the functional role of that part of the cortex in which the seizure discharge begins. Such seizures may also be associated with postictal focal disturbances (for example, Todd's phenomenon). These are differentiated from primarily generalized seizures which commence bilaterally and in which consciousness is lost suddenly and the

**Table 17.1.**   Classification of seizures

**Partial seizures** (seizures beginning locally)

*Simple* (consciousness not impaired)
  a with motor symptoms
  b with somatosensory or special sensory symptoms
  c with autonomic symptoms
  d with psychic symptoms

*Complex* (with impairment of consciousness)
  a beginning as simple partial seizures (progressing to complex seizure)
  b impairment of consciousness at onset
      i) impairment of consciousness only
      ii) with automatism

*Partial seizures becoming secondarily generalized*

**Generalized seizures**

*Absence seizures*
  a simple (petit-mal)
  b complex

*Myoclonic seizures*

*Clonic seizures*

*Tonic seizures*

*Tonic–clonic seizures*

*Atonic seizures*

patient therefore experiences no significant aura. Any partial seizure may spread to become generalized with a secondary tonic–clonic (grand mal) seizure.

Electroencephalographic (EEG) findings help differentiate partial and generalized seizures. Interictal EEGs tend to show focal spikes, and, on occasion, associated focal slow waves in patients with partial seizures, but synchronous, high amplitude, generalized spike and wave discharge in patients with generalized seizures. Recordings taken during a seizure will show either an initial localized onset in a partial seizure, or a generalized onset. Postictally localized or generalized slowing of activity will be seen depending on whether or not the seizure remained focal.

### Simple partial seizures

The symptoms described during partial seizures are of prime importance in neurology and neurosurgery as they provide valuable information as to the site of origin of seizure discharge.

The most common origins for simple partial seizures are within the frontal or temporal lobes.

Frontal seizures most commonly manifest as *adversive attacks*. These comprise tonic or clonic deviation of the head and eyes away from the side of the discharging focus, often associated with jerking of the arm of that side or the adoption of a raised flexed posture of the arm. On occasion, seizures may begin similarly in the leg. Penfield and Rasmussen (1950) found that conjugate deviation of the eyes and less frequently turning of the head, resulted only from stimulation of the precentral cortex, at the junction of the hand and face areas. It may be that when tonic posturing of the limbs is associated with such head and eye movements, that this has a different significance. Foerster (1936) obtained such mass movements by stimulating areas of frontal, parietal and temporal cortex. Such movements can persist after ablation of the motor cortex or section of the pyramidal tracts. Indeed they may even occur with ipsilateral stimulation (Denny-Brown 1966).

Penfield and Rasmussen comment upon immediate loss of consciousness with either generalized convulsion, or adversion, which occurred in a proportion of patients with a frontal cortical lesion. It is tempting to correlate the facility with which frontal epileptogenic lesions cause generalized seizures with the observation that status epilepticus is more commonly associated with lesions of this area of the brain than elsewhere (Janz 1964).

Adversion as a form of frontal lobe seizure is more common than the classically described Jacksonian seizure with a recruiting march over the motor cortex. Both types of motor seizure may be followed by a Todd's hemiparesis. Involvement of the frontal speech areas may give rise to sudden speech arrest, or unintelligible muttering, associated with, or independent of, other motor features.

*Epilepsia partialis continua* represents a rare form of frontal seizure. It consists of repetitive rhythmic jerking of groups of muscles in the arm, leg or face, originally described in association with epidemic encephalitis in Russia. However, the syndrome is seen most frequently in association with vascular disease, and with tumours. The jerking may last for hours or days at a time and tends to be highly refractory to conventional anticonvulsant drugs.

A greater variety of simple partial seizures occur due to temporal lobe disturbance. When the uncus is involved the patient may experience abnormalities of taste or smell, usually of an unpleasant nature. Epigastric disturbances are common and it is increasingly recognized that pallor, flushing, and changes in heart rate and other autonomic features may accompany temporal lobe disturbances making their differentiation from syncopy at times difficult. A variety of psychic phenomena may be experienced in seizures with temporal lobe origin without consciousness being impaired. *Déjà vu* and *jamais vu* phenomena are common but patients may also perceive auditory or visual hallucinations which seem to represent some form of 'memory playback'. Commonly these experiences may be 'indescribable'.

Other types of simple partial seizures are less common. Those arising from the parietal region are characterized by positive sensory disturbance and paraesthesiae. They may be difficult to differentiate from sensory ischaemic symptoms of migrane and transient ischaemic attacks. Occipital scizures are even more uncommon and cause the perception not of formed images, but of balls of light, flashes or colours usually confined to the contralateral half visual field.

### Complex partial seizures

Complex partial seizures (psychomotor seizures) are differentiated from simple partial seizures by varying degrees of impairment of consciousness. This impairment of consciousness may be preceded by symptoms of a simple partial type usually those associated with a temporal lobe origin (*see* above). However in some instances consciousness may be impaired at the outset of the seizure, and thus an aura (the usually characteristic feature of a partial seizure) may be absent.

Complex partial seizures are more commonly associated with complex visual and auditory hallucination than are simple temporal seizures. They may include perceptual illusion with objects appearing larger or smaller or distorted. There may be perseveration of images. There is often an emotional component to seizures, most commonly a feeling of fear and foreboding, but occasionally anger, depression or even elation.

Complex partial seizures are not infrequently associated with ictal automatism which is usually crude in type (smacking of the lips, facial movement, or fidgeting and picking at the clothes). Occasionally more complex behaviour is seen which may lead to arrest for shoplifting, indecent exposure or other antisocial acts. Complex partial seizures are frequently succeeded by postictal confusion.

Whilst automatism is a hallmark of complex partial seizures, it may also occur in association with generalized absence seizures and as a postictal phenomenon.

On occasion, complex partial status epilepticus may occur, in which patients exhibit a prolonged abnormal mental state with confusion and disorientation which is frequently associated with automatic behaviour and with subsequent amnesia for the entire period of time during which these events occurred.

## Generalized seizures

The most common form of generalized seizure (whether this occurs in a primary fashion or following a partial seizure), is the tonic–clonic or grand-mal attack. When of primary origin the patient experiences no aura but may describe a more nonspecific and longer lasting prodrome of general malaise. The patient initially demonstrates a tonic phase with extension and opisthotonus associated with respiratory arrest and cyanosis. Emptying of bladder and bowel may occur. Subsequently the patient enters a clonic phase of rhythmic generalized jerking lasting for a variable length of time. (Less commonly only tonic or clonic phases may be seen.) This is followed by deep coma with an ascending conscious level which usually includes a postictal phase of confusion and sometimes automatic behaviour. On becoming fully conscious, usually within 15–60 minutes, the patient may experience generalized aches and pains consequent on uncoordinated muscle activity, become aware of a bitten tongue and have a generalized headache and feeling of lethargy with a desire to sleep.

Other types of generalized seizure always occur on a primary basis, and are characterized by briefer attacks which invariably begin during childhood, and rarely persist into adult life.

The most classical, but probably the rarest type of such childhood generalized seizures, is the petit mal seizure. This is characterized by sudden, usually momentary, absence during which a child loses contact with its surroundings. There may be some minor myoclonic activity around the eyelids. These attacks may occur very frequently during the course of the day and the child is frequently unaware of their occurrence. This form of epilepsy may declare itself as learning difficulty at school due to the effect that frequent seizures have on concentration.

Atypical (complex) absences are more common, and usually occur as part of a symptomatic epilepsy in children with pre-existing brain damage. The absences are more prolonged, and frequently associated with myoclonic activity, or atonic attacks both of which may result in the child being thrown to the ground, frequently suffering trauma.

Brief myoclonic jerks occur in a number of differing epileptic syndromes. They may be associated with absence (as in complex absences) or more commonly occur without impairment of consciousness. The arms tend to be most frequently involved in a sudden flexion movement.

## Status epilepticus

This is a state of recurrent tonic–clonic seizures without recovery of consciousness between attacks. It represents a medical emergency with a high morbidity and mortality. Status may occur in approximately 3% of epileptic patients but is most common in patients with severe epilepsy, who are noncompliant with drug therapy. It may also occur following alcohol withdrawal, as well as in acute meningitis or encephalitis or other metabolic disturbance. An initial presentation with status epilepticus is particularly common with frontal lobe lesions such as tumour or abscess.

## Relative frequency of seizures types

Data on the relative frequency of seizure types is unsatisfactory as it is largely based on populations of patients with relatively severe epilepsy which include large numbers of patients with partial epilepsies. With this in mind most series would suggest that approximately one third of epilepsies may be of a generalized type whilst

Table 17.2.  Incidence of seizure types. Taken from a population of 1505 patients with nonfebrile seizures from Aarhus, Denmark (Juul-Jensen & Foldspang 1983).

| Type of seizure | % |
| --- | --- |
| Primary tonic–clonic | 25.6 |
| Petit-mal | 3.9 |
| Myoclonic epilepsies | 3.1 |
| Simple partial seizures | 4.9 |
| Complex partial seizures | 17.9 |
| Partial + tonic–clonic | 14.4 |
| Alcohol-induced seizures | 6.3 |
| Stress-induced seizures | 8.0 |
| Drug-induced seizures | 1.3 |
| Isolated unprovoked seizures | 13.4 |
| Unclassified | 1.2 |
| | ____ |
| | 100 |

two thirds are partial (most commonly with a temporal lobe origin) (Table 17.2).

## Epilepsies

Seizures of similar types occur in differing clinical settings where they carry varying significance. Alternatively specific seizure types may only be seen in one epileptic syndrome. Clearly the management of epileptic patients must be geared to their epilepsy, in its broadest terms and as it affects their lives, rather than simply the management of their seizures.

It will be recognized that three major factors interact in an individual patient to determine the manifestation of seizure disorder. These are:

1  the genetic predisposition towards seizures;
2  the age of the patient;
3  underlying cerebral pathology.

Thus similar degrees of head injury may or may not be complicated by post-traumatic epilepsy depending on the presence of absence of a family history of epilepsy. The presence of a similar cerebral pathology may result in a sec-

ondarily generalized epilepsy should the pathology be present from early life, or a partial epilepsy should the pathology develop in later life. In some patients the only abnormality may be a family history of epilepsy, in others a specific pathology such as cerebral abscess will result in epilepsy irrespective of genetic factors.

The classification of epileptic syndromes presents formidable problems. Inevitably there are patients whose epilepsy fails to correspond to rigid classification, but the following represents a description of the more common epileptic syndromes, their prognosis and their significance.

### The partial epilepsies

These epilepsies are characterized by the occurrence of partial seizures with or without secondary tonic–clonic seizures. They develop at any age but become proportionately more common with increasing age. Partial epilepsies are often symptomatic of structural brain disease. This is most clearly demonstrated by findings from studies of CT scanning in epileptic patients. Gastaut and Gastaut (1976) studied 401 patients, and found abnormalities in 63% of patients with partial seizures, compared to 11% of patients with generalized seizures.

Whilst partial epilepsy in childhood may be symptomatic of structural disease, this is by no means inevitable. Simple motor seizures are commonly seen in benign focal motor epilepsy of childhood. In this syndrome, which is more common than petit mal epilepsy, simple motor seizures commence between the ages of 8 and 12 years in an otherwise normal individual. Seizures tend to be few in number, occur mainly during sleep and rarely progress to grand-mal seizures. They remit, usually in adolescence, without a risk of later epilepsy (Louiseau & Beaussart 1973). The EEG shows the presence of well localized Rolandic area spike discharge. Similar forms of benign focal epilepsy in childhood may more rarely result in somatosensory or visual seizures.

Other simple partial epilepsies, commencing in childhood, may be associated with structural disease, but this is usually of a nonprogressive nature. Tumours are rarely a cause of partial epilepsy before adulthood (Yang *et al.* 1979).

The significance of partial epilepsy commencing in adult life is the relatively high expectation of finding a tumour. Approximately 10% of patients with late onset epilepsy (over the age of 25 years) have brain tumours (Raynor *et al.* 1959, Juul-Jensen 1964). This incidence rises to 30–40% where there is a clear history of partial seizures (Raynor *et al.* 1959, Sumi & Teasdall 1963).

The likelihood of finding a neoplastic basis for epilepsy during adult life is strongly influenced by partial seizure type. In a representative series of 1685 patients with partial epilepsy commencing after 25 years, tumours were identified in 21% of 1211 patients with simple motor epilepsy, 56% of 98 patients with somatosensory epilepsy, 24% of 148 patients with other simple sensory seizures (auditory, visual, olfactory, gustatory) and 13% of 228 patients with complex partial epilepsy (Mauguirre & Courjon 1978). Tumours arising in parietal and frontal lobes seem most frequently to be complicated by epilepsy (Penfield & Jasper 1954).

Obtaining an adequate clinical description of seizures is the single most important step towards identifying a neoplastic basis for epilepsy. The finding of focal slow wave disturbance on the EEG, and the presence of localizing neurological signs, further increases the probability of a positive result from CT scanning (Young *et al.* 1982).

*Complex partial epilepsy*

Complex partial epilepsy (CPE) demands particular discussion because of its significance, associations, and its poor response to medical therapy. In this syndrome complex partial seizures occur with or without tonic–clonic seizures, and present the most frequent management problem for the adult neurologist. Whilst associated tonic-clonic seizures are usually suppressed by anticonvulsant therapy, complex partial seizures often continue, with a tendency to show

clustering in time. Neurological clinics are full of patients with continued complex partial seizures in spite of large and frequently changed doses of anticonvulsants. It is thus in this disorder that selection of patients for neurosurgical treatment is of greatest importance.

The aetiology of complex partial epilepsies remains obscure in the majority of patients. Before the advent of CT scanning, Currie *et al.* (1971) found tumours in 9.5% of 666 patients with temporal lobe epilepsy (7% gliomas). With CT scanning Gastaut and Gastaut (1976) found tumours in 16% of patients with late onset complex partial epilepsy. The latter authors found an abnormal CT scan in 60% of patients with CPE, but generalized and localized atrophy were by far the most common radiological findings.

This is very much in keeping with histological findings derived from more highly selected cases subjected to temporal lobectomy. Mathieson (1975) has reported findings in 857 such cases. In 40% little or no abnormality was detected. Some form of atrophic or gliotic lesion was found in 36% (hippocampal sclerosis in 15%), gliomas accounted for 12%, and other tumours and hamartomas for 3%.

Thus the chances of finding a surgically treatable tumour in patients with late onset complex partial epilepsy is remote. Again further help in this respect can be obtained from the EEG. Bitemporal abnormalities are common in complex partial epilepsy (25–30%), but do not seem to occur with neoplasia, where it is usual to see strictly unilateral disturbance (Klass 1975, Engel *et al.* 1975).

Particular interest has been aroused in the relationship between complex parial epilepsy and Ammon's horn (mesial temporal) sclerosis. This consists of loss of neurons from the $H1$ sector of the hippocampus (Fig. 17.1). It was found in 50% of Falconer's temporal lobectomy specimens (Falconer & Serafetinides 1963). Accumulating evidence suggests that this results from prolonged seizures affecting the immature brain, often in the presence of hyperpyrexia (Meldrum 1975). In such circumstances relative hypoxia

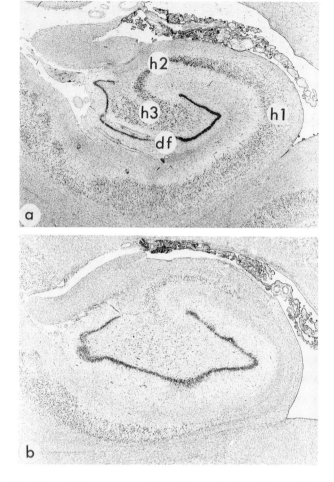

**Fig. 17.1.**(a)   A section of normal hippocampus stained with cresyl violet and magnified 13 times. The picture shows the traditional diversion of the cortical ribbon into the 3 fields: h1 or Sommer sector, h2 or resistant part and h3 or end folium. df indicates the dentate fascia.

(b)   The staining and the magnification are the same as in (a). In the classical hippocampal sclerosis of the epileptic patient the neuronal population in the h1 field is almost totally destroyed. There is also a marked loss of nerve cells in the end folium and to a lesser extent in the dentate fascia. Some neurons always survive in the resistant part.

This specimen came from a mentally subnormal woman of 48 who had suffered from epilepsy since infancy. (Kindly provided by Dr J. A. N. Corsellis.)

may occur due to the excess metabolic activity of discharging neural tissue, even in the presence of artificially maintained respiration and perfusion (Meldrum *et al.* 1974). However, it remains uncertain how specific the abnormality is for complex partial epilepsy, and whether it represents a cause, or a consequence of the dis-order. Margerison and Corsellis (1966) found the lesion 36 of 55 unselected epileptic patients coming to autopsy, and in 72% it was associated with a clinical history temporal lobe seizures, and temporal EEG changes. Similar hypoxic damage was however, apparent in the cerebellum, amygdala, thalamus and cerebral cortex.

## Mental disturbance and CPE

Psychiatric abnormality is a common accompaniment of epilepsy. This relationship has been recognized for many years. Hughlings Jackson was impressed by this and stated that 'epilepsy was the cause of insanity in 6% of insane persons'. Whilst the definitions and percentages may have changed in subsequent years, a large literature exists to support this bald statement.

Rutter *et al.* (1970) in a study of the school population of the Isle of Wight found that behavioural disorders were approximately four times more frequent in children with uncomplicated epilepsy than in the general population. They were two to three times more common than in children with physical disability that did not involve the brain. Patients with complex partial epilepsies suffer the highest incidence of psychiatric abnormality. Pond and Bidwell (1959) found evidence of psychological disorder in 29% of epileptic patients in general practice population, but in 50% of patients with temporal lobe epilepsy.

However the range of abnormalities found is wide. It encompasses personality disorder, affective illness, psychoses and intellectual impairment. In no case is there good evidence for specificity in the clinical manifestations of these abnormalities.

## Personality disorders and CPE

It is a commonly held belief that patients with complex partial epilepsy exhibit specific personality traits. They are said to be irritable, impulsive and bad tempered and to show unusual degrees of egocentricity, religiosity and perseveration. In short, they have an unparalleled talent for annoying people.

How close to the truth this is remains controversial. Bear and Fedio (1977) have recently studied 27 patients with temporal lobe epilepsies (15 with right sided abnormalities, 12 with left sided abnormalities) and compared these with a control group without epilepsy. They found that humourless sobriety, dependence and circumstantiality most strongly characterized the epileptic patients. Patients with left sided abnormality more frequently showed abnormalities of personality than those with right sided changes, and tended to be more angry, paranoid and dependent. Others have suggested that patients with temporal lobe epilepsies exhibit a triad of religiosity, hypergraphia and hyposexuality (Waxman & Geschwind 1975). However, this evidence can be balanced by an equal volume of evidence which refutes these ideas (Tizzard 1962, Small *et al.* 1966).

One very commonly held belief is that epileptic patients exhibit violent and antisocial behaviour, and that in particular violent crime may be committed during the course of ictal or postictal automatism. Gunn has shown that epilepsy is three times more common in the male prison population than in the community as a whole (Gunn 1977), and that the prevalence is highest in violent offenders. However, such crude observations may well be artifactual, reflecting that epileptic patients are more likely to come from deprived socioeconomic backgrounds (Treiman & Delgado-Escueta 1983). Furthermore, exhaustive search amongst the prison population reveals very few cases in which violent crime can be directly linked to either ictal or postictal automatism (Gunn & Fenton 1971). In spite of this overall negative evidence, some proponents would still suggest that rage reactions and episodic discontrol syndromes may result from unrecognized subclinical temporal lobe seizures (Rodin 1982).

## Psychosis

Not only do epileptic patients have a higher than expected incidence of psychotic illness (Gundmundsson 1966), but epilepsy is itself unexpectedly common in psychotic patients. This association has fascinated psychiatric observers, and stimulated a number of detailed studies (Trimble 1983). Once again these disorders are most common in patients with CPE. Psychotic episodes may be brief, or prolonged. The psychotic symptoms reported had no specific features, and there was a mean difference in onset of 14 years between epilepsy and psychosis (Slater *et al.* 1963). In some instances brief psychotic episodes appeared to follow seizures, in others more chronic psychoses became less severe than when seizures occurred. Flor-Henry (1969) suggested that the association of complex partial epilepsy and psychosis was much more common when the dominant lobe was involved.

*Affective and neurotic disorders*

Depression, of an endogenous type, is perhaps the most common psychiatric disorder in epileptic patients (Betts 1974). It has been suggested that this is most common in patients with non-dominant temporal lobe lesions (Flor-Henry 1969). Suicide is also common in epileptic patients (Rodin 1968), as is selfpoisoning with anticonvulsant drugs. Pond and Bidwell (1959) found that neurotic symptoms accounted for half the psychiatric disturbances in epileptic patients in a general practice.

*Cognitive function*

Patients with epilepsy are often held to be retarded or show intellectual deterioration. Such problems are most commonly seen in patients with brain damage acquired prior to the onset of epilepsy, and who suffer additional psychosocial isolation, as well as the often insidious adverse effects of anticonvulsant drugs (Trimble 1980). Epilepsy *per se* only rarely contributes directly to mental deterioration, and it must be remembered that populations of noninstitutionalized epileptic patients have I.Q.s within the range of normal.

The association between epilepsy in general, and complex partial epilepsy in particular, and psychiatric disturbance has been a great stimulus to speculation about the role of the temporal lobe in the production of mental symptoms.

Clearly the temporal lobe has important functions in both emotion and perception due to its association with the primitive limbic system. The possibility that temporal lobe pathology may directly cause both complex partial epilepsy and psychiatric symptoms, or that persisting temporal lobe epileptic disturbances may cause secondarily disturbance of other temporal lobe functions is an intriguing possibility.

*Primary generalized epilepsies*

It is important to consider the primary generalized epilepsies to contrast them with more neurosurgically relevant partial epilepsies. They occur in subjects without neurological disease on an apparently genetic basis. The prime EEG characteristic is the generalized spike and wave discharge. Onset before the age of 3 years is uncommon, and after the age of 25 years these epilepsies progressively decrease in incidence.

Most commonly primary generalized epilepsy presents with tonic–clonic seizures beginning in childhood or adolescence. There is no aura, although myoclonus may precede seizures (*see* below). Seizures tend to be infrequent, respond well to therapy, and become less frequent with maturity. Less commonly more clearly defined primary generalized epileptic syndromes are encountered.

*Petit mal epilepsy*

This is a relatively rare syndrome which occurs in the absence of identified cerebral disease. There is a positive family history in up to 40% of cases (Metrakos & Metrakos 1961). Twin studies have shown a concordance rate as high as 75% (Lennox 1960). Siblings of children with true petit mal have the characteristic EEG disturbance of 3 Hz spike and wave in up to 80% of cases even in the absence of clinical seizures.

Simple absences begin between the ages of 3 and 15 years. They rarely persist into adult life, and only 30–50% of patients develop grand mal seizures during early or later life.

A prime requirement for the diagnosis of true petit mal is the observation of classical generalized 3 Hz spike and wave pattern on the EEG.

It must be emphasized that this is a rare syndrome. It is still true that any minor seizure may be described by non-neurologists as petit mal. The diagnosis can practically be excluded if the attacks are occurring in adult life, when minor seizures are invariably a form of partial epilepsy.

### Benign myoclonic epilepsy of adolescence

A benign myoclonic epilepsy is seen developing in adolescence, characterized by early morning myoclonic jerks mainly of the upper limbs which occur without obvious alteration in consciousness, and which may on occasion build up in frequency prior to a generalized tonic–clonic seizure. The disorder is most commonly seen commencing in adolescence and the EEG shows spike and wave activity often associated with a myoclonic response that is particularly easily induced by photic stimuli, but which may also occur in response to other sensory stimuli, for example sudden noise and movement. The syndrome frequently has a familial basis, and responds well to anticonvulsant drugs with a good longterm prognosis. Valproate seems particularly effective but withdrawal of drug treatment, even after long periods of remission almost always results in relapse.

### The secondary generalized epilepsies

These syndromes commence in young children who frequently, but not always, have pre-existing cerebral damage or disease. They are characterized by the occurrence of more complex absence seizures frequently interspersed with tonic, clonic or tonic–clonic seizures and myoclonus.

### The Lennox–Gastaut syndrome

This syndrome has also been called 'petit mal variant' (Gibbs & Gibbs 1952) and myoclonic–astatic petit-mal (Doose et al. 1970). Fits most commonly commence before the age of 2 years and onset is extremely uncommon after the age of 7 or 8 years. It may account for up to 10% of all epilepsies (Gastaut 1973), i.e. it is twice as common as true petit mal epilepsy. It may develop in infants with a wide variety of cerebral pathology, including perinatal trauma, tuberous sclerosis, inborn errors of metabolism, and microcephaly. Less commonly it may develop in apparently normal children.

Children suffer frequent seizures of diverse symptomatology, but most often characterized by absence with brief massive bilateral myoclonus, tonic seizures or atonic drop attacks resulting in numerous falls causing multiple injuries particularly to the head and necessitating the wearing of a protective helmet. More conventional tonic–clonic, simple motor and complex partial seizures may occur. Absence status is much more common in this disorder than in true petit mal.

The interictal EEG typically shows bilateral synchronous spike and wave complexes between 1 and 2.5 Hz.

The prognosis for both development and seizure control is poor in contrast to true petit-mal. Retardation is present from the onset in up to half of the patients and may be severe. Where the disorder has been present for some time retardation can be seen in up to 90% of patients. Seizures usually persist into adult life, but change in character, often with the development of more typical complex partial seizures.

### Infantile spasm (West syndrome)

This represents the most severe part of the spectrum of secondary generalized epilepsy in childhood. The disorder is almost universally associated with severe pre-existing cerebral damage (prenatal or perinatal). Up to 25% of cases may be caused by tuberous sclerosis.

Onset is between the ages of 4 and 7 months in half the cases and onset is rare after one year. The clinical hallmarks of the syndrome are spasms consisting of sudden massive forward flexion of the head associated with bending of the knees and flexion and abduction of the arms. This may result in brief lightning spasms or more sustained movements. Other seizure types include simple motor and tonic seizures.

Retardation is often obvious before the onset of the disorder but even in apparently previously well infants behavioural regression is frequently seen.

The interictal EEG shows a severe disturbance devoid of normal background activity, consisting of chaotic high amplitude asynchronous slow waves mixed with multifocal sharp waves and spikes (hypsarrhythmia).

Conventional anticonvulsant drugs have little effect on infantile spasms, but treatment with ACTH (20–60 units per day) appears to be helpful particularly when commenced early in the course of the disorder. However, up to 90% of patients show severe mental retardation and death may occur in up to 20%.

## The investigation of epilepsy

The investigation of epilepsy is undertaken, to add weight to the clinical diagnosis, to aid classification of seizures and epilepsy, and to define any underlying pathology that may require additional or alternative treatment.

It is relatively uncommon for physicians to witness seizures or be able to record an EEG during one. Therefore the diagnosis of epilepsy is ultimately a clinical one based on the history obtained from patients and their relatives. Electroencephalographic recording can however be a useful procedure in adding weight to a clinical diagnosis, although it can never prove or disprove the clinical diagnosis of epilepsy.

Major problems arise in the interpretation of EEG recordings because mild nonspecific abnormalities may occur in up to 10% of the population without a history of epilepsy, and because many patients with mild epilepsy have normal interictal records. Furthermore in patients with complex partial seizures, medial temporal foci may be remote from conventional EEG electrode placements so that focal spike activity may not be recorded from other than sphenoidal or nasopharyngeal leads, even during a clinically obvious seizure.

In addition to conventional EEG recording, recent technological advances have allowed the recording of EEG in combination with video tape of the behavioural responses of patients over prolonged periods. Less cumbersome ambulatory monitoring can also be undertaken on an outpatient basis (Binnie 1983). With the increasing periods for which these techniques allow monitoring, it is hoped that increased numbers of clinically relevant EEG abnormalities may be detected.

As well as helping to confirm a clinical diagnosis of epilepsy the EEG may be of value in determining the type of epilepsy suffered by the patient. The differentiation of absence seizures due to generalized spike wave abnormalities, and complex partial seizures associated with temporal lobe spikes may allow a differing and more appropriate therapeutic approach.

The necessity for investigation other than with an EEG in patients presenting with epilepsy will vary with the age of the patient, the type of epilepsy, and the presence or absence of neurological signs. It can be argued that all patients presenting with epilepsy require biochemical and haematological screening, and exhaustive neuroradiological investigation to determine a cause for their epilepsy. This may be economically wasteful in view of the very low rate of detection of conditions demanding a treatment other than by the prescription of anticonvulsant drugs. It is more important to recall, however, that careful physical examination may well reveal a cause for epilepsy, for example skin lesions of adenoma sebaceum in tuberous sclerosis, the port wine stain of Sturge-Weber syndrome, the finding of multiple neurofibromatosis, the characteristic facial skeletal abnormalities that may be seen in association with a variety of metabolic storage diseases.

Biochemical and haematological screening rarely discloses a cause for epilepsy. Exceptions to this are in neonates where hypoglycaemia and hypocalcaemia are particularly important, and in middle age where the finding of an elevated mean cell volume, and abnormal liver function tests may confirm the clinical suspicion of alcohol-induced seizures. Routine serogical testing for syphilis is more difficult to justify as neurosyphilis now represents an exceedingly uncommon cause of epilepsy.

Skull X-rays are routinely ordered in patients presenting with epilepsy. They may rarely disclose evidence of raised intracranial pressure, intracranial calcification or abnormal vascular markings from a meningioma. However, it is relatively rare for patients with such abnormalities on the skull X-ray to be free of abnormal neurological signs or symptoms of raised intracranial pressure which should have already alerted the clinician. It is thus debatable whether a skull X-ray is a necessary routine investigation in new cases of epilepsy.

The place of CT scanning, which has largely replaced radioisotope scanning in neurological centres, in the investigation of epilepsy remains controversial. Some have suggested that every patient with epilepsy should have a CT scan. The economics of such a policy are difficult to support. A number of studies of the results of CT scanning in epilepsy have been published. Overall they would indicate that CT scans are abnormal in approximately 40–50% of patients with epilepsy. However, the most common abnormalities are atrophic and tumours are found in only 8–10% of patients. The percentage of patients with tumours rises to 16% in patients over the age of 20, and to 22% when only partial seizures are examined. In adult patients with late onset epilepsy it is rare to detect tumours by CT scanning in the absence of partial seizures, focal neurological signs or a focal EEG abnormality (Young et al. 1982). When all three of these features are present CT scanning will reveal a tumour pathology in up to 70% of cases.

This provides a potent argument for restricting CT scanning in epilepsy to a selected group of patients with the onset of partial epilepsy in adult life who also have symptoms and signs indicating progressive cerebral disease. This policy is also supported by the realization that early and unselective CT scanning may give rise to a number of false negative scans and an erroneously optimistic prognosis. Furthermore it is sanguine to recall that up to 90% of tumour epilepsies are due to gliomas or metastases, i.e. lesions which are rarely curable, even by a radical surgical approach.

## Causes of epilepsy and seizures

Seizures and epilepsy may be symptomatic of a wide variety of systemic and neurological disease. The former causes (Table 17.3) usually

**Table 17.3.** Systemic disturbance causing seizures.

Fever
Hypoxia
Hypoglycaemia
Electrolyte imbalance

Renal failure
Hepatic failure
Respiratory failure

Drugs
Drugs withdrawal
Toxins

Pyridoxine deficiency
Porphyria
Inborn errors of metabolism

result in generalized tonic–clonic seizures, whilst the latter (Table 17.4) cause partial, or if the pathology is present from early life, secondary generalized epilpsies.

Two specific causes of epilepsy are particularly relevant to neurosurgical practice; post-traumatic and postoperative epilepsy.

**Table 17.4.** CNS disease causing seizures and epilepsy.

| | |
|---|---|
| *Congenital* | Birth trauma, tuberous sclerosis, arteriovenous malformation, lipid storage diseases, leucodystrophies, Down syndrome. |
| *Infective* | Meningitis, encephalitis, abscess, syphilis. |
| *Trauma* | Diffuse brain injury, haematoma (extradural, subdural, intracerebral), depressed fracture, penetrating (missile) wound. |
| *Tumour* | Glioma, meningioma, secondary carcinoma, etc. |
| *Vascular* | Atheroma, arteritis, aneurysm, embolism. |
| *Degenerative* | Alzheimer, Pick, Creutzfeld–Jacob |
| *Miscellaneous* | Demyelination |

## Post-traumatic epilepsy

Much has been written about epilepsy following head injury; Jennett (1975) consulted some 500 publications but listed less than 100 because of 'serious deficiency in the information' given in the others. A number of criteria are essential to studies of the subject.

Observation over a sufficiently long period of time is essential, for in at least one-fifth of all the patients with epilepsy the first fit is delayed for 2 or more years after the injury. Most figures quoted for the risk of post-traumatic epilepsy are related to an arbitrary period of follow-up. Actuarial probabilities, derived from lifetable analysis are more meaningful in defining risk on a per annum basis. Large numbers are necessary to give significance to subgroup analysis for patients with differing degrees of severity, type, locations and complications of injury. The bald statement that the incidence is 5% in a series is of little practical value, for according to the factors operating in an individual case it varies from no more than that of the general population to nearly 100%. The information required when considering a particular patient is the incidence in that subgroup which most closely matches the circumstances of the case. Even that item of information provides only an estimate of probability, for as yet there is no method accurately of predicting whether the patient will or will not develop epilepsy. Statistical studies have their most practical application in litigation.

If epilepsy is to be linked to a preceding head injury, it is necessary to lay down criteria to characterize the nature and severity of the injury. There may be primary brain injury resulting in either concussion, which may be defined in terms of amnesia for and succeeding the event (retrograde and post-traumatic amnesia) or the quantitatively more severe diffuse white matter (axonal) injury. The duration of post-traumatic amnesia (PTA) gives an indication of the severity of primary injury. In addition secondary brain damage may result, which may be either generalized, for example raised intracranial pressure complicating haematoma, or localized resulting, for instance, from a depressed fracture with dural laceration.

The definition of the term epilepsy also requires comment. Some investigators have excluded cases of solitary post-traumatic seizures on the grounds that this does not constitute epilepsy in the accepted sense of a predisposition to recurring seizures, but difficulty arises in agreeing upon the minimum number of seizures which constitutes a persistent susceptibility; this is avoided by including every case in which a fit occurs after a head injury. A solitary fit is, however, uncommon. In their series of cases of post-traumatic epilepsy, Walker and Jablon (1959, 1961) found that 13% had only one attack throughout the period of follow-up (6–9 years).

In the following brief account, post-traumatic epilepsy will be discussed emphasizing particularly the factors modifying its incidence, its time of onset and the likelihood of its cessation. Evidence concerning the prophylactic and therapeutic value of drugs is discussed in the section on treatment (*see* below).

*Brain wounds due to missiles*

Although the brain may sustain severe and localized damage as a result of a closed depressed fracture of the skull, with or without dural penetration, wounds of the brain caused by missiles which penetrate the dura mater at high velocity provide a well defined and homogenous group. In many the localization and the extent of the injury are anatomically precise and the relationship between the incidence of epilepsy and such factors as retention of foreign bodies, haematoma, brain infection and associated primary damage can be determined. This group of head injuries has rightly received special attention in the literature and has been reviewed by Walker and Jablon (1961). Some of these figures and those from subsequent reports are summarized in Table 17.5.

**Table 17.5.** Incidence of epilepsy following missile injuries.

|  | % |  |
|---|---|---|
| Wagstaffe (1928) | 19 | World War I |
| Credner (1930) | 50 | World War I |
| Ascroft (1941) | 45 | World War I |
| Russell & Whitty (1952) | 43 | World War II |
| Walker & Jablon (1959) | 36 | World War II |
| Caveness & Liss (1961) | 40 | Korean War |
| Caveness et al. (1979) | 33 | Vietnam War |

It is likely that 50% represents a best estimate of the risks of epilepsy, for the figure of Russell and Whitty (1952) was calculated on a 5 year follow-up after wounding and takes no account of the subsequent development of fits. In Ascroft's series (1941), 13% of the patients with epilepsy had their first fit more than 5 years after the injury.

Experimental studies in epilepsy have shown that the epileptic threshold differs from one part of the brain to another. The careful scrutiny of charts depicting the site of injury has shown that, consonant with experience in cerebral tumour, wounds in the vicinity of the central fissure carry the greatest probability that epilepsy will develop. In Russell and Whitty's series, wounds of the motor and premotor cortex were followed by epilepsy in 55% of cases; the incidence after wounds elsewhere was around 38%. The figures of Walker and Jablon (1961) however do not give much support to this, possibly due to a failure to discriminate between 'prefrontal' and 'motor and premotor'.

The extent of the cerebral wound, which may be increased by surgical intervention, increases the liability to epilepsy. If the presence and severity of hemiparesis is taken as a criterion of extent of the injury, 66% of cases with persistent hemiplegia had fits and 47% of those with persistent monoplegia (Russell & Whitty 1952). Walker and Jablon (1961) also found an association between the risk of epilepsy and extent of wound as judged by both surface and depth measurements and by neurological deficit, though hemianopia was associated with a lower incidence than sensory or motor paresis, perhaps attributable to the lower incidence of epilepsy after occipital injury.

Walker and Jablon (1961) did not find that removal of intracranial metal and bone fragments affected the incidence of epilepsy except where in-driven fragments were exclusively bone. In the latter group epilepsy occurred in 25% and in the former it occurred in approximately 40%. One explanation may be that indriven fragments of bone alone may have been due to injuries other than missile induced ones and that they were less extensive injuries. An interesting finding in Ascroft's series was a higher incidence (53%) when metal had been removed than when it remained indwelling (38%). Possibly this was due to extension of damage by the manoeuvres necessary for removal.

Infection exerts an important influence on the incidence of epilepsy. Ascroft found that when the wound had healed within 15 days the incidence was 36%; when it had remained unhealed after 60 days it was 57%. After abscess formation the incidence increases to 73% (Walker & Jablon 1961). Epilepsy is almost an inevitable sequel of brain fungus, occurring in 86 and 92% of cases in two series (Caveness et al. 1962). Against these figures must be set those of Russell and Whitty who found that in such cases the incidence of persistent epilepsy was no higher than 54%. Infection may encourage the development of epilepsy simply by increasing the extent of brain damage, or by promoting the formation of a perimeter of partially damaged brain cells, resulting in a mixed glial and fibrous scar.

Although missile wounds of the brain tend to produce localized damage (though it may be extensive) compared with the diffuse neuronal damage of primary injury, the patterns of resultant epilepsy are similar. Only a minority suffer exclusively from focal attacks, the figure varying from 13 to 31% in different series.

*Blunt injuries of the head*

In this category are included all injuries not caused by high velocity missiles; i.e. the vast majority of civilian injuries. The incidence of epilepsy is much lower than in the cases of penetrating missile injury and there is a wide variation in the reported figures because this group is not homogenous. Walker (1964) gives a list of published figures, in which the incidence varies between 0.75% and 20%. The incidence figures found by Penfield and Shaver (1945) and Phillips (1954) are in close accord, 5 and 6% respectively and include early and late fits. Jennett (1975) reported that epilepsy starting within the first week occurred in 5% of unselected head injuries. Also the incidence of late epilepsy in the same series was 5%. Studies of the population of Olmstead County, Minnesota (Annegers *et al.* 1980) revealed that in patients sustaining a minor head injury (no fracture or loss of consciousness or post-traumatic amnesia of less than 30 minutes) there was no statistical increase in the incidence of epilepsy over and above that prevailing in the general population. These differences undoubtedly reflect artifacts created by the manner of selection of patients included in the former studies.

*Time of onset*

There is general agreement that approximately 75% of patients developing post-traumatic epilepsy have their first fit within a year of injury. This is so both for missile (Russell & Whitty 1952, Ascroft 1941) and for blunt injuries (Phillips 1945, Jennett 1975). Russell and Whitty

excluded cases in which fits in the first month were not repeated later, and the figure of Phillips was recalculated by Jennett to include early fits; that of Jennett included early fits. Jennett emphasized that the percentage figures would be modified by inclusion or exclusion of fits which occur soon after the injury and by the length of the follow-up. In his series 19% of patients who developed late epilepsy had their first fit after the fourth year and 3% more than 10 years after injury. Partial and generalized attacks showed no difference in time of onset.

There has long been an opinion among clinicians that fits which arise within the first few weeks of an injury do not carry the same prognostic significance as do those with a later onset: that they are related only to the acute damage sustained by the brain and do not necessarily precede persistent epilepsy. Denny-Brown (1943) was apprehensive that such patients, having had an early fit, might be labelled epileptic when the likelihood of further fits was remote. Jennett arbitrarily divided his cases into 'early' epilepsy (those with seizures within the first week), and 'late' epilepsy (those who had fits after that week). Although the separation into groups of early and late has been valuable for the purposes of statistical study, it has a disadvantage in that it is arbitrary. Providing this is recognized no harm follows. It is erroneous to infer that there is a sudden reduction in the day-to-day incidence of the first seizure at the end of the first week. Jennett and Lewin (1960) point out in an earlier study, that in the period from the second to tenth week after injury, a first fit was recorded for only one patient out of 64 who had fits, early or late. Subsequently, a number of cases were discovered in which the first fit occurred in this apparently latent period. Calculations based on the figures which Phillips (1954) gave of the intervals of time after the injury at which the first fit occurred shows that the average daily incidence steadily declines after the first 24 hours, which exhibited the highest daily incidence in his series (7% of the 190 cases with epilepsy). Calculations made from Jennett's (1975) figures put the first day's incidence much higher (17%), though it is not possible to construct a curve of daily incidence: of patients with epilepsy within 8 weeks of injury, 80% had their first fit within the first week (Jennett 1969).

## Early epilepsy

Early epilepsy after minor injury is more common in children under the age of 5 years than in adults. After severe injuries there was no difference. This is the basis for the belief that a fit in a child soon after an injury is not of serious import, which can be erroneous. As might be anticipated, severity of injury as judged by fracture, long PTA, neurological deficit and haemorrhage was found to be associated with a higher incidence of seizures within the first week (and, as will be seen, fits developing later). It is important to note that approximately one-quarter of the cases of intracranial haematoma suffered fits. Of those who died after injury and who had fits, two-thirds proved to have an intracranial haematoma (Jennett 1975). Though early epilepsy is associated with a higher mortality (9% as opposed to 5%), this is almost all due to the increased mortality associated with intracranial haematoma.

The important question which an arbitrary division into 'early' and 'late' should answer is whether a fit in the first week predisposes to later fits. Follow-up of patients with early seizures disclosed that late fits ensued in 25%, compared with an incidence of 3% of late epilepsy in the absence of early fits. In adults only the respective incidences were 33% and 3% whereas in children they were 17% and 4% (Jennett 1975). The nature of the investigation was such that the cases of late post-traumatic epilepsy were loaded with certain factors (for example depressed fracture or haematoma) which predispose to epilepsy. When cases with these complications were eliminated, later epilepsy occurred overall in only 1.2% but if there had been an early fit the incidence rose to 51%. The behaviour of early epilepsy following brain wounds was studied by Whitty (1947); the follow-up covered periods of

2.5–3 years after the injury and 'early' meant within 10 days of wounding. He found that in 52% the fits recurred later. These figures dispose of the general notion that fits occurring within a short time of a head injury are of little prognostic significance and one must agree with the conclusion of Jennett (1975) that early epilepsy is an important predictor of late epilepsy, particularly in the absence of haematoma or a depressed fracture.

## Late epilepsy

Late epilepsy was calculated by Jennett (1975) to be anticipated in about 5% of the survivors of head injuries (including those who had also had early fits but excluding those in whom the fits did not recur after the first week). This compares with 6% in the 500 cases of Phillips (1954). Both these series were confirmed to patients seen in hospital. Annegers et al. (1980) found the incidence of late epilepsy to be 1.8% in a community based study.

The importance of an early fit in determining later epilepsy has already been noted. What other factors may increase the liability? A correlation between incidence of epilepsy and severity of a brain wound or its complication has been shown to exist. In closed injuries Phillips found a long PTA to be associated with a high incidence; about half the patients with post-traumatic epilepsy had a PTA of over 24 hours, compared with about one-quarter of the whole series of head injuries. Jennett (1975) found a somewhat similar preponderance in favour of prolonged PTA but when cases with early epilepsy, depressed fracture and haematoma were excluded, a long PTA had no significant effect upon the incidence of late epilepsy, the incidence being 1%. In patients who did not have an early fit, a depressed fracture or an intracranial haematoma increased the incidence of epilepsy to 15 and 31% respectively.

Phillips found an incidence of epilepsy of 68% in patients with depressed fractures. Jennett (1975) found that in cases with dural laceration the incidence was 24%. This doubled in the presence of focal signs or a PTA exceeding 24 hours. In the presence of focal signs late epilepsy occurred in a quarter of cases and this incidence was increased by a PTA greater than 24 hours, by dural tearing, but not by the presence of early seizures. Children less frequently developed late seizures after depressed fracture than adults.

Epilepsy in the first week occurred in 25% of patients with haematoma. It appeared most frequently in cases of multiple intradural haematomata or subdural collections. The initial fit did not occur until after the first 24 hours in 70%. Late epilepsy occurred in one-third of the patients who survived a haematoma. Jennett makes the important practical points that a fit was never the only indication of a developing haematoma, nor does it alone provide an indication for exploration; these accord with clinical experience.

The relative frequency of partial and of generalized tonic–clonic seizures (presumably developing due to secondary generalization from a focal onset) following blunt injuries varies with different observers. Phillips recorded 16 and 84% respectively, though it is not made clear whether these are exclusive because he provided no figures for a mixed group. Jennett (1975) states that in 43% of the patients with early epilepsy at least some of the fits were 'focal motor' whilst in late epilepsy though 40% have focal features at some time during the attack, many become generalized. Hoff and Strotzka (1951) found in patients with focal epilepsy, a steady increase over the years in the number who developed generalized attacks. Temporal lobe seizures were exceedingly rare in the early cases: their complex nature and the descriptions required to identify them would in any case militate against their recognition at this stage of recovery. In late epilepsy temporal lobe patterns were observed in 19% of all the patients with post-traumatic epilepsy. A somewhat similar incidence was found by Vitale et al. (1953), who approached the subject from a different angle, deriving their cases from an EEG departmental index, though the diagnosis of temporal lobe seizure was a clinical one.

*Remission of epilepsy*

The question whether early epilepsy (arising within 7–10 days of the injury) is liable to persist has already been alluded to: nonpersistence may be viewed as remission and the quoted figures show that this happens in about 50–75% of cases depending on their nature and complications. Walker and Jablon (1961) plotted the curves of persisting epilepsy in three groups of cases: (1) those with the first attack within a week of injury; (2) those within the interval 1–13 weeks; (3) those between 3 and 12 months. In the second year, about 65% of the first group remitted, about 15% of the third group and the second group were intermediate. The three curves steadily declined in the succeeding years keeping their relative positions. Caveness (1963) reported a remission rate of 53% and no significant difference between early and late epilepsy. The remission rate in Jennett's series of late onset was 25% but one-third of cases continued to have frequent fits. If the first seizures occurred four or more years after the head injury the epilepsy was less likely to remit. Temporal lobe seizures were more likely to persist than other types. The dependence or otherwise of remission in post-traumatic epilepsy on anti-epileptic therapy is uncertain, but general considerations would indicate that patients with post-traumatic epilepsy are likely to run a high risk of relapse should drug treatment be withdrawn after a period of remission (Chadwick 1984).

*Predisposition*

From the few cases of previously diagnosed epilepsy which came to light in his enquiry Jennett formed the opinion that there was little predisposition to early seizures following head injury. Walker and Jablon (1961) examined the incidence of epilepsy in the immediate relatives of head-injured men who developed epilepsy, and of those who did not. The family incidence was slightly higher (1 in 107) in those with post-traumatic epilepsy than in those without (1 in

191). The incidence was higher still (1 in 64) in those in whom fits were frequent and were generalized. The conclusion is drawn that 'genetic predisposition may have played a role in at least some of the veterans who developed recurrent epilepsy of the focal type' though the conclusion cannot be justified in any statistical sense. Whatever may be the precise role of constitutional factors, it must be relatively unimportant as epilepsy may follow certain types of injury in 50% of patients. Walter (1942) pointed out that there is a great individual variation in the convulsant threshold to electrical stimulation as revealed by electroconvulsant therapy. He thought that the genetic background may act to discourage the spread of the fit. Potter (1978) suggested that there may be a personal metabolic factor involved in the maturation of brain scars. This variant might not only explain why some patients develop seizures, but also the variable time of onset in different patients.

*Value of electroencephalography*

The clinical application of EEG was developing rapidly when the Second World War started and interest in head injury and the organization of centres for the treatment of such patients provided this investigation with a fresh and enlarging field. It was hoped and anticipated that serial observations on these patients would reveal those which were destined to develop epilepsy. Unfortunately the EEG has not supplied the information necessary for this prediction. Williams (1941) was one of the earliest to study the EEG following head injury. The main features in the early records are depression or loss of alpha rhythms and appearance of slow waves of theta or delta frequencies, focal, unilateral or generalized. Spike discharge may appear in the vicinity of local damage, but rarely in the case of a closed head injury (Bickford & Klass 1966). Williams (1941) found that abnormalities tend to diminish within 2 months and the record shows little further change after 6 months. He could not predict epilepsy from the early records. In a later

paper Williams (1944b) drew attention to the occurrence of 'larval' discharges, spike and wave complexes, similar to those he had described (1944a) in interseizure records in idiopathic epilepsy. These paroxysmal discharges were encountered in 27% of the records of idiopathic epilepsy, but not in nonepileptics, nor after head injury if there were no fits. In post-traumatic epilepsy he found them in 8.6% of cases; in 5% he noted them before epilepsy had developed. They were more frequent after penetrating than after closed injury. Williams concluded that the appearance of larval episodes at an interval after a head injury would very probably herald the development of epilepsy. But the low incidence of this abnormality, and the relatively high incidence of normal records in post-traumatic epilepsy (40%, Williams 1944b) renders prediction impossible in most cases. In a discussion on this problem Williams (1955) stated that 'the likelihood of the development of epilepsy is not consistently reflected in the post-traumatic EEG Marshall and Walker (1961) provide convincing evidence to confirm this. They compared the early EEG records of head-injured men, who 5 years later were or were not suffering from epilepsy. There was no significant difference in the characteristics of the early records of the two groups. Examination of the recent records in the two groups also revealed no distinguishing features. It is remarkable in how large a proportion of those with active epilepsy the current EEG was normal or borderline. Contrary findings were reported by Hoff and Strotzka (1951) in a study confined to penetrating wounds. They found that if the EEG was normal after the injury fits developed within 6 months in only 2.4%; if abnormal in 76%.

Jennett (1975) studied 1,000 records taken from 722 patients; 80% showed abnormalities in the first week. This declined to 60% over a few months and then remained static. Patients experiencing early seizures more often had abnormal records in the first week when compared with those who did not have a fit in this period, but after this period there was no difference between the groups having late seizures and those who did not. Even serial records on individual patients did not help to predict which of the patients would eventually have a late seizure.

The question of whether prophylactic anticonvulsant therapy is of value in the management of head-injured patients is discussed in the section of this chapter on the treatment of epilepsy (*see* below).

### Postoperative epilepsy

Recently interest in the question of seizures arising after craniotomy for supratentorial conditions has been stimulated because such patients may have to modify their lifestyle, for example stop driving at least temporarily on the basis that they have a prospective disability even though they may not yet have experienced a seizure (Pond & Espir 1978). Data from Rochester (Hauser & Kurland 1975) suggests that between 20 and 59 years there is a 0.02% risk of developing epilepsy de novo per year. The overall incidence of seizures occurring after supratentorial craniotomy is 17% during a minimum follow-up period of 5 years (Foy *et al.* 1981a). The actual incidence varied from 3% to 92% depending upon the condition for which the craniotomy was undertaken.

Over one-fifth of patients undergoing aneurysm surgery will develop postoperative seizures (Cabral *et al.* 1976a, North *et al.* 1983). The incidence varies according to the site of the aneurysm: 7.5% for internal carotid, 21% for anterior communicating and 38% for middle cerebral aneurysms (Cabral *et al.* 1976b, Foy *et al.* 1981a). Additional adverse factors include; intracerebral haematoma, cortical damage, splitting the Sylvian fissure, cerebral swelling and perioperative rupture of the aneurysm. That at least part of the risk of epilepsy associated with aneurysm is generated by the surgical procedure is suggested by the 8.3% incidence in 261 conservatively managed survivors following aneurysmal subarachnoid haemorrhage reported by Storey (1967). Arteriovenous malformations

and spontaneous intracerebral haematomata from other causes carry incidences of epilepsy of 50% and 20% respectively.

The incidence of epilepsy following tumour surgery is more difficult to assess since it occurs at an arbitrary point in time during the natural history of the disease process. Cortical damage would seem to be important, as is suggested by Cabral *et al.*'s study (1976a) of acoustic neuromas in which only those cases approached transtentorially experienced seizures (22%) and by the higher incidence of seizures (20%) following craniotomy for glioma as compared with burr hole biopsy (9%) (Foy *et al.* 1981a). These authors agree with North *et al.* that the incidence of seizures commencing *de novo* following surgery for meningioma is 22%. The incidence is higher for parasaggital lesions than for convexity or basal tumours. Some 44% of patients who have preoperative seizures do not have any further seizures postoperatively. Both groups of authors record low incidences (5–6%) for explorations of the suprasellar region, mainly for pituitary adenomas and craniopharyngiomas. Other authors (Cast & Wilson 1981) have found a higher incidence of epilepsy (15%) following the subfrontal approach to pituitary adenomas.

Supratentorial abscesses carry a very high incidence of postoperative seizures. With sufficiently long follow-up virtually all developed this problem (Legg *et al.* 1973, Foy *et al.* 1981b). Surprisingly however, the overall incidence of seizures following indwelling ventricular shunting is 24% (Copeland *et al.* 1982). Multiple revisions marginally increased the chance of developing seizures but the occurrence of a complicating infection, no matter whether it manifested itself as a wound infection or meningitis, resulted in a statistically significant increase in the incidence.

Thirty seven per cent of all patients who experience postoperative seizures do so within the first week and over 40% of this group continue to experience seizures later. The only common exception to this appears to be patients with anterior cerebral artery complex aneurysm, of whom only 13% continue to experience further episodes. By the time one year has elapsed 77% of those who will experience a seizure have done so and by two years this figure had reached 92% (Foy et al. 1981b). Once two years have elapsed the chance of a patient who has had an aneurysm clipped developing seizures for the first time is virtually zero. The only group with a continuing high risk of this at five years are patients who have had a supratentorial abscess.

In patients with early seizures the risk of developing further seizures is very high (70%) if the generalized component was preceded by a focal element, and only 5% of those patients developing seizures later than one week postoperatively have a single seizure.

There is some evidence (Cabral & Scott 1977, Legg et al. 1973) that although the presence in a postoperative EEG of spikes, sharp components and slow waves alone does not act as a prognostic indicator that seizures will occur, these abnormalities are seen more frequently in those going on to develop seizures when compared with those who did not.

## The medical treatment of epilepsy

The management of the patient with epilepsy comprises a number of aspects, including counselling and social support. However, the major aim will always be to render the patient free of seizures.

The first line of treatment in epilepsy will usually be with drugs. As neurosurgeons frequently institute and supervise anticonvulsant therapy the following review of the pharmacology of antiepileptic drugs may be of value. The subject has been well reviewed by Richens (1982).

### When to start anticonvulsant drugs

There is no clear evidence available to the clinician to indicate whether anticonvulsant drugs should be started after one, two, three or more seizures.

The frequency with which an isolated seizure in adult life is followed by recurrent fits is controversial. In a recent community survey in general practice (Goodridge & Shorvon 1983) the lifetime prevalence of epilepsy including single seizures was 20.3 per thousand but after excluding single seizures was 17 per thousand. A single seizure was followed by recurrence in 80% of patients.

Hospital based studies, however, suggest a lower recurrence rate. Clelland et al. (1981) noted a recurrence of seizures in 39% of 70 patients referred to an adult neurological clinic during a mean follow-up of 4 years 9 months. A larger study from the United States (Hauser et al. 1982) found that the risk of recurrence was 18% at 1 year and 21% at two years and 27% at three years, with little subsequent increase in risk with longer periods of follow-up.

The very different outlook between this general practice survey and hospital based populations may well reflect referral patterns. Clearly all patients with epilepsy initially have a single seizure but in the majority of cases subsequent seizures occur within a short period of time. By the time they reach a neurological clinic they are diagnosed as having epilepsy rather than a single isolated seizure.

At present most neurologists in the United Kingdom do not treat a single isolated seizure and will await the occurrence of a second or subsequent seizure. In the United States there is a greater tendency to treat a single seizure (Hauser et al. 1982). However this policy has no definite effect in reducing the risk of subsequent seizures even in those patients at higher risk, for example those with previous neurological insults. Clearly there is a need for further information concerning the prognosis of an isolated seizure and the possible effects of early treatment.

It is generally accepted that at least two seizures should occur within a relatively short period (1–2 years) before drug treatment is commenced.

There has been an increasing practice over recent years to begin anticonvulsant treatment before the onset of seizures in neurosurgical patients who are at a high risk of developing epilepsy, for example patients with severe head injury or following supratentorial craniotomy. The rationale for such preventive treatment is uncertain, and it is impossible to know for how long preventive treatment should be continued.

### Head injuries

The evidence as to whether prophylactic anti-convulsants are of value in preventing seizures in groups of head-injured patients with a high risk of epilepsy remains controversial.

One problem in attempting to solve this question is that this population of patients tends not to take their prescribed medication. This clearly emerged from a study reported by McQueen *et al.* (1983) in which the incidence of late seizures was similar in the treatment and placebo groups. Young and his colleagues also found that pro-phylactically administered phenytoin failed to reduce the incidence of both early (1983a) and later (1983b) seizures. Caveness *et al.* (1979) had a similar experience with a prophylactic anti-convulsant programme carried out during the Vietnam War. In contrast, North *et al.* (1983) found in a mixed study of post-traumatic and postoperative cases that there was a significant reduction in the incidence of seizures in the treated group during the period 7–72 days post injury, but not outside this time interval. Other reports have indicated the effectiveness of prophylaxis (Servit & Musil 1981). Janz (1983) has reviewed the subject and suggested that though there might be marginal benefits to such a policy, there is, to date, little statistical evidence to support the case for prophylactic anti-convulsants in the head-injured patient. If there is a marginal benefit to be gained, this will have to be set against the undoubted complication rate in patients who are loaded rapidly with anti-convulsants (Chadwick *et al.* 1984). The answer to this problem must await the completion of a large, well controlled trial.

### Postoperative seizures

Whether anticonvulsants given prophylactically following supratentorial procedures, which are known to carry a high incidence of postoperative seizures, significantly influence that incidence has not yet been determined. Fabiny and Fortuny (1980) reported that in a series of patients with operated intracranial aneurysms treated with prophylactic anticonvulsants the incidence of seizures was 4.5%. Shaw *et al.* (1983) reported on a prophylactically treated series of high risk patients and found no significant difference in the incidence of epilepsy during the first six post-operative months when compared with a pre-vious retrospective study (Foy *et al.* 1981a, 1981b). However, within the treated group there was a suggestion that those patients who com-plied with the drug regimen experienced fewer seizures than those who did not, but there were considerable problems with side effects, par-ticularly skin rashes (Chadwick *et al.* 1984). A recent controlled trial from Australia (North *et al.* 1983) has reported that prophylaxis with phenytoin is effective from the end of the first week to the completion of the tenth week, but that there was no difference between the treated and control groups outside this time period. They also found that seizure control was maximal when therapeutic serum levels were achieved and suggested that where possible anti-convulsant therapy should be started one week before surgery.

Whether and when a patient suffers seizures following injury to the brain is dependent upon the maturation characteristics of the cortical brain scar in the particular patient (Potter 1978). This led to the suggestion that anticonvulsants given for a period of time during which scar maturation would occur, might prevent seizures even following cessation of the treatment. The second possibility was that the prophylactic medication might merely defer the onset of the seizures for the duration of the treatment. The data of North *et al.* (1983) suggests that the second possibility is correct, as there was a greater incidence of seizures during the second year in patients who had received twelve months prophylaxis as opposed to those given placebo.

## Choosing an anticonvulsant drug

Monotherapy with anticonvulsants given in optimal doses, is satisfactory for the majority of patients with epilepsy. There is little evidence to indicate that additional drugs significantly improve seizure control, whilst polytherapy commonly leads to increased chronic toxicity and drug interaction. Single drug therapy is to be preferred wherever possible (Reynolds & Shorvon 1981).

Data on the comparative efficacy of anticonvulsant drugs is extremely sparse and all randomized studies in adult patients fail to differentiate between the comparative efficacy of drugs tested, possibly because the numbers of patients studied have been too small to achieve the necessary statistical power (Chadwick & Turnbull 1985).

Absence seizures in children are responsive to ethosuximide and valproate but unresponsive to drugs effective against tonic–clonic and partial seizures, for example phenytoin and carbamazepine. ACTH is of particular value in the management of the infantile spasm syndrome and valproate as well as benzodiazepines (clonazepam and nitrazepam) may have a specific role in the management of myoclonic epilepsies.

Porter (1982) has recently suggested a decreasing likelihood of effectiveness against varying seizure types (Table 17.6). This table illustrates accepted clinical practice but is not yet supported by data from any randomized comparative anticonvulsant studies.

The management of status epilepticus presents frequent problems in neurosurgical practice. Even in the absence of neurosurgical disease or intervention, the condition has a mortality of up to 21% (Rowan & Scott 1970). In neurosurgical patients this may be even higher, and in addition there may be considerable morbidity.

Drugs of value must be rapidly acting and available for administration by an intravenous route. Chlormethiazole, thiopentone and benzodiazepines (diazepam and clonazepam) are most commonly used. The aim must be to give sufficient drug in order to suppress seizures quickly and effectively, and respiration may have to be supported whilst this achieved. Bolus injections may be used initially, but, in the absence of a prompt response, an intravenous infusion should be commenced. There is no place for the intramuscular administration of any anticonvulsant other than paraldehyde (*see* below). It is important to initiate or maintain longer term anticonvulsant therapy, by an intravenous route if this is possible, or nasogastric tube. Treatment of any underlying cause of status epilepticus must be sought and treated urgently (abscess, encephalitis, frontal tumour), but the commonest cause is probably inadequate or irregular compliance in patients with chronic severe epilepsies.

**Table 17.6.** Order of efficacy of antiepileptic drugs.

| Decreasing likelihood of effectiveness | Tonic–clonic seizures | Simple partial seizures | Complex partial seizures |
|---|---|---|---|
| 1 | phenytoin | phenytoin | carbamazepine |
| 2 | carbamazepine | carbamazepine | phenytoin |
| 3 | phenobarbitone | primidone | primidone |
| 4 | valproate | phenobarbitone | phenobarbitone |

Data from Porter 1982.

## Pharmacokinetics of anticonvulsant drugs

Pharmacokinetics define characteristics of drug absorption, distribution and elimination. The fact that anticonvulsant drug concentrations can be estimated in body fluids has lead to a widespread use of anticonvulsant level monitoring in clinical practice. In spite of this, many important clinical phenomena are poorly appreciated, and, paradoxically, the importance of monitoring is often over emphasized. It is most important to remember when measuring plasma or serum drug concentrations that one is sampling a physiological compartment far removed from the site of therapeutic drug action (Fig. 17.2).

Some of the more important pharmacokinetic data on commonly used anticonvulsants are summarized in Table 17.7.

*Absorption of drugs*

Anticonvulsants vary in their rate of intestinal absorption, as judged by the time to peak concentration after a single oral dose. Phenytoin, and carbamazepine are relatively insoluble and are slowly, and incompletely absorbed. pH may influence significantly the availability of phenytoin, which is insoluble at acid pH in the stomach and depends largely on duodenal absorption (Dill *et al.* 1956). The bio-availability of phenytoin may also be influenced by the pharmaceutical presentation of the drug. An outbreak of phenytoin intoxication occurred in Australasia due to a change in the excipient of phenytoin capsules from calcium sulphate to lactose (Tyrer *et al.* 1970). Phenytoin bio-availability can thus be variable and it may be important to specify a pharmaceutical preparation rather than using the generic name.

In contrast, other anticonvulsants such as valproate, ethosuximide, barbiturates and

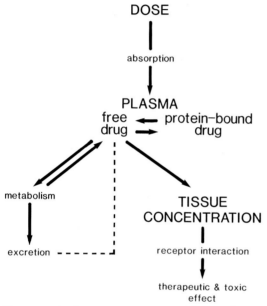

**Fig. 17.2.** A schematic representation of pharmacokinetics of anticonvulsant drugs.

**Table 17.7.** Pharmacokinetics of anticonvulsants.

| | Absorption | | Metabolism | |
| Drug | Time to peak serum conc. (hrs) after oral dose | Protein binding % | Active metabolites | Half-life (hrs) |
|---|---|---|---|---|
| Phenytoin | 4–12 | 90 | – | 9–140 |
| Phenobarbitone | 1–6 | 45 | – | 50–160 |
| Primidone | 2–5 | 20 | Phenobarbitone Phenylethylmalonamide | 4–12 |
| Carbamazepine | 4–24 | 75 | 10,11–epoxide | 8–30 |
| Valproate | 1–4 | 90 | – | 8–20 |
| Ethosuximide | 1–4 | – | – | 40–70 |
| Diazepam | 0.5–2 | 97 | N–desmethyldiazepam oxazepam | 20–60 |
| Clonazepam | 1–3 | 85 | – | 20–60 |

benzodiazepines are quickly and completely absorbed by the oral route.

Particular problems occur when anti-convulsants are administered parenterally. Prep-arations of phenytoin recommended for intramuscular administration are very alkaline, and when buffered to physiological pH in muscle tissue, become less soluble and are very slowly absorbed. Transfer from oral to intramuscular administration may lead to falling serum levels (Wilensky and Lowden 1973). Similar con-siderations apply to the intramuscular absorp-tion of diazepam (Hillstad et al. 1974) and to a lesser degree phenobarbitone. Intramuscular administration of these drugs should never be used in the management of status epilepticus, although in the case of diazepam, rectal admin-istration sometimes may be adequate. Intra-venous administration of all anticonvulsant drugs is preferable in order to obtain a rapid onset of action, and oral administration (via a nasogastric tube) preferable for maintaining serum levels of routinely administered anti-convulsants. The ECG should be monitored during intravenous administration of anti-convulsant drugs, particularly phenytoin because of the risk of cardiac arrhythmias.

*Protein binding*

It is usual to measure total serum or plasma concentrations of anticonvulsant. However phenytoin, valproate and benzodiazepines are heavily protein bound and only a small portion of the measured concentration is phar-macologically active as free drug. For phenytoin and carbamazepine, but not valproate and phenobarbitone, it is possible to monitor activity from salivary concentrations of the drugs; the salivary glands act as a simple dialysis membrane across which free drug equilibrates (Reynolds et al. 1976). However, there are practical problems in the collection of specimens (for example pres-ence of recently ingested food) and in the fact that lower concentrations of drug are present for

assay. The approach has not been widely used in clinical practice.

Protein binding of drugs has several important clinical implications. Renal, and hepatic failure, and other hypoalbuminaemic states may con-siderably increase the ratio of free to bound drug. Bilirubin may compete for albumin binding sites with phenytoin (Hooper et al. 1973), whilst val-proate is bound to albumin free fatty acid binding sites and interaction between drug and these endogenous substances may occur (Patel et al. 1980). Protein binding of anticonvulsants may also cause drug interactions. In particular, the administration of valproate may decrease the binding of phenytoin to plasma protein (Perucca et al. 1980). Carbamazepine itself is strongly protein bound (Table 17.7) but its metabolite 10,11-epoxide is only 50% protein bound. Both are anticonvulsant but the lesser binding of the metabolite may increase its contribution to the pharmacological activity of the drug.

A further factor complicating the relationship of total plasma or serum concentrations of drug to tissue concentrations is the degree of tissue binding. Lipophilic drugs such as phenytoin and carbamazepine diffuse into brain tissue rapidly and are heavily bound there, leading to brain concentrations of the same order as total plasma concentrations (Houghton et al. 1975). However, valproate distribution is largely restric-ted to extra cellular fluid, and brain con-centrations of this drug are thus considerably less than total plasma concentration.

*Drug metabolism*

Anticonvulsants are usually extensively metab-olised by hepatic enzymes before excretion. This is the rate-limiting step in the elimination of the drug. Rates of elimination vary and are usually expressed in terms of drug half-life (Table 17.7), which is important in determining:

1   the interval between doses of the drug (ideally equal to the drug half-life),
2   the time required to reach a new steady state

after alterations in drug dosage (usually five times the half-life),

3 the timing of sampling for drug level estimation.

Phenytoin and phenobarbitone have long half lives and can satisfactorily be administered as a single daily dose without there being large diurnal fluctuations in drug level. Up to 14–30 days may elapse before steady state levels are achieved following alteration in dosage, although when initiating phenytoin therapy, intravenous loading regimes will produce earlier steady-state concentrations (Cranford *et al.* 1978). Because of the nonlinear metabolism of phenytoin (*see* below) half-life increases with increasing serum levels and at toxic concentrations the rate of elimination and time to steady-state may be unexpectedly prolonged. Rechecking serum levels after a change in dosage may therefore have to be delayed in patients taking phenytoin and phenobarbitone but a single sample is an accurate reflector of serum levels throughout the day.

Drugs with shorter half lives (for example carbamazepine and valproate) may need to be given two or three times daily in order to maintain reasonably consistent serum levels through the day. It is less clear how total plasma concentrations of shorter acting drugs are related to therapeutic effect. The anticonvulsant action of valproate develops slowly after a single dose of the drug, and may be maintained for a prolonged period after drug withdrawal (Rowan *et al.* 1979a). Peak serum levels of valproate may be more important in determining anticonvulsant effect than trough levels, and valproate is clinically effective when administered once or twice daily (Rowan *et al.* 1979b).

Within individual patients, there is a linear relationship between dose and serum level over the clinical dosage range for most anticonvulsant drugs. The important exception to this is phenytoin, which is metabolized to 5-(p-hydroxy-phenyl)-5-phenylhydantoin (p-HPPH) by microsomal liver enzymes which are saturable within the therapeutic range of serum levels.

Thus with increasing doses of phenytoin a smaller proportion of the drug is metabolized and serum levels rise quickly (Fig. 17.3). Small increments in phenytoin dosage may lead to large increases in serum level, and clinical intoxication, therefore it may be necessary to use small increments of 50 or 25 mg per day. Unfortunately the optimal range for the drug lies on the steep part of the curve, so that minor changes in the bioavailability of phenytoin, and drug interactions have major clinical effects.

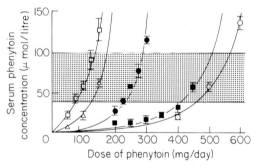

**Fig. 17.3.** Relationship between phenytoin dose and serum level in five patients in whom steady state concentrations were measured at several different doses. Each point represents the mean ± SD of 3–8 separate estimations of the serum level. The curves were fitted by computer using the Michaelis–Menten equation. The stippled area indicates the 'therapeutic range' of serum levels but is more generous than the usually quoted 40–80 $\mu$mol/1 (note: 4 $\mu$mol/1/1 = 1 $\mu$g/ml). (Reproduced from Richens & Dunlop, 1975, by kind permission of the Editor.)

For all anticonvulsant drugs there is a wide interpatient variation in the relationship between dose and serum level. This is largely attributable to varying rates of drug metabolism, determined in turn by a number of factors, the most important of which are genetic factors, age and enzyme induction.

Individuals differ in drug metabolizing capacity, and some are unable to deal with phenytoin because of deficient parahydroxylation. In children, with the exception of neonates, the half-life of anticonvulsants is shorter than that in adults and larger doses, on a weight basis, are usually necessary. With increasing age, rates of metabolism decrease and elderly patients may be particularly sensitive to conventional adult doses of anticonvulsant drugs.

Phenytoin, phenobarbitone and carbamazepine are potent inducers of hepatic enzymes. Carbamazepine induces its own metabolism, so that serum levels tend to fall with time, which may account for the high incidence of adverse reactions if this drug is not introduced slowly. When multiple drug regimes are used anticonvulsants usually interact so as to speed the rate of metabolism of other drugs. In particular it may be very difficult to attain optimal serum levels of carbamazepine and valproate in patients who are receiving other anticonvulsant drugs. Larger doses of these drugs are required in patients receiving polypharmacy. This applies not only to anticonvulsants but is also responsible for increased metabolism of oestrogen preparations which leads to a higher incidence of breakthrough bleeding, and contraceptive failure in epileptic patients.

In contrast, the metabolism of phenytoin is frequently impaired by the presence of other drugs (Perucca 1982). The most clinically important of these is sulthiame which has a potent inhibitory effect on the metabolism of phenytoin and may account for the anti-epileptic action of this drug.

Anticonvulsant drug metabolism is also important because in some cases active metabolites are produced (Table 17.7). Primidone, carbamazepine, and diazepam all have active metabolites which probably contribute to the therapeutic effect of the drug. Whilst it is accepted practice to measure serum phenobarbitone levels derived from primidone, phenylethylmalonimide (PMA) its other active metabolite, and 10,11-epoxide the active metabolite of carbamazepine are not routinely measured. Therefore monitoring serum levels of carbamazepine and primidone gives only a partial picture of active anticonvulsant substances in serum or plasma. Protein-binding and metabolism of active metabolites may differ considerably from those of the parent drug. Thus the half-life of phenobarbitone is of greatest importance in determining the dosage interval for primidone.

## Drug levels and therapeutic effect

Many laboratories offer a routine service for the estimation of commonly used anticonvulsant drugs. They frequently quote therapeutic ranges of serum or plasma concentration (Table 17.8),

Table 17.8.  'Therapeutic' serum concentrations.

| Drug | Plasma/serum concentration ($\mu$g/ml) |
|---|---|
| Phenytoin | 10–20 |
| Phenobarbitone | 15–35 |
| Carbamazepine | 4–8 |
| Valproate | 50–100 |
| Ethosuximide | 40–120 |

which are largely arbitrary and have, with the possible exception of phenytoin, little or no basis in controlled clinical studies (Turnbull et al. 1984). Whilst the upper limit of the therapeutic range is easily defined in terms of the appearance of toxic effects (nystgamus, dysarthria, ataxia and drowsiness in the case of phenytoin, barbiturates, carbamazepine), the serum level at which these occur can be very variable. The most consistent relationship between serum level and toxic effects is for phenytoin, but even with this drug many patients may tolerate, and indeed require, serum levels greater than 20 $\mu$g/ml for seizure control. For phenobarbitone and carbamazepine there is a wider variation in individual tolerance to serum concentration.

The lower limit to the therapeutic range is extremely difficult to define. It is evident that in many patients epilepsy is controlled with serum levels of anticonvulsants that are below published optimal ranges. A major determinant of the best therapeutic level would appear to be the type and severity of the underlying epilepsy. It would be absurd to suggest that a patient presenting at the age of twelve with three or four primarily generalized tonic–clonic seizures, and who has no neurological disease, requires a similar serum level of anticonvulsant to control his seizures as a patient presenting at the age of forty with complex partial seizures due to a cerebral glioma. Unquestioning acceptance of 'therapeutic ranges' can lead to a patient whose seizures are satisfactorily controlled on a low dose and serum level having his dose of anti-convulsant needlessly increased, thereby running an increased risk of adverse reactions; conversely patients who tolerate and need high serum levels may have their dose needlessly reduced, thereby running the risk of further seiz-ures. It is of great importance to treat the patient rather than the serum level.

*Indications for monitoring of serum level of anticonvulsants*

A number of factors influence the need for anti-convulsant monitoring (Table 17.9). It is of par-ticular importance with phenytoin, because of the nonlinear relationship between dose and serum level and the sensitivity that many patients show to small increments in dosage.

Table 17.9.  Indications for anticonvulsant monitoring.

1.  Use of phenytoin
2.  Polypharmacy
3.  In patients in whom assessment of toxicity is difficult
4.  In patients with renal/hepatic disease
5.  Assessing compliance
6.  During controlled studies of anticonvulsants

It will rarely be necessary in patients receiving monotherapy with the other drugs, pheno-barbitone, carbamazepine or valproate. In patients who require polypharmacy, serum level monitoring becomes essential and it may be par-ticularly helpful in patients of low intelligence in whom the detection of toxicity presents par-ticular problems and as a check on compliance with the therapeutic regimen.

## Prognosis of epilepsy

There is a considerable amount of data con-cerning the prognosis of epilepsy. The majority of studies have been hospital based. This has an adverse effect on the outcome, patients with more severe and refractory epilepsy being more likely to be referred to specialist centres. In this respect the study of Annegers *et al.* (1979) is of particular importance as a unique, community based study; 457 patients were followed for at least 5 years, and 141 for 20 years. The prob-ability of being in a remission lasting for 5 years or more was 61% at 10 years, and as high as 70% at 20 years. These figures are considerably more favourable than other studies, reflecting the community basis of the study.

In the majority of other studies remission rates are consistently between 20 and 30% despite the fact that they include periods before the advent of modern anticonvulsant therapy (Rodin 1968). This suggests that remission in epilepsy largely reflects the natural history of the disease rather than the influence of anticonvulsant medication, a suggestion which receives some support from Annegers *et al.* (1979) who were unable to show major changes in remission rates in patients diagnosed with epilepsy between the years of 1935 and 1959 and those diagnosed between 1960 and 1974.

A number of factors influence the prognosis for remission of seizures (Table 17.10). The age of onset of epilepsy is perhaps one of the most important. There is general agreement that the commencement of seizures within the first year of life (when it is usually symptomatic of cerebral

Table 17.10.  Factors influencing the remission of epilepsy.

1.  Age of onset
2.  Seizure classification
3.  Duration and severity of epilepsy
4.  Whether symptomatic or idiopathic

pathology), carries an adverse prognosis. However, apart from this exception, childhood epilepsy is more likely to remit than adult onset epilepsy.

Whatever the age of onset, the duration of epilepsy prior to treatment and remission is an important prognostic factor. Annegers *et al.* (1979) showed that most patients who achieve remission do so early during the course of treatment. With continuing seizures and the passage of time it becomes progressively less likely that an individual patient will enter remission. Thus there is a plateau in the number of patients in remission 15–20 years after the onset of epilepsy.

Seizure type is of major importance. Remission rates are approximately 60% for patients with only tonic–clonic seizures, and between 20 and 40% in patients with complex partial seizures. The combination of complex partial seizures with secondary generalized tonic–clonic seizures seems to have a particularly adverse prognosis. In such patients it is common to find that whilst the tonic–clonic seizures come under control, partial seizures remain resistant to anti-convulsant drug therapy (Turnbull *et al.* 1985). Other generalized epilepsies of childhood carry varying prognoses. Between 80 and 90% of patients with simple absences (petit mal) are likely to enter remission. Patients with the West and Lennox syndromes or complex absences show a lower remission rate (33–65%).

Symptomatic epilepsy, especially when complicated by an associated neuro-psychiatric deficit carries a poorer prognosis than epilepsy of unknown aetiology.

Although the overall prognosis of epilepsy and its response to drug therapy is excellent, neurosurgeons will be less impressed as most of the patients they see with epilepsy have partial seizures, often related to structural cerebral pathology (trauma, tumour, operative scarring), all of which may show relative drug resistance. Neurosurgeons may also be asked to help treat that most resistant epilepsy of all, complex partial epilepsy.

## Surgery for epilepsy

### Indications for further investigation

The indications for consideration of surgery can be stated briefly although their application to a particular patient may be difficult.

1   The failure of optimal medical treatment to provide adequate control of the fits. The operative words here are 'optimal' and 'adequate'. Modern drugs must be exhibited in sufficient dosage over a period of time long enough to prove their failure, and the patient must have con-scientiously taken them. An occasional fit does not mean inadequacy of control; interpretation will be coloured by the nature of the seizure, the amount of upheaval it causes in the patient's life and, therefore, by assessment of the individual patient, and of his or her work and environment. One motor seizure without loss of consciousness each month may be no more than an incon-venience; on the other hand a complex partial seizure with postictal confusion every 3 months may debar a patient from employment.

2   Intellectual and psychological sequelae have developed, of a nature thought to be reversible if the fits can be abolished.

3   Evidence, which may be derived from a variety of sources, that the epilepsy is due to a neoplasm and on which assumption operation is advisable at that time, quite apart from the question of relieving the epilepsy. The phrase 'at that time' is an important qualification because in some cases of neoplasm, operation immedi-ately after a tentative diagnosis is made is not necessarily a wise decision. This judgement lies in the realm of tumour surgery and is dealt with elsewhere.

If these obligatory preliminary enquiries reveal that operation may be entertained, the surgeon must be able to answer further questions before being able to make a decision. The answers to these questions are provided by investigations which must be undertaken, both before and after admission to hospital.

1   Where is the abnormal area or 'focus' which originates the seizure discharge? The patterns of the attacks, the past history and a careful examination may provide suggestive evidence as to the locality of a potential lesion (for example meningocerebral cicatrix, healed brain abscess, hemiatrophy).

2   Is the epileptogenic area surgically accessible and could it be excised without inflicting a

serious neurological penalty, in terms of loss or impairment of function?

These questions can often be answered in out-patient visits, with skull X-rays, CT and EEG examinations. In certain cases the surgeon can be quite sure that surgery will not help and admission to hospital for fuller investigation is unnecessary. But if the patient passes this preliminary screening further questions need to be answered.

3   Is there more than one epileptogenic focus? If so, is one dominant and the other secondary, or are the foci independent of one another (autonomous)? These questions are particularly important, and frequently difficult to answer in temporal lobe epilepsy, when one side may be 'leading', in an epileptic sense, the other providing a mirror image though of slightly diminished brilliance and clarity.

4   Is the rest of the brain healthy or is there evidence of widespread disturbance of neuronal activity? This may be suggested by the past history, the physical findings or the EEG.

5   Is there a macroscopic lesion which might be responsible for the epilepsy?

6   Is the intellectual and educational background such that the patient can benefit from a successful operation?

**Special investigations**

*Radiology*

Examination of the skull may reveal indirect evidence of a space-occupying lesion, or of raised intracranial pressure. Pathological deposits of calcium may be due to a tumour, to an angiomatous malformation, or healed inflammatory disease. Asymmetry of the skull may suggest hemiatrophy of the brain. It may amount to diminution in size of one-half, or to underdevelopment of one middle fossa as shown by a raised petrous ridge, a sphenoidal ridge lying in too posterior a plane and flattening of the temporal squame. The vault may be thicker on

this side. An old depressed fracture may be detected, indriven fragments of bone or a foreign body.

Computerized tomographic scanning allows detection of smaller quantities of calcification, haemorrhage, atrophy (focal or general), dysplastic lesions, for example tuberous sclerosis, and mass lesions such as tumours. However, in a small group of patients Polkey (1982) found that although only 50% of his patients undergoing surgery had an abnormality, none of the patients with a tumour were missed by enhanced CT scanning.

High definition CT in planes along the axis of the temporal lobe with intravenous and, if necessary, intrathecal contrast media can replace satisfactorily air encephalography in the identification of atrophic lesions of the temporal lobe, such as mesial temporal sclerosis.

Angiography should be employed if there is any reason to suspect a vascular anomaly or occlusion. In addition, it is important in stereo-electroencephalography to ensure that no major vessel is perforated during insertion of the electrodes, and in conjunction with Wada testing (*see* below).

Positron emission tomography (PET) has been used in some specialist centres to aid the localization of epileptogenic foci; [18]fluoride-oxyglucose is administered to a patient and the positron emissions displayed as an index of local brain glucose metabolism. The gliosis of epileptogenic regions usually causes reduced emissions in the interictal state, but increased metabolism may be evident during seizures (Mazziotta & Engel 1985).

Magnetic resonance imaging of phosphate spectra may in the future become a valuable investigational tool.

*Electroencephalography*

Electroencephalography is of such importance that it requires the services of a highly skilled staff experienced in the interpretation of epileptic records, and laboratories equipped to carry out specialized tests. The surgeon may easily be led astray by enthusiastic and uncritical opinions on the mass of accumulated information. Past records should be reviewed for chronological comparison which may provide valuable indications as to the primary focus. Routine examinations should be repeated several times in order to confirm the constancy of an abnormality. Further information may be gained from records during sleep (occurring naturally, or induced by quinalbarbitone, or seconal) and during the graduated intravenous injection of thiopentone sodium (pentothal). Brazier *et al.* (1976) have used diazepam. These accentuate or bring out (latent) spike and sharp wave abnormality and healthy brain responds by an increase in fast activity. An absence of, or diminution in drug-induced fast activity suggests the presence of damaged tissue and is helpful in the investigation of temporal lobe epilepsy (Kennedy & Hill 1958).

Further EEG examinations should take account of the clinical localization and abnormalities already revealed. Thus scalp electrodes should be grouped more closely about the scar of a head injury in order to determine as precisely as possible the relevant area of the scar involved in discharge. If temporal lobe epilepsy is suspected electrodes may be inserted into the infratemporal fossa to pick up discharges from the inferior surface of the lobe. Such sphenoidal leads and were first described by Jasper (1949) and Jones (1951) and the technique was elaborated by Pampiglione and Kerridge (1956).

Interical recordings of sharp waves and spikes are important and correlate well with the site of origin of seizures in most patients. On occasion, however, seizures may arise at some distance from, and even contralateral to interical focal spikes (Engel *et al.* 1981). For this reason, every effort should be made to verify the site of origin of seizures by ictal recording. This can usually be achieved by surface recording during prolonged monitoring by telemetry or ambulatory monitoring at a time when drug therapy is reduced or stopped. Even so, artifact can obscure the onset of the seizure discharge, in which case the use of implanted electrodes should be considered.

In some patients there may be doubt as to which hemisphere is dominant for speech, which is of obvious importance if temporal lobectomy is contemplated on what may prove to be the dominant side. Wada found that the injection of amylobarbitone sodium (sodium amytal) into the internal (or common) carotid artery caused a transient paralysis of the functions of the ipsilateral cerebral hemisphere; aphasia accompanied flaccid hemiplegia when the injection was made on the dominant side. This useful discovery was elaborated into a formal test (Wada & Rasmussen 1960) and was then further refined by Serafetinides *et al.* (1965). Rovit *et al.* (1961) have found that if the EEG is recorded at the same time the test can be used for distinguishing secondary from primary bilateral synchrony. The former is abolished when the injection is ipsilateral to a cortical lesion; the latter persists during the injection although it may be modified.

The investigation in animals of epileptic discharges and of other electrophysiological phenomena has shown that fine wire electrodes inserted into the brain may be left *in situ* for a considerable time without harm and that valuable information can be derived from them. The first application in man was probably that of Bickford and Cairns, who in 1944 left a multistrand electrode within the track of an intracerebral battle injury for several days and obtained good recordings (Woltman 1953). Delgado *et al.* (1952) described their use in psychiatric patients and since then they have been used extensively in selected cases of epilepsy. Their value lies in the fact that electrical abnormality of an epileptic nature may be taking place in a deeply placed mass of grey matter without being revealed in the simultaneous scalp record, but can be sampled by an electrode inserted into it. Under a small covering dose of antibiotic, electrodes can be left in the subdural space and in the brain for several weeks with little risk of infection. Histological examination has only occasionally revealed the site previously occupied by a wire. Abnormal potentials which can be ascribed to the injury of insertion subside within 1–3 days (Fischer-Williams & Cooper 1963, Bates 1963, Marsan & Abraham 1966). The areas of the brain which may require investigation by these delicate techniques are the frontal and the temporal lobes. In the former situation they may provide means of determining epileptic discharges arising from the orbital or the medial surfaces, in which the scalp records reveal secondary projected synchrony. Electrodes may be inserted to sample the activity of the medial and of the orbital cortex; in these situations the introduction can be performed freehand with sufficient accuracy provided the position of the frontal and occipital horns have been identified by pneumoencephalography or CT. Subdural plates can sometimes be inserted either side of the falx, but adhesions frequently prevent this. In the case of temporal lobe, one or more subdural plates can be placed over the convexity cortex and leashes inserted into the uncus, the amygdalum and the hippocampus. For these structures accuracy of implantation can only be achieved by stereotaxic technique after identifying the temporal horns. Both hemispheres should be investigated with symmetrically implanted electrodes and the EEG examinations should include concurrent recordings from scalp electrodes.

Indwelling electrodes carry some risk but provide an opportunity to study deep electrical activity. As well as providing more information about the interictal EEG, implanted electrodes can also be used in the study of spontaneously occurring seizures. No ethical problems arise if the use of the technique in a particular patient is governed by the need to obtain information for management decisions which cannot be obtained by more conventional methods. Such information includes detection of discharges not revealed by scalp electrodes, more precise localization and identification, if there is more than one focus, of their autonomy or otherwise. These data may be crucial in the decision for or against operation.

'Parasagittal high-voltage electrical potentials of almost any form or frequency may be considered epileptiform from the EEG point of view'

(Jasper 1954). Certainly the most dramatic, obvious, and perhaps the most frequent of these in partial epilepsy are random (sporadic) spikes. To qualify as a criterion of an epileptic focus they should be seen against an abnormal background and should be consistently present at approximately the same site in several records. The same holds good for sharp waves which are thought to originate as spikes but modified by conduction through or across brain tissue. Abnormality of background comprises a diminution of such activity and the presence of irregular slow waves (of delta and theta frequencies). The spikes which are seen in contralateral homologous areas are often of lesser amplitude, slightly slower (more broadly based) and less frequent in repetition. Hill (1963) states that the ratio of random spikes in the dominant focus to those in the secondary focus may vary between 4 to 1 and 100 to 1. Spikes and sharp waves may be intermingled with slow waves or linked with them to form repetitive irregular patterns, often referred to as complexes; when highly organized and rhythmical they become 'spike and wave' discharges and constitute the secondary bilateral synchrony which Jasper described in relation to certain frontal lesions. By concentrating the scalp electrodes and rearranging their connections it may be possible to localize the discharge more precisely by the phenomenon of phase reversal. If these discharges are arising from a small superficial site, they should be restricted to an area of scalp some 5 cm across and beyond this should be found a normal record. The abnormalities seen in the records that are derived from implanted electrodes are of a similar order, though the spike discharges are of a much greater magnitude and may be barely or not at all represented in the overlying scalp record.

When large areas of the hemisphere are atrophic, as in children with hemiplegia, epilepsy and behaviour disorders, the EEG record on the relevant side shows much more diffuse abnormality; spikes, sharp waves, slow activity particularly in the delta frequencies, are widely dispersed in the various channels. There may be areas of isopotential (absence of recognizable activity) which usually indicate a subjacent porencephalic cyst. The contralateral (apparently healthy) side also shows similar changes but of lesser degree, though lack of activity would suggest bilateral disease. It sometimes happens that spike or sharp wave discharges appear to be more pronounced on the side which by clinical judgement is the healthy side. This may indeed be the case, on the grounds that such discharges occur more readily or are better conducted in the healthy tissue, and that they are secondarily projected from the abnormal other side. This may be ascertained by scrutinizing the amount of slow activity which is a better criterion of degree of brain damage. The distinction may be sharpened by the effect of a barbiturate which activates fast activity in normal tissue but fails to do so, or to the same extent, in the diseased zone.

The EEG manifestations of a clinical seizure have already been described. The general pattern is of a rapidly progressive development of waves of increasing amplitude regularly repeated; the rhythmic discharge gradually slows, stops suddenly and is followed by a brief period of extinction of activity. Of special importance when bilateral abnormalities are present in the interictal record, is the mode of onset of the seizure record in some cases. The random spikes may increase somewhat in frequency but then disappear and other activity is so reduced that the traces are virtually flat in the affected area or over much of that side of the head. During the period of suppression, a matter of some seconds, high voltage sharp waves may be seen in the opposite homologous area; these may be mistaken for the seizure discharge and lead to wrong lateralization (Hill 1963).

## Psychiatric, psychological and social assessment

Although the diverse physical investigations may favour operation, no decision can be made without a thorough examination of the psychiatric and psychological state of the patient and the social background. This requires professional advice, appropriate tests, interviews with relatives and if appropriate a visit to the home by a psychiatric social worker. The decision about surgical treatment should be arrived at after discussion with those concerned.

All patients require full neuropsychological appraisal. The Wechsler Adult Intelligence Scale (WAIS) provides overall assessment of intelligence, and performance patterns on the subtests of the Scale can help to localize areas of cortical dysfunction. Because of the importance of the temporal lobes in memory functions, more detailed testing of verbal and visual memory is important, and may indicate which temporal lobe (dominant or nondominant) is more affected (Luria 1980). Agreement between the lateralization of the maximal EEG disturbance and an appropriate impairment of verbal and visual memory is in favour of a decision for surgical treatment, whilst evidence of bilateral or multilobar disfunction is a contraindication.

Further testing to determine the lateralization of speech and memory, and therefore the risks of temporal lobectomy, will usually be needed. Wada testing can be undertaken in conjunction with cerebral angiography (Wada & Ramussen 1960). With a catheter in the internal carotid artery 50–100mg amylobarbitone is injected until contralateral weakness occurs, at which point testing of language function and memory is undertaken. After recovery, the contralateral artery can be injected and the tests repeated. If memory is severely impaired by unilateral carotid injection, this indicates some dysfunction of the contralateral temporal lobe structures, and a significant risk to memory if ipsilateral temporal lobectomy is carried out.

## Decision to operate

Various questions must be answered in order to decide whether operation is advisable. Operation is justified if it can be shown that:

1   All the investigations concur with the clinical picture in incriminating a particular portion of brain.

2 The area is accessible for extirpation without inflicting significant functional deficit, or significant additional deficit.

3 EEG evidence of epileptiform activity elsewhere in the brain indicates that it is of a secondary nature.

4 Psychiatric and intellectual handicaps present no bar to operation, with the proviso that cure of epilepsy may in some patients lessen the handicap.

Provided that the data are favourable, the decision about surgery is rarely difficult in patients with a convexity focus, for example meningocerebral cicatrix, or a focus due to healed abscess, or if a macroscopic lesion had been identified. Candidates for temporal lobectomy provide most problems in decision making.

## Operation

Operative treatment can be divided into two types, resective and functional.

### Resective surgery

*Lobectomy*

For details of the technique of temporal lobe resection the reader should refer to Penfield and Jasper (1954), Falconer *et al.* (1955) and Falconer (1971), and for frontal lobectomy to MacCabe (1971). Certain general principles govern the procedure. With the discovery of anaesthetic agents which produce little more than deep sleep and do not inactivate the observable electrical activities of the brain, an increasing number of surgeons employ general anaesthesia. It has its advantages in convenience to the surgeon and oblivion for the patient and it is clearly the method of choice in children, in uncooperative patients and in most cases of temporal lobectomy. Nevertheless it denies both surgeon and patient the great advantage of conscious responses to electrical stimulation which

may prove of importance in accurate assessment of the site and extent of the extirpation. When operating on the dominant hemisphere under general anaesthesia there is no method of determining the precise site and boundaries of areas necessary for speech. It is possible to combine the advantages of both methods, by employing a short lasting intravenous drug (for example sodium thiopentone) during the preliminary stages, discontinuing this when the brain is exposed, and reverting to it for the closure. But there is no doubt that local anaesthesia with premedication is to be preferred. The requirements are copious amounts of dilute local anaesthetic solution, repeated if necessary as the deeper tissues are reached, and injected into the dura mater when it is exposed; absolute quiet in the theatre; reassurance of the patient by the surgeon, and warnings of any immediate unpleasant or unusual events (for example breaking the bone flap, electrical stimulation). The scar which follows a penetrating head wound binds together skin, brain and its membranes; consequently care must be exercised during the exposure stage of the craniotomy that the various layers are reflected and the intervening scar tissue divided without the transmission to the brain of any traction; not an easy exercise. The size of the craniotomy will be governed by the site and the extent of the lesion and the EEG abnormality. In the case of the temporal lobe, the opening should extend to the floor and the anterior wall of the middle fossa, so as to provide easy access to the temporal pole for electrocorticography (ECoG) and to facilitate the extirpation of the lobe without unnecessary traction or other manipulation. During this examination the brain must be kept moist and at normal temperature, otherwise its electrical activities will be affected. To effect this, those parts of the cortex not immediately required for testing (for example by stimulation or ECoG) should be protected. The brain should be scrutinized for evidence of abnormality and very gently palpated to detect undue firmness of consistency.

Electrocorticography is carried out by applying

recording electrodes to the brain, in a systematic sequence of patterns. The abnormalities revealed by ECoG are of the same order as those derived from the scalp, but the potential changes are at least four times as great. Detection of electrical artifact is important and may arise from imperfect contact with the cortex, arterial pulsation, cortical irrigation, respiration, movement of electrically charged objects or persons and variation in temperature. ECoG was originally used to define the site of electrical abnormality and hence the area to be excised. Too rigid pursuit of these abnormalities can lead to increased postoperative neurological defects (Polkey 1982). In particular it does not help in determining the extent of a temporal lobe resection. In resections of areas of the cortical mantle ECoG may be of great value particularly in lessening the risk of dysphasia in the dominant hemisphere.

The technique of extirpation follows normal neurosurgical practice with the proviso that lines of incision should have particular regard for the blood supply of adjacent brain. This means the preservation of major arteries and veins, modifying the resection if necessary, lest ischaemia of surrounding tissue give rise to further epileptogenic areas. Marginal grey matter is removed by suction so that a narrow fringe of pia mater is preserved, ensuring the blood supply of the subjacent cortex. Histological studies have shown that removal of brain by suction gives rise to less gliosis than the use of endothermy and ligation (Steelman 1949). Temporal lobectomy should include the uncus, the amygdalum, hippocampus and hippocampal gyrus. The amygdalum can be sucked away gently after the lobectomy is completed if the site of the uncus and the tip of the temporal horn have been carefully noted. The posterior limit of the resection will be governed by the situation of speech function (identified by speech arrest following stimulation) and by the increasing probability of hemianopia as the extent of the resection is pushed posteriorly. Some useful anatomical details of the temporal lobe have been described by Penfield and Baldwin (1952) but studies of the resultant visual field defects have shown considerable variations between extent of resection and extent of field defect (Marino & Rasmussen 1968). In general the more posterior the resection the more likely is the defect to approach full hemianopia, though this rarely occurs. The lack of strict correlation may be due to individual variation in the position of the inferior fibres of the optic radiation as they sweep around the temporal horn (Meyer's loop). An alternative and perhaps as likely cause is variation in the degree of ischaemic damage to these fibres following interruption of small deep branches from the middle cerebral artery. Great care is required during the removal of the uncus and the hippocampal gyrus owing to their close proximity to structures bearing medial (i.e. deep) relationship; these include the third and fourth cranial nerves, the posterior cerebral artery, veins, and the brain stem. The integrity of these structures can be best respected by peeling the medial temporal portions of brain tissue out of their pial investment, which then remains as a protective covering. They are often firm, almost rubbery, which facilitates this manœuvre. It is also notable that often they partly lie over the free edge of the tentorium as though displaced medially by past herniation. If it is possible to do so without risk of functional deficit further brain should be removed; hippocampus and its gyrus are easily reached with a sucker. Often another centimetre or so will abolish the unwanted discharges. Opinions differ as to the importance of removing portions of the insula; the risks of causing hemiparesis by damaging perforating branches of the middle cerebral artery are considerable (Penfield et al. 1961). An incidence of 20% for neurological complications after insulectomy has been reported (Silfvenius et al. 1964). Orbital cortex may be safely removed provided it is not taken so far back or so deeply as to damage vessels entering the anterior perforated substance. It must be emphasized that the removal of all tissue from which spikes have been recorded is often impracticable and the late results show that what appears to have been an ineffective operation as judged by the final ECoG control may nevertheless prove very successful. Avoidance of major functional deficit must always determine the surgeon's judgement.

The pre-operative anticonvulsant drugs should be resumed forthwith. Fits which occur after the operation should be carefully recorded by the nursing staff and if they are similar to pre-operative patterns the advisability of early re-exploration and further excision must be seriously considered; it will depend upon whether the surgeon was radical or conservative in his extirpation. Fits of a different pattern result from the activating effects of trauma, either directly or indirectly as a consequence of disturbed blood circulation; venous occlusion is probably the commonest sequel. The administration of a short-acting anticonvulsant, for example diazepam or chlormethiazole, may be necessary for a short period in addition to the usual regime. The fits usually subside within a few days.

### Results of operation

Mortality for these operative procedures is now very low. Penfield (1958) reported a death rate of 1.5% in 470 patients (includes all types of operation). At the London Hospital there was only 1 death among 63 patients submitted to temporal lobectomy and that was due to pulmonary embolus; Rasmussen and Jasper (1958) reported 2 deaths following 217 operations for temporal lobe epilepsy and Jensen (1975) a mortality of 0.5%. Rasmussen (1983) records a

similar mortality (0.4%) in 1,034 in non-tumoural cases, with only one operative death in the last 950 cases. Sixteen patients died from a variety of causes in the first 2 postoperative years. There was a 1.7% mortality for frontal lobectomy (Rasmussen 1975).

The effects upon the patients can be considered under several headings; the epilepsy, the psychiatric aspects, the penalties in terms of neurological function and social rehabilitation;

### Epilepsy

For some time there has been uncertainty whether initial relief from seizures persists, or whether, as years pass, an increasing number of patients will relapse. Operations for epilepsy have now been practised with modern techniques for a length of time sufficient to provide prolonged observations. After the second year there is very little decline in the percentage of good results (Rasmussen & Branch 1962, Falconer & Serafetinides 1963).

Table 17.11 sets out some published results. Rasmussen (1983) discussed the results of temporal lobectomy in 1034 cases without a tumour but in 120 of these there was less than 2 years follow-up information. The prognosis for temporal lobe epilepsy is somewhat better than that for frontal lobe epilepsy. It is encouraging that in some of these patients a second operation was undertaken with a similar ratio of successful

Table 17.11. Results of operations for epilepsy.

| Source | Localization | No fits or very few % | Improved % | Failure % | Number of points |
|---|---|---|---|---|---|
| Rasmussen & Branch (1962) | Temporal | 43 | 25 | 32 | 389 |
| Rasmussen (1963) | Frontal | 33 | 30 | 36 | 168 |
| Falconer & Serafetinides (1963) | Temporal | 53 | 30 | 17 | 100 |
| Green & Schutz (1964) | Temporal | 12 | 57 | 31 | 60 |
| Paillas et al. (1963) | Mixed | 39 | 27 | 34 | 100 |
| Northfield (1965) | Temporal | 62 | 18 | 20 | 58 |
| Jensen (1975) | Temporal | 42 | 22 | 36 | 831 |
| Rasmussen (1975) | Frontal | 23 | 32 | 45 | 236 |
| Rasmussen (1983) | Temporal | 37 | 26 | 37 | 894 |

results. The criteria for 'cure' and for improvement vary; in some reports 'cure' includes only those patients in whom there were no seizures after the operation; in others it includes those patients who had fits in the first year or so but none thereafter. Columns 1 and 2 together indicate clearly whether the operation was worthwhile; in column 3 are the failures which speak for themselves. In temporal lobe tumours (Rasmussen 1983) there were 2 operative deaths in 174 cases. Thirteen died in the first 2 postoperative years, 144 survived, and in those with follow-up data 52 died between 2 and 18 years later; 46% became seizure free and in 76% the seizure frequency was greatly reduced.

It is important to ascertain to what degree prognosis depends upon the elimination of electrical signs of epileptic discharge, as judged by the postexcisional ECoG or by the postoperative EEG. There are two groups of cases: (1) those in which there were bilateral abnormalities before operation, (2) those in which abnormality in the field of operation could not be entirely eradicated.

1  Bengzon et al. (1968) found that in about one-half (55%) of their unsuccessful cases bilateral abnormalities were present before operation, whereas in successful cases the figure was 30%. The experience of Falconer and Serafetinides (1963) was similar. They also made the cogent points that a strictly unilateral EEG focus is no guarantee for success, and that bilateral EEG abnormalities by no means preclude it, provided the predominant side can be determined and that lobe removed. Bloom et al. (1960) isolated 29 cases of epilepsy with independent bitemporal EEG abnormality treated by unilateral lobectomy; in 19 there was predominance and 6 of these had a successful result; in the other 10 both temporal lobes seemed equally abnormal and in only one was operation successful.
2  Successful results can follow what appears to have been an incomplete operation by the ECoG criterion. An ECoG abnormality of the insula provides a problem. In 106 such cases Silfvenius et al. (1964) found no significant evidence that a persistent abnormality in this area of cortex

militated against success. Rasmussen (1983) had similar findings but Bengzon et al. (1968) found that the postexcisional ECoG was free from discharge in 64% of the successful results and in only 28% of the unsuccessful. Scalp records after operation showed no epileptiform features in three quarters of the successes, and in less than half of the unsuccessful cases. This proportion of good records dwindles in later examinations. Falconer and Serafetinides (1963) reported on the EEG findings 3 years after operation; no epileptic activity was found in 81% of the successful and in 8% of the unsuccessful cases. A number of patients remain free from fits in spite of persistent EEG abnormalities. Rasmussen (1983) assumed that the remaining focus represented a lower order of epileptogenicity.

Other factors which might influence prognosis were examined by Bengzon et al. (1968), two of which will be considered. It might be assumed theoretically that the longer a patient suffers epilepsy prior to operation, the less the hope of success. This assumption is false and long duration of epilepsy prior to operation does not necessarily militate against success. The other influence upon prognosis is the nature of the pathological lesion. Here it is important to recall the dictum of Penfield, that the removal of normal tissue is useless (Penfield & Jasper 1954, Penfield 1958). In 100 specimens of temporal lobe removed for epilepsy Falconer and Serafetinides (1963) found medial temporal sclerosis in 47 and small tumours or hamartomas in 24, the others containing miscellaneous or equivocal lesions; the most successful results occurred in the first two groups.

*Psychiatric aspects*

The behaviour disorders associated with epilepsy, aggressiveness and tantrums, improve considerably in accordance with the degree of success in abolishing fits. Falconer and Serafetinides (1963) reported that of 19 aggressive patients who were virtually free of fits, 16 showed improvement in behaviour compared with only one showing lessening of aggression amongst 10 whose fits persisted unabated. In Northfield's (1965) series, 13 of 25 aggressive patients showed improvement (Paillas *et al.* 1963). Where there is a general improvement in behaviour, cooperation and attentiveness, some recovery of educability may be anticipated (Liddell & Northfield 1954). Psychosis may also improve, particularly where the disorder has taken an episodic course. James (1960) assessed on a numerical basis the social adjustment of 72 patients with temporal lobe epilepsy, before and after lobectomy. For aggressiveness, the pre-operative degree of adjustment was 5% and the final assessment after operation was 73%, for psychotics the relative figures were 14 and 66%. Operation does not have a beneficial effect upon those firmly established psychoses which resemble schizophrenia, even though the fits may be cured (Slater *et al.* 1963). Hill (1958) considered that patients with hysterical or inadequate personalities were not suitable for operation and little improvement in these symptoms was noted by Falconer and Serafetinides (1963).

*Morbidity*

Visual field defects can result from temporal lobe resection. If the limit is between 5 and 6 cm from the temporal tip the incidence of a complete homonymous hemianopia is approximately 5%. This is due to variations in Meyer's loop (Falconer & Wilson 1958). As the extent of the resection increases so does the risk of a homonymous hemianopia, until it is almost certain beyond 7 cm. An upper quadrantanopia is more common, occurring in nearly two thirds of patients, but frequently recedes during the first postoperative year (Polkey 1982). Marino and Rasmussen (1968) found that the defects were frequently incongruous, the larger loss being in the field of the ipsilateral eye. The changes in the visual fields are rarely a disability; indeed loss of up to a quarter of the visual field is usually not appreciated by the patient until tests are carried

out, though a similar loss in the lower instead of the upper field would probably be immediately perceived (*see also* Van Buren & Baldwin 1958, Falconer & Wilson 1958). Extension into the lower field on either side may cause difficulty in negotiating obstructions, doorways and traffic. A right hemianopia interferes with reading because scanning the lines is difficult and the whole word or phrase is not immediately perceived. The patient requires instruction and usually rapidly accommodates.

Other signs of focal damage to the brain consequent upon extirpation of an epileptogenic lesion will depend upon its situation. Hemiplegia and dysphagia are more likely if corticectomy is carried out in or near the insula. They usually resolve unless a major branch of the middle cerebral artery is damaged. Jensen (1975) found incidences of 2% for permanent hemiparesis and 5% for dysphasia. Hearing is unaffected by temporal lobectomy although Heschl's gyrus is often so close to the margin of resection; Paillas *et al.* (1963) thought that there might be some impairment to vocal compared with tonal tests and found an impaired reaction to provoked vertigo. Disturbances of evoked nystagmus in patients with temporal lobe lesions have been studied by Carmichael *et al.* (1961).

In contrast to the psychiatric benefits, certain psychological penalties may be exacted by temporal lobectomy. The most serious is impairment of recent memory. In its most severe degree it was previously found as a regular sequel to bilateral selective extirpation of the hippocampal formation and to bilateral temporal lobectomy which included these deep structures. These early operations were carried out in an attempt to alleviate certain intractable mental disorders (Terzian & Ore 1955, Scoville & Milner 1957). The failure of memory was for current and recent events and appeared to depend upon the extent to which the hippocampus on each side was destroyed; removal of uncus and amygdalum, sparing the hippocampus, did not have this effect. In its severest form the memory loss was still evident several years after the operation. There was no impairment of intelligence. There are other sporadic records of similar severe memory defects and it is clear that bilateral temporal lobectomy is absolutely contraindicated. Unfortunately the sequel has been encountered after unilateral operations; in these it is assumed that on the unoperated side pre-existing disease (Ammon's horn sclerosis) has so damaged the deep temporal structures that healthy tissue has been reduced below the minimum necessary to subserve function.

Horel (1978) reviewed the neurology of memory and mentioned cases of encephalitis involving the limbic system and associated with severe memory loss. Jones (1974) demonstrated the need for mnemonic aids in the learning process after left but not right temporal lobectomy. Apart from these severe disturbances, more subtle impairment of mental function has been observed after temporal lobectomy, mostly related to removals on the dominant side. Meyer and Yates (1955) found a significant difficulty in learning; Hill (1958) noted it particularly in relation to auditory information, and he emphasized that this proved a serious handicap in certain occupations, for example a telephone operator. Milner (1958) carried out detailed psychological tests before and after temporal lobectomy in 100 patients and noted similar and other disorders and showed in addition that they were to a slight degree present before the operation, presumably due to the lesion causing the epilepsy or to the epileptic discharges. These auditory learning defects gradually improve (Blakemore & Falconer 1967). The special role which the left temporal lobe may play in preserving the correct 'timing' of stimuli derived from each hemisphere is the subject of a fascinating study by Efron (1963).

### Social rehabilitation

This depends not only upon the success of the operation in abolishing fits, but also upon any psychiatric disorder which might have been present, the social and home background, whether the patient had lived in hospital for some time, and the availability of a rehabilitation service, both psychiatric and physical. The operation is only one stage in the return to a useful and happy life (James 1960). There may be an interval of a year or so before psychiatric improvement is such as to permit satisfactory employment. During this time aftercare and guidance are essential. A small proportion of patients pass through a stage of depression which may require treatment. In his survey of frontal lobe resections for epilepsy, Rasmussen (1963) stated that of those patients whose fits were greatly reduced, about 90% achieved a satisfactory social result (i.e. working and domestic duties) but in the failures this proportion was only 37%. In the 60 patients with temporal lobe epilepsy reported by Green and Schutz (1964), all of whom were dependent (unemployed) prior to operation, 60% subsequently became self-supporting. In a detailed analysis of 'clinical socioeconomic and psychological changes after temporal lobectomy' in 100 patients Taylor and Falconer (1968) found a net gain in employment of 24. Jensen (1976) states that social adjustment is most likely if operation was undertaken before 15 years of age in patients with normal intelligence and good postoperative seizure control.

### Other cortical resections

Removal of other parts of the cortex which are mainly central or parietal (rarely is the occipital cortex a focus of epileptigenic activity) is undertaken rarely. It is undertaken under local anaesthesia with ECoG and stimulation control. Rasmussen (1975) and Talairach et al. (1974) have reported 64% and 67% respectively in which the seizures were abolished or substantially controlled. Bhatia and Kollevold (1976) however achieved this in only 30%.

*Hemispherectomy*

A group of young patients can be defined in whom hemiplegia during infancy is followed by intractable epilepsy and later by serious mental disorder. The hemiplegia may be the result of a birth injury or may develop suddenly in infancy during a febrile illness, often with severe convulsions. The causes of this hemiplegia, hemiconvulsion, epilepsy (HHE) syndrome are discussed by Gastaut *et al.* (1960). Part or most of one cerebral hemisphere atrophies, sometimes to a degree that the brain tissue over the dilated lateral ventricle is reduced to a filmy translucent membrane. The epilepsy shows a variety of patterns, partial and generalized. Behaviour disorders are usually the most obvious and distressing of the mental disturbances: tantrums, violence and general indiscipline. Education becomes irregular and often impossible, there being both dulling of intelligence and an inability to attend, to cooperate and to mix with other children. The EEG shows a wide range of paroxysmal and slow wave abnormalities diffusely scattered over both hemispheres. On the atrophic side the EEG is generally of lower voltage and with more slow waves; an area of relative EEG silence may be found indicating absence of subjacent cortical neuroelectrical activity. Radiological examination may reveal asymmetry of the skull and marked dilatation of all or of part of the lateral ventricle on the relevant side: the contralateral ventricle commonly shows slight but sometimes considerable dilatation. Although McKenzie appears to have performed the first hemispherectomy for hemiplegia and fits (Williams & Scott 1939), Krynauw (1950) placed the operation on a firm basis when he reported the results in 12 patients.

Selection of patients is made on clinical and radiological grounds rather than on the EEG examination; bilateral abnormality is no bar to operation and the EEG of the healthier hemisphere usually improves after operation. But radiological examination is important, because considerable dilatation of the 'healthy' ventricle shows that brain damage is present bilaterally and that hemispherectomy is inadvisable. In HHE patients the 'dominant' hemisphere for speech is the healthy one.

The technique of the operation has been described by Krynauw (1950), McKissock (1953) and Laine and Gros (1956). The usual practice is to remove all that remains of the hemisphere including medial and inferior cortex, temporal lobe and its deep structures, down to the plane of the body of the ventricle, but to spare the basal ganglia; particular care is taken to avoid damage to the central branches of the anterior and the middle cerebral arteries. The mortality rate is comparatively low, between 5 and 10%. Wilson (1970) has analysed the results in McKissock's 50 cases. There was 1 postoperative death, though 15 patients died later from haemorrhagic complications, some many years after the operation (*see* below). Of the survivors 68% remained free from fits and 14% were much improved. Behaviour disorders were abolished or lessened in 93% and nearly one-half showed psychological improvement (*see also* White 1961, Rasmussen & Gossman 1963, Laine *et al.* 1964). Cairns and Davidson (1951) published a careful description of the changes in intellect and behaviour after hemispherectomy in 3 patients, with dramatic improvement in the rate of learning in one case. Hemispherectomy adds nothing to the neurological deficit when cerebral atrophy is already severe and extensive. Indeed, improvement has been noted in speech (Basser 1962) and in the performance of the paralysed limbs. Some have suggested that the latter is due to a lessening of spasticity. Denny-Brown and Chambers (1958) considered that such 'improved function following removal of brain can only mean that unrestrained activity of avoiding mechanisms in man, as in monkey, can prevent function for which an alternative coarser mechanism is nevertheless present'. The popularity of the operation has waned in recent years; Griffith (1967) reviewing the Oxford results in 18 cases, pointed out that these operations had taken place between 1950 and 1961 and there had been none since. Late sequelae may be the reason for this (Carmichael 1966). Griffith *et al.* (1969) draw attention to an unusual delayed complication which may prove fatal. It develops some years ( a maximum of 12 years was reported) after the hemispherectomy during which time health is good, and takes the form of insidious general deterioration, headaches, recurrence of mental disturbance and progressive lethargy. The cause is repeated haemorrhage into the hemicranial cavity and CSF pathways with consequent fibrosis and obstructive hydrocephalus (*see also* Hughes and Oppenheimer 1969). The cavity is found to be lined with a vascular granular membrane similar to that of a chronic subdural haematoma. Removal of the membrane and the insertion of a ventriculoatrial shunt has cured some cases. Now that this serious complication has been recognized its earlier diagnosis should be possible and effective treatment practicable.

### Functional surgery

In view of the predominant role which the amygdaloid nucleus may play in the genesis or elaboration of the seizures of temporal lobe epilepsy, tentative attempts have been made to excise or destroy it, in some cases including the hippocampus. Excision by formal craniotomy is difficult because of the deep situation of the nucleus. It can be reached and removed by suction, after opening up and separating the margins of the Sylvian fissure and identifying the uncus, or by an approach through the temporal horn after incising the middle temporal convolution. These manœuvres inevitably involve much trauma to superficial structures. The idea that intractable epilepsy requires electrical propagation over neural pathways, irrespective of the basic pathology underlying the epileptogenic focus led to the idea that sterotactic interruption of the fibres in these pathways might control seizures. Some evidence for this was forthcoming from the production of such lesions to control aggressive behaviour (Narabayashi *et al.* 1963) which incidentally reduced the seizure frequency. In addition McLardy (1969) had sug-

gested that temporal lobe surgery was effective because it interrupted the connections between the amygdala and the hippocampus.

Stereotactic amygdalotomy has been noted (Narabayashi & Shima 1973) to improve uncontrolled seizures in 50% of cases, whereas Vaernet (1972) found it to be effective in only one sixth of cases. Mundinger *et al.* (1976) felt that unilateral foci were more likely to respond than bilateral ones and that fornicotomy and commissurotomy should be combined with amygdalotomy.

Turner (1963) has described three operations for temporal lobe epilepsy, in which fibre pathways are cut at certain well-defined sites. The lesion is a leucotomy (lobotomy) made through a burr hole with a special leucotome, usually under stereotactic control. Three sites were chosen:

1   A quadrantic cut in the coronal place, in the roof of the temporal horn about 1 cm posterior to its tip. This divides what is called the isthmus of the temporal lobe.
2   A quadrantic cut in the same plane as in 1, but downwards through the hippocampus, behind the uncus.
3   A cut to divide 'fibres sweeping backwards and upwards from the orbital surface of the frontal lobe'. It constituted a basal frontal leucotomy.

A lesion at site 1 was used in all cases, and an additional lesion at sites 2 and 3, either unilaterally or bilaterally in some of the cases. The results in 38 patients were as follows; fits were abolished or frequency or severity reduced in nearly 70%, and mental disorders improved in 67%. Turner concluded that operation at site 1 was indicated for major psychomotor epilepsy and behavioural disturbances, that bilateral operations were more successful than unilateral, and that basal anterior leucotomy (site 3) relieved depression. The results encourage the use of these operations in cases of temporal lobe epilepsy unsuitable for lobectomy because of bilateral and equally active EEG abnormality.

An example of interruption of the limbic lobe 'circuit' at a more distant point than Turner's operations is that of Umbach (1966) who had divided the fornix (fornicectomy) at the level of the anterior commissure. In some cases this had been done bilaterally (at intervals of 6–8 months), and in some combined with destruction of the amygdalum and hippocampus. The technique is by sterotaxis and 18 patients have been observed for periods of 3–11 years; 5 have been rendered fit free, and grand mal abolished in 11 of the 13 who suffered that type in addition to temporal lobe fits. Behaviour improved and no persistent adverse effects were encountered after the bilateral operations.

Lesions more centrally situated have also been employed. Wycis et al. (1966) have placed these in the pallidum on one or both sides and in some cases in conjunction with a lesion in the amygdalum. Observations on 11 patients cover 6–10 years, and in about one-third the fits (of minor, salaam and grand mal patterns) were abolished. A few patients with various types of seizure have been treated by lesions in the thalamus with some successful results (Mullan & Penfield 1959). Experimental observations on induced cortical epilepsy led Jinnai to the conclusion that the corticofugal pathways became closely approximated in the brain stem in the region below the thalamus and above the red nucleus; a lesion here appeared to raise the threshold of convulsive cortical activity (Jinnai & Nishimoto 1963). He has published the results of lesion made in the Forel-H field in 59 epileptic patients. At the end of 1 year 36% were still free from fits and about one quarter had not been improved but later reports from the same group (1976) reflect disappointment in the overall results.

### Cerebral commissurotomy

There is evidence that the commissures, particularly the corpus callosum, are of prime importance in the spread of seizure discharge (see above). For this reason, a number of surgeons have undertaken division of the forebrain commissures in the belief that confining a seizure discharge to one hemisphere should restrict generalized seizures developing after a partial onset in one hemisphere (Van Wagenen & Heuren 1940, Luessenhop 1970, Wilson et al. 1977).

The numbers of patients treated by this means remains small and the results are difficult to assess. Certainly the operation has been more important for our understanding of cerebral disconnection syndromes than for the treatment of epilepsy. Some have claimed benefit in seizure control for some patients, but this has been at the expense of not inconsiderable morbidity, and even mortality which has been due to the development of complicating hydrocephalus and ventriculitis (Wilson et al. 1978). For this reason a more restricted approach has been suggested, confining the operation to section of the corpus callosum, leaving the anterior and hippocampal commissures and fornix intact, and avoiding the necessity of opening the ventricles at operation. It has been claimed that this modification is as successful as the more extensive procedure in the control of seizures, and to carry fewer complications (Wilson et al. 1978). The place of the operation in the surgical treatment of epilepsy awaits the publication of a larger series of patients.

The diversity of human disease raises the difficulty of selecting a specific target in a particular patient. This has led Talairach et al. (1974) and Ojemann and Ward (1975) to conclude that functional stereotactic surgery directed at the subcortical structures is less effective than resective surgery and is largely applied empirically.

## References

ANNEGERS J. F., GRABOW J. D., GROOVER R. V., LAWS E. R., ELVEBACK L. R. & KURLAND L. T. (1980) Neurology, 30, 683.
ANNEGERS J. F., HAUSER W. A. & ELVEBACK L. R. (1979) Epilepsia, 20, 729.
ASCROFT P. B. (1941) Brit. med J., 1, 739.
BASSER L. S. (1962) Brain, 85, 427.
BATES J. A. V. (1963) In Electroencephalography, 2nd edn. (Eds HILL D. & PARR H.) p. 429. Macdonald, London.
BEAR D. M. & FEDIO P. (1977) Arch. Neurol., 34, 454.

BENGZON A. R. A., RASMUSSEN T., GLOOR P., DUSSAULT J. & STEPHENS M. (1968) Neurology, 18, 717.
BENNET F. E. (1953) Neurology, 3, 668.
BETTS T. A. (1974) In Epilepsy—Proceedings of the Hans Berger Centenary Symposium, pp. 326–338.
BHATIA R. & KOLLEVOLD (1976) Epilepsia, 17, 61.
BICKFORD R. G. & KLASS D. W. (1966) In Head injury Conference Proceedings, (Eds CAVENESS W. F. & WALKER A. E.) Lippincott, Philadelphia.
BINNIE C. D. (1983) In Recent Advances in Epilepsy (Vol. 1), (Eds PEDLEY T. A. & MELDRUM B.) Churchill Livingstone, Edinburgh.
BLAKEMORE C. B. & FALCONER M. A. (1967) J. Neurol. Neurosurg. Psychiat., 30, 304.
BLOOM D., JASPER H., RASMUSSEN T. (1960) Epilepsia, 1, 351.
BRAZIER M. A., CRANDALL P. H. & WALSH G. O. (1976) Exp. Neurol., 51, 241.
CABRAL R. J., KING T. T. & SCOTT D. F. (1976a) J. Neurol. Neurosurg. Psychiat., 39, 663.
CABRAL R. J., KING T. T. & SCOTT D. F. (1976b) J. Neurol. Neurosurg. Psychiat., 39, 1052.
CABRAL R. J. & SCOTT D. F. (1977) J. Neurol. Neurosurg. Psychiat., 40, 97.
CAIRNS H. & DAVIDSON M. A. (1951) Lancet, ii, 411.
CARMICHAEL E. A. (1966) Clin. Proc. Children's Hospital. D. C., 22, 285.
CARMICHAEL E. A., DIX M. R., HALLPIKE C. S. & HOOD J. D. (1961) Brain, 84, 571.
CAST I. P. & WILSON P. J. E. (1981) J. Neurol. Neurosurg. Psychiat., 44, 371.
CAVENESS W. F. (1963) J. Neurosurg, 20, 57.
CAVENESS W. F. & LISS H. R. (1961) Epilepsia, 2, 123.
CAVENESS W. F., WALKER A. E. & ASCROFT P. B. (1962) J. Neurosurg., 19, 122.
CAVENESS W. F., MEIROWSKY A. M., RISH B. C., MOHR J. P., KISTLER J. P., DILLON J. D. & WEISS G. H. (1979) J. Neursurg., 50, 545.
CHADWICK D. (1985) In Recent Advances in Epilepsy, (Eds PEDLEY T. A. & MELDRUM B. S.) pp. 111–25 Churchill Livingstone, Edinburgh.
CHADWICK D. & TURNBULL D. M. (1984) J. Neurol. Neurosurg. Psychiat., 48, 1073.
CHADWICK D., SHAW M. D. M., FOY P. M., RAWLINS M. D. & TURNBULL D. M. (1984) J. Neurol. Neurosurg. Psychiat, 47, 642.
CLELLAND P. G., MOSQUERA J., STEWARD W. P. & FORSTER J. B. (1981) Brit. med. J., 283, 1364.
COPELAND G. P., FOY P. M. & SHAW M. D. M. (1982) Surg. Neurol., 17, 279.
CRANFORD R. E., LEPPIK I. E., PATRICK B., ANDERSON C. B. & KOSTIK B. (1978) Neurology (Minneap.), 28, 874.
CREDNER L. (1930) Zbl. ges. Neurol. Psychiat., 126, 721.
CURRIE S., HEATHFIELD K. W. G., HENSON R. A. & SCOTT D. F. (1971) Brain, 94, 173.
DELGADO J. M. R., HAMLIN H. & CHAPMAN W. P. (1952) Confin. Neurol., 12, 315.
DENNY-BROWN D. (1943) Amer. J. Psychiat., 100, 585.
DENNY-BROWN D. (1966) The Cerebral Control of Movement. Liverpool University Press.
DENNY-BROWN D. & CHAMBERS R. A. (1958) Res. Pub. Ass. Res. Nerv. Ment. Dis., 36, 35.
DILL W. A., KAZENKO A., WOLFF L. M., GLAZKO A. J. (1956)

Journal of Pharmacology and Experimental Therapeutics, 118, 270.
DOOSE H., GERKEN H., LEONHARDT R., VOLZKE E. & VOLZ C. (1970) Neuropaediatrie, 2, 59.
EFRON R. (1963) Brain, 86, 403.
ENGEL J., DRIVER M. V. & FALCONER M. A. (1975) Brain, 98, 129.
ENGEL J., RAUSCH R., LIEB J. P., KUHL D. E. & CRANDALL P. H. (1981) Ann. Neurol., 9, 215.
EVARTS E. V. (1964) J. Neurophysiol, 27, 152.
FABINY G. C. A. & FORTUNY L. A. (1980) Lancet, 1, 1299.
FALCONER M. A. (1971) In Operative Surgery, Vol. 14 Neurosurgery (LOGUE V. Ed.) p. 142, Butterworth, London.
FALCONER M. A. & SERAFETINIDES E. A. (1963) J. Neurol. Neurosurg. Psychiat., 26, 154.
FALCONER M. A., HILL D., MEYER A., MITCHELL W. & POND D. A. (1955) Lancet, 1, 827.
FALCONER M. A. & WILSON J. L. (1958) Brain, 81, 1.
FISCHER-WILLIAMS M. & COOPER R. A. (1963) Electroenceph. clin. Neurophysiol, 15, 568.
FISHER R. S. & PRINCE D. A. (1977) Electroenceph. clin. Neurophys., 42, 608.
FLOR-HENRY P. (1969) Epilepsia, 10, 363.
FOERSTER O. (1936) Brain, 59, 135.
FOY P. M., COPELAND G. P. & SHAW M. D. M. (1981a) Acta. Neurochir., 55, 15.
FOY P. M., COPELAND G. P. & SHAW M. D. M. (1981b) Acta. Neurochir., 55, 253.
GASTAUT H. (1973) In Evolution and Prognosis of Epilepsy. (Eds LUGARASI E., PAZZAGLIA P. & TASSINARI C. A.) Aulo Gaggi, Bologna.
GASTAUT H. & GASTAUT J. L. (1976) Epilepsia, 17, 377.
GASTAUT H., POIRER F., PAYAN H., VIGOUROUX M. H., SALAMON G., TOGA M. (1960) Epilepsia, 1, 418.
GIBBS E. A. & GIBBS E. L. (1952) Atlas of Encephalography. Vol. 2: Epilepsy. Addison-Wesley, Reading.
GOODRIDGE D. M. & SHORVON S. D. (1983) Brit. med. J., 287, 645.
GOWERS W. R. (1885) Epilepsy and other chronic convulsive diseases. American Acad. Neurol. Reprint Series, vol. 1, 1964. Dover Publications, New York.
GREEN J. R. & SCHUTZ D. G. (1964) Arch. Neurol., 1, 135.
GRIFFITH H. B. (1967) Ann. roy. Coll. Surg. Eng, 41, 183.
GRIFFITH H. B., FALCONER M. A. & WILSON P. J. E. (1969) J. Neurosurg, 30, 413.
GUNDMUNDSSON G. (1966) Acta neurol. Scand., Suppl. 25.
GUNN J. (1977) Epileptics in Prisons. Academic Press, London.
GUNN J. & FENTON G. W. (1971) Lancet, 1, 1173.
HAUSER W. A., ANDERSON V. E., LOEWENSON R. B. & McROBERTS S. M. (1982) New Engl. J. Med., 307, 522.
HAUSER W. A. & KURLAND L. T. (1975) Epilepsia, 16, 1.
HILL D. (1958) Proc. roy. Soc. Med., 51, 610.
HILL D. (1963) In Electroencephalography, 2nd edn. (Eds HILL D. & PARR G.) Macdonald, London.
HILLESTAD L., HANSEN T., MELSOM H. & DRIVENESS A. (1974) Clin. Pharmacol. Ther., 16, 479.
HOFF H. & STROTZKA H. (1951) Wiener med. Wsch., 101, 767.
HOOPER W. D., BOCHNER F., EDIE M. J. & TYRER J. H. (1973) Clin. Pharmacol. Ther., 15, 276.
HOREL J. A. (1978) Brain, 101, 403.
HOUGHTON G. W., RICHENS A., TOSELAND P. A., DAVIDSON S. & FALCONER M. A. (1975) J. Clin. Pharmacol, 9, 73.

HUGHES J. F. & OPPENHEIMER D. R. (1969) Acta Neuropath, 13, 56.

JACKSON J. H.  Selected Writings, Ed. TAYLOR J. (1931) Vol 1: On epilepsy and epileptic convulsions. Hodder & Stoughton, London.

JAMES I. P. (1960) J. Ment. Sci., 106, 143.

JANZ D. (1964) J. Neurol. Sci, 1, 446.

JANZ D. (1983) In Research Progress in Epilepsy, Chapter 18. Pitman, London.

JASPER H. H. (1949) Electroenceph. Clin. Neurophysiol., 1, 11.

JASPER H. H. (1954) In Epilepsy and Functional Anatomy of the Human Brain. (Eds PENFIELD W. & JASPER H. H.) p. 586. Churchill, London.

JASPER H. H. & DROOGLEEVER-FORTUYN J. (1946) Res. Pub. Ass. Res. Nerv. Ment. Dis., 26, 272.

JENNETT W. B. (1962) Epilepsy after blunt head injuries. Heinemann, London.

JENNETT W. B. (1969) Lancet, 1, 1023.

JENNETT W. B. (1975) Epilepsy After Non-Missile Head Injuries, 2nd Edn. Heinemann, London.

JENNETT W. B., LEWIN W. (1960) J. Neurol. Neurosurg. Psychiat., 23, 295.

JENSEN I. (1975) Acta Neurol. Scand., 52, 354.

JENSEN I. (1976) Acta Neurol. Scand., 54, 22.

JINNAI D., MUKAWA J. & KOBAYASHI K. (1976) Acta Neurochir. Suppl., 23, 159.

JINNAI D. & NISHIMOTO A. (1963) Neurochirurgia, 6, 164.

JONES D. P. (1951) Electroenceph. clin. Neurophysiol., 3, 100.

JONES M. K. (1974) Neuropsychologia, 12, 21.

JUUL-JENSEN P. (1964) Acta Neurol. Scand., 40, Suppl. 5, 1.

JUUL-JENSEN P. & FOLDSPANG A. (1983) Epilepsia, 24, 297.

KENNEDY W. A. & HILL D. (1958) J. Neurol. Neurosurg. Psychiat., 21, 24.

KLASS D. W. (1975) In Complex Partial Seizures and their Treatment. (Eds PENRY J. K. & DALY D. D.) pp. 163–181, Raven Press, New York.

KRYNAUW R. A. (1950) J. Neurol. Neurosurg. Psychiat., 13, 243.

LAINE E. & GROS Q. (1956) L'Hemisphectomie. Masson, Paris.

LAINE E., PRUVOT P. & OSSON D. (1964) Neurochirurgie, 10, 507.

LEGG N. J., GUPTA P. C. & SCOTT D. F. (1973) Brain, 96, 256.

LENNOX W. G. (1960) Epilepsy and Related Disorders. Little & Brown, Boston, .

LIDDELL D. W. & NORTHFIELD D. W. C. (1954) J. Neurol. Neurosurg. Psychiat., 17, 267.

LLOYD K. G., MUNARI C., BOSSI L. STOEFFELS C., TALAIRACH J., MORSELLI P. (1981) In Neurotransmitters, Seizures and Epilepsy. (Eds MORSELLI P. L. et al.) pp. 325–334. Raven Press, New York.

LOISEAU P. & BEAUSSART M. (1973) Epilepsia, 14, 381.

LOWRIE M. B., MACCABE J. J. & ETTINGER G. (1978) Electroenceph. clin. Neurophysiol, 44, 23.

LUESSENHOP A. J. (1970) J. Amer. med. Ass., 213, 1630.

MACCABE J. J. (1971) In Operative Surgery Vol. 14 Neurosurgery (LOCUE V. Ed.) p. 58. Butterworth, London.

LURIA A. R. (1980) Higher Cortical Functions in Man, 2nd. ed. Basic Books, New York.

MAUGIERRE F. & COURJON J. (1978) Brain, 101, 307.

MARCUS E. M. & WATSON C. W. (1966) Arch. Neurol., 14, 601.

MARCUS E. M. & WATSON C. W. (1968) Arch. Neurol., 18, 88.

MARGERISON J. H. & CORSELLIS G. A. N. (1966) Brain, 89, 499.

MARINO R. & RASMUSSEN T. (1968) Neurology, 18, 825.

MARSAN A. J. & ABRAHAM K. (1966) Confin. Neurol., 27, 95.

MARSHALL C. & WALKER A. E. (1961) Epilepsia, 2, 138.

MATHIESON G. (1975) In Complex Partial Seizures and their Treatment, (Eds PENRY J. K. & DALY D. D.) pp. 163–181. Raven Press, New York.

MAZZIOTTA J. C. & ENGEL J. (1985) In Recent Advances in Epilepsy, vol. 2 (Eds PEDLEY T. A. & MELDRUM B. S.) pp. 65–101. Churchill Livingstone, Edinburgh.

MELDRUM B. S. (1975) In Modern Trends in Neurology. (Ed. WILLIAMS D.). Butterworths, London.

MELDRUM B. S., HORTON R. W. & BRIERLEY J. B. (1974) Brain, 97, 407.

METRAKOS K. & METRAKOS J. D. (1961) Neurology (Minneap.), 11, 474.

MEYER V. & YATES A. J. (1955) J. Neurol. Neurosurg. Psychiat., 18, 44.

McKISSOCK W. (1953) Proc. roy. Soc. Med., 46, 431.

McLARDY T. (1969) Nature, 221, 877.

McQUEEN J. K., BLACKWOOD D. H. R., HARRIS P., KALBAG R. M. & JOHNSON A. L. (1983) J. Neurol. Neurosurg. Psychiat., 46, 899.

MILNER B. (1958) Res. Publ. Ass. Res. Nerv. Ment. Dis., 36, 244.

MORRELL F. (1960) Epilepsia, 1, 538.

MULLAN S. & PENFIELD W. (1959) Arch. Neurol. Psychiat., 81, 269.

MUNDINGER F., BECKER P., GROLKNER E. & BACHSCHMID G. (1976) Acta Neurochir. Suppl., 23, 177.

NARABAYASHI H., NAGAO T., SAITO Y., YOSHIDA M. & NAGAHATA M. (1963) Arch. Neurol, 9, 11.

NARABAYASHI H. & SHIMA F. (1973) In Surgical Approaches in Psychiatry (Eds LAITINEN L. V. & LIVINGSTONE K. E.) p. 129. MTP, Lancaster.

NORTH J. B., PENHALL R. K., HANIETH A., FREWIN D. B. & TAYLOR W. B. (1983) J. Neurosurg., 58, 672.

NORTHFIELD D. W. C. (1965) In Second Symposium on Advanced Medicine. (Ed. TROUNCE J. R.) p. 161. Pitman Medical, London.

NORTHFIELD D. W. C. (1968) Brit. med. J., 2, 471.

OJEMANN G. A. & WARD A. A. (1975) In Neurosurgical Management of the Epilepsies: Advances in Neurology Vol. 8 (Eds PURPURA D. P., PENRY J. K. & WALTER R. D.) p. 241. Raven Press, New York.

PAILLAS J. E., DARCOURT G., RIGHINI C. & HEVITIER A. (1963) Presse Med., 71, 1169.

PAMPIGLIONE G. & KERRIDGE J. (1956) J. Neurol. Neurosurg. Psychiat., 19, 117.

PATEL I. H., LEVY R. H., VENKATARAMANAN R., VISWANATH C. T. & MORETTI-OJEMANN L. (1980) Clin. Pharmacol. Cher., 27, 277.

PENFIELD W. (1958) Brit. med. J., 1, 669.

PENFIELD W. & BALDWIN M. (1952) Ann. Surg., 136, 625.

PENFIELD W. & JASPER H. H. (1954) Epilepsy and the Functional Anatomy of the Human Brain. Little Brown & Co., Boston.

PENFIELD W., LENDE R. A. & RASMUSSEN T. (1961) J. Neurosurg., 18, 760.

PENFIELD W. & RASMUSSEN T. (1950) The Cerebral Cortex of Man. Macmillan, New York.

PENFIELD W. & SHAVER M. (1945) Res. Pub. Ass. Res. Nerv. Med. Dis., 24, 620.

PEROT P. (1963) Phd Thesis, McGill University.

PERUCCA E. (1982). In A Textbook of Epilepsy (Eds. LAIDLAW J. & RICHENS A.) pp. 358. Churchill Livingstone, Edinburgh.

PERUCCA E., HEBDIGE S., GATTI G., LECCHINI S., FRIGO G. M., CREMA A. (1980) *Clin. Pharmacol. Ther.*, **28**, 779.

PHILLIPS D. G. (1945) *J. Neurol. Neurosurg. Psychiat*, **8**, 79.

PHILLIPS G. (1954) *J. Neurol. Neurosurg. Psychiat.*, **17**, 1.

POLKEY C. E. (1982) In *A Textbook of Epilepsy*. (Eds LAIDLAW J. & RICHENS A.) Chapter 10. Churchill Livingstone, Edinburgh.

POND D. A. & BIDWELL B. H. (1959) *Epilepsia*, **1**, 285.

POND D. A. & ESPIR M. (1978) *Medical Aspects of Fitness to Drive*. Medical Commission on Accident Prevention p. 22.

PORTER R. J. (1982) In *Antiepileptic Drugs* (Eds WOODBURY D. M., PENRY J. K. & PIPPENGER C. E.) Raven Press, New York.

POTTER J. M. (1978) *J. Neurol. Neurosurg. Psychiat.*, **41**, 265.

PRINCE D. A. (1968) *Exp. Neurol.*, **21**, 467.

PRINCE D.A. & FARRELL D. (1969) *Neurol. (Minneap.)*, **19**, 309.

RASMUSSEN T. (1963) *Epilepsia*, **4**, 181.

RASMUSSEN T. (1975) In *Neurosurgical Managements of the Epilepsies. Advances in Neurology Vol. 8.* (Eds PURPURA D.P., PENRY J. K. & WALTER R. D.) p. 197. Raven Press, New York.

RASMUSSEN T. (1983) *Epilepsia*, **24 (Suppl. 1)**, 567.

RASMUSSEN T. & BRANCH C. (1962) *Postgrad. med. J.*, **31**, 9.

RASMUSSEN T. & GOSSMAN H. (1963) *Neurology*, **13**, 659.

RASMUSSEN T. & JASPER H. (1958) In *Temporal Lobe Epilepsy* (Eds BALDWIN M. & BAILEY P.) p. 440. Thomas, Springfield, Illinois.

RAYNOR R. B., PAINE R. S. & CARMICHAEL E. A. (1959) *Neurol. (Minneap.)*, **9**, 11.

REYNOLDS E. H. & SHORVON S. D. (1981) *Epilepsia*, **22**, 1.

REYNOLDS F., ZINOYAMIS P., JONES N., SMITH S.E. (1976) *Lancet*, **2**, 384.

RIBAK C.E., HARRIS A.B., VAUGHAN J.E., ROBERTS E. (1981) In *Neurotransmitters, Seizures and Epilepsy*. (Eds MORSELLI P. L. *et al.*) pp. 11–20. Raven Press, New York.

RICHENS A. (1982) In *A Textbook of Epilepsy* (Eds LAIDLAW J. & RICHENS A.) Churchill Livingstone, Edinburgh.

RICHENS A. & DUNLOP A. (1975) *Lancet*, **2**, 247.

RODIN E. A. (1968) *The Prognosis of Epileptic Patients*. Thomas, Springfield, Illinois.

RODIN E. A. (1982) In *Pseudoseizures* (Eds RILEY T. L. & ROY A.) pp. 185–212. Williams and Wilkins, Baltimore.

ROVIT, R. L., GLOOR P. & RASMUSSEN T. (1961) *Arch. Neurol.*, **5**, 606.

ROWAN A. J., BINNIE C. D., WARFIELD L. A. & MEIJER J. W. A. (1979a) *Epilepsia*, **20**, 61.

ROWAN A. J., BINNIE C. D., BEER-PAWLOWSKI N. R. B., GOEDHART D. M., GUTTER T., VAN DER GEEST P., MEINARDI H. & MEIJER J. W. A. (1979b) *Neurology (Minneap.)*, **29**, 1450.

ROWAN A. J. & SCOTT D. F. (1970) *Acta neurol. Scand.*, **46**, 573.

RUSSELL W. R. & WHITTY C. W. M. (1952) *J. Neurol. Neurosurg. Psychiat.*, **15**, 93.

RUTTER M., GRAHAM P. & YULE W. (1970) In *Clinics in Developmental Medicine*, No 35. Spastics International Press, London.

SCHEIBEL M. E. & SCEIBEL A. B. (1973) *Epilepsy: its Phenomena in Man*. pp. 315–335. Academic Press, New York.

SCHWARTZKROIN P. A. & WYLER A. R. (1980) *Ann. Neurol.*, **7**, 95.

SCOVILLE W. B. & MILNER B. (1957) *J. Neurol. Neurosurg. Psychiat.*, **20**, 11.

SERAFETINIDES E. A., HOARE R. D. & DRIVER M. W. (1965) *Brain*, **88**, 107.

SERVIT Z. & MUSIL F. (1981) *Epilepsia*, **22**, 315.

SHARPLESS S. K. (1969) In *Basic Mechanisms of the Epilepsies*. (Eds JASPER H. H., WARD A. A., POPE A.) pp. 329–348. Little & Brown, Boston.

SHAW M. D. M., FOY P. M. & CHADWICK D. W. (1983) *Acta Neurochir.*, **69**, 253.

SILFVENIUS H., GLOOR P. & RASMUSSEN T. (1964) *Epilepsia*, **5**, 307.

SLATER E., BEARD A. W. & GLITHEROE E. (1963) *Brit. J. Psychiat.*, **109**, 95 & 150.

SLOPER J. J., JOHNSON P., POWELL T. P. S. (1980) *Brain Res.*, **198**, 204.

SMALL J., HAYDEN M. & SMALL I. (1966) *Amer. J. Psychiat.*, **123**, 303.

STEELMAN H. F. (1949) *Arch. Neurol. Neurosurg. Psychiat.*, **62**, 479.

STOREY P. B. (1967) *Brit. med. J.*, **3**, 261.

SUMI S. M. & TEASDALL R. D. (1963) *Neurology (Minneap).*, **13**, 582.

TALAIRACH J. *et al.* (1974) *Neurochirurgie*, **20**, Suppl. 1.

TAYLOR D. C. & FALCONER M. A. (1968) *Brit. J. Psychiat.*, **114**, 1247.

TERZIAN H. & ORE G. D. (1955) *Neurology*, **5**, 373.

TIZZARD B. (1962) *Psychological Bulletin*, **59**, 196.

TREIMAN D. M. & DELGADO-ESCUETA A. V. (1983) *Recent Advances in Epilepsy*, (Eds PEDLEY T. A. & MELDRUM B. S.) pp. 179–209. Churchill Livingstone, Edinburgh.

TRIMBLE M R (1980) In *Current Developments in Psychopharmacology* (Eds ESSMAN W. B. & VALZELLI L.).

TRIMBLE M.R. (1983) In *Recent Advances in Epilepsy*. (Eds PEDLEY T. A. & MELDRUM B. S.) pp. 211–229. Churchill Livingstone, Edinburgh.

TURNBULL D. M., RAWLINS M. D., WEIGHTMAN D. & CHADWICK D. (1984) *J. Neurol. Neurosurg. Psychiat.*, **47**, 231.

TURNBULL D.M., HOWEL D., RAWLINS M.D. & CHADWICK D. (1985) *Brit. med. J.* **290**, 815.

TURNER E. (1963) *J. Neurol. Neurosurg. Psychiat.*, **26**, 285.

TYRER J.H., EDIE M.J., SUTHERLAND J.M. & HOOPER W.D. (1970) *Brit. med. J.*, **4**, 271.

UMBACH W. (1966) *Confin. Neurol.*, **27**, 121.

VAERNET K. (1972) *Confin. Neurol.*, **34**, 176.

VAN BUREN J. M. & BALDWIN M. (1958) *Brain*, **81**, 15.

VAN GELDER N. M., SHERWIN A. L., RASMUSSEN T. (1972) *Brain Res.*, **40**, 385.

VAN WAGENEN W.P. & HEUREN R.U. (1940) *Acta Neurol. Psychiat.*, **44**, 740.

VITALE A., DONDY M. & REMOND A. (1953) *Rev. Neurol.*, **88**, 374.

WADA J. & RASMUSSEN T. (1960) *J. Neurosurg.*, **17**, 266.

WAGSTAFFE W. D. (1928) *Lancet*, **2**, 561.

WALKER A. E. (1964) In *Acute Injuries of the Head* (4th ed.) (Ed. Rowbotham G. F.) Livingstone, Edinburgh.

WALKER A. E. & JABLON S. (1959) *J. Neurosurg.*, **16**, 600.

WALKER A. E. & JABLON S. (1961) *A Follow-up Study of Head Wounds in World War II*, V. A. Medical Monographs. U. S. Gov. Printing Off., Washington D. C.

WALTER W. G. (1942) *Proc roy. Soc. Med.*, **35**, 777.

WARD A. A. (1969) In *Basic Mechanisms of the Epilepsies*. (Eds JASPER H. H., WARD A. A., POPE A.) pp. 263–268. Little & Brown, Boston.

WARD A. A. (1978) In *Dynamic Properties of Glial Cells*. (Eds SCHOFFENIELS F., FRANCK G., HERTZ L.) pp. 413–427. Pergammon Press, Oxford.

WAXMAN S. G. & GESCHWIND N (1975) *Arch. gen. Psychiat.*, **32**, 1580.

WHITE H. H. (1961) *Confin. Neurol.*, **21**, 1.

WHITTY G. W. M. (1947) *Brain*, **70**, 416.

WILENSKY A. J. & LOWDEN J. A. (1973) *Neurology (Minneap.)*, **23**, 318.

WILLIAMS D. (1941) *J. Neurol. Neurosurg. Psychiat.*, **4**, 107.

WILLIAMS D. (1944a) *Brain*, **70**, 416.

WILLIAMS D. (1944b) *J. Neurol. Neurosurg. Psychiat.*, **7**, 103.

WILLIAMS D. (1955) *Electrenceph. clin. Neurophysiol.*, **7**, 495.

WILLIAMS D. J. & SCOTT J. W. (1939) *J. Neurol. Psychiat.*, **2**, 313.

WILSON D. H., REEVES A., GAZZANIGA M. (1977) *Neurology (Minneap.)*, **27**, 708.

WILSON D. H., REEVES A., GAZZANIGA M. (1978) *Neurology (Minneap.)*, **28**, 649.

WILSON P. J. E. (1970) *Brain*, **93**, 147.

WOLTMAN H. W. (1953) *Proc. Mayo Clin.*, **28**, 313.

WOODBURY D. M. (1980) In *Antiepileptic drugs: Mechanisms of Action.* (Eds GLASER G. H., PENRY J. K., WOODBURY D. M.) pp. 249–303. Raven Press, New York.

WYCIS H. T., BAIRD H. W. & SPIEGEL E. A. (1966) *Confin. Neurol.*, **27**, 114.

WYLER A. R., FETZ E. E. & WARD A. A. (1973) *Exp. Neurol.*, **40**, 567.

WYLER A. R., OJEMANN G. A. & WARD A. A. (1982) *Ann. Neurol.*, **11**, 301.

YANG P. J., BERGER P. E., COHEN M. E. & DUFFNER P. K. (1979) *Neurology*, **29**, 1084.

YOUNG A. C., COSTANZI J. B., MOHR P. D. & FORBES W. S. (1982) *Lancet*, **1**, 1446.

YOUNG B., RAPP R. P., NORTON J. A., HAACK D., TIBBS P. A. & BEAN J. R. (1983a) *J. Neurosurg.*, **58**, 231.

YOUNG B., RAPP R. P., NORTON J. A., HAACK D., TIBBS P. A. & BEAN J. R. (1983b) *J. Neurosurg.*, **58**, 236.

# Chapter 18
# Surgical treatment of pain

J. B. MILES

A number of clinical observations and animal experiments during the latter part of the last century gradually provided indirect evidence that a small discrete unilateral lesion of the spinal cord could render the opposite side of the body below the level of the lesion oblivious of stimuli which elsewhere caused pain, while other forms of sensibility might remain unaffected. Gowers (1886) stated that 'it seems to be almost certain that the anterolateral ascending tract constitutes the path for sensibility to pain'.

These observations culminated in the decision by Spiller that an anterolateral incision in the cord might be therapeutically beneficial. His colleague Martin performed the first cordotomy in 1911 (Spiller & Martin 1912). Frazier (1920) put the operation on a firmer basis by drawing attention to certain technical details. Since that time anterolateral cordotomy has become a recognized and valuable operation and surgeons have explored the possibilities of extending the scope of operations at ever higher levels, in the brain stem, in the diencephalon, and in sub-cortical and cortical zones. These surgical procedures have been based on the assumption, firmly held at any rate until recent years, that the pain evoked by organic lesions depends exclusively on the transmission of nerve impulses along the spinothalamic tracts, and above the thalamus on a notional interaction between specific sensory nuclei and the cortex. The various operations will be described later; here it is necessary to review briefly current views on the neurophysiology of 'pain'. This is because widening experience has shown that the basic assumption referred to above is not valid; it naïvely ignores the intricate pathways and activities involved in the appreciation of a noxious stimulus. It provides no explanation for certain facts that are a matter of observation among all neurosurgeons who have had experience in this field; some 20% of spinal cordotomies fail to relieve pain, although as judged by clinical tests (level and density of analgesia) there appears to be no anatomical reason for this failure; cordotomy which abolishes satisfactorily the pain for which it was performed may not block appreciation of other noxious stimuli (for example, strong electrical stimulation, White & Sweet 1955); immediately or later, pain may appear elsewhere, inexplicable by extension of the primary disease, and painful sensations may develop within the analgesic area; the level of analgesia resulting from the cordotomy normally falls in patients who survive several years, when pain may recur. Finally, and perhaps a significant contribution to pain physiology from this branch of 'experimental' human surgery, these disadvantages and failures are more frequent and more severe when the tractotomy is carried out within the brain stem.

No attempt will be made to define pain; it would be out of place, the writer is not qualified to embark on such metaphysical exercises and he assumes that the reader fully understands what is generally meant. Moreover, his patients will reply to questions on an equal level of mutual understanding. Whether the sensations of which some patients complain, perhaps with unusual flights of imagery, qualify as pain must be left to the observer's clinical experience and judgment; if uncertain he should seek psychiatric advice about the patient before embarking upon any surgical treatment. The problem of separating complaints of an emotional nature, requiring their own treatment, from that of organic origin, can even occur when there is an unequivocally physical cause, particularly when the pain, by virtue of its duration, has become chronic.

Here, we will consider the pathways and mechanisms invoked by nervous impulses which arise from lesions and stimuli known to evoke pain consistently. But, as Noordenbos (1959) so lucidly pointed out, emphasis must be placed upon the accurate use of words, for example sensation, sensibility (or sensitiveness), pain-tracts, fibres, terminals and so forth. 'Sensation' refers to the interpretation of stimuli by the conscious subjects, whether a flash of light or a dart of what they call pain. 'Sensibility' is the property or characteristic of skin (or an internal organ) to react to a stimulus (whether physical and applied externally or the violent contraction of smooth muscle of a viscus).

Nociception, a term now commonly used, and approved by the International Association for the Study of Pain Nosological Sub-Committee, is similar to, but an expansion of, sensibility. Iggo (1981), uses it as referring to the peripheral and spinal processes that precede and underlie the sensation of pain. There are no pain nerve endings, fibres or tracts; the intention is to state that these normal structures react to certain stimuli by transmitting nerve impulses. It is still common however to refer to the neurons involved in the process of nociception as being 'nociceptors'.

The translation of a stimulus (whatever its nature) into a nerve impulse is the function of the nerve terminal, highly organized for instance like a Pacinian corpuscle or the simple ubiquitous unmyelinated free nerve ending (see Symposium on Touch Heat and Pain 1966). These and others constitute the biological transducers which in applied physiology provide electrical methods for measuring and recording changes in various body systems. Proximal to the peripheral nerve terminal, communications through fibres, pathways, tracts, nets are through trains of nerve impulses characterized by time-course, amplitude, frequency, modified by summation, inhibition, facilitation, and by speed of transmission, this being dependent upon nerve fibre diameter.

At no point are they 'pain' or 'touch' impulses; labels of specificity and of point of origin are added at a 'high' cerebral level; in the case of 'pain' the whereabouts of this level is unknown and it may well be multiple or diffuse. It is generally conceded that many parts of the brain are involved in or may modify the appreciation of pain: the thalamus, the limbic system, the hypothalamus, the reticular formation, parietal and frontal cortex; consequently to speak of a 'terminal centre is meaningless' (Melzack & Wall 1965, see also Keele & Smith 1962).

Views on the mechanism of cutaneous sensibility have fluctuated and conflicted to a remarkable degree in the last quarter of a century and unanimity is still lacking. There is no dispute over the anatomy of the diverse receptor structures, some highly complex, around and within which afferent nerve fibres terminate, nor over the presence of fine unmyelinated free nerve endings 'the most widely distributed receptors in the body' (Truex & Carpenter 1969). Nor have the observations of Weddell (1941 a and b) been controverted, that the terminal arborizations of afferent nerves form a fine mesh, providing multiple innervation of the receptors and so branching that minute areas of skin are innervated from all directions. But opinions diverge acutely on the manner in which this remarkably complicated sensory organ (in the skin and deep tissues) and its no less complicated central connections operate. The classical theory and one which is still held in some quarters maintains that four basic forms (modalities) of sensation can be recognized: touch, pressure, variation of temperature, and pain; that each modality depends upon a specific receptor and that when this is activated by the appropriate (adequate) stimulus the resultant nerve impulse is transmitted through nerve fibres of particular size (which determines speed of transit) to a particular termination in the brain. This scheme envisages a rigid modality-specific pathway from end-organ to cerebral termination and the labelling and localization depend upon this link. Diametrically opposed to this theory is that which denies specificity to the peripheral nerve endings, but views them as responsive to a variety of stimuli, though with a lower threshold to a particular parameter. The complexity of the peripheral transducers and their mesh of interlocking and overlapping innervation is an essential element of such a system whereby a great variety of impulses passes centrally, providing a spectrum or pattern of information which is decoded and interpreted at a high cerebral level. Goody (1957) in a general review of the nature of pain has emphasized that all sensations depend upon the pattern of afferent stimuli and that pain is the result of a departure from normally experienced patterns. 'The pattern of excitation of the skin will be carried more or less faithfully to the central nervous system by a large group of afferent fibres and the contribution of any one fibre will be relatively unimportant. In the whole sensory message describing the touch, the time element will be as important as the spatial; the rate of rise and fall of the excitation in different regions will show whether the body has been touched by something hard or soft, moving or stationary. And since 100 nerve fibres can send in more than 10,000 impulses per second the means of communication will be quite adequate to convey the information in considerable detail' (Adrian 1949). An excellent review of earlier theories and of the evidence favouring the 'pattern' theory is provided by Weddell (1955), one of its presenters.

Recent technical developments have allowed microelectrode recording of single nerve fibres in the human peripheral nerve (Torebjork et al. 1970). Perhaps surprisingly, the exploration using this technique has revealed a degree of specificity of stimulus to threshold and response that rekindles the specific theory of pain sensitivity, at least to the peripheral nerve (Ochoa & Torebjork 1983). Jasper (1966) pointed out that thalamic cells are constantly recording the arrival of impulses activated by peripheral stimuli of which the subject may or may not be aware, though other cells of the thalamus respond briefly to new stimuli and rapidly cease to do so on repetition; this perhaps provides a glimpse of the mechanism of attention. The

theory of modality-specific pathways, includes the correlation of modality-impulse transmission with the diameter of the relevant axones. The belief in such strict correlation has also been subjected to severe criticism, lone reason being that C-fibres are said also to respond when the stimulus is light touch. Very recent human recordings using this microelectrode technique have revealed distinct correlation between evoked responses in the fine, poorly myelinated C-fibres of the human peripheral nerve with the sensation described by the patient as pain (Torebjork et al. 1984).

Using a microrecording technique Wall (1960) examined the activity of cells in the posterior horn of the spinal cord consequent upon cutaneous stimulation; all the cells examined responded briefly to light touch, to prolonged heavy pressure and to temperature change. They responded to all modalities; the difference in pattern depended on the nature of the stimulation. Noordenbos (1959) draws attention to the analysis of fibre diameters in the white matter of the cord undertaken by Haggquist (1936). This work showed that there is no segregation into tracts according to fibre size, but an intimate mixture, although the relative richness of large and of small fibres varies.

The anterolateral cord contained a high proportion of fine fibres but not to the exclusion of coarse fibres and a smaller ratio of fine fibres was encountered in the posterior columns. Large diameter axons within the posterior columns ascending as first order fibres make connection with the dorsal column nuclei. Only largest diameter (A) fibres make this contact, although fibres of all diameters connect with cells in the dorsal horn (Melzack & Wall 1962). Thus the medial lemniscus carries only information derived from large fibres, believed to be concerned with discrimination qualities, for example touch, joint movement. Mountcastle (1966) states that this system is highly specific for place and for quality, in sharp contrast to the spinothalamic system whose impulses are widely dispersed and whose specificity for place and quality is negligible 'and is concerned with the maintenance of general levels of awareness'. That large diameter fibres exert influence in the 'appreciation of pain' is suggested by the following observations. The spontaneous discharge activity of single secondary afferent neurons in the dorsal horn was greatly modified and even extinguished by regular repetitive stimulation of A fibres in the relevant peripheral nerve, whereas repetitive stimulation of the C fibres (after blocking the A fibres) resulted in a gradually increasing though delayed activity. White and Sweet (1969) draw attention to the similarity between this and the characteristics of hyperpathia (allodynia): high threshold, long latency and prolonged discharge. These experiments had led them to a clinical application, by attempting to relieve pain with electrical stimuli appropriate to the activation of large diameter fibres. The second observation is that of Noordenbos (1959) who found that in peripheral nerves affected by herpes zoster which had given rise to severe post herpetic neuralgia, there was a great reduction of large medullated nerve fibres and an increase in the number of fine nonmedullated fibres. Noordenbos (1959) also quotes observations, experimental and clinical, that damage to posterior columns may give rise to unpleasant paraesthesiae of spontaneous pain.

Melzack and Wall (1962) specify five effects of dividing a neural pathway: (1) particular fibres cannot transmit centrally; (2) the total number of responding neurons is decreased; (3) the temporal and spatial patterns of impulses attaining the brain are altered; (4) feedback is disturbed; (5) the relationship between ascending sensory systems is altered. They propose a theory which includes an element of specificity, such as Mountcastle and others hold to prevail in the medial lemniscal system, and a dominant role for the influence of spatial and temporal pattern. In a subsequent, imaginative and greatly influential paper (Melzack & Wall 1965) this theory was developed in respect particularly of pain mechanisms. They point out that a rigidly specific theory cannot account for the failure of a proportion of operations to abolish permanently pain of nonmalignant origin and following

which pain may occur in the analgesic areas and may even be worse: for the common experience that in some conditions, for instance causalgia, non-noxious stimuli may trigger pain although cutaneous thresholds are raised: for the irradiation of certain classes of pain and for its delay in some instances for many seconds which implies 'unusual summation of input'. They proposed that at the segmental level there is a 'gate-control system' in which two tiers of cells in the posterior horn modulate in various ways the afferent input while discharge patterns in the posterior columns provide a central controlling influence.

The barrage of input impulses evoked by the stimulus is determined by the total number of active fibres and the frequencies of impulse and by the balance of large and small fibres. Melzack and Wall consider that pain results only after monitoring of the afferent input by central cells. They suggest that this cerebral control exerted on the segmental selection is a function of first-order fibres in the dorsal columns made possible by their high speed of conduction and by other dorso-lateral pathways suggested by the work of Morin (1955) and others, which transmit at even faster speeds. The descending selective or modulating impulses may be transmitted by established corticofugal (Dawson 1958) and by reticulospinal pathways. These theories are valuable in that they contain without conflict undeniably credible observations of earlier workers and plausibly explain some of the unusual features of pain following lesions in the peripheral and central neural pathways. Support for this view is provided by the experiments of Hagbarth and Kerr (1954). They showed in cats that the afferent volley evoked by dorsal root stimulation, recorded from dorsal and ventral columns and at higher levels, is inhibited by stimulating various central structures including the reticular formation and certain areas of cortex. The primary afferent spike in the dorsal column (in the first order sensory neuron) is unaffected but other responses and those in the anterior column are all depressed. This depression of activity is abolished by general anaesthesia and by high transection of the cord; the conclusion is that ordinarily there is a constant or tonic descending inhibitory activity, playing on the synaptic afferent transmission.

For the neurosurgeon seeking ways of relieving pain, it is apparent that too many consistent and contrary observations have been made to accept the view that the highly complex pattern of afferent communication from the peripheral sensory organ can be served by a simple modality-fibre size-specific system. Although the success of anterolateral cordotomy in relieving pain in a high proportion of patients cannot be denied, this should not be adduced as evidence that the sensation of pain depends simply on the integrity of the spinothalamic tracts. The possibility that inhibitory influences play a role in controlling afferent patterns of impulses which excite the sensation of pain have led to novel approaches to its relief. These have included peripheral nerve stimulation, sometimes called transcutaneous nerve stimulation (TNS), spinal column stimulation or dorsal column stimulation (DCS) and deep brain stimulation (DBS). Usually this stimulation has been to points on the somatosensory pathway, but, in the brain, other points, such as the deep central grey areas surrounding the third ventricle and the aqueduct have been stimulated and may prove to be having an effect through a descending inhibitory system or systems.

To conform with the original scope of this book, operations on the sympathetic and peripheral nervous system are largely excluded. They are diverse in their location and extent and in appropriate circumstances have proved valuable. Their indications, technicalities and results are excellently described in the monumental volumes of White and Sweet (1955, 1969) and in more recent, specialized books on pain (*Persistent Pain* Vol 1, 1977, and Vol 3, 1981).

The conditions to be discussed might well have already failed to respond to surgical procedures to the peripheral nervous system. They will include a high proportion of pain associated with malignant disease, but also conditions totally unconnected with malignancy, such as painful amputation stumps, phantom limb pains, post herpetic and other inflammatory conditions, and central pain syndrome, associated with intrinsic disease to the brain or spinal cord, such as stroke or trauma.

The separation into malignant and non-malignant aetiologies is important for several reasons. In the former, physical health may be so poor that major operation would not be tolerated even though desirable on anatomical grounds, yet the pain may demand the relief which certain minor procedures can offer, and their limited duration may be adequate. The intensity of pain and the shortened expectancy of life may justify an operation which has side-effects that would be intolerable in a patient with a normal expectancy (for example thalamotomy). In malignant disease the severity of pain and its anatomical origins are easier to define. The dysaesthesiae and other unpleasant complications of tractotomies are usually of small consequence if the primary pain is satisfactorily abolished. In any case these tend to be more a consequence of repeated tractotomies, less likely with the reduced life expectation in this group.

When the aetiology of pain is nonmalignant and the expectation of life is normal or at least many years, the decision to operate and the choice of operation must become more difficult and requires greater discrimination.

Whether the patient has reached the limit of toleration of pain depends upon opinion rather than assessment against criteria; upon the degree of drug dependence and upon individual reaction to pain; it is often difficult to correlate the degree of complaint with the presumed aetiology. As noted in the opening review, it is an unhappy general experience that, with the passage of years, pain-relieving operations tend to lose their earlier beneficial effect and unpleasant sequelae are more likely to appear or to get worse, though fortunately occasionally they gradually lessen, or at any rate become more tolerable. The immediate complications of paresis and impaired sphincter control, which are more likely to occur the more efficient and drastic the operative section, will, if persistent, constitute a serious disability for a patient who would otherwise expect to enjoy years of healthy activity. Interference with sexual intercourse, particularly the sensory aspects, is an adverse sequel of cordotomy that should not be minimized. The replacement of pain (which perhaps was not intolerable) by a fresh handicap may not meet with the patient's approval. It is important for any procedure applied for treatment of nonmalignant pain, to have low morbidity. Unfortunately, many of these techniques also have low efficiency. In this group it is important to be able to apply a range or spectrum of treatments, any of which might turn out to be applicable to the individual. This range of treatment might include psychotherapy, hypnotherapy, meditation, biofeedback, acupuncture, or electrical stimulation (Miles 1983).

In performing pain relieving operations it is of the greatest importance to inform the patient in the fullest way possible about the nature of the operation and its possible consequences. Often these patients are driven to desperation by their longstanding pain and commonly have recognizable psychogenic traits, such as depression and suspicion.

These, together with the psychotrophic effects of prescribed drugs, might well render communication difficult. Wherever possible it is important to have a close relative present at such discussions.

*Peripheral nerve blockade*

Although of limited value in the overall management of pain such percutaneous techniques have the considerable advantage of being immediately available, even at the time of the first interview. In the patient with very advanced malignancy, even if this does not provide longstanding pain relief it may greatly improve the morale by indicating that the pain is not completely intractable. It can also serve to give the patient experience of the 'numbness' that might

be obligatory with a more permanent denervation.

*Posterior spinal root blockade*

In 1931 Dogliotti showed that the introduction of a judicious amount of absolute ethyl alcohol into the spinal subarachnoid space would damage the adjacent sensory rootlets sufficiently to block afferent impulses for several months. The hypobaric nature of the alcohol required careful positioning of the patient so that the spirit bathed the anatomically appropriate nerve roots. If minimal quantities were injected pain was relieved without significant sensory or motor loss. A more reliable modification was introduced by Maher (1955, 1957) by the substitution of phenol for alcohol. A 5% solution of phenol in glycerin has been found to give the most consistent results and the details of its preparation have been given by Maher (1960). These are important, for any contamination of either constituent by water renders the preparation highly irritating, also emphasized by Nathan and Scott (1958); this effect is probably the result of too rapid a liberation of the phenol into the spinal fluid. Phenol in pantopaque (myodil) may be used to provide radiological control of the level of injection.

These solutions are hyperbaric compared with cerebrospinal fluid and accurate placement depends upon a careful adjustment of the patient's position and selection of the site of injection. The technique is fully described in Maher's papers and, provided that only a small amount (0.1–0.2 ml) is injected at a time and its effect on sensory and motor systems determined before instilling a further increment, uncontrolled damage will be avoided. Nevertheless, if the anatomical distribution of the pain requires a block of the second, third and fourth sacral nerves, there is inevitably risk of spincter disturbance. If bilateral block is necessary, this should be undertaken at separate sessions. Subarachnoid injections are most effective and successful for blocking the roots from the low thoracic level downwards. At higher levels Maher recommends extradural instillation, but these are less effective. Brown (1961) reported the results in a large series of patients: 80% of those suffering from malignant disease were completely relieved; urinary retention and muscular weakness were transient complications in a very small proportion. Serious complications occurred in two patients as a result of water contamination of the phenolglycerin preparation.

It has been assumed that the relief of pain with little or no sensory or motor loss depended upon a special susceptibility of fine (C) fibres to the toxic quality of the phenol; the observations of Iggo and Walsh (1960) gave support to this view. Nathan and Sears (1960) carried out more searching electrophysiological tests which showed that depending upon concentration, duration of exposure and solvent, phenol could cause reversible or irreversible block, the order of block being the same as for local anaesthetics, small fibres before large; recovery takes place in the reverse order.

Smith (1964) examined the histology of spinal roots and cords of patients treated with phenol injections. Degeneration was constantly present in fibres of all diameters, with no selectivity. An interesting disclosure was degeneration in the posterior columns, attributable to that in the posterior roots; posterior root ganglia were affected little or not at all. There were no signs of irritative effects on the leptomeninges of spinal cord. These workers (Nathan et al. 1965) conclude that the immediate effect of phenol on the posterior roots is that of a local anaesthetic, to which fibres are selectively vulnerable according to diameter and lasting some 20 minutes. The permanent effects are due to degeneration, to which fibres of all diameters are equally susceptible. Relief of pain was attributed to destruction of an adequate number of afferent fibres, not to a selective effect. In this context it is well to recall a quotation made by Melzack and Wall (1962) from Sherrington that 'pain is summation' and the concluding remark of Noordenbos (1959) that 'pain is too much'.

*Posterior rhizotomy*

Theoretically, if the cause of the pain can be accurately delineated by segmental boundaries and is limited to but a few, division of these sensory roots should provide permanent relief of pain. Such conditions might include traumatic lesions of peripheral nerves, operation scars, intercostal or occipital neuralgias and root pain persisting after protrusion of intervertebral discs. In practice, while posterior rhizotomy can prove useful, the results are unfortunately erratic and unpredictable; it has rarely proved satisfactory for the treatment of painful amputation stumps or phantom limb pain, especially when there has been plexus avulsion, with spinal cord injury.

Perhaps the simplest explanation for failure of rhizotomy is anatomical, relating to failure to identify the appropriate nerve roots and to divide a sufficient number. Equally important is the intradural microanatomy with considerable wandering of root filaments, sometimes over several segments. There is also recognition that up to 15% of sensory fibres, although having their cell body in the dorsal root ganglion eventually enter the spinal cord via the ventral root (Coggleshall et al. 1975, Hosobuchi 1980). This means that dorsal root section might not be sufficient and ganglionectomy is necessary.

The massive intramedullary segmental connections in the region of the dorsal horns (Lissauer's tracts) must also mean that while a peripheral nerve might still have a moderately discrete area to serve, when it comes to central connections, major segmental overlap results. Segmental overlap in deep tissues (scleratomes) is much more extensive than in skin (dermatomes) and probably accounts for the failure of rhizotomy to relieve the pain of deep or widespread tumours.

'Posterior rhizotomy has for the most part proved an unsatisfactory operation and is being abandoned' (Northfield 1948). If dorsal rhizotomy is to be tried, it is recommended that at least three and preferably five adjacent roots are cut out and the dorsal root ganglia excised (Miles

1977). This entails an extensive laminectomy and the biological resilience of the patient to withstand such a procedure must be in question.

*Anterolateral cordotomy*

The anterolateral quadrant of the spinal cord is commonly called 'the spinal thalamic tract', but these two terms are not synonymous. The majority of the fibres in the anterolateral tract are in fact spinoreticular (Bowsher 1957) and take part in a polysnaptic, slowly propagating sensory pathway of perhaps greater relevance to the reception of pathological pain than the true spinothalamic fibres. The latter are probably responsible for the rapid awareness of a noxious stimulus and involved in accurate localization of that threat. Attempts to differentiate anatomically between the two forms of ascending fibre tracts have proved fruitless. The spinoreticular fibres probably originate from the deepest laminae of the posterior grey horn numbered 7 and 8 by Rexed (1952), while the true spinothalamic fibres, ascending to the ventroposterior thalamus, probably originate from the slightly more superficial layers of the posterior grey horn laminae 4, 5 and 6 (Bowsher 1977).

It is commonly held that the fibres cross to the opposite side of the spinal cord within one or two segments, but in man the evidence of surgical incisions suggests that crossing occupies more than this length of cord and that a minimum of six segments should be allowed above the upper limit of the segmental level of the pain when planning the site of the incision. The fibres take up positions in the periphery of the anterolateral quadrant. The observations of Smith (1957) show that in the cervical region there is considerable variation in their distribution in depth; they may occupy a compact zone just below the pia mater, or they may be situated more deeply. This is in accordance with operative experience, for in some patients an incision in the upper thoracic region only 3–4 mm in depth may provide a satisfactory high level of analgesia,

though in most the incision must reach a depth of 5 mm. Variability and probably some interweaving of position may account for the retention of islands of normal sensibility within the otherwise analgesic zone.

Suggestions that there are in fact two separate ascending tracts with differing function (Truex & Carpenter 1969) are not supported by operative experience. Dissociation of loss of sensibility for pain and for temperature may be seen following cordotomy, but without its presenting any regular pattern; dissociation is also seen in intramedullary tumours and other lesions, notably syringomyelia. Loss of appreciation of light touch is often difficult to detect, though loss of tickle and of the special sensations of the genitalia are generally demonstrable. This makes it likely that different fibres are involved but not that they are segregated into identifiably separate bundles. The disposition of the spinothalamic fibres accumulating from successive segments is of great importance to the surgeon. Operative experience indicates that the fibres from lower segments are displaced by those from higher segments (i.e. of more recent entry) towards the periphery of the quadrant and somewhat in a posterior direction. It is what one might anticipate would occur on anatomical grounds as the fibres emerge from the anterior commissure. Thus in the highest level of the spinal cord the sacral fibres will be closest to the surface, with a greater bulk posteriorly near the equator of the cord, and the lumbar thoracic and cervical fibres are found at respectively deeper levels. This laminar distribution accords with the findings of Walker (1940) and Glees (1953). Lahuerta (1984a) in his doctorate thesis beautifully illustrates the same tendency, his evidence being gleaned from clinical and autopsy correlations in 38 cases (Fig. 18.1).

It is stated commonly that the anterior limit of the spinothalamic fibres corresponds to the line of emergence of the most anterior (motor) rootlets, and that the posterior limit is marked by the equator of the cord and coincides externally with the attachment of the ligamentum denticulatum. There is no developmental reason

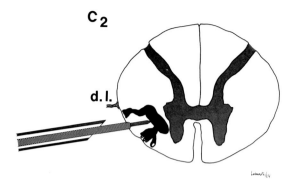

**Fig. 18.1.** Distribution for fibres ascending in the anterolateral spinal cord at the second cervical segmental level, as elucidated from correlations between the analgesia after percutaneous cordotomy and the position of the lesion discovered at autopsy (Lahuerta 1984a). (d.l. = dentate ligament; the estimated line of the cordotomy electrode is shown diagramatically).

why such rigid limits should define the extent of these fibres, histological findings do not support the teaching, and it is at variance with operative experience which constitutes evidence more reliable than any derived from animal experiments. Surgical observations show that to obtain the highest possible level of analgesia at any given level of incision into the cord, it may be necessary to extend it virtually to the midline anteriorly and to include all the distal segments it is necessary sometimes to extend it a millimetre or so posterior (i.e. dorsal) to the attachment of the ligamentum denticulatum. On the other hand the ligamentum denticulatum is occasionally attached to the pia posterior to the equator; if unrecognized this may lead to an incision that extends too far dorsally. Furthermore, to achieve a consistently dense universal analgesia below the desired level, it may be necessary to incise deeply into the cord, to a depth which in places may reach the grey matter. Extension of the incision in these directions carries inevitable risks; extension anteriorly may damage the pyramidal tract. Ipsilateral paralysis may in some cases be ischaemic, from damage to penetrating branches of the anterior spinal artery. Variation in the level at which the spinothalamic fibres decussate may lead occasionally to surprising effects of unilateral cordotomy. Thus French and

Peyton (1948) reported entirely ipsilateral analgesia in one case; the desired effect was obtained only when a cut was also made on the other side. Relief of unilateral pain may require a bilateral cut as a result of incomplete decussation. These anomalies are due to decussation taking place at an unusually high level in the cord.

One of the reasons for percutaneous cordotomy replacing open surgical cordotomy is the opportunity to explore the anatomy of the anterolateral quadrant of the spinal cord and by test stimulation to identify the positions of the relevant fibre tracts. This is undoubtedly of greater practical value than depending on predicted anatomy.

*Open cordotomy*

Anterolateral open cordotomy is usually performed at one of two levels; about the third thoracic segment for pain below the midthoracic level, including the lower limb; in the region of the first or second cervical segments for pain above the level of the mid thorax. (When the percutaneous technique is preferred for unilateral pain, pain may be at any level). The size of the cervical enlargement, the multitude of, bulk and eloquence of its roots render section at this level more hazardous with an increased risk of undesirable sequelae including weakness, anaesthesia and dysaesthesia. In the upper thoracic region the size of the cord is such that a cut of up to 5 mm depth at the equator can be tolerated with little risk of pyramidal damage. In the high cervical region the depth may be up to 8 mm. It must be noted that it is easy to make confident and glib statements concerning the depth of a cut, but an error of 1 mm is probably very common. Once the pia has been incised its contents tend to bulge and the incision to gape, rendering depth measurement only approximate.

To achieve the best result during open surgical cordotomy the patient should be wakened from the anaesthetic after the initial cut and tested for both motor deficit and level of analgesia. However, few would conduct the whole procedure under local anaesthetic as has been advocated by Diemath *et al.* (1961).

Division of and traction on the ligamentum denticulatum at the desired level will usually provide sufficient access to the anterolateral quadrant. Section of the adjacent posterior sensory roots will afford greater mobility should it prove necessary. Division of the tract is usually painless, though pain can be appreciated if the knife emerges anteriorly pressing on the dura and certainly a small, but sharp pain is encountered as the pia mater is punctured, using the percutaneous technique.

High cervical cordotomy, probably performed first in 1923 by Bromley (1930) has been said to have some advantages over thoracic cordotomy, the suggestion being that the relevant fibres were present in a more compact bundle at this level (Brihaye & Retif 1961). White and Sweet (1969) did not accept the anatomical basis for high cervical cordotomy being superior. The operation is however, technically more difficult with an increased mortality rate due in part to respiratory complications as will be discussed later.

*Percutaneous cordotomy*

This highly ingenious and skilful method of interrupting fibres in the anterolateral quadrant in the cervical spine was devised by Mullan (Mullan

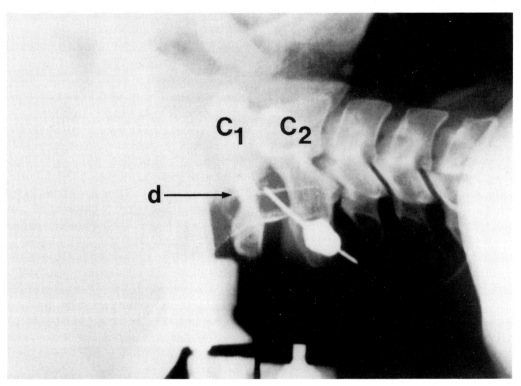

**Fig. 18.2.** Lateral radiograph during C1–2 percutaneous cordotomy. The dentate ligament (d) has been outlined by radio contrast injection. The cordotomy electrode will be advanced into the cord immediately anterior (above) this line, in order to achieve anterolateral cordotomy.

*et al.* 1963). Local anaesthesia was used at the site of puncture below the mastoid process. Percutaneous entry of a needle into the cervical theca between the first and second vertebrae was achieved using biplane radiographic control. They originally used a radioactive strontium-yttrium-beta emitting source at the tip of the needle which was placed immediately adjacent to the anterolateral quadrant of the spinal cord.

Rosomoff *et al.* (1965) described an important modification of the method using electrocoagulation. Since then and with but minor modifications this technique has proved increasingly preferable to open surgical cordotomy (White & Sweet 1969) (Fig. 18.2).

Because of the risk of respiratory failure from this high cervical lesion, Lin *et al.* (1966) and Lipton *et al.* (1974) developed anterior approaches to the lower cervical spine through the intervertebral discs. These techniques are laborious and probably have little practical advantage over an upper thoracic surgical cordotomy. Attempts to employ stereotactic techniques have been described by Hitchcock (1969) and by Todd *et al.* (1969).

## Complications of anterolateral cordotomy

### Respiratory failure

That respiratory function was at risk in these operations has been recognized for many years, even by Foerster as quoted by Peet *et al.* (1933). It is most likely to occur in patients whose pulmonary efficiency is already impaired by disease and in this respect a patient with cancer of the lung infiltrating the chest wall or brachial plexus, which would be efficiently treated by percutaneous high cervical cordotomy, might perish as a result of the combination of pulmonary infiltration on one side and ventilatory dysfunction due to interruption of the descending autonomic fibres on the other. Similarly, bilateral anterolateral sections of the cord at the same session is likely to prove dangerous. Another expression of the same complication has been the sudden

death of the patient during sleep in the first few postoperative days and in whom the cause of death could not be explained, the so-called 'Ondine's Curse'.

Nathan (1963a & b) carried out investigations from which he concluded that the descending pathways subserving ipsilateral respiratory movement are concentrated in the ventrolateral part of the spinal cord, between the lateral part of the ventral horn and the periphery of the cord. Belmusto *et al.* (1963) and Hitchcock and Leece (1967) studied pulmonary function during anterolateral cordotomy and the effects upon it of selective extensions of the cut. Their observations suggest a more extensive distribution of the relevant pathways than were defined by Nathan. Two important points emerge from this paper, elaborating previous clinical experience. The first is the apparent relationship between ventilation and the level of consciousness or alertness, and that respiratory activity was helped by the patient's attentiveness; the converse of this is implicit in the sudden death which may occur during sleep. The second is the gradual recovery of respiratory movement which occurs spontaneously in the course of several weeks after operation. The lessons here are clear: that nursing attention must be of the highest order, particularly at night and that apparatus capable of supporting ventilation must be immediately available. An apnoea monitoring and warning device is invaluable in these circumstances. It has been commonly stated that the threat exists for only a day or so after the operation, but this is somewhat optimistic and potential danger may exist for a week or so, particularly if respiratory infection develops.

Another aggravating factor has recently become more likely: this is persistence of pharmacological respiratory depression due to prolonged pre-operative narcotic analgesics. Since the introduction of sustained release morphine, examples of postoperative respiratory failure seem to have been more frequent; it is now policy to recommend stopping such analgesics at least 48 hours before cordotomy. Satisfactory relief of pain probably aggravates the tendency to sleep apnoea, by the removal of the powerful stimulus of pain. Routine blood gas analysis, twice daily for the first two postoperative days, may also alert the clinician to incipient respiratory failure.

In overt respiratory depression Naloxone can prove lifesaving by antagonizing the central respiratory depressant effect, while Doxapram hydrochloride can give a more prolonged respiratory stimulating effect.

*Arterial hypotension*

A sudden drop in blood pressure is often recorded immediately after incision into the spinal cord, moderate and evanescent when the incision is unilateral and in the thoracic region, more severe and protracted if bilateral, or if unilateral at the high cervical level. In practice its effects are rarely noted and this is particularly obvious in the case of percutaneous cordotomy in the cervical region when the patient is awake; recumbency and elevation of the foot of the bed are usually all that is necessary in the way of treatment.

Awareness of the possibility of this complication, albeit transitory, is more important regarding avoidable secondary effects. Patients undergoing cordotomy are commonly elderly and frail, and ischaemic complications such as myocardial infarction can result from significant arterial hypotension. The precise situation in the human cord of the descending pathways which subserve sympathetic nervous activity is not known. Belmusto *et al.* (1963) noted that the blood pressure fell when the incision was deepened to 4–5 mm concurrent with changes in the respiratory tidal volume. In the cat and monkey Kerr and Alexander (1964) found pathways serving autonomic function which were situated superficially in the lateral columns. They were identified by stimulation which elevated the arterial blood pressure and the intravesical pressure. Cordotomy in the cervical region gives rise to a Horner syndrome, which of course may also be encountered in cases of intramedullary lesions, such as tumour and syringomyelia, in

which the interruption is in the grey matter containing the intermediolateral nucleus.

*Disturbed sphincter control*

The function of micturition is delicately balanced and retention of urine is common after any operation involving manipulation of the spinal cord; the disturbance usually persists for only a day or so and responds readily to treatment. Following cordotomy at any level a similar disturbance is common and consistent with the effects on control of the bladder sphincter of tumours which compress the spinal cord at various levels; thus thoracic cordotomy is more likely to be associated with disturbance of sphincter function rather than cervical cordotomy.

Persistent urinary retention after unilateral cordotomy occurs in less than 5% of cases (Lipton 1979), but this figure increases to as much as 20% when bilateral incisions have been made (White & Sweet 1969).

It is of course more likely to occur if there is already some peripheral neurological deficit in the control of sphincter function such as with infiltrating intrapelvic tumours when, ipsilateral, central, autonomic dysfunction is combined with contralateral, general, peripheral nerve dysfunction.

Although on theoretical grounds bowel disturbance might be expected as commonly as that of the bladder, experience shows that this is not so. Constipation occurs as a result of loss of sensation of rectal fullness and may bring about recurrent attacks of diarrhoea that may lead to incontinence. White and Sweet (1969) drew attention to the lack of abdominal pain in bowel obstruction following bilateral cordotomy and that patients are unable to distinguish between faeces and flatus.

Valuable contributions on the physiology of micturition and of defecation and their disturbance after cordotomy have been made by Nathan and Smith (1951, 1953 and 1958) and briefly summarized by Nathan (1963) in the study of the results of cordotomy. These observations have included cystometrographic records during and after operation, tests of bladder and rectal sensibility and correlation with post-mortem findings in the spinal cord. They conclude that the descending fibres which control the voluntary initiation of micturition and defecation, and the ascending fibres responding to distention and the desire to relax sphincters are assembled at all levels of the spinal cord (including the cervical) in a narrow band across its equator opposite the central canal. They are most concentrated at depth near the grey matter. Patients are therefore at great risk if destruction is being conducted deeply in this region of the spinal cord as is often the case for sacral pain. They distinguish between the entirely automatic function which develops after total division of the cord (as in traumatic paraplegia) and the disturbance after anterolateral cordotomy. In the latter, the posterior columns are preserved and it is suggested that these are the substate for the vague abdominal sensations, which for many postcordotomy patients, provide substitute information of the state of the bladder and bowel (Nathan 1956a).

## Paresis

The incidence of ipsilateral paresis following unilateral cordotomy varies greatly in the reported series and has been reviewed in depth by White and Sweet (1969). Though some claim not to have seen it, Lipton (1979) suggests that if carefully looked for there is some detectable weakness in 90% of patients after percutaneous cervical cordotomy, though this will prove significant in less than 40%, and a handicap in only 20%. In percutaneous cordotomy the clinician is able to test both the arm and leg for power during the procedure; this should afford a degree of protection against a major motor deficit.

While minor degrees of hemiparesis may be of little practical consequence in advanced malignancy, it can prove a major drawback when this technique is applied to benign conditions, particularly for phantom leg pain when the limb

under threat is the sole support for the body, and it is of great concern when there may be a need to repeat the lesion in the future.

## Dysaesthesiae

Under this heading there are at least two varieties. The first consists of a soreness of the skin and sometimes pain at or about the segmental level of the cordotomy with a girdle distribution. Happily, this tends to be temporary. Its cause is uncertain, though because it is thought that excessive rotation of the spinal cord is associated with an increased incidence and severity, therefore its cause is associated with traction on peripheral nerves. Against this hypothesis, rhizotomy has not proved an effective manœuvre in preventing this type of dysaesthesiae.

Dysaesthesia below the level of the cordotomy constitutes a more serious complaint. The onset is usually delayed and it is encountered more frequently when the procedure has been undertaken for benign lesions and even more often following repetition of the cordotomy. It emerges as simultaneous with return of sensation, and may take the form of tingling, 'pins and needles', or other sensations, be described as extremely painful with a sensation of heat, cold, rawness or be of relatively ill-defined localization. This form of dysaesthesiae comes into the category of 'central pain' so clearly described by Riddoch (1939). Nathan (1963) described how these dysaesthesiae were abolished by spinal anaesthetic, suggesting their dependence upon an input from the peripheral nerves. White and Sweet (1969) have, like many others, found a second and higher cordotomy to be unhelpful in relieving the symptoms. In the light of modern research on pain mechanisms it is more likely that these abnormal sensations are related to disturbances of the pattern of ascending impulses. The delay in their appearance is due to chemical or physiological modification constituting a change in segmental function in the spinal cord.

Referred sensations, sometimes called allachesthesia, noted by Ray and Wolffe (1945) have been particularly studied by Nathan (1956b). Noxious stimulation on the skin or deep tissues within the analgesic area is felt by the patient, but is referred after unilateral cordotomy to the opposite (normal) side, though not necessarily to the homologous position: the referred sensation is poorly localized and it usually has an unpleasant or painful quality. After bilateral cordotomy the sensation may be referred to an area above the level of the analgesic. Repetitive noxious stimuli appear to have a summating effect with a delayed diffuse response.

When unilateral cordotomy has been performed for the relief of strictly unilateral pain due to a malignant growth, it is a not infrequent experience for the patient to complain of similar pain on the other side within a few days of the operation. This disturbing and disappointing outcome is usually interpreted as indicating a pre-existing extension of growth to implicate structures on the other apparently sound side; pain on that side was not appreciated by the patient because of the intensity of pain in the area of complaint. This may be an example of diffuse noxious inhibition (Le Bars et al. 1979) a well-known phenomenon in the human. Nathan (1956b) considers that development of contralateral pain of this type is an example of reference. Whether or not this is the correct explanation, the pain can be relieved by a second operation converting the unilateral to a bilateral section.

*Recurrence of pain*

A falling level of analgesia and gradual return of pain sensibility, within a few days of operation suggests that insufficient spinothalamic fibres have been divided. If the procedure has been an open surgical one the unsatisfactory decision to perform early revision of the incision has to be undertaken. The same can occur after a percutaneous destruction, but less often. If the level of analgesia holds firm both by level and completeness of analgesia, for the first few days after operation it is likely to be associated with relief of pain, sufficient to cover the life expectancy associated with malignant disease. Experience of applying the technique to benign persistent pains has clearly shown the tendency for the analgesia to diminish and for pain to return. White (1962) was able to observe a considerable number of patients for many years and found that in about one half there was recovery of pain sensibility to a lesser or greater degree. Subsequent cordotomy at a higher level generally proved unsuccessful in providing further relief. Very few could continue to advance the recommendation of cordotomy for the treatment of benign persistent pains even though in a small proportion of cases the effect can be prolonged. The morbidity of the first lesion and even more of subsequent lesions make it an unsatisfactory procedure for benign pain (Evans & Lloyd 1968).

Two explanations have been made for delayed recovery from the effects of anterolateral tractotomy. One possibility is that a sufficient number of fibres regenerate. Although sprouting of dividing axons within the central nervous system has been observed, reformation of a long fibre and formation of its synapses on an appropriate cell has never been demonstrated; until then the possibility cannot be accepted.

The other, and more likely possibility, is the development of alternative pathways. Nathan (1963) points out that the posterior columns contain, in addition to the first order neurons ascending to the gracile and cuneate nuclei, other neurons which originate from cells in the segmental grey matter. He suggests that these may be partly responsible for conducting those impulses which are concerned in the abnormal reference of pain. Painful or unpleasant sensations when the posterior columns are mechanically stimulated have been reported (Sourek 1969). During the operation of myelotomy, pricking of the dorsal columns with a fine needle has given rise to pain felt on the homolateral side of the body or lower limb, in a pattern which corresponds with the lamination of segmental fibres in the column. An alternative pathway may also be provided by multisynaptic segmental

change of neurons, by collaterals of spinothalamic fibres which are centred on the
reticular formation and which may separate
early from the main tract and thus escape
division. The part played by spinothalamic fibres
in activating reticular formation is summarized
by Rose and Mountcastle (1959) and the evidence for a multisynaptic ascending spinal
pathway by Noordenbos (1959). No final conclusions can be drawn, but the theory of 'alternative pathways' is more plausible than that of
'regeneration' (*see also* Bishop 1962).

### Results of anterolateral cordotomy

Table 18.1 records the experience from open,
surgical cordotomy; the results from White and
Sweet (1969) dominate because of their great
experience: their two volumes provide a valuable
store of information.

*Relief of pain and mortality (Table 18.1)*

**Comment** The category 'relieved' includes both
total and partial relief of pain because a more
accurate assessment cannot always be extracted
from the information supplied: about twice as
many patients obtain total relief as obtain partial
relief.

Mortality in patients with cancer is higher
than those with a benign lesion. For cervical
cordotomy, the mortality is higher if the cancer
affects the upper part of the body than if the
cancer is in the lower part of the body: the overall
mortality is very high, almost certainly related
to the high proportion of bilateral cordotomies
undertaken during this period.

*Complications and sequelae (Table 18.2)*

**Comment** 'Abnormal sensations' include par-
aesthesae, dysaesthesiae, painful or otherwise
and 'reference of pain'. A high figure in Nathan's
cases due to his special investigations into 'reference of pain', the incidence being 28%; this
leaves the incidence of dysaesthesiae at 6%,
similar to the series of White and Sweet. 'Paresis'
comprises severe and lasting weakness or paralysis, the direct consequence of operation.

'Bladder disturbance' includes only persistent
dysfunction, possibly aggravated by the causative lesion in some, but precipitated by operation.

An expectation of over 80% total pain relief
following cervical cordotomy was described by
White and Sweet (1969); in a review of over
3,000 recorded cases Lorenz et al. (1975)
reported excellent or good results ranging from
75 to 96% in various series.

Lahuerta et al. (1984b) have described complete pain relief in 64%, partial relief in 23% and
no relief in 13% and reviewed many of the recent
reports regarding percutaneous cervical cordotomy. The mortality of this procedure is low.

**Table 18.1.** Relief of pain and mortality following anterolateral cordotomy.

| Reference | Total patients | Nature of disease | Level of operation | Relieved (%) | Mortality (%) |
|---|---|---|---|---|---|
| Brihaye & Retif (1961) | 74 | malignant | cervical | 77 | 11 |
| | 7 | benign | cervical | 85 | no deaths |
| | 20 | malignant | thoracic | 65 | no deaths |
| | 8 | benign | thoracic | 62 | no deaths |
| Nathan (1963) | 104 | all cases | cervical & thoracic | 77 | 3 in first week |
| | 21 | malignant | cervical | 70 | no deaths |
| White & Sweet (1969) | 28 | malignant | cervical | 54 | 21 |
| | 30 | benign | cervical | 70 | 3 |
| | 271 | malignant | thoracic | 77 | 8 |
| | 70 | benign | thoracic | 86 | no deaths |

Table 18.2. Complications and sequelae following anterolateral cordotomy.

| Reference | Description of cases | | Abnormal sensations (%) | Paresis (%) | Bladder Disturbance (%) |
|---|---|---|---|---|---|
| Brihaye & Retif (1961) | cervical | all cases | 2.4 | 4.9 | 8.6 |
| | thoracic | all cases | 29.0 | 21.0 | 32.0 |
| McKissock (1961) | same material as Nathan 1963 | | | | |
| | successful | bilateral | | | invariable |
| | successful | unilateral | | | never |
| Nathan (1963) | cervical | unilateral | | 14.0 (upper limb) | |
| | cervical + thoracic | unilateral | 34.0 | 10.0 (lower limb) | |
| | cervical + thoracic | bilateral | | 24.0 (lower limb) | |
| White & Sweet (1969) | cervical | unilateral | 8.8 | 2.0 | 2.0 |
| | thoracic | unilateral | 6.0 | no cases | 1.6 |
| | thoracic | bilateral | 7.0 | 13.0 | 20.0 |

White and Sweet (1969) reported a mortality of 1.7% while Lahuerta et al. described a mortality of 6%. Selection of cases will determine, to a large extent, the risk of mortality from this procedure. In the Liverpool series described by Lahuerta et al. (1984b) five of the six deaths occurred in patients with extensive lung destruction due to carcinoma, who died from respiratory failure following unilateral high cervical cordotomy. The threshold for acceptance of patients for cordotomy in this unit is low, such that any patient expected to live more than a few weeks would be considered for cordotomy.

Because of the acknowledged risk of fatal sleep apnoea following bilateral cervical percutaneous cordotomies (Mullan & Hosobuchi 1963) various tactics have been employed to minimize this threat. Lin et al. (1966) developed an anterior approach allowing the second lesion to be made in the lower cervical cord, below the outflow of the phrenic nerve on that side. The electrode is inserted through a lower cervical intervertebral disc (C5–6 or C6–7) diagonally so as to penetrate the opposite anterolateral cord quadrant. Lipton et al. (1974) designed and described a similar stereotaxic approach. However, in practice this technique is difficult, particularly in the rather decrepit patient group under consideration, in whom extensive cervical disc degeneration is common. Lipton (1979) would attempt bilateral

selective cordotomy at two stages, but at the same level approached laterally in preference to anterior cordotomy. Great care is taken to keep the upper level of the sensory deficit on one side as low as possible, in an attempt to maintain diaphragmatic innervation.

The low mortality and potential for selectivity in the awake patient, mean that percutaneous cordotomy can be more extensively applied to patients with advanced disease. The technique however does require practice and some sophisticated equipment, including radiographic screening facilities.

Its application to benign persistent pain confers no advantage over that of open cordotomy and it suffers the same likelihood of delayed failure, paresis, dysaesthesia and bladder disturbance (Lahuerta et al. 1984b). Levin and Cosman (1981) propound the advantages of lesion making using temperature control, a technique that has been adopted by many.

### Commissural myelotomy

Spinothalamic fibres can be interrupted as they cross the anterior commissure by a vertical incision in the median plane of the spinal cord. This was the basis of an alternative operation for the relief of pain suggested by Greenfield and put into practice by Armour (1927). The result is a bilaterally symmetrical area of analgesia whose upper and lower limits will be dependent upon the levels of the cord segments incised and upon the particular pattern of decussation for any given patient. It is the latter which renders the results of this operation somewhat unreliable; to provide a good allowance for delayed sensory decussation demands more extensive laminectomy than for cordotomy. The operation has found little support beyond a few centres. Wertheimer and Lecuire (1953) have described their experience in 107 patients of which 80 were available for follow-ups. The mortality in the first week was 7%. In most cases pain was due to malignant growth and in all the pain was situated below the umbilicus. The pain was totally relieved in one third of cases and partially relieved in another third. Dense analgesia was achieved in about one third; temporary dysaesthesiae, painful and otherwise, were frequent, but permanent in only two patients. Limb weakness occurred temporarily, never permanently and disturbance of micturition was persistent in only two patients. The technique as described by Wertheimer and Lecuire had the interesting feature of a relatively shallow incision, to a maximum of 4 mm, thus making it unlikely that all anterior commissural fibres could have been divided, although the instance of pain relief was considerable. Sourek (1969) described in valuable detail the technique, and the correlation between segmental levels of pain, myelotomy and resultant analgesia in 25 patients. Pain relief occurred in each in spite of the lack of correlation between the segmental extent of the pain and the cutaneous analgesia resulting. No paresis or sphincter disturbance was described. Sourek described a method of determining the midline by pricking the posterior column while the patient was awake and able to recognize a sharp, painful sensation on one or other side of the body usually in the legs. Using the more modern advantages of operative microscopy and microneurosurgical instrumentation it is usually clearly evident that a fine septum of dense pia mater constitutes the midline and that frequently

perforating draining veins pass down in this septum between the posterior columns, again indicating the correct line for incision. Of considerable recent interest has been the suggestion that extensive midline commissurotomies are not needed in order to provide a major relief of pain over large areas of the body. This approach is associated with the suggestion that, in the deep medial portions of the posterior columns, an extralemniscal system of fibres associated with pain conduction, is to be found, particularly in the high cervical region and that destruction of these rather than the crossing spinothalamic fibres is what produces pain relief. Hitchcock (1969) described a stereotactic method of achieving this in the high cervical region, as has Schwartz (1976), and the anatomical background has been thoroughly explored by Smith and Deacon (1984). Gildenberg and Hirshling (1981) have, on a similar basis, performed limited myelotomy at the thoracolumbar area of the cord. The duration and frequency of satisfactory pain relief following these limited procedures have been questioned (Papo 1979). As a surgical procedure for the relief of intractable pain, this operation remains to be proven.

*Spinothalamic tractotomy in the brain stem*

The difficulty of obtaining a sufficiently high level of analgesia by cervical cordotomy and the attendant risks, together with the need for procedures to relieve pain from malignant growths involving the trigeminal and glossopharyngeal distribution, have persuaded surgeons to attempt destruction of the spinothalamic pathways at higher levels, in the medulla, pons, and midbrain.

Medullary tractotomy was first undertaken by Schwartz and O'Leary (1941). The tract occupies a fairly superficial restricted area bounded dorsally by the corpus restiforme and delimited by the emerging vagus and glossopharyngeal rootlets and anteriorly (that is ventrally) by the bulge of the olive. Caudally to this bulge, at or below the level of the obex of the fourth ventricle, the anterior limit is marked by the rootlets of the hypoglossal nerve. The technique is difficult, demanding a posterior fossa exploration and some degree of rotation of the medulla and with the risk of ataxia resulting from damage to the restiform body. White and Sweet (1969) record the experience from the literature of 69 such operations. Mortality was high at 20% and dysaesthesiae occurred in two patients.

*Pontine and mesencephalic tractotomy*

Pontine tractotomy, pioneered by Dogliotti (1938), is rarely performed, due to the operative risks. Mesencephalic tractotomy was proposed by Walker (1942) as an alternative to Dogliotti's operation because of the easier access. The section is made at the intercollicular level where the tract lies fairly superficial, though somewhat overlayed by the brachium of the inferior colliculus, extending posteriorly from the lateral sulcus. Division of the outflow of the inferior colliculus appears not to cause significant deafness, though this would be complete if a bilateral section was performed. Again, White and Sweet (1969) have assembled the experience from the literature. The serious disadvantage of the operation is the incidence of dysaesthesae, and other neurological deficits are common.

Stereotaxic techniques to interrupt the spinothalamic tracts in the brain stem have been described (Wycis & Spiegel 1962), but again there is a high incidence of neurological morbidity with a 15% incidence of dysaesthesiae. The most successful results appear to be those briefly reported by Mazars *et al.* (1960) but detail is insufficient in this report.

*Dorsal root entry zone cordotomy*

This is a procedure by which a destructive lesion is created in the posterolateral sulcus of the spinal cord at the point of entry of the dorsal (sensory) roots. The technique was introduced with the intention of treating the burning dysaesthetic pain associated with brachial plexus avulsion syndrome. Nashold and Ostdahl (1979) presented an initial experience of 21 patients treated by this technique; two thirds achieved good pain relief, i.e. greater than 75%. In view of the deficiencies of anterolateral cordotomy in providing longterm pain relief, it is somewhat surprising to hear descriptions of pain relief continuing for more than eight years following this procedure.

In addition to its application in the cervical region, it has also been used to treat leg pain syndromes following trauma which Nashold considers may also be a form of avulsion, and post herpetic neuralgia. In the latter condition it would appear to be more successful in removing the hypersensitivity than the background burning discomfort.

The initial high incidence (66%) of unwanted neurological morbidity following dorsal root entry zone lesions (Nashold & Ostdahl 1979) has been reduced by modifying the output current of the radiofrequency generator used to deliver the punctate coagulation (Nashold 1981), but a risk of neurological deficit remains, particularly where there has already been spinal cord injury (Thomas & Sheehy 1982).

The theoretical basis for this technique is to be found in the experimental animal studies of Albe-Fessard and Lombard (1981) who, in attempting to replicate the painful state associated with cervical plexus injury, used preganglionic dorsal root section in the rat as the experimental technique. Microelectrode recordings from the region of the dorsal horn and from thalamic centres showed that following this procedure neurons around the dorsal horn became hyperactive, suggesting epileptic or discharge-generating pools of neurons. Attempts were therefore made to extend these studies by producing destructive lesions in the vicinity of the discharge pools. The effect of the original dorsal root sections in the rat was to promote, in a high proportion of animals, limb autotomy. Following dorsal root entry zone coagulation this autotomy rate was grossly reduced (Albe-Fessard 1984). These studies have involved two major assumptions, the first being

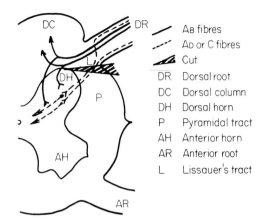

AB fibres — Aᴅ or C fibres ---- Cut DR Dorsal root DC Dorsal column DH Dorsal horn P Pyramidal tract AH Anterior horn AR Anterior root L Lissauer's tract

**Fig. 18.3.** Diagrammatic representation of the position of the cut recommended by Sindou, which might also be the area of destruction achieved by Nashold.

that sectioning the dorsal root replicates the human syndrome associated with avulsion of the dorsal roots, and the second that the phenomenon of autotomy equates to the human brachial plexus avulsion pain syndrome.

Approaching the area by an entirely different experimental route Sindou *et al.* (1974), in investigating the fibre pattern in the dorsal root at its entry to the spinal cord, showed quite clearly the anatomical re-alignment of the A delta and C fibres to the axilla (lateral aspect of) the dorsal root; on the basis of this information they performed selective knife cut destruction into the cord at the dorsal root entry zone (Fig. 18.3). Sindou *et al.* (1976) described the efficiency of this technique in relieving cancer pain and pain associated with spasticity.

The lesions created by these techniques are so close topographically as to suggest that they are perhaps achieving the same result. There remains doubt as to what functional interruption is being achieved and there must also remain doubt as to the longterm effectiveness of these procedures. At the same time it is clear that there are sufficient, otherwise intractable, painful conditions, particularly that of brachial plexus avulsion syndrome that have failed to respond to less risky procedures and for which this technique is acceptable.

*Stereotaxic Lesions in the Thalamus**

Concurrent with the use of stereotaxic procedures in the treatment of involuntary movements has been an attempt to define and interrupt nuclei or pathways within the thalamus essential for the perception of pain. Hecaen *et al.* (1949) provided one of the earliest reports; lesions were made in the ventral posterior medial, centromedian and basal dorsal medial nuclei in six cases of thalamic syndrome of Dejerine and Roussy (1906). Pain was relieved to some extent, but only temporarily. The lesions in the ventral posterior medial and posterior lateral nuclei have frequently been made, but it is generally conceded that the results have been disappointing; some three-quarters of the patients obtain considerable immediate benefit, but the pain soon returns in about one half (Riechert 1960). It was understandable that the nuclei of the thalamus first to be attacked should be the known sensory relay stations, the so-called 'specific' nuclei. To quote Brodal (1969) 'it is unanimously agreed that the nucleus ventralis lateralis posterior (VPL) receives fibres from the medial lemniscus and the spinothalamic tract', though he disapproves of the division of the thalamic nuclei into nonspecific and specific. Stimulation within this nucleus gives rise to sensations of diverse quality which confirm anatomical studies that the fibres are arranged in a somatotopical pattern, caudal segments being represented most laterally and the higher segments progressively more medially. Apart from its connections with the reticular system, the medial lemniscus terminates in the lateral portion of the nucleus.

Both lateral and medial nuclei receive spinothalamic fibres; the extreme medial or arcuate tail of the nucleus receives those from the head (VPM). More recent studies have made it certain that spinothalamic fibres, in the diencephalon

* The naming of thalamic nuclei remains a problem (*see* Chapter 19); in an attempt to simplify understanding, but not to solve the problem, generally accepted initials will often be used.

are more diffusely distributed than this. Noordenbos (1959) has estimated that although several thousand fibres must arise in each cord segment, only 50 of these attain the thalamus. Bowsher (1957) in studies of human material following anterolateral cordotomy, found terminal degeneration bilaterally in the reticular formation of the medulla, pons and midbrain in the region of all four colliculi, bilaterally in the ventral posterolateral, and ipsilaterally in the centromedian nucleus of the thalamus. However, Mehler (1966a) is critical of the evidence that the centromedian and intralaminar nuclei play a significant role as relay stations on the spinothalamic pathways. The rostral connections of the spinothalamic fibres are highly complex and appear increasingly so with each fresh study; it is uncertain to what extent this complexity is related to the reticular formation and its 'activating' functions and to its excitation of affective responses which are such a rich, though variable, component of pain. Concise summaries of these problems are provided by Brodal (1969), Truex and Carpenter (1969) and Bowsher (1977).

These anatomical and physiological developments have led to a shift of stereotaxic lesions away from the ventral lateral (specific) nuclei to the ventral posterior medial and intralaminar (nonspecific) nuclei. Bilateral lesions are frequently needed for even pain that appears to be felt entirely unilaterally.

Mark *et al.* (1963) and Mark and Ervin (1969) have noted that the results of thalamic lesions for the relief of pain correlated with post-mortem verification and can be roughly divided into three categories:

1  Lesions in the ventral posterior lateral nucleus cause profound somatosensory loss, but provide little or no relief of pain.
2  Lesions including parafascicular, intralaminar and median nuclei cause little or no sensory loss and give good pain relief.
3  Those which involve the dorsal medial and anterior nuclei give rise to a severe alteration of affect, pain is ignored, but its perception seems undiminished; this resembles the effect of leucotomy which will be mentioned later.

The results described were that pain was relieved in one half of the 38 patients treated by thalamic lesions in various nuclei; in six patients with parafascicular or centromedian nuclei lesions, relief was good in five and fair in one. Bettag (1966) obtained good results for combined lesions in the centromedian and caudal ventral nuclei; half the patients were entirely free from pain and in another one third the pain was greatly lessened. Fairman (1976) reported the results of unilateral lesions in the intralaminar and centromedian nuclei: in all 30 patients pain was due to malignant disease and in 27 it was abolished during the period of survival, up to one year. Hankinson (1969) employed similar targets and in 10 patients with bilateral lesions he noted considerable improvement: the cases included examples of the thalamic syndrome and postherpetic pain. Lesions of the centromedian nucleus alone have been made by Watkins (1972) and of 14 patients with malignant disease pain was alleviated in all but one; bilateral lesions were necessary in only three; all died within a year. In a group of 20 patients suffering from pain of nonmalignant origin the operation proved completely successful in 15, though it was necessary to perform bilateral operations in 12 of these in order to achieve total relief. The longest period of relief was six years and in eight patients has exceeded four years. However, more sanguine results are described by Bouchard *et al.* (1977) who illustrated clearly that which is now almost universally agreed regarding thalamotomy for pain, namely, that when applied for persistent pain associated with malignancy, good pain relief is limited to periods of survival not more than six months: the operation is therefore both effective and appropriate for the patient with advanced malignancy. When applied to benign persistent pain the overall success rate, even with bilateral lesions, is much lower and with less persistence of effect.

Variability in the results of what are assumed to be anatomically similar lesions is doubtless associated with uncertainty as to the uniform nature of the location and extent of the lesions due to anatomical variations. There is also a lack of post-mortem verification of location of lesions. Reports on the ability to provoke pain by stimulating in these target zones are even more discordant (Ervin & Mark 1960, Hankinson 1960, Hassler & Riechert 1959, Sano *et al.* 1966). Finally, it is to be noted that bilateral lesions in areas which anatomically might be expected to involve the rostral connections of the reticular formation have little or no effect upon the state of consciousness. The explanation probably resides in the distinction between 'reticular formation' and 'activating system'. Brodal (1969) emphasizes that the terms are not synonymous, the former referring to morphology and the latter to function.

Since the introduction of such sophisticated techniques as percutaneous cordotomy most neurosurgeons have shown a marked disinclination to perform thalamotomy even for advanced malignancy. This has coincided with the overall reduction in the use of stereotaxic surgery which has followed the introduction of L-Dopa in the treatment of parkinsonism. It is useful at this time to emphasize the efficiency with which unilateral thalamotomy can relieve contralateral pain of malignancy when this arises from the head and neck and to state that the quality of pain relief, without detectable sensory or other deficit, provides for a comfortable short-term survival.

*Pituitary destruction*

Endocrine ablative techniques for cancer were initiated by Beatson (1896) directed at the ovaries, then by Huggins and Hodges (1941) directed at the testes, and by Huggins and Bergenstahl (1952) directed at the adrenal glands.

In 1953 Luft and Olivecrona reported the successful application of transcranial hypophysectomy for the treatment of pain associated with advanced carcinoma of the breast and prostate. Olivecrona noted that in some patients the pain relief associated with a hypophysectomy

had occurred by the time the patient had recovered from the anaesthetic and the same phenomenon was noted following transsphenoidal hypophysectomy (Hardy 1971), transsphenoidal percutaneous radiofrequency coagulation (Zervas 1969) and other techniques. Greco *et al.* (1957) and, later, Moricca (1974) described pituitary destruction by injection of alcohol into the gland by the transsphenoidal route, defined the pain relief that resulted and confirmed sporadic reports by others, that pain relief can also occur when the malignancy is other than that normally considered to be hormonally influenced, namely from the breast or prostate.

This simple technique has now been used throughout the world and numerous reports confirm its efficiency (Moricca 1977, Lipton *et al.* 1978). More than 75% of patients obtain pain relief, but in the majority relief does not last more than three months; furthermore, the technique is not without risk (Lipton *et al.* 1978).

The means by which destruction of the pituitary gland, or structures close to it, relieves pain is not understood and have been debated at some length (Miles 1983, 1984b). The extent of pituitary endocrine dysfunction following destruction is not associated with the degree of pain relief (Williams *et al.* 1980). Anterior hypothalamic injury can follow the alcohol injection technique as recorded *post mortem* (Lipton *et al.* 1978) and on experimental cadaveric injection (Miles 1979) but this form of damage does not correlate with the degree of pain relief (Miles 1984b). Studies of neuropeptides in CSF and blood, while fragmentary, have provided no clue as to the mechanism of pain relief (Miles 1984b). A recent suggestion by Yanagida *et al.* (1984) that electrical stimulation of the pituitary gland also relieves pain complicates the explanation, but while it allows for the construction of hypotheses of releasing and inhibiting circuitry between the pituitary gland and the hypothalamus, it does not as yet provide a solution. This is clearly an area for exploration and discovery.

*Operations on the cortex and subcortical white matter*

The role played by the cortex in the perception of pain remains unsolved. It may be restricted to the function of localization of the noxious stimulus; pain arising from stimulation of skin and joints is accurately localized as are innocuous stimuli. Stimuli arising in the deeper tissues and viscera do not emerge into the consciousness, except for the normal calls of physiological activity such as distension of the bladder. Noxious adequate stimuli in these parts give rise to pain which, in general, is poorly localized. The localization at the point of origin of the stimulus requires the use of the body image (schema) as a form of reference map. The body image is gradually built up during the early years of development, from a summation of experiences. The intimate relation between the constant stream of afferent stimuli from receptors and this 'central map' is very close and the 'map' remains intact and unaltered, even if a projecting portion of the body, is removed (Riddoch 1941). The brain continues to register a 'whole' image. This is exemplified in the remarkable phenomenon of phantom limb, a normal sequel to amputation that may persist for years or even permanently. The gradual diminution in size and length, particularly of the proximal part of the phantom limb, is described with great clarity by Henderson and Smyth (1948).

Electrical stimulation of the cortex rarely evokes the sensation of pain; in Penfield's experience sensations of pain comprised little more than 1% of the sensory responses (Penfield & Boldrey 1937). Durable cutaneous analgesia is rarely caused by surgical excision of sensory cortex (White & Sweet 1969). Marshall (1951) provides fascinating data correlating injuries to the brain and the subsequent sensory disturbances including hyperpathia (allodynia).

An entirely novel surgical approach to the problem of pain relief was reported by Talairach *et al.* (1960). This was based on the theory that the perception of pain depends on the integrity of the thalamocortical connections, in which the secondary sensory cortex plays an important role. The operation aims at creating lesions deep to the secondary sensory area which sever its links with the thalamus. Poggio and Mountcastle (1960), Truex and Carpenter (1969) and Brodal (1969), have all emphasized the significance of S2 cortex in the appreciation of pain, while Penfield and Rasmussen (1950) in man and Hassler (1960) in monkeys, have tended to refute its significance. Talairach's operation is now undertaken only rarely.

*Leucotomy for pain relief*

Early experience of leucotomy for mental disorder included the observation that the patient became more tolerant of pain. In due course therefore, leucotomy came to be used for patients with severe pain resistant to other forms of treatment and who might be psychiatrically healthy except for the direct consequences of the pain (Freeman & Watts 1946). The effect appears to be one of diminution of apprehension, anxiety and concern about the pain, in the same way that these reactive and excessive emotional states are relieved in mental illness. The patient becomes relaxed and unconcerned, puts on weight and pain is no longer a preoccupation of the mind. Nevertheless to direct enquiry, it is clear that the pain is usually still present though no drugs may be needed to deaden it. A series of tests carried out by Elithorn *et al.* (1955) on patients before and after leucotomy showed that the autonomic responses, which were taken as criteria of anticipatory fear of a painful stimulus, were reduced, but there was no consistent elevation of threshold for pain. It has therefore been stated that leucotomy relieves the suffering though not the pain.

The great disadvantage of leucotomy is the degradation of personality which follows this operation; this may prove a major disaster in the family circle. Elithorn *et al.* (1958) studied in detail a series of patients in whom leucotomy had been performed for pain and came to the conclusion that in order to provide relief from the anguish of severe organic pain, some personality change is a necessary price. The advantages and otherwise of the variety of operations that have been designed to achieve leucotomy will be discussed in the chapter on psychosurgery.

The more limited brain lesions which are produced, for instance, by cingulotomy (Foltz & White 1962), inferior medial quadrant frontal section and unilateral frontal leucotomy (Scarff 1950) have proved helpful in diminishing suffering with fewer sequelae. The scope of these 'disconnecting' operations in the relief of pain, however, has always been a subject of dispute. The efforts of the pharmaceutical industry in designing psychotropic drugs, suitable for all occasions, have proved most successful and this, together with the threat of an unwanted change in personality, has meant that leucotomy for the relief of pain is now undertaken extremely rarely.

## The paroxysmal neuralgias

### Trigeminal neuralgia

Pain in the face may arise from a great variety of causes and may show diverse characteristics. The area of its distribution may be recognizably limited to the distributions of a major nerve trunk, or to one or more of its branches, or the pain may be of regional distribution, affecting an area without respect for nerve boundaries and involving other parts of the head and neck. At times it may be difficult to decide whether to classify the complaint as facial pain or as headache. The term neuralgia is restricted to a pain which conforms to the anatomical boundaries of the nerve, which is persistent or recurrent and maintains a fairly constant pattern. The term 'facial pain', by its imprecision, includes a regional as well as a nerve distribution. There would appear to be no justification for the use of the term 'atypical facial pain' when 'facial pain' is specific only to region and not to the character of the pain.

It has been usual to subdivide trigeminal neur-

algia into primary (idiopathic) and secondary (symptomatic) by virtue of the establishment of a demonstrable cause in the latter. Current therapy (to be described later in this chapter) challenges the validity of this classification. Until it is generally accepted that a demonstrable cause can always be found, subdivision along traditional lines will, however, continue to be used.

One of the various patterns of trigeminal pain stands out by reason of its constancy and ease of recognition: paroxysmal trigeminal neuralgia (synonyms: *tic douloureux*, trigeminal tic). This form of neuralgia has been recognized for centuries. Harris (1937) states that it was described by Avicenna 900 years ago and that the term *tic douloureux* was applied by Andre in 1756. The Shorter Oxford English Dictionary defines 'tic' as 'a disease or affection characterized by spasmodic twitching of certain muscles, especially of the face'. The contortion gives the expression of great pain. Treatment of this condition has, for the greater part of the twentieth century, been a major concern of neurosurgeons, in spite of its relative rarity. Olivecrona (1961) estimated that in Sweden it arises in about one of every 70,000 individuals.

*Clinical features*

1   The pain is strictly limited to the distribution of one or more branches of the trigeminal nerve.
2   The pain is sudden and short-lived, commonly lasting seconds or at the most a few minutes (hence 'paroxysmal').
3   It is frequently provoked by light mechanical stimuli within the trigeminal area, the so-called 'trigger-points'.
4   There is usually no detectable abnormality of function of the trigeminal nerve.

Of these characteristics 1 and 2 are considered essential, although it is now clear that when the pain is partially suppressed by Carbamazepine the normally brief flashing pains can be replaced by a more constant dull ache. The untreated pain is usually unbearably intense, even in the first attack which the patient experiences, though it becomes even worse in degree, in duration, in frequency and often more liable to spread to other branches of the same trigeminal nerve as the years pass. It is described as a 'red-hot needle', 'a shoot of pain', 'an electric shock'. It is evident that the sensation is one of pain and the patient often declares it worse than any previously endured. Its duration is brief and between attacks there is usually no pain. After many attacks or many years, the paroxysms may last longer, may comprise bouts of rapidly recurrent brief bursts; pain lasting several hours is atypical. Between severe paroxysms there may be a persistent dull ache in the area affected. Although the pain may start superficially, say in the gum or facial skin, its spread is usually deep so that the patient describes it as within the jaw or the tongue and spreading upwards into the temple or orbit. It is rarely described as residing in the skin. Diagnosis is aided if the effect of pain is witnessed: the patient is commonly immobilized though sometimes the features of the side affected are distorted; there may be suffusion of the skin and of the conjunctiva and tears may appear in the ipsilateral eye; the episode lasts for seconds or a minute or so, when the patient relaxes and continues the conversation. It is rare for the patient to press the hand to the face. In general the pain does not awaken the patient at night.

Frequently recurring bouts of pain may be followed by a remission of many months, but these periods of freedom gradually shorten.

The pain is entirely confined to the trigeminal territory and starts with fair consistency at one point, the entry of the 'stab'. In a detailed analysis of 650 cases, Henderson (1967) found this to be within the territory of the third division of the trigeminal nerve in 35%, of the second division in 36% and of the first division in 12%; the pain originated simultaneously in the upper and lower gums in only 12%. This conforms with the experience of Harris. Occasionally the site of onset may vary from one division to another; more usually the pattern is constant, or occasionally the paroxysm may involve all three trigeminal divisions. In about 5% of cases the neuralgia affects each side of the face, but apparently never simultaneously, so that each individual bout of pain remains strictly unilateral. The second side becomes affected usually after an interval of some years; in some three of the 32 bilateral cases of Henderson's series the interval was between 20 and 30 years and Harris records an interval of 37 years. Bilateral trigeminal neuralgia should suggest the probability of symptomatic tic due to multiple sclerosis.

*Precipitation of pain*

Lightly touching the skin, gum or mucosa in the majority of affected patients is likely to provoke the pain. So adequate a stimulus is this that some patients will immediately flinch if the examiner even begins to make the attempt to do this. The area, usually quite small, from which the pain is so easily and regularly triggered is commonly served by the same trigeminal division as that embracing the pain and it may coincide with the point of onset of pain. But not infrequently, the trigger area is in a separate division; it has occasionally been recorded remote from the trigeminal field.

It is entirely characteristic and probably of aetiological significance, though in what way is unknown, that light touch is more likely to provoke pain than heavier stimulus. Pain may be provoked by cold wind blowing on the face, and by any cause for startle. The sensitiveness of the trigger mechanism is often rendered evident to the examiner's eye by a small patch of unshaven skin, by the dirty greasy appearance of one side of the face owing to the total abstention from washing or by the failure to keep one side of the oral cavity clean. This is particularly clearly seen when the trigger area is on the tongue. Loss of weight may result from the inability to take food or to masticate it because of pain.

*Objective findings*

The finding of any neurological deficit within the trigeminal distribution, particularly if this should persist during remissions from the pain, suggests that the neuralgia is symptomatic of a progressive disease for which a search may then be appropriate. Usually no neurological deficit is found. However, one does encounter patients who suffer frequent paroxysms of great severity in whom slight degrees of objective sensory disturbance can be detected. Hyperaesthesia (distinct from the trigger area) is a more common finding, while slight sensory impairment is sometimes also seen. This most commonly takes the form of corneal insensitivity, but whether or not this merely reflects an age-related phenomenon rather than something specific to the condition, is unknown. Symptomatic or secondary trigeminal neuralgia can undoubtedly have the same clinical characteristics as those described as typical for primary, or idiopathic trigeminal neuralgia (Miles 1980). However, if the disease process, of which the pain is symptomatic, progresses, then the character of the pain will change to that of a more constant type and neurological deficit will become recognizable.

John Hunter realized that trigeminal neuralgia might erroneously be considered of dental origin and sound teeth removed because of it. He stated that the pain was 'entirely a nervous affliction' (Henderson 1965). It is still not uncommon to encounter patients who have had numerous dental extractions in an attempt to abolish the pain. Active, quiescent, or healed lesions of the jaws, paranasal sinuses and nasal cavities and of the anterior cranial fossa have been implicated. More commonly, however, it is the ganglion or the sensory root of the trigeminal system that has been the site of causative disease. This may be an intrinsic tumour (schwannoma) or adjacent epidermoid, meningioma, acoustic schwannoma, malignant disease of the base of skull, chordoma, aneurysm or invasive pituitary tumour. A very unusual form of symptomatic trigeminal neuralgia is seen in association with longstanding intracranial pressure, in which it is believed that herniation of brain through fenestrations in the dura of the floor of the middle fossa, in the vicinity of Meckel's cave, is responsible for the pain. Jefferson and Schorstein (1955) found persistent trigeminal pain to be an infrequent sequel to trauma and it usually took the form of a dysaesthesia. Paget disease of the base of the skull and even fibrous dysplasia can, presumably by stenotic compression, precipitate trigeminal pain.

Rapidly spreading numbness associated with pain has been described, but its cause not determined (Harris 1935, Hughes 1958, Spillane & Wells 1959). Trigeminal pain associated with herpes zoster will be described in more detail later. Evidence of disseminated (multiple) sclerosis is found in an appreciable proportion of patients with paroxysmal trigeminal neuralgia, estimated by White and Sweet (1960) to be 1.7%. They have also estimated the incidence of trigeminal neuralgia in patients with disseminated sclerosis to be 1%.

## Idiopathic trigeminal neuralgia

The implication of this label has been that, in addition to the classical clinical picture of *tic douloureux* and with absence of neurological deficit, this form of trigeminal neuralgia has no obvious cause. However, as early as 1934, Dandy challenged its occult nature and by posterior fossa exploration in 215 cases described unequivocal pathology in the vicinity of the sensory root in 10%, a suspect physical contact usually by an artery, in a further 30% and various other suspect structures, such as veins and adhesions bringing the total percentage of suspected structural abnormality up to 60%. After many years of disbelief, Jannetta has rekindled the general interest in structural abnormality as the basis for trigeminal neuralgia, usually by compression at the trigeminal root entry zone in the posterior fossa. In 100 consecutive patients explored for *tic douloureux* using the operating microscope he described some form of physical cause in all (Jannetta

1976). The most common finding was indentation or distortion of the trigeminal root zone at its point of entry into the brain stem by a loop of the superior cerebellar, the anterior inferior cerebellar or the basilar artery or occasionally other vessels.

Electron microscopic studies of the trigeminal ganglion have shown some degenerative changes in nerve fibre and ganglion cells (Beaver 1967, Kerr 1967) similar to, but much more marked than those found in 'normal' controls (Moses 1967). Kerr stated that the myelin changes were unlike any reported in other disease states. The significance of these findings is uncertain, but proof of pathological changes in this distressing disorder is, of itself, important.

## Treatment

While all known analgesics, including morphine, have been used to suppress this most severe pain, it was only when King (1958) showed that anticonvulsants such as sodium hydantoinate reduced the triggered responses in certain experimental models of trigeminal neuralgia, that effective progress began. Carbamazepine (Tegretol), another anticonvulsant, has proved so effective in suppressing the pain as to almost constitute a diagnostic test of trigeminal neuralgia. Relief, particularly in the early stage of the condition, is prompt, often total, and its use may only need to be periodic, taking advantage of the natural remissions that occur at this early stage. However, there is no doubt that with time and more frequent episodes of pain, the quantitative relief of pain reduces, in spite of increasing dosage (up to a gram a day), and with this increase in dosage the unwanted neurotropic effects of ataxia, dizziness, mental blunting and even frank sedation, appear. There is no doubt as to the usefulness of carbamazepine in relieving the acute pain and in managing the, sometimes, extremely elderly or infirm patient with trigeminal neuralgia, but there are many who would suggest that longterm exposure to this powerful drug is perhaps less satisfactory than

a surgical attempt to suppress the pain, either permanently or for a long period, by one of the invasive techniques to be described later. There are no figures to indicate the number of patients with idiopathic trigeminal neuralgia who remain satisfactorily relieved of pain by longterm carbamazepine, to compare with the number who eventually come to more definitive procedures.

Interventional methods tend to be directed either to destruction of some part of the trigeminal sensory system or to decompression of the sensory root in the posterior fossa, along the lines advocated by Dandy (1927).

### Interruption of trigeminal sensory pathways

One of the major dilemmas in the understanding of trigeminal neuralgia is the equal facility with which destructive procedures of either the peripheral nerve or its central connections may relieve the pain. Peripheral procedures have the advantage of ease of technique and expediency, not to be forgotten in the debilitated elderly patients with such severe pain that they cannot eat, but also carry the disadvantage of inevitable return of pain and sensation usually from 3 to 6 months later. Destruction of the ganglion provides a more uncertain period of relief, perhaps due to the anatomical considerations to be detailed later. Destruction of the sensory root often provides permanent pain relief, which usually correlates with the totality of this destruction. Destruction to central connections, trigeminal tract, nucleus or thalamus is more erratic, and often short lived in its effect.

### Neurolytic injection

The injection of absolute alcohol into a peripheral nerve has the advantages mentioned above. This procedure can be performed to the supraorbital nerve in its foramen, the infraorbital nerve in its foramen or, more rarely, to the mental nerve at its foramen. The mandibular division can be reached without much difficulty as it exists from the base of skull.

By passing a needle through the foramen ovale under radiographic control it is possible to enter and inject the Gasserian ganglion or its sensory root in Meckel's cave. The earliest injections of the trigeminal ganglion were performed by Harris in 1910 (Harris 1912), by Taptas (1911) and Hartel (around 1912). As neurosurgical techniques have improved so alcohol injections have become less popular (Penman 1949).

Henderson (1965) made a detailed study of the anatomy of the ganglion, its branches and its sensory root with the aim of explaining some of the anomalous results of alcohol injection. The paper deserves careful attention for it appears to be a unique study. Important points are the variations in length of the three primary divisions and of the sensory root of the trigeminal nerve, so that one can regard the ganglion as having pre- and postfixed positions; these will affect the depth beyond the foramen ovale to which the needle must be thrust in order to reach the ganglion. The ganglion measures some 4–5 mm in width, 2–4 mm in thickness and 15–25 mm in length, that is, in its semilunar diameter, mediolaterally. Consequent upon its narrowness and thinness, an injection into its substance almost invariably breaks through into Meckel's cave where the injected medium will bathe the sensory root fibres. Thus a 'ganglion' injection is probably a misnomer and total trigeminal denervation is probably always due to a root lesion. This is in keeping with the work of Penman and Smith (1950) who examined material from a patient dying from a lung cancer some months after a ganglion injection for *tic douloureux* which resulted in total trigeminal analgesia. Histological examination revealed extensive destruction of the sensory root fibres whereas in the Gasserian ganglion there was 'no extensive loss of neurons'. Their examination also showed degeneration of the primary pathways in the pons, of the pontine and spinal nuclei and of the secondary trigeminal neurons, the quinto- or bulbothalamic tract. Henderson ascribed return of sensation, following what was

supposedly an injection into the ganglion, to escape of alcohol around the divisions, the tip of the needle having failed to reach the ganglion. This escape of injected alcohol is aided by the frequent presence of a small emissary vein which connects medially with the cavernous sinus and pterygoid plexus (Henderson 1966).

Two routes are available in order to traverse the foramen ovale for injecting the ganglion or its sensory root. The lateral route was simultaneously introduced by Harris in 1910 (Harris 1912, 1937) and Taptas (1911). The needle is inserted into the skin of the cheek below the middle of the zygomatic arch and advanced so that it passes over the sigmoid notch of the mandible in an obliquely ascending direction to enter the foramen approximately in the coronal plane. In successful cases the point will traverse the ganglion from lateral to medial boundaries and theoretically permits differential destruction: in practice the results seem to confirm this desirable quality, since sparing of ophthalmic sensation renders the likelihood of keratitis remote. Irger (1930) also describes a lateral approach. The anterior approach was described by Hartel (1912) in a well illustrated paper. The needle is inserted into the cheek just above and lateral to the angle of the mouth and directed upwards, medially and backwards, aiming at a point posterior to the pupil in the mid zygomatic plane (tubercle of zygoma). The foramen ovale lies with its long axis directed forwards and consequently more in the axis of the needle introduced by the anterior approach; thus it is more easily traversed, though the point of the needle tends to pass through the narrow width of the ganglion and to enter Meckel's cave. The foramen is in fact shaped more like a canal with its central axis directed laterally to varying degrees.

Early operators used free-hand penetration. Kirschner (1933) mentions radiological assistance and Penman (1949) strongly advocated it. Radiographic screening, or a series of still pictures, is now the usual practice and undoubtedly minimizes the anguish of this otherwise sometimes stressful procedure, undertaken largely under local anaesthesia (Delfino 1983).

Various neurolytic materials have been used, of which alcohol has been most universal, with attempts made to contain its injection to the ganglion or divisions and to minimize leakage into the subarachnoid space. Phenol in glycerine was introduced by Jefferson (1963) and is still preferred (1966). With the patient in the sitting position and the needle almost vertical, the hyperbaric solution is injected into Meckel's cave. More recently Hakansson (1981), described the use of glycerol to achieve the same effect. This interesting technique involved temporary exposure of the sensory root to the neurolytic substance which was then withdrawn. This is somewhat different from other techniques in providing gradual relief of pain with minimal or no neurological deficit. As with all other methods advocated over the years, only prolonged follow-up data will determine whether pain relief proves as satisfactory in the longterm as in the immediate effect.

### Percutaneous coagulation

Kirschner (1931, 1933) introduced electrocoagulation of the Gasserian ganglion, but until recently the method gained only limited support because of the high incidence of complications. White and Sweet (1969) modified the technique so that (1) electrical stimulation allows localization of the electrode tip to the particular fibres subserving the area of pain, and (2) temperature recognition and therefore control, so as to limit the spread of heat coagulation and thereby to minimize the former complications of unwanted cranial nerve palsies. Temperature control also allows for differential fibre destruction with some preservation of light touch, a most invaluable asset in those patients suffering first division trigeminal neuralgia (Sweet & Wepsic 1974).

The recurrence rate following this technique is of the order of 20–25% in the first five years (Miles 1980). The recurrences of pain following trigeminal neurolytic injection for similar periods of follow-up were around 30%, as described by

Harris (1940) from a series of 1,433 patients of whom 457 could be traced. Stender (1961) reported a 24% recurrence of the same form of pain while only 53% of patients were ever totally painfree.

### Open surgical operation

A great number of open procedures have been used. All can relieve pain, but with varying ease and risk, and the duration of pain relief tends to parallel the amount of sensory deficit following the procedure. The earliest operation consisted of division of the extracranial branches, causing relief of pain for several months. John Lizars of Edinburgh (1787–1860) divided the mandibular nerve in the infratemporal fossa on 15 March 1821. Rose (1890) avulsed part of the Gasserian ganglion after excising the maxilla and enlarging the foramen ovale. Horsley made a pioneering attempt on the sensory root of the ganglion 'I thought one might be able to remove the Gasserian ganglion or divide the fifth nerve behind it' (Horsley et al. 1891). He made some dissections and came to the conclusion that its intimate connection to the cavernous sinus would render complete removal of the ganglion impracticable. On 11 December 1890 he operated on a physically frail patient and through a temporal craniectomy incised the dura mater, elevated the temporal lobe, opened the roof of Meckel's cave and avulsed the root. Unfortunately, the patient died some hours later, probably from shock, for post-mortem examination revealed no compression of haematoma. Cushing (1900) reported four cases of total extirpation of the ganglion without a death. He performed 30 procedures on cadavers in order to familiarize himself with the various steps prior to performing it on patients.

Spiller and Frazier (1901) recorded the first case of successful division of the sensory root of the Gasserian ganglion. Later, Frazier refined the operation by preserving the fibres destined for the ophthalmic division and by avoiding damage to the motor root. In 1928 he was able to report on 500 cases and his operation was accepted as a standard procedure in neurosurgery. This procedure was undertaken through a temporal craniectomy and extradural approach along the floor of the middle cranial fossa with incision of the infralateral dura of Meckel's cave and thus exposure of the sensory root and ganglion.

An intradural approach, very similar to that undertaken by Horsley, was introduced in 1938 by Wilkins (1966) in order to avoid traction damage to the greater superficial petrosal nerve and the resultant dry eye and risk of ulceration that was a feature of the extradural technique. The comparative values and risks of the two procedures have been studied by Pennybacker (1961). Facial paralysis occurred in 1.8% after the intradural approach compared with 11% after an extradural approach. Likewise keratitis occurred in 5% of cases following intradural exploration compared with 42% of cases after extradural exposure.

The sensory root can also be divided as it lies in the cerebellar pontine angle through a small unilateral suboccipital craniectomy. This method was initiated by Dandy (1929) for three reasons. One was on the presumption that there might be a local causative lesion, such as a tumour. The second was to avoid facial paralysis, while the third was on the logic that division of the lateral part of the sensory root close to the pons resulted in dissociated relative analgesia over the whole of the trigeminal field with preservation of some light touch and lessened postoperative incidence of unpleasant dysaesthesia.

Dandy (1932) considered that as the sensory fibres coursed towards the pons a rearrangement took place, so that those concerned with pain were grouped in its lateral border, while those associated with light touch often constituted a separate root or roots superomedially, and if preserved allowed a degree of preservation of light touch sensation throughout the face. Olivecrona (1947), in describing that little sensory loss could be detected if only the lateral half of the root was cut, tended to support Dandy's contention. Sjöqvist (1938) found no segregation of fine

diameter fibres in the lateral aspect of the root. Jannetta (1967) concluded that there was support for the presence of 'accessory' sensory fibres as described by Dandy (1932) lying between the motor and sensory roots near the pons.

An early disadvantage of the posterior fossa approach appeared to be the increased risk of this procedure under the surgical conditions of that time. Olivecrona (1947) described a comparison of mortality following the Frazier operation of 0.4%, compared with that after the Dandy operation of 3.3%. Dandy himself described no death in 150 consecutive posterior fossa explorations for trigeminal neuralgia (1932). The vast improvement in anaesthetic techniques and the consequent ease of access to the posterior fossa together with the considerable safety afforded by the use of the operating microscope and the advanced instrumentation for use with the microscope have greatly reduced the surgical hazard of this approach, but it does remain greater than that for most percutaneous techniques. There remains, however, the considerable advantage to be gained by correcting causative pathology.

*Trigeminal sensory root decompression*

Few supported Dandy in his surety that a cause for trigeminal neuralgia could often be found in the posterior fossa in the form of contact with or compression of the sensory root (1934) but recent advocates have described even higher proportions of such pathology (Jannetta 1976). The duration of pain relief following such procedures again, has yet to be defined. It is now known that pain relief can persist for many years, but whether this will be in the majority of cases or not has yet to be established.

It would seem reasonable to approach the problem of trigeminal neuralgia with the knowledge that a range of techniques are available and that no single technique may be optimal for all cases. Where there may be a suggestion of a disease process with perhaps local or distant neurological symptom or sign then thorough investigation of this by computerized tomography or nuclear magnetic resonance scanning may indicate a line of treatment specific to the disease process. In the relatively young and fit patient there would seem to be considerable encouragement toward recommending posterior fossa exploration with a view to excluding pathology such as tumour and affording relief from pain by its removal, or by decompression of the nerve from surrounding structures such as loops of the superior cerebellar artery. In the old or infirm patient there would seem to be good justification for employing a less invasive technique. The appropriateness of any specific percutaneous technique will be determined by the experience of the particular surgeon. At present percutaneous, temperature controlled, radiofrequency coagulation of the sensory root is the most popular procedure, but percutaneous neurolytic injection of alcohol, phenol or glycerol can be equally effective.

*Trigeminal tractotomy*

In the preface of his monograph, *Studies on Pain Conduction in the Trigeminal Nerve*, Sjöqvist (1938) explains that these anatomical studies were undertaken to determine 'the distribution of pain conducting fibres of the sensory trigeminal root'. They led him to examine the bulbospinal tract and finally to a new operation for the relief of facial pain. He concluded that fibres transmitting impulses concerned with pain sensibility from the entire trigeminal distribution were assembled in the bulbospinal tract, descending to the medulla and upper cervical segments and terminating in the spinal sensory trigeminal nucleus. This nucleus is continuous with the substantia gelatinosa of the posterior horn, reaching as low as the second cervical segment. Rostrally, it is continuous with the main trigeminal sensory nucleus. These findings were in keeping with clinical observations of cases of infarction in this area. Later observations on patients who had had division of the descending

spinal tract led to the assumption that the fibres of the tract terminated in reverse order of their distribution on the face, the ophthalmic fibres most caudally, the maxillary and the mandibular division successively at higher levels. However, these opinions are not totally accepted. Many would suggest that the only topographical arrangement is in a plane transverse to the long axis of the medulla and spinal cord with the ophthalmic fibres lying ventrally to the maxillary and then mandibular fibres. Kunc (1961, 1966) concluded that all three divisions terminated at all levels of the spinal nucleus, but he found that fibres from the peripheral part of the trigeminal field appeared to descend the lowest, while those from the central (around the mouth and tip of the nose) terminated more rostrally. This would be in keeping with the onion-skin pattern of trigeminal analgesia which is said to characterize certain central lesions of the medulla oblongata and spinal cord (Dejerine 1914). Brodal (1969) provides a worthwhile review of this complex matter.

The spinal trigeminal tract (syn. bulbospinal, descending trigeminal) lies superficial in the medulla, accessible to the surgeon at the level of the middle and lower one third of the inferior olive and remains superficial for the rest of its course.

It lies splayed over the spinal nucleus, which forms a prominence, the tuberculum cinereum; this may aid in identifying the site of the tract. The tract is bounded dorsally by the cuneate nucleus and fasciculus, and ventrally by the plane of the emerging fibres of the vagus nerve, and ventral to this plane by the spinothalamic fibres. Rostral to this position the tract is buried under the inferior and middle cerebellar peduncles.

Sjöqvist first performed his operation for sectioning this tract on 10 May, 1937; later experience caused him to recommend that the incision should be made at the level of the most caudal rootlet of the vagus, 3 mm deep and extending 3–4 mm dorsally. He felt that this level was at the junction of the middle and lower one thirds of the olive which is about 8–10 mm rostral to the inferior limit of the fourth ventricle (the obex). Because of the high incidence of complications of ataxia, impairment of position sense and two point discrimination, Grant and Weinberger (1941) recommended a lower incision, 5 mm caudal to the level of the obex and claimed they still obtained analgesia in all divisions. Imperfect knowledge of divisional representation in the tract, together with the high incidence of complications, particularly dysaesthetic, led to different recommended sites for sectioning and also intraoperative localizing tests (Falconer 1949, Kunc 1961, 1964) by which the patient (under local anaesthetic) indicates the site of sensation on the face that results from sharp needle pricking of the surface of the exposed medulla. Further details on the anatomical debate are to be found in White and Sweet (1969, p. 241), McKenzie (1955) and Truex and Carpenter (1969).

Stereotactic approaches to destruction of the descending trigeminal tract in the spinal cord have also been designed (Hitchcock & Schvarcz 1972) but the same problems of anatomical localization and neurological complications obtain, and these operative approaches have found progressively less favour in the management of trigeminal neuralgia.

## Results

Table 18.3 contains a selection of results from the extensive literature on the subject of treatment of trigeminal neuralgia. Northfield (1961) reviewed in detail 272 patients operated on by various forms of rhizotomy, with follow-up observations available on 221. There was a case mortality of 3.7% and an operational mortality of 3.1%. After the primary fractional rhizotomy

**Table 18.3.** Results of treatment of paroxysmal trigeminal neuralgia.

| Reference | Freedom from original pain (%) | Mortality (%) | Ophthalmic complications (%) | Paraesthesiae (%) | Anaesthesia dolorosa (%) | Facial palsy (%) |
|---|---|---|---|---|---|---|
| Injection | | | | | | |
| Jefferson (1966) | 72 up to 4 years | — | — | — | — | — |
| Henderson (1967) | 65 for 1 to 17 years | — | 19 | — | — | — |
| Hakansson (1981) | 86 for $1\frac{1}{2}$ years | — | — | — | — | — |
| Electrocoagulation | | | | | | |
| Schurmann & Butz (1968) | 98 up to 5 years | — | 0 | — | — | — |
| Sweet (1976) | 72 | 0 | 5 | — | 1.2 | 0 |
| Compression, neurolysis and similar operations | | | | | | |
| Taarnhoj (1961) | 60 | 0.5 | — | 5 | — | — |
| Rhizotomy—temporal | | | | | | |
| Olivecrona (1947) | 91 | 0.4 | 1.3 | 11.0 | 3.0 | 11.0 |
| Pennybacker (1961) | 96 | 1.4 | 6.0 | — | 2.0 | 5.0 |
| Rhizotomy—suboccipital | | | | | | |
| Olivecrona (1947) | 82 | 3.3 | 2.0 | 3.2 | 0 | 0 |
| Walker et al. (1966) | 80 | 2.0 | 0.0 | 27.0 | — | — |
| Decompression suboccipital | | | | | | |
| Jannetta (1976) | 95 | 1 | — | — | — | — |

Bulbospinal tractotomy
  derived from the analysis by White & Sweet of published series
  Recurrent pain (%): mild 24, severe 14. Mortality 1.7.
  Paraesthesiae: mild 24, severe 0.5.

there was a recurrence of pain in 50%, while after primary total rhizotomy the recurrence rate was 34%; after secondary total rhizotomy the recurrence was 61% and after tertiary total rhizotomy 50%. With this high incidence of recurrence Northfield emphasized that in only three patients was the continuing pain similar to that of the original. More common was a form of anaesthesia dolorosa. Miles (1980) describes a comparative series from the Centre for Pain Relief, Walton Hospital, Liverpool with details on recurrence rates and complications indicating the high recurrence rate to be expected after neurolytic injection, even of the ganglion, the high morbidity particularly to trigeminal function after surgical root section, and the superiority of radiofrequency coagulation in respect of recurrence and morbidity. However, radiofrequency coagulation is not the complete answer to the problem of treating trigeminal neuralgia in respect of either duration of relief or freedom from complications.

## Complications and sequelae

### Ophthalmic

All methods of treating trigeminal neuralgia associated with any degree of denervation of the ophthalmic division may lead to keratitis and even ulceration. Particular care must be taken when the vision of the contralateral eye has become impaired or lost for some reason. Selection of the operation for such an instance might have posterior fossa decompression as the preferred procedure, with glycerol instillation or radiofrequency coagulation as the next choice.

If the corneal reflex is found to be absent, precautions should be taken, involving at the least a transparent cover to the eye and tarsorrhaphy if the ophthalmic divisional loss is profound. Rhizotomy procedures associated with loss of lacrimation are particularly threatening in this respect.

Ocular palsies, of which an abducent nerve palsy is the most common, usually relate to spread of neurolytic fluid either in the subarachnoid space or in the layers of dura. With temperature control, coagulation techniques are unlikely to cause this.

Facial paralysis was not uncommon with procedures for sensory root section, by the extradural (Frazier) approach (Pennybacker 1961) but are extremely rare with any of the preferred current procedures. Dysaesthesiae seem to accompany all techniques save (to date) that of posterior fossa microsurgical decompression. The common incidence for this complication following surgical section of the root has been around 4%; Sweet (1976) compiled figures from many different series of radiofrequency electrocoagulation when the most common incidence was around 2%. In many series there has been a tendency to separate dysaesthesiae into painful or uncomfortable dysaesthesiae and 'simple' dysaesthesiae. In another series there has been a tendency to have some kind of separate category between recurrence of the original kind of pain and that of anaesthesia dolorosa and whether this is a 'simple' or painful dysaesthesia is impossible to determine. Miles (1980) noted on retrospective scrutiny, the tendency for the original pain to be not typical of trigeminal neuralgia in patients who later developed anaesthesia dolorosa, after various destructive techniques.

Anaesthesia dolorosa is a syndrome of poorly localized pain, sometimes described as burning, but more often in less well identified terms, such as 'like worms under the skin', and is usually within the trigeminal distribution, but can overlap onto the neck. It is usually associated with a redness and often a coarsening of the skin or puffiness. It is rarely present immediately after the destructive lesion, but gradually builds up, from quite innocuous-sounding paraesthesiae to a full blown picture, over months. It is commonly associated with psychiatric overtones, particularly depression. Additional destructive techniques are not to be recommended. Psychotropic medication particularly in the form of antidepressant therapy is commonly useful; the current drug of choice is probably Clonazepam (Rivotril). In addition to its tranquillizing effect it would appear to be specifically useful for facial pain. Electrical stimulator implant in the somato-sensory pathways, at the thalamic level, has also proved useful in the short-term at least (Hoso-buchi *et al.* 1973).

## Nasal ulceration

This is an infrequent sequel. Ulceration of the skin usually begins on or close to the nares and gradually expands over the cheek, always in an area of anaesthesia. Schorstein (1943) described in detail eight examples with illustrations. It is not uncommon for some form of sensation akin to dysaesthesia to be present in the vicinity of the ulceration and it is likely that self mutilation occurs as a result of unconscious scratching.

Herpes simplex affecting the lips is a common event after procedures on the trigeminal path-ways at peripheral nerve ganglion and sensory root level, but has also been seen following stimu-lation of VPM, the thalamic relay area for facial sensation (Miles, personal observation).

## Selection of treatment

It is clear from the foregoing that no single form of treatment is likely to be optimal for all patients suffering trigeminal neuralgia. Where there may be a hint from the clinical picture, either by the painful symptoms not conforming to the classical as previously described, or when neurological deficit is recognized either within the territory of the trigeminal nerve or elsewhere, a search for a causative disease process is necessary. This should include computerized tomography and, if an intrinsic lesion of the brain stem is to be excluded, nuclear magnetic resonance imaging. Vertebrobasilar angiography may also be con-sidered necessary, but this may be considered an unjustified risk in the main group of patients presenting with trigeminal neuralgia, who will be very old and often very infirm. In the younger and fit person there now seems to be every indi-cation for posterior fossa exploration with the

hope of curing the disease process or at least of relieving pain by decompression of the nerve root without neurological deficit. In the older or infirm patient less invasive investigation and treatment may be indicated and efforts directed merely towards relieving the pain rather than coagulation or curing the disease process. Per-cutaneous radiofrequency coagulation or gly-cerol instillation may be preferred. If there is doubt as to the categorization of the pain, for instance whether it is glossopharyngeal or tri-geminal neuralgia, there is still a place for local anaesthetic blockade. Test neurolysis by alcohol injection as practised by Northfield and Cairns (Northfield 1973) is probably no longer justified.

## Geniculate neuralgia

Intense attacks of pain may occur in the somatosensory distribution of other cranial nerves, but are rare as compared with the fre-quency of *tic douloureux;* like that disorder, they are distinguished by an absence of neurological deficit although similar pain may be caused by tumours. Geniculate neuralgia was described by Hunt (1907, 1937) who, from a study of the eruption when herpes zoster affects this ganglion predicted a cutaneous distribution to the external meatus.

The first case of geniculate neuralgia to be treated by operation was reported by Clark and Taylor (1909). The pain was immediately in front of the external auditory meatus, in the anterior wall and in its depths; at first in brief stabs, it later became continuous and was pre-cipitated by placing a finger in the meatus. It was totally abolished by intracranial division of the nervus intermedius, the facial nerve and part of the auditory nerve; a remarkable feat for that time. White and Sweet (1969) list details of nine published cases, in each of which the pain was centred in the ear, either deeply or in the external auditory meatus with a varying degree of spread to the neighbouring structures. A trigger area was detected in only two. In some the pains were brief and paroxysmal, while in others more continuous, even for hours. In all but one the pain was eventually abolished by division of the nervus intermedius. In the exception, the pain was cured by a later bulbar tractomy, although this was followed by burning dysaesthesiae. With the advent of microsurgical approach to the cerebellar pontine angle, section of nervus intermedius is not difficult, even though in its position between the 7th and 8th nerves, great care is required and even though it commonly adopts a plexiform nature, it is usually clearly seen and can be safely divided.

*Glossopharyngeal neuralgia*

This was first described by Sicard and Robineau (1920) who treated three patients successfully by extracranial division of the glossopharyngeal nerve, branches from the vagus and the cervical sympathetic area. Harris (1921) described cases and named the condition; Weisenberg (1910) drew attention to the distribution of pain sometime earlier and in his case the cause was a cerebellar pontine angle tumour. White and Sweet (1969) briefly list information concerning 275 published cases and include those in which the pain is primarily in the larynx. Because of the accepted overlap in the distribution of glossopharyngeal and vagus sensory fibres they prefer the term vagoglossopharyngeal neuralgia. The pain may start anywhere in these territories, but tonsil, root of tongue and ear are favourite sites. It is often precipitated by the act of swallowing and examination may reveal a trigger zone in the pharyngeal area. If anaesthetizing this locally renders the patient painless, the diagnosis is established. Diagnostic blockade of the trigeminal mandibular nerve may be necessary to differentiate between trigeminal neuralgia in that nerve territory and glossopharyngeal neuralgia. The pain may be lancinating or continuous and the syndrome as a whole is much less discrete than trigeminal neuralgia. Curious associated disturbances have been described; uncontrolled coughing, a feeling of cramp or obstruction of the throat and cardiac symptoms.

The usual manifestations of the latter can be dramatic and frightening and include asystole, syncope and even convulsions. Such syndromes are well described in association with infiltrating cancer in the neck with presumed involvement of the extracranial glossopharyngeal nerve (Patel *et al.* 1979). Cardiac phenomena are presumably effected by a mechanism similar to stimulation of the carotid sinus. White and Sweet (1969) discuss this problem in detail.

Dandy (1927) reported two successful intracranial sections of the glossopharyngeal nerve and thereafter this approach superseded the extracranial. It is now usual to section the upper part of the vagal rootlets at the same time as sectioning the 9th nerve.

Percutaneous radiofrequency coagulation with insertion of the electrode through the neurogenic notch (pars nervosa) has been undertaken and has proved successful, both for idiopathic glossopharyngeal neuralgia and that associated with infiltrating malignancy (Broggi & Siegfried 1979).

Medullary tractotomy has also been employed for glossopharyngeal pain by Kunc (1966), who had become convinced that there was a specific bundle between the cuneate fasciculus, and the dorsomedial margin of the spinal root of the trigeminal nerve. This operative approach is now rarely, if ever, used.

*Relief of pain due to head and neck malignancies*

It will be clear that surgical section of the primary sensory pathways of the 5th, 7th, 9th and 10th cranial nerves is applicable to the relief of pain from invasive neoplasms of the head and, if extended to the upper cervical roots, to those involving the neck also. As ulceration and secondary infection is a common association with such tumours the risks of open operative section via the posterior fossa, even using modern microsurgical techniques, must be significant. Percutaneous radiofrequency coagulation of the trigeminal and glossopharyngeal and upper vagal fibres can be very effective as long as the tumour does not obstruct the access for the needle (Broggi & Siegfried 1979). However, there can be a marked discrepancy between nerve territories and infiltration by the tumour might well mean incomplete relief of pain by nerve destruction. There is much to be said for preferring medial thalamotomy to multiple attempts at root section. The duration of effect in relieving pain by each of these procedures is likely to be similar and of the order of six months.

### Non-destructive surgery for the relief of pain: electrical stimulation

The importance of whether or not a pain is due to an uncontrolled malignant process with the obligatory limitation in capacity and life expectancy, has been emphasized earlier in this chapter. Although destructive techniques directed to the central nervous system might prove effective in relieving some benign persistent pain such as phantom limb pain or thalamic pain syndrome, they are usually not appropriate by virtue of the limited period over which they effectively relieve pain, and the incrementally more troublesome neurological morbidity that results from repeated destruction.

As a result, many widely differing, non-destructive, methods of suppressing pain have been explored. These have included the psychological, such as psychotherapy, hypnosis, meditation and biofeedback; the ill understood, such as acupuncture; the mechanical such as physical rehabilitation and combining many of these with behavioural therapy, the holistic approach. These techniques are clearly outside the remit of this book, but electrical stimulation is one other approach that can be made to the problem of benign persistent pain.

### Transcutaneous Neural Stimulation (TNS)

Melzack and Wall (1962, 1965) proposed that incoming traffic in the small C and A delta fibres, entering the spinal cord could be suppressed by 'competing' traffic entering via larger fibres. This formed the basis of the Gate Control Theory and helped explain why vibration and friction applied to a limb can appear to ease pain in the same member.

Externally applied electrical stimulation has been used extensively for many years and undoubtedly has a place in controlling benign persistent pain, albeit only a small proportion. It is sufficiently effective to be used over the long-term (Long 1974). When the site of pain is too extensive or bilateral, then it becomes impracticable to maintain surface contact sufficient to achieve effective TNS and stimulation to the central nervous system becomes necessary.

### Dorsal column stimulation

It was quickly recognized that while the Gate Control Theory was derived from experimental peripheral nerve stimulation, it could equally well apply to stimulation of the spinal cord when the same effect was achieved antidromically by stimulation of the posterior column of the spinal cord. Shealy et al. (1967) and Nashold and Friedman (1972) reported the effectiveness of dorsal column stimulation in relieving pain.

In order to provide for longterm, repeated or continuous stimulation of the spinal cord an implanted circuit was necessary and the design and engineering necessary for this was initiated by William Sweet and the manufacturer Roger Avery, in Boston in the mid 1960s. The original circuits were 'dead', being activated by an external transmitter or induction source. (Fig. 18.4.)

The systems have now become more complex and some have their own power sources, in a manner similar to those used in cardiac pacemakers. The early electrode implantations were made without attempt at selection, save that the patient had suffered pain of a chronicity of at least six months. Initial results clearly revealed that spinal cord stimulation did not relieve all pain (Miles et al. 1974) and that assessment protocols were necessary in order to predict favourable responses and minimize failures

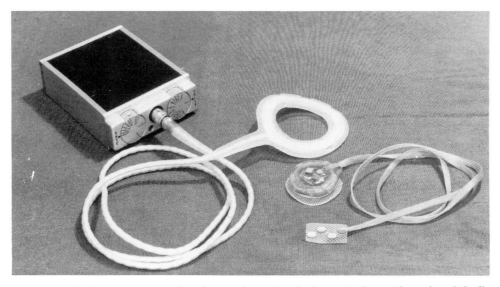

**Fig. 18.4.** Radiotelemetric equipment for achieving chronic dorsal column stimulation. The implanted 'dead' circuit is on the right and the external transmitter on the left.

(Miles 1984a). A period of preliminary percutaneous spinal cord stimulation proved to be an important part of any assessment protocol (Hosobuchi *et al.* 1972). The immediate enthusiasm for this technique has been tempered by the unsatisfactory results of poor selection and also by the less exciting experience of needing to modify and repair the implants when therapeutic effect has deteriorated. Such deterioration can be related to biological factors and involves an increased threshold to stimulation or to more mechanical factors, such as electrode movement or implant material failures. There is no doubt that in spite of the accepted reduction in effect with time (Kranick & Toden 1984) worthwhile pain relief can be obtained in many examples of benign persistent pain and without harm to the nervous system.

It is currently more common to perform the implantation as a two-stage procedure with the addition of a receiver system or power pack, to the preliminary percutaneous electrode, after the pain relieving effect has been established. The alternative is that of two completely separate stages, the first of which is the percutaneous

trial, which if effective is followed by an open surgical implantation. There are advantages and disadvantages to each of these methods (Miles 1984a).

The way in which electrical stimulation relieves pain is not established. Although minor neurological deficits presumably related to myelopathic electrical blockade, has been noted (Lindblom & Meyerson 1975), it has not been a regular observation and there is no noted permanent dysfunction. When successful the pain relief is almost instantaneous with the production of paraesthesiae in the area concerned; although in some patients the effect ceases immediately stimulation is stopped, more often, the pain relief extends long after the cessation of stimulation, even for days. Attempts to correlate the stimulation pain relief with neurochemical changes have largely failed. All that seems sure, is that to be effective the projection paraesthesiae must cover the area of pain, mix in with the pain syndrome and, best of all, appear pleasant in character, that is, a pleasurable substitute for the pain.

## Deep Brain Stimulation (DBS)

For benign persistent pains high in the body, such as in the head and neck, stimulation of the somatosensory pathways can be undertaken within the brain; favourite sites are in the medial lemniscus, in the ventral lateral thalamus (VL) and in the internal capsule. Mazars *et al.* (1974) have practised such stimulation with apparently remarkable efficiency since the early 60s. Similarly Fairman (1976) had apparently long-standing success in the field of thalamic and hypothalamic brain stimulation. Again such chronic and repeated stimulation requires an implanted circuit with the electrode being inserted using stereotaxic guidance. A trial period of percutaneous stimulation is usually employed before the electrode is converted to a permanent implant by the addition of a receiver system, usually placed subcutaneously on the anterior chest wall, at a second operation.

The resulting pain relief from such stimulation appears to vary greatly. Siegfried (1982) obtained excellent relief of pain in de-afferentation pain syndromes, though these results have not been shared by others (Miles 1984a).

A different form of DBS has evolved from the experimental animal studies into electrical anaesthesia carried out by Reynolds (1969). He illustrated that it was possible to perform surgical procedures on rats during chronic stimulation of the deep central grey matter around the aqueduct of the mid brain. Heath and Mickle (1960) had already studied anterior and presumably hypothalamic (septal) stimulation in an attempt to reduce various forms of suffering both psychological and associated with malignancy. It was Richardson and Akil (1977) who combined the knowledge of both these forms of stimulation and implanted chronic deep brain electrodes to the junction of the peri-aqueductal and paraventricular grey matter of patients and achieved significant pain relief, but of a different form from that associated with stimulation of the deep brain somatosensory pathways. This form of stimulation provokes no paraesthesiae, but instead produces a gradual relief of pain, often taking 20

minutes to achieve and usually associated with a prolonged poststimulation analgesic effect. This form of pain relief has been reported to be associated with recognizable neuropeptide changes in the CSF involving release of beta-endorphin (Hosobuchi *et al.* 1979). It has also proved possible, partially to reverse this form of stimulation analgesia by the use of Naloxone, an opiate antagonist. These facts clearly seem to implicate chemical generation as a result of the stimulation and coincided with the important discoveries of endogenous opioids in the deep brain structures by Hughes *et al.* (1975). Again, however, this technique has not proved applicable to all forms of pain and suffers, even more than dorsal column stimulation, because of problems of patient selection. To date, the only sure method of knowing whether DBS will relieve pain is by trial implantation using stereotaxic surgical techniques.

The technical details and verified results of stimulation techniques have not been quoted in detail as the techniques are relatively new and still undergoing such considerable surgical and material design modifications as to make critical assessment of results uncertain for the moment. The efficiency, and especially the durability, of these stimulation techniques is by no means perfect, but with the speed of technological advance, it is clear that at least some patients may be kept comfortable for many years. Those patients that have proved unsuitable for these techniques may be sustained by the reasonable hope that as a result of studying patients being treated by these sophisticated techniques, the great deal of basic neuroscientific information, particularly in the area of neurotransmitters or neuromodulators, that is resulting might provide further answers to the continuing problems of persistent pain.

## Post herpetic neuralgia

This most distressing disorder tends to be an affliction of the older person. While it is generally thought that a higher percentage of older patients suffer persisting pain from their herpes zoster infection there are no accurate epidemiological data to confirm this, or to establish the exact percentage of patients with herpes zoster who suffer persistent post herpetic pain. It can afflict the trigeminal nerve, when it is the ophthalmic division that is particularly likely to suffer, but also any other sensory nerve in the body. Head and Campbell (1900) first recognized the ganglion of the afflicted nerve to be the main site of herpetic damage. Like the patient with anaesthesia dolorosa, the patient with post herpetic neuralgia, particularly in the trigeminal distribution, often seems particularly miserable with a high incidence of associated psychiatric disturbance, usually depression.

There is no analgesic preparation specifically effective in this condition, though if shooting pains become dominant, in addition to the background burning pain and hyperaesthesia, then Carbamazepine is often useful. Anti-depressant psychotropic medication is probably of greater value than any other medication.

Surgical treatment of post herpetic neuralgia has on the whole proved quite unsuccessful, in spite of the great range of procedures that have been tried. Excision or undermining of the scarred skin has been tempting, particularly when the area is small or convenient for spontaneous healing or grafting. While some patients may have been improved as a result of this technique, it is only a small minority (White & Sweet 1969).

Destruction of the peripheral nerve, its ganglion or sensory root, has likewise been advanced, but is of distinctly uncertain value. It seems likely that the small proportion of cases responding are those in which significant sensation has been retained in the scarred area, while those with marked anaesthesia in the area of pain have been unaffected.

Regional sympathetic denervation has been tried to relieve post herpetic pain in the head and that originating from the spine, without effect. Hindbrain tractotomies have proved useless; anterolateral cordotomy has proved effective in a small proportion of cases, but not over the longterm (White & Sweet 1969 p. 475). More recently the Nashold dorsal root entry zone coagulation procedure has been applied to post herpetic neuralgia, but Nashold himself has suggested that again it is the hyperaesthetic element of the pain that is suppressible, while the background constant burning pain tends to remain (Nashold 1984).

Electrical stimulatory techniques should be applicable to this benign persistent pain; TNS has proved useful, but again only in a small proportion of cases (Nathan & Wall 1974). There has been no reported success for dorsal column stimulation in post herpetic neuralgia. Deep brain stimulation to VPM, that part of the ventral lateral thalamus (VL) associated with relay of sensations from the face, has proved useful in a minority of cases, but the technique is perhaps particularly difficult to apply to the population of elderly infirm patients that tend to suffer post herpetic trigeminal neuralgia.

There is fairly general agreement that surgical techniques of all kinds are best avoided, unless out of desperation, in this extremely refractory pain syndrome.

# References

ADRIAN E. D. (1949) *Sensory Integration. The First Sherrington Lecture.* Liverpool University Press.
ALBE-FESSARD D. (1984) Personal communication.
ALBE-FESSARD D. & LOMBARD M. C. (1981) *Pain,* (Suppl.) 1, 580.
ARMOUR D. (1927) *Lancet,* 2, 691.
BEATSON G. T. (1896) *Lancet,* 2, 104 162.
BEAVER D. L. (1967) *J. Neurosurg.,* 26, 138.
BELMUSTO L., BROWN E. & OWENS G. (1963) *J. Neurosurg.,* 20, 225.
BETTAG W. (1966) *Proc. Third Int. Cong. Neurol. Surg. 791.* Exerpta Medica Foundation, Amsterdam.
BISHOP G. H. (1962) In *Neural Physiopathology* (ed. Grenell R. G.) p. 95. Harper and Row, New York.
BOUCHARD G., MAYANAGI Y. & MARTINS L. F. (1977) In *Neurosurgical Treatment in Psychiatry, Pain and Epilepsy,* p. 693–698. Eds. W. H. Sweet, S. Obrador J. G. Martin-Rodriguez) University Park Press, London.
BOWSHER D. (1957) *Brain,* 80, 606.
BOWSHER D. (1977) In *Persistent Pain,* Vol. I, pp. 1–20. (Ed. S. Lipton) Academic Press, London.
BRIHAYE J. & RETIF J. (1961) *Neurochirurgie,* 7, 258.
BRODAL A. (1947) *Arch. Neurol. Psychiat.,* 57, 292.
BRODAL A. (1969) *Neurological Anatomy in Relation to Clinical*

*Medicine*, 2nd edn. Oxford University Press, London.

BROGGI G. & SIEGFRIED J. (1979) In *Advances in Pain Research and Therapy*, Vol. II, pp. 469–473. (Eds J. J. Bonicca, V. Ventafridda) Raven Press, New York.

BROMLEY L. (1930) *Guy's Hosp. Reps.*, **80**, 234.

BROWN A. S. (1961) *Second Int. Cong. Neurol. Surg. Int. Cong. Series No. 36, E59*. Excerpta Medica Foundation, Amsterdam.

CLARK L. P. & TAYLOR A. S. (1909) *J. Amer. med. Ass.*, **53**, 2144.

COGGLESHALL R. E., APPLEBAUM M. L., FACEM M., STUBBS T. B. & SYKES M. T., (1975) *Brain*, **98**, 157.

CUSHING H. (1900) *J. Amer. med. Ass.*, **34**, 1034.

DANDY W. E. (1927) *Arch. Surg.*, **15**, 198.

DANDY W. E. (1929) *Arch. Surg.*, **18**, 687.

DANDY W. E. (1932) *Ann. Surg.*, **96**, 787.

DANDY W. E. (1934) *Amer. J. Surg.*, **24**, 447.

DAWSON G. D. (1958) *Proc. roy. Soc. Med.*, **51**, 531.

DEJERINE J. (1914) *Semiologie des Affections du Systeme Nerveux*. Masson, Paris.

DEJERINE J. & ROUSSY G. (1906) *Rev. Neurol.*, **14**, 521.

DELFINO U. (1983) In *Persistent Pain*, Vol. IV pp. 145–158. (Eds. S. Lipton & J. B. Miles) Academic Press, London.

DIEMATH H. E., HEPPNER F. & WALKER A. E. (1961) *Postgrad. med. J.*, **29**, 485.

DOGLIOTTI M. (1931) *Presse Med.*, **39**, 1249.

DOGLIOTTI M. (1938) *Anaesth. Analg.*, 143.

ELITHORN A., GLITHEROE E. & SLATER E. (1958) *J. Neurol. Neurosurg. Psychiat.*, **21**, 249.

ELITHORN A., PIERCY M. F. & CROSSKEY M. A. (1955) *J. Neurol. Neurosurg. Psychiat.*, **18**, 34.

ERVIN F. R. & MARK V. H. (1960) *Arch. Neurol.*, **3**, 368.

FAIRMAN D. (1976) In *Advances in Pain Research and Therapy*. (Eds. J. J. Bonicca & D. Albe-Fessard) Raven Press, New York.

FALCONER M. A. (1949) *J. Neurol. Neurosurg. Psychiat.*, **12**, 297.

FOLTZ E. L. & WHITE L. E. (1962) *J. Neurosurg.*, **19**, 89.

FRAZIER C. H. (1920) *Arch. Neurol. Psychiat.*, **4**, 137.

FRAZIER C. H. (1928) *Ann. Surg.*, **88**, 534.

FREEMAN W. & WATTS J. W. (1946) *Proc. roy. Soc. Med.*, **39**, 445.

FRENCH L. A. & PEYTON W. T. (1948) *J. Neurosurg.*, **5**, 403.

GILDENBERG P. L. & HIRSHLING R. M. (1981) *Medical Journal, St Joseph's Hospital, Houston*, **16**, 199.

GLEES P. (1953) *Acta Neurosurg. Wien.*, **7**, 160.

GOODY W. (1957) *Brain*, **80**, 118.

GOWERS W. R. (1886) *Diseases of the Nervous System. Vol. 1: Diseases of the Spinal Cord and Nerves*. Churchill, London.

GRANT F. C. & WEINBERGER L. M. (1941) *Surg. Gynaec. Obstet.*, **72**, 747.

GRECO T., SBARAGNI F. & CAMMILLI L (1957) *Septimana Medicale*, **45**, 355.

HAGBARTH K. E. & KERR D. I. B. (1954) *J. Neurophysiol.*, **17**, 294.

HAGGQUIST G. (1936) *Z. mikr.-anat. Forsch.*, **39**, 1.

HAKANSSON S. (1981) *Neurosurgery*, **9**, 638.

HANKINSON J. (1960) *J. Neurol. Neurosurg. Psychiat.*, **23**, 352.

HANKINSON J. (1969) In *Recent Advances in Neurology and Neuropsychiatry*, 8th edn. (eds. Lord Brain & Wilkinson M.) p. 147. Churchill, London.

HARDY J. (1971) *J. Neurosurg.*, **34**, 582.

HARRIS W. (1912) *Lancet*, **I**, 218.

HARRIS W. (1921) *Brain*, **44**, 557.

HARRIS W. (1935) *Brit. med. J.*, **I**, 1112.

HARRIS W. (1937) *The Facial Neuralgias*. Oxford University Press, London.

HARRIS W. (1940) *Brain*, **63**, 209.

HARTEL F. (1912) *Arch. Klin. Chirurg.*, **100**, 193.

HASSLER R. (1960) *Acta Neurochirurg.*, **8**, 353.

HASSLER R. & RIECHERT T. (1959) *Arch. Psychiat. Nervenheilk*, **200**, 93.

HEAD H. & CAMPBELL A. W. (1900) *Brain*, **23**, 353.

HEATH R. G. & MICKLE W. A. (1960) In *Electrical Studies in the Unanaesthetised Brain*. (Eds. Ramsey E. R. & O'Doherty) Paul B. Hoebuer, New York.

HECAEN H., TALAIRACH J., DAVID M. & DELL M. B. (1949) *Rev. Neurol.*, **81**, 917.

HENDERSON W. R. (1965) *Ann. roy. Coll. Surg. Eng.*, **37**, 346.

HENDERSON W. R. (1966) *J. Anat.*, **100**, 905.

HENDERSON W. R. (1967) *Brit. med. J.*, **1**, 8.

HENDERSON W. R. & SMYTH G. E. (1948) *J. Neurol. Neurosurg. Psychiat.*, **11**, 88.

HITCHCOCK E. (1969) *J. Neurosurg.*, **31**, 386.

HITCHCOCK E. (1970) *J. Neurol. Neurosurg. Psychiat.*, **33**, 224.

HITCHCOCK E. & LEECE B. (1967) *J. Neurosurg.*, **27**, 321.

HITCHCOCK E. & SCHVARCZ J. R. (1972) *J. Neurosurg.*, **37**, 412.

HORSLEY V., TAYLOR J. & COLMAN W. S. (1891) *Brit. med. j.*, **2**, 1249.

HOSOBUCHI Y. (1980) *Pain*, **8 (2)**, 167.

HOSOBUCHI Y., ADAMS J. E. & RUTKIN B. (1973) *Arch. Neurol.*, **29**, 158.

HOSOBUCHI Y., ADAMS J. E. & WEINSTEIN P. R. (1972) *J. Neurosurg.*, **37**, 242.

HOSOBUCHI Y., ROSSIER J., BROOM F. E. & GUILLEMIN R. (1979) *Science*, **203**, 279.

HUGGINS C. & BERGENSTAHL D. M. (1952) *Cancer Res.*, **12**, 131.

HUGGINS C. & HODGES C. V. (1941) *Cancer Res.*, **1**, 293.

HUNT J. R. (1907) *J. nerv. ment. Dis.*, **34**, 73.

HUNT J. R. (1937) *Arch. Neurol. Psychiat.*, **37**, 253.

HUGHES B. (1958) *Proc. roy. Soc. Med.*, **51**, 529.

HUGHES J., SMITH T. W., KOSTERLITZ H. W., FOTHERGILL L. A., MORGAN B. A. & MORRIS H. R. (1975) *Nature*, **258**, 549.

IGGO A. (1981) In *Persistent Pain*, Vol. III, p. 1–16. (Eds. S. Lipton & J. B. Miles.) Academic Press, London.

IGGO A. & WALSH E. G. (1960) *Brain*, **83**, 701.

IRGER J. M. (1930) *Ann. Surg.*, **92**, 984.

JACK T. M. & LLOYD J. W. (1983) *Ann. roy. Coll. Surg. (Eng.)*, **65 (2)**, 97.

JANNETTA P. J. (1967) *J. Neurosurg.*, **26**, 109.

JANNETTA P. (1976) In *Progress in Neurological Surgery*, Vol 7 (Part 1) pp. 180–200. (Eds. H. Krayenbuhl, P. E. Maspes & W. H. Sweet) Karger, Basel, Switzerland.

JASPER H. H. (1966) In *Brain and Conscious Experience*, (Ed. Eccles J. C.) p. 256. Springer, Berlin.

JEFFERSON A. (1963) *J. Neurol. Neurosurg. Psychiat.*, **26**, 345.

JEFFERSON A. (1966) In *Pain*, (eds. Knighton R. S. & Dumke P. R.) p. 365. Little, Brown & Co., Boston, Massachussetts.

JEFFERSON G. & SCHORSTEIN J. (1955) *Brit. J. Surg.*, **42**, 561.

KEELE C. A. & SMITH R. (1962) *The Assessment of Pain in Man and Animals: An International Symposium*. U.F.A.W. Livingstone, Edinburgh.

KERR F. W. & ALEXANDER S. (1964) *Arch. Neurol.*, **10**, 249.

KERR W. L. (1967) *J. Neurosurg.*, **26**, 132, 151. 1865

KING R. B. (1958) *J. Neurosurg.*, **15**, 290.

KIRSCHNER M. (1931) *Arch. Klin. Chirurg.*, **167**, 761.

KIRSCHNER M. (1933) *Arch. Klin. Chirurg.*, **176**, 581.

KRANICK J. U. & THODEN U. (1984) In *A Textbook of Pain* (Eds. P. D. Wall & R. Melzack) pp. 701–705. Churchill Livingstone, London.

KUNC Z. (1961) *Second Int. Cong. Neurol. Surg. Int. Congress*, Series No. 36, E107. Excerpta Medica Foundation, Amsterdam.

KUNC Z. (1964) *Tractus Spinalis Nervi Trigemini*. Naklad. Ceskeslovak. Akad. Ved., Praha.

KUNC Z. (1966) In *Pain* (eds. Knighton R. S. & Dumke P. R.) p. 351. Little, Brown & Co., Boston, Massachussetts.

LAHUERTA J. (1984a) Doctorate thesis to the University of Pamploma.

LAHUERTA J., LIPTON S. & WELLS J. C. D. (1985) Percutaneous cordotomy: results and complications in a recent series of 100 patients. *Ann. roy. Coll. Surg. (Eng.)* **67**, 41.

LE BARS D., DICKENSON A. H. & BESSON J. M. (1979) *Pain*, **6**, 283.

LEVIN A. B. & COSMAN E. R. (1981) In *Persistent Pain*, Vol. III pp. 259–264. (Eds. S Lipton & J. B. Miles) Academic Press, London.

LIN P. M., GILDENBERG P. C. & POLAKOFF P. P. (1966) *J. Neurosurg.*, **25**, 553.

LINDBLOM U. & MEYERSON B. A. (1975) *Pain*, **1**, 257.

LIPTON S. (1979) In *Advances in Pain Research and Therapy*, p. 425–437. (Eds. J. J. Bonicca & V. Ventafridda) Raven Press, New York.

LIPTON S., DERVIN E. & HEYWOOD O. B. (1974) In *Advances in Neurosurgery*. Ed. J. J. Bonicca. Vol. 4, pp. 689–694. Raven Press, New York.

LIPTON S., MILES J. B., WILLIAMS N. & BARK-JONES N. (1978) *Pain*, **5**, 75.

LIZARS J. (1821) *Edin. Med. Surg. J.*, **17**, 529. (See also *Brit. med. J.*, 1960, **2**, 1665).

LONG D. M. (1974) *Minn. Med.*, **57**, 195.

LORENZ R., GRUMME T., HERMANN D., PALLESKE H., KUHNER A., STENDE U. & ZIERSKI J. (1975) In *Advances in Neurosurgery*, Vol. 3 (Eds. H. Penyholy, M. Brock, J. Hamer, M. Klinger and O. Spoerri) pp. 178–185. Springer, Berlin.

LUFT R. & OLIVECRONA H. (1953) *J. Neurosurg.*, **10**, 301.

MAHER R. M. (1955) *Lancet*, **I**, 18.

MAHER R. M. (1957) *Lancet*, **I**, 16.

MAHER R. M. (1960) *Lancet*, **I**, 895.

MARK V. H. & ERVIN F. R. (1969) In *Pain and the Neurosurgeon*, (Eds. White J. C. & Sweet W. H.) p. 856. Thomas, Springfield, Illinois.

MARK V. H., ERVIN F. R. & YAKOVLEV P. I. (1963) *Arch. Neurol.*, **8**, 528.

MARSHALL J. (1951) *J. Neurol. Neurosurg. Psychiat.*, **14**, 187.

MAZARS G., MERIENNE L. & CIOLOCA C. (1974) *Neurochirurgie.*, **20**, 117.

MAZARS G., ROGE R. & PANSINI A. (1960) *J. Neurol. Neurosurg. Psychiat.*, **23**, 352.

MCKENZIE K. G. (1955) *Clin. Neurosurg.*, **2**, 50.

MEHLER W. R. (1966a) In *Pain* (Eds. Knighton R. S. & Dumke P. R.) p. 11. Little, Brown & Co., Boston, Massachussetts.

MEHLER W. R. (1966b) *Confin. Neurol.*, **27**, 18.

MELZACK R. & WALL P. D. (1962) *Brain*, **85**, 331.

MELZACK R. & WALL P. D. (1965) *Science*, **150**, 971.

MILES J. B. (1977) *Persistent Pain*. Ed. S. Lipton, Vol. I, pp. 129–148. Academic Press, London.

MILES J. B. (1979) In *Advances in Pain Research and Therapy*, Vol. 2, pp. 373–380. (Eds. J. J. Bonicca & V. Ventafridda) Raven Press, New York.

MILES J. B. (1980) In *Persistent Pain*, Vol. II, pp. 223–248. (Ed. S. Lipton) Academic Press, London.

MILES J. B. (1983) *Brit. Journal. hosp. Med.*, **30**, 348.

MILES J. B. (1984a) In *A Textbook of Pain*, p. 656–665. (Ed. P. Wall & R. Melzack) Churchill Livingstone, London.

MILES J. B., LIPTON S., HAYWOOD M., BOWSHER D., MUMFORD J. & MOLONY V. (1974) *Lancet*, **1**, 777.

MORIN F. (1955) *Amer. J. Physiol.*, **183**, 245.

MORRICA G. (1974) In *Advances in Neurology*, Vol. IV, pp. 707–714. (Ed. J. J. Bonica) Raven Press, New York.

MORRICA G. (1977) In *Persistent Pain*, Vol. I, pp. 149–174. (Ed. S. Lipton) Academic Press, London.

MOUNTCASTLE V. B. (1966) In *Brain and Conscious Experience* (Ed. Eccles J. C.) p. 85. Springer, Berlin.

MULLAN S. & HOSOBUCHI Y. (1968) *J. Neurosurg.* **28**, 291.

MULLAN S., HARPER P. V., HEKMATPANAH J., TORRES H. & DOBBIN G. (1963) *J. Neurosurg.*, **20**, 931.

NASHOLD B. C. (1981) *J. Neurosurg.*, **55**, 1012.

NASHOLD B. C. (1984) *Neurosurgery*, **6**, 942.

NASHOLD B. S. & FRIEDMAN H. (1972) *J. Neurosurg.*, **36**, 590.

NASHOLD B. S. & OSTDAHL R. H. (1979) *J. Neurosurg.*, **51**, 59.

NATHAN P. W (1956a) *J. Neurol. Neurosurg. Psychiat.*, **19**, 101.

NATHAN P. W. (1956b) *J. Neurol. Neurosurg. Psychiat.*, **19**, 88.

NATHAN P. W. (1963a) *J. Neurol. Neurosurg. Psychiat.*, **26**, 353.

NATHAN P. W. (1963b) *J. Neurol. Neurosurg. Psychiat.*, **26**, 487.

NATHAN P. W. & SCOTT T. G. (1958) *Lancet*, **1**, 76.

NATHAN P. W. & SEARS T. A. (1960) *J. Physiol.*, **150**, 565.

NATHAN P. W. & SMITH M. C. (1951) *J. Neurol. Neurosurg. Psychiat.*, **14**, 262.

NATHAN P. W. & SMITH M. C. (1953) *J. Neurol. Neurosurg. Psychiat.*, **16**, 245.

NATHAN P. W. & SMITH M. C. (1958) *J. Neurol. Neurosurg. Psychiat.*, **21**, 177.

NATHAN P. W. & WALL P. D. (1974) *Brit. med. J.*, **3**, 645.

NATHAN P. W., SEARS T. A. & SMITH M. C. (1965) *J. Neurol. Sci.*, **2**, 7.

NOORDENBOS W. (1959) *Pain*. Elsevier, Amsterdam.

NORTHFIELD D. W. C. (1948) In *Recent Advances in Surgery*, 3rd edn. (Ed. Edwards H. C.) p. 313. Churchill, London.

NORTHFIELD D. W. C. (1961) *Second Int. Cong. Neurol. Surg. Int. Cong. Series No. 36, E23.* Excerpta Medica Foundation, Amsterdam.

NORTHFIELD D. W. C. (1973) *The Surgery of the Central Nervous System*. p. 611. Blackwell Scientific Publications, Oxford.

OCHOA J. & TOREBJORK E. (1983) *J. Physiol.*, **342**, 633.

OLIVECRONA H. (1947) *Acta Psych. Scand. Suppl.*, **46**, 268.

OLIVECRONA H. (1961) *Triangle*, **5**, 60.

PAPO I. (1979) In *Advances in Pain Research and Therapy*, pp. 439–447. (Eds. J. J. Bonicca & V. Ventrafridda) Raven Press, New York.

PATEL A. K., VICENTE U., YAP M. D., FIELDS J. & THOMPSEN M. D. (1979) *Arch. intern. Med.*, **139**, 1281.

PEET M. M., KAHN E. A. & ALLEN S. S. (1933) *J. Amer. med. Ass.*, **100**, 488.

PENFIELD W. & BOLDREY E. (1937) *Brain*, **60**, 389.

PENFIELD W. & RASMUSSEN T. (1950) *The Cerebral Cortex of Man*. Macmillan, New York.

PENMAN J. (1949) *Lancet*, **2**, 268.

PENMAN J. & SMITH M.C. (1950) *J. Neurol. Neurosurg. Psychiat.*, **13**, 36.

PENNYBACKER J. B. (1961) In *Scientific Aspects of Neurology* (Ed. Garland H.) p. 153. Livingstone, Edinburgh.

POGGIO G. F. & MOUNTCASTLE V. B. (1960) *Bull. Johns Hopk. Hosp.*, **106**, 266.

RAY B. S. & WOLFF H. G. (1945) *Arch. Neurol. Psychiat.*, **53**, 257.

REXED B. (1952) *J. comp. Neurol.*, **96**, 415.

REYNOLDS D. V. (1969) *Science*, **164**, 444.

RICHARDSON D. E. & AKIL U. (1977) *J. Neurosurg.*, **47**, 178.

RIDDOCH G. (1941) *Brain*, **64**, 197.

RIECHERT T. (1960) *Acta Neurochirurg.*, **8**, 136.

ROSE J. E. & MOUNTCASTLE V. B. (1959) In *Handbook of Physiology*. Section I. Neurophysiology (Eds. Field J., Magoun H. W. & Hall V. E.) Vol. I, p. 387. Williams and Wilkins, Baltimore.

ROSE W. (1890) *Lancet*, **2**, 914.

ROSOMOFF H. C., CARROLL F., BROWN J. & SHEPTAK P. (1965) *J. Neurosurg.*, **23**, 639.

SANO K, YOSHIOKA M., OGASHIWA M., ISHIJIMA B. & OHYE C. (1966) *Confin. Neurol.*, **27**, 63.

SCARFF J. E. (1950) *J. Neurosurg*, **7**, 288.

SCHORSTEIN J. (1943) *J. Neurol. Neurosurg. Psychiat.*, **6**, 46.

SCHWARTZ H. D. & O'LEARY J. L. (1941) *Surgery*, **9**, 183.

SCHWARTZ J. R. (1976) *J. Neurol. Neurosurg. Psychiat.*, **39**, 53.

SHEALY C. N., MORTIMER J. T. & RESWICK J. B. (1967) *Anaesth. Analg. Cleveland*, **46**, 489.

SICARD R. & ROBINEUA (1920) *Rev. Neurol.*, **27**, 256.

SIEGFRIED J. (1982) *Appl. Neurophysiol.*, **45**, 143.

SINDOU M., FISHER G. & MANSUY L. (1976) In *Progress in Neurological Surgery*, Vol. 7, Part I, pp. 201–259. (Eds. H. Krayenbuhl, P. E. Maspes & W. H. Sweet. Karger, Basel, Switzerland.

SINDOU M., FISHER G., GONTELLE A. & MANSUY L. (1974) *Neurochirurgie*, **20**, 391.

SJÖQVIST O. (1938) *Acta Psychiat. Neurol. Scand.*, Suppl. **17**.

SMITH M. C. (1957) *Brain*, **80**, 263.

SMITH M. C. (1964) *Brit. J. Anaesth.*, **36**, 387.

SMITH M. C. & DEACON P. 1984) *Brain*, **197**, 671.

SOUREK K. (1969) *J. Neurosurg.*, **31**, 524.

SPILLANE J. D. & WELLS C. E. C. (1959) *Brain*, **82**, 391.

SPILLER W. G. & FRAZIER C. H. (1901) *Phil. med. J.*, **8**, 1039.

SPILLER W. G. & MARTIN E. (1912) *J. Amer. med. Ass.*, **58**, 1489.

STENDER A. (1961) *Second Int. Cong. Neurol. Surg. Int. Cong.* Series No. 36, E25. Excerpta Medica Foundation, Amsterdam.

SWEET W. H. (1976) In *Progress in Neurological Surgery*, Vol. 7, pp. 153–179. (Eds. H. Krayenbuhl, P. E. Maspes & W. H. Sweet) Karger, Basel, Switzerland.

TALAIRACH J., TOURNOUX P. & BANCAUD J. (1960) *Acta Neurochirurg.*, **8**, 153.

TAPTAS N. (1911) *Presse Med.*, **80**, 798.

TEW J. (1977) In *Current Techniques in Operative Neurosurgery*, p. 409–426. (Eds. H. H. Schmidek & W. H. Sweet) Grune & Stratton, New York.

THOMAS D. C. & SHEEHY J. (1982) *J. Neurol. Neurosurg. Psychiat.*, **45**, 949.

TODD E. M., CRUE B. C., & CARREGAL E. J. A. (1969) *Confin. Neurol.*, **31**, 106.

TOREBJORK H. E., HALLIN R. G., HONGELL A. & HAGBARTH K. E. (1970) *Brain Res.*, **24**, 443.

TOREBJORK H. E., LAMOTTE R. H. & ROBINSON C. J. (1984) *J. Neurophysiol.*, **51 (2)**, 325.

TRUEX R. C. & CARPENTER M. B. (1969) *Human Neuronanatomy*, 6th edn. Williams and Wilkins, Baltimore.

WALKER A. E. (1940) *Arch. Neurol. Psychiat.*, **42**, 284.

WALKER A. E. (1942) *Arch. Surg.*, **44**, 953.

WALL P. D. (1960) *J. Neurophysiol.*, **23**, 197.

WATKINS E. S. (1972) Personal communication.

WEDDELL G. (1941a) *Proc. roy. Soc. Med.*, **34**, 776.

WEDDELL G. (1941b) *J. Anat.*, **75**, 441.

WEDDELL G. (1955) In *Annual Review of Psychology*, **6**, 119, (Ed. Stone C. P. & McNemar Q.) Annual Review Inc., Stanford, California.

WEISENBERG T. H. (1910) *J. Amer. med. Ass.*, **54**, 1600.

WERTHEIMER P. & LECUIRE J. (1953) *Acta Chirurg. Belg.*, **52**, 568.

WHITE J. C. (1962) *Neurol. Med. Chirurg.*, **4**, 1.

WHITE J. C. & SWEET W. H. (1955) *Pain; its mechanisms and neurosurgical control*. Thomas, Springfield, Illinois.

WHITE J. C. & SWEET W. H. (1969) *Pain and the Neurosurgeon*. Thomas, Springfield, Illinois.

WILKINS H. (1966) *J. Neurosurg.*, **25**, 370.

WILLIAMS N. E., MILES J. B., LIPTON S., HIPKIN L. & DAVIS J. C. (1980) *Ann. roy. Coll. Surg. (Eng.)*, **62**, 203.

WYCIS H. T. & SPIEGEL E. A. (1962) *J. Neurosurg.*, **19**, 101.

ZERVAS N. (1969) *N. Engl. J. Med.*, **280**, 429.

# Chapter 19
# Surgery of functional disorders

## J. B. MILES

## Mental disorders

In the early years of this century, when neurosurgery was developing as a specialized subject, little attention was paid to the possibility of relieving mental disorder by operation. The neurosurgeon was too busy evolving techniques, seeking answers to the problems of localization of tumours, studying their natural history and grappling with the control of raised intracranial pressure. Nevertheless, observations on persons suffering from accidental brain damage and experimental observations were accumulating and were to be the basis of a revolutionary form of treatment in certain varieties of mental illness. As early as 1875, some 10 years after Lister introduced his antiseptic technique, Ferrier observed that after the removal of portions of its frontal lobe a monkey still retained many of functions, but he concluded that a decided change was produced in the animal's character and disposition. Some years later Bianchi also performed frontal lobe ablations and noted a suppression of feeling or sentiment similar to that seen in human beings who had suffered severe frontal lobe damage (Bianchi 1922). He also described a lack of self-restraint and of initiative. Bianchi's resections were polar and did not include the orbital surface of the frontal lobe; with prescience he said (page 135) that this area, the orbital surface, would provide a good field for experiment in the future, but this invitation was not taken up for many years. In 1891 Burkhardt reported the results of operation upon 6 patients suffering from schizophrenia; the operations were cortical resections in various areas of the brain, designed to render the patients less difficult to nurse. All were somewhat improved.

It is clear that Burkhardt was the first surgeon to design and to execute a definitive brain operation to allay mental disorder. The next attempt was by Puusepp in 1910 and in these operations incisions were made into the brain on one side; they were precursors of leucotomy as Burkhardt's were of topectomy. Puusepp was not impressed by his results (he did not publish them until 1937) and a quarter of a century was to elapse before further operations were carried out on humans for this purpose. Bianchi had stressed the value of critically observing behavioural changes in animals brought about by excising portions of brain and Sherrington (1906) thought that these were 'new methods of promise'. In order to study the results of frontal lobe lesions as fruitfully as possible, animals were trained to carry out complicated tests and procedures and a critical comparison made of their performances before and after operation: these techniques were at that time novel, but are now commonplace. Such a programme was designed by Fulton and Jacobsen in 1933, when two chimpanzees were given an intensive training for 6 months. Early in 1934 bilateral frontal ablations were carried out on both animals in two stages. After recovery from these operations, 'on superficial inspection their cage behaviour did not seen to have altered particularly, but careful observation revealed certain behavioural changes. Before operation, when as a result of a wrong choice in their tests they were unrewarded, both animals displayed frustration by exhibiting temper tantrums; after the operations the animals no longer showed this emotional response' (Fulton 1949).

## Prefrontal leucotomy

At the Second International Neurological Congress in 1935, when these experiments were reported, Professor Moniz of Lisbon enquired whether, such an operation having prevented experimental neurosis and frustrational behaviour in animals, it would not be feasible to relieve anxiety states in man by similar surgical means. For several years Moniz had been seriously contemplating the value of damaging frontal lobe connections as a method of dealing with severe mental disorder. These experiments on the chimpanzees, Lucy and Becky, provided the final encouragement. On his return to Lisbon a series of patients were operated upon by his associate Lima (who subsequently succeeded to the Chair of Neurology). The technique consisted of injecting small quantities of absolute alcohol into the white matter of the anterior part of the frontal lobe. This proved unpredictable in its effect (as with alcohol injections for Parkinsonism) and an instrument was devised which, when rotated on its axis, cut a spherical core of white matter 1 cm in diameter. Six of these lesions were made on each side. In some patients these operations were dramatically beneficial and when the results were published in 1936 the new operation of leucotomy was rapidly taken up by Freeman and Watts in the United States (where it was called lobotomy) and more gradually in other countries. Freeman and Watts (1942) modified Lima's technique. A small burr hole was made on each side of the head 6 cms above the zygomatic arch and 3 cms posterior to the external angular process of the frontal bone and a spatulate instrument was introduced into the frontal lobe to a depth just short of the midline (so that the anterior cerebral artery and its branches were not damaged) in order to divide the central core of white matter, just in front of the tip of the frontal horn. The operation had a mortality of up to 3% and was followed by epilepsy in about 3%. Mental confusion and urinary incontinence tended to persist for several weeks.

In a study of 'Prefrontal Leucotomy in a Thousand Cases' (Freeman & Watts 1947), nearly two-thirds of the patients suffered from schizophrenia, and of these only 16% were discharged recovered, while 36% were improved, but had to remain in hospital.

In a critical survey of the results in one hospital five or more years after operation, Robin (1959) found no convincing evidence that leucotomy provided any better longterm results in a group of schizophrenic patients, when assessed against a comparable control group, and McKenzie and Kaczanowski (1964) arrived at this similar conclusion.

In nonpsychotic illness however, such as obsessional and compulsive neurosis, depression, hypochondriasis, melancholia, anxiety states and drug addiction, there was general agreement that leucotomy usually gave much relief. Strom-Olsen and Tow (1949) found that three-quarters of a group of patients with such illnesses were relieved of their symptoms by leucotomy and this was twice the proportion of psychotics relieved by the same operation. The relief of pain was recognized as being similar to the freedom from frustration of the chimpanzees Becky and Lucy. The patient was released from the sense of mental tension, from anxiety and from feelings of guilt. Although emotions are flattened, the abatement of such symptoms might well have the most profound value to a patient, for whom life is rendered once more endurable and even pleasant.

### Adverse effects of leucotomy

The undesirable effects from leucotomy represent an exaggeration or excessive degree of the desirable qualities induced by the operation. These might include a lack of consideration for others and an inability to foresee the consequences of one's actions; habitual remarks, activities and attitudes not acceptable by the ordinary social standards of the community; apathy, lack of initiative and lack of self respect leading even to personal slovenliness.

One of the difficulties in assessing neuropsychological or behavioural defects after leucotomy has been that of obtaining a reliable control for comparison. This was overcome by Tow (1955) in a valuable and time-consuming research study in which the patient provided his own control, as in the experiments with Lucy and Becky. Tow selected 36 patients of average intelligence with well preserved personality who fully cooperated. Each was subjected to a battery of tests by Tow himself, under conditions as similar as possible before and about one year after the standard leucotomy operation. It is not possible to quote his results in full, but they clearly demonstrated an impaired performance 'in tests which measure predominantly cognitive functions needing powers of logical thinking, reasoning, perception of relations, and planning. This is an important finding in view of the belief still widely held that the frontal lobes subserve only those functions which are primarily emotional or temperamental.'

*Causes of postleucotomy disablement*

The post-mortem studies of many observers have revealed that the variability in the results has been largely attributable to differences in the size of the cut in the brain, the extent of the lesion, and its situation particularly in respect to its location in the anteroposterior axis of the cerebrum.

Another unpredictable factor is the extent of the secondary damage resulting from haemorrhage, thrombosis, necrosis and oedema of the brain beyond the slit-like cavity produced primarily by the surgeon's instrument (Yakovlev *et al.* 1950). In a series of 122 post-mortem specimens examined by McLardy (1950) cerebral haemorrhage from the operation appeared to be the cause of death in approximately 25% and these all occurred within 14 days. In another 22 cases death had occurred within 6 months of the operation and in some of these the posterior orbital cortex had been damaged, while in others there had been damage to the head of the caudate nucleus.

It is now recognized that if the cut is too far back, or gives rise to necrosis of the anterior part of the basal ganglia or the posterior orbital cortex, it is likely to lead to profound intellectual and personality damage and even to be fatal.

**Modifications in operative technique**

Many modifications of leucotomy have been made in an attempt to avoid the serious disadvantages and these are now of historic interest only (McKissock 1951, Grantham 1951, Penfield 1948, Heath & Pool 1948, and Le Beau 1951).

Others have devised techniques whereby gradual, incremental leucotomy could be achieved. White *et al.* (1960) and White & Sweet (1969) used an indwelling electrode into the ventromedial part of each frontal lobe and gradually enlarged a thermocoagulation lesion until the desired effect could be obtained (most of their cases were of leucotomy for uncontrolled pain). Crow *et al.* (1961, 1963) used a technique of stereotaxic implantation of multiple fine electrodes in a fanwise manner into the depths of frontal lobes and on the basis of temporary blocks induced by polarization gradually built up a leucotomy effect by coagulation, using the same electrodes.

They maintained their electrodes in a percutaneous mode for prolonged periods of time, in some cases for as long as one year.

Scoville (1949) introduced a method of undercutting of the frontal basal cortex that Knight (1964) modified in order to avoid excessive basal ganglia damage, by making the destructive lesions using radioactive yttrium, inserted stereotaxically. In Britain, this technique, with minor modifications, has been the method used in the small number of centres still performing this procedure (Bartlett *et al.* 1981).

**Cingulotomy as a variation of leucotomy**

Based on the observations of Smith (1944) and Ward (1948) Cairns became interested in ablations of the anterior cingulate cortex and achieved some success with nonpsychotic patients, in a manner very similar to that following standard leucotomy, but with very little damage to personality (Whitty *et al.* 1952). Lewin (1961) also reported improvement in neurotic patients which was marked in 11 out of 26 and moderate in 10 out of 26. This type of lesion can be achieved stereotaxically with little morbidity and with a quoted significant improvement in between 70 and 80% of disabling mental disorders as reported by Ballantine *et al.* (1977). Stereotaxic cingulotomy can be combined with medial frontal leucotomy with good effect on obsessional neuroses, with greater accuracy and greater safety (Mitchell-Heggs *et al.* 1977).

### Physiological basis for success of leucotomy

Post-mortem studies have confirmed the opinions based upon clinical observation, that the further rostral the lesion was made, the less its effect and the more caudal, the greater the effect; patients who had succumbed with severe mental deterioration and vegetative disorders were usually found to have lesions sufficiently posterior to encroach upon the basal ganglia. Likewise, the size of the lesion was important, allowing major rostral lesions to be successful while much smaller bilateral caudal lesion could be disastrous. The contributions by Meyer and his associates on the changes found in the brain following leucotomy have been assembled by Meyer and Beck (1954) and the following conclusions drawn. The lesion must be of adequate size to be effective; those in the mid central, orbital and cingulate regions were more effective than those in the dorsolateral parts of the frontal white matter. Where these latter areas were damaged, and particularly if the cortex was included, personality changes were more severe.

The desirable changes achieved by leucotomy in the form of modification of excessive emotional behaviour implies an association with the function of the hypothalamus, the 'primary centre of integration for emotional expression' (Fulton 1951).

Le Gros Clark and Boggon (1933) had already shown in animals that the frontal cortex received projections from the dorsomedial nucleus of the thalamus, and this state was confirmed in necropsy specimen studies following leucotomy operations (Meyer *et al.* 1947, Freeman & Watts 1947). A pathway continuity was also shown from the dorsomedial nucleus to the hypothalamus, together with the known frontal lobe/hypothalamic connection through the anterior nucleus of the thalamus. The latter receives afferent fibres from the mammillary body and sends efferents to the cingulate gyrus.

Later work revealed evidence of a direct corticofugal pathway from the posterior orbital cortex to the hypothalamus (Le Gros Clark & Meyer 1950, Wall *et al.* 1951). The anatomical and physiological evidence of free provision for the transmission of hypothalamic impulses to the prefrontal cortex have thus provided the basis for a theory that the desirable effects of leucotomy are due to interruptions of these pathways. Further support for this theory is gained from the successful abandonment of the standard, more gross, operations for the smaller, selective, and anatomically more specific procedures with equally good clinical effects and reduction of unwanted, complicating intellectual disturbance. Cingulectomy, which probably also damages the cingulum bundle, is in the region of arrival of the projection from the anterior nucleus of the thalamus, while limited leucotomies aimed at central, medial and orbital segments are well placed to interrupt the outflow from the dorsomedial nucleus of the thalamus in the anterior segment of the internal capsule. In this respect the findings of Crow *et al.* (1963) showing that the distribution of the most effective lesions coincided with this area, is highly significant.

Little attention has been paid to the possibility that benefit derives from dividing the corticofugal pathways to the thalamus such as those arising from the posterior part of the orbital cortex and passing without relay to the hypothalamus. It is these that Knight (1964) thought may be selectively damaged by his technique of yttrium implant.

The extent to which intelligence suffers as a result of prefrontal lesions has been a matter for considerable debate, acrimony and even legislation. For the assessment of the results of leucotomy an endeavour should be made to differentiate between intelligence in all its levels, and the affective aspects of personality. In some aspects this may prove difficult or impossible because of mutual influences over performance. Failure to return, after the operation, to the same employment may be the result of intellectual dulling, but it may be due to dulling of interest and consequent lack of application and drive from impairment of affect.

### Present status of leucotomy

From an exciting and scientifically sound origin, leucotomy is being increasingly rejected as an appropriate or acceptable method of treating mental disorders. In England and Wales during the years 1942–1954 about 10,000 patients underwent leucotomy or one of its modifications (Tooth & Newton 1961). By 1976 this figure had reduced to around 150 per annum (Bartlett *et al.* 1981) and has continued to reduce. In part the procedure has become obsolescent due to the massive improvement in the psychotropic pharmacopoeia. In addition, however, public opinion, led by powerful pressure groups, often not well informed, has resulted in a definite and possibly inappropriate disinclination for neurosurgeons to become involved in its practice. Seriously interested workers have become overwhelmed by the practical difficulties resulting from the Mental Health Act Commission Report, section 57, by which clinical and possibly moral responsibility appears to be shifted from the doctor towards a lay committee, with decisions resulting that may not always be in the best interests of the patient (Bridges 1984).

### Temporal lobectomy and mental disorders

Temporal lobectomy for epilepsy may be followed by gratifying improvement in the associated behaviour disorder and temporal leucotomy has been undertaken for the same purpose. In infantile hemiplegia, hemispherectomy has proved highly successful in abolishing uncontrollable temper tantrums. It is tempting to seek a common physiological basis for an explanation of the success of these anatomically distinct operations, frontal, temporal and hemisphere, the common and desirable effect of which is to modify the abnormal or excessive influence of the affect on behaviour. In some patients this disorder of function appears to have no structural basis; in others the disorder of function appears to be the result of its distortion by epileptic discharges arising usually from a structural abnormality. The hypothesis that there is a common link between lobectomy and the leucotomies, mentioned previously, in attenuating a link between the hypothalamus and other parts of the brain, is an attractive one and is supported by present knowledge of cerebral anatomy and function. Lesions in the frontal lobes appear to be successful in so far as they diminish known connections with the hypothalamus. In temporal lobectomy and in hemispherectomy the hypothalamus and its ramifications in the limbic lobe are freed from the noxious influence of a bombardment by abnormal neuronal discharge. Interruption of the limbic circuit by temporal lobectomy may act in a similar way. Such an explanation is a gross oversimplification of the complexities of the subject, but provides a working hypothesis by which to seek further information.

## References

BALLANTINE H. T., LEVY B. S., DAGI T. F. & GIRIUNAS I. B. (1977) In *Neurosurgical Treatment in Psychiatry, Pain and Epilepsy*, pp. 333–54. (Eds. W. H. Sweet, S. Obrador, J. G. Martin-Rodriguez) University Park Press, Baltimore, U.S.A.
BARTLETT J., BRIDGES P. & KELLY D. (1981) *Contemp. Indic. Psychosurg*, **138**, 507.

BIANCHI L. (1922) *The Mechanism of the Brain.* E. S. Livingstone, Edinburgh.

BRIDGES P. K. (1984) *Bull. roy. Coll. Psych.,* **8**, No. 8.

BURKHARDT G. (1891) *Allg; Z. Psychiat.,* **47**, 463.

CROW H. J., COOPER R. & PHILLIPS D. G. (1961) *J. Neurol. Neurosurg. Psychiat.,* **24**, 353.

CROW H. J., COOPER R. & PHILLIPS D. G. (1963) *Progressive leucotomy.* Current Psychiatric Therapies, vol. 3. Grune and Stratton, New York.

FREEMAN W. & WATTS J. W. (1942) *Psychosurgery.* Thomas, Springfield, Illinois.

FREEMAN W. & WATTS J. L. (1947) *J. comp. Neurol.,* **86**, 65.

FULTON J. F. (1949) *Functional Localisation in the Frontal Lobes and Cerebellum.* Clarendon Press, Oxford.

FULTON J. F. (1951) *Frontal Lobotomy and Affective Behaviour.* Chapman and Hall, London.

GRANTHAM E. G. (1951) *J. Neurosurg.,* **8**, 405.

HEATH R. G. & POOL J. L. (1948) *J. nerv. ment. Dis.,* **107**, 411.

KNIGHT G. (1964) *Brit. J. Surg.,* **51**, 114.

LE BEAU J. (1951) *J. ment. Sci.,* **97**, 480.

LE GROS CLARK W. E. & BOGGON R. H. (1933) *Brain,* **56**, 83.

LE GROS CLARK W. E. & MEYER M. (1950) *Brit. med. Bull.,* **6**, 1536.

LEWIN W. (1961) *J. Neurol. Neurosurg. Psychiat.,* **24**, 37.

McKENZIE K. G. & KACZANOWSKI G. (1964) *Canad. med. Ass. J.,* **91**, 1193.

McKISSOCK W. (1951) *Lancet,* **2**, 91.

McLARDY T. (1950) *J. Neurol. Psychiat.,* **13**, 106.

MEYER A. & BECK E. (1954) *Prefrontal Leucotomy and Related Operations.* Oliver and Boyd, Edinburgh.

MEYER A., BECK E. & McLARDY T. (1947) *Brain,* **70**, 18.

MITCHELL-HEGGS N., KELLY D. & RICHARDSON A. E. (1977) In *Neurosurgical Treatment in Psychiatry, Pain and Epilepsy.* pp. 367–80. (Eds. W. H. Sweet, S. Obrador, J. G. Martin-Rodriguez). University Park Press, Baltimore, U.S.A.

MONIZ E. (1930) *Tentatives Operatoires dans le Traitement de Certain Psychoses.* Masson, Paris.

PENFIELD W. (1948) *Res. Publ. Ass. nerv. ment. Dis.,* **27**, 519.

PUUSEPP L. (1937) *G. Accad. Med. Torino,* **100**, 3.

ROBIN A. A. (1959) *J. Neurol. Neurosurg. Psychiat.,* **22**, 132.

SCOVILLE W. J. B. (1949) *J. Neurosurg.,* **6**, 65.

SHERRINGTON C. S. (1906) *The Integrative Action of the Nervous System,* p. 307 (reprinted Camb. Univ. Press 1947).

SMITH W. K. (1944) *Fed. Proc.,* **3**, 42.

STROM-OLSEN R. & TOW P. M. (1949) *Lancet,* **1**, 87.

TOOTH G. C. & NEWTON M. P. (1961) *Leucotomy in England and Wales: 1942–1954.* HMSO, London.

TOW P. M. (1955) *Personality Changes following Frontal Leucotomy.* Oxford University Press, London.

WALL P. D., GLEES P. & FULTON J. F. (1951) *Brain,* **74**, 66.

WARD A. A. (1948) *J. Neurophysiol,* **11**, 13.

WHITE J. C. & SWEET W. H. (1969) *Pain and the Neurosurgeon.* Thomas, Springfield Illinois.

WHITE J. C., SWEET W. H. & HACKET, T. P. (1960) *Arch. Neurol.,* **2**, 317.

WHITTY C. W. M., DUFFIELD J. E., TOW P. M. & CAIRNS H. (1952) *Lancet,* **1**, 475.

YAKOVLEV P. I., HAMLIN H. & SWEET W. H. (1950) *J. Neuropath. exp. Neurol.,* **9**, 250.

# Chapter 20
# Surgery of movement disorders

## J.B. MILES

Operative procedures for the control of involuntary movement occupied much neurosurgical attention in the 1950s and 60s. Great expertise was achieved from the widespread application of stereotaxic techniques for suppressing the shake and the rigidity of Parkinsonism. This expertise was accompanied by considerable equipment development making the technique safe and its application to many other, though perhaps less amenable, involuntary movements was thus justified. The advent of more effective and specific medical treatment for parkinsonism in the 1970s immediately and drastically obviated the need for surgery with the effect that only a very small number of neurosurgeons continued stereotaxy and the number of procedures for all kinds of involuntary movements dropped. Recently, it has been recognized that L-Dopa does not provide the complete answer for all aspects of Parkinsonism. The more florid movement disturbances, particularly shake, are sometimes only poorly suppressed and, increasingly, it is being recognized that a disabling dyskinetic movement of the face and limbs can result from the toxic effects of high dosages of the drug. As a result there has been a gradual revival of interest in thalamotomy for some patients with Parkinson disease, particularly when shake is unilateral and gross, and the patient relatively young.

The involuntary movements and dystonias are a consequence of disease, either of the basal ganglia themselves, or of other cerebral structures having intimate connection with the basal ganglia. With the exception of hemiballismus, the pathology is usually diffuse affecting nuclear concentrations and communicating pathways.

*Athetosis* is a relatively slow movement with a sinuous or writhing character and most easily recognized in the upper limb. The movement is a combination of the involuntary adoption of one or other of two opposing postures. In the one flexor activity predominates: the arm is drawn towards the body, the fingers and wrist flex in supination. The other is characterized by extension and abduction at the shoulder, extension of elbow and wrist with pronation and extension and abduction of digits. In the foot the movements are from flexion of toes to their extension and fanning, with the ankle usually in plantar flexion. In lesser degrees of athetosis the movements are largely restricted to the wrist and fingers; when severe the whole limb is wildly active and in double athetosis both sides are involved. The movements are aggravated by external stimuli and by attempted voluntary action. Denny-Brown (1962a) considered that these two opposed postures to represent exaggerated forms of the basic reactions of exploration and of avoiding. Degeneration is found in the putamen, alone or most severely. The disorder usually arises in childhood.

*Chorea* is characterized by rapid, jerky irrelevant, assymmetrical movements which are irregular in repetition and in amplitude, and in which it may be difficult to detect any pattern. It occurs when the subject is otherwise at rest and during willed movements and then 'produces a typical clownish effect. The patterns of chorea are extremely diverse and bizarre' (Mettler 1967; this paper provides very useful definitive descriptions of all forms of involuntary movement, using the description in its broadest meaning and provides a valuable review of the results of animal experiments designed to reproduce these movements). Denny-Brown (1962a) made the point that in chorea there is a 'continual flow of motion without the irregular alternation that characterizes athetosis'. Posture is lost in a choreiform movement, whereas two or more attitudes can be distinguished in athetosis. The outstanding degenerative changes in chorea are found in the caudate nucleus and in the frontal cortex.

*Hemiballismus*, as its name implies, affects the limbs of one side only and is characterized by irregular proximal flinging movements that tend not to affect the face, that subside in sleep and that seem to be triggered or aggravated by movement of the affected limb. It is not always possible clearly to differentiate between severe hemichorea and hemiballismus (Martin 1967, Mettler 1967).

Hemiballismus is unique amongst the involuntary movement in usually having a sudden onset and also commonly being found to be due to a discrete lesion in or close to the subthalamic nucleus (of Luys). This can be due either to haemorrhage or to infarction. The condition is particularly prone to occur in diabetics. Similar movements have been produced in monkeys by a lesion in the subthalamic nucleus: at least 20% of the nucleus must be destroyed, but excessive destruction of adjacent structures, particularly when provoking hemiplegia, will not be associated with production of the abnormal movement. In some cases the subthalamic nucleus has been found intact and in these cases the lesion is thought to have interrupted the pathways connecting it to the pallidum (Martin 1967).

*Tremor* derives from the rhythmical alternating contractions of opposing groups of muscles. It is commonly divided into two varieties. That which occurs when the limb is at rest is called postural or simple tremor, and is typical of Parkinson disease. The other common variety of tremor is evoked by active movement and is called action or intention tremor and is seen in some cases of multiple sclerosis, or in laterally placed cerebellar lesions.

*Parkinsonian tremor* is of low frequency (between 4 and 8 beats per second). A pill rolling movement between thumb and index finger is classical. The lips and tongue may be involved and although the tremor may be restricted to one side of the body initially, being a generalized disease, there is a tendency for all limbs eventually to be affected. The movement may, at times, become so violent as to rock the bed or even to render the patient into exhaustion.

Parkinsonism may arise as a late sequel of encephalitis lethargica or as a result of cerebral degeneration, whether this be idiopathic or associated with arterial ischaemic disease. Degeneration is found in the globus pallidum and in the subtantia nigra. Smith (1966) considered that degeneration in the substantia nigra was the commonest pathological finding. Loss of pigment and specific neurochemical depletion may be fundamental in the etiology of Parkinson disease (Cotzias 1967).

*Rigidity* of muscles is also a feature of disease of the basal ganglia. In parkinsonism it may prove more disabling than the tremor and as the disease advances tremor tends to diminish with the increase of rigidity. Immobilization by rigidity in a posture of generalized flexion may be the ultimate result; Denny-Brown calls this the 'pallidal' syndrome. The rigidity is described as plastic (lead pipe), for the muscles provide a steady resistance against passive movement; this distinguishes it from the clasp-knife resistance of spasticity in which the stretched muscles suddenly give way as a result of lengthening. Electromyography reveals the essential difference in the reactions to stretch. In spasticity, an increasing number of motor units fire in response to the stretch, in rigidity units cease firing as others become active so that the total number contracting remains about the same. If tremor is present or is evoked in the rigid muscle when stretched, the resistance acquires a jerky quality, the cogwheel phenomenon.

*Dystonia* is the name given to an attitude or posture adopted as a result of maintained muscular rigidity. The abnormal posture may be forcibly corrected (except for soft tissue contracture and joint stiffness) but it immediately returns when the force is removed. In mild parkinsonism, dystonia is commonly seen in the hands; the metacarpophalangeal joints are somewhat flexed and the interphalangeal joints extended (Gortvai 1965), and is often relieved by operation. The terminal pallidal syndrome described above is one of generalized flexor dystonia. Dystonia may occur with lesions causing athetosis and the attitude is of flexion of the upper and extension of the lower limbs; Denny-Brown calls this the hemiplegic posture of the 'striatal syndrome'. The recognition of minor degrees of dystonia is particularly important, as evidence of an organic cause for unusual limp, abnormal habitual posture of a hand and finger which might be otherwise considered 'hysterical' or due to some obscure local lesion. The patient should be watched when walking, wearing only a pelvic triangle, in order that asymmetry and minor involuntary movements can be detected. It is during active movement that the earliest stage of dystonia may be evoked.

*Dystonia musculorum deformans* is a condition in which writhing movements of the trunk and limbs cause slow semipatterned and often grotesque postural distortions primarily of the trunk and head and less frequently of the limbs. There has been a tendency by some to include torticollis, under its title of torsion dystonia, in this group, but so little is known about its aetiology and whether, indeed, there is any evidence of an organic basis, that it is probably unjustified.

*Myoclonus* is defined as exhibiting sudden contractions of muscles or parts of muscles and the more generalized form is most commonly seen after cerebral injury due to hypoxia (Hallet *et al.* 1977). A form of myoclonus particularly precipitated by motor activity is called action myoclonus and is being increasingly recognized as a complication of severe head injury (Andrew *et al.* 1982).

## Physiology

Denny-Brown devoted much study to the physiology of movement and its disintegration as a result of disease. His experiments were based on the Sherringtonian technique of analysis of the reactions and spontaneous activity remaining after section of the neuroaxis at progressively higher anatomical levels, and of destructive lesions and extirpations of basal areas and of the cerebral cortex. In his writings (1962a, 1962b, 1966) he had emphasized the importance of projections from the cerebral cortex to the pallidum and to the striate region. 'The contribution of the Rolandic and pyramidal system to movement provides a more delicate type of projected stereotaxic exploratory reaction for which the extrapyramidal reactions are a necessary substrate' (1966).

Denny-Brown considered chorea and parkinsonian tremor to be closely related to the fundamental disorder athetosis, representing an instability of attitude, a conflict between the coarse antagonistic reflex reactions of exploration and of avoiding which are released by basal ganglia disease. He showed that symmetrical lesions in thalamic nuclei in monkeys abolished either one or other of the basic reaction patterns of grasping and avoiding (1966). No changes in posture occurred however, while thalamic lesions for parkinsonism in man are often followed by an apparent, temporary, difficulty in maintaining posture.

Martin (1967) from an extensive personal experience of postencephalitic parkinsonism describes the clinical phenomena as either positive (rigidity and involuntary movements) or negative (functions lost or defective, such as the poverty of movement called akinesia).

In general, neurosurgical ablative procedures are more likely to benefit the positive features of the disease than the negative. However, even to this rule there are exceptions such as the considerable improvement in facility and strength of, particularly hand movement, that is to be seen after effective reduction in rigidity by thalamotomy.

## Anatomy

The anatomy of the basal ganglia and its connections is complex and only the surgically important features can be mentioned here. The most readable accounts are those of Crosby *et al.* (1962), of Hassler (1959) and of Jung and Hassler (1960).

It is unfortunate that the difficulties in understanding the subject are aggravated by differences in terminology. The cortical areas may be indicated by either Brodmann's or Vogts' terminology. The ventral nuclei of the thalamus (with which neurosurgeons are particularly concerned) are given one set of names in the English language literature, derived largely from the work of Le Gros Clark and Walker, and a different set in the European literature largely based on the work of Hassler. In their study of the thalamic nuclei, Andrew and Watkins (1969) undertook to indicate the limits of variability of these structures, and while their general findings agree most closely with Hassler, there is further modification of the nomenclature. In Table 20.1 are set out what appear to be the equivalent thalamic nuclei

**Table 20.1.** Nomenclature of thalamic nuclei.

| German | English |
| --- | --- |
| Lateropolaris (Lp) | Ventral anterior (VA) |
| Ventro-oral anterior (Voa) | Ventral lateral (basal anterior portion) (VL) |
| Ventro-intermedius (Vim) | Ventral lateral (lateral portion) |
| Ventro-oral posterior (Vop) | Ventral lateral (basal posterior portion) (VL) |
| Ventrocaudal (Vc) (divided into four portions) | Ventral posterior lateral (subdivided) (VPL) |
| | Ventral posterior medial (subdivided) (VPM) |
| | Ventral posterior, inferior (VPI) |

with different names, but identity is said not to be exact. The derivations are from Carpenter (1967), Crosby *et al.* (1962) and Hassler (1959).

The ventral posterior (ventrocaudal) group is at times referred to as the ventrobasal complex; the medial apex (pars parvocellularis) of the ventral posterior medial nucleus corresponds to the nucleus semilunaris.

The nomenclature is also confusing regarding

the basal ganglia which formerly included the thalamus, but now, usually do not. Likewise it is common for the corpus striatum to compromise the caudate nucleus, the putamen and globus pallidus (the last two forming the lenticular or lentiform nucleus). However, Ranson and Clark (1947) label the caudate nucleus and putamen as 'striatum' which becomes the 'corpus' striatum when the pallidum is added. The basal ganglia is now usually meant to include the subthalamic nucleus and the substantia nigra.

The extrapyramidal terminology has little semantic justification as it refers to the descending pathways concerned with the organization or control of muscular movement reaching the spinal cord by a route other than through the medullary pyramids. It implied the absence of association with the pyramidal cells of the cortex, thought incorrectly to be totally responsible for the pyramidal fibre tracts.

Following Martin (1967) the main connections of the basal ganglia can be conveniently grouped as internal, afferent and efferent. Internal fibres link together the caudate and putamen and these with the pallidum, which has strong two-way connections with the subthalamic nucleus and the substantia nigra. Afferent fibres to the corpus striatum come from all parts of the cerebral cortex and in particular from the motor and premotor areas. Other afferents are received from the central median and intralaminar nuclei of the thalamus. The major efferent pathway of the corpus striatum flows from the pallidum, much of it passing to the thalamus in two bundles, the fasciculus lenticularis, comprising fibres which transverse the internal capsule, and the ansa lenticularis which takes a looped medial course anterior and ventral around the internal capsule. The fasciculus is sometimes referred to as the dorsal division of the ansa.

In the subthalamic region, between the caudal boundaries of the thalamus above and the subthalamic and red nuclei below, known as the field of Forel, the fasciculus (H2 bundle of Forel) and the ansa (H1 bundle or thalamic fasciculus) combine to traverse the H field and enter the basal aspect of the thalamus to end in the ventral oral anterior nucleus (Voa). Immediately behind them are the thalamic fibres of the brachium conjuctivum which terminate in the ventral oral posterior (Vop).

In the outflow of the pallidum are reciprocal connections linking the basal ganglia, the red nucleus and the reticular formation. Links with the reticular formation are also provided by the connections from the central median and intralaminar nuclei to the striatum. Several thalamocortical projections are recognized, particularly to the precentral cortex (areas 4 and 6). (Carpenter 1967 gives a clear summary of the connections of the ventral thalamic nuclei). The stated connections remain horribly confusing and their accuracy may still be in question.

Brodal (1963) emphasized three possible circuits:

1 Precentral cortex—striatum—pallidum—thalamic nucleus ventral lateral—precentral cortex
2 Precentral cortex—pons—cerebellar cortex—nucleus dentatus—brachium conjunctivum—thalamic nucleus ventral lateral—precentral cortex
3 Pallidum—subthalamic nucleus—substantia nigra—pallidum

## Evolution of surgical treatment

The early attempts to abolish involuntary movements were directed at the corticospinal motor system, on the grounds that wherever they originated the movements finally depended upon the integrity of these pathways. Excision of the motor cortex was performed on several patients with athetosis by Horsley (1890 and 1909), a clinical application of the newly won knowledge in physiology and further experiences were reported by Bucy and Buchanan (1932). The pyramidal tracts were divided in the cervical spinal cord by Putnam (1940) and Oliver (1949) and in the cerebral peduncle by Walker (1949) and others (Broager 1955, Meyers 1956). In all

these operations a price had to be paid for the relief of unceasing and fatiguing movements in the form of paralysis of varying intensity; in general, a successful result ran parallel with the degree of permanent loss of voluntary power. Such operations were appropriate for only the most severely afflicted patients. A more selective approach was used by Putnam (1933), who restricted the cervical cordotomy to the anterior columns, which was successful for athetosis but not for parkinsonian tremor. Credit must be given to Meyers (1942) for turning his attention to the basal ganglia and its connections; by this he became a forerunner, opening up the field for modern methods. His first operation was carried out in 1939, when a postencephalitic tremor was abolished by excising the anterior two-thirds of the caudate nucleus (Meyers 1940; in the discussion which follows, it was reported that the idea came to Meyers as a result of the observed loss of tremor in a patient after a frontal lobectomy in which the line of resection included part of the caudate nucleus; the discussion includes no denial from Meyers). Other operations were tried and in due course Meyers found that section of the pallidal outflow, ansotomy, was the most effective. These operations were formidable and carried a high mortality rate of about 15%, because they required an osteoplastic craniotomy and intraventricular manipulation; they were performed in 54 patients and included cases illustrating all the chief forms of hyperkinesia (Meyers 1951 contains a full review). The significance of this new approach, in particular to Parkinson disease of which the rigidity was relieved in addition to the tremor, was noted by other surgeons who devised technically easier routes to the pallidal outflow (Fenelon 1950, Guiot & Brion 1953). Concurrent with these developments were the experiences of Cooper. In 1952 during the course of an attempted pedunculotomy for involuntary movements, he experienced severe bleeding and was compelled to occlude the anterior choroidal artery. In an inspired moment he decided to abandon the operation, to await the effects of infarction. The patient recovered and tremor and rigidity were cured. It was assumed that the infarcted area included the pallidum. Thereafter, occlusion of the anterior choroidal artery was frequently performed for parkinsonism, though with unpredictable success, because of the inconstant pattern of vessel distribution (Cooper 1958). These diverse operations established the principle that destruction of the pallidum or its outflow provided a selective method of relieving certain symptoms of basal ganglia disease, but the techniques were crude, uncertain of success and carried too high a mortality.

In the course of his animal experiments on the cerebellum Horsley (Clarke & Horsley 1906) realized that a technique was needed for making small lesions in predetermined sites, in the depths of the brain, of a controllable size, but essential for scientific accuracy was the avoidance of unwanted superficial damage, such as accompanies a preliminary craniotomy. For this purpose he (or Clarke) conceived the brilliant notion that any chosen point in the brain could be precisely related by measurement to three planes perpendicular to one another. By choosing constant positions for the planes, constant relationship to readily identifiable points on the animal's skull and an accurate anatomical atlas of brain and skull, navigational measurements in three planes would identify the position of a deep target within the skull. The three planes chosen were: the midsagittal; the horizontal, lying 10 mm above and parallel to a plane passing through the inferior orbital margins and the middle of the external auditory meatus; the coronal, passing through the midmeatal points perpendicular to the horizontal. These planes provided zeros from which measurements were taken. This stereotaxic (this word was used by Clarke & Horsley 1906) system required for its application an apparatus, rigidly and accurately constructed, which could be fixed to the skull in the horizontal plane, bearing a movable carriage which could lower into the brain, through a small hole in the skull, an appropriate thin instrument, for stimulating the brain electrically or for creating a lesion. The movements available to the instrument were in directions parallel to the

three zero planes and all could be accurately measured. The instrument was a fine example of precision engineering and was the responsibility of Clarke. The classical paper by Horsley and Clarke (1908) in which the system and instruments are fully described and illustrated should be studied by all interested in the subject, as an example of lucid and simple exposition and of thoroughness in solving intricate problems. One of these was the method to be used for creating the deep lesion. The latter was to be small, of controllable size, uncomplicated by distant effects and accompanied by minimal or negligible damage to superficial tissue, particularly cortex. The reason for this lay in the anatomical problem to be solved; to trace the degeneration consequent upon destruction of the cerebellar nuclei and significant amounts of cortical damage might nullify the observations. As a result of critical experiments, anodal electrolysis was chosen, the current being introduced through a fine platinum wire insulated with glass. It is noteworthy that half a century later, the best means of creating a lesion of controllable size and shape are still under discussion (see below).

No apology is necessary for this preoccupation with these creative activities of Horsley, for they constitute an epoch in the development of neurosurgery. It was a remarkable observation by Clarke (1920) when he prophesied that the stereotaxic instrument might be used on humans for the making of lesions in the thalamus in order to relieve pain. Nevertheless, although frequently used in neurophysiological laboratories, a quarter of a century passed before it was suitably modified for operations on the human brain by Spiegel et al. (1947) and then first for the purpose of relieving certain mental disorders by damaging the dorsomedial nucleus of the thalamus. Thereafter, the value of the stereotaxic technique for interrupting deeply situated pathways in the treatment of certain symptoms of basal ganglia disease, of intractable pain and for other purposes was rapidly and widely appreciated.

As already mentioned, a significant lapse has occurred in the use of stereotaxic surgery with the advent of effective pharmacological treatment for involuntary movements, particularly those of parkinsonism. Many of the specialist stereotaxic surgeons have since used the opportunity of applying their skills for the implantation of deep brain electrodes after the usefulness of this technique had been advocated by Richardson and Akil (1977). More recently there is clear evidence of a return of interest in the technique of stereotaxic surgery for the more suitable cases of parkinsonism, namely, young, fit patients with unilateral disease poorly controlled by L-Dopa and usually with a dominance of shake. The recent design of stereotaxic equipment suitable for linking the technique to the investigatory potential of computerized tomography has undoubtedly further promoted stereotaxic surgical approaches (Boetius *et al.* 1980, Roberts & Brown 1980, Thomas *et al.* 1984).

## Stereotaxic systems

No attempt will be made to cover in detail the many instruments designed and the critical bases for their accuracy as details can be found in specialized texts (*Stereotaxy of the Human Brain*, edited by G. Schaltenbrand and A. Earl Walker [1982], *Neurosurgical Treatment in Psychiatry, Pain and Epilepsy*, edited by W. H. Sweet, S. Obrador and J. G. Martin-Rodriguez [1977]). All systems, however, attempt to solve a specific set of problems.

1   The patient should be awake, able to provide information by exploratory stimulation techniques, both to aid the physiological accuracy and to avoid unwanted complications. Local anaesthesia is therefore used. The calibrated apparatus which establishes the space within which the target is to be located, must be rigid and capable of rigid fixation to the skull, yet at the same time be light in weight and as free from psychological threat as possible.

2   Radiographic scrutiny of the frame and the head contained by it involving divergence of rays, either requires specific and often fixed alignment techniques or actually takes advantage of

the divergent phenomenon. (Dawson *et al.* 1969). If computerized tomographic radiography is employed a new set of problems arises, involving radio compatability, tomographic section identification and pixel size (Dervin & Miles 1984).

3   The zeroing for coordinates which, in laboratory animals, were based on the skull have not proved applicable to man.

When axial radiographic scrutiny is used it has been the practice to identify the third ventricle by contrast ventriculography and to use such landmarks as the anterior and posterior commissures or the lateral ventricular foramen. When using computerized tomography, the target is perhaps less distinct, but is probably still preferable to an indirect internal landmark such as the third ventricle.

### Anatomical targeting

It was recognized in the early stages of stereotaxic surgery that human brains showed great individual variability in the size and relative positions of the central structures. This prompted the creation of brain atlases, usually based on fairly small numbers of specimens of normal brain (Spiegel & Wycis 1952, Schaltenbrandt & Bailey 1959, Delmas and Pertuiset 1959, Van Buren and Maccubbin 1962). Variations in size and location of key central structures may be much greater in the diseased human brain (Andrew & Watkins 1969). Care must still be taken in differentiating between the high degree of accuracy theoretically assured by the precision instrumentation and the innate variability in anatomy and function of the individual brain, particularly when diseased.

Physiological targeting with exploratory techniques such as depth EEG recording, electrical stimulation (Hassler *et al.* 1960) and micro-electrode recordings of spontaneous and evoked action potentials (Albe-Fessard *et al.* 1962, 1967, Giuot *et al.* 1962, Gaze *et al.* 1964, Jasper & Bertrand 1966), is widely used. Cryogenic lesion making allows the production of a temporary neurological dysfunction at the target, so that an assessment can be made of the therapeutic effect and any neurological deficit prior to the creation of a permanent lesion.

## Methods of lesion making

Various devices have been invented, and although a spectrum of techniques are still in use, radiofrequency coagulation, appears to many to be the superior. Certain common requirements of the technique are to be considered:

1   The instrument should be thin, but rigid.
2   The lesion should be of predictable and consistent size and shape.
3   There should be minimal surrounding or delayed reaction.
4   The risk to adjacent blood vessels and the subsequent possibility of haemorrhage should be minimal.

'Electrolysis' was used by Horsley and Clarke, later by Spiegel and Wycis (1952) and Spiegel (1966) and was shown to be unpredictable and with a definite haemorrhagic risk by Sweet and Mark (1953). Cutting of the brain by special instruments was undertaken for a limited time. Tissue freezing by liquid nitrogen, with the definite advantage of target production of preliminary, reversible dysfunction at the site was introduced by Cooper (Cooper & Lee 1961), and has had both its critics (Coe & Ommaya 1964) and its supporters (Hankinson 1965, 1969).

'Electrocoagulation' was introduced by Cushing using the diathermy machine designed by Bovey; subsequent studies of the lesions created by lateral coagulation have been made by Wyss (1945), Hunsperger and Wyss (1953), Watkins (1965), Yasargil et al. (1959), Mundinger et al. (1960), Aronow (1960) and Tasker (1980). A widespread conversion to radiofrequency generated heat coagulation has now occurred, and the advantages of this technique in producing a discrete and predictable lesion, particularly when the tip temperature is controlled, have been advocated by Cosman (personal communication) and others (Mundinger et al. 1960).

## Size of lesion

Considerable and fascinating work was undertaken by Smith (1962, 1966, 1967) who studied autopsy specimens of brain obtained from patients with movement disorders treated by stereotaxic surgery and who had died some years later from other causes. She provided many illustrations showing the considerable variation in the size of lesions produced by earlier techniques. In these important studies she showed that despite variations in location of the lesions, good control of tremor could be obtained; the size of the lesion appeared to be as important as its location. A conclusion was reached that $50\,mm^3$ was the minimal size of lesion which would prove effective in controlling tumour. Walsh (1966) considered $60-120\,mm^3$ to be optimal.

## Choice of target

In the early years of stereotaxic surgery for involuntary movements the aim was destruction of the medial part of the contralateral pallidum or closely related ansa lenticularis and, as mentioned earlier, a lesion in this location was found to be less effective against tremor than rigidity. Attention was then directed towards the basal part of the lateral mass of the thalamus. Hassler and Riechert (1954) pointed out that destruction of the thalamic nucleus ventralis–oralis would destroy the terminals of the pallidothalamic fibres and the origins of the thalamic projections to the precentral cortex; Cooper (Cooper & Bravo 1958) had independently noted that large (double) lesions in the vicinity of the pallidum giving good results involved the ventral lateral thalamus. Thereafter, the ventral lateral nucleus (VL) became increasingly the preferred target and remains the usual location for lesions today. Post-mortem findings by Hassler et al. (1965) in a small series of specimens correlated relief of rigidity with a lesion in Voa and Forel's bundle H, and of tremor with a lesion in Vop. Lesions in the centromedian nucleus have also proved effective (Rand *et al.* 1962, Markham *et al.* 1966). Vim has been the preferred target for some other investigators (Narabayashi & Ohye 1978, Andrew 1981).

The internal capsule is closely adjacent to these pallidal and thalamic targets and its implication was at one time feared as likely to cause hemiplegia. The anatomical investigations of Smith (1967) showed that in humans the corticospinal projection lies further back in the posterior limb of the internal capsule than is usually pictured; consequently it generally escapes injury when the aim is pallidum or ventral lateral nucleus, even if the aim is inaccurate or the lesion excessively large. Although in her experience lesions in the neighbouring internal capsule were frequent (and frequent also in the specimens of Norholm & Tygstrup 1963), nevertheless, pyramidal tract involvement, as proven by degeneration studies, was rare (the crucial piece of evidence in her work). Bertrand (1966) plotted the results of electrical stimulation during stereotaxic operations and found pyramidal responses limited to a zone of about 8–9 mm in the middle one-third of the posterior limb of the capsule. Some surgeons have deliberately made lesions in that portion of the capsule adjacent to the pallidum, having found by experience that such involvement improved their results and were unattended by hemiparesis (Guiot *et al.* 1969, Gillingham 1962). The fasciculus lenticularis, part of the pallidal outflow, traverses this portion of the capsule and its destruction may account for the added effectiveness of the capsular lesion.

In recent years surgeons have been exploring the possibilities of lesions immediately ventrocaudal to the thalamus, in the field of Forel (Andy *et al.* 1963, Spiegel *et al.* 1963, Mundinger 1965). In this area are packed both the ansa and the fasciculus lenticularis, shortly before entering the thalamus; thus a small lesion here might more fully interrupt the pallidothalamic pathway

than a larger one in either pallidum or thalamus. Also in this area are dentato- and rubrothalamic links, disconnection of which it was thought might be helpful. Apart from a more effective relief of rigidity and tremor, it was hoped that the drowsiness and psychic disturbances which may follow thalamotomy would be avoided.

Many believe that this target has little advantage over that in the ventral lateral thalamus and also that the incidence of complications such as hemiballismus and ocular motor disturbance from the close proximity of the subthalamic nucleus and the oculomotor nucleus respectively, as reported by Andy *et al.* (1963) and Spiegel *et al.* (1963), militate against safe lesion making in the subthalamic areas.

To recapitulate, lesions may be made in the globus pallidus, in the ansa lenticularis, in the anterior part of the posterior limb of the internal capsule where the fasciculus lenticularis is involved, in the field of Forel interrupting the pallidodentato- and rubrothalamic fibres, or in the ventral anterior and ventral lateral nuclei of the thalamus (Poa, Voa, Vop and Vim). In general, lesions in the nuclei and in the capsule need to be larger than those in the field of Forel. Smith (1967) found that although lesions targeted at the pallidum tend to involve more of the capsule than lesions targeted at the thalamus, it is the latter that is more likely to damage corticospinal fibres, but even then there was no correlation between corticospinal fibre destruction and the success of the operation.

Even more remarkable is the diversity of movement disorders that would appear to be amenable to lesion making in a limited and standard target area. The common factor may be the protection which the lesion affords to the premotor and motor cortex or the interruption of one of the neuronal circuits described by Brodal. Denny-Brown (1962a) felt that the success of ventral lateral thalamotomy depended upon the division of the thalamopallidal connections.

## Indications for operation

*Parkinsonism* has been the condition most commonly treated by stereotaxic procedures; most stereotaxic neurosurgeons 'cut their teeth' in treating this condition, but since the advent of effective pharmacological treatment of many of the generalized features of parkinsonism, a major reduction in the number of patients treated surgically has ensued. Tremor and rigidity have been the symptoms most effectively treated, though oculogyric crises have also proved amenable (Gillingham & Kalyanaram 1965). When rigidity has been a major problem, bradykinesia has been relieved consequent to the reduction of this hypertonia.

Other (negative) features have proved resistant to surgical treatment. These include akinesis, titubation, festination, pro- and retropulsion, drooling, dysphagia and dysphonia. The severity of these features would determine whether they constituted relative or absolute contra-indications to surgery.

The ideal case is a relatively young and otherwise fit patient with unilateral shake and/or rigidity, but patients with these symptoms bilaterally might well benefit from at least a unilateral lesion. Krayenbühl *et al.* (1961) showed that bilateral thalamotomy was both permissible and effective. Bilateral thalamotomies were formerly undertaken often, but the subsequent incidence of aggravation of the 'negative' features have generated a distinct disinclination to make bilateral stereotaxic lesions.

*Intention tremor* whether due to multiple sclerosis or trauma has been less satisfactorily treated possibly due to the associated and widespread disease or injury. *Hemiballismus* has been effectively treated (*see* Results), but debate continues as to the natural history of this condition.

*Athetosis* and *dystonia* due to perinatal or degenerative factors have also been treated with various degrees of success and, in truth, more out of desperation than of enthusiasm.

*Spasmodic torticollis* likewise has gone through a phase of treatment by thalamotomy with distinctly dubious results (Hankinson 1969). The relatively recently recognized condition of post-traumatic action myoclonus is, at present, being actively and effectively treated by thalamotomy (Andrew *et al.* 1982, Bullard & Nashold 1984).

## Results of operation

*Parkinsonism* is a progressive disease affecting wide areas of the deep brain structures and the success obtained by stereotaxic surgery in such patients can be realistically assessed only against the background of the natural history of the disease. Hoehn and Yahr (1967) carefully reviewed a large series of patients with a mean age of onset for the primary form of the disease of 55 years, and 25 years for the encephalitic variety.

Of those with the primary form of parkinsonism, within 5 years of onset one quarter were severely disabled or dead and within 9 years this was so for two-thirds; on the other hand the disease may be so slow in some patients as to take 20 or more years to effect disablement. In a later paper (Hoehn & Yahr 1969) the same authors analysed in detail the effects of operation and the progress of disease in 150 patients observed for a mean postoperative period of 4.4 years. They showed that in 90% of patients, tremor and/or rigidity could be abolished, though one quarter developed recurrence. The success, however, depended mainly on the stage of the disease process at which surgical intervention occurred. In the early stages removal of the unilateral shake might well be associated with a return to complete normality; whereas in a later stage of the disease process, removal of the same feature might afford little change in the capacity of the debilitated patient.

The effectiveness of L-Dopa in relieving some of the 'negative' features of parkinsonism has however resulted in a tendency to delay consideration of surgery for such signs as unilateral shake, which is still optimally to be treated by thalamotomy. With increasing awareness that the dyskinesis associated with L-Dopa over-dosage may prove as embarrassing or disabling as the original symptoms, an increasing number of physicians are now prepared once again to consider surgical intervention as a treatment modality other than as a last resort. Thalamotomy may well allow a reduction of the dosage of L-Dopa and so reduce its overdosage effects and timely thalamotomy can protect the patient from the development of overdosage dyskinesis (Narabayashi *et al.* 1984).

Intention tremor, whether post-traumatic or associated with multiple sclerosis, has been treated with success with stereotaxic surgery by a small number of enthusiasts (Cooper 1960). Most people have experienced less success and a definite tendency to aggravate the incapacity due to extension of neurological deficit. Brice and McLellan (1980) experienced some success in treating intention tremor due to multiple sclerosis by deep brain stimulation and reported the results. However, in subsequent cases they have been unable to recapture the initial success (personal communication).

Hemiballismus was first treated successfully by Martin and McCaul (1959). McCaul (1961) advocated a lesion much larger than that used in parkinsonism, a point also made by Hankinson (1969). There is considerable emphasis amongst those surgeons who have had experience of these rare conditions, that operation should not be deferred too long. The patients are usually elderly, commonly suffer from diabetes mellitus, usually also have generalized vascular disease and they can become physically exhausted by the wild energetic movements. This opinion, however, conflicts with the experience quoted by Hyland and Forman (1957) who reported good resolution of symptoms either spontaneously or by appropriate medication in 12 out of 14 cases. The discrepancy is almost certainly a reflection of the severity of the cases quoted. When the movement is severe and exhausting the likelihood of spontaneous resolution would seem to be low and urgent thalamotomy should be considered. When the movement is only mildly incapacitating it would seem quite appropriate to manage the movement conservatively, allowing time for spontaneous resolution. It is also worth

bearing in mind that anterolateral cordotomy devised by Putnam (1938) might still have a place in the treatment of this disorder if pallidal and/or thalamic lesions prove ineffective (Strain & Perlmutter 1957).

Athetosis and dystonia, unlike other forms of involuntary movement, comprise a distinct category, for they develop for the most part in young people as a result of perinatal damage. The pathological cerebral changes are self limiting, not of a progressive degenerative nature and do not occur when the brain has become the seat of senile and atheromatous changes. In a personal study of 73 cases afflicted by choreo-athetoid 'cerebral palsy' Polani (1959) found a history of severe neonatal jaundice in approximately one half, and of neonatal respiratory difficulties in the others. The abnormal movements made their appearance between the ages of one year and three and a half years. Attempts to abolish athetosis and to relieve dystonia have not met with such a high rate of success as in parkinsonism (Cooper 1965, 70%, Riechert 1962, 40%). It has been found necessary in many cases to make multiple or extensive lesions, sometimes involving pallidum, ventral lateral, ventral posterior lateral, posterior medial and central median nuclei of the thalamus, and the internal capsule. Such extensive lesioning could be tolerated without major deficit only in this relatively young category. Whether such extensive lesions have a specific effect or whether many of the lesions are in nonfunctioning pathological tissue is uncertain. It is also difficult to correlate the results of Cooper (1965) and the size of the lesion he claims to produce, with those of Narabayashi *et al.* (1960), who effected improvement in two thirds of their cases by lesions up to 1 cm in diameter in each pallidum.

Spasmodic torticollis is regarded by some as a local form of dystonia and it has been treated by stereotaxic surgery using pallidal and ventral lateralthalamic lesions. Handa *et al.* (1962) reported 'remarkable' improvement in six out of twelve cases and Cooper (1965) 'excellent' results in a large series. Hankinson (1969), however, expressed the unsatisfactory experience of most neurosurgeons who find little permanent advantage following thalamotomy. A temporary effect is often achieved but this commonly lasts only weeks or months. Cooper (1965) has a large experience of these cases and considers that massive thalamic lesions give the best treatment and that occasional success can even be achieved by a simple unilateral lesion. Perhaps the only justification for considering stereotaxic thalamotomy for this condition is the acknowledged unpredictability of the response to other procedures such as anterior cervical rhizotomy or spinal accessory nerve section (Dandy 1930, Putnam et al. 1949, McKenzie 1955).

Action myoclonus following head trauma is a relatively recently recognized form of involuntary movement, though it seems to be effectively removed by thalamotomy (Andrew et al. 1982, Bullard & Nashold 1984). It is suggested that the traumatic injury is to the region of the red nucleus and that while the jerky aspect of the movement initiated or aggravated by activity can be successfully reduced, other aspects of the overall post-traumatic neuropathology, such as dysarthria, uncoordination or simple tremor, may not be reduced and may even be aggravated (Andrew et al. 1982). One major difficulty in assessing the effect of surgical treatment on this type of movement disorder is that the abnormal movements may vary so much in frequency over time and may even disappear spontaneously.

## Complications and sequelae

Cerebral haemorrhage is probably the commonest cause of death after stereotaxic operation. It probably results from the approximation of the coagulating electrode tip to a vessel with disruption of the vessel when the electrode is withdrawn. A CT scan illustrates very clearly this type of unfortunate complication (Fig. 20.1b). Reduction in the volume of the coagulating electrode tip probably reduces this risk and control of electrode tip temperature is also said to reduce the likelihood of complicating

haemorrhage. Since stereotaxic thalamotomy has ceased to be employed for the more disabled and advanced cases of parkinsonism, postoperative complications of a general nature, such as chest infection, and pulmonary embolism are unlikely to be seen. Also specific complications encountered during the period of enthusiastic surgery for all kinds of parkinsonism, such as dysarthria, dysphagia or pseudobulbar palsy, are unlikely. Akinetic mutism is a complication of pallidal destruction and thought to be similar to that encountered in connection with many different conditions in the vicinity of the third ventricle (Denny-Brown 1962a). It is not produced by the thalamic lesion.

Hemiparesis is the commonest single neurological abnormality, but occurs probably in less than 1%. As a temporary phenomenon it may be due to perifocal oedema, particularly when cryosurgical lesions have been used. Steroid therapy is helpful in these cases.

Hemiballismus is an alarming complication of lesion making in Forel's field. The abnormal movements start usually at the time of operation or immediately afterwards, rarely a day or so later, though in a few cases the onset is thought to have been delayed several years.

They affect the contralateral limbs, usually the upper. The hyperkinesis varies in degree and usually subsides within a week or so and only occasionally are such new formed abnormal movements severe and persistent like the dramatically occurring spontaneous type. Chorea, athetosis, tremor and myoclonic jerks have all been described following thalamotomy. Hughes (1965) recorded a 3% incidence of these surgically precipitated involuntary movements and reviewed the literature. Both of two examples of athetosis and three of four examples of hemiballismus subsided spontaneously within a few weeks. It is generally accepted that it is inadvertent involvement of the subthalamic nucleus that causes the hemiballismus. If further operation appears advisable, a lesion in the ventral lateral thalamus (Vop or Vim), pallidotomy or a lesion in the internal capsule may be undertaken.

For a detailed and numerical analysis of mor-

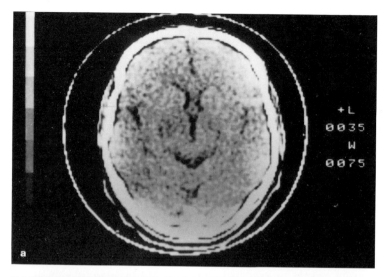

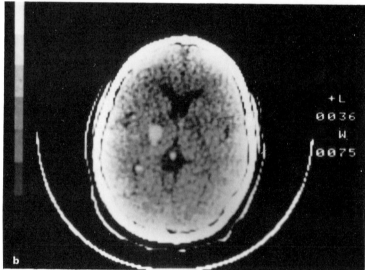

**Fig. 20.1.** Post thalamotomy CT scans showing (a) the expected localized oedema and infarction after a successful and complication free lesion, and (b) a localized intrathalamic haematoma in a patient who suffered a temporary hemiparesis.

tality, morbidity and cause of death in a large series of cases of Parkinson disease treated by cryothalamectomy, see Stellar and Cooper (1968).

## References

ALBE-FESSARD D., ARFEL G., GUIOT G., HARDY J., VOURCH G., HERTZOG E., ALLONARD P. & DEROME P. (1962) *Rev. Neurol.*, **106**, 89.

ALBE-FESSARD D., ARFEL G., GUIOT G., DEROME P. & GUILBAUD G. (1967) *Clin. Neurophysiol.*, **Suppl. 25**, 132.

ANDREW J. & WATKINS E. S. (1969) *A Stereotaxic Atlas of the Human Thalamus and Adjacent Structures.* Williams & Wilkins, Baltimore.

ANDREW J., FOWLER C. J. & HARRISON M. J. G. (1982) *J. Neurol. Neurosurg. Psychiat.*, **45**, 815.

ANDY O. J., JURKO M. F. & SIAS F. R. (1963) *J. Neurosurg.*, **20**, 860.

ARONOW S. (1960) *J. Neurosurg.*, **17**, 431.

BERTRAND G. (1966) *J. Neurosurg.*, **24**, 419.

BOETIUS J., BERGSTROM, M., GREITZ, T. & RIBBET C. T. (1980) *Applied. Neurophysiol.*, **43 (3–5)**, 164.

BRICE J. & McLELLAN L. (1980) Suppression of intention tremor by contingent deep brain stimulation. Lancet I: 1221–1222.

BROAGER B. (1955) *Acta Psychiat. Neurol. Scand.*, **30**, 107.

BRODAL A. (1963) *Acta Neurol. Scand.*, **39**, Suppl. 4, 17.

BUCY P. C. & BUCHANAN D. N. (1932) *Brain*, **55**, 479.

BULLARD D. E. & NASHOLD B. S. (1984) *J. Neurosurg.*, **61**, 316.

CARPENTER, M. B. (1967) In *Modern Trends in Neurology, No. 4*, (Ed. Williams D.) p. 1. Butterworth, London.

CLARKE R. H. (1920) *Johns Hopk. Hosp. Reps, Spec. Vol.*, p. 8. Johns Hopkins Press, Baltimore.

CLARKE R. H. & HORSLEY V. (1906) *Brit. med. J.*, **2**, 1799.

COE J. & OMMAYA A. K. (1964) *J. Neurosurg.*, **21**, 433.

COOPER I. S. (1958) *Proc. roy. Soc. Med.*, **52**, 47.

COOPER I. S. (1960) *New Engl. J. Med.*, **263**, 441.

COOPER I. S. (1965) *J. Neurol. Sci.*, **2**, 520.

COOPER I. S. & BRAVO G. J. (1958) *Neurology*, **8**, 701.

COOPER I. S. & LEE A. ST J. (1961) *J. nerv. ment. Dis.*, **133**, 259.

COTZIAS A. C., VAN WOERT M. H. & SCHIFFER L. M. (1967) *New Engl. J. Med.*, **276**, 374.

CROSBY E. C., HUMPHREY T. & LAVER E. W. (1962) *Correlative Anatomy of the Nervous System*. Macmillan, New York.

DANDY W. E. (1930) *Arch. Surg.*, **20**, 1021.

DAWSON, B. H., DERVIN E. & HEYWOOD O. B. (1969) *J. Neurosurg.*, **31**, 361.

DELMAS A. & PERTUISET B. (1959) *Topometrie Cranio-encephalique chez l'Homme*. Masson, Paris, and Blackwell, Oxford.

DENNY-BROWN D. (1962a) *The Basal Ganglia and their Relation to Disorders of Movement*. Oxford University Press, London.

DENNY-BROWN D. (1962b) *Proc. roy. Soc. Med.*, **55**, 527.

DENNY-BROWN D. (1966) *The Cerebral Control of Movement*. Liverpool University Press, Liverpool.

DERVIN J. & MILES J. B. (1984) *Neurochirurgia*, **27**, 162.

FENELON M. F. (1950) *Rev. Neurol.*, **83**, 437.

GAZE, R. M., GILLINGHAM F. J., KALYANARAM S., PORTER, R. W., DONALDSON A. A. & DONALDSON I. M. C. (1964) *Brain*, **87**, 691.

GILLINGHAM F. J. (1962) *Confin. Neurol.*, **22**, 385.

GILLINGHAM F. J. & KALYANARAM S. (1965) *Confin. Neurol.*, **19**, 237.

GORTVAI P. (1965) *J. Neurol. Neurosurg. Psychiat.*, **26**, 33.

GUIOT G. & BRION S. (1953) *Rev. Neurol.*, **89**, 578.

GUIOT G., HARDY J. & ALBE-FESSARD D. (1962) *Neurochirurgia*, **5**, 1.

HALLETT M., CHADWICK D., ADAM J. & MARSDEN C. D. (1977) *J. Neurol. Neurosurg. Psychiat.*, **40**, 253.

HANDA H., ARAKI C., MORE K., MIZAWA I. & ITO M. (1962) *Confin. Neurol.*, **22**, 393.

HANKINSON J. (1965) *J. Neurol. Neurosurg. Psychiat.*, **28**, 184.

HANKINSON J. (1969) In *Recent Advances in Neurology and Neuropsychiatry*, 8th edn. (Ed. Lord Brain & Wilkinson M.) p. 147. Churchill, London.

HASSLER R. (1959) In *Introduction to Stereotaxic Operations with an Atlas of the Human Brain* (Eds. Schaltenbrandt G. & Bailey P.) vol. 1, p. 230. Thieme, Stuttgart.

HASSLER R. & RIECHERT T (1954) *Nervenarzt*, **25**, 441.

HASSLER R., RIECHERT T., MUNDINGER F., UMBACH W. & GANGLBERGER J. A. (1960) *Brain*, **83**, 337.

HASSLER R., MUNDINGER F. & RIECHERT T. (1965) *Confin. Neurol.*, **26**, 282.

HOEHN M. M. & YAHR M. D. (1967) *Neurology*, **17**, 427.

HOEHN M. M. & YAHR M. D. (1969) In *Third Symposium on Parkinson's Disease*, p. 274. E. S. Livingstone, Edinburgh.

HORSLEY V. (1890) *Brit. med. J.*, **2**, 1286.

HORSLEY V. (1909) *Brit. med. J.*, **2**, 125.

HORSLEY V. & CLARKE R. H. (1908) *Brain*, **31**, 45.

HUGHES B. (1965) *J. Neurol. Neurosurg. Psychiat.*, **28**, 291.

HUNSPERGER R. W. & WYSS O. A. M. (1953) *Helv. physiol. pharmacol. Acta*, **II**, 283.

HYLAND H. H. & FORMAN D. M. (1957) *Neurology*, **7**, 381.

JASPER H. H. & BERTRAND G. (1966) In *The Thalamus* (Eds. Purpura D. P. & Yahr M. D.) p. 365. Columbia University Press, New York.

JUNG R. & HASSLER R. (1960) In *Handbook of Physiology. Section I. Neurophysiology* (Eds. Field J, Magoun H. W. & Hall V. E.) vol. 2, p. 863. Williams & Wilkins, Baltimore.

KRAYENBUHL H., WYSS O. A. M. & YASARGIL M. G. (1961) *J. Neurosurg.*, **18**, 429.

MARKHAM C. H., BROWN W. J. & RAND R. W. (1966) *Arch. Neurol.*, **15**, 480.

MARTIN J. P. (1967) *The Basal Ganglia and Posture*. Pitman Medical, London.

MARTIN J. P. & McCAUL I. (1959) *Brain*, **82**, 104.

McCAUL I. (1961) *Proc. roy. Soc. Med.*, **54**, 378.

McKENZIE K. G. (1955) *Clin. Neurosurg.*, **2**, 37.

METTLER F. A. (1967) In *Neurophysiological Basis of Normal and Abnormal Motor Activities* (eds. Yahr M. D. & Purpura D. P.) p. 445. Raven Press, New York.

MEYERS H. R. (1940) *Arch. Neurol. Psychiat.*, **44**, 455.

MEYERS H. R. (1942) *New York State J. Med.*, **42 (i)**, 317 and 535.

MEYERS H. R. (1951) *Acta Psychiat. Neurol. Scand.*, **Suppl. 67**.

MEYERS R. (1956) *Surg. Forum.*, **6**, 486.

MUNDINGER F. (1965) *Confin. Neurol.*, **26**, 222.

MUNDINGER F., RIECHERT T. & GABRIEL E. (1960) *Zbl. Chirurg.*, **85**, 1051.

NARABAYASHI H. & OHYE C. (1978) *Proc. clin. neurophysiol.*, **5**, 165.

NARABAYASHI H., SHIMAZU H., FUJITA Y., SHIKIBA S., NAGAO T. & NAGAHATA M. (1960) *Neurology*, **10**, 61.

NARABAYASHI H., YOKOCHI F. & YASOICHI N. (1984) *J. Neurol. Neurosurg. Psychiat.*, **47**, 831.

NORHOLM T. & TYGSTRUP I. (1963) *Acta Neurol. Scand.*, **39**, Suppl. 4, 196.

OLIVER L. C. (1949) *Lancet*, **I**, 910.

POLANI P. E. (1959) *Guy's Hosp. Reps.*, **108**, 32.

PUTNAM T. J. (1933) *Arch. Neurol. Psychiat.*, **29**, 504.

PUTNAM T. J. (1938) *Arch. Neurol. Psychiat.*, **39**, 258.

PUTNAM T. J. (1940) *Arch. Neurol. Psychiat.*, **44**, 950.

PUTNAM T. J., HERZ E. & GLASER G. H. (1949) *Arch. Neurol. Psychiat.*, **61**, 240.

RAND R. W., CRANDALL P. H., ADEY W. R., WALTER R. D. & MARKHAM C. H. (1962) *Neurology*, **12**, 154.

RANSON S. W. & CLARK S. L. (1947) *The Anatomy of the Nervous System*, 8th edn. Saunders, Philadelphia.

RICHARDSON D. E. & AKIL H. (1977) *J. Neurosurg.*, **47**, 178.

RIECHERT T. (1962) *Confin. Neurol.*, **22**, 356.

ROBERTS T. S. & BROWN R. (1980) *Appl. Neurophysiol.*, **43** **(3–5)**, 170.

SCHALTENBRANDT E. & BAILEY P. (1959) *Introduction to Stereotaxic Operations with an Atlas of the Human Brain*, 3 vols. Thieme, Stuttgart.

SMITH M. C. (1962) *Brit. med. J.*, **1**, 900.

SMITH M. C. (1966) *J. Neurosurg.*, **25**, part 2, 247.

SMITH M. C. (1967) In *Modern Trends in Neurology, No. 4*, (Ed. Williams D.) p. 21. Butterworth, London.

SPIEGEL E. A. (1966) *J. Neurosurg.*, **24**, 433.

SPIEGEL E. A. & WYCIS H. T. (1952) *Stereoencephalotomy*, part 1. Heinemann, London.

Spiegel A. A., Wycis H. T., Marks M. & Lee A. J. (1947) *Science*, **106**, 34.

Spiegel E. A., Wycis H. T., Szekely E. G., Adams J., Flannagan M. & Baird H. W. (1963) *J. Neurosurg.*, **20**, 871.

Stellar S. & Cooper I. S. (1968) *J. Neurosurg.*, **28**, 459.

Strain A. E. & Perlmutter I. (1957) *J. Neurosurg.*, **14**, 332.

Sweet W. H. & Mark V. H. (1953) *Arch. Neurol. Psychiat.*, **70**, 224.

Thomas D. G., Anderson R. E. & DuBoulay G. H. (1984) *J. Neurol. Neurosurg. Psychiat.*, **47**, 9.

Van Buren J. M. & Maccubbin D. A. (1962) *J. Neurosurg.*, **19**, 811.

Walker A. E. (1949) *Acta Psychiat. Neurol. Scand.*, **24**, 723.

Walsh L. S. (1966) *J. Neurosurg.*, **24**, 440.

Watkins E. S. (1965) *J. Neurosurg.*, **23**, 319.

Wyss O. A. M. (1945) *Helv. physiol. pharmacol. Acta*, **3**, 437.

Yasargil M. D., Wyss O. A. M. & Krayenbuhl H. (1959) *Schweiz. Med. Wochscht.*, **89**, 143.

# Chapter 21
# Compressive and vascular disorders of the spinal cord

G. F. G. FINDLAY

## Introduction

Several forms of pathology, including some vascular lesions, produce their clinical effects by compressing the spinal cord either from without or from within its substance. Spinal cord compression as an aspect of spinal degenerative disease in the cervical and thoracic areas will be discussed in the following chapter.

The clinical manifestations of a tumour (using the term in the broadest sense) affecting the spinal cord are ascribed to the consequences of compression, hence the term 'compression paraplegia'. Increase in the bulk of the lesion inherent in its nature, whether neoplastic, inflammatory, or cystic, will occupy space progressively within the limited capacity of the spinal canal: if the lesion is extramedullary such occupation will be first at the expense only of extradural fat, venous blood volume and cerebrospinal fluid, but later at the expense of the spinal cord. In the early stages the lesion may manifest its presence by the involvement of extramedullary structures, for example the root pain of a neurofibroma or the bone pain of a vertebral metastasis, while the cord is yet uninvolved. If the lesion is intramedullary, manifestations will be from the onset compatible with disturbance of cord function.

The great variety of clinical patterns which are encountered in cases of spinal cord compression show that the processes involved are complex; The use of the word 'compression' may give rise to a naïve notion that the effect is a simple one of nerve dysfunction spreading evenly across the transverse plane of the cord. Factors which will determine the clinical picture include the following:

1   The position of the tumour in the horizontal plane relative to the anatomical components of the spinal cord at that level.
2   The topography of anatomical components.
3   The varying susceptibility to pressure and to ischaemia displayed by white and grey matter and by different fibres within the white matter.
4   The derivation and peculiarities of the blood supply of the spinal cord at that level.
5   The nature of the lesion.
6   The speed of compression.

*1. Position of lesion.* Clinical methods often achieve a considerable degree of accuracy in diagnosing the site of compression, in the transverse plane and in the longitudinal, segmental, level. There is usually some concordance between the site, the anatomical components which are put at risk and the abnormalities of neural function. Pressure on the posterior aspect of the cord is likely to affect first and more severely the posterior columns; on the lateral aspect, ipsilateral spastic weakness from impaired conduction of the subjacent pyramidal tract is often combined with contralateral impairment of perception for pain and for temperature, the Brown–Séquard syndrome; on the anterior aspect of the cord, an early, often transient, symptom may be ataxia of the leg due to interference with spino-cerebellar pathways at a time when weakness is a lesser disability, and hypoalgesia and therm-analgesia may be restricted to more proximal segment for the pathways subserving such function from lumbar and sacral segments lie in the dorsolateral part of the anterior quadrants. These simple patterns become less clearly defined as compression increases because displacement of the cord brings it against the diametrically

opposed dural sheath which exerts counterpressure on the cord with extension of neurological disturbance; later, pressure and
counterpressure mount when the theca is so distended that the bony confines of the spinal canal
are reached. It used to be thought that the ligamentum denticulatum modified the effect of cord
compression by an anteriorly placed tumour, by
limiting the mobility of the cord in an anteroposterior direction and by conducting stress to
the part of the cord to which it is attached,
namely the coronal equator and the closely subjacent pyramid tract (Kahn 1947). The argument in support of such an effect seems
complicated and unconvincing and is invalidated
by the observations of Stoltman and Blackwood
(1966). They found that the ligamentum effectively limits the movement of the cord in its long
axis within the theca, but not at all in the anteriorposterior direction.

It is important to realize that this stylized progression of disorder may be greatly modified by
other factors to be discussed. For example, the
early onset and the frequency with which spastic
weakness is encountered in all forms of compression is probably the result of a selective vulnerability to pressure of large diameter fibres.

2. *Topography.*   Compression arising from within the substance of the cord may be expected
to give rise to a picture of disturbance com-
mensurate with symmetrical centrifugal expansion, modified by the precise point of origin,
direction and speed of growth and its expansile
or invasive characters. These factors appear to
exert a greater influence over the evolutionary
pattern than in extramedullary compression and
probably account for difficulties in achieving an
early clinical diagnosis in some cases. Early
involvement of grey matter and of decussating
spinothalamic pathways may explain the frequency of pain of a particular quality often
termed 'central' and of its regional rather than
segmental distribution, of relatively symmetrical
cuirasse distribution of impairment of pain and
temperature sensibility, and of bilateral involvement of long tracts. When the lesion is in seg-

ments providing the limb outflow its effect upon
the anterior horn cells is detectable as a lower
motor neuron palsy, in company with upper
motor neuron effect upon lower segments. The
former is recognized by the marked muscle
atrophy, flaccidity, absence of tendon reflexes
and muscular fasciculation.

This general correlation of site of compression
with anatomical structure provides an unduly
optimistic view of the ease of clinical diagnosis,
but other factors may modify the clinical evolution. An intramedullary lesion may be relatively silent for many years prior to manifesting
a recognizable neurological deficit; or may
present so rapidly that the lesion could be due to
ischaemia or acute demyelination.

3. *Selective vulnerability to pressure.*   Interruption of axonal conduction by pressure partly
depends upon fibre size; large diameter fibres
are more susceptible (Gasser & Erlanger 1929,
Tarlov 1957). This may account for the dominance of spastic weakness in compression, particularly by extradural lesions and, although
subjectively weakness may be unilateral, careful
examination commonly provides evidence of
abnormality on the apparently healthy side. Grey
matter appears to be more resistant to pressure
than the white matter (McAlhaney & Netsky
1955). The reflection of this is seen in the different effects of extra- and intramedullary tumours
of the cervical and lumbar enlargements. Atrophic flaccid weakness, fasiculation and loss of
tendon reflexes are distinctive characteristics of
intramedullary tumour because of early and
direct involvement of anterior horn cells; such
findings are slight if the lesion is extramedullary,
unless it also involves nerve roots.

4. *Blood supply of the spinal cord.*   The extent to
which changes in the function and structure of
the spinal cord resulting from compression are
actually due to ischaemia is a matter of uncertainty. In contrast to the effect of compression,
the grey matter is more susceptible to hypoxia
than white matter (Krogh 1950). In general,
grey matter is better vascularized than white

matter although to a lesser extent in the thoracic area (Craigie 1972). If circulatory deficiency were a predominant influence in producing the clinical effects of extramedullary compression, this would lead one to expect much greater evidence of anterior horn cell loss than is actually found. Tarlov (1957) concluded from his experiments that the mechanical effects of pressure on the neural structures was all important though he did not deny that anoxia may also play a part. The relative susceptibility of axis cylinders to anoxia was studied by Heinbecker (1929) who found that the smallest diameter fibres are more readily effected than larger; again in contrast to the effects of pressure. The work of Gelfan and Tarlov (1955) suggests that the afferent systems within the spinal cord are more resistant to anoxia than the motor pathways thus perhaps explaining the early appearance of motor weakness.

Although it seems likely that compression is the dominant factor, the rapidity with which physiological cord transection can occur as a terminal event in a more slowly progressing pathology (such as extradural metastasis) certainly suggests that ischaemia can also play an important role.

The anatomy of the spinal vasculature is of an unusual pattern, in both longitudinal and transverse distribution and good accounts are given by Romanes (1965), Djindjian et al. (1969) and Aminoff (1976). The blood supply of certain regions of the cord is particularly at risk from interference by extrinsic lesions and ischaemia induced by pressure may produce remote effects.

The general pattern of the superficial vascular network is fairly constant, consisting of one anterior and two posterior spinal arteries with incremental supplies of blood derived from feeding vessels entering along the segmental roots. There is, however, great individual variation in detail, particularly of the calibres of the three longitudinal arteries at different segments, the number and size of the feeding vessels and the location of those delivering a major contribution of blood. These are most frequently in the lower cervical segment, C6 or C7 and in the lower thoracic or upper lumbar region. The dominant cervical and lumbar tributaries may be derived from the right or left side with equal frequency but in the thoracic region the majority are left sided. Each ventral root is accompanied by a vessel but the majority of these supply only the nerve root. Only between 6 and 10 of these vessels are true radiculomedullary arteries with branches which join the anterior spinal artery (Gillilan 1958). Nevertheless, no radicular vessel should be sacrificed and, if a nerve root has to be divided, its accompanying vessel should be separated and preserved. A more constant feature is the large size of one of the thoracolumbar feeding arteries. This is the artery of Adamkiewicz and its supplies the lumbar enlargement and ascending part of the anterior spinal artery. In 75% of people it enters the canal along the ventral root of T10, T11, or T12 on the left side but occasionally it may enter in the upper lumbar area. When its origin is more rostral, another lower branch will supply the conus and lumbar enlargement (Lazorthes et al. 1966).

The points of entry into the spinal canal of the blood supply and its arrangement on the cord are such that the upper thoracic cord around D4 possesses the most precarious blood supply, lying in a vascular boundary zone between areas supplied by feeders coming rostrally from the branches of the subclavian artery and caudally from the descending aorta. An unexpected paraplegia may follow aortic surgery or cardiac arrest and is presumably due to profound local ischaemia in these boundary areas.

Wasting of the intrinsic muscles of the hands may be encounted in compressive lesions of the cervical cord situated at levels higher than the segment which innervates those muscles (T1) and has even been observed in foramen magnum tumours (Symonds & Meadows 1937). This false localizing sign is attributed to ischaemia of the anterior spinal artery or an important radicular artery. Similarly, pressure on the artery of Adamkiewicz or other large feeding vessel in the lower end of the spinal canal may give rise to signs of a cord lesion at a level too high or too low and of a distribution discrepant with the tentative diagnosis.

The final distribution of blood is by two systems, superficial and deep. The superficial network is made up of fine branches from the anterior and posterior spinal arteries which pass transversely around and ramify on the surface of the cord, irrigating a collar of superficial fibres. The deep circulation depends upon the sulcal arteries, branches given off from the anterior spinal artery as it lies on the anterior sulcus of the cord. The sulcal arteries enter the cord through the sulcus and turn to either side to supply one half of the central core; they rarely divide to supply both sides. Their territory includes the anterior and central part of the grey matter and the deeper parts of the long tracts including the pyramidal fibres. These important deep branches are most numerous in the cervical and lumbar enlargements, where they may number 3–7 per centimeter length of cord. In the thoracic segment they are sparse, 1–2 per centimeter (Lazorthes 1962). The tips of the posterior horns and a varying extent of the posterior columns are supplied by penetrating branches of the posterior spinal arteries. Pressure upon the anterior aspect of the cord, by restricting the blood flow through the anterior spinal artery or its sulcal branches may play a part in the production of pyramidal damage and evoking lower motor neuron damage. This mechanism has been held responsible for the severe signs of myelopathy in some cases of cervical spondylosis in which postmortem examination reveals a distribution of cord degeneration compatible with such an ischaemic origin. However, in experimental work on the effect of anterior extradural masses, Doppman and Girton (1976) showed the anterior spinal artery to be somewhat resistant to occlusion by pressure and the first vascular event which they identified was occlusion of the posterior spinal veins. The removal of anteriorly placed compressing lesions via a posterior approach carries a grave risk of inflicting severe and often permanent damage on the spinal cord. This is partly explained by the difficulty of access and by mobilization of the already compressed

cord; but the proximity of the lesion to the anterior spinal artery makes this structure highly vulnerable. In addition, the thoracic vascular boundary zones make anterior lesions, such as protruded thoracic disc, even more dangerous to approach by laminectomy and the modern trend towards anterior spinal approaches for anterior disease has done much to lower morbidity. The rich anastomosis of vessels on the anterolateral surface of the vertebral bodies allows the safe ligation of segmental vessels during such anterior surgery as they arise from the aorta but coagulation of a vessel within the intervertebral foramen itself is more dangerous.

5. *Character of the compressing lesion.* Although so many factors influence the clinical picture that generalizations based on individual cases are liable to be misleading, it seems likely that the consistency of the indenting mass is of importance, related as this is to its rate of expansion. At comparable sizes, a hard lump such as a disc protrusion or a tough meningioma tends to produce more pronounced neurological deficit than a soft tumour or a cyst. Intramedullary gliomas greatly vary in their effects; as with the cerebral gliomas their increase in size may be expansive or invasive. Slowly growing ependymomas compress the surrounding cord tissue and may cause little disability for a long time and may closely mimic extramedullary compression. Even the character of extradural tumours is of importance as it is recognized that cord compression due to certain metastases, especially lung, carries a worse prognosis with respect to recovery of neurological function following threapy (Black 1979, Constans *et al.* 1983).

6. *Speed of compression.* In general, the more rapid the rate of compression, the more intense are the effects on neurological function. Stages of neurological deficit coalesce so that a clear evolutionary picture cannot be discerned. In extradural spinal abscess, total physiological cord transection may develop in a few hours. With such rapid compression there is a greater liability to concomitant vascular occlusion,

because no opportunity is given for accommodation. The damage sustained by the cord in traumatic paraplegia from a fracture dislocation of the spine, may be regarded as compression with a time course shortened to fractions of a second. The effect on the cord is that of disruption of its elements. On the other hand compression which develops over the course of months and years provides an opportunity for the cord to be slowly displaced, deformed and flattened while retaining neuronal activity to a remarkable degree. Presumably the blood vessels in that portion of the cord also accommodate to the abnormal anatomy. The obverse of these facts is that, again in general, neurological recovery of much greater degree can be anticipated when the time course of compression has been slow. A severe or even total neurological deficit, if produced over a long time, can still be compatible with full recovery after decompression.

## Pathophysiology of the compressed spinal cord

Little progress has been made in understanding the apparent anomalies which occur in spinal cord compression. Established total paraplegia mitigates against recovery, yet this can occur if the time scale of the compression has been slow, even when the spinal cord has been reduced to a distorted ribbon of tissue. In rapid compression the cord at operation may seem grossly normal yet little recovery occurs.

Purves-Stewart & Riddoch (1923) studied 106 cases of compression of the cord. They noted that the microscopic changes might be relatively slight even when paraplegia had been severe. Slight changes comprised perivascular cellular infiltration and obliteration of the Virchow–Robin space with little evidence of oedema. In severe cases there were areas of necrosis which they consider corresponded to the distribution of pial or radicular arteries which had been obliterated. In the grey matter there were degenerate nerve cells; in the white matter the myelin was oedematous, axis cylinders were destroyed and

glial cells had proliferated. These changes were more marked near the site of compression. The leptomeninges were thickened, veins distended and the walls of veins and capillaries were thickened. They observed that degeneration in descending tracts was more severe than in the ascending tracts but less than the degree of paresis might warrant. They further suggest that the recoverable structural change corresponded to myelin damage and debated whether this was a simple effect of mechanical pressure but concluded that a nutritional disturbance resulting from interference with circulation was more important. On the arterial side they thought this followed occlusion of terminal vessels rather than segmental: areas of necrosis corresponded to this pattern and small vessels were found to be obliterated. They also considered that venous congestion played an important part in damaging the nutrition of the cord below the lesion.

McAlhany and Netsky (1955) examined 19 specimens of compressed cord. They noted similar changes, more marked in the white than the grey matter. The interest of their studies lies in the distribution of white matter damage which they observed. Demyelination or necrosis occurred in small scattered foci, bands or wedges or larger confluent areas. Necrotic areas were deemed infarcts and in these areas blood vessels were collapsed though none were thrombosed; radicular and sulcal arteries were patent. Infarcts were rare in the grey matter. They emphasized the disparity in the degrees of damage noted in the anterior columns, compared with that in the lateral and posterior; there was always a relative sparing of the anterior columns, even when the compressing agent was anterior to the cord. They wondered whether the anterior sulcus gave a measure of protection, its structure acting as a support. (An alternative explanation might be the greater resistance to compression of fibres of small diameter, of which the anterior columns contain a higher proportion than elsewhere).

Tarlov (1957) studied the effects of experimental compression and extrapolated the changes to the human. Although certain features of the experimental material were dissimilar to human pathological material, several microscopic features similar to human changes were produced. They consisted of: swelling of myelin sheaths above and below the point of compression; later myelin breakdown and Wallerian degeneration of the axons; cavitation and haemorrhagic extravasation in cases subjected to more severe and lengthier compression.

It is probably a mistake to attempt to isolate the causal factors of mechanical and vascular disturbance, since it is inconceivable that long standing pressure will not affect the nutrition of nervous tissue. The use of the word 'nutrition' by Purves–Stewart and Riddoch emphasized the fact that, although blood vessels may not be obliterated, nevertheless free diffusion of essential requirements through the compressed tissue is probably hindered. Sufficient evidence is available to show that vascular obstruction, arteriolar and venous, indubitably plays an important role in acute compression, in lesions of inflammatory nature, and in long standing cases.

The experimental work of Doppman and Girton (1976) suggested that there was indeed microcirculatory failure within a compressed segment of the cord. However, mechanical pressure is responsible for the deformity, the approximation of nerve fibres and myeline sheaths, and for the shrinkage of the bulk of the cord. This apparent loss of cord substance must be a late event as Ushio *et al.* (1977) have shown that extradural compression induces oedema in the cord, probably of vasogenic type. The oedema involves primarily white matter, though grey matter eventually becomes involved in the swelling process which can eventually lead to diminished blood supply within the affected areas. It is likely that it is only following the breakdown of myelin and its removal that the loss of bulk within the cord occurs. The possible disturbance of conduction in the nerve fibre due to deformity, loss of water, narrowing of myelin sheath (all functions of abnormal focal pressure) and whether they interfere with ion changes across the axon membrane are conjectural. That axis cylinder disruption within the central nervous system and permanent interruption of con-

duction may be equated is axiomatic. Apart from the nonspecific changes of congestion and cellular reaction, alterations in the myelin sheath varying from narrowing, swelling and interruption to dissolution, provide the other clue. Is demyelination alone sufficient to interrupt conduction? Is failure of conduction due to an accompanying injury to the axon which is not shown by current histological techniques? Is demyelination recoverable? Answers to these questions would correlate the degrees of cord damage with potential for clinical recovery.

In the early part of this century, Purves–Stewart and Riddoch put forward the suggestion that the recoverable element in compressive lesions corresponded to areas of myelin damage. McDonald and Sears (1970) established a technique by which they were able to create discrete areas of demyelination in the posterior columns of cats by direct application of diphtheria toxin; the damage to axons being minimal. They confirmed that loss of myelin completely blocked conduction in large lesions and that, in smaller lesions, conduction velocity was reduced, the refractory period prolonged and there was an inability to transmit high frequency trains of impulses. They thought that the latter abnormality might be important in the genesis of symptoms such as increasing weakness during exercise. Alteration in the temporal sequence of arrival of stimuli along diverse fibre systems must greatly disorganise integration and the pattern of stimuli subsequently dispatched. This may account for some neurological disturbances, for instance on the afferent side, paraesthesiae, dysaesthesiae and central pain. Proof that remyelination can occur in the spinal cord has been produced by Harrison *et al.* (1970) but the completeness and time-course of such recovery remain unclear.

Recovery from cord compression and indeed from all central nervous lesions is greatly influenced by the state of physical health. Sepsis, from urinary tract infection or from decubitus ulceration, dehydration and electrolyte disturbances, anaemia, tissue wasting, low plasma proteins, all postpone or delay neurological recovery. In addition, acute infection or development of a pressure sore can cause deterioration of neurological function; with resolution of the infection, progress is resumed.

Some prognostic significance has been attached in the past to the state of muscular tone: the opinion has been held that a flaccid spinal paralysis is less likely to improve than one which is spastic. This belief takes no account of the causes of flaccidity. Flaccid palsy may be due to involvement of the lower motor neuron in the lesion and so far as this is the result of damage or death of anterior horn cells prognosis is poor; this is well exemplified by the central damage which may occur in injury to the cervical spine and in the lesions of the lumbar enlargement. If due to damage to the peripheral axon recovery may occur. In acute cord compression such as occurs with collapse of a diseased vertebra, flaccidity is evidence of spinal shock which may endure for days and until it passes voluntary movement is unable to develop. Immediately after the removal of a spinal tumour, pre-existing spasticity may be replaced by flaccidity for a few days, also the results of a transient degree of spinal shock. The factors mentioned above which militate against recovery also contribute to flaccidity as part of the depression of neuronal activity. Correction of these disorders will promote the natural processes of recovery. In some respects therefore the passing of flaccidity is a good omen, denoting a reassertion of nervous activity, whether of a normal kind (voluntary movement), or with abnormal consequences (reflex movement and spasticity). Misinterpretation of flaccidity in a patient with acute cord compression may cause diagnostic confusion because of the erroneous assumption that the presence of a lower motor neuron sign such as flaccidity implies that the lesion cannot be located within the spinal cord.

## Aetiology of compression

Many different types of lesion can cause compression of the spinal cord and nerve roots. The following broad classes of pathology may be implicated:

1   neoplasms: intradural, extradural, vertebral
2   cystic: congenital, meningeal, parasitic
3   infective: acute, chronic
4   spinal deformity and Paget disease
5   vascular lesions
6   degenerative disease in cervical and thoracic areas (Chapter 22)
7   Inflammatory: rheumatoid arthritis in cervical spine (Chapter 22)

A simple method of classifying these lesions is to study the relationship which they bear to the various compartments within the spinal canal, and this has practical surgical implications: *extradural*, including tumours arising from the vertebrae or entering the canal through the intervertebral foramina; *intradural*, but extrinsic to the cord and *intramedullary*, arising within the spinal cord.

The relative frequency with which these various groups present varies for reasons as diverse as geographical situation and local referral policy. With regard to spinal neoplasia, Percy *et al.* (1972) estimated the annual incidence of spinal cord tumours to be 1.3 cases per year per 100,000 people as compared to an incidence of 12.5 for primary brain tumours. Sloof *et al.* (1964) found that over 50% of the patients in their extensive series had benign extramedullary tumours but they excluded all metastatic and vertebral tumours, which in everyday practice account for the majority of spinal neoplastic lesions. Glioma is the commonest childhood intraspinal tumour; the next commonest lesion being dermoid cyst. However, spinal cysts of clinical importance are rare, as is spinal compression from deformity or Paget disease. Spondylotic disease of the spine (to be discussed in the following chapter) is widespread, but severe myelopathy due to it is less common. Tuberculous and bacterial osteitis associated with spinal compression is common in many areas and occurs in western practice.

## Symptoms and signs

A general clinical syndrome can be discerned when the spinal cord is compressed by a tumour or other expanding process. Early symptoms may arise from the involvement of structures other than the spinal cord itself, for instance the bone pain of a metastasis, the root pain of a neurofibroma on a thoracic nerve root, the 'sciatica' of a tumour of the filum terminale: the neurological disturbances of an angiomatous malformation may be due to ischaemia from an arteriovenous shunt. For the sake of simplicity such symptoms are included in the pattern of the syndrome; special or distinguishing features will be considered as they arise.

The symptoms and signs of a spinal tumour originate in one of two ways: firstly from the disordered function of the segment (or segments) directly involved; and, secondly from the disorder of function of the spinal cord below this level, that is from the (relatively) isolated portion of the cord. Successful diagnosis depends upon their recognition and upon their correct interpretation in terms of the two groups of disorder. They are considered under the headings of sensory and motor.

## Segmental sensory disturbances

Pain is the commonest first symptom and it is unusual for compression to evolve entirely without pain. Various types of pain can be distinguished and some are reliable indicators for localization.

1. *Pain of spinal root origin* is described as shooting, stabbing, burning, electric shocks, the epithets indicating its severity, its repetitive nature and its tendency to radiate. The distribution of the pain conforms to that of a spinal root, partially or wholly and one or more roots may be involved although at first unilateral. Pain may be projected to a digit, or area of skin or group of muscles. In the latter cases the pain may have a peculiarly intense and nauseating quality and tends to be long lasting; it is notice-

able in the pain associated with root compression from disc protrusions and spondylosis. An important symptom is aggravation of the pain by coughing and other forms of straining and by changes in the position of the vertebral column; in some positions the pain may noticeably be less. The skin and deep tissues in the distribution of the pain are often sore to touch and to pressure. The recognition of pain of radicular origin is of great importance for diagnosis; its correct anatomical interpretation provides the best clinical evidence of localization. When pain is absent, perhaps after a severe bout, there may be paraesthesia in the affected areas, consisting of subjective numbness, tingling, or a sensation of 'pins and needles'.

2. *Pain with quite different characteristics arises from disturbed function within the spinal segment.* It is more continuing, less paroxysmal, often described with difficulty and of an aching, dull or burning nature; it may be of a severity equalling radicular 'neuralgia', but uninfluenced by straining and movement of the spine. The distribution of the pain is not strictly radicular but is more widespread. It may conform to a region affecting part or whole of a limb, to one side of the body including its limbs, or to the whole body below the affected level. The wide diffusion of the pain and its remote occurrence, for example in a lower limb from a cervical lesion may mislead with regard to level and to longitudinal extent. Although the reference of the pain is dependent upon the anatomy of the spinal pathways, it originates from the diseased segment(s). It is encountered in both intra- and extramedullary tumours. The pain is termed 'central' and has much in common with the spontaneous pain of thalamic lesions. Compressing lesions in the thoracic portion of the spinal canal are liable to produce pain or unpleasant paraesthesiae as a band around the trunk, so-called girdle pain. The description sometimes makes it clear that this is radicular in origin: at other times the abnormal sensation appears to be segmental. A symptom which is of segmental origin is the sudden occurrence of tingling and widespread paraesthesia evoked by extremes of flexion or extension of the

neck and rapidly radiating from the region down through the body perhaps to the extremities of all limbs. It was described by Lhermitte (1934) and named after him, although it had been recorded earlier by Babinski and Dubois (1918).

3. *Pain of a third variety can be distinguished and is of spinal origin.* It is located in or about the vertebral column, on one or both sides, generally of a dull quality, continuous and of variable degree. Not infrequently there is slight tenderness of the area affected and percussion of the spinous processes may show localization to one vertebra. The pain may or may not respond to change in posture. Intense pain is more likely to be a signal of bony pathology, especially infection, but severe and prolonged lumbar pain without objective signs has been encountered in large ependymomas of the cauda equina.

Although the symptoms evoked by pressure upon a single sensory root may be pronounced, often there is little or no objective abnormality. Owing to the overlapping of dermatomes, the extent and degree of impairment of cutaneous sensibility is slight and may be difficult to identify. In these circumstances it may be possible to demonstrate defects of discriminative sensibility; for instance two-point discrimination and awareness of the lightest of touches may be impaired in a digit in root compression by a prolapsed disc, when sensation in the limb is otherwise intact. The development of a clear cut area of anaesthesia and analgesia of radicular pattern will occur when the tumour is large enough to interfere with the adjacent nerve roots or cord segment above and below. Impairment of joint position sense also requires dysfunction of more than one root. As opposed to loss of cutaneous sensibility, it may be possible to define hyperaesthesia and hyperalgesia in the appropriate dermatome.

### Sensory disturbances arising in the spinal cord

These arise as a result of interference with the conduction of the ascending pathways. Some neurologists place central pain in this category but such a positive reaction is more easily understood if it is regarded as a segmental disturbance, as described above. Impaired conduction may be manifest as a loss of feeling, numbness, sense of 'walking on cotton wool'. Appreciation of heat and cold may be impaired so that the patient may burn a finger without feeling the pain, or the heat of bath water may be felt with one foot but not with the other. The sense of temperature may be perverted, cold or heat provoking an excessive and painful response. Complaint of lack of knowledge of the whereabouts of a foot when walking, of ataxia particularly in the dark, suggests loss of postural sensibility. Loss of pelvic sensation may reveal itself as an unawareness of a full bladder or rectum and a lack of the sensation of the passage of urine and of faeces. These sensory deficits are usually coupled with disturbed sphincter control.

The abnormal signs which develop will depend upon the degree to which the various columns of ascending fibres are affected. Predominant involvement of the dorsal columns shows itself by impairment of touch, joint position and vibration sense, two-point discrimination and stereognosis; involvement of the anterolateral columns by impairment of pain and of temperature sensibility, other forms of cutaneous sensibility being preserved, a state of 'dissociated' sensory loss. The intensity and the pattern of these sensory deficits are determined by the degree of interruption of conduction and its extent in the transverse plane of the spinal cord. In the early stages of compression the deficits may be slight and misleading because they reveal disturbed function only in the parts of the cord remote from the lesion, that is to say at low level. Later the levels rise and provide an accurate indicator. At the upper margin of analgesia, which is usually most accurately determined by lightly dragging the point of a pin upwards over the trunk from the numb to the normal area, a zone of hyperalgesia may be detected which is a reliable sign of the segmental level of the lesion.

## Segmental motor disturbances

In contrast to the pain of a root lesion, muscular weakness usually appears relatively late. Muscles, like dermatomes, receive an overlapping innervation; nevertheless from the cervical and the lumbosacral enlargements certain roots arise which are predominant in the muscle groups which they supply. Analysis of the weak movement will identify the root affected. Extension of the compression to more than one root and to the cord so that the anterior horn is involved accentuates the weakness. Whether root or grey matter is affected, the weakness has the characteristics of a lower motor neuron lesion and it is important for the diagnosis that this is recognized and distinguished from the effects of an upper motor neuron lesion. Muscle tone is flaccid, wasting is marked, the appropriate tendon reflex is diminished or destroyed, and fasciculation occurs. When a mixed upper and lower motor neuron lesion is present the loss of the tendon reflex and the identification of muscular fasciculation enables one to be certain that lower motor neurons are involved thus indicating segmental (i.e. root or anterior horn) damage. In the absence of root pain and when cutaneous sensory loss is slight, the sign of lower motor neuron damage may be the clinical evidence of the longitudinal level of the lesion and the number of segments through which it extends. Owing to the great development and functional complexity of the limb muscles, a careful search will usually reveal such signs if the lesion involves the cervical or the lumbosacral enlargements. By contrast segmental motor disturbance is difficult to detect with lesions above C5 and between T1 and L1. Slowly growing lesions within these areas may remain undiagnosed for a long time, perhaps being erroneously diagnosed as disseminated sclerosis or hysteria. If compression involves the second and third sacral segments or nerve roots, micturition is affected. The bladder detrusor is paralysed and distends; retention is accompanied by overflow incontinence, a frequent or constant dribbling of urine. The reflexes of the sexual

orgasm are also destroyed. Faecal incontinence may occur.

## Motor disturbances arising in the spinal cord

These arise below (caudal to) the lesion as a consequence of interruption of descending pathways; they reflect the distorted function of a partially isolated cord. The legs are first affected. The patient complains of stiffness of the muscles, often more noticeable or more disabling than the weakness which gradually develops. There is difficulty in mounting and descending steps, in folding the legs to sit down, catching the feet and stumbling, ataxia and unsteadiness. In the upper limbs movements are difficult to perform because of weakness, stiffness, clumsiness and slowness. Trembling may be mentioned, which proves to be clonus and the legs may involuntarily stiffen or bend or jump, often with cramp like pains. Undue local fatiguability may be noticed before weakness is appreciated. Micturition is affected sooner or later but only when both sides of the cord are compressed. Normal control depends upon an unconscious, or when the urge to micturate is marked, upon a conscious and willed, inhibition of the reflex mechanism of bladder evacuation; voluntary micturition abolishes inhibition of the reflex. Interference with descending pathways of control shows itself as a difficulty in starting the act, precipitancy owing to the brevity of warning and episodes of incontinence due to automatic evacuation. Sometimes disturbance ends in acute retention but more commonly in the gradual release of an automatic bladder in which the patient cannot control the expulsion of urine when the intrevesical pressure reaches a certain level, so called 'overflow incontinence'. Sufficient intravasical pressure may be suddenly attained by alterations in abdominal pressure as a result of coughing or changing position and the reflex may also be excited by the sensory stimulation of areas served by the 'isolated' cord. The effect on bowel activity is usually severe constipation though if the motion is loosened by the use of an aperient or as a result of mucosal irritation by faecal impaction, an incontinent action occurs. Reflex penile erection and ejaculation may develop, in contra-distinction to their abolition when the lesion directly involves the midsacral segments or roots.

## Regional diagnosis

The features of diagnostic importance in compression in certain spinal regions will be emphasized.

### Cervical

The first and second segments may be involved in tumours straddling the foramen magnum. Tumours caudal to this level but rostral to the cervical enlargement may be difficult to detect. Pain is in the nape of the neck and occipital region and is commonly aggravated by movement of the head which may compel the patient to hold the head stiffly awry, resisting passive movement. This is particularly common in children. Muscular wasting of the suboccipital muscles is not apparent unless unilateral but weakness of shoulder elevation may be present. Involvement of the fourth segment may affect the main contribution to the phrenic nerve; only bilateral phrenic paralysis is likely to be detected clinically and radiological examination of the diaphragm is more reliable. Impairment of sensation in the trigeminal area may be encountered in high cervical tumours, due to involvement of the descending (spinal) root and pain, simulating trigeminal neuralgia, has been reported (Webb et al. 1953). Nystagmus may also occur, but its mechanism is unknown. Tenderness of spinous or transverse processes is a useful localizing sign. The sensory level to pin prick in high lesions may be posteriorly above the occiput and anteriorly along the margin of the mandible, at the junction of the second cervical dermatome and the trigeminal field. Lower levels run around the neck at collar level; the lower border of C4 passes across the acromion process and down over the chest anteriorly to the second intercostal space, where it adjoins that of T2, but may extend to the nipple line. In the early stages, spastic weakness usually affects only the legs but in the arms all the tendon jerks are likely to be exaggerated. Later the complete picture of spastic quadriparesis emerges. If the lesion extends downwards with involvement of C5 and C6 segments the biceps jerk will be abolished; such an isolated sign reliably indicates the lower extent of the lesion.

Tumours compressing the cervical enlargement or its roots usually provide conspicuous symptoms and signs, partly because the enlargement occupies proportionately more space in the spinal canal and partly because of the highly organized function of the upper limb. The longitudinal display of sensory and motor function facilitates their neurological analysis. Radicular pain is recognized if the description is accurate and its anatomical localization is readily identified if the patient is made to trace its course with a finger. Muscular pain and tenderness is usual when nerve roots are affected; this is noticeable not only in the limb muscles but also in the posterior scapular muscles, particularly medial to the vertebral border in C6 and C7 lesions. Muscular weakness is flaccid, atrophic, fasciculating and restricted to a pattern determined by root distribution, in contradistinction to spastic weakness which affects the limb diffusely and does not cause wasting. Changes in the tendon jerks are important, for the reflex is abolished if the relevant root or segment is involved and those dependant upon the segment immediately below are increased. Thus the biceps jerk may be abolished and the triceps increased; or the triceps lost and finger jerks all exaggerated. Weakness and wasting of the intrinsic muscles of the hand may occur as a result of pressure on the cord at a higher level; as mentioned earlier it is thought to be a remote ischaemic effect on the anterior horn cells. Horner syndrome due to interruption of the cervical sympathetic outflow may be observed in tumours at the cervicothoracic junction. The causes may be an intramedullary lesion blocking the anterior horn cells of spinal nerves of T1 and T2, or an extraspinal extension of tumour blocking the stellate ganglion, the rami communicantes or their upward extension.

**Thoracic**

Pain is the most important symptom, whether of root, central or spinal variety. It calls for relief which cannot be effective without accurate diagnosis of the cause and in slowly growing tumours it may be the only symptom or disability until the emergence of spastic paraparesis. Without pain, segmental evidence of progressive compression may be absent, slight, or overlooked and the spastic weakness is attributed to a degenerative process. Focal wasting and weakness cannot readily be detected in the intercostal muscles though lesions extending over several segments may produce such weakness of the paraspinal muscles that a paralytic scoliosis ensues, especially in children. Abdominal reflexes may be difficult to elicit in the obese and in those with lax abdominal muscles. They are lost when the lesion is above T6 as a part of the abnormal activity of the 'isolated cord'; also as a result of lower motor neuron damage at lower levels between T6 and T12. The evidence of compression and of its level is more solid when cutaneous sensory impairment is manifest, often more easily demonstrable on the trunk than on the limb, owing to the regular band-like arrangements of the dermatomes which facilitates testing by dragged pin-point. It should be noted that C4 dermatome is contiguous with T2 over the front of the chest and that T2 and T3 send tail-like prolongations into the axilla. The nipples lie within the fourth, and the umbilicus within the tenth, thoracic dermatomes.

**Lumbosacral**

As in the lower cervical region and for similar reasons, the symptoms and signs are usually conspicuous and their anatomical analysis straightforward. In addition to pain of radicular distribution, which as a consequence of the crowding together of nerve roots may have a multiple origin, pain in the back may be severe. In part this is due to the frequency of large tumours which expand the spinal canal, to the bodyweight and transmission of mechanical stresses. The elongated distribution of the dermatomes down the leg is such that L1 lies just below the inguinal ligament, L3 includes the front of the knee, L5 most of the dorsum of the foot except the lateral border which is S1 territory together with most of the sole and all the heel. The saddle area and perineum are supplied by the lower sacral segments, S2 sending a narrow band of varying width down the back of the thigh on to the calf. The muscles moving the hip-joint receive a rather broad motor innervation, the flexors from upper lumbar and the extensors from upper sacral roots. The third lumbar root is of particular importance for the quadriceps extensor and its impairment will abolish the knee jerk; L4 for inversion and L5 for eversion and dorsiflexion of the foot; standing tip-toe, and plantar flexion of the toes, foot and ankle all require an intact S1 supply. The ankle jerk is lost in S1 lesions. The hamstrings also depend heavily upon S1.

**Cauda equina**

Compression of the cauda equina may offer difficulty in localization. Since the lesion lies below the termination of the spinal cord, the clinical picture is one of root involvement, consequently weakness is of a lower motor neuron type; flaccid atrophy, fasciculation and loss of tendon reflexes. The plantar response is lost if the sensory deficit includes S1 and if the flexors and extensors are too weak to activate the joint. The commonest cause of cauda equina compression is an acutely ruptured lumbar disc and is discussed in Chapter 22. Some lesions, for example ependymoma, may affect both the conus of the spinal cord and the cauda equina giving a mixed picture of upper and lower motor neuron changes. Some tumours arise on the periphery of the leash of roots, for instance with a neurofibroma of L3 the pain and sensory loss may for some time remain restricted to one limb, involving only the adjacent nerve roots. Others arise within the leash, as in the case of ependymoma, the commonest intradural neoplasm in this region, and will affect roots bilaterally from the outset. At first the affected roots are the most central which are also the most caudal. Pain of radicular type and pain in the lumbar spine are usually prominent features of a cauda equina lesion, though the ependymoma may reach a large size before causing significant symptoms whilst a much smaller neurofibroma will often give very severe pain. Cauda equina tumours are liable to extend upwards so as to press upon or invade the conus medullaris; some arise from the conus or are adherent to it from the outset, for example a dermoid or similar cyst. In these cases disturbance of control of the bladder will be evident, and of the type characterized by a paralysed detrusor. The same type of incontinence arises whether the lesion is primarily in the conus or the cauda equina, but its place in the chronological sequence of symptoms may provide the clue; conus lesions and those involving S1–4 roots on both sides, i.e. centrally placed in the cauda, will affect micturition early but lesions arising in the periphery of the leash affect micturition later or not at all. Impotence is often the earliest indication of a lesion of the cauda equina in a male subject, but this information will seldom be volunteered by the patient. He should always be asked specifically about the capacity to achieve and sustain penile erection and ejaculation. Localization of level may prove difficult owing to the length of the nerve roots between their attachment to the lumbrosacral enlargement and their departure from the spinal canal. Thus L3 radicular pain may be due to a lesion on that root under the third lumbar lamina, where it will expand to compress only the cauda equina. However, the pain may equally well be due to a lesion on the root at, or close to, the L3 spinal segment under the twelfth thoracic lamina and here it will cause compression of the spinal cord; the sensory level may be similar in each

example, but the rest of the clinical picture very different. Cutaneous sensory loss from centrally situated cauda lesions is usually typical; it is bilateral though often not precisely symmetrical and may show patches of escape and conforms to the so-called saddle area, namely the buttocks, perineum, posterior aspect of the thighs and perhaps extending down over the calves. It is worth noting that the penis and scrotum derive their cutaneous nerve supply from S2 and 3, and consequently are involved in the area of sensory loss, but the adjacent groin is not.

The clinical localization of the level of a tumour provides an answer expressed in relation to a spinal cord segment. For the purpose of a surgeon planning the position of incision and bone removal, this must be translated into vertebral levels. In the upper cervical region cord segment and vertebra are numerically similar for practical purposes, but as levels move lower there is an increasing discrepancy. The lower cervical cord segments lie opposite 1 vertebra higher, and the upper 9 thoracic cord segments 2 vertebrae higher; lower segments are situated at increasing intervals above the vertebra of the same number so that L1 cord segment is opposite T10 vertebra and the sacral segments opposite L1 vertebra. Identification of spinous processes by palpation and counting is often difficult; to procure accuracy for the surgeon, it is the usual practice for the radiologist to indicate with an indelible mark on the skin of the back the level of the myelographic abnormality at the time of his examination. The actual numerical identity of a spinous process obtained by palpation and counting can be confirmed or corrected radiologically: an opaque marker is affixed with adhesive to the patient's back opposite the selected spinous process and radiographed. In the cervical region the most accurate method is to identify the spinous processes by palpation after they have been exposed by the incision which must extend virtually always from the external occipital protuberance to C7 or lower. Skin markers in this region are separated too far from the spinal canal by the thick mass of muscle to be a reliable guide.

## Vertebral column and integuments

A careful examination of the whole length of the spine may uncover clues to both localization and pathology. Shortness of the neck, abnormal position of the head and excessively restricted mobility of the neck occur in congenital malformations and acquired deformities which may compress the spinal cord at the level of the foramen magnum or atlanto-axial junction such as basilar impression. Arnold–Chiari malformation and atlantoaxial subluxation and Klippel–Feil deformity. Observation and palpation may reveal deformity at any level, congenital or acquired, paralytic, neoplastic or inflammatory in origin. Local paravertebral swelling may be detected. Tenderness on percussion of one particular spinous process is a useful localizing pointer, but it has no special pathological significance. A scoliotic deformity may be present due either to paraspinal muscular paralysis or sometimes, when seen in conjunction with severely restricted movement, to muscle spasm. Disease and collapse of vertebral bodies may cause an obvious kyphosis or gibbus. The presence of sinuses, dimples or abnormal hairy patches, especially over the occiput or lumbar spine, suggests a developmental abnormality and raises the likelihood of an intraspinal dermoid or lipoma in conjunction with spina bifida occulta. Much may be learnt by the examination of the spine column, an aspect which is sometimes neglected due to the enthusiastic search for neurological signs.

## Investigation of spinal compression

### Plain radiology

A common and barely understandable error which occurs is that following a correct clinical diagnosis of spinal cord compression, only the lumbar spine is X-rayed thus missing the area of the cord involved. Obviously, the whole vertebral column should be X-rayed even in cases in which the clinical level of the suspected lesion is evident because there may be multiple lesions and because diffuse changes may be present. Radiological abnormalities comprise: 1 deformities and malformations, 2 disease arising primarily in the bones or intravertebral discs, and 3 the secondary effects of an intraspinal tumour causing pressure erosion of bone.

1 Radiological examination may well clarify the nature of any spinal deformity which may be present: congenital malformations such as block or hemivertebra; scoliosis or kyphoscoliosis; and vertebral collapse of varying aetiology.

2 Bone destruction is most commonly due to metastatic carcinoma producing as the earliest sign destruction of a pedicle (Fig. 21.1). Disease in the vertebral body will lead to destructive collapse and angulation of the spine (Fig. 21.2) and there will often be a paravertebral shadow due to extraspinal tumour mass. Primary tumours of the vertebrae are infrequent. The commonest is chordoma which usually arises in

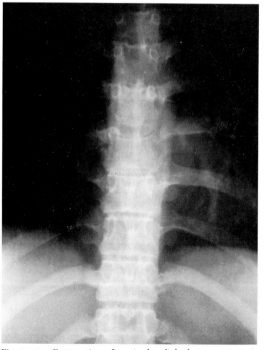

**Fig. 21.1.** Destruction of a spinal pedicle due to metastatic tumour.

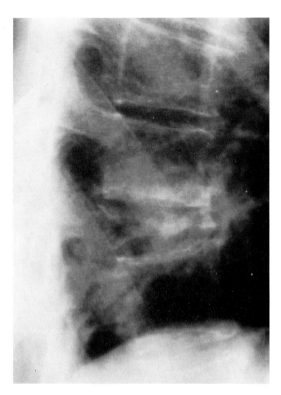

**Fig. 21.2.** Collapse of vertebral body due to metastatic tumour.

the sacrum but may affect other areas. Osteosarcoma and chondrosarcoma are fortunately rare lesions as are the more benign lesions such as aneurysmal bone cysts. Non-neoplastic diseases which cause cord compression may be seen to produce changes visible on plain X-ray; for example, degenerative disc disease, ankylosing spondylitis and Paget disease (Miller 1967).

3 A proportion of primary intraspinal tumours betray their presence by pressure erosion of adjacent bone. Localizing radiological evidence is highest for the neurofibromas and lowest for the meningiomas, 45% and 10% respectively in Bull's (1953) series, and intermediate for intramedullary tumours 32% according to Lombardi and Passerini (1964). Erosion may be recognized in three places:

(a) The margins of an intervertebral foramen which is thereby enlarged. This is typical of a neurofibroma and in the thoracic region the large extraspinal extension of a dumb-bell shaped tumour may also erode adjacent ribs.

(b) The medial aspect of corresponding pedicles, thereby causing a widening of the spinal canal. In well centred and good quality anteriorposterior radiography, the normal pedicle can be identified by the oval or round annular shadow cast by its dense cortical layer. The minimum distance between pedicles can be measured with fair accuracy and this interpedicular distance, the transverse (coronal) diameter of the spinal canal, varies at different levels, being wide to accommodate the cervical enlargement narrowest at the midthoracic level and wide again in the lumbar region. Widening of the interpedicular distance is unusual in tumours restricted to one or two vertebral levels and thus is rare in the presence of meningiomas and neurofibromas (Selosse and Granieri 1968). However, more extensive lesions such as an intramedullary tumour, are likely to show increase in the interpedicular distance (Fig. 21.3). An earlier and more prevalent sign is the appearance of thinning of the medial aspects of the pedicles also seen in Fig. 21.3. Pedicular changes and spinal canal widening is also seen in non-neoplastic disorders such as syringomyelia and sometimes merely represents a congenital malformation with dysplasia of the posterior elements.

(c) The posterior surface of the vertebral body may be hollowed out by the pressure of the tumour (Fig. 21.3). The discs resist this erosion and maintain the integrity of the upper and lower surfaces of the contiguous bodies; consequently when several vertebrae are affected, their posterior surfaces in the lateral X-ray projection cast a series of concavities, described as 'scalloping'. This may occur at any level but, is most usual in lower thoracolumbar or sacral regions. The tumour is generally massive and has been present for a long time with minimal symptoms. This is most commonly seen in neurofibromas or ependymomas of the cauda equina. However, scalloping has been reported in cases of communicating hydrocephalus without a spinal tumour being present (Shealy et al. 1964) and in cases of dural dilation or ectasia, an uncommon

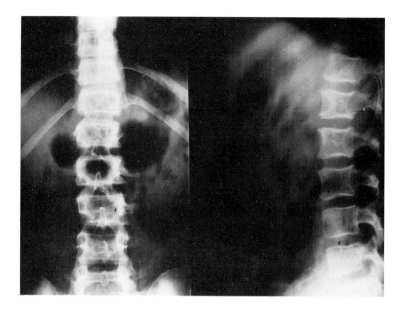

**Fig. 21.3.** Thining of pedicles and scalloping of vertebral bodies associated with an intramedullary tumour.

finding in neurofibromatosis again in the absence of a spinal tumour (Heard & Payne 1962).

### CSF examination

Lumbar puncture in a patient with spinal tumour must not be regarded as an innocuous procedure. Not infrequently it is followed within a few hours by an aggravation of the symptoms and signs of cord compression. This may be no more than an increase of pain, or ascent or deepening of relative sensory loss but occasionally the aggravation is much more severe. Total paraplegia may rapidly develop. This is attributable to shift in the tumour as a result of the loss of fluid below the block, partial or complete, causing an imbalance of pressure above and below the tumour. According to shape and mobility, preponderant pressure above the tumour may rotate it so that it is wedged more forcibly against the cord. Other mechanisms which may effect the integrity of the cord are a sudden increase in the size of the tumour as a result of haemorrhage into its substance and ischaemia of the cord consequent upon compression of an entering arterial radical or of adjacent veins. For these

reasons, CSF sampling is best done at the time of myelography, if this is to be performed, as this avoids two lumbar punctures. Should deterioration then occur, the information necessary for surgical exploration is available and this can and should proceed forthwith. For much the same reasons, it is now accepted that the Queckenstedt test to assess the presence or absence of a spinal block is potentially dangerous and that it should no longer be performed. In any event, much more accurate information is gained from myelography.

Loculation of fluid below a total spinal subarachnoid block leads to an increase in its protein constituents derived partly from the transudation of plasma from congested veins and partly from the lesion itself if it lies intradurally. The amount of protein varies widely from relatively moderate to massive increases in the CSF protein according to the totality of the block, its nearness to the level of puncture and its duration. With high concentrations the fluid is yellow-brown in colour and coagulates. The combination of high CSF protein but a normal cell count is commonly referred to as Froin syndrome.

In the majority of cases of spinal tumour there

is no increase in the number of cells in the cerebrospinal fluid. A minor increase in the number of cells per cubic millimeter to about ten or more suggests the possibility of an intradural tumour or that metastatic invasion has occurred though usually the dura mater resists this. Occasionally a slight increase of cells (and of protein) is seen in cases of root compression by a prolapsed intervertebral disc, due it is believed to an active inflammatory response in the root sheath. A considerable pleiocytosis and raised protein content in conjunction with subarachnoid obstruction is suggestive of an inflammatory aetiology: granuloma, tuberculosis, parasitic cyst or epidural abscess.

Though not actually causing cord compression, a very similar clinical picture can result from carcinomatous invasion of the meninges (Boyle *et al.* 1980). In this situation examination of the cytology of any cells found after centrifugation may show malignant cells. A considerable advance in the diagnosis of intradural tumours may well accompany current interest in the use of monoclonal antibodies as markers for tumour cells even when present in only extremely small numbers (Hancock & Medley 1983, Coakham *et al.* 1984).

## Myelography

The introduction by Sicard and Forestier (1922) of a method of radiological examination of the spinal subarachnoid space by the instillation of a (relatively) inert radio-opaque medium was a milestone in the history of the surgery of the spinal cord. Within its special field of diagnosis it was an event as important as Dandy's development of air ventriculography.

Various media have been used as contrast agents but for many years the mainstay was myodil. This is an oily substance which is not water-soluble and will remain intact in the patient for many years. Unfortunately myodil and similar agents have proved to have irritant qualities and, especially in the presence of blood or previous surgery, can lead to an adhesive

arachnoiditis with the clinical consequences of persistent and often severe pain. Oily substances have largely been replaced by water-soluble agents. The early types were also capable of producing reactions and were painful on injection. Newer reagents such as Iopamidol and Iohexol have proved much safer so far. Water-soluble agents allow improved definition, especially of nerve roots; but dilution of the dye can make full examination of the entire cord difficult. Because of this, it is usual for the dye to be injected via cervical puncture when the area of interest lies in the cervical cord. A further indication for cervical puncture occurs when a total block to the flow of contrast is seen following a lumbar injection. If the extent or nature of the rostral side of the block has to be seen, then dye must also be injected via cervical puncture.

From the nature of the deformity produced in the dye column it is usually possible to deduce whether the lesion is extradural or intradural, either extra- or intramedullary. An extradural obstruction (Fig. 21.4) creates an irregular,

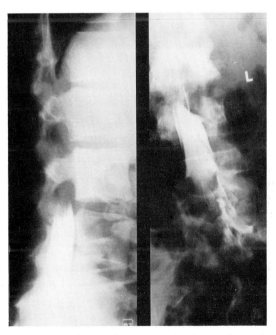

**Fig. 21.4.** Myelogram showing extradural mass effect with complete obstruction, due to lymphoma extending from the sclerotic body of L3.

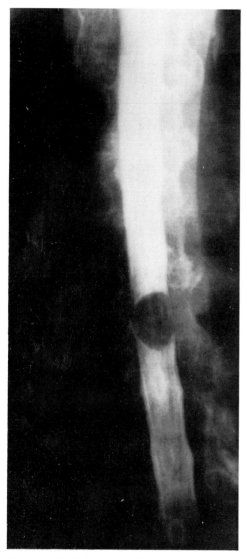

**Fig. 21.5.** Typical myelographic appearance of an intradural, extramedullary tumour, for example meningioma.

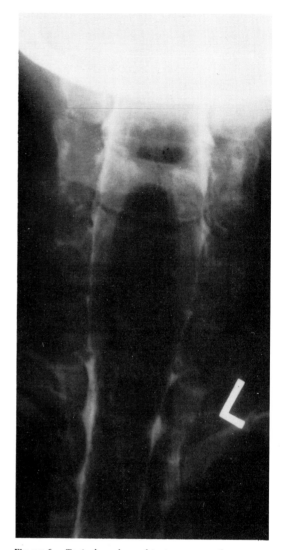

**Fig. 21.6.** Typical myelographic appearance of an intramedullary tumour.

serrated or brush-like margin at the margin of an approximately transverse filling defect and, of course, is often seen with some of the plain X-ray changes referred to previously if due to a metastasis. An intradural (but extramedullary) tumour such as meningioma, causes a rounded filling defect (Fig. 21.5) which usually can be seen to be displacing to one side the ribbon-like cord which shows as a relatively translucent area within the dye column. In intramedullary tumours, (Fig. 21.6) the medium divides into two columns which flow either side of the swollen cord; the effect is a deep blunt-nosed filling defect in the end of the dye column. On the antero-posterior projection, a central protrusion of a cervical disc can mimic this appearance.

Occasionally, the traverse of the dye in one direction appears normal and abnormality is only discovered when either the dye is run caudally again or the patient is screened in the supine position. Enlarged vessels within the subarachnoid space may show as serpentine filling defects or irregular channels of relative translucency which run through the dye column in a generally longitudinal direction. These may represent obstructed veins either above or below a total block and are particularly common around an intramedullary haemangioblastoma. Equally, they may, of course, be due to an arteriovenous malformation.

The development of spinal angiography has provided a means whereby vascular lesions seen on myelography can be further elucidated. The earliest application was in the gross assessment of the extent and the feeding vessels of the spinal arteriovenous malformations (Djindjian *et al.* 1962). At first the irrigation of the abnormal portion of the spinal cord depended upon overflow from a large dose of medium injected into the aorta itself under high pressure. Much improved definition resulted from the refinement of selective catheterisation of intercostal and lumbar arteries (DiChiro *et al.* 1967, Doppman *et al.* 1969, Djindjian *et al.* 1970). This selective technique allows a smaller quantity of medium and a slower injection pressure to be used, thus rendering the technique safer. Apart from the investigation of arteriovenous malformation, spinal angiography is of use in the identification of the blood supply of certain vertebral tumours, such as aneurysmal bone cyst, and of vascular intradural tumours such as haemangioblastoma.

Other investigative techniques are useful in the assessment of cord compression which is not of acute onset. Computerized tomography and magnetic resonance imaging are discussed elsewhere. Radioisotope bone scanning can give information of bone metastases even in the absence of plain X-ray changes. It can also be effective in bone infection, especially if early 'blood-pool' images are used (Gilday *et al.* 1975). Electromyography and evoked potentials seem likely to play increasing roles and the use of evoked potential monitoring is under evaluation as an intraoperative monitoring technique (Grundy 1982).

Prior to discussion of individual lesions in detail, some consideration of the general aspects of the surgical approaches used in the treatment of cord compression is appropriate. For many years, the standard approach has been that of laminectomy. Laminectomy remains essential if exposure of the cord is necessary over several segments such as when dealing with an intramedullary tumour. However, there has been in recent years an increasing awareness of the problems of this approach. Laminectomy especially in children or if involving the facet joints, carries a risk of progressive kyphotic deformity which approaches 100% in the cervical spine of children (Yasouka *et al.* 1982). Much greater awareness of the structural aspects of the spinal disease and the consequences of bone removal is necessary for neurosurgeons who understandably give their main attention to the neural elements. Experimental evidence (Doppman & Girton 1976) has shown conclusively that laminectomy fails to provide adequate decompression of large anteriorly situated masses. Equally, clinical experience shows that attempts to remove such anterior masses from a posterior approach is fraught with hazard. Accordingly, an increasing use of anterior or anterolateral approaches to the spine involving thoractomy or thoraco-abdominal exposures in addition to anterior cervical surgery is developing and will be referred to further.

## Intradural tumours

### Extramedullary tumours

Tumours of the spine which arise intradurally may be extra- or intramedullary. The commonest intradural but extramedullary tumours are the neurofibromas and meningiomas.

*Neurofibromas* (Schwannomas) are the commonest benign spinal tumours, arising from any of the spinal nerves. They originate almost invariably from the posterior roots and this may account for the high incidence of radicular pain as a presenting symptom. The histological appearance is the same in both intracranial and spinal tumours. To the naked eye at operation it commonly presents as a round lesion with a smooth yellow or pink glistening surface. It lies relatively mobile under the arachnoid but firmly attached to the parent nerve root which is incorporated in its capsule. The consistency of a neurofibroma is usually softly elastic; the tumour may be cystic and sometimes contains recent or old haemorrhage. Size varies according to the space within the spinal canal available before severe compression of the cord demands attention and to the presence or otherwise of extension beyond the confines of the canal. A common size for an entirely intradural thoracic tumour is about 2 cm. They are often larger in the upper cervical region and in the lumbosacral region they may be much larger, at times practically filling the canal and 5 cm or more in length. The tumour may extend within an expanded root sheath into and through the relevant intervertebral foramen, to form another mass outside the spinal column. This may be palpable in the neck in cervical tumours; thoracic tumours may form a large mass casting a radiological shadow in a chest X-ray film. The extraspinal portion of a dumb-bell tumour may be discovered by the thoracic surgeon before its intraspinal portion has given rise to spinal symptoms. Dumb-bell tumours are uncommon in the lower part of the spinal canal, though many of the tumours in this region extend into the intervertebral foramina. There is variation in the use of the term 'dumb-bell'; some writers limiting the name to tumours which extend within and without the spinal canal while others include a tumour which is merely intra- and extradural, the constriction being imposed by the dura mater of the root sheath. Gautier-Smith (1967) reported a series of 115 cases of spinal neurofibroma of which 26 were of the dumb-bell variety, the majority in the cervical region. In 4 patients, chest X-rays showed the soft tissue shadow of the extraspinal portion of a thoracic tumour. Twelve of these patients had some cutaneous stigmata of neuro-

fibromatosis and the occurrence of single or multiple neurofibromas, with or without cranial lesions, in patients with neurofibromata may occur at any age, though they are rare in the first decade and usually present between the ages of 30 and 60 years. They affect the sexes equally. The commonest presenting symptom is radicular pain which may have been present for years. The spacious lumbosacral canal often permits a longer duration of root pain before other symptoms and signs make it clear that the cause is not a prolapsed intervertebral disc, although the constant nature of the pain in the cases of a neurofibroma should alert suspicion. Paradoxically, some tumours arising from cervical roots may present with myelopathy and no root pain (Gautier–Smith 1967). Evidence of the effects of cord compression develop gradually in general and because of the lateral position of the tumour presentation may be initially as a Brown–Séquard syndrome, except of course in the cauda equina. Almost half the patients are diagnosed within two years of onset (Nittner 1976) but very long histories are not uncommon (Elsberg 1925).

Neurofibromas cause radiological evidence of bony erosion more frequently than any other variety of primary intraspinal tumour with changes being found in nearly half the cases (Bull 1953, Gautier–Smith 1967). Enlargement of the intervertebral foramen is typical and a large tumour may erode the adjacent vertebral body. Increase of the interpedicular distance is uncommon except in the lumbosacral region, where extensive erosion can accompany large tumours. Myelography shows either the typical changes of an intradural, extramedullary lesion or, if the tumour is large enough, a complete block.

The detailed account of the clinical features and operation make it likely that the spinal tumour removed by Horsley (Gowers & Horsley 1888), the first ever to be removed, was a neurofibroma. The removal of a small, accurately localized neurofibroma can be one of the simplest operations in the neurosurgical range, resulting in complete cure. By contrast those extending through the intervertebral foramen and the large cauda equina tumours can prove tedious and risky tests of neurosurgical skill. The difficulties are troublesome haemorrhage from extradural veins and the fixity of the tumour by its extra-dural extension along the course of the issuing nerve root; while contending with these the surgeon must constantly bear in mind the imperative need to avoid damage to the spinal cord, whose nourishment has already been jeo-pardized by the tumour. This problem is some-times best resolved by excising first the intradural portion, so that subsequent manipulations will not be transmitted to the cord. This is not an easy procedure if the tumour is wedged against the cord, or has extended anteriorly but intra-capsular piecemeal removal will diminish its bulk, and thus facilitate withdrawal of the capsule and remaining fragments without dis-turbing the cord. Unroofing the intervertebral foramen allows the removal of foraminal tumours. When the extraspinal portion of a dumb-bell tumour is large, it may be better to defer its removal to a second operation through an extraspinal approach. The operative mortality when performed in reasonably fit patients is extremely low. With regard to results, the extent to which neurological function recovers has been considered in general terms in the earlier part of this chapter. Fortunately in the majority of cases of neurofibroma, a high degree of recovery can be anticipated even in cases of established para-plegia. However, functional recovery may be dis-appointing in large lumbosacral neurofibromas because a number of roots may be involved and removing tumour from them may increase the neurological deficit. The sacrifice of the posterior spinal root to which the tumour is attached is of no consequence to the patient, at whatever level this happens to be. When the tumour is attached to several posterior roots their division would lead to demonstrable loss of cutaneous (and deep) sensibility; the resultant disability would depend upon localization. sensory impairment over the trunk and the parts of the limb is uncomfortable but of no other importance. If the digits of the hand are affected, the disability may be severe, if the foot is rendered analgesic, there is a risk of

pressure ulceration and walking may be abnor-mal. Impairment of penile, urethral, vaginal or anal sensibility may impair sphincter control and sexual sensation. When important multiple pos-terior roots are involved, every effort should be made to preserve as many filaments as possible. Tumours extending into the intervertebral foramen are inextricably bound with the motor fibres of the mixed nerve and the resultant loss of muscular power may be important. Fortunately, the overlapping supply from adjacent roots, ensured by the limb plexuses usually prevents severe disability. The patient should be warned of these possible sequelae in the routine pre-operative discussion.

Recurrence of a neurofibroma is likely only in tumours with extradural extensions or in large cauda equina tumours. In such, it may not be possible to be certain that extirpation is total. Intradural tumours are unlikely to present this difficulty. Recurrence of compression due to fresh tumour arising on a different nerve is very uncommon, other than in neurofibromatosis.

Radicular pain may occasionally persist after operation and should not lead to the assumption of recurrence. Its quality is generally different from pre-operative pain, being duller, more diffuse, associated with cutaneous hyperalgesia and reminiscent of postherpetic neuralgia. It is probably the result of abnormal impulses arising in the stump of the affected sensory root, or in the compressed cord.

*Meningiomas* occur with equal or perhaps slightly less frequency than neurofibromas. They have a predilection for the thoracic canal and are very rare in the lumbosacral canal. Spinal meningiomas are much more common in women with some 80% occurring in females (Nittner 1976). The tumour may arise from any point of the circumference of the theca though it often lies close to the exit of a nerve root, where it may lie anterior to the cord. They are firmly attached to the overlying arachnoid and dura and in consequence do not have the mobility of an entirely intradural neurofibroma. At oper-ation the tumour, of round, oval or somewhat lobulated shape has usually a finely granular surface, pink or pinkish-red in colour. The consistency is firm and tough and on incision gritty particles may be felt. Cystic degeneration or haemorrhage is rare. By these features it is usually possible to guess its nature correctly although the two tumours are sometimes quite indistinguishable. The meningeal attachment of a spinal meningioma closely resembles its intracranial counterpart. It may be broad, rendering the tumour sessile, or much narrower being much smaller than the size of the tumour. Through the attachment the tumour usually receives its major blood supply, consequently the dura mater in this area is often thickened and vascular and there is an increase of extradural vessels; the extradural venous plexus may be particularly rich and individual veins much enlarged. Although the dura is firmly involved, spread external to the membrane is uncommon. Primary extradural meningioma is rare, though it was described by Elsberg in 1928.

The peak age incidence of presentation occurs in the sixth decade, somewhat later than a neurofibroma, but there are no essential features in the clinical picture which differentiate the two lesions. Although initial radicular pain occurs less frequently this is of little help in the individual case. A combination of age and sex of the patient and situation of the tumour may allow a shrewd guess. Thoracic cord compression over the course of several years in a woman above middle age is more likely to be due to a meningioma than anything else. The same may be said if she presents the picture of a cervical cord syndrome, provided spondylosis is excluded; anteriorly placed meningiomas are not uncommon in this situation and may present a picture resembling an intramedullary glioma or syringomyelia. A diagnosis of meningioma is most unlikely in lumbar or sacral lesions. Plain radiography is usually unhelpful with only 10% of Bull's series (1953) showing changes; usually pedicular erosion. It should be noted that hyperostosis does not occur with spinal meningiomas as is so common with the intracranial variety because the spinal dura mater is a single entity separate from the periosteum of the vertebrae.

Another difference is the rarity of radiological evidence of calcium deposits within the tumour although these may be present microscopically; it showed radiologically in only 2 of Bull's 59 cases, and 4 of the 84 of Lombardi and Passerini (1964). Myelography confirms the presence of an intradural, extramedullary tumour but does not differentiate between meningioma and neurofibroma. Tumours high in the cervical area may show filling defects resembling other conditions especially when they are situated anteriorly and cause splaying of the cord when the myelographic appearance may be mistaken for an intramedullary lesion.

The removal of a meningioma differs from that of a neurofibroma in some respects. Even a small tumour is not mobile like a neurofibroma because of dural attachment. Occasionally, small posteriorly sited tumours may be delivered *in toto* and their dural origin excised. However, in large tumours, rather than risk bruising the cord, it is safer to exenterate the centre of the tumour as is the common practice with intracranial meningiomas. Once the centre has been decompressed, the capsular fringe can be safely delivered and the dura origin excised. Tumour exenteration is an essential step in the surgery of anteriorly based tumours but in such cases dural excision may be impractical. In such cases the origin may be diathermized to reduce the risk of recurrence. It should be borne in mind that unlike a neurofibroma, a meningioma tends to engulf structures which lie in the direction of its growth and so it may surround a nerve root or important artery. When the dural origin has been excised, watertight closure of the dura usually necessitates the use of an artificial dural patch.

The results of surgical removal of spinal meningiomas parallel those of neurofibromas save in respect of recurrence. Recurrence is more likely with meningiomas lying anterior to the cord, due to the deficiencies of dealing with the dura attachment. On occasion, it may prove unwise to attempt radical tumour excision of a large, anterior high cervical tumour from behind. A transoral approach may be safer in such cases rather than risk cord retraction, though such an approach has its own major hazards (Mullan *et al.* 1966).

## Intramedullary tumours

Intramedullary tumours are rare, representing less than 5% of all spinal tumours, including metastases (Simeone & Lawner 1982). Of nearly 9000 primary tumours of the nervous system analysed by Sloof *et al.* (1964), only just over 300 were intramedullary; 90% of which were gliomas of one type or other. Nearly 50% of intramedullary tumours arise in the conus or cauda equina, while the remainder are spread through the remaining regions. Exceptionally, a glioma may occur in an extramedullary site probably arising from heterotopic glia (Cooper *et al.* 1950).

The peak age incidence for the clinical onset of spinal cord gliomas is between the second and fourth decade, somewhat younger than for neurofibroma and meningioma. The incidence of spinal tumours in children is less than the adult; in children, there is a 1:4 ratio of spinal/cranial tumours as opposed to 1:2 in adults (Simeone & Lawner 1982). However, when they do occur in children they are likely to be intramedullary gliomas or dermoids (Ingraham & Matson 1954). Interestingly, Fortuna and Giuffre (1971) found that in children less than 14 years of age there was a strong female preponderance but that in older children males were predominantly affected. Overall, the male:female ratio is 7:5 (Sloof *et al.* 1964).

All the varieties of glioma found intracranially can occur in the cord, though medulloblastoma occurs only as secondary seedlings and oligodendrogliomas of the cord are rare. The nature of the cord gliomas, however, show a different distribution to those of the brain. The commonest is the ependymoma due to its preponderance amongst cauda equina tumours. Astrocytomas account for the bulk of the remainder. There is, however, a small but important group of more rare intramedullary tumours such as: lipoma; haemangioblastoma; teratoma; dermoids and epidermoids; melanoma; and metastasis.

With regard to spinal astrocytoma, many authors have followed the lead of Kernohan *et al.* (1949) by grading the tumours into four grades with grade I representing low-grade tumours and grades III and IV the malignant glioblastomas. With increasing appreciation of the fact that this merely represents a spectrum of disease, there is a tendency to consider tumours as being benign or malignant depending on the histology. This recognizes a trend for more aggressive tumours to progress more quickly but should not lead one to suspect that all tumours labelled benign will have an insidious course. Russell and Rubinstein (1971) further described astrocytomas with regard to morphology; the vast majority of those which occur in the cord are of the fibrillary type.

Macroscopically, an intramedullary astrocytoma can be recognized by causing a fusiform swelling of the cord within an expanding bony canal. The swelling may extend through several, sometimes many, segments. At its maximum diameter, the swollen cord may completely fill the dura to the exclusion of cerebrospinal fluid and the spinal rootlets are closely applied to its surface. Where tumour is more superficial, the columns of rootlets may be seen to be more widely separated though only the dorsal and lateral surfaces can be so fully inspected. The appearance of the cord is in other ways obviously abnormal in large gliomas. The colour is often yellow or pink, the tissue appears more opaque; although some tumours close to the surface may present as a greyish translucent area. The pial blood vessels follow a different pattern from the adjacent normal areas and the posterior spinal arteries may be displaced from their usual position; the more central part of the affected cord is often less vascular while the more peripheral cord is congested with a richer network of contorted visible arteries and dilated veins.

Although the majority of astrocytomas extend through only a limited extent, they can occupy the entire spinal cord. Sloof *et al.* (1964) demonstrated two astrocytomas which ran from C3 to L1 and from C7 to L5. These holochord tumours are rod-shaped and have rounded ends which indent fluid cavities at either end. Epstein and Epstein (1982) have emphasized the frequency with which large caudal and rostral cysts can occur in children, sometimes in the presence of only a very small solid component to the apparently holochord tumour. Barnett and Newcastle (1974) when studying the relationship of syringomyelia to tumour have also described extensive cysts. Their work, however, suggests that the frequency of finding large cysts in adults (30%) may be less than in children (75%; Epstein & Epstein 1982). The fluid in these cysts has a high protein content and is yellow; the walls are smooth and apparently non-neoplastic. The aetiology of such cysts is not clear. They could be due to exudation from the tumours but the polar placing of the cysts suggest that they are more likely to be due to an embryonic fault, whereby in part of the cord a solid tumour forms, and in other parts fluid dissects up and down the line of least resistance around the central canal. There may be small cysts within the tumour due to necrosis, a finding which is commoner in the more aggressive lesions. Astrocytomas, in general, do not have clear planes of cleavage from the surrounding cord and are locally infiltrative.

As a presenting symptom, pain is not as common as it is in extramedullary tumours but occurred in 68% of the series presented by Sloof et al. (1964) and sooner or later proves a major complaint in about two thirds (Austin 1961). The pain is less often radicular and more regional in distribution. If bilateral at the onset, or becoming so early in the history, a glioma is probable. Central pain is more frequent, as is spinal or paraspinal pain. Cutaneous sensory loss is likely to be of bilateral distribution and a Brown–Séquard pattern is unlikely except in the earliest stages. A cuirasse pattern may be seen early, but later in evolution the loss is liable to envelope all segments including sacral, whereas sacral escape is usual in extramedullary compression; the state of sensibility in the perineal region should be carefully sought. Dissociated impairment of cutaneous sensibility is not a reliable discriminating sign, though if of suspended distribution it is suggestive of a lesion within the cord. Broager (1953) comparing the clinical pictures of glioma, neurofibroma and meningioma noted that in cervical region the level of cutaneous sensory loss rarely reached as high a segmental level as the tumour, when this was a glioma.

On the motor side, conspicuous signs indicating a lower motor neuron type weakness, particularly if they are bilateral or originate from several segments, favour a glioma. In this respect, the importance of muscular fasciculation has already been emphasized. As explained above, the signs of a lower motor neuron lesion are more difficult to detect when the lesion is in parts of the cord not serving the limb outflow.

The duration of history and age of the patient are not good diagnostic guides in the individual cases. This is due to the considerable overlap of the ranges of age at presentation for all spinal tumours. Equally a very short length of history may be seen in both astrocytoma and meningioma, and both these lesions also occur with very long histories. Following the clinical presentation of an intramedullary astrocytoma nearly all patients deteriorate further. The rate of such deterioration is very variable and many patients with virtually static or very slowly progressive clinical courses have been seen. However, the clinical histories of the patients in the series of Epstein and Epstein (1982) show that a more rapid deterioration occurred in many of their patients subjected only to biopsy and decompression.

Myelography in a case of astrocytoma will show the typical appearance of an intramedullary lesion within an expanded bony canal. There may be a total block to the contrast necessitating cervical puncture to delineate the upper end of the lesion which may extend over a great distance. The experience of Epstein and Epstein (1982) in their series of 19 patients under the age of 16 years suggests that, in children at least, the solid component of the tumour is likely to correspond to the areas of maximum bony changes on plain X-ray. Much greater localization of the solid portion can be potentially achieved by the technique of endomyelography (Quencer *et al.* 1976) in which contrast is introduced percutaneously into the cysts within the cord. Such information is important in cases undergoing radical excision and it is to be hoped that this information may be reliably forthcoming from CT or magnetic resonance imaging which allow a noninvasive delineation of the cystic and solid components.

The earliest attempts at surgical excision of intramedullary tumours involved a two-stage technique (Elsberg 1911). At the first operation, a posterior midline myelotomy was performed and some ten days later the wound was re-explored. On some occasions the tumour had partially extruded through the myelotomy and could be removed. However, for many years the standard practice on discovering an intra-medullary astrocytoma was merely to provide a wide bony and dural decompression and to restrict the actual intradural surgery to a biopsy or needle aspiration of any cystic component. These patients were usually given radiotherapy and many went on to do very well with longterm survival of 30 years being reported (Sloof *et al.* 1964). However, not all patients fare so well and many of these long survivors do so with a marked neurological deficit and may be paraplegic for many years prior to their death. Some deteriorate rapidly following decompression (Arendt 1976) and others deteriorate over a few months as described above.

This has led some surgeons to attempt total macroscopic removal of astrocytomas. Some of these tumours do seem to be expansive rather than infiltrative and so potentially removable. Apparent total removal of relatively localized astrocytomas has been reported (Garrido & Stein 1977, Malis 1978) but it is only with developments in technology that radical excision has been attempted in holochord tumours. Epstein and Epstein (1982) have reported their experience of radical removal aided by an ultrasonic aspirator and it seems likely that the combination of this tool with a laser to perform the initial myelotomy as atraumatically as possible fol-

lowed by coagulation of the residual tumour cavity with the defocused laser will lead to even greater versatility. Of the 14 patients in their series with holochord tumours, total macroscopic removal was achieved in them all, the longest extending from C2 to L1. Whether such a radical approach will actually achieve cure remains to be seen as the follow-up period of patients so treated is not long enough to know what the recurrence rate will be. Nevertheless, it has been shown that radical removal can be achieved without neurological damage and in many cases with recovery of a deficit which was progressing despite previous decompressive surgery and radiotherapy.

The role of radiotherapy in cord astrocytomas is not clear and no trial has given definitive results. There is some suggestion that radiotherapy is beneficial following simple decompression (Sloof *et al.* 1964). It is debatable whether radiotherapy should be given following radical excision in an attempt to destroy any residual cells or to withhold it pending a possible recurrence. Due to the vulnerability of the neur-axis of children to radiotherapy it is wisest not to irradiate children following total excision.

It is appropriate at this stage to mention the problem of postlaminectomy deformity that is a particular hazard in children. Laminectomy that includes the facet joint may produce kyphotic deformity in adults (Verbiest & Paz y Geuse 1966). However, in growing children even laminectomy with preservation of the joints has an incidence of kyphosis approaching 50% (Yasuoka *et al.* 1982), with an incidence of nearly 100% if performed over the cervico-thoracic junction. It is important, therefore, to limit the extent of bony removal and, hence, the need for greater pre-operative localization of the solid part of astrocytomas, mentioned above. Following laminectomy, children must be placed in an orthopaedic brace as soon as serial X-rays have identified a developing kyphus, and prophylactically if the laminectomy is in the cervical or cervical–thoracic area. As compliance with rigorous spinal bracing in children is far from universal, attempts to preserve the posterior spinal structures by laminotomy and recon-stitution of the spine have been made (Raimondi 1976) but this still requires temporary bracing.

Spinal ependymomas pose a problem similar to the astrocytomas, though there are important differences. The ependymoma accounts for a majority of intramedullary tumours, especially in the caudal area. They have the same slight male predominance as gliomas overall and tend to present in the same age range. Approximately one-half of all spinal ependymomas arise in the cauda equina; the remainder being truly intra-medullary (Fischer & Tommasi 1976). Ependy-momas have a greater tendency to present on the cord surface than do astrocytomas and they tend to grow along and between the posterior columns. They also show a greater tendency to have better planes of demarcation and to appear encapsulated. This, in conjunction with the fact that they tend to be more localized, enhances the ability of the surgeon to achieve total macro-scopic resection.

Ependymomas of the cauda equina can some-times present as discrete masses attached to the filum terminale (Wortzmann & Botterell 1963) but more frequently appear as large masses filling the lumbosacral canal, either pressing the roots outwards or invaginating them within the tumour mass. Such tumours frequently show mucinous changes and are histologically des-cribed as myxopapillary. 'Metastatic' spread through the CSF from spinal ependymomas has been observed (Watt 1968) but this 'upward' spread seems to be less common than downward dissemination from cranial ependymomas or medulloblastomas. Extraspinal metastases have been described (Watt 1968, Rubinstein 1970) but only after surgical intervention.

The mode of presentation depends primarily on the site of the lesion and there are really no clinical features which accurately differentiate ependymomas from astrocytomas. However, presentation with a conus or cauda equina syn-drome would certainly favour an ependymoma, especially if this is associated with marked exca-vation of the lumbosacral canal (Lombardi and Passerini 1964) Total macroscopic removal of an ependymoma can be achieved with greater frequency and ease than in astrocytoma, though regrettably not in every case. As with astro-cytomas, long survival following treatment is possible but, in the series presented by Sloof et al. in 1964, the overall results were somewhat disappointing with only about 50% of patients surviving 5 years. There is general agreement that total macroscopic removal improves the chance of survival but little information exists about the quality of such survival. Many sur-geons advocate radiotherapy following incom-plete excision but there is some evidence, albeit inconclusive, that radiotherapy may para-doxically shorten survival (Barone & Elvidge 1970). It seems reasonable if radiation is to be used, that postoperative CSF is examined cyto-logically in order to identify those patients with free malignant cells present who can then undergo neuraxis irradiation.

Intramedullary haemangioblastoma is a rare vascular tumour of the spinal cord; whereas those of the posterior fossa are relatively common. In 1966, Kendall and Russell could find only 70 previously reported cases. The intradural spinal variety is usually solitary but can occur with other lesions in the cord or brain or as part of the von Hippel–Lindau complex. Spinal haemangioblastomas usually lie on the surface of the cord, embedded within it to a greater or lesser extent. They usually have a pink, highly vascular appearance with the grossly enlarged feeding and draining pial vessels resembling an arteriovenous malformation. This resemblance may be further enhanced if the actual hae-mangioblastoma is concealed within the cord as occasionally happens (Krishnan & Smith 1961). Like their posterior fossa counterparts, spinal haemangioblastomas may have an associated cystic component.

Clinical presentation is usually that of an expanding intramedullary lesion but may be more abrupt with subarachnoid haemorrhage. Myelography may suggest the diagnosis, if an intramedullary lesion surrounded by serpiginous defects due to the associated vasculature is shown. Spinal angiography is necessary to accurately delineate the vascular supply (Di Chiro & Doppman 1969).

The treatment is primarily surgical, as total removal will result in cure. Decompression laminectomy is not effective and radical removal should always be attempted (Guidetti & Fortuna 1967). Usually a good plane of cleavage will be found allowing separation from the surrounding cord tissue. Although radiotherapy may slow the rate of tumour growth it is generally accepted that it is not curative.

## Extradural and vertebral metastases

Although other neoplasms occasionally occupy the extradural space, for example lipoma, neurofibroma, neuroblastoma, by far the commonest extradural and indeed spinal tumour is a metastasis from a distant or haematological primary source. Metastases may either arise purely in the extradural space or more commonly invade into that space from an adjacent vertebral metastasis. Gilbert et al. (1978) found pure extradural metastases in 15% of their cases, all the remainder being related to a vertebral deposit. They develop usually by haematogenous spread, although in certain cases this may occur on a local basis via the vertebral venous plexus such as is thought to be the case in prostatic secondaries. Occasionally extraspinal primary tumours may invade the spine by direct spread and the commonest example of this occurrence is renal carcinoma.

The frequency with which tumours metastasize to the spine is highly variable. Studying a wide range of primary tumours at autopsy, Barron et al. (1959) found that myeloma had the greatest tendency to seed to the spine, followed by prostate and kidney. Cobb et al. (1977) systematically followed over 12,000 patients with breast cancer and found an incidence of radiologically proven spinal metastases of 20%. Although certain tumours may have a propensity to disseminate to the spine, the tumours which present most commonly with cord compression are, by and large, those which occur with greatest frequency in the community. Thus,

lung and breast cancers dominate most unselected series (Brice & McKissock 1965, Gilbert et al. 1978, Constans et al. 1983). The other primaries which are frequently seen with spinal metastases are kidney and prostate and the tumours of haematopoietic tissue such as lymphoma. Most general series report significant numbers of cases where the site of the primary lesion is unknown. Shaw et al. (1980) reporting 120 cases presenting to a neurosurgical unit, found that a primary site was known in only 52% of their patients at the time they presented and that even after further investigation and biopsy, the primary remained occult in 28%. The commonest site in the spinal column to be affected is the thoracic spine with only 26% of the remainder appearing in the lumbosacral area and 15% in the neck (Törma 1957). Most vertebral body and purely extradural metastases occupy between one and three segments. Many patients may have multiple spinal deposits but multiple sites of compression are unusual in most experience, Gilbert et al. (1978) found them in nearly 20% of their patients. The most common part of the vertebral body to be affected is the pedicle, but extensive involvement of the body is also common and causes vertebral collapse. The adjacent discs are unaffected, in contrast to vertebral collapse due to infective agents.

Spinal pain is the earliest feature in most patients and is rarely absent. The pain may be localized to the midline over the affected area of the spine or, if a nerve root is involved by tumour or collapse, may be radicular. The persistence of spinal or radicular pain in the absence of an adequate explanation (such as supporting signs of disc prolapse), especially in a patient with known malignancy, should raise the suspicion of a spinal metastasis. Only by such awareness and early diagnosis can the disastrous effects of cord compression by prevented or alleviated. Only occasionally does the onset of neurological disease coincide with the onset of pain. In most instances, pain precedes the onset of neurological symptoms by some days or more commonly weeks. Gilbert et al. (1978) found a median delay of 7 weeks in their patients and, although the figures of Shaw *et al.* (1980), correspond with this order of delay, they found that in 18% of their patients there was an interval of greater than six months between onset of pain and neurological deficit.

Unfortunately, the majority of patients present only after the onset of neurological deficit, usually with muscle weakness. By the time the patients are referred to the neurosurgeon, the motor deficit is often advanced. In an extensive literature review, Findlay (1984a) found that only one quarter of over 1800 cases presented to a neurosurgical unit whilst still able to walk, even with an aid such as a walking-frame. In addition, 14% were totally paraplegic. Some comment on the use of the word 'paraplegic' is appropriate; the use of this term in a loose manner to indicate profound weakness is to be deprecated. Paraplegia should be used only as it is used here, to imply total loss of motor and sensory function. This allows more precise comparison of results.

Sensory symptoms and signs are important primarily as indicators of the level of compression. Only approximations to level can be made; but a pin-prick level at the nipple line suggests compression around T4, and at the umbilicus at around T10. Examination of the sensory level on the back of the trunk may be slightly more sensitive in localization. Such rough localization of level is important in directing attention to the appropriate area of the spine during clinical and radiological examination. Sphincteric disturbance was present in 57% of the patients studied by Gilbert *et al.* (1978) and was found to be an unfavourable sign. Occasionally, when the site of compression is at the conus or cauda, sphincteric disturbance may be early clinical feature.

The mode of onset of neurological deficit is important. Usually, there is an antecedent history of increasing difficulty with walking for a few days or weeks followed, if not diagnosed earlier, by a more rapid decline leading up to the presentation. Occasionally, the onset of weakness can be dramatic in which case the mechanism is likely to be vascular due to thrombosis of an important vessel within the tumour mass or even more occasionally, due to sudden pathological fracture of a diseased vertebral body. This type of dramatic onset is associated with a poor prognosis for neurological recovery. The duration of history has been claimed by many to influence recovery; longer histories are associated with a more favourable outlook (for example Brice & McKissock 1965, Chade 1976). However, a similar number of reports claim that the length of history did not influence outcome (for example Hall & Mackay 1973, Dunn *et al.* 1980). There is overall agreement that paraplegia of greater than 24 hours duration is very unlikely to recover, although occasional successes have been reported (Halnan & Roberts 1967). The nature of the primary tumour has great bearing in recovery potential; metastases from the breast and haematopoietic tumours are favourable, whereas the outlook from bronchogenic lesions is very poor. There are, however, exceptions to these general statements. One of the most powerful predictors of neurological recovery is the neurological status at the time of presentation. Findlay (1984a) has shown that of patients ambulant at the time of treatment, approximately 70% will remain able to walk and of those whose weakness was severe enough to prevent ambulation but were not paraplegic, only one-third walk again despite treatment by laminectomy, radiotherapy alone or in combination. Several authors have commented on the fact that vertebral collapse carries a poor prognosis but very few have produced sound evidence of this claim (Brice & McKissock 1965). In recent study, Findlay (1984b) has shown just how poorly patients with vertebral collapse fare. In comparison with a group of 39 patients without vertebral collapse, the pretreatment state of the 41 with collapse showed no overall difference but the outcome of the vertebral collapse group was much worse with only 15% able to walk following laminectomy as opposed to 33% in those with no collapse. Further, 22% of the vertebral collapse group developed spinal instability following laminectomy. The final factor of importance in prognostic terms is the level of compression. Livingstone and Perrin (1978), confirmed that cauda equina compression carried the most favourable outcome in terms of recovery. Tumours compressing the thoracic cord had the worst outlook though there is debate as to whether the lower thoracic cord (Livingstone & Perrin) or the upper thoracic area (White et al. 1971) is the most vulnerable area.

Plain radiology of the clinically suspected part of the spinal column will show evidence of metastasis in approximately 60% of patients (Black 1979). Black stresses, however, the importance of viewing the whole spine, to which one should add a chest film, to seek for multiple deposits. The most characteristic signs are loss of a pedicle, vertebral collapse and a paravertebral soft tissue mass (Figs. 21.1 and 21.2). In cases of collapse of the vertebral body it is extremely important to be aware of the possibility of an infection rather than neoplastic causes of collapse; in the former cases, the intervening disc is likely to be destroyed and the bony disease is maximal in the vertebral endplate area. It is usual practice to confirm that the site of cord compression corresponds to the vertebral lesion by myelography where usually a complete extradural block is seen (Fig. 21.4). On occasion, the block may be incomplete and this carries a favourable effect on outcome (Young et al. 1980). Isotope bone scanning may be useful in that it can identify metastases at a stage where plain X-ray is still normal, but other causes of positive uptake such as infection or degenerative change can lead to a mistaken diagnosis. CT investigation of spinal metastases is not commonly undertaken but Sartor (1983) felt that CT was 'superior to conventional methods'. Many patients present with metastasis from an unknown primary tumour and in such cases investigation should be undertaken to reveal the source if not obvious from clinical examination and chest radiography. Usually, the clinical urgency of the cord compression precludes such investigation prior to treatment, and the biopsy of the tumour may add histological clues to the origin of the tumour.

Assessment of the efficacy of differing modes of treatment has been complicated by the widely differing types of populations studied and by the lack of agreement on how to judge the success of treatment. Many authors merely comment on the number of patients whose neurological deficit 'improves' without indicating whether this is of minor or major degree. In his review of the effects of standard treatment, Findlay (1984a) suggested that the only criterion of success was the restoration or retention of the ability to walk, arguing that more minor improvement did not alter the quality of survival. It is accepted that restoration of sphincter control is of importance but for this to occur in the absence of motor recovery sufficient to allow ambulation is unusual. Because of the sources of data used in that review, direct comparison of the results of differing treatments could not be made, but some general conclusions were drawn. The results of laminectomy alone were found to be very poor; whereas, laminectomy with follow-up radiotherapy and primary irradiation with steroid cover gave closely similar results. These results, however, were somewhat disappointing showing that, with 25% of the patients still ambulant prior to treatment, only considerably less than one-half were able to walk following treatment. From this and other series it is clear that one way to improve results is to diagnose and treat patients at a very early stage. Cobb et al. (1977) followed a group of people with breast cancer and irradiated them when skeletal spinal metastases became apparent on routine films and prior to neurological deficit. None of these cases subsequently developed evidence of cord compression. Further reasons for not being complacent comes again from Findlay (1984a) who showed that, of the people still walking before treatment, only some 70% were able to continue doing so afterwards; in other words, treatment failed in very nearly one-third.

For many years the customary treatment for malignant spinal cord compression has been by emergency laminectomy, although Elsberg (1941) felt that in some cases the morbidity and mortality involved were prohibitive. There has been greater consideration of other therapies in recent years and this is still under debate. The advantages cited for laminectomy are that it provides: urgent relief of spinal compression in deteriorating cases; diagnostic confirmation by biopsy; and that it is less likely to cause further deterioration than radiotherapy. These opinions may not be as valid as has been widely accepted.

Few details exist as to the efficacy of laminectomy in the small group of patients whose cord function is rapidly deteriorating. However, Smith (1965) found that rapidly progressive disease had the poorest prognosis and did not respond to surgery. Gilbert et al. (1978) had 22 patients with rapidly developing weakness; 9 underwent laminectomy and none improved, while 7 of the 13 treated by urgent radiotherapy improved, but to what extent is not recorded. The belief that radiotherapy cannot produce immediate relief is erroneous. There are several studies (for example Kahn et al. 1967, Gilbert et al. 1978) which show that radiotherapy alone applied to a mixed group of tumours can produce clinical success. Rubin (1969) in clinical and experimental work showed that, provided the initial dose of radiation was large enough, the tumours immediately shrank without swelling in the way which occurred with earlier, lower dose regimes. The role of steroid therapy as a means to gain time and as an adjunct to the radiotherapy is important (Ushio et al. 1977). The dramatic effect of irradiation on certain haematopoietic tumours is well known (Friedman et al. 1976) but it is important to emphasize that throughout this section reference is being made to the usual highly varied histological types of tumour which present to the neurosurgeon, and not selected radiosensitive tumours.

The diagnostic confirmation obtained by biopsy during laminectomy is a most important factor. Effective management of the whole patient can be based only on a firm tissue diagnosis. Even with a high index of suspicion, the clinician may misdiagnose as a secondary a more benign lesion such as infection or lymphoma. If laminectomy is not performed, and this is becoming more common, and the patient treated by

irradiation, a tissue diagnosis remains essential. Occasionally, this can be achieved without involving the spine; for example bronchoscopic diagnosis of a lung primary. More often the site of biopsy remains the spinal lesion. In cases without collapse, diagnosis can be achieved by a mini-hemilaminectomy approach via a very small posterior incision. Tumour is often found in the extraspinal soft tissues or can be obtained by a fenestration-type procedure with minimal bone removal. The importance of such a conservative surgical approach will become clear. In the presence of vertebral collapse, tissue diagnosis can be obtained by percutaneous needle biopsy. Using a posterolateral approach to avoid the facet joint and transverse process, a needle can be guided under X-ray control into the affected body and multiple core biopsies obtained. The technique was originally described by Robertson and Ball (1935) and refined by Ottolenghi (1955). A full description of the approach, also used for lumbar discography and injection of lytic enzymes, is given by McCulloch and Waddell (1978). By bringing the point of the needle insertion slightly closer to the midline as one ascends rostrally, biopsy up to the level of T4/5 can be made. Fyfe et al. (1983) have compared the diagnostic yields of such biopsies using either a fine-needle or trephine needle of 3 mm diameter and showed conclusively that needle biopsy must be performed with the large needle. This technique give a correct diagnosis in 90% of cases but a pathological answer may require several days if the specimen has to be decalcified. However application of the techniques of histological smears can often give an immediate diagnosis.

The use of radiotherapy as a primary treatment has always raised fears that neurological deterioration will follow unless surgical decompression precedes irradiation. Just under 20% of all patients treated by radiotherapy alone showed a major functional deterioration (Findlay 1984a). However, what has not been widely appreciated, is that an equivalent proportion of patients undergoing laminectomy followed by radiotherapy also show such deterioration. Such patients probably represent treatment failures with progression of the disease process rather than being directly made worse by the treatment. It, therefore, appears that treatment by laminectomy or by primary radiotherapy offer the same somewhat limited hope of success and similar chances of failure. Irradiation is the simpler procedure with less morbidity; laminectomy has been shown to carry a mortality rate in the order of 10% and a high risk of producing painful spinal instability especially when performed in a patient with vertebral collapse (Wright 1963, Brice and McKissock 1965, Findlay, 1984a, 1984b).

The traditional role of laminectomy as the initial therapy in malignant cord compression is now open to question and its place was debated by Black (1979) in an excellent review. Overall, even in rapidly deteriorating cases, it seems to be no more effective in terms of either success or failure than radiotherapy. Such radiotherapy must be urgently available and lack of early availability of this resource may still leave a place for surgery. However, modern evidence is that laminectomy performed on cases with vertebral collapse is unlikely to be effective and can have disastrous morbidity.

The management of such patients with anteriorly sited spinal metastases produces a major problem due to the fact that, in addition to the poor surgical results, radiotherapy seems to have a very poor chance of allowing ambulation in a patient with collapse and severe deficit. Doppman and Girton (1976) showed in experimental material that laminectomy failed to decompress the cord compressed by an acutely expanding ventral extradural mass as judged by angiographic displacement and clinical results. More relevant is the work of Bennett and McCallum (1977) who showed that laminectomy in cats with a slowly expanding anterior mass resulted in worsening of somatosensory evoked potentials and clinical outcome. Work such as this, realization of the limitations of existing laminectomy and radiotherapy, and the greater safety and wider use of surgical techniques involving an anterior approach to the cervical and thoracic spine via anterior neck incision or thoracotomy for diverse pathologies has led some surgeons to operate directly on the collapsed vertebra and its tumour mass (for example Harrington 1981, Siegal et al. 1981, Siegal & Siegal 1985). This approach, allowing dural decompression supplemented by spinal fusion has given encouraging results but no wide-scale evaluation has yet been performed. The place of this radical approach will be limited in malignant disease but the poor results of existing therapy justify attempts to improve the success rate. In patients unsuitable for such radical surgery because of old age or widespread disease, considerable improvement in postlaminectomy morbidity and reduction of pain can be gained by combining laminectomy with a posterior stabilization of the type employing a rigid segmental fixation rather than distraction. Examples of such techniques are given by: Cusick et al. (1983), Harrington rods with segmental wiring and acrylic fusion; Allen and Furguson (1982), L-shaped Luque rods with segmental wiring; or by Miles et al. (1984), segmental fixed laminar bar.

Mention must finally be made of two other types of therapeutic approach in malignant disease. Firstly is the use of chemotherapy, occasionally as a prime agent but usually as an adjunct. Tumours where this may be especially helpful are those with endocrine relations such as breast and prostate where hormonal manipulation by drugs or surgery (for example hypophysectomy or orchidectomy) may produce a clinical response. It is of paramount importance not to entirely focus attention on the spinal metastasis itself but to treat the whole patient. Thus, if any therapy is possible for the primary disease, this should be given whenever appropriate. Finally, this leads to the place of inactive management. When one considers the many adverse effects of the treatments discussed above and their low success rate, it becomes clear that there are certain instances where aggressive therapy is contraindicated. Nothing can be worse than subjecting an ill patient with vertebral collapse to injudicious laminectomy which may leave him not only unable to walk but with a chronically painful and unstable spine.

## Primary tumours of the spinal column

Tumours arising primarily from the spinal column only rarely present to a neurosurgeon unless he has a particular interest in spinal disease. The most commonly seen tumour of this group is the chordoma. The nature of this tumour and its prevalence in and about the spheno-occipital portion of the skull is described in Chapter 10. It is also encountered in the vertebral column, usually sacrococcygeal, next in frequency in the cervical region, and rarely elsewhere. Its main incidence is thus at the extreme limits of the notochord; sacrococcygeal examples roughly equal in numbers all others put together. Windeyer (1959) analysed the records of others and of 29 personal cases, totalling 478; sacrococcygeal constituted 53%, spheno-occipital 33% and intermediate vertebral only 13%.

The biology of chordoma in the spine is similar to that in the skull. Of slow growth, it invades and destroys bone irregularly and forms smooth exuberant masses in adjacent soft tissues. It spreads to contiguous vertebrae, destroying intervening discs and collapse is common. By the time of neurological presentation there may be a sizeable mass. Remote metastases by lymphatic and vascular systems have been noted and local recurrence is common. Presentation may occur over a wide age range but it is rare for the tumour to occur at less than 20 years of age. Chordomas arising in the more unusual sites (cervical, thoracic or lumbar) usually present with progressive cord compression, though those in the neck may present with a mass. The patient with a sacrococcygeal chordoma is more likely in the first instance to attend a general surgical rectal or genitourinary clinic than a neurosurgical clinic. The early symptoms are pain in the low back or sacrum and disturbance of rectal and bladder function. These develop as a result of the pelvic mass of tumour. Later symptoms may be swelling over the sacrum and radicular pain of lumbar and sacral distribution, associated with evidence of motor and sensory deficit.

Radiological appearance of chordoma in the cervical and thoracic parts of the spine does not usually provide a pathological diagnosis. But if several contiguous vertebrae are affected and a long history excludes the likelihood of metastases, chordoma should be suspected. Sacrococcygeal chordoma causes great expansion of the sacral canal and destruction of its walls in accordance with the major direction of spread, irregular areas of erosion, formation of trabeculae in unaffected bone and sometimes calcification.

By the time of presentation, most tumours are beyond the stage of reasonable resection. However, in the case of sacral tumours, Stener and Gunterberg (1978) have described a method of radical sacral amputation which can be performed in tumours which are not high enough to involve the S1 root foramina. This resection leaves enough of the body of S1 to allow normal weightbearing but does result in permanent sacrifice of sphincter control which, however, has already been lost in many cases. Radical resection of chordoma in other areas of the spine may also be technically feasible (Fielding et al. 1979). Despite these approaches, the majority of surgical treatment is palliative with repeated posterior debulking procedures being necessary. This approach may have beneficial results as tumour growth is usually slow and patients may be kept ambulant for a considerable time (Windeyer 1959). The same caveats remain, however, with respect to laminectomy in the presence of vertebral body collapse as were discussed in the section on metastic disease. Chordomas are not radiocurable although most patients are treated with postoperative irradiation to try to delay recurrence following incomplete resection.

Other primary tumours have a more malignant tendency than chordoma. Primary spinal osteosarcoma is rare and tends to develop in areas of Paget disease. Metastatic deposits from an osteosarcoma elsewhere are more common. Radical resection by synchronous or staged anterior and posterior surgery is feasible but should be supplemented with radiotherapy and chemotherapy. Survival rates and results of such surgery are not yet available as the lesions are fortunately rare. Other tumours of malignant nature are chondrosarcoma and Ewing's sarcoma. The former can have a very varied rate of progress but can undergo rapid deterioration in the final-stages. The primary therapeutic approach is of surgical ablation. On the other hand, Ewing's sarcoma is a childhood lesion in which reasonable results with irradiation and chemotherapy are being obtained. Although reasonably considered as primary spinal tumours, the behaviour, features and therapy of myeloma and lymphoma affecting the vertebrae have so much in common with metastic disease that they are considered in that section.

With regard to the more benign primary spinal tumours, osteoid osteoma can cause diagnostic difficulty in young people presenting with protracted back pain who may be misdiagnosed as due to lumbar disc protrusion. The appearance of marked stiffness and scoliosis is very suggestive of the lesion which is best identified by bone or CT scanning rather than plain radiography (Kirwan et al. 1984). However, a similar syndrome can be seen in children with 'adolescent' disc syndrome, but in such cases a lumbar radiculogram will reveal the protruded disc. Larger than normal osteoid osteomas tend to be termed osteoblastoma but carry the same benign connotation. Aneurysmal bone cysts are also benign lesions which occur in the young. They present with pain and occasionally cause neurological deficit when of large size. They are ideally treated by radical excision and grafting though in certain areas of the spine curettage and packing with bone can be a reasonable alternative (Hey et al. 1978). Other lesions such as osteochondroma or giant cell tumours (which occasionally have malignant potential) occur and interested readers are referred to the brief review of Friedland and Southwick (1982).

## Intraspinal cysts

Cysts which arise in the spine fall into three categories, according to the nature of their lining membrane. Each category includes several groups with distinctive features and the origin of

some cysts is clear whilst in others their origin may be obscure. Their total number represents only a small proportion of lesions giving rise to spinal cord compression. The groups are:

1 Epithelial: epidermoids, dermoids, teratomas, enterogenous (neuroenteric).
2 Endothelial: arachnoid, extradural, perineural and sacral.
3 Parasitic: echinococcus, cysticercosis, schistosomiasis.

The congenital lesions of meningocele and myelomeningocele are not included in this section.

### 1a. Epidermoid, dermoid and teratoma

They are very infrequent occupants of the spinal canal; they take seventh place in the list of intraspinal tumours of the Mayo Clinic (Sloof et al. 1964) with an incidence of only 1.4%. They occupy a higher place amongst children's tumours, coming third at 17% in Hamby's (1944) cases. The majority of these cysts give rise to symptoms in adulthood. Morbid anatomy and the characteristics by which they are divided into epidermoid, dermoid, teratoid and teratoma have been described in the chapter dealing with intracranial examples. Strictly speaking the teratoma should be considered by itself for it is commonly more solid than cystic.

The ratio in which epidermoid and dermoid cysts occur within the cranium and within the spinal canal is roughly 3 to 1 according to Tytus and Pennybacker (1956). They arise from an error of development with the exception of one particular group. Choremis et al. (1956) drew attention to the occurrence of lumbar epidermoid cysts in children who some years previously had been treated for tuberculous meningitis; in some there were several cysts. Other similar cases have been reported, for instance by Blockey and Schorstein (1961) in which pyogenic meningitis was the preceding complaint. The contention is that in these cases the cyst originated by dermal implantation on the end of a needle. Blockey and

Schorstein identified the problem as being the open-ended needle used prior to the introduction of disposable needles with stylettes. The incidence of this complication of lumbar puncture has fallen dramatically.

Epidermoids and dermoids occur throughout the length of the spine, but are rare in the cervical region and most frequent in the lumber. They may lie within the cord or subdurally. Examples lying anterior to the cord have been reported and those within the roots of the cauda equina commonly abut on, or are partially within, the conus medullaris. Excluding implantation cysts, they occur at all ages but the majority present in adults. There may be a connection between the intraspinal cyst and the skin surface where a sinus or a dimple a hairy naevus may be evidence of congenital spinal deformity such as an occult spina bifida. The surface connection may allow penetration of infection and subsequent meningitis; rarely the cyst itself may rupture liberating its contents into the CSF to cause a sterile chemical meningitis.

Radiological examination is likely to show evidence of a longstanding intraspinal mass by reason of local erosion and expansion of the spinal canal. This alone will not distinguish an epidermoid or dermoid cyst but associated spinal malformation points to the diagnosis, particularly if the patient is a child and if there is some external stigma such as dimple, sinus, naevus or hairy tuft. Occult spinal bifida may be associated with a fibrolipomatous mass or with a dermoid.

If they do not involve the spinal cord most of the cysts can be totally removed. On theoretical grounds it should be possible to extirpate intramedullary cysts but as in the cerebral examples, the wall may be so filamentous that its removal damages the adjacent cord. Preliminary evacuation of the contents may help in the withdrawal of the cyst lining but if this is adherent it is wise to desist. Although recurrence is to be anticipated, this may not occur for many years during which time the patient may enjoy good function.

Teratomas are rare; from the literature and their own experience Sachs and Horrax (1949)

could collect only 25 examples compared with 62 epidermoids and dermoids. They are somewhat more common in children than adults and in the lumbosacral than higher regions of the spine. Usually extramedullary though attached by a pedicle to the cord, they may arise within the cord. The cystic element may predominate or the tumour may be entirely solid; it may be malignant and give rise to subarachnoid and remote metastases (Rand and Rand 1960). Ossification may occur within the solid portion, large enough to cast an intraspinal 'shadow' in the radiograms. The rarity of radiological opacities in this situation lends a diagnostic importance to this finding; otherwise the radiological signs are those of a longstanding expanding mass in the spinal canal. In the majority of cases a correct diagnosis of the nature of the lesion is unlikely to be achieved, but one feature is emphasized by those who have had personal experience, namely marked fluctuations in the severity of the clinical picture; but such fluctuations do occur in other cystic forms of cord compression. Prognosis after removal of a teratoma is good provided there has been no histological evidence of malignancy. Occasionally the teratomatous 'sacrococcygeal tumour' of infants and children may have an intraspinal tongue of tumour.

## 1b. Enterogenous cysts

These cysts are encountered mainly in the thoracic area and their distinctive macroscopic common feature lies in the consistency of their contents which is mucoid or stringy. They may lie ventral or dorsal to the cord or within its substance. Similar cysts have also been found lying ventral to the pons, in front of the cervical cord and in the conus (Small 1962). The cyst wall is usually lined by a low columnar or cuboidal celled and sometimes ciliated epithelium with mucus-containing cells. Many thoracic enterogenous cysts are associated with extensive malformation of the adjacent vertebrae: ill formed or bifid neural arches, widening of the canal, diastematomyelia, hemivertebra. There may be malformation elsewhere; Arnold–Chiari, lumbar spina bifida, diverticula from the oesophagus passing into the spinal canal through or between vertebral bodies and mediastinal cysts (Rhaney and Barclay 1959). To describe these cysts as neurenteric implies their origin from remnants of the neurenteric canal. Bremer (1952) pointed out that the neurenteric canal runs from the yolk sac cavity through the primitive knot (Hensen's node) to the amniotic cavity: remnants must lie immediately caudal to the coccyx. Malformations or residual communications between intestine and dorsal surface at higher levels he called accessory neurenteric canals; he suggested that they arise at an early stage when the yolk sac is shrinking and lateral compression forces it dorsally to protrude through the developing notochord. It is to this mechanism that he ascribes the bony spur and split spinal cord of diastomatomyelia. Bentley and Smith (1960) elaborated this thesis further in explanation of enterogenous cysts, complex malformations in the posterior mediastinum and anterior meningocele. Rhaney and Barclay (1959) considered adherent growth of notochord to be the predisposing factor. Removal of these cysts via an intraspinal approach can be difficult as the walls are often tightly adherent to neural tissue. Although complete removal is ideal, drainage and wide opening of the cysts can produce dramatic neurological recovery. However, recurrence is not uncommon and may require re-operation or perhaps percutaneous aspiration of the cyst under ultrasonic guidance. If the presence of an anterior intrathoracic connection is shown, a further transthoracic procedure should be performed to remove this part.

## 2. Endothelial cysts

A considerable group of intraspinal cysts are lined by endothelium, contain clear watery contents resembling or identical to cerebrospinal fluid and are often termed meningeal. Their aetiology in many cases is obscure, though some probably arise from a developmental error and

their enlargement is due to hydrostatic factors. It is convenient to consider them in two groups according to their anatomical position, intradural and extradural. The former are commonly referred to as 'arachnoid cysts'.

(a) *Arachnoid cysts* or more accurately, leptomeningeal cysts are found as sausage-shaped collections of cerebrospinal fluid sequestered within a compartment of arachnoid. This portion of meninx may appear transparent and entirely normal, or may show the thickening and opacities of fibrosis. The cysts may be single or multiple, most commonly occurring in the thoracic region posterior to the cord. They may be found accidentally at operation or post-mortem and be inferred from myelography, without giving rise to symptoms of cord compression. On the other hand large loculations of fluid may give rise to symptoms which resolve following surgical intervention.

Arachnoid cysts, into which contrast medium cannot enter and which give a filling defect or nonspecific block on myelography, may be aetiologically related to arachnoidal diverticula or pouches which are sporadically encountered during radiological examination. These are commonly multiple and lie posterior to the cord; the medium flows into the pouch and is retained in the erect position, flowing out when the patient lies down (Teng & Rudner 1960). It is likely that these pouches are developmental, due to excessive trabeculation in the leptomeningeal space. Complete isolation of a pouch by increase in size from pulsation, by gradual closure of its mouth as a result of wedging between cord and theca or by adventitious adhesions may account for the rare arachnoid cyst.

(b) *Extradural cysts* are more common than the intradural variety. Gortvai (1963) culled the literature of 56 cases and added 5 personal ones and several more have since been reported. The cyst lies in the epidural space posterior to the theca, is of cylindrical shape, and usually extends under several neural arches. It has a pale, firm, thin wall which may resemble dura but is a fibrous capsule for the inner lining layer of endothelium, which may show areas of proliferation like an arachnoid granulation. The cyst is easily separable from the dura mater except at an extremity, usually the upper, where a small isthmus or pedicle fuses with the dura. This may be in the midline or at the junction of a dura sheath with the theca. The pedicle may be solid or may contain a small canal by which the cyst communicates directly with the subarachnoid space. The general view is that these represent a pulsion diverticulum through a small dural deficiency, though the description of very similar lesions arising in the lumbar spine and described as ganglion cysts from the facet joint is of interest (Kao *et al.* 1968).

Extradural cysts may present at all ages but do so most frequently in patients between 10 and 15 years old. They can arise anywhere in the spine, most commonly in the thoracic area. As in other cystic lesions, periodic clinical improvement followed by deterioration is common. The radiological examination shows an expanded spinal canal. Dastur (1963) reported the usual presence of paravertebral soft tissue shadows with erosion of adjacent ribs. Myelography may merely demonstrate a block compatible with an extradural lesion, but the medium may occasionally enter the cyst identifying its nature and situation. In Dastur's cases it entered the paravertebral shadows and operation confirmed that they were diverticula of extradural cysts.

There is no particular difficulty in excising these cysts but the pedicle should be examined carefully for a communication with the subarachnoid space. This may be only of pinhole size, but it should be obliterated by a clip or ligature to guard against a leak of cerebrospinal fluid possibly causing a recurrence. A large dural defect should be closed with a fascial graft. The prognosis is excellent.

(c) *Perineural cysts* (root cysts). Cystic swelling in the course of the spinal nerve roots after their enclosure by the sheath of dura mater are occasionally encountered. They lie within the root sleeve, between the pial sheath and the surrounding arachnoid, involving the posterior root or the ganglion or both. It is thought that such cysts result from adhesions causing loculation

between these layers. Tarlov (1953) found degenerative changes in nerve fibres and ganglion cells within the cysts. He formed the opinion that they might occasionally be the cause of radicular symptoms and published his experiences with several cases and further details of the morphology of these cysts. Rexed and Wennström (1959) studied the pathology of these cysts and were unsure as to whether there was communication with the subarachnoid space. However, Holt and Yates (1964) confirmed the subarachnoid communication which allows these cysts to fill with contrast during radiculography. Tarlov (1961) reviewed 32 cases, all but 2 arising on sacral roots. Symptoms included backache, radicular paraesthesiae or impaired sensibility, limb weakness and urinary difficulty, but there was no characteristic clinical picture. Operation was performed in 30 patients, complete symptomatic relief resulting in half. Tarlov recommended total excision of the posterior root and its ganglion, which was carried out in 15 patients with complete relief in 12.

Extradural cysts may occur in the lumbosacral region, and should not be confused with perineural cysts. Confusion arises because both are occasionally referred to as 'sacral cysts' and the same name is loosely used also for sacral meningoceles.

## 3. Parasitic cysts

Parasitic cysts within the dural tube are exceedingly rare in this country. There are a few records of intramedullary cysticercosis (Singh *et al.* 1966) and the literature records a limited number of cases of schistosomiasis. The reader, however, is directed to the account of parasitic diseases of the spinal cord by Hughes (1966). Intradural hydatid cysts are thought only to occur as seedlings from a cerebral primary cyst but the extradural variety are considered here for convenience. Hydatid disease is commoner in some sheep-farming regions of the British Isles (such as South Wales) but remains a rare disease. On the contrary, Talib (1968) reported some 100 cases per year in an Iraqi hospital, though few involved the spine. Hydatid infestation of bone differs from that of other tissues by the absence of the formation of the external fibrous membrane or ectocyst within which forms the main and the daughter cysts. Spillage from these during removal reinfests the operation site. The lack of ectocyst is attributed to a failure of reaction by the bone; in consequence daughter cysts spread widely into the bone and their eradication is possible only by resection of the whole bone, or amputation. The impracticability of this in the case of the spine prevents surgical eradication of the disease, although a few cases have been reported in which the cyst has been solitary and its removal has resulted in cure. Robinson (1959) has reviewed the spinal form of the disease in the light of his experiences and the literature.

Spinal manifestations occur more commonly in early middle age, rarely in the young or the old. The thoracic vertebrae are more commonly infested and next commonest. The vertebral body becomes honeycombed with cysts and adjacent vertebrae may be involved though the intervertebral disc is spared. Collapse and the formation of a gibbus is common but later for the compact shell of the body tends to resist erosion while the cysts spread into the cancellous tissue of the pedicles and neural arches. Invasion of the paravertebral tissues causes soft tissue shadows in the X-rays; the outer edge may show calcification. Robinson points out that these radiological changes are similar to those of spinal tuberculosis; distinction may be made by the destruction of the disc in the latter disease. Paraplegia develops in about one-quarter of the cases. This may be due to the extrusion of material into the spinal canal if collapse occurs, or to the cysts eroding into the walls of the canal and infesting the extradural tissue, where they spread widely. Invasion of the dura mater is apparently very rare.

The evolution of compression is undistinguished: pain of spinal and radicular distribution and the development of the signs of neurological deficit. The course may cover months or even several years. Special tests (Casoni, complement-fixation, eosinophilia) are of value if the results are positive, but the diagnosis is not excluded if they are negative.

Treatment consists of laminectomy and removal of as many of the cysts as possible. Long periods of palliation have been achieved but the ultimate prognosis is bad. It has been observed in the operative treatment of hydatid disease elsewhere that if the wound becomes secondarily infected and the patient recovers, a recurrence of cysts is less likely to occur.

# Spinal cord compression of infective origin

The spinal cord may become compressed by an extradural infective process which may be acute, as in extradural abscess, or chronic, as in a low-grade pyogenic or tuberculous process. Subdural abscess is rare and clinically indistinguishable from the extradural variety. Intramedullary abscess is exceedingly rare.

## Acute extradural spinal abscess

Dandy (1926) was perhaps the first to emphasize the serious nature of this illness and the necessity of urgent therapy to avoid permanent paraplegia. It is not a common disease and although the clinical picture is dramatic, delayed diagnosis has disastrous consequences. The majority of the collections of pus which develop do so in the thoracic area. They usually remain localized to a few segments but may spread the full length of the spine, though they are prevented from extending intracranially by the attachment of the dura to the margins of the foramen magnum. Infection is haematogenous from an obvious or occult focus elsewhere in the body or it invades the extradural tissues from a vertebra, usually pedicle or neural arch. Osteomyelitis of the vertebral body is less likely to infect the extradural space for anterior to the dura there is no loose fatty areolar tissue; the posterior longitudinal ligament helps to restrain the intraspinal spread of infection. Whether blood-borne infection or spread from osteitis is the more frequent cause is uncertain. Browder and Meyers (1941) reported that in 14 cases there was unequivocal evidence of vertebral bone infection in 12 (post-mortem examination, operation findings, radiological changes), on the other hand Hulme and Dott (1954) could prove bone or joint infection in only one quarter of their cases. The commonest organism is the *staphylococcus aureus*. Disorders which contribute to this type of infection are diabetes mellitus and intravenous drug abuse.

Inflammatory swelling, pus and granulation tissue lead to compression of the spinal cord. Involvement of the extradural spinal veins causes thrombophlebitis which is liable to spread into the veins of the spinal cord and the radicular arteries may be the seat of arteritis and thrombosis. Thus the cord is at risk by both compression and infarction; in some cases at operation or post-mortem it appears to be little compressed but extensively softened. The dura is fortunately remarkably resistant to infection. The cerebrospinal fluid may remain entirely free from pleiocytosis which may lead to the false assumption that an inflammatory process cannot be the cause of the illness. If intrathecal infection occurs, it is more likely to be due to spread along thrombosed veins. Acute extradural abscess is a fulminating disease in which paraplegia may develop in hours or a few days.

Excruciatingly severe pain in the spine is the first and most important symptom, its site corresponding to the level of the extradural infection. Although backache is a banal symptom of many illnesses, rarely is it so severe and localized, and accompanied by such paravertebral muscle spasm, except in an acute exacerbation of a prolapsed intervertebral disc from which the absence of systemic disorder and the later course of events makes distinction clear. Concurrent with the pain, acute extradural abscess is accompanied by the toxic symptoms of infection, malaise, fever and raised pulse rate. Painful stiffness of the neck may simulate acute meningitis. The syndrome of the spinal cord com-

pression usually commences within a day or so and spread of the spinal pain in radicular pattern should immediately arouse suspicions of an intraspinal lesion. The motor and sensory disturbances indicating failure of spinal cord function commonly start distally rising steadily as compression increases and as purulent exudate spreads upwards and downwards. As mentioned earlier, paraplegia may be total within a day or so; the final stages are often abrupt consonant with the vascular occlusions that may be found post-mortem. In 7 of the 25 cases reported by Hulme and Dott (1954) the interval between the onset of symptoms of impaired cord function and total paraplegia was 24 hours or less. The rapid evolution may induce a state of spinal shock characterized by flaccidity of the paralysed muscles and absence of reflexes, as seen in traumatic paraplegia. Retention of urine is common. The spine is usually tender at the site of the initial pain, though if upward extension of the abscess has lifted the sensory level above this area, tenderness may have been abolished. Careful inspection in a good light, or palpation may reveal the presence of a slight fullness or swelling over, or to one side of, of the affected area. Rarely and in more subacute cases, there may be redness and fluctuation. An important sign is painful rigidity of the neck and spine.

Many false diagnoses have been made in cases of acute extradural spinal abscess usually because it is relatively uncommon and consequently its possibility has not been entertained. Little harm is done if the urgency of relieving a rapidly progressive spinal compression is recognized and prompt action taken; operation will reveal the pathological nature of the lesion so that appropriate treatment is instituted. However, the consequences for recovery of function and for life are grave if the developing neurological disturbance is not quickly recognized as spinal compression. Erroneous diagnoses include intra-abdominal suppuration, multiple sclerosis and transverse myelitis, but the severity and persistence of the pain should lead one to suspect extradural abscess as the cause.

Investigations are directed towards confirmation of pyogenic infection, radiological evidence of bone disease and lumbar puncture. A polymorphonuclear leucocytosis is commonly present and the sedimentation rate may be high though this may be due to a concurrent infection. X-rays of the spine are unlikely to show osteitis in the early stages of the acute disease and confusion with malignant infiltration is more likely in subacute cases. Myelography is of prime importance in order to detect obstruction of the subarachnoid space by compression. The question has been raised as to the danger of infecting the leptomeninges by the lumbar puncture if an abscess is present. Occasionally the needle will traverse a pool of pus before penetrating the dura mater; therefore aspiration should be repeatedly attempted as the point of the needle passes through the extradural space. In any case spreading the infection has less serious consequences than has failure to make the correct diagnosis. A complete extradural block will be present if there is paraparesis, except in the rare fulminating case in which spinal infarction precedes compression, and then there is likely to be partial obstruction. The cerebrospinal fluid contains an increased amount of protein and sometimes a mild pleiocytosis, usually polymorphonuclear; but as noted earlier, the cell count may be normal. Very occasionally an abscess and suppurative meningitis are both present.

Cure of an acute extradural abscess probably cannot be achieved by antibiotic therapy alone and, in any event, surgery is needed to relieve the tension of the abscess and to allow bacteriological examination of the pus. In the case of an extradural abscess, the best surgical approach is via laminectomy as the main collection of pus may extend posteriorly over several segments. In many cases, the amount of frank pus actually obtained from the extradural space is minimal; the infective process being present as adherent granulation tissue with small pockets of pus. Provided that appropriate antibiotic therapy in adequate parenteral dosage is commenced, it is unnecessary to expose the entire extent of the purulent exudate. The major

pockets of pus should be drained and the extradural space running caudal and rostral to the laminectomy irrigated via a soft catheter. The dura should not be opened in the presence of an extradural abscess as it provides a fairly effective barrier to the spread of infection when intact. There is debate as to whether to close the wound without drainage or to leave drains down the extradural space for postoperative irrigation. Very occasionally, in a panspinal abscess it may be necessary to perform two small laminectomies, one in the cervical area and one lumbar, to allow effective drainage. Mortality has been dramatically decreased with modern antibiotic therapy. Nevertheless, acute extradural abscess remains a grave disease with high morbidity. Cases which have been diagnosed at an early stage with only minor neurological deficit have a good prognosis but, due to the rapidity with which the disease progresses, great clinical awareness is necessary to make such an early diagnosis. The development of paraplegia is a very ominous sign and recovery from this state of complete paralysis is rare.

## Chronic pyogenic infection of the spine

The vast majority of low-grade pyogenic infections of the spine originate *de novo* or postoperatively as an area of vertebral osteitis and pus and granulation tissue invade the extradural space as a secondary event only. However, pure chronic extradural infection can occur and syphilitic gummae used to be the commonest cause of such infection (Fisher 1963). Chronic extradural abscesses with organisms which more usually cause acute infection were seen by Hulme and Dott but in such cases the true diagnosis is likely to be discovered only at laminectomy.

Intradural infection is rare. Pyogenic acute intramedullary abscesses vary rarely follow meningitis and the development of paraparesis during a bout of meningitis should lead to suspicion of this diagnosis. However, the progression of the disease may be very slow in the cases reported by Betty and Lorber (1983). Chronic intradural infection is more likely to be due to fungi, tuberculoma or gummae.

The organisms responsible for low-grade spinal osteitis are usually staphylococci, although brucella, coliforms and pseudomonas are sometimes responsible. The disease may present acutely but more usually there is a history of several weeks of spinal pain and radicular pain. If untreated the disease leads to bony destruction and angulation which may narrow the spinal canal. This, in conjunction with invasion of the epidural space by pus, leads to the clinical syndrome of cord or cauda equina compression. Sudden deterioration due to infarction of the cord consequent upon thrombosis in blood vessels within the pus may occur. Chronic spinal osteomyelitis is most commonly seen in the thoracolumbar area. It may affect only the posterior elements of the spinal column but more usually the infection develops in the vertebral body. Penetration along the blood-vessels passing into the disc in young people or interference with the blood supply of the end-plate and its consequent destruction allows the infective process to involve the disc. Thus, vertebral collapse and blurring of the end-plate area of the vertebra adjacent to a narrow disc space is highly suggestive of infection. Such changes are usually present on plain radiographs by the time the patient presents. However, they do take some weeks to develop and, in an early case, radiology may be normal. Bone scanning especially with early 'blood-pool' imaging may be positive in early disease (Gilday et al. 1975). The disease process is usually localized but occasionally several segments of the spine may be involved.

Treatment in a case with little or no neurological deficit consists of bed rest and antibiotics.
However, prior to commencing treatment the diagnosis should be confirmed by needle biopsy which will also allow culture of any pus obtained for antibiotic sensitivity. Not all of these cases of low grade infection will yield actual pus therefore the biopsy procedure should include lavage of the disc space and the removal of some cores of

adjacent bone for pathological evaluation looking for organisms. The efficacy of treatment can be judged by the subsidence of pain, restoration of erythrocyte sedimentation rate (ESR) to normal, and eventually radiological signs of bony fusion. Once pain and the ESR are subsiding, the patient can be mobilized in a close fitting spinal support jacket. Antibiotic therapy has to be given over a lengthy period, often lasting some months. In cases with significant signs of cord compression and those with increasing kyphotic deformity, surgical measures in addition to antibiotics are necessary. The poor results, limitations and dangers of laminectomy in the presence of anterior spinal disease are best recognized in the realm of infection and have been so for many years (Seddon 1935). Radical anterior debridment of the abscess and infected bone is necessary to decompress the dura. Spinal stability can then be achieved following prolonged recumbency but application of the surgical techniques developed for tuberculous disease (see below) allows much better management. The insertion of strut bone grafts in infected areas does not impede their incorporation into bony fusion and early mobilization with supporting jacket can be performed (Kemp et al. 1973). Severe kyphotic angulation or anterior strut grafting over a lengthy spinal segment may require additional posterior support by segmental spinal instrumentation but it is important to stress that this is performed on top of the laminae and that laminectomy is not performed.

Infection of the disc space alone is rare in adults but does occur in children (Spiegel et al. 1972). By far the commonest cause of discitis in adults is as a complication of surgery or discography. After an initial period of postoperative improvement of usually 6–8 weeks, there is a recrudescence of back pain which is often severe. There is virtually no systemic evidence of infection but the ESR is usually markedly elevated. Occasionally, blood cultures can be positive but usually organism identification is dependant on disc aspiration though even this can be negative in the presence of infection. Plain radiology only shows changes in later stages and bone scanning is unhelpful due to postoperative changes. Treatment consists of rest and antibiotics (the organism is almost always staphylococcal) until the pain and ESR have subsided. The final result of the discectomy operation is not usually compromised following a successfully treated postoperative discitis, despite the intervening period of pain and immobility.

**Tuberculous spinal disease**

Tuberculous involvement of the spine typifies those areas of spinal disease where there is considerable overlap between orthopaedics and neurosurgery. The bony destruction which occurs demands understanding of the problems of instability and fusion techniques whilst dural compression especially in cases with bony kyphosis, demands considerable neurosurgical expertise to allow safe decompression. Ideally, this calls for a team approach combining both disciplines, and any neurosurgeon dealing with such problems alone must acquire experience and understanding of spinal fusion by anterior routes.

Spinal tuberculosis is most common in the thoracic followed by the cervical and lumbar regions. Neurological compromise is mostly the result of compression by intrusion of disease products into the spinal canal. The agent may be tuberculous granulation tissue and pus, extruded sequestra or fragments of intervertebral disc; factors which produce slow changes in the course of progressive disease. More sudden deterioration may result from pathological fracture and sudden vertebral collapse. Paraplegia from these causes is of 'early' onset, that is to say during the active stages of the disease, and forms a distinct clinical group. Compression may also be caused by the sharp apex of an angular bony kyphus which may occur late in the disease providing the other clinical group of paraplegia of 'late' onset. In 'late' cases clinical manifestations are delayed until after the spinal disease appears to have entirely healed; the interval may be one of years. Late paraplegia may also be due to a recrudescence of tuberculous activity within the spinal canal. The two groups of cases, early and late, are of about equal magnitude and the disease, although uncommon, is by no means rare in this country. Neither is it confined to immigrant populations, being seen not infrequently in people from Caucasian backgrounds.

The occurrence of neurological involvement in spinal tuberculosis (Pott's paraplegia) is actually uncommon (Cholmeley 1959) but it is these cases that tend to present to a neurosurgeon. Pain is often the presenting symptom and paraparesis usually evolves slowly with severity fluctuating in the early stages. Sensory disturbance is often mild or absent. In advanced cases, a paravertebral abscess may erupt onto the surface as a discharging sinus. Occasionally, plain radiography may not be grossly abnormal especially in cases where the infective focus is in the neural arch. More commonly there is severe destructive disease of the anterior spinal column with kyphotic angulation and the radiographic appearances are similar to those described for chronic pyogenic infection. It is important to stress that patients with tuberculous spinal disease do not normally have active pulmonary disease. The main diagnostic confusion arises with metastatic disease and here the role of needle biopsy becomes of paramount importance as, on the one hand, laminectomy in tuberculosis is disastrous and, on the other, radiotherapy in tuberculosis is obviously ineffective. During placement of the guiding needles during needle biopsy, a paravertebral abscess is often found and aspiration of the slightly bloodstained, thin pus will give the diagnosis.

Several therapeutic approaches have been used following the introduction of effective antibiotic therapy which has allowed the expansion of surgical techniques. Laminectomy is contraindicated because it merely destabilizes the spine. Costotransversectomy is less destructive but poses problems if the disease extends over many segments. Griffiths *et al.* (1956) felt that this approach only produced neurological recovery if pus was found under tension. Wilkinson (1955) extended this procedure to a two-level approach that allowed packing the cavity of the empty abscess with bone chips but effective strut-grafting is impractical through this approach. Dott and Capener (Alexander 1946) devised a more extensive procedure termed anterolateral decompression which gave a better access by a retropleural approach following excision of the heads and necks of several ribs. Hodgson and Stock (1956) pioneered the radical anterior approach via thoractomy or thoracoabdominal operation which has now been adapted to other anterior spinal disorders. This approach allows radical decompression of the spine over many segments, if necessary. Additionally, the defect so created can be stabilized by a bone graft from either iliac crest or fibula. The use of this technique gives superior results both from the point of stability and neurological recovery (MRC Working Party on Tuberculosis of the Spine 1982) and it also allows a safer approach to patients with late paraparesis due to acute bony angulation, where the kyphus can then be stabilized with anteriorly placed strut grafts.

A mainstay of treatment is effective antibiotic therapy. In patients who do not have neurological deficit, or only a very minor one, chemotherapy alone has been shown to give acceptable results and the addition of bed rest or plaster jacket did nothing to improve such results (MRC Working Party on Tuberculosis of the Spine 1976, 1978). However, patients so treated take longer to achieve spinal fusion and have an increased incidence of late bony kyphosis and paraparesis. For this reason, the MRC Working Party reported in 1982 that the approach of radical resection of the lesion with autologous bone grafting of Hodgson and Stock (often referred to as the 'Hong Kong' procedure) was the treatment of choice in spinal tuberculosis, wherever the facilities and expertise for such procedures were available. It should be stressed, however, that all the patients studied in these MRC reports were still able to walk the length of a room prior to treatment. Those with more severe neurological deficits should all be treated by urgent radical anterior surgery.

## Intraspinal lipoma

Lipomas account for 1% of intraspinal tumours. They may lie in the extradural tissue and here their presence is understandable in view of the considerable amount of fatty tissue normally present. Others lie within the arachnoid, attached loosely or, more commonly firmly, to the spinal cord and may be embedded within it; emerging nerve roots may pass through the lipomatous tissue. The aetiology of these lesions is obscure and there is some debate as to whether they are neoplastic or hamartomatous. It is probably significant that in an appreciable proportion there are associated congenital abnormalities elsewhere in the body (Caram et al. 1957). They also occur as part of a spina bifida occulta, may extend within the theca and be incorporated in the conus; such lesions are part of the dysraphic malformations and are considered elsewhere.

Whether extra- or intradural, they lie on the posterior aspect of the cord; the former are more limited in extent, generally under one or two laminae, the latter may be much longer and some are recorded to have covered practically the whole length of the spinal cord (Talbert & Simmons 1961). They occur at all ages though the majority of middle-aged patients who present give an account of a long history reaching back into early life (Giuffré 1966). The clinical course is usually slow and often entirely painless with gradually evolving cord compression. Marks et al. (1984) have reported extradural lipomata mimicking the features of lumbar disc prolapse. Extradural lipomas have a predilection to appear in the thoracic area whilst the intradural variety often develop in the neck. Those arising in the conus and cauda equina area are usually associated with dysraphic states. Intradural lipomas are invariably juxtamedullary and intimately related to the pia. On the first exposure there may be the appearance of a plane of cleavage from the adjacent cord but trial dissection soon reveals that there is none and that neural elements traverse the lipoma. Radiology may show evidence of expansion of the canal and myelography may show the appearance of an intramedullary tumour. The fatty composition is revealed on CT as an area of very low density, lower than CSF.

## Kyphosis and kyphoscoliosis

Severe spinal deformities may themselves ultimately give rise to paraplegia. This develops slowly, the earliest sign being a spastic weakness of the legs often accompanied by numbness or tingling of the feet which can eventually lead to paraplegia. Deformities which act thus are midthoracic in which region the tight fit of the cord in the spinal canal and the pattern of the blood supply to the spinal cord renders it susceptible to interference. Apart from this common factor, the causes of paraplegia from kyphosis and kyphoscoliosis are probably different. In the former the deformity of the spinal cord makes an acute angle which deeply indents the spinal cord; it may be thinned to a ribbon. The extent to which the theca and its contents are stretched over the apex of the deformity perhaps determines which cases become paraplegic, for if the vertebral bodies are considerably reduced in height as a result of collapse, angular deformity will not necessarily stretch the cord. In kyphoscoliosis, the deformity is sinuous and the kyphotic element less acutely angulated though the total deformity may still be severe. The spinal cord is affected over a greater number of segments and is usually not flattened to a ribbon-like structure. The scoliosis adds two other stresses to the cord, lateral flexion and rotation along its axis. The cord is drawn against the pedicles of the concavity and the roots in their dural sheaths on the convexity of the deformity are put on the stretch. Vertebral, and therefore cord, rotation may be so marked that the roots of the convexity aspect lie almost posterior and those of the concavity almost anterior to the cord. These multidirectional distortions of the long tracts may impair their conduction. In addition, tension in the convexity roots and approximation of the intervertebral foramina of the concavity may obstruct blood flow through the radicular arter-

ies which are particularly important in this junctional zone of vascular supply. Winter and Hall (1978), in an extensive review have discussed the various aetiological factors involved. These can range from congenital (hemivertebrae and failure of anterior segmentation) to postoperative, following laminectomy or thecoperitoneal shunting and each category may pose different problems.

Surgical treatment is indicated at the earliest sign of cord involvement. Indeed, proper early treatment of many aetiological factors can prevent neurological involvement. Surgical correction after severe cord compression has occurred is not only more hazardous but also allows less chance of recovery. The surgical correction has to be carefully planned and tailored to each individual. It may well require staged surgery which essentially consists of excision of the kyphotic and compressing segment via an anterior approach with strut grafting followed by posterior segmental stabilization. Indeed, during the correction of kyphotic deformity in ankylosing spondylitis it is necessary to perform a wedge osteotomy of the spine to allow correction. This was initially described by Smith-Peterson et al. in 1945, and has been reviewed more recently by Simmons (1977).

## Paget disease of the spine

The changes induced in the vertebral column in Paget disease (osteitis deformans) may be such that neurological deficit can arise as first reported by Wyllie (1923). Paget disease itself is not uncommon especially with increasing age. Involvement of the spine, especially lumbosacral, is common but spinal cord dysfunction is rare (Miller 1967). The aetiology of the neurological deficit is unclear. It may be related to genuine compression by hyperplastic bone or to a vascular steal related to the grossly hyperaemic bone. The disease passes through alternating resorptive and proliferative phases which alter the bone structure with the result that there is some vertebral body collapse and transverse expansion associated with pedicular and laminar thickening. Neurological deficit is commonest in the thoracic area and is occasionally related to sarcomatous change in adjacent Paget bone. Clinical features are often slow to evolve and pain is unusual in the absence of sarcomatous changes.

Standard treatment prior to the medical advances discussed below was by laminectomy. This could be an extremely hazardous procedure due to the intense vascularity of the bone. Sadar et al. (1972) reported on 64 of their patients who had undergone laminectomy. Eighty-five per cent of them improved but 6 patients had to have more than one laminectomy. More recently, Douglas et al. (1981) reviewed the results of medical therapy with calcitonin and diphosphonates showing results identical to those of surgery. They felt that the rapid neurological response seen in many patients was due to the reduction in bony blood flow obtained by these drugs and that progress could be monitored by following the levels of serum alkaline phosphatase.

## Vascular disorders of the spine

### 1. Arteriovenous malformations

From approximately 1960 onwards there has been an increasing awareness of the potential for treatment which exists in the management of patients with spinal arteriovenous malformation (AVM). Such lesions were formerly considered as rare, surgically untreatable abnormalities of, in particular, the thoracolumbar cord. However, increasing knowledge of the natural history and vastly improved diagnostic techniques have led to more frequent diagnosis and better understanding, although there is still considerable debate of the underlying pathological anatomy and physiology. With this has come realization that the majority of such lesions can be removed with considerable benefit to the patient. Frequency is still difficult to assess. In their monograph on myelography Lombardi and Passerini

(1964) reported 317 spinal tumours and 34 AVMs, an incidence of 10%; but the majority of series give an incidence of between 4 and 5% for the ratio of spinal AVM to tumour (for example Krayenbühl et al. 1969). Higher incidence figures tend to reflect the personal interest of certain authors such as Pia in 1975 (10.5%). Surgical interest is reflected by the increasing number of patients reported, with Pennybacker (1958) reporting on 16 cases found in the course of 390 spinal explorations for focal disease, then the reports of Krayenbühl et al. in 1969 (43 cases), R. Djindjian et al. in 1969 (50 cases), Pia in 1978 (60 cases) and R. Djindjian again in 1978 (now with 150 cases.). It seems that the history of cerebral AVMs has been repeated; an increasing number of spinal cord examples being discovered as the cause of obscure progressive paraparesis and of sub-arachnoid haemorrhage by heightened awareness and the use of modern diagnostic techniques, with a large proportion becoming amenable to excision. Although arteriovenous malformations may occur throughout the length of the spinal cord, they occur more frequently in the caudal area. In the series reported by R. Djindjian et al. in 1969, 12% of cases were in the cervical area, 28% were upper thoracic and 60% were in the thoracolumbosacral area. The remarkable series of selective arteriography studies from authors such as R. Djindjian et al. (1966) and DeChiro et al. (1967) have shown that some malformations may have multiple feeding vessels from enlarged radicular arteries in differing spinal areas.

When displayed at operation a spinal AVM can present an intimidating appearance. The cord may be entirely concealed by grossly dilated and convoluted blood vessels: some with well formed walls, containing red blood and pulsating vigorously which appear to be arteries; others with thin walls, larger size and also containing oxygenated blood which appear to be veins distended with blood from the arteriovenous communication; yet others are veins distended with dark blood. Between the vessels there may be a highly visible feltwork of pial vessels. In lesser specimens there may be only a few tortuous vessels, which may be seen to rest in dents on the posterior aspect of the cord. By inspection alone, it can be very difficult to ascertain how much of the lesion lies within the cord. The classification of M. Djindjian (1978) of true intramedullary AVM's show that undoubtedly lesions do involve the tissue of the cord and are supplied by feeders which penetrate the cord coming often from the anterior spinal circulation, though such findings do not necessarily imply that the lesion is unresectable (Cogen & Stein 1983). However, the majority of AVMs arise from posterior circulation and in many of these the site of the true fistula may not even be intradural (Symon et al. 1984) with fistulous communication in the extradural space and the cord vessels merely being draining veins. Even true posteriorly sited juxtamedullary AVMs do not necessarily penetrate the cord or implicate its blood supply but rather seem to invaginate it (Shephard 1963). Indeed, the surrounding, immediately adjacent cord shows a layer of gliosis just as is found in the cerebral variety (Bergstrand et al. 1964).

Attempts by different authors to classify spinal AVMs by their site and architecture has lead to a confusing situation not helped by disagreement on the significance of the exact site of the fistula. Early attention was centered on the position and extent of all abnormal vessels discovered; whereas more recently, there has been concentration on defining the exact 'nidus' of the arteriovenous fistula as distinct from its feeding arteries and draining arterialized veins all of which can extend over segments (Doppman 1971). There is more consensus over the true intramedullary lesion fed by mixed anterior and posterior supplies as described by Michel Djindjian; the debate primarily centres on the posterior lesions. All authors agree on the occurrence of posteriorly sited and supplied AVMs but disagree on their relative frequency and nomenclature. M. Djindjian found that 40% of his 150 patients had what he termed retromedullary AVMs. It is clear that this group corresponds closely to that of Aminoff (1976) but he felt that they constituted 80% of cases. Logue (1979) reported on 24 cases, all of which were retromedullary. He stressed that this type of spinal AVM tends to present in elderly males. Further, he showed that although abnormal vessels were present on the back of the cord sometimes with small branches which penetrated the cord, the lesion really consists of a single feeding artery in 90% of cases with the nidus of the fistula lying on or outside the dura near the entry of the nerve root. This work has recently been updated by Symon et al. (1984).

As a result of such work, Aminoff et al. (1974) suggested that one explanation of the development of neurological damage in the presence of a spinal AVM was that of the effect of a prolonged rise in the venous pressure transmitted back to the cord. They argued that in the case of these retromedullary or extradural lesions that the only contact between the fistula near the root and the cord was via the arterialized draining vein and that, therefore, 'a steal' effect could not be responsible. Following this to its conclusion, it was suggested that all that was necessary for successful treatment was the disconnection of the fistula by division of the draining vein which had often previously been described erroneously as a 'feeder'. Though Logue still recommended obliteration of the fistula which was surgically easy to perform Symon et al. go so far as to suggest that this may be unnecessary. On the contrary, Hurth et al. (1978) felt that a 'steal' mechanism by which blood was shunted away from the cord through the fistula was the most likely explanation of an evolving deficit. There does seem little doubt that when the precarious nature of the cord blood supply is considered, part at least of the effects of the cord of an intramedullary lesion may be mediated by such a shunting mechanism.

Although other mechanisms for producing neurological deficit have been suggested, for example cord compression (Shephard 1963) and thrombosis of vessels (Wyburn–Mason 1943), there is one mechanism which is accepted by all authors; that of subarachnoid haemorrhage. Haemorrhage is unusual in the retromedullary or dural type and its occurrence suggests a lesion with an intramedullary component. Aminoff and

Logue found that subarachnoid haemorrhage occurred in 10% of their patients; though R. Djindjian *et al.* (1969) reported an incidence of 30%. Aminoff and Logue reported cervical AVMs to carry twice the risk of haemorrhage than those of other regions. This probably represents the fact that true retromedullary AVMs are less common in the cervical area. Aminoff (1976) found that one half of patients with subarachnoid haemorrhage had at least one recurrent haemorrhage which proved fatal in 18% of those patients. A further one-half of those surviving their second haemorrhage went on to have at least one other bleed. Fortunately, haematomyelia appeared to be rare.

Clinically, arteriovenous malformations may present at any age. Intramedullary varieties tend to present early and have a higher incidence of subarachnoid haemorrhage whereas the retromedullary, dural or extradural types tend to present later in life with a progressive neurological deficit. The incidence of subarachnoid haemorrhage has been discussed. Clinically, it presents in much the same way as the cerebral variety although an onset of the pain over the spine is suggestive of spinal origin. Marked radicular pain in association with subarachnoid haemorrhage also suggests a spinal origin. Odom (1960) observed that the source of spinal subarachnoid haemorrhage was not necessarily an AVM but that on occasion it could be a neoplasm and aneurysms arising from spinal vessels do occur, albeit rarely (Leech *et al.* 1976). Spinal subarachnoid haemorrhage may be associated with signs of spinal cord dysfunction and such signs do not necessarily imply the occurrence of haematomyelia.

The commonest clinical presentation of a spinal AVM, however, is with a progressive, usually episodic, spastic paraparesis (or quadriparesis). This was present in 86% of the patients reviewed by R. Djindjian *et al.* (1969). The episodes comprise a sudden development over the course of hours or days of symptoms and signs of a partial lesion of the spinal cord, which as rapidly improve, occasionally completely but usually only partially. A feature

which distinguishes them from multiple sclerosis or other intrinsic disease is that the recurrent episodes occur at the same anatomical level. The recurrence, failure to resolve, or progression of such episodes lead to an increase in neurological deficit which will eventually lead to paraplegia or quadriplegia. Sensory disturbances accompany the motor and may be of diverse distribution: Brown–Séquard; suspended; and generalized. Pain is frequently radicular, affecting more than one dermatome in the back, and of the central types; dysaethesiae also occur. Loss of sphincter control complicates the more severe episodes. When the lesion occupies the cervical or lumbar enlargements the signs indicate more clearly that the paresis affects both upper and lower motor neurons. Since vascular malformations are most frequent in the lower part of the spinal cord, the pattern of radicular pain and of mixed upper and lower motor neuron weakness is the commonest clinical picture. Recurrences gradually lead to severe or total motor and sensory paraplegia and reflex emptying of the bladder. The course of the disease varies, so that severe disability may be present within a year or may be postponed for 20–30 years. However, progression is usually more rapid and Aminoff *et al.* (1974) found that 19% developed severe gait disturbance within six months and that 50% were chairbound within only three years. Episodic changes in the degree of paraparesis may take another form; the patient finds that after walking a short distance, a few hundred yards or for 10 minutes or so, he is compelled to stop because of weakness of the legs or of intense muscular fatigue; having rested, he can again proceed. This phenomenon, first described by Dejerine (1906) and which he called 'intermittent claudication of the spinal cord' is a striking symptom and Dejerine noted that in some cases it led to a spastic paraplegia. He presumed it was due to inadequate circulation in the spinal cord and compared it to the experiments of Stenson in 1667 in which temporary paralysis of an animal's hind limbs followed a few minutes of digital compression of the abdominal aorta. It is encountered also in spinal atherosclerosis (Hughes & Brownell 1966) and more commonly with exercise-induced radicular pain of spinal stenosis.

Differential diagnosis lies between spinal tumour, demyelinating disease, protruded cervical or thoracic disc, polyarteritis nodosa and spinal thrombophlebitis; the latter being a difficult area perhaps related to the necrotic myelitis reported by Foix and Alajouanine (1926) though some have deemed this to be merely a cryptic intramedullary AVM. Many patients with a spinal AVM will have been labelled as hysterical or at least psychologically over-reacting before the AVM is correctly diagnosed. Two important physical signs may aid clinical diagnosis. There may be a vascular naevus in the dermatomes corresponding to the angiomatous spinal segments. This association was first recorded by Cobb (1915). The patient was seen by Cushing who appreciated the significance of the naevi (there were four) and made a correct diagnosis of the nature of the spinal lesion, subsequently confirmed at operation. The incidence of cutaneous vascular abnormalities is low, but it is likely that a careful search is not always made. They were present in 20% of the cases of Ommaya et al. (1969). It should be noted that cutaneous naevi may accompany vertebral vascular lesions and are not necessarily confined to the corresponding dermatomes (Wyburn–Mason 1943). The second valuable sign is a bruit audible over the spine; it is however an infrequent finding (Matthews 1959).

The cerebrospinal fluid taken during an acute episode of deterioration may be bloodstained; at other times it usually contains an increased amount of protein. The cell count is commonly normal, though a mild pleiocytosis may be found after a relapse.

Plain radiography usually shows no abnormality, but widening of the spinal canal due to erosion of the pedicles is occasionally encountered. The finding of an angioma of a vertebral body will suggest that the vascular anomaly is extradural, for the association of bone and spinal cord vascular lesions appears to be exceptional.

Myelography presents a typical appearance in many cases, provided the examination is carried out with sufficient contrast medium and includes screening in both the prone and the supine positions and of the full extent of the theca. In the experience of Djindjian et al. (1970) myelography was abnormal in over 90% of cases but only just over half of these showed the specific appearance of tortuous vessels. As pointed out by Lombardi and Passerini (1964) the appearance on myelography of enlarged, tortuous blood vessels above or below a block may merely represent congested but normal vessels in the area of a tumour. A spinal haemangioblastoma can give a very similar picture.

The advent of safe and selective spinal arteriography has been a major advance in the management of these lesions. The details have been extensively described, primarily by Djindjian, Di Chiro and other groups, but with this technique it is possible to localize precisely the fistulous nidus of the malformation identify all feeding vessels, and usually to determine the presence or absence of supply coming from the anterior spinal arterial system. The technique requires painstaking attention to detail and selective catheterization of all intercostal and lumbar vessels (and vertebral arteries in cervical cases), although there is a possibility that the technology of digital subtraction angiography may allow the use of 'scout' mainstream films to limit the number of selective catheterizations necessary to delineate a malformation. The procedure is now comparatively safe with permanent neurological deterioration being a rare complication (Di Chiro & Wener 1973). The earlier higher risks of mainstream aortography resulted from the older and stronger contrast media then used along with the much greater volumes and injection pressures necessary when selective catheterization is not used.

The first attempt at surgical treatment of a spinal arteriovenous malformation was made by Krause in 1906 and reported in 1911. From that time, sporadic attempts at treatment primarily by ligation of feeding vessels were made but success was rare and failure common, with the result that many regarded these lesions as inoperable.

Radiotherapy was tried and found useless. De-compression alone produced some response but led to an average improvement in only 20% with deterioration in 40% (Yaşargil, quoted by Pia 1978). With greater experience it has become clear that total extirpation of the fistula gives the best results. These results are well summarized up to the late 1970s by Pia (1978) and further results have been published by Logue (1979), Cogen and Stein (1983), Oldfield et al. (1983) and Symon et al. (1984). The earlier attempts at total excision (for example Bassett et al. 1949, Shephard 1963, 1965) involved extensive lami-nectomy and removal of all abnormal vessels. With modern angiography however, surgery has centered on excision of only the actual fistula itself, leaving the extensive draining veins in situ (Doppman 1971, Logue 1979, Symon et al. 1984). Advances in operative microsurgery have increased the surgical accessibility of intra-medullary malformations such that even in the cervical area these lesions can be successfully removed from within the spinal cord (Yaşargil 1975). The final place of embolization in the treatment of spinal AVMs is not yet clear. Any-thing less than the total occlusion of all feeding vessels, no matter how small, will result in the eventual refilling of the lesion (Doppman 1978). The use of embolization in lesions fed by the anterior spinal artery is hazardous due to lack of control of the emboli but total occlusion of a posterior AVM with a single feeding vessel has been reported (R. Djindjian 1978b). Doppman et al. (1971) speculated on the possibility of embol-ization with a polymerizing agent which has been put into practice on limited scale by Hilal and Michelson (1975). Embolization as a pre-operative procedure to reduce blood flow in large intramedullary lesions may be a useful adjunct and it may also be of use in the paraplegic patient with severe pain as a palliative measure.

## 2. Vertebral angioma

Angioma is a chance radiological finding in many parts of the skeleton but most frequently it occurs in the vertebrae and next so in the skull. Schmorl and Junghans (1932) in their classical treatise on the spine found an incidence in the spine of 10%. Clinical symptoms developing from purely vertebral angiomas are rare and are related to pathological fracture. However, the majority of the vertebral angiomas have an extradural component (Pia 1978) and these lesions may produce cord compression. Symp-toms usually do not arise until middle age.

The tumour is of the cavernous type and usually originates in the body, gradually involv-ing the whole vertebrae. The body diminishes little in height, but may expand somewhat; col-lapse is not common, perhaps because pressure on the spinal cord is likely to occur before this event. Compression may be due to bulging of the body into the spinal canal, or extension of the vascular growth into the extradural space. Occasionally the tumour spreads into the para-vertebral tissue giving rise to a paravertebral soft tissue shadow in the X-ray films. Extensive paravertebral angiomatosis may be dem-onstrated by angiography. More than one ver-tebra may be affected, contiguously or at intervals.

The majority of cases present with a straight-forward history of spinal and root pain followed by symptoms and signs of cord compression. The duration of symptoms may be a few months to many years. Occasionally, the picture is one of progressive sensory and motor paraparesis with virtually no pain. Pregnancy is liable to aggra-vate symptoms which may subside after delivery, as with intradural angiomatous malformations. Vertebral collapse, uncommon in angioma as compared with myeloma and metastasis, leads to rapid development or worsening of spinal cord compression.

The radiological signs of angioma of the ver-tebra are usually typical (Figure 21.7). The sagit-tal and coronal diameter of the body may be slightly increased while the height is slightly diminished. There is a general diminution in bone density and texture is diffusely softened; against this background is seen well marked ver-tical trabeculation which imparts the charac-

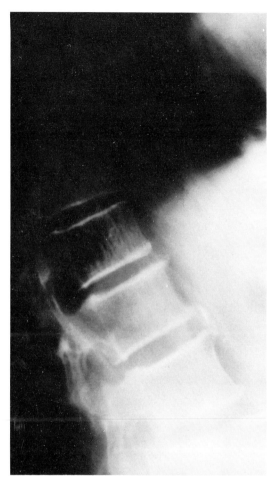

**Fig. 21.7.** Appearance on plain spinal X-ray of an angioma of the vertebral body.

teristic striation. Occasionally, the vertical trabeculae are poorly developed and the appearance is then of reticulation or honeycombing. Angiography is advisable in order to assess the blood supply and also the extent of any extradural, or indeed, intradural, communication which may occur.

At one time laminectomy to relieve compression was associated with a very high mortality from haemorrhage. This resulted in many people using radiotherapy. Modern operative techniques allow much safer and more radical surgery and preoperative embolization should reduce haemorrhage. Excellent results have been reported with over 80% being improved by surgery (Kreuger *et al.* 1961, Pia 1978). However, Kreuger *et al.* also reported similar results in those of their patients who were treated solely by radiotherapy but the selection for each treatment was unclear. On the contrary, Pia felt that radiotherapy was useless.

## 3. Spinal extradural haematoma

A comparatively rare cause for acute compression of the spinal cord is extradural haemorrhage. No cause is found in some, in others the bleeding is derived from an extradural angiomatous mass, rarely it is traumatic in origin. It has been reported in haemophilia, in polycythaemia (Odom 1960) and during anticoagulant therapy (Cloward & Yuhl 1955, Connolly 1965). It is likely that an angiomatous mass is the commonest cause and that the vascular tissue evades detection when the clot is evacuated, or it is destroyed by the haemorrhage, as sometimes happens to the cryptic variety in the brain. Extradural vascular malformations are less common than intradural ones; they may occur alone, or in association with a similar lesion of the cord, or in association with or as an extension of an angioma of the vertebra. In a series of 8 cases of extradural vascular lesion described by Guthkelch (1948) 3 were extensions from vertebral angiomas, 3 were haemangioblastomas or allied tumours and 2 were cavernous angiomas. In none had there been spontaneous haemorrhage and the course of events was a fairly rapid march of sensorimotor paraparesis over periods of a week to a few months, and root pain was conspicuous only in those with vertebral involvement. By contrast, extradural haemorrhage usually gives rise to initial pain and stiffness of the back and progresses to compression paraplegia within hours or days. Odom (1960) traced 32 cases including 4 personal ones and he noted that in a considerable number the pain due to the bleeding came on immediately after stretching or stooping. The relationship between trauma, direct and indirect, and rupture of an extradural angiomatous lesion has also been examined by Dawson (1963). The clinical picture of compression paraplegia from an extradural haematoma resembles that due to an acute spinal extradural abscess. Both diseases are comparable in their surgical urgency with intracranial examples. Operative relief must be prompt or the spinal cord will suffer irreparable damage. Myelography is necessary to localize the site of compression accurately and plain film should be taken to exclude pathology such as a vertebral angioma. Evacuation of a spinal extradural haematoma is effected by laminectomy and may prove a simple operation. Fragments of clot should be preserved for examination and the dura mater and the walls of the spinal canal scrutinized for evidence of a vascular abnormality. If there is an angioma of bone, or an extensive extradural vascular malformation, haemorrhage may render the operation difficult and a hazard to life; although the operation is undertaken as an emergency, an adequate reserve of blood for transfusion should be ensured. In the series of 32 cases analysed by Odom (1960) operation was carried out in 26 and 3 died. Complete functional recovery took place in 9 (40% of the survivors) only slight recovery in 9, but in 5 there was no recovery of function. Lepoire et al. (1961) reported a higher mortality: 10 of 28 cases died, while the proportion who recovered function was roughly similar to Odom's series.

#### 4. Spinal cord infarction

As has been discussed in this chapter, the blood supply of the spinal cord is precarious in certain regions and the effects of any vascular occlusion can be catastrophic. The cause of such occlusive episodes may be due to disease in a vital feeding vessel usually the anterior spinal artery. However, other causes may be due to: involvement of vessels by malignant tumours; dissecting aortic aneurysm or to arteriosclerosis of the aorta with subsequent embolism (Wolman & Brad-

shaw 1967). Henson and Parsons (1967) felt that transient ischaemic attacks similar to those which occur in the brain could affect the spinal cord perhaps eventually causing permanent deficit.

The clinical onset is of sudden, unheralded loss of function. There is often some spinal pain but severe pain should suggest an aortic aneurysm. The paralysis is flaccid and there is loss of spinothalamic sensation but, due to their supply from the posterior spinal arteries, the posterior columns are relatively spared. Thus, there may be some retention of proprioceptive sensation. Loss of sphincteric control is usual. Treatment, other than supportive care, is unfortunately ineffective. Spontaneous recovery may occur but if the deficit is severe and there are no signs of improvement in the first 24 hours the prognosis is grave.

## References

ALEXANDER G. L. (1946) Proc. roy. Soc. Med., **39**, 730.
ALLEN B. L. & FERGUSON R. L. (1982) Spine, 7, 276.
AMINOFF M. J. (1976) Spinal Angiomas. Blackwell Scientific Publications, Oxford.
AMINOFF M. J., BARNARD R. D. & LOGUE V. (1974) J. Neurol. Sci., **23**, 255.
ARDENT A. (1976) In Handbook of Clinical Neurology (Eds. Vinken P. J. & Bruyn G. W.) Vol. 20, pp. 323–352. North Holland, Amsterdam.
AUSTIN G. (1961) The Spinal Cord. Thomas, Springfield, Illinois.
BABINSKI J. & DUBOIS A. (1918) Presse. Med., **26**, 64.
BARNETT H. J. & NEWCASTLE N. B. (1974) In Syringomyelia, (Ed. Barnett H. J., Foster J. B. & Hudgson P.) pp. 261–300. Saunders, Philadelphia.
BARONE B. M. & ELVIDGE A. R. (1970) J. Neurosurg., **33**, 428.
BARRON K. D., HIRANO A., ARAKI S. & TERRY R. D. (1959) Neurology (Minneap.). **9**, 91.
BENNETT M. H. & McCALLUM J. E. (1977) Surg. Neurol., **8**, 63.
BENTLEY J. F. & SMITH J. R. (1960) Arch. Dis. Chidh., **35**, 76.
BERGSTRAND A., HÖÖK D. & LIDVALL H. (1964) Acta Neurol. Scand., **40**, 169.
BETTY M. & LORBER J. (1963) J. Neurol. Neurosurg. Psychiat., **26**, 236.
BLACK P. (1979) Neurosurgery, **5**, 726.
BLOCKEY N. J. & SCHORSTEIN J. (1961) J. Bone Jt. Surg., **43b**, 556.
BOYLE R., THOMAS M. & ADAMS J. H. (1980) Postgrad. med. J., **56**, 149.
BREMER J. L. (1952) Arch. Path., **54**, 132.
BRICE J. & McKISSOCK W. (1965) Brit. med. J., **1**, 1341.
BROAGER B. (1953) Acta Psychiat. Neurol. Scand., Suppl. 85.

BROWDER J. & MEYERS R. (1941) *Surgery*, **10**, 296.

BULL J. W. (1953) *Acta. Radio.*, **40**, 283.

CARAM P. C., SCARCELLA G. & CARTON C. A. (1957) *J. Neurosurg.*, **14**, 28.

CHADE H. O. (1976) In *Handbook Of Clinical Neurology* (Eds. Vinken P. J. & Bruyn G. W.) Vol. 20, pp. 415–434 North Holland, Amsterdam.

CHOLMELEY J. A. (1959) In *Modern Trends in Diseases of the Vertebral Column* (Eds. Nassim R. & Burrows J.) p. 137. Butterworth, London.

CHOREMIS C., ECONOMOS D., PAPADATOS C. & GARGAILAS A. (1956) *Lancet*, **2**, 437.

CLOWARD R. B. & YUHL E. T. (1955) *Neurology*, **15**, 600.

COAKHAM H. B., GARSON J. A., BROWNELL B. *et al* (1984) *Lancet*, **2**, 1095.

COBB S. (1915) *Ann. Surg.*, **62**, 641.

COBB C., LEAVENS M. & ECKLES N., (1977) *J. Neurosurg.*, **47**, 653.

COGEN P. & STEIN B. M. (1983) *J. Neurosurg.*, **59**, 471.

CONNOLLY R. C. (1965) *Riv. Pat. nerv. ment.*, **86**, 225.

CONSTANS J., DE DIVITIS E., DONZELLI R., *et al* (1983) *J. Neurosurg.*, **59**, 111.

COOPER I. S., CRAIG W. McK. & KERNOHAN J. W. (1950) *Collected Papers Mayo Clinic*, **42**, 492.

CRAIGIE E. H. (1972) In *The Spinal Cord: Basic Aspects and Considerations*, ed. Austin, G., pp. 59–87. Thomas, Springfield, Illinois.

CUSIK J. F., LARSON S. J., WALSH P. R. *et al* (1983) *J. Neurosurg.*, **59**, 861.

DANDY W. E. (1926) *Arch. Surg.*, **13**, 477.

DASTUR H. M. (1963) *J. Neurol. Neurosurg. Psych.*, **26**, 231.

DAWSON B. H. (1963) *J. Neurol. Neurosurg. Psych.*, **26**, 171.

DEJERINE J. (1906) *Rev. Neurol.*, **13**, 341.

DI CHIRO G., DOPPMAN J. & OMMAYA A. K. (1967) *Radiology*, **88**, 1065.

DI CHIRO G. & DOPPMAN J. (1969) *Radiology*, **93**, 25.

DI CHIRO G., & WENER L. (1973) *J. Neurosurg.*, **39**, 1.

DJINDJIAN M. (1978) In *Spinal Angiomas* (Eds. Pia H. W. & Djindjian R.) pp. 75–83. Springer-Verlag, Berlin.

DJINDJIAN R. (1978a) In *Spinal Angiomas* (Eds. Pia H. W. & Djindjian R.) pp. 98–136. Springer-Verlag, Berlin.

DJINDJIAN R. (1978b) In *Spinal Angiomas*, (Eds. Pia H. W. & Djindjian R., pp. 189–200, Springer-Verlag, Berlin.

DJINDJIAN R., DURNESNIL M., FAURE C., LEFEBURE J. & LEVÈQUE B. (1962) *Rev. Neurol.*, **106**, 278.

DJINDJIAN R., FAURE C., HOUDART R. *et al.* (1966) *Acta Radiol. Diagn.*, **5**, 145.

DJINDJIAN R., HOUDART R. & HURTH M. (1969) *Les Angiomas de la Moelle Epiniere.* Masson, Paris.

DOPPMAN J. L. (1971) *Brit. J. Radio.*, **44**, 758.

DOPPMAN J. L. (1978) In *Spinal Angiomas* (Eds. Pia H. W. & Djindjian R.) pp. 201–208. Springer-Verlag, Berlin.

DOPPMAN J. L. & GIRTON M. (1976) *J. Neurosurg.*, **45**, 195.

DOPPMAN J. L., DI CHIRO G. & OMMAYA A. K. (1969) *Selective Arteriography of the Spinal Cord.* Green, St. Louis.

DOPPMAN J. L., DI CHIRO G. & OMMAYA A. K. (1971) *J. Neurosurg.*, **34**, 48.

DOUGLAS D. L., DUCKWORTH T., KANIS J. A. *et al* (1981) *J. Bone Jt. Surg.*, **63**, 495.

DUNN R., KELLY W., WOHNS R. *et al* (1980) *J. Neurosurg.*, **52**, 47.

ELSBERG C. A. (1916) *Diagnosis and Treatment of Surgical Diseases of the Spinal Cord and its Membranes.* Saunders, Philadelphia.

ELSBERG C. A. (1925) *Ann. Surg.*, **81**, 1057.

ELSBERG C. A. (1928) *Surg. Gynaec. Obstet.*, **46**, 1.

ELSBERG C. A. (1941) *Surgical Disease of the Spinal Cord Membranes and Nerve Roots: Symptoms, Diagnosis and Treatment.* Hoeber, New York.

EPSTEIN F. & EPSTEIN N. (1982) *J. Neurosurg.*, **57**, 685.

FIELDING J. W., PYLE R. N. & FIETTI V. G. (1979) *J. Bone Jt. Surg.*, **61a**, 251.

FINDLAY G. F. (1984) *J. Neurol. Neurosurg. Psychiat.*, **47**, 761.

FINDLAY G. F. (1987) *J. Neurol. Neurosurg. Psychiat* **50**, 151

FISCHER G. & TOMMASI M. (1976) In *Handbook of Clinical Neurology* (Eds. Vinken P. J. & Bruyn G. W.) pp. 353–388. North Holland, Amsterdam.

FISHER A. (1963) *Proc. Aust. Ass. Neurol.*, **1**, 31.

FOIX C. & ALAJOUANINE T. (1926) *Rev. Neurol.*, **2**, 1.

FORTUNA A. & GIUFFRE R. (1971) *Neurochirurgia (Stuttg.)*, **14**, 14.

FRIEDLANDER G. E. & SOUTHWICK W. D. (1982) *The Spinc.* (Eds. Rothman R. H. & Simeone F. A.) pp. 1022–1040. Saunders, Philadelphia.

FRIEDMAN M., KIM T. H. & PANAHON A. M. (1976) *Cancer*, **37**, 1485.

FYFE I. S., HENRY A. P. & MULHOLLAND R. C. (1983) *J. Bone Jt. Surg.*, **65b**, 140.

GARRIDO E. & STEIN B. M. (1977) *Surg. Neurol.*, **7**, 215.

GASSER E. H. & ERLANGER J. (1929) *Amer. J. Physiol.*, **88**, 581.

GAUTIER-SMITH P. C. (1967) *Brain*, **90**, 359.

GELFAN S. & TARLOV I. M. (1955) *J. Neurophysiol.*, **18**, 170.

GILBERT R. W., KIM J. H. & POSNER J. B. (1978) *Ann. Neurol.*, **3**, 40.

GILDAY D. L., PAUL D. J. & PATERSON J. (1975) *Radiology*, **117**, 331.

GILLILAN L. A. (1958) *J. Comp. Neurol.*, **110**, 75.

GIUFFRÉ R. (1966) *Acta Neurochir.*, **14**, 69.

GORTVAI P. (1963) *J. Neurol. Neurosurg. Psychiat.*, **26**, 223.

GOWERS W. R. & HORSLEY V. (1888) (Reprinted 1963) *J. Neurosurg.*, **20**, 815.

GREENWOOD J. (1963) *J. Neurosurg.*, **20**, 668.

GRIFFITHS D. L., SEDDON H. J. & ROAF R. (1956) *Pott's Paraplegia.* Oxford University Press, London.

GRUNDY B. L. (1982) *Neurosurgery*, **11**, 556.

GUIDETTA B. & FORTUNA A. (1967) *J. Neurosurg.*, **27**, 530.

GUTHKELCH A. N. (1948) *J. Neurosurg.*, **11**, 199.

HALL A. & MACKAY N. (1973) *J. Bone Jt. Surg.*, **55b**, 497.

HALNAN K. & ROBERTS P. (1967) *Brit. med. J.*, **3**, 534.

HAMBY W. B. (1944) *J. Neuropath. exp. Neurol.*, **3**, 397.

HANCOCK W. M. & MEDLEY G. (1983) *Lancet*, **2**, 739.

HARRINGTON K. D. (1981) *J. Bone Jt. Surg.*, **63a**, 36.

HARRISON B. M., McDONALD W. I., OCHOA J. & SEARS T. A. (1970) *J. Neurol. Sci.*, **10**, 409.

HAY M. C., PATERSON D. & TAYLOR T. K. (1978) *J. Bone Jt. Surg.*, **60b**, 406.

HEARD C. & PAYNE E. E. (1962) *J. Neurosurg. Psychiat.*, **25**, 345.

HEINBECKER P. (1929) *Amer. J. Physiol.*, **89**, 58.

HENSON R. A., PARSONS M. (1967) *Quart. J. Med.*, **36**, 205.

HILAL S. K. & MICHELSON J. W. (1975) *J. Neurosurg.*, **43**, 275.

HODGSON A. R. & STOCK F. E. (1956) *Brit. J. Surg.*, **44**, 266.

HOLT S. & YATES P. O. (1964) *Brain*, **87**, 481.

HUGHES J. T. (1966) *The Pathology of the Spinal Cord.* Lloyd-Luke, London.
HUGHES J. T. & BROWNELL B. (1966) *Arch. Neurol.,* **15,** 189.
HULME A. & DOTT N. (1954) *Brit. med. J.,* **1,** 64.
HURTH M., HOUDART R., DJINDJIAN R. *et al.* (1978) *Prog. neurol. Surg.,* **9,** 238.
INGRAHAM F. D. & MATSON D. D. (1954) In *Neurosurgery of Infancy and Childhood* (Ed. Thomas C. C.) pp. 345–362. Thomas, Springfield, Illinois.
KAHN E. A. (1947) *J. Neurosurg,* **4,** 191.
KAHN F., GLICKSMAN A., CHU F. *et al* (1967) *Radiology,* **89,** 495.
KAO C. C., UIHLEIM A., BICKEL W. H. *et al* (1968) *J. Neurosurg.,* **29,** 168.
KERNOHAM J. W., MABON R. F., SVEIN H. J. *et al* (1949) *Proc. Mayo Clin.,* **24,** 71.
KEMP H. B., JACKSON J. W., JEREMIAH J. D. *et al* (1973) *J. Bone Jt. Surg.,* **55b,** 715.
KENDALL B. & RUSSELL J. (1966) *Brit. J. Radiol,* **39,** 817.
KIRWAN E. O'G, HUTTON P. A., POZO P. L. *et al.* (1984) *J. Bone Jt. Surg.,* **66b,** 21.
KRAUSE F. (1911) *Chirurgie des Gehirns und Rückenmarks.* Berlin.
KRAYENBÜHL H., YASARGIL M. G. & McCLINTOCK H. G. (1969) *J. Neurosurg.,* **30,** 427.
KREUGER E. G., SOBEL G. L. & WEINSTEIN C. (1961) *J. Neurosurg.,* **18,** 331.
KRISHNAN K. R. & SMITH W. T. (1961) *J. Neurol. Neurosurg. Psychiat.,* **24,** 350.
KROGH E. (1950) *Acta. Physiol. Scand.,* **20,** 263.
LAZORTHES G. (1962) *Rev. Neurol.,* **106,** 535.
LAZORTHES G., GOUAZE A., BASTIDE G. *et al* (1966) *Rev. Neurol.,* **144,** 109.
LEECH P. J. (1976) *J. Neurosurg.,* **45,** 331.
LEPOIRE J., TRIDON P., MONTANT J. & GERMAINE F. (1961) *Neurochirurgie,* **7,** 298.
LHERMITTE J. (1934) *Rev. Neurol.,* **41,** 148.
LIVINGSTONE K. & PERRIN R. (1978) *J. Neurosurg.,* **49,** 839.
LOGUE V. (1979) *J. Neurol. Neurosurg. Psychiiat.,* **42,** 1.
LOMBARDI G. & PASSERINI A. (1964) *Spinal Cord Diseases.* Williams & Wilkins, Baltimore.
McALHANY H. J. & NETSKY M. G. (1955) *J. Neuropath. exp. Neurol.,* **14,** 276.
McCULLOCH J. A. & WADDELL G. (1978) *Brit. J. Radiol.,* **51,** 498.
McDONALD W. I. & SEARS T. A. (1970) *Brain,* **93,** 575 and 583.
MALIS L. I. (1978) *Clin. Neurosurg.,* **25,** 512.
MARKS S., MILES J. B. & SHAW M. D. (1984) *Surgical Neurology,* in Press.
MATTHEWS W. B. (1959) *Lancet,* **2,** 117.
MILES J. B., BANKS A., DERVIN E. *et al* (1984) *J. Neurol. Neurosurg. Psychiat.,* in Press.
MILLER J. D. (1967) *Scot. med. J.,* **12,** 441.
MRC Working Party on Tuberculosis of the Spine (1976) *J. Bone Jt. Surg.,* **58b,** 399.
MRC Working Party on Tuberculosis of the Spine (1978) *J. Bone Jt Surg.,* **60b,** 163.
MRC Working Party on Tuberculosis of the Spine (1982) *J. Bone Jt. Surg.,* **64b,** 393.
MULLAN S., NAUNTON R., HEKMAT-PANAH J. *et al.* (1966) *J. Neurosurg.,* **24,** 536.

NITTNER K. (1976) In *Handbook of Clinical Neurology,* (Eds. Vinken P. J. & Bruyn G. W.) Vol. 20. pp. 177–322. North Holland, Amsterdam.
ODOM G. L. (1960) *Clin. Neurosurg.,* **8,** 197.
OLDFIELD E. H., DI CHIRO G., QUINDLEN E. A. *et al.* (1983) *J. Neurosurg.,* **59,** 1019.
OMMAYA A. K., DI CHIRO G. & DOPPMAN J. (1969) *J. Neurosurg.,* **30,** 679.
OTTOLENGHI C. E. (1955) *J. Bone Jt. Surg.,* **37a,** 443.
PENNYBACKER J. (1958) *Proc. roy. Soc. Med.,* **51,** 547.
PERCY A. K., ELVEBACK L. R., OZAKAZI H. *et al* (1972) *Neurology (Minneap.),* **22,** 40.
PIA H. W. (1975) *Dtsch. Ärztebl.,* **72,** 727.
PIA H. W. (1978) In *Spinal Angiomas* (Eds. Pia H. W. & Djindjian R.) pp. 48–74. Springer-Verlag, Berlin.
PURVES-STEWART J. & RIDDOCH G. (1923) *Rev. Neurol.,* **1,** 565.
QUENCER R. M., TENNER M. S. & ROTHMAN L. M. (1976) *Radiology,* **118,** 637.
RAIMONDI A. J., GUTIERREZ F. A. & DI ROCCO C. (1976) *J. Neurosurg.,* **45,** 555.
RAND R. W. & RAND C. W. (1960) *Intraspinal Tumours of Childhood.* Thomas, Springfield, Illinois.
REXED B. A. & WENNSTRÖM K. G. (1959) *J. Neurol. Neurosurg. Psychiat.,* **40,** 1067.
RHANEY K. & BARCLAY G. P. T. (1959) *J. Path. Bact.,* **77,** 457.
ROBERTSON R. C. & BALL R. P. (1935) *J. Bone Jt. Surg.,* **17b,** 749.
ROBINSON R. G. (1959) *Brit. J. Surg.,* **47,** 301.
ROMANES G. J. (1965) *Paraplegia,* **2,** 119.
RUBIN P. (1969) *Radiology,* **93,** 1243.
RUBINSTEIN L. J. (1970) *Arch. Path.,* **90,** 35.
RUSSELL D. S. & RUBINSTEIN L. J. (1971) *Pathology of Tumours of the Nervous System.* Arnold, London.
SACHS E. & HORRAX G. (1949) *J. Neurosurg.,* **6,** 97.
SADAR E. S., WALTON R. J. & GOSSMAN H. H. (1972) *J. Neurosurg.,* **37,** 661.
SARTOR K. (1983) In *Whole Body Computerised Tomography* (Ed. Wegener O. H.) S. Karger, Basel.
SCHMORL G. & JUNGHANNS H. (1932) *Die gesund und kranke Wirbelsäule im Roentgenbild.* Thieme, Leipzig.
SEDDON H. J. (1935) *Brit. J. Surg.,* **22,** 769.
SELOSSE P. & GRANIERI U. (1968) *Neurochirurgie,* **14,** 135.
SHAW M. D., ROSE J. E. & PATERSON A. (1980) *Acta Neurochir.,* **52,** 113.
SHEALY C. N., LEMAY M. & HADDAD F. S. (1964) *J. Neurol. Neurosurg. Psychiat.,* **27,** 567.
SHEPHARD R. H. (1963) *Neurochirurgia,* **6,** 58.
SHEPHARD R. H. (1965) *Riv. Pat. nerv. ment.,* **86,** 276.
SICARD J. A. & FORESTIER A. (1922) *Bull. Mem. Soc. Med. Hop. Paris,* **46,** 463.
SIEGAL T. & SIEGAL T. (1985) *Neurosurgery,* **17,** 424.
SIEGAL T., SIEGAL T., ROBIN G. *et al* (1981) *Ann. Neurol.,* **11,** 28.
SIMEONE F. A. & LAWNER P. M. (1982) In *The Spine* (Eds. Rothman R. & Simeone F. A.) pp. 1041–1054. Saunders, Philadelphia.
SIMMONS E. H. (1977) *Clin. Orthop. Rel. Res.,* **128,** 65.
SINGH A., AGGARWAL N. D., MALHOTRA K. C. & PUTRI D. S. (1966) *Brit. med. J.,* **2,** 684.
SLOOF J. L., KERNOHAN J. W. & MacCARTY C. S. (1964) In *Primary Intramedullary Tumours of the Spinal Cord and Filum Terminale.* Saunders, Philadelphia.

SMALL J. (1962) *J. Neurol. Neurosurg. Psychiat.*, **25**, 184.

SMITH R. (1965) *J. Neurol. Neurosurg. Psychiat.*, **28**, 152.

SMITH-PETERSEN M. N., LARSON C. B. & AUFRANC O. E. (1945) *J. Bone Jt. Surg.*, **27**, 1.

SPIEGEL P. G., KENGLO K. W., ISSACSON A. S. *et al.* (1972) *J. Bone. Jt. Surg.*, **54a**, 284.

STENER B. & GUNTERBERG B. (1978) *Spine,*, **3**, 351.

STOLTMAN H. F. & BLACKWOOD W. (1966) *J. Neurosurg.*, **24**, 43.

SYMON L., KUYAMA H. & KENDALL B. (1984) *J. Neurosurg.*, **60**, 238.

SYMONDS C. P. & MEADOWS S. P. (1937) *Brain*, **60**, 52.

TALBERT O. R. & SIMMONS C. N. (1961) *Neurology (Minneap.)*, **11**, 645.

TALIB H. (1968) *Brit. J. Surg.*, **55**, 576.

TARLOV I. M. (1953) *Sacral Nerve-root Cysts.* Thomas, Springfield, Illinois.

TARLOV I. M. (1957) *Spinal Cord Compression.* Thomas, Springfield, Illinois.

TARLOV I. M. (1961) *Second Int. Cong. Neurol. Surg. Int. Cong. Series*, No. 36, E. 147. Excepta Medica Foundation, Amsterdam.

TENG P. & RUDNER N. (1960) *Arch. Neurol.*, **2**, 348.

TÖRMA T. (1957) *Acta. Chir. Scand.*, (Suppl.) **225**, 1.

TYTUS J. S. & PENNYBACKER J. (1956) *J. Neurol. Neurosurg. Psychiat.*, **19**, 241.

USHIO Y., POSNER R., POSNER J. B. *et al.* (1977) *Neurology (Minneap.)*, **27**, 422.

VERBIEST H. & PAZ Y GEUSE H. D. (1966) *J. Neurosurg.*, **25**, 611.

WATT V. (1968) *J. Neurosurg.*, **29**, 424.

WEBB J. H., CRAIG W. McK. & KERNOHAN J. W. (1953) *J. Neurosurg.*, **10**, 360.

WHITE W. A., PATTERSON R. H. JR & BERGLAND R. M. (1971) *Cancer*, **27**, 558.

WILKINSON M. C. (1955) *J. Bone Jt. Surg.*, **37b**, 382.

WINDEYER B. W. (1959) *Proc. roy. Soc. Med.*, **52**, 1088.

WINTER R. B. & HALL J. W. (1978) *Spine,*, **3**, 285.

WOLMAN L. & BRADSHAW P. (1968) *Paraplegia*, **6**, 32.

WORTZMANN G. & BOTTERELL E. H. (1963) *J. Neurosurg.*, **20**, 164.

WRIGHT R. (1963) *Ann. Surg.*, **157**, 227.

WYBURN-MASON R. (1943) *Vascular Abnormalities and Tumours of the Spinal Cord and its Membranes.* Kimpton, London.

WYLLIE W. G. (1923) *Brain*, **46**, 336.

YAŞARGIL M. G., DE LONG W. B. & GUARNASCHELLI J. J. (1975) *Surg. Neurol.*, **4**, 211.

YASUOKA S., PETERSON H. A. & MacCARTY C. S. (1982) *J. Neurosurg.*, **57**, 441.

YOUNG R., POST E. & KING G. (1980) *J. Neurosurg.*, **53**, 741.

# Chapter 22
# Spinal degenerative disease

## F. G. FINDLAY

In the early part of this century, the role of degenerative changes in the spinal column and their clinical effects were hardly recognized. Isolated early reports of massive traumatic disc disruption (Middleton & Teacher 1911) did appear and Elsberg (1928) and Stookey (1928) des-described 'chondromas' arising from cervical discs and causing neurogenic compression. At the same time, Schmorl was working on the morbid anatomy of intervertebral discs, work which was made more widely known by Beadle (1931). This stimulus led Mixter and Barr (1934) to review their combined experience thus heralding full recognition of the significance of lumber disc protrusion.

The recognition that degeneration of structures other than the intervertebral disc could cause compression of neural structures followed the work of Verbiest (1954) who highlighted the problem of spinal stenosis and neurogenic claudication of nerve roots. However, the fact that reactive bony and ligamentous changes in the spine occurred in response to disc degeneration had been realized for many years (Lane 1885, Schmorl & Junghanns 1932).

In 1940 Stookey identified the clinical syndromes which occur in relation to degenerative disease of the cervical spine. The importance of cervical spondylotic myelopathy was emphasized by Brain (1948), and Wilkinson (1967) reviewed the pathological changes seen in the cord and the natural history of the disease at this spinal level.

## Intervertebral disc: normal anatomy and function

The normal disc consists of three parts: the cartilaginous end plates, the nucleus, and the annulus. Opinions vary as to whether the cartilaginous plates should be considered as part of the disc or the vertebral body but they serve functions important to both tissues. In any event, present attitudes are directed away from viewing the disc in isolation, but rather to study the entire moving segment involving the disc, joint, bones and ligamentous structures at each level.

The hyaline cartilage plates are in contact on one side with cancellous vertebral bone and with the annulus on the other side. They cover the upper and lower vertebral surfaces except at the peripheral margins which are derived from a separate, annular epiphysis.

The nucleus is derived from embryonic notochordal tissue and consists of a gelatinous matrix. In the lumbar region, it lies slightly eccentrically, being situated nearer the posterior margin of the disc. It contains a loose network of fine fibrous strands with a cartilaginous cellular matrix. The normal nucleus is deformable but incompressible and behaves hydrostatically (Virgin 1951, Nachemson 1981). The more peripheral fibres near the cartilaginous plates are embedded into its substance, so allowing fixation.

The annulus surrounds the nucleus, adhering closely to the vertebral bodies. It is a structure composed of strong, interconnected fibrous tissue whose purpose is to resist horizontal and torsional stress. Inspection reveals the layers to run concentrically but none entirely completes the circle, and in successive layers the fibres run in different oblique directions. The deeper layers of the annulus are of great strength and pass into the epiphyseal ring of the body. The more superficial layers spread on to the surface of the body fusing with the periosteum and anterior longitudinal ligaments. The texture and density of the annulus is less posteriorly, as the posterior longitudinal ligament is less strong than the anterior. It is likely that this is because the tensions put on these posterior structures in flexion are largely absorbed by the paraspinal muscles, the ligaments between the neural arches and the zygoapophyseal joints.

Although it is possible to distinguish various portions in an intervertebral disc, it may be emphasized that in health there is no discontinuity. The intervertebral disc is a functioning unit. However, an important aspect of Schmorl's investigations was the study of the spine as a whole; a structure in which flexibility and strength have been attained by the combination of bone and fibrocartilage. The vertebral column consists basically of an anterior stable column composed of vertebral bodies and their intervening discs with a posterior column composed of the posterior bony elements, ligaments and muscles. On a cross sectional plane, the bony, articular, ligamentous and muscular structures at each spinal level form an integrated unit which has been termed the motor segment (Junghanns 1929, Schmorl & Junghanns 1959).

The nourishment of the intervertebral disc is largely by diffusion. In health, only the most superficial layers are penetrated by blood vessels. The remainder of the disc is supplied by diffusion through the cartilage plates from the adjacent cancellous bone. The avascularity of the interior of the healthy disc is an inevitable consequence of the high intrinsic pressure of the nucleus (Nachemson 1966, 1981). The dependance on diffusion is responsible for the radiological changes seen in the disc when chronic infection such as tuberculosis affects the vertebral endplates, thus stopping the nourishment of the disc.

There has been debate as to whether the disc has a nerve supply. Von Luschka (1858) identified what is now termed the sinuvertebral branch of the spinal nerve. This enters the spinal canal through the intervertebral foramen to supply articular structures, ligaments, meninges and blood vessels. It is now recognized that, while the deeper parts of the annulus and the nucleus are not innervated, the superficial lamellar layers are supplied by filaments of the sinuvertebral nerves (Bowden *et al.* 1967).

The function of the intervertebral disc is, along with other pliable spinal structures, to render the spine flexible, resilient, and strong. The amount of mobility at each motor segment is relatively small compared with the total spinal range of movements. Cervical and lumbar segments are more mobile but the planes of the lumbar articular facets limit rotation, thus increasing the torsional stress on the annulus of the disc. The disc alters shape in response to the stresses imposed upon it and the relative incompressibility of the nucleus enables the disc to transmit and dissipate force, such as the superimposed body weight, through the axis of the spine.

The physical characteristics of the disc alter with ageing due to a loss of the initial high degree of hydration present in the young healthy nucleus. Nevertheless, the nucleus possesses an intrinsic degree of turgor, being an inherent state of expansibility. This turgor is due also to a degree of counter pressure induced by the concentric fibres of the annulus. The actual intradiscal pressure has been measured *in vivo* by Nachemson and his associates. Their results have been published in a series of papers, principally Nachemson (1959), Nachemson and Morris (1964) and more recently summarized by Nachemson in 1981. These workers have shown that changes in posture greatly affect the pressure within, and load on, a lumbar intervertebral disc. As compared to the situation in recumbency, the load increases by: a factor of two in the standing position; a factor of three when sitting; and a factor of eight when lifting with the back bent. In his study of pressures in abnormal discs, Nachemson (1965) showed the increase in load with postural changes to be even further exaggerated.

## The pathophysiology of degeneration

The description by Schmorl of vertical prolapse of the nucleus into the cancellous bone of the vertebral body through a defect in the cartilaginous endplate coupled with Von Luschka's observation of posterior protrusions into the canal (though wrongly interpreted as notochordal remnants) stimulated interest in the pathology of the intervertebral disc. Saunders and Inman (1940) made extensive studies, determining that the discs were subject to progressive change throughout life. They found these changes to be so widespread in the population that they had difficulty in determining what could be accepted as normal and what was pathological.

The nucleus is the first part of the disc to deteriorate. It loses its glistening, resilient appearance and becomes dull and leathery. Progressive changes cause small cracks and cavities, and the nucleus develops a fibrillary structure reminiscent of cooked lobster, readily recognizable when a pathological disc is removed at operation. The cartilage plates are more resistant to change but become thinned and cracked. This allows the degenerate nucleus to become vascularized, a condition entirely incompatible with normal disc. The annulus develops radiating fissures which appear at areas where the normally incomplete fibres fail to meet. This is most likely to occur in the posterolateral part of the disc and is worsened by repeated torsional stress. The collapse of the height of the nucleus further loosens the annular fibres, exacerbating this process.

The actual cause of the primary changes in the nucleus is not clear. There is no doubt that the degree of hydration of the nucleus decreases with age and that degenerate discs have less water content and a decreased ability to bind water than normal discs. Hendry (1968) reviewed the mechanism whereby a disc can hold water and rejected theories of osmotic pressure in the preference of actual binding of water by the gel. This property is due to the acid aminoglycan content of the nucleus which decreases

and deteriorates with age. Bobechko and Hirsch (1965) suggested that the avascularity of the developing disc would prevent its recognition by the immune system. If the disc were to become exposed to blood, it could incite an autoimmune response. Certain workers have produced supportive evidence but no conclusive involvement of either cellular or humoral immune mechanisms has been identified as yet.

The alteration in nuclear mechanics throws excessive stress on the annulus thus encouraging the annular changes described above. The direct consequence of degeneration of the disc as a whole is protrusion beyond its normal perimeter and failure of its normal physiological function. The former induces reactive changes in the adjacent vertebral body and nerve roots, whilst the latter throws an additional strain on adjacent motor segments inducing changes in those structures. In all but the most acute disc rupture, these changes occur simultaneously but may be of varying degree producing either predominately the problems of disc prolapse or of spondylosis.

Prolapse of the disc beyond its normal contour may occur in the anterior, lateral or posterior direction. Anterior and lateral protrusions are of no consequence in the lumbar spine though the reactive changes they excite may be visible radiologically. Rarely anterior protrusion with reactive changes in the neck may be florid enough to cause dysphagia. Posterior protrusion of the disc, especially posterolateral, is common and is of most importance as it may cause neural compression.

Once protrusion of the disc becomes established, the load-bearing characteristics of that disc become further compromised, with nuclear material being extruded along any lines of annular weakness. This produces a dome-shaped eminence in the spinal canal which may be unimpressive in the prone position. Further changes may lead to a diffuse bulge causing a bar across the canal, a condition more commonly found in the neck though also seen in lumbar stenosis. More usually, however, the dome enlarges and if the annulus finally gives way free fragments of nuclear and annular material can leave the disc space assuming a place deep to the posterior longitudinal ligament (subligamentous extrusion) or rupture through the ligaments, becoming a free intraspinal fragment. Such free fragments remain as an intraspinal mass irrespective of position, whereas recumbency may allow a mere protrusion to reduce its intraspinal component to some degree. A disc protrusion may evoke considerable fibroblastic reaction in the extradural tissue which exaggerates the height of the protruding portion of the disc. This process may become adherent to the dura of the root sleeve.

Protrusion of a disc can occur at any spinal level and many do not elicit clinical symptoms. Some prolapses may diminish in size perhaps due to further dehydration. Lindblom and Hultqvist (1950) have shown that fragments of fibro-cartilage can be destroyed by reactive granulation tissue. Clinical instances of thoracic disc protrusion are fortunately rare but when present show very severe disc changes including the development of calcification. Clinical herniations in the cervical and lumbar areas are much more frequent, though Lombardi and Passerini (1964) reviewing 669 operated cases found that 93.5% were lumbar discs. Most modern practices would identify a much greater frequency of cervical disc disease.

As a result of disc degeneration, an increase in mobility between adjacent vertebrae develops and great strain is thrown on the other parts of each motor segment. Schmorl termed the changes as 'spondylosis deformans' and Lane (1885) ascribed them to adaption of the spinal column to occupational stress. The bone of the vertebral body itself is no longer cushioned against the stresses, strains and shocks of physical activity. The vertebral body tends to expand perhaps aided by osteoporotic changes and its surface becomes irregular and sclerotic. The periphery develops outgrowths of bone, initially as a lip but then as spurs due to periosteal activity excited by the abnormal stresses induced by the annular fibres. Adjacent spurs, if very large, may join and fuse, further limiting motion at that

level. Such spurs occur in conditions other than degenerative disease, in particular ankylosing spondylitis. Macnab (1977) described a particular spike of bone found on the front of the vertebral body about 3 mm from the disc space as a 'traction spur' and thought it arose from stresses around sites of ligamentous insertion.

Such osteophyte formation rarely occurs posteriorly into the lumbar canal but is commonplace in the neck. The greater frequency in the cervical area may be due to the increased mobility of that area. The uncovertebral joints whereby the posterolateral aspects of adjacent cervical vertebral bodies articulate are thought by Töndury (1961) to develop during life, starting as a fissure in the lateral part of the disc and are a common site of degenerative changes. Plain radiographic appearances of these degenerative changes are very common in asymptomatic patients. Friedenberg and Miller (1963) showed that over 70% of asymptomatic people over the age of 70 years had degenerative changes on their cervical spine X-ray.

These reactive and degenerative changes occur also in the posterior spinal elements. The ligamentum flavum can hypertrophy and become a compressive agent in its own right. The ligaments and capsules of the facet joints become stretched; allowing increased mobility in the joints. This causes osteophytic changes in the facet with resulting overgrowth of the bone and intrusion into the canal. The facet joints then may sublux not only in an axial but also a rotational plane. This process has been eloquently summarized by Brown (1982) who shows that the end result is narrowing of the lateral recess of the spinal canal, producing the classic trefoil canal of spinal stenosis on cross-section. This process may be asymmetrical. If this occurs there may be malalignment in rotation with shortening of the distance between the spinous process and the facet on that side as described by Forfar (1977). This not only deranges the mechanics of that segment but may stretch the nerve root around the pedicle especially during rotatory movements. In addition, reactive changes in a single facet joint may cause bony entrapment of a single root by encroaching on the root foraminal tunnel. This characteristically produces radicular pain for the first time in a more elderly patient than is usual with simple nuclear herniation (Macnab 1977).

The final factor to be discussed in the pathophysiology of spinal degeneration is the significance of the anteroposterior diameter of the canal. This measurement varies, not only in different parts of the canal, but also within normal individuals at the same level. The role of a congenitally stenotic canal in encouraging the clinical features of superimposed degenerative disease has been shown using ultrasound techniques by Porter *et al.* (1980). They measured the sagittal diameter of the lumbar spine in over 700 people, many of whom were miners. Their study showed that, in those people within the study who had disabling disc symptoms, 56% of them had sagittal lumbar canal diameters less than the tenth percentile of the normal range. They also showed that women tend to have larger diameters than men and point out that this may be advantageous in order to withstand the stresses of pregnancy.

Such congenital predisposition to narrowing of the canal is distinct from the degenerative stenosis described above. Acquired stenosis of the canal is probably most common in the cervical area due to degenerative processes therein and the role of such changes will be discussed below. Certain diseases also are associated with narrowing of the canal, the principal one being achondroplasia.

## Clinical features of lumbar disc disease

The cardinal symptoms of lumbar disc protrusion are backache and pain which radiates along the distribution of the roots involved by the protrusion. Since about 90% arise from the lowest two discs, therefore involving the fifth lumbar and first sacral roots, the pain is distributed along the sciatic nerve. Pain of that description has long been called 'sciatica' and it is generally accepted that its commonest cause is a prolapsed lumbar intervertebral disc.

The association of back pain and sciatica was recognized by generations of physicians before Mixter and Barr drew attention to the role of the disc in 1934. Prior to that time, they were ascribed to a process known as 'fibrositis' which commenced in the spinal muscles and spread to the leg. It was recognized that prolonged rest would lead to remission and it is perhaps salutary to remember in this day and age that prior to 1934 no patients underwent discectomy and that the long term tendency is for the clinical features of a prolapsed disc to gradually subside.

From a diagnostic and therapeutic point of view, it is essential to separate true 'sciatica' from other types of pain as stressed by Waddell (1982). Pain in the distribution of the nerve root such as 'sciatica' is best termed radicular pain. Back pain itself is obviously pain experienced over the midline spinal structures and the term 'referred pain' should be reserved for the relatively ill-defined sensations which spread from the back into the buttock or thigh on stimulation of certain spinal tissues other than the nerve root. It is important to recognize that all pain felt in the leg is not due to a prolapsed disc. Equally, many other more sinister pathologies can produce back pain, referred pain or radicular pain.

The condition of back pain and referred pain due to degenerative rather than other spinal pathology is often referred to as 'mechanical back pain'. The origins of such pain are not clear, however. The nucleus itself is not innervated and presumably cannot produce pain directly. Other structures do have a nerve supply: notably, the outer annulus, posterior longitudinal ligaments, joint capsule and periosteum. Abnormal stimulation of these structures by either stretching, electrical stimulation or the injection of hypertonic saline produces pain of an aching character in the back, buttock or thigh (Mooney & Robertson 1976) and this constitutes referred pain. Protrusion of an intervertebral disc may disturb some of these structures but the loss of height and abnormal stresses of the collapsing disc strain the facet joints, eliciting pain from these structures.

Acute or severe disturbance of these areas may elicit spasm of the erector spinae muscles producing further distortion of the joints and causing more pain and a list. It is likely that most conservative therapeutic manoeuvres such as rest, heat, support and local injection relieve pains in these areas and reduce the paraspinal spasm.

Pain produced by direct stimulation of the nerve root produces a much sharper, lancinating pain which is more localized than referred pain. Such pain radiates down the posterolateral aspect of the leg below the knee and often into the foot. It is frequently associated with paraesthesiae. Radicular pain is worsened by the increases of intraspinal pressure associated with coughing and straining and may be alleviated by postures which relax the affected nerve root such as lying with hips and knees flexed. It is important to note in passing that the rare prolapse of a high lumbar disc may produce a true radicular pain but which is felt in an area similar to referred pain.

Prolapse of a lumbar disc usually occurs in the posterolateral area close to the entry of the nerve root canal. However, the compressed root is not the one which passes through that particular foramen as the root enters its canal rostral to the disc. The affected root crosses the disc and descends under the next lamina to leave the spinal canal below the pedicle supporting that lamina. Since there are 8 cervical nerves but only 7 cervical vertebrae, the segmental root leaves caudal to the pedicle of the same numerical value; T1 root leaving at T1/T2 and L5 at L5/S1. Therefore, the customary L5/S1 disc prolapse involves the S1 root as it passes over the L5/S1 disc to the first sacral foramen. On occasion, however a large lateral prolapse can occlude the foramen sufficiently to involve the L5 root at lumbosacral space. The affected nerve root usually comes to lie on or slightly medial to the dome of the prolapse but less commonly the prolapse can present in the axilla of the root.

The involvement of a nerve root by a disc protrusion produces radicular pain. This may be due to one of several reasons:

1   Tension due to displacement, which makes the nerve take a longer course and more susceptible to trunk or lower limb movement. Straight leg raising to 90° causes a descent of the lower lumbar roots into the root canals of about 5 mm. Flexion of the neck has been shown to produce movement of the dural tube by up to 5 cm (O'Connell 1946). The roots of the cauda equina are slack in the neutral position but straighten in spinal flexion. O'Connell (1943) considered axial tension in the root as the most important factor in the production of pain and showed that such tension is more easily produced when the root is in its dural sheath rather than in its thecal course.

2   Pressure by displacement. It is disputed whether pressure causes pain, because it stops nerve conduction if it is sufficient and constant and would produce numbness. However, the pressure induced in a root fluctuates with movement and the degree of oedema in the surrounding structures. This may elicit pain if it causes ischaemia of the root. The clinical picture of relief of pain at the time of onset of a major neurological deficit is well recognized and corresponds to the cessation of neuronal conduction.

3   Swelling of the nerve root, with resulting fixation by adhesions both within, and without, its dural sheath, aggravates the effects of physical stresses.

The great majority of disc prolapses requiring operation occur during early middle age and are commoner in males by a factor of two to one. This tendency to affect young wage-earning people was emphasized by O'Connell in 1951 and put in its more modern day perspective by the Cochrane report (DHSS 1979). It must be realized however, that those coming to operation represent only a small minority of those who suffer from backpain in general. Waddell (1982) estimated that only 5000 operations on the back are performed per annum in the UK, but that over one million people actually consult their family doctor on account of backache each year. In a fascinating study, Kane (1980) showed that people in the USA are six times more likely than Britons to have a back operation, with the rate fluctuating even more dramatically in certain areas of the USA.

Accurate diagnosis of the clinical features of a prolapsed lumbar disc is essential as the first step in planning treatment, as removal of abnormal but incidental disc protrusions not causative in the pain syndrome will produce poor results. An accurate and detailed history is essential as it forms the basis of diagnosis. Factors of importance include: the mode of onset of pain and its periodicity; aggravating and relieving factors; nature of employment; history of trauma; and the previous attempts at treatment and the response to such treatment. The most important task is to decide whether the pain represents back, referred or radicular pain.

Back pain is felt in a fairly wide distribution in the midline and usually felt to be deep seated. More localized pain is suggestive of more sinister spinal pathology such as infection or neoplasm. Referred pain again is of aching nature distributed to the buttocks and thighs. Radicular pain, on the contrary, is a sharp localized pain involving a part or whole of the territory of the affected nerve root. Radicular pain usually occurs in association with back pain and O'Connell (1951) in his review of 500 cases found root pain alone in only 13%.

Other factors may be present in the history which suggest dysfunction of the root. There may be complaints of paraesthesiae or of actual motor weakness. Thus, pins and needles over the dorsum of the foot would implicate the fifth lumbar root, whereas over the lateral border of the foot they would suggest involvement of the first sacral. Equally, a foot drop implicates dysfunction of the muscles served by L5. Control of sphincters is usually disturbed only when multiple roots are compressed as in the cauda equina syndrome but Ross and Jameson (1971) have described disturbance of micturition as the sole symptoms of a large prolapsed disc.

Clinical examination commences with observing the patient's gait. The painful stiffness of the back and leg give the patient a characteristic limp. Movement is slow, the trunk dips to the affected side as the limb takes weight and the actual transfer of weight is for a minimum time. The patient's back is then viewed from the rear whilst standing. The pelvis is commonly tilted down on one side due to slight flexion of his hips and knee to relieve pain. This imparts a flattening to the lumbar spine and may produce a list to either side. Palpation of the paraspinal muscles may reveal spasm or an area of local tenderness. Spinal movements are restricted. This is poorly assessed by the commonly used test of forward bending with outstretched fingers. Placing the fingers on the toes involves not only spinal movement but hip flexion and can even be achieved by patients with ankylosed spines. A better test is to measure movements between skin marks placed on the lumbar spine during flexion as described by Macrae and Wright (1969). Waddell et al. (1982) have shown this to be a reproducable and reliable test.

Signs of root irritation selectively aggravate an irritable root and reproduce radicular pain. Straight leg raising (Lasègue's test in meningitis) is performed with the patient in a relaxed, supine position. With the knee remaining in extension, the leg is slowly raised by the examiner. In the presence of a disc protrusion affecting either the L5 or S1 roots the test provokes radicular pain which limits the straignt leg raising. Dorsiflexion of the ankle increases the pain; flexion of the knee will relieve pain. It is only in the midrange of straight leg raising between about 30° and 60° that the root is actually stretched over a disc protrusion (Fahrni 1966). Production of pain at less than 30° is unlikely to be genuine. Edgar and Park (1974) showed that the most specific root irritation sign was production of pain in the affected limb during raising of the good leg. Apparent abnormalities of the straight leg raising test can be confirmed as being functional by distracting the patient and getting him or her to sit up on the bed with legs stretched out in front; effectively showing 90° of straight leg raising.

Signs of root compression indicate neural dysfunction. Most commonly this shows as depression or loss of the ankle jerk indicating S1 root compression. A normal knee and ankle jerk will often be seen in L5 compression; and the knee jerk is abolished by pressure on the L3 root. A diminished ankle jerk seldom recovers even after many years and may only signify previous root compression rather than active disease. Of root compression signs, reflex changes, therefore, are not the strongest predictors of disc disease; sensory or motor changes are more reliable.

Sensory impairment in a dermatomal pattern is a sign of root compression and does not occur in referred pain, though that symptom may be associated with an enhanced response to cutaneous stimuli. Affected areas tend to be smaller than the entire dermatome and total anaesthesia and analgesia are very rare. Hypo-aesthesia in the lateral aspect of the calf and on the dorsum of the foot suggest a L5 lesion; whereas loss on the outside and underside of the sole suggests S1. Sacral sensation is usually unimpaired other than in a cauda equina syndrome.

Motor weakness with wasting and fascic-ulation are unusual and are more suggestive of neuropathy or motor neuron disease. Weakness does occur, however, and is a sign of severe root compression. Tests for weakness of the following movements may indicate the root affected: extension of the knee (L3 and L4) dorsiflexion and eversion of the foot (L5); plantarflexion and inversion of the foot (S1).

These clinical factors provide only a guide to localization and do not take account of multiple or anomalous innervation. Localization is particularly awkward in the presence of bony segmental anomalies such as lumbarization of a sacral vertebra. In this situation, Waddell (1982) has suggested the identification of the lowest level with a fully formed disc space and two free, unarticulated transverse processes as the 'last fully mobile level'. The L5 root emerges through the root canal at the last fully mobile segment in 75% of these patients with segmental anomalies.

## Patterns of presentation

The commonest pattern of presentation is of a gradual onset of back pain followed by the development of radicular pain and progressive disability as a result of pain rather than any neurological deficit. Many episodes commence with an episode of trauma or sudden, unprotected muscular effort; especially if combined with spinal rotation. The vast majority of such acute episodes will settle within 6 weeks irrespective of any type of treatment. Because of this, a history of recurring episodes is characteristic and indeed a history of continuous, unremitting pain should be viewed with suspicion as either being of a nonorganic or neoplastic nature. More occasionally, an initial episode of radicular pain will fail to settle and the patient will present to the surgeon during this initial episode.

In a small but highly important group of cases, a lumbar disc lesion may be acute and large enough to cause compression of the cauda equina. The incidence of this is about 3% of all operated lumbar discs. Diagnosis may be difficult and, if operation is delayed, permanent disability may result from paralysis of sphincters and distal muscles. There may be a long history suggestive of disc trouble; while in other cases a cauda equina syndrome is the first evidence of spinal disease. Compression develops abruptly, with the onset typically of bilateral radicular pain, and progresses rapidly; it may be precipitated by strain but may also develop overnight, as in 4 of 25 cases reported by Jennett (1956). The abruptness and severity of the pain is not typical of disc disease and may pose diagnostic difficulties. Another misleading feature is the diminution or disappearance of pain as paralysis develops indicating cessation of neuronal function. Defective control of sphincters is often the final and compelling reason for referral to a neurosurgeon. Diagnosis and immediate operation must not be delayed if maximum potential for recovery is to be allowed, as emphasized by Shephard in 1959. O'Laoire et al. (1981) suggested that the prognosis for recovery of sphincters was not as gloomy as is generally accepted. However, of their 29 patients, 16 had at least some residual sphincteric function present at the time of operation.

## Investigation

It should be stressed at this point that general examination of the patient, other than just the back and legs, is imperative. It is necessary to exclude other disease such as breast neoplasm or intra-abdominal pathology which could be significant in causing back pain either directly or indirectly.

As an absolute minimum, the patient should have an estimation of the erythrocyte sedimentation rate (ESR) and plain films of the chest and lumbar spine. The former may alert one to unsuspected pathology if raised to abnormal levels. Plain radiology is necessary in the first place to exclude gross destructive lesions but more importantly to identify any bony segmental anomaly which might be present. Degenerative changes in the discs and facet joints will be seen along with reactive changes in the vertebral body such as osteophyte formation. These changes, however, are not in anyway diagnostic of disc protrusion. Plain films are important also because they allow identification of patients with spondylolisthesis of varying severity and type.

### Radiculography

Soon after the definitive paper by Mixter and Barr, Hampton and Robinson (1936), in a beautifully illustrated and equally valuable paper, showed that with appropriate projections radiculography would reveal disc prolapses. Radiculography using oil-based substances such as Myodil has now been almost universally replaced by newer water-soluble contrast agents. These have the advantage of allowing easier and improved filling of the nerve root sleeve with a resultant increase in the diagnostic yield (Hirsch *et al.* 1969). Water-soluble agents are also associ-

ated with a lower rate of complications, in particular arachnoiditis (Grainger *et al.* 1976).

If there is a clear clinical diagnosis of disc prolapse but nonoperative therapy is planned there is no absolute need to confirm diagnosis by radiculography. Although opinions differ, the commonest attitude is, on the other hand, to perform radiculography prior to surgery if this is planned (Fig. 22.1). This is recommended

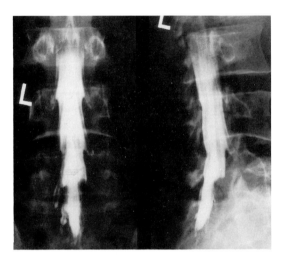

**Fig. 22.1** Lumbar radiculogram showing right L5/S1 disc protrusion.

because clinical diagnosis, although effective at diagnosing disc prolapse, is poor for localization of level. Edgar and Park (1974) were only able to localize the correct level in 50% of their patients. This is due to variation in nerve root arrangement, the exact position of herniations, and the siting of nerve fibres in roots other than those in which they normally exit the canal. With pre-operative radiological localization surgical exploration can be limited to a single space. An additional reason for radiculography is that in rare instances, a pre-operative radiculogram may display an unsuspected neoplasm, such as an ependymoma or neurofibroma.

It is well recognized that radiculography is not always accurate but accuracy with the newer forms of water-soluble contrast media now available is better. Genuine protrusions may still be missed, especially those lying laterally in a capacious canal at the lumbosacral level. Alternatively, root cut-off may be due to hypertrophy of a facet joint rather than disc protrusion. Even when a genuine disc protrusion is found it may merely be an incidental finding. Hitselberger and Witten (1968) found that 24% of 300 patients undergoing posterior fossa myelography for the investigation of acoustic tumours showed asymptomatic lumbar disc lesions. However, the age range of their patients was older than those normally presenting with disc lesions. Wilberger and Pang (1983) have recently suggested that many patients showing a so-called incidental, asymptomatic prolapse will develop symptoms in the near future.

## Discography

In the monograph of Schmorl and Junghanns (1932) are reproductions of radiographs of spines in which the discs have been injected with a radio-opaque medium. The injected healthy nucleus pulposus gives a well defined globular shadow but in the degenerative disc the medium forms an irregular, flattened shadow. Several routes are available for discography but the safest is the lateral approach (McCulloch & Waddell 1978). The finding of a radiologically abnormal disc is not confirmation that this is the source of the patient's pain but reproduction of radicular pain during the injection is thought by some to be significant.

Discography has not been very popular as a diagnostic test and probably has only a limited place in the investigation of difficult cases. It has, however, a place as the first stage of chymopapain injection and in the planning of the extent and suitability of spinal fusion.

## Computed tomography

The arrival of newer generation CT scanners has opened new possibilities in imaging the lumbar canal. It also has limitations, however, due to the fact that the scanning must be selective to a restricted area. To take multiple slices through the entire lumbar canal would be a lengthy procedure and involve excessive irradiation.

A herniated disc shows on a CT scan as an area of abnormal increased density lying in the canal and indenting the low density epidural fat. In comparison between CT and radiculography, Haughton et al. (1982) found that the accuracy of each technique appeared to be comparable but, of course, the CT method was noninvasive. Difficulty is still encountered with CT scanning in the diagnosis of recurrent disc prolapse as the radiological densities of scar tissue and degenerate disc are very similar.

## Other imaging techniques

Epidurography (injection of contrast into the extradural space) may be helpful in cases where a root lesion is suspected but the radiculogram is normal. Using this technique and concentrating on one or two roots only on the affected side it is possible to delineate the root sleeve further distally than by intradural injection. It has a higher false positive and false negative rate than modern radiculography and has a somewhat limited place restricted to the difficult diagnostic problem.

Similarly, epidural venography has been advocated by many as a primary investigation. It relies on showing the disc protrusion by its compressive effect on adjacent epidural veins. Justification for its use came primarily from comparison with myodil radiculography where epidural venography was claimed to be more accurate (Macnab et al. 1976). However, as has been shown above, modern radiculography is more accurate and the place of venography now is similar to epidurography, namely as an adjunct rather than a primary test.

Injection of the root sleeve with radiopaque material followed by local anaesthesia has been advocated (Macnab 1971) but has failed to find widespread use.

Magnetic resonance imaging (MRI) produces excellent evidence of degenerative changes in discs (Modic *et al.* 1984). However, it is not yet clear exactly what the role of MRI will be in the display of actual disc protrusion as opposed to simple degeneration. It is likely that with the development of cross-sectional images displaying the prolapse against the highlighted CSF that this will become the investigation of choice where available. It is also likely that it will replace discography in the assessment of degeneration prior to fusion.

Radionuclide bone scanning has no place in the diagnosis of disc lesions. It does, however, have a very important role in the exclusion of more sinister spinal pathology such as infection or neoplasia. The bone scan becomes positive in any area of increased vascularity or metabolic activity. It may often show pathology when plain radiographs are normal (Galasko & Doyle 1972) but it is totally lacking in specificity, being positive not only in infection and tumours but also in osteoarthritic areas.

**Electrophysiology**

Electromyography (EMG) can show the effect of denervation on specific muscles and this produces corroborative evidence of root compression. Leyshon *et al.* (1981) have recommended the use of EMG in patients who have had previous surgery or who have bony entrapment. Although not all their patients had clinical signs of root compression, they did not correlate the findings of electrical abnormality with the presence of such signs. This makes assessment of the role of EMG difficult as many feel that this investigation will only be sufficiently positive to allow diagnosis in cases with detectable clinical signs of root compression and that it fails to help patients without clinical signs, in whom diagnosis is most difficult. Due to variation in the

motor supply of extensor digitorum brevis, EMG is not helpful in localization (Young, quoted by Leyshon *et al.* 1981). It is possible that the use of spinal evoked potentials may be more precise than EMG in cases without clinical signs (Feinsod *et al.* 1982).

## Differential diagnosis

A list of ailments, trivial and serious, which may give rise to persistent low backache and to lumbar and sacral root pain, separately or in combination, would be tedious, of little value and probably incomplete. On the one hand, it would include hysterical states and, on the other hand, malignant growths within the pelvis. Armstrong (1965) does list many of the causes of back and root pain. Careful attention to history, clinical and radiological examination rules out many alternatives and, since this subject forms part of orthopaedic as well as neurological surgery, an opinion from each specialist is valuable in obscure cases.

It is possible to predict accurately the presence of a protruded lumbar disc. Waddell *et al* (1979) have adapted the criteria used by McCulloch (1977) in his study of chemonucleolysis. These were derived from analysis of data in series, published previously (Hirsch & Nachemson 1963, Hudgins 1970, Macnab 1977). Waddell's eventual criteria are composed of a quartet of clinical factors, namely: a predominant complaint of radicular rather than back pain; signs of root irritation; signs of root compression; and positive radiculography. In his series, Waddell found that the presence of any three or four of these factors accurately predicted the presence of a disc protrusion in all cases. When only one factor was present, no patient was found to have a protrusion, although other pathology could be present. This reinforces the fact that back pain on its own, or even in association with an abnormal disc, will not respond to surgery restricted to excision of that disc.

Several conditions may simulate some, but not

all, of the cinical features of a prolapsed disc in a patient:

1 *Bony nerve entrapment.* Hirsch (1948) and Briggs (1948) had each observed that roots could be trapped far laterally in the foramen. Schlesinger (1955) reviewing over 600 laminectomies for disc disease, identified 43 cases where the root was compressed by bone in the foraminal canal. Macnab (1971) postulated that narrowing of the disc could lead to descent of the pedicle which could kink the root. Further changes result in subluxation of the facet joints and increased root entrapment. More severe degeneration produces the changes of a unisegmental lateral recess stenosis.

The onset of radicular pain for the first time in a patient over 40 years old may well be due to bony entrapment. In Waddell's series described above, the finding of radicular pain with nerve root compression but not irritation signs (i.e. normal straight leg raising) was highly suggestive of bony entrapment.

2 *Primary spinal pathology.* Bony disease commonly produces back pain but only rarely elicits radicular involvement. Benign tumours, such as osteoma, and malignant lesions, such as metastases, may cause diagnostic difficulty. Infection of the disc and surrounding endplates is usually pyogenic or tuberculous, although other organisms may be causative. When present the radiological appearance of destruction of the disc and endplates may be suggestive and the infective diagnosis can often be confirmed by needle aspiration of the disc. Postoperative discitis may be extremely difficult to distinguish from recurrence of a disc prolapse. Acute extradural abscess causes intense pain and rapid development of neurological signs.

3 *Intradural tumour.* Very occasionally, an intradural nerve root tumour such as a neurofibroma may mimic disc prolapse. Tumours of the conus may present with back pain which may be particularly troublesome at night, and radiculography should always include the conus area to exclude such pathology.

4 *Extraspinal disease.* Infiltration of the sciatic plexus in the pelvis or buttock by neoplasia produces severe, boring, unremitting radicular pain. The lack of periodicity of the pain should separate it from disc disease. In addition, some authors postulate entrapment of the sciatic nerve by aberrant muscles or fibrous tissue in the sciatic notch.

5 *Neurological disease.* The signs of root compression may be apparent in any neurological disease affecting the lower motor neuron, such as peripheral neuropathy. The changes, however, are often more widespread and pain is usually not as predominant as in disc disease.

6 *Conjoint lumbar root.* An abnormal conjunction of two lumbar roots leaving the dural canal in the same root sleeve can cause radiological and operative confusion (White *et al.* 1982). It is possible for the upper part of such a root to be tightly compressed around the pedicle.

## The role of illness behaviour

The behaviour of any normal person who becomes ill will alter. This is particularly so if the illness is painful and prolonged. Certain people, especially if their character shows a tendency to neuroticism or hypochondriasis, will so exaggerate their behaviour that it becomes abnormal. It is vital to the management of such patients that it is understood that such changes are not intentional or conscious and that they should be seen as separate from the much less common malingerer or psycatric disturbance. The presence of nonorganic physical signs was recognized in the early part of this century (Collie 1913, Jones & Llewellyn 1917) but were largely interpreted as evidence of intentional malingering.

The role of illness behaviour in the evolution of lumbar spine disease has been greatly clarified by a group of workers who initially reviewed the results of operation on Workmen's Compensation Board patients in Canada (Waddell *et al.* 1979, McCulloch 1977), and emphasized the influence of a psychogenic component on the results of chemonucleolysis, showing that the presence of a significant psychological component lowered the success rate from 74% to 11%. The assessment of such a 'psychogenic component' is open to many forms of bias. Waddell *et al.* (1980) attempted to standardize the interpretation of nonorganic physical signs in back pain by evaluating the signs of illness behaviour. From a much larger group, they eventually chose five signs which were reliable and reproducible both between examiners and temporally. Essentially, four of these signs depend on the apparent production of pain by manoeuvres which only simulate spinal movement and which would not normally cause pain either in a normal subject or in a patient with genuine disc prolapse. The final sign was that of patient overreaction which, although the most accurate predictor, was the least reproducible sign.

The presence of three out of five of the factors should suggest a significant nonorganic factor to the illness but by no means excludes genuine organic pathology as both may co-exist. Their presence, however, indicates that surgery is much less likely to provide satisfaction to both patient and surgeon and that, if undertaken, surgery will need to be supplemented with considerable psychological support and treatment.

## Operative treatment

Symonds (1939) wrote that 'if prolapsed intervertebral disc is anything but a rare cause of sciatica it is a lesion which is in most cases capable of spontaneous repair'. The great majority of patients suffering from an episode of nonspecific back pain will be better within six weeks regardless of any type of therapy (Rowe, 1969). If, however, only patients shown to have disc protrusion present are considered, only 30% respond to conservative therapy (Collona and Friedenberg 1949). In a study performed in Scandinavia (Weber 1973), it was shown that surgical treatment produced better results at one year but, that at four years, there was no difference between the surgically and conservatively treated groups. The long term tendency for such

symptoms is for them slowly to improve. The ability of disc surgery to provide 'success' depends clearly on what the patient expects from operation. Patients expecting total freedom from pain will most often be disappointed and eventually have to accept a lesser outcome (Crawshaw *et al.* 1984).

These factors must be clearly in the neurosurgeon's mind when deciding whether or not to operate and in what to advise the patients as to the expected outcome. Assuming a confident diagnosis of disc protrusion as earlier described, there are broadly four categories of indication for operation:

1  Acute cauda equina syndrome. An absolute indication for immediate surgery.
2  Signs of severe root compression; such as foot drop.
3  Failure of complete rest to relieve severe radicular pain whether in the first or subsequent attack.
4  Recurring episodes of radicular pain; which limit the patient's lifestyle or ability to work.

Recent advances have broadened the scope for operative intervention in the management of disc protrusion. It must be emphasized, however, that each of the techniques to be described should be considered as an operative procedure, including enzymatic injection. The indication for each technique are as described above and each technique is designed to alleviate problems caused by disc protrusion and not other types of spinal pathology.

The aims of the procedures are to relieve pressure on the nerve root by reducing or removing the disc protrusion and to weaken the spine by as little as possible. To achieve this during open operation the removal of bone, muscle and ligamentous attachments should be minimized, but at the same time adequate exposure must be obtained to identify and adequately remove the pathology.

## Open discectomy

This is usually performed prone using various positions to ensure that the abdomen is not compressed so as to avoid dural and venous congestion. Formal laminectomy is unnecessary except in cases of massive prolapse as found in acute cauda equina syndrome. Laminectomy aggravates spinal instability, as this procedure is being performed in a spine with degenerative discs, unlike the multiple laminectomies performed for intradural tumour in a relatively normal spinal column. Sufficient exposure can usually be achieved by reflecting that part of the ligamentum flavum which overlies only the appropriate interspace on the affected side. Only minimal parts of the contiguous hemilaminae and lateral bony recess need be removed. The nerve root may then be identified and retracted medially to allow the disc prolapse to be inspected. If there is no free fragment the annulus must be incised to allow removal of the degenerative disc material. Most surgeons then proceed to exenterate as much disc material as possible, although others have shown that the amount and the weight of the removed disc material does not correlate with results (Nashold & Hrubec 1971, Shannon & Paul 1979).

The postoperative management of patients following discectomy varies. In previous years, many patients were kept recumbent for several weeks. It is more usual now to encourage earlier mobilization, although some surgeons still keep patients in bed for one or two weeks. Recent wide experience of immediate mobilization starting on the first postoperative day suggests that it is psychologically better for the patient, causes no more discomfort than at one week, and perhaps lessens the chance of deep venous thrombosis. Sitting and driving should be discouraged for the first two to three weeks and to return to light work is possible at six weeks. All patients should be instructed in ongoing back care, such as correct bending and avoiding lifting, which is necessary during their remaining life span.

## Microdiscectomy

Williams (1978) devised a microsurgical approach whereby a disc protrusion could be removed via a one inch incision. The original stimulus was a cosmetic consideration. This, however, led to an appreciation of the advantages of the technique with respect to minimal tissue disturbance and improved visualization of both root and disc. The intraspinal part of the operation is very similar to open discectomy except that no bone at all is removed and extradural fat is preserved. In addition, the nerve root canal can be decompressed well laterally with experience, if necessary. It is not surprising, therefore, that long-term results in terms of success and recurrence are identical to open operation (Wilson Harbaugh 1981). The advantage lies in the limited disturbance of soft tissue allowing less postoperative pain, earlier discharge from hospital and return to work. Whilst the latter two of these factors were shown to be true in the study of Wilson and Harbaugh, no study has actually demonstrated the improvement in postoperative pain attributed to this procedure. The earlier discharge from hospital, however, does support the fact that mobilization is easier in patients treated by microdiscectomy.

## Chymopapain injection

The technique of injecting an enzyme directly into the nucleus pulposus in order to dissolve its substance was developed by Lyman Smith (Smith et al. 1963, Smith 1964). Subsequent refinements in the chymopapain enzyme have reduced the previously worrying incidence of anaphylaxis to very low levels which now approximate the mortality of surgical discectomy. The procedure is most safely performed under local anaesthesia but the reproduction of pain during disc injection can be disturbing. Though there are exceptions (for example Ejeskar et al. 1983) many authors report similar efficacy to open discectomy (Smith 1964, McCulloch 1977, Nordby & Brown 1977). However, with increasing usage it has become apparent that there may be an appreciable relapse rate, with surgical therapy then becoming necessary. In a recent study, Crawshaw *et al.* (1984) found that 12 of the 25 patients in their chymopapain group required surgical treatment at a mean interval of 5 months following the injection. Bradford *et al.* (1983) have reported experimental evidence that the disc can recover its normal histology and chemical state within one year of injection with restoration of the disc height to normal. It may be, therefore, that chymopapain can only produce short-term benefit in many cases.

## Results of surgery

The results of operation are best considered under three headings: the effect on back pain; the effect on root pain; and the recovery of impaired neurological function.

1  *Back pain.* Back pain alone is not an indication for discectomy. However, back pain commonly occurs along with radicular pain, 89% of DePalma and Rothman's patients (1969), and patients will expect it to disappear unless appropriately counselled. Although 60% of the patients in this large series reported by DePalma and Rothman achieved complete relief of both back and leg pain, many patients had persistent back pain following surgery. This is not surprising as the function of the disc is not restored by its exenteration and the affected motor segment does not become normal. Most patients who are warned that they may be left with some degree of back pain following surgery are able to accept this and accommodate accordingly.

2  *Root pain.* The surgical relief of radicular pain is much more successful. Most authors quote acceptable relief of pain in between 75 and 90% of cases. The relief is not always total and many patients may still get 'twinges' of radicular pain which serve to remind them of the necessity of ongoing back care.

3  *Impairment of nerve root function.* It is uncommon for there to be permanent disability due to muscular weakness or cutaneous sensory loss from the involvement of a single root. A lost tendon reflex seldom returns and marked sensory loss may remain as a permanently numb area but this is usually small and of no great significance. Motor recovery may be very slow and a drop foot can take more than a year to recover but total motor recovery did occur in 50% of patients with a pre-operative deficit in DePalma and Rothman's series.

There are many possible causes of failure. Martin (1981) has described some of the pain syndromes which occur in failed back surgery. Waddell *et al.* (1979) found that inadequate pre-operative diagnosis of the cause of back or leg pain accounted for the majority of operative failures. Other causes of failure could be technical (for example incorrect level explored), psychological, and recurrence of disc prolapse. They showed that repeated operations (especially, third and fourth) were seldom likely to succeed and, that repeat operation was associated with a considerably increased chance of the patient being made worse. They did, however, identify factors which were compatible with good results for repeated operation. The factors were: at least six months relief of pain following first operation; limb pain worse than back pain; and a herniation at a new level. If the first operation has failed to produce any relief at all, repeat surgery should be considered only if an identifiable factor can be proved and corrected.

The place of spinal fusion in the surgery of lumbar disc disease is not clear. Many more fusion procedures were performed twenty years ago than at present. Persistent, severe and disabling mechanical back pain may require spinal fusion but the success rate is not high. In a few situations, such as at the time of disc removal in a young patient with spondylolisthesis, fusion is mandatory. The addition of fusion at the time of disc removal has been said to improve results marginally (Nachlas 1952) but to an extent insufficient to warrant performing it routinely. It is clear, however, that performing a fusion when discectomy alone has failed is unlikely to succeed and that fusion is best performed as a combined procedure with discectomy, if specified indications are appropriate.

Spinal fusions fall into two broad categories: the interbody fusion when bone graft is placed into the cleared disc space from either an anterior or posterior approach; and only fusions of either the neural arch or transverse processes. Early mobilization is now accepted and the previous prolonged periods of recumbency following fusions are now no longer required. Fusion from the sacrum to higher than L4 is unlikely to succeed and a fusion of only L5 to S1 will be ineffective if the L4/5 disc is degenerate. It is, therefore, advisable to perform discography prior to deciding the extent of fusion.

## Lumbar spinal stenosis

Diffuse degenerative and reactive changes in the spine may lead to canal narrowing in all directions. This causes the syndrome of spinal stenosis, first emphasized in English literature by Verbiest (1954) and must be separated from the forms of congenital stenosis discussed in the section on the pathophysiology of degeneration. The effects of repeated rotational strain on a motor segment is to induce, amongst other changes, degenerative changes in the neural arch and facet joints which lead to overgrowth of the joint into the canal. This, in time, causes stenosis in the lateral recess and entrapment of nerve roots (Forfar 1977, Kirkaldy-Willis et al. 1978). Patients presenting with spinal stenosis are usually over 60 years of age, and complain almost universally of back pain. In addition, one third will have radicular pain and one third, neurogenic claudication. (Getty 1980). This latter term refers in this context to radicular pain which is exacerbated by activity and subsides with rest as distinguished from the much more common exacerbation of back pain with activity. Neurogenic claudication is worsened or induced by an extended lumbar spine (Wilson 1969) and the patient may start to walk with an increasingly stooped posture to flex the spine, thereby increasing its anteroposterior diameter (Dyke 1979). Signs of root irritation are often missing, but compression signs are common, especially after exertion (Getty 1980). The treatment of this condition too often results in multiple-level midline laminectomies which fail to decompress the lateral recess. It is now generally accepted that more attention should be paid to localizing the root or roots involved and to decompress them by an undercutting facetectomy which preserves some of the integrity of the facet joint (Getty et al. 1981, Venner & Cook 1981).

## Thoracic disc prolapse

Although radiological signs of degenerative changes in thoracic discs are not uncommon, the clinical effects of compression of either spinal cord or nerve root are rare. The reported percentage of all disc lesions coming to operation is usually less than 1% (Love & Kiefer 1950, Larson et al. 1976). The lower 6 thoracic discs account for three-quarters of the cases, and the last two discs for one-quarter. The majority of patients present in middle age (Lombardi & Passerini 1964).

The clinical features of thoracic disc disease are protean and diagnosis is often delayed (Otani et al. 1982). It is possible, however, to discern three clinical groups according to the presentation.

1  *Typical compression syndrome.* Symptoms and signs evolve in a manner simulating an intraspinal neoplasm: root and back pain; progressive paraparesis; impairment of sensation and loss of sphincters. A Brown-Séquard syndrome may be seen.

2  *Painless progressive paraparesis.* In perhaps half the cases, root and back pain are minimal. Spastic weakness develops slowly and may be asymmetrical. Occasionally, the onset is acute (Otani et al. 1982). Symptoms may fluctuate and objective signs of sensory loss may be absent for years, during which time a diagnosis of demyelinating disease may have been considered.

3  *Radicular.* Back pain with pain of intercostal distribution is not uncommon and is due to a laterally placed protrusion. Progression of the protrusion may well lead to the onset of myelopathy.

**Investigation**

The radiological identification of symptomless degenerative changes in thoracic discs is not uncommon but, where these changes are severe and restricted to a disc level consonant with the clinical features, the association is suggestive. Thoracic disc protrusions themselves may become densely calcified for reasons which are not clear (Fig. 22.2).

Myelography is essential for diagnosis and accurate localization. Defects lying opposite the disc space on lateral and anteroposterior radiographs are typical. The examination may be technically difficult and repeat examinations may be necessary to confirm a clinically suspected lesion. This point merits repetition; that a single negative examination in a case with suggestive clinical picture should be repeated. Sekhar and Jannetta (1983) found CT scanning following myelography to be useful in confirming the local abnormality. These authors felt that spinal angiography to identify the point of entry of the artery of Adamkiewicz was unnecessary.

**Treatment**

Radicular pain is only a relative indication for surgery as other means of pain relief such as facet block may be effective. If decompressive surgery is not performed, however, the patient must be closely followed in case myelopathy develops. The onset of myelopathy is an absolute indication for surgery, as the more advanced the deficit the greater the risks and less the chances of improvement become (Otani *et al.* 1977). The removal of a thoracic disc prolapse is technically difficult for the following reasons:

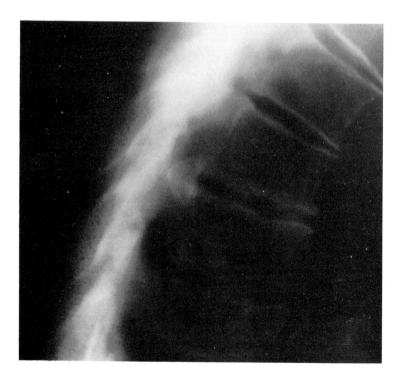

**Fig. 22.2** Lateral tomogram showing calcified protruded thoracic disc.

1 The small size of the spinal canal; the presence within it of the spinal cord and the protrusion leaves no room for manoeuvre;
2 The anterior situation of the hard fibro-cartilaginous mass renders operating space essential; particularly so, as the dome of the protrusion may perforate the dura and embed itself in the cord;
3 The viability of the spinal cord is already jeopardized by the compression and the relative vascular insufficiency of that area.

Early attempts at treating thoracic discs by laminectomy led to very disappointing results (Love & Kiefer 1950, Logue 1952). Indeed, all of Logue's patients were neurologically worse postoperatively, with only four showing eventual improvement. In 1969, Perot and Munro reviewed the results of laminectomy from the available literature. Of the 91 patients treated, 40 either failed to improve, were made paraplegic or died; and, if only centrally placed protrusions were considered, 32 of the 57 patients were in these categories. Laminectomy for disc protrusion above the T10/11 level was particularly dangerous, with only 11 of the 34 patients showing any improvement at all.

Due to these poor results, Hulme (1960) modified the procedure of costotransversectomy which had been used by Alexander (1946) and others for tuberculous spinal disease. This had the advantage of producing a more oblique approach to the anterior aspect of the cord and the disc. A small cavity was then drilled out in the adjacent vertebral bodies into which the disc could be mobilized. This dramatically reduced the numbers of patients who were made worse by operation, but the procedure still had limited access and disasters still could occur. Some other variations of this technique are available (for example transpedicular; Patterson and Arbit 1978) but several people following Hulme's principle of a more anterior attack on the disc opted for a transthoracic route. Craaford et al. (1958) were the first intentionally to approach a thoracic disc protrusion via thoracotomy, but several other reports of this approach, either extrapleural or transpleural, have appeared (Ransohoff et al. 1969, Perot & Munro 1969, Otani et al. 1982) and the results of these studies offer a vastly improved chance of neurological recovery over other methods. Again following the original lead, Findlay has modified the radical anterior spinal operation for tuberculosis (Hodgson & Stock 1956) to use in thoracic disc prolapse. This entails a transthoracic removal of a major part of the contiguous vertebral bodies to produce a much larger cavity into which the disc may be more safely mobilized and delivered, the defect being made good by iliac crest bone graft. Early mobilization is still possible and of the initial eighteen patients so treated all have shown dramatic neurological improvement and all but one have been able to return to full functional activity (Findlay 1985).

## Cervical spondylosis

An early description of a cervical disc prolapse causing quadriparesis was that of Walton and Paul (1905). Stookey (1928) described the clinical patterns of compression by 'chondromas' some years before Mixter and Barr's paper clarified the role of disc protrusion in the lumbar spine. Much less progress was made in correlating similar changes in cervical discs with their much greater variety of associated neurological disturbance. However, Stookey (1940) in a further contribution described the types of neurological compromise which a cervical disc could cause:

1 Compression of a cervical root alone; now commonly referred to as cervical radiculopathy.
2 Compression of roots and spinal cord; causing myeloradiculopathy.
3 Compression of cord alone; referred to as cervical spondylotic myelopathy. Brain (1948, Brain et al. 1952) was largely responsible for recognizing that myelopathy could be due to cervical spondylotic changes without necessarily causing neck or arm pain. Brain and Wilkinson (1967) reviewed much of what was known

about the pathology and natural history of this disease in their book.

It has been emphasized in the section on pathophysiology that intervertebral disc protrusion is but an incident in the course of a degenerative process which leads ultimately to the changes of spondylosis. This is particularly true in the cervical spine where the reactive changes are much more likely to cause neural compression than the disc. This may reflect only the relatively small volume of cervical discs (Bull 1948).

## Pathophysiology of cervical spondylosis

Symptomatic cervical disc prolapse is much more common than prolapse of thoracic discs but less common than in the lumbar area. The most frequently affected level is C5/6 (DePalma & Rothman 1970). As in the lumbar spine, degenerative changes readily occur in those mobile parts adjacent to a rigid area such as a congenital block vertebra or an operatively fused level. Trauma or severe muscular effort plays a less important role than in lumbar prolapse but flexion or hyperextension may acutely damage a cervical disc causing abrupt neurological deficit. A history of minor trauma as an exacerbating factor for the clinical syndrome is, however, not uncommon (Wilkinson 1967).

A general account has already been given of the manner in which reactive spondolytic changes occur in response to the results of disc degeneration. Certain features with regard to this process in the cervical spine deserve emphasis. Loss of disc substance causes shortening with resulting flattening of the normal curve. In severe cases this may lead to a tendency for the head to be flexed downwards. In order to look forward, the patient must then exaggerate the normal cervical lordosis with resulting crowding of the laminae. The shortening of the spine disturbs the normal alignment of the zygoapophyseal articular surfaces, leading to secondary osteoarthritic changes which can encroach on the intervertebral foramen causing nerve root compression. Shortening also alters the normal downward oblique course of the spinal root in the foramen causing it to run more horizontally, or even in a cranial direction (Adams & Logue 1971a). Bulging of the annulus in the cervical area due to nuclear degeneration tends to happen in several places across the posterior part of the disc producing a bar-like transverse ridge across the canal, 5 mm or more high. The bulging and reactive changes which arise from the region of the neurocentral joint of Luschka are particularly important as they jut into the intervertebral foramen immediately anterior to the root, compressing it against the facet joints behind.

Commonly in the lumbar spine, disc degeneration affects only one level but in the cervical area it is much more commonly multiple. Of the 17 patients examined at necropsy by Wilkinson (1960), only in two were the changes restricted to a single level; the C5/6 disc was affected in all but one. Disc degeneration allows an abnormal degree of mobility to develop between adjacent vertebrae. Subluxation and degenerative spondylolisthesis are more commonly seen in the cervical area, probably due to the relatively less powerful musculotendinous support in this region.

The anterior dura is commonly thickened and adherent to the floor of the spinal canal. Adhesions may also be found around the root sleeves which may anchor them to the intervertebral foramina, and intradural adhesions between dura, arachnoid and pia are common over segments affected by cervical spondylosis.

Frykholm (1951) studied the anatomy of cervical nerve roots, their dural coverings and the changes seen in spondylosis, which he aptly termed 'root sleeve fibrosis'. The mouth of the sleeve is wide, funnel shaped and smoothly rounded as it leaves the theca. Each dorsal and ventral rootlet passes into a separate compartment, in which it is freely mobile, formed by a septum across the distal root sleeve. This maintains the identity of each until beyond the dorsal root ganglion where they fuse to form the segmental nerve. In spondylosis, the sleeves become thickened and anchored to the disc and foramen. At operation, the root may appear noticeably swollen corresponding probably to the regenerative fibres seen by Greenfield (1953) in histological preparation. In addition to the root being swollen, reactive changes may narrow the root canal thus exacerbating the compression.

Although the root is tethered distally, there is considerable movement of the tissues within the spinal canal when the neck moves. O'Connell (1946) estimated that, during flexion, the posterior contour of the canal increased by up to 5 cm, while the anterior contour increased by up to 2 cm. Adams and Logue (1971a) showed that this movement occurred by a combination of upward dural displacement and stretching. They confirmed also that the roots moved in proportion to the dural displacement but that, in view of their distal fixation, this induced tension in the root which was pronounced if the root took a descending course to exit the spinal canal.

The spinal cord itself may be severely compressed and thinned when it passes over an osteophytic bar. The cord becomes widened by this compression; a feature which can mimic an intramedullary tumour on an anteroposterior film during myelography. The ventral aspect may show a number of impressions corresponding in number and situation to the spondylotic bars. Hughes (1966) in his review of the pathological changes noted that the cord is indented in all cases of myelopathy although indentation could also occur without clinical or pathological changes. The pathological changes seen in the spinal cord varies greatly in degree and in extent, but could include:

1 In the anterior horns of the grey matter there was loss of some neurons, degeneration of others, glial cavitation and proliferation, attributable to ischaemia. These changes were most severe at the level of indentation but could be widespread (Mair & Druckman 1953)
2 Demyelination of the corticospinal tract and posterior columns.
3 Wallerian degeneration in ascending tracts

above and descending tracts below the site of compression.
4 Proliferation of small blood vessels and intimal thickening.

## The aetiology of the myelopathy

Two main factors may be responsible for the development of myelopathy in cervical spondylosis, mechanical compression leading to deformation of the cord, and ischaemia due to interference with spinal cord bloodflow. The problem of aetiology is complex because of the diffuse and patchy extent of the pathological changes in the spinal cord itself, the diversity of the clinical presentation and the variable incidence of myelopathy in patients with radiological evidence of spondylosis.

It is difficult to avoid the conclusion that pressure deformation plays an important and direct role, distinct from possible ischaemic effects. It is difficult, however, to explain the relative sparing of the anterior columns which must bear the brunt of the pressure. Cervical myelopathy has been simulated experimentally by compressing the cord (Gooding et al. 1975) and it has been shown that sagittal compression is more likely to cause myelopathy than coronal (Doppman 1975).

Examination of the dimensions of the spinal canal radiologically and *post mortem* makes it clear that the occurrence of myelopathy is related to the size of the spinal canal, a basic factor being the natural sagittal diameter of the canal. Several studies of the canal dimensions have been made but Payne and Spillane (1957) were the first to study post-mortem dimensions in normal and spondylotic patients. Radiographic studies have established a range of normal values for the sagittal diameter at each cervical level (Logue 1957, Burrows 1963, Wolfe et al. 1965, Nurick 1975). The techniques vary slightly in the points of measurements but most agree that a sagittal diameter of the cervical canal of less than 13 mm in the midcervical area is abnormal. The average diameter of the spinal cord in the cervical area has been shown to average 10 mm (Penning & Van der Zwagg 1966), thus congenital stenosis, is associated with further encroachment by degenerative changes, can easily compress the cord. The association of sagittal stenosis with the clinical syndrome of cervical spondylotic myelopathy is well established (Burrows 1963, Bradley & Banna 1968, Nurick 1972).

Soft tissue changes during extension of the neck aggravate canal narrowing. Taylor (1953) and Stoltmann and Blackwood (1964) demonstrated that in flexion the ligamenta flava and superior margins of the laminae form a smooth roof to the spinal canal; in extension, approximation of the laminae causes buckling of the ligamenta flava so that they present a series of corrugations in the dorsal wall which form characteristic notch-like filling defects on myelography. The effects of this narrowing are accentuated by the increased diameter of the cord which shortens on extension of the neck (Breig 1960). Although the canal diameter is effectively increased during flexion, the consequences of flexion cannot be ignored. During flexion the canal lengthens and the spinal cord is drawn out. As described above, this puts tension on the nerve roots but Breig did not feel that the cord itself was under tension but rather adapted in length by a 'concertina' effect. However, he did show that in the flexed spondylotic spine the cord was indented and attenuated by the bars and was widened transversely. This distortion was most apparent in the anterior horns and microangiography revealed defective filling of vessels in these areas.

The distribution of the focal degeneration affecting the anterior horns and basal (ventral) portion of the posterior columns, lies within the territory of the penetrating branches of the anterior spinal artery (Mair & Druckman 1953) and it may be assumed that compression of that artery is an important cause of the apparently ischaemic histological changes in the grey matter. However, Hughes and Brownell (1964) showed that thrombosis of the anterior spinal artery was rare in cervical spondylotic myelopathy; nevertheless this does not exclude inter-

mittent obstruction or impairment of blood supply as a cause. Other features suggest an ischaemic aetiology: hyperplasia of small arteries and thickening of their walls; extension of degeneration into segments below the level of compression on the basis that bloodflow in the anterior spinal artery is caudal; and spastic paraparesis being one of the earliest signs of myelopathy with the relevant pyramidal fibres at the boundary zone of the anterior spinal artery supply.

Ischaemia of the spinal cord at C5 and 6 could be produced in other ways. Radicular arteries of supply may be compressed or occluded within the intervertebral foramina (Frykholm 1951). Waltz (1967) showed that the cross-sectional areas of the foramina were reduced by about 20% in passing from flexion to extension. This is of no consequence in health, but in a spondylotic intervertebral foramen, obstruction of radicular blood flow could occur during extension which could be significant if the artery was a major contributor to spinal cord blood flow or if several foramina were affected.

Taylor (1964) felt that the variable and fluctuating signs in cervical spondylotic myelopathy could best be explained by intermittent vascular occlusion of the arterioles supplying the cord. He also showed that the clinical effects of spinal cord anoxia due to major vessel occlusion were similar to those found in myelopathy due to spondylosis. However, Brieg et al. (1966) felt that compromise of the intrinsic blood supply of the cord itself was more likely to be the cause than compression of the arteries of supply. They also observed that patients who have a tenuous radicular supply to the cervical cord on grounds of anatomical variance would be more at risk of developing critical ischaemia.

Some more recent experimental and pathological studies (Gledhill et al. 1973, Gooding et al. (1975) have emphasized the significance of demyelination in the cord raising the possibility that it is the myelin sheaths which are predominately affected by either pressure or ischaemia. Overall, it appears fairly certain that both compression and ischaemia play important roles in the pathogenesis of cervical spondylotic myelopathy and, indeed, these are brought together by Doppman (1975) who showed that cord compression could obliterate blood flow in the sulcal artery of the cord whilst leaving the anterior spinal artery patent.

## Clinical features

Due to the multiplicity of the factors which influence the location and extent of the lesions in the spinal cord and roots, and not least among these are the level and number of segments involved, the clinical manifestations of cervical spondylosis are extremely variable. The length of history may be very short, especially if associated with trauma, or may stretch over many years with many unsuccessful attempts at treatment. Although isolated cervical radiculopathy is common, pure myelopathy is rare and more usually presents as a myeloradiculopathy with features of both problems. However, the clinical features of radiculopathy and myelopathy will be described as separate entities.

### Radiculopathy

Pain is usually felt initially in the neck and may radiate out over the shoulders. The onset of brachalgia (radicular pain) brings pain in the arm spreading distal to the elbow. The distribution is widespread and conforms to scleratomes (segmental distribution to muscles and bones) rather than to dermatomes, although there may be dermatomal sensory changes. The widespread distribution of pain has been ascribed to compression of nerves of the brachial plexus due to secondary spasm of the scalenus anterior muscle (Spurling & Scoville 1944) or it may be due to traction on the roots of the brachial plexus caused by dropping of the shoulder due to muscle atony. More usually, however, the affected shoulder is held in an elevated attitude. The pain has the same characteristics as in lumbar disc

prolapse; deep, boring, even nauseating, pain aggravated by activity of the arm and by coughing or straining. The periodicity of the pain with relapses and remission is not as striking as in the lumbar area. Relief may be obtained by shoulder abduction with a flexed elbow, such as placing the affected hand on the head, as this manoeuvre reduces the length and tension of the cervical roots (Davidson et al. 1981).

Muscular weakness and wasting with fasciculation may be seen if root compression is severe. The affected muscle may suggest which root is compressed but anomalous supply and multiple innervation sometimes render precise localization inaccurate (Brendler 1968). Sensory changes such as paraesthesiae and numbness are common. Frequently they form a subjective complaint but no objective deficit can be elicited; though in many such cases diminution of pinprick sensation and 2-point discrimination will be found. The dermatome affected is, again, an aid to localization but, as in the motor changes, may be relatively imprecise. Depression of the biceps, triceps or supinator jerk is often found.

### Myelopathy

Pain is a variable symptom in cervical spondylotic myelopathy. Neck and radicular pain may be present, especially in patients with myeloradiculopathy but it is important to note that many patients suffer no pain whatsoever. Motor weakness is the commonest initial symptom, usually starting in the lower limb. Spasticity of the lower limbs is noted as a shuffling or dragging of the feet and the gait is often ataxic when the paraparesis is slight. In the later stages, spasticity with spontaneous clonus may be extreme and the patient eventually becomes unable to walk. The distribution of weakness is usually uneven between the upper and lower limbs and between the two sides. Sphincter disturbance occurs late. In the upper limb the patient may notice clumsiness of the hands and fingers, particularly for fine skilled movements which may be due as much to proprioceptive loss as to loss of power. Paraesthesiae are common in the upper limbs comprising sensations such as numbness and tingling. They may be of an unpleasant dysaesthetic nature and occur in the digits or in a radicular distribution.

Even with advanced spondylosis, neck movements may be painless and only mildly restricted and the cervical curve may appear flattened. According to the level and extent of the lesion, signs in the upper limb will be predominantly of a lower or an upper motor neuron type. In general, the proximal musculature is more affected by atrophic weakness (LMN) and the distal by spastic weakness (UMN). Wasting of the shoulder girdle, biceps and triceps muscles may be pronounced. Wasting of the intrinsic muscles of the hand is not a good segmental localizing sign for it may be present when the principal zone of the cord compression is several segments above the first thoracic level. It is likely to result from the anterior horn changes already alluded to. Fasciculation is often present but is rarely severe in degree and extent, an important point for the distinction between spondylotic myelopathy and motor neuron disease. The tendon reflexes in the arm will depend upon the extent to which the segmental LMN is damaged which impairs or destroys them. They will be exaggerated as a result of UMN interruption if the relevant segment is caudal to the level of cord involvement. A frequent finding is normal or exaggerated biceps jerk, an absent triceps jerk and exaggerated finger jerks; a combination suggesting a myelopathy maximal at the C7 level. The behaviour of the supinator (radial) jerk may be helpful if, when it is absent, a tap on the radius elicits flexion of the digits or biceps. This phenomenon is known as an 'inverted supinator jerk' and is regarded as evidence of a lesion in the C5 segment.

The weakness of the trunk and lower limbs is entirely of UMN type; spasticity may be more disabling than loss of power. The gait is of a broad-based ataxic or spastic type and lower limb reflexes are exaggerated with clonus and extensor plantar responses. The degree of limb involvement in cervical spondylotic myelopathy is

variable; some patients having a spastic paraparesis, others a quadriparesis.

Impairment of cutaneous sensibility can be demonstrated in the majority of cases, though its distribution varies markedly and is commonly asymmetrical. It may be limited to the upper limbs and be dermatomal or peripheral in type affecting only the finger tips. Loss of deep sensibility (joint movement and vibrations) is an important sign, commonly seen in the toes. Loss of proprioception more rarely affects the upper limb when the resulting deficit can be grossly disabling and is usually associated with high cervical compression.

The natural history of cervical spondylotic myelopathy is highly variable. Lees and Turner (1963) found that 50% of their patients improved, at least temporarily without treatment. However, DePalma et al (1972) followed for 5 years those patients who had failed to respond to conservative treatment but who had refused surgery and found that only 45% of them achieved a tolerable level of symptomatic relief. A few patients will experience an initial deterioration and go on to a fairly stable neurological state. Others experience a fluctuating but slowly deteriorating course; while a significant number (20%) will deteriorate relentlessly (Clark & Robinson 1956). Attempts have been made to predict those in the latter category. Lees and Turner (1963) thought that neither age nor number of levels affected were important, while DePalma et al (1972) found a history of industrial compensation or hyperextension injury to be adverse factors. Adams and Logue (1971b) emphasized the role of excessive cervical mobility and, more recently, Barnes and Saunders (1984) found this to be the only factor associated with deterioration.

The syndromes discussed above are those associated with chronic spondylotic changes. However, as in the lumbar spine, acute disc rupture may occur, especially if associated with trauma. An acute prolapse which normally presents in a younger age group may produce a radiculopathy affecting the root compressed or more rarely can cause an acute, or subacute myelopathy. The symptoms of the radiculopathy may or may not settle with time, rest and conservative therapy; myelopathy is almost universally progressive.

## Differential diagnosis

1 *Disseminated sclerosis* is perhaps the most difficult differential diagnosis. The presence of signs in the cranial nerves and disturbance of micturition early in the course of the disease or abnormal visual evoked responses are suggestive of demyelination. The problem is made more difficult by the fact that the presentation of disseminated sclerosis in older patients tends to be in a spinal rather than cranial form (Brain 1977). Diagnosis is not helped by conventional radiology as the presence of spondylotic changes in the cervical spine are of course common and do not confirm the existence of cervical spondylotic myelopathy. The importance of examination of the cerebrospinal fluid in all cases studied by myelography must be emphasized. This should include measurement of the IgG fraction of the CSF protein. Equally, there is no doubt that both diseases may coexist and indeed there is cause to suspect that the compression and/or the ischaemia of the degenerative process may predispose or enhance the effects of areas of demyelination in the cervical cord. Appropriate surgical therapy may produce considerable benefit though unfortunately this does not often last.

2 *Motor neuron disease* may be difficult to distinguish from cases of myelopathy in which sensory symptoms and signs are inconspicuous or absent. Dysarthria and other signs of bulbar palsy along with severe muscle wasting and pronounced fasciculation should suggest motor neuron disease. The presence of marked lower motor neuron signs in the lower limbs or on electromyography are very suggestive of this disorder.

3 *Spinal tumours*, either intra- or extramedullary, may present a similar picture. Severe, constant radicular pain may suggest a neurofibroma and the Brown-Séquard syndrome is commoner in the presence of a tumour though it can be due to spondylosis (Nurick 1975). Myelography should always be sufficiently complete to exclude this possibility.

4 *Malignancy.* Malignant processes may mimic cervical spondylosis either by producing a nonmetastatic neuropathic syndrome, or by carcinomatous meningitis (Boyle *et al.* 1980).

5 *Rheumatoid arthritis.* Cervical involvement occurs in up to 25% of patients with rheumatoid arthritis (Conlon *et al.* 1966). Involvement at the C1/2 level produces atlanto-axial subluxation while disease at the midcervical level causes problems identical to cervical spondylotic myelopathy but with a much higher incidence of instability.

Cervical radiculopathy may also be mimicked by various disorders:

1 *Neuralgic amyotrophy.* This is an acute disorder often related to immunization or a flu-like viral illness. The onset is with intense pain followed by a neurological deficit which usually outlasts the pain before resolving (Tsairis *et al.* 1972).

2 *Thoracic outlet syndrome.* Compression of the brachial plexus in or proximal to the thoracic outlet will produce many of the features of radiculopathy. The finding of vascular bruits or variations in the radial pulse with arm movement suggests this diagnosis.

3 *Pancoast tumour.* An apical lung tumour can invade the brachial plexus producing severe, unremitting pain with gross loss of function.

4 *Peripheral nerve compression neuropathy.* Entrapment of the median nerve in the carpal tunnel or the ulnar nerve at the elbow may mimic radiculopathy because pain may extend well proximal to the site of compression. Careful examination, especially of the sensory findings, supplemented by nerve conduction studies, should exclude these diagnoses.

## Investigations

Plain radiological examination of the cervical spine in the anteroposterior and lateral projection will reveal any bony spondylotic changes present such as osteophytosis or disc narrowing. Equally, the role of a congenitally stenotic canal or localized degenerative narrowing has been emphasized and plain radiology may suggest the presence of either of these entities. The loss of the normal cervical lordosis with straightening of the cervical spine may be seen and suggests relatively acute pathology with reflex muscular spasm. The routine examination often includes oblique views to show the intervertebral foramina but McPherson and McPherson (1981) suggest that this addition is unhelpful for routine screening. However, the addition of flexion and extension views performed under controlled conditions in patients with proven disease may yield valuable evidence of subluxation and instability.

The presence of an abnormal radiograph must be interpreted with great care as such changes are extremely common with aging and do not necessarily confirm the clinical diagnosis as being due to the effect of cervical spondylosis. Several surveys, such as that of Lawrence et al. (1966) have shown the prevalence of degener-

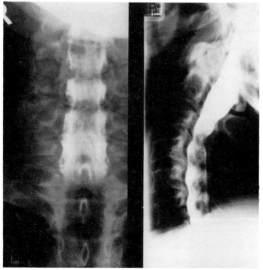

**Fig. 22.3** Cervical myelogram showing cervical spondylosis with multiple indentations of the dural sac due to disc protrusion, osteophytes and ligamentous thickening.

ative changes on plain X-ray in the general population to be great; over 80% of people over 55 years had abnormal radiographs.

Myelography (Fig. 22.3) with examination of the CSF is essential for: furthering the diagnosis, determining the degree of encroachment upon the spinal canal, and establishing the number of levels involved. With modern water-soluble contrast media, better definition is gained if the puncture is performed in the cervical area to aid the concentration of the dye within the area of interest. The chief abnormalities on anteroposterior views are:

1  Absence of filling of one or more root pouches;
2  A transverse bar indicating a ridge running across the back of the disc space;
3  Apparent widening of the cord shadows when stretched across osteophytes;
4  Obstruction to the flow of dye at levels of severe disease, an obstruction which can sometimes be overcome by changing the neck posture.

On the lateral view there may be:

1  Evidence of indentation anteriorly by osteophytic spurs or 'soft' disc material;
2  Evidence of posterior compression due to hypertrophy or buckling of the ligamenta flava and indentation by the lamina.

Several of the other investigative procedures described under lumbar disc disease are applicable to the cervical area. For example, Kikuchi et al. (1981) strongly advocated discography and root sleeve injection in the investigation of radiculopathy. CT scanning, especially in conjunction with subarachnoid contrast material, will undoubtedly play an increased role. Electrophysiology may have a role to play but unfortunately there is considerable overlap between normal and abnormal cases in respect of the amplitude and latency of evoked responses which make assessment difficult (El Negamy & Sedgwick 1979, Silvola et al. 1981). Abnormal visual evoked responses may suggest that a myelopathy is due to neurological (for example, disseminated sclerosis) rather than spondylotic causes.

## Management

### 1. Radiculopathy

As in the cases of the lumbar spine, the vast majority of acute episodes or exacerbations of neck pain and radiculopathy will respond satisfactorily to rest and analgesics. Some may require further conservative measures such as axial traction in slight flexion. Chiropractic manipulation has often been performed at some time before the patient presents to a neurosurgeon but, although this technique is sometimes successful, from a safety point of view it should be performed only after plain radiology has shown that there is no cervical instability. A mainstay of conservative therapy has always been the immobilization of the neck in some form of collar. Whilst this may meet with success by allowing natural resolution of the acute attack, it must be appreciated that only the most rigid types of fixation limit cervical movement to any real extent and that the commonly prescribed soft-collar has only minimal effect, especially on lateral bending and rotation (Johnson et al. 1981). Advocates of collars say that their presence reminds the patients to limit their activities; critics feel that such reminders may reinforce a pattern of illness behaviour and delay recovery.

Occasionally, acute disc rupture may lead to an acute myelopathy or nerve root compression causing abrupt and pronounced neurological deficit. Either of these entities are indications for urgent surgical treatment. A large laterally-placed disc rupture may cause both root and cord compression or merely compress the side of the spinal cord producing a Brown-Séquard syndrome. Very occasionally, acute disc ruptures may transgress the dura and lie partly or entirely in an intradural position.

A small percentage (although in clinical practice a large number due to the frequency of the disease) of patients with radiculopathy will fail to settle on conservative therapy, develop evidence of severe root compression, or suffer frequent relapse which interferes with normal work and activities. Such patients merit consideration for surgical treatment. Although, several different techniques of surgery are available, the essence of obtaining good surgical results lies, not so much with choice of techniques, as selection of patients. Patients suffering only from neck pain have a relatively low chance of being improved regardless of approach; those with radicular pain in the arm are considerably more likely to benefit (Connolly et al. 1965, White et al. 1973).

The main debate in realms of surgical techniques is whether the surgical approach should be anterior or posterior to the spine, or indeed, lateral (Verbiest 1968). The original moves towards anterior cervical surgery consisted of techniques to remove the degenerate disc with its associated osteophytes and then perform a bony fusion at that level (Robinson & Smith 1955, Cloward 1958). The fusion was performed not only to give immediate stability thus terminating the spondylotic process at this level, but also to slightly distract the vertebrae and open the intervertebral foramen thus relieving distortion on the nerve root. In 1960 Hirsch reported equally good results by performing only a simple discectomy without performing a fusion. As it was realized that the good results of the anterior fusion procedures did not strictly depend on achieving bony fusion, many other excellent results of disc excision without fusion have been reported, including those of Robertson (1973), Robertson and Johnson (1980), Martin (1976), Wilson and Campbell (1977), Rosenørn et al. (1983). The vast majority of cases where simple disc excision has been performed go on to solid fusion between the contiguous bodies in any event. Variations of the procedures of disc excision with or without fusion include whether or not to open the posterior longitudinal ligament or whether to excise or leave bony osteophytes. Surgeons who do not excise osteophytes claim, with some justification, that the presence of a bony fusion will stop stress across the joint and the spurs will gradually disappear. However, all exponents of disc excision without fusion remove these spurs so as to open the foramen because there will be no distraction of the disc space.

Whichever technique is used, it is fair to state that the results appear to be equally good. It is probably true that patients in whom fusion has been omitted experience more neck pain in the first few postoperative weeks but they are spared the discomfort and relatively high complication rate of the donor iliac crest wound. Alternative graft materials are available such as cadaver bone or treated allograft material but they are not universally accepted. Kiel (allograft) bone alone has been shown not to be incorporated into a true bony fusion (McMurray 1982) and probably should no longer be used. The newly developed ceramic grafts injected with the patient's own bone marrow may prove more acceptable.

Review of papers reporting results of anterior cervical surgery of any type give reasonably consistent results between 70 and 90% of patients being improved. The reporting of 'excellent' results, i.e. total relief of symptoms, produces a much wider reported range but on average some 60 to 70% of patients return to their previous activity with only minimal discomfort. Fewer than 5% are reported as worse. Many authors claim that the presence of soft disc material rather than osteophyte is a favourable sign but Lunsford et al. (1980) found no difference in their results whether 'hard' or 'soft' discs were found. The presence of disease at multiple levels has been claimed as an adverse prognostic factor (Robinson et al. 1962, Jacobs et al. 1970); however, others found no difference in results regardless of the number of operated levels (De Palma et al 1972, Lunsford et al. 1980).

Anterior cervical surgery however, does have some disadvantages. Amongst these are:

1   The operation is definitive, not exploratory, and is unsuitable if there is doubt either of diagnosis or level involved.
2   There is a risk of damage to the recurrent laryngeal nerves, producing postoperative hoarseness and dysphonia.
3   Visualization of the affected root is poor and decompression is confirmed more by feel than vision.

4   Fusion of the disc space (either intentional or as a late result of simple discectomy) subjects surrounding motion segments to increased strain and can accentuate further degeneration.

Posterior procedures for the treatment of radiculopathy largely comprise attempts to unroof the nerve root foramen by partial facetectomy. This approach ordinarily leaves the disc intact unless a free fragment is found which should be removed piecemeal. It has the advantage that the first stage can to some extent be exploratory with probing of several levels in the lateral angles via the ligamenta flava. When the abnormal disc is discovered, the foramen is opened by drilling. Frykholm (1951) recommended that the dural root sleeve should be incised to liberate the nerve root. This is now seldom performed but it is often necessary to incise the overlying fibrous sheath to mobilize the root so as to expose underlying disc material. Occasionally, extensive laminectomy is performed in patients with radiculopathy (Alsharif et al. 1979) but this is usually reserved for patients who have evidence of a myelopathy in addition.

Reports of the results of posterior foraminotomy for radicular pain are not common. Frykholm reported improvement in 66% of patients treated by his procedure. Higher rates of success have been reported, with over 90% of patients being improved (Spurling 1956, Knight 1964, Casotto & Buoncristiani 1981). The posterior approach like the anterior, does, however, have some disadvantages:

1   Anterior midline disc protrusions cannot be approached directly with absolute safety.
2   Extensive facetectomy and laminectomy impairs stability and can lead to deformity (Verbiest and Paz y Geuse 1966).
3   Postoperative discomfort is considerable.
4   Unless combined with fusion, the procedure does not stabilize and therefore does not terminate the spondylotic process.

No adequate comparison between the results of anterior and posterior techniques exists but it seems likely that the overall success rate is comparable for either approach. Pending such a controlled comparison, the choice of approach remains the preference of the surgeon based on individual cases.

## 2. Myelopathy

When considering either an ischaemic or a compressive aetiology for myelopathy the ideal operation should remove all proliferative disc tissue and osteophytes which impinge upon neural tissue. This has been done through a laminectomy (Allen 1952) but has been abandoned because of the disastrous quadriplegia which often followed such a procedure. There is little room via laminectomy for the manoeuvres necessary to remove bony excrescences lying anterior to the root or cord and the cord is likely to suffer from direct trauma or from ischaemia. Less aggressive posterior procedures designed simply to decompress the cord from behind can be successful, but anterior surgery does allow direct access, with low morbidity, to the areas of reactive spondylosis so intimately concerned in the aetiology of cervical spondylotic myelopathy.

The anterior surgical procedures used in the treatment of myelopathy are fundamentally the same as those used for radiculopathy. The same argument relating to whether or not to fuse exists, although most surgeons would opt for some type of bony fusion when operating at more than two levels. Anterior techniques are not very amenable to the therapy of multiple level disease, although up to 4 levels can be treated. The main place of anterior surgery lies in patients with marked disease at one or two levels. Multiple level disease, especially in a stenotic cervical canal, has usually been taken as an indication for a laminectomy approach but recent experience with selective anterior operation at the worst level in cases with multiple level disease has been encouraging.

When considering posterior approaches, foraminotomy alone as used for radiculopathy has no place in the surgery of myelopathy; the surgery must be more extensive as it is primarily a decompressive procedure. Scoville (1961) felt that laminectomy should extend to one level above and below the extent of the disease and Taylor (1964) felt that opening the foramina was essential in an attempt to improve blood flow in the radicular arteries. This approach has been reemphasized by Epstein et al. (1982) who further suggested that the laminectomy should be performed with a high speed drill to avoid the danger of impinging on the theca with the blade of a rongeur introduced under the lamina. This is a particular hazard as the cord is often so displaced by the anterior spondylotic bars that little intervenes between it and the undersurface of the lamina.

Other types of posterior procedure exist; division of the dentate ligaments was suggested by Kahn (1947) and by Rogers (1961) in an attempt to release the cord but this is no longer practised. More extensive procedures have been advocated, such as total cervical laminectomy with limited foramen magnum decompression (Aboulker et al. 1965, Alsharif et al. 1979) but do not find widespread acceptance. In summary, it may be said that the most common posterior procedure used for the treatment of myelopathy at this time is a laminectomy extending from C3 to C7, inclusive, often accompanied by foraminotomy, and leaving the dura mater intact.

Operation by either approach in cases with myelopathy may be immediately followed by neurological deterioration. The cause of this may be intraoperative trauma and the greatest care and gentleness is necessary during surgery; but other potential causes exist and must be avoided. The cervical cord in cervical spondylotic myelopathy is already compressed and further extension of the neck under anaesthesia, during endotracheal intubation, may cause damage. Equally the transfer and positioning of the patient prior to and after operation require great care. Rigorous avoidance of even minimal arterial hypotension should be observed in these patients who may be elderly, hypertensive and intolerant of reduced arterial pressure.

With this factor in mind, the selection for

surgery of patients with myelopathy is not easy. The best surgical results are obtained in patients with a history of less than one year, as in patients with long-established myelopathic deficit dramatic improvement cannot be anticipated on a regular basis (Phillips 1973). As a majority of patients only present to the neurosurgeon later than one year, operation is often undertaken in order to prevent further deterioration. As has been discussed earlier the natural history of cervical spondylotic myelopathy is highly variable and this makes selection of patients and assessment of results very difficult. It is usual, however, to offer surgery when confronted with a patient giving a definite history of progression of the myelopathy even though the condition of a few of these patients would stabilize even without surgery. The justification of this approach comes from the fact that the less severe the neurological deficit is at the time of surgery, the greater is the chance of good recovery.

Unlike the situation with cervical radiculopathy where there appear to be equally good results with either anterior or posterior approach, in myelopathy there is evidence to favour an anterior approach. Laminectomy however, has its strong advocates who achieve excellent results with the technique (Fager 1977, Epstein *et al.* 1982) but the majority of papers presenting results of laminectomy show improvement in only 50–60% (Northfield & Osmond-Clarke 1967, Bishara 1971, Gorter 1976) results which are not dissimilar to the natural history. Laminectomy will retain a role in the management of patients with widespread spondylotic disease but it also has a disconcerting tendency towards late neurological deterioration some years after the procedure, a complication unusual following anterior operation (Crandall & Gregorius 1977). It is contraindicated in patients with marked evidence of segmental instability and subluxiation, as this may well be increased following posterior decompression.

Phillips (1973) reviewed his experience with both anterior and posterior approaches. He found a greater rate of improvement in those undergoing anterior interbody fusion with 74% being improved (86% if the history was less than one year). The study was not, however, randomized or controlled and, in fact, no such study has been reported. Gorter (1976), reviewed several series, found that the number of patients cured by anterior operation (34%) was twice that of laminectomy although similar numbers were either cured or improved (74% anterior, 70% posterior). Robertson and Johnson (1980) reported results of anterior surgery in different clinical situations; in those with myelopathy, 85% were dramatically improved. Several other authors have produced results approaching this figure, amongst them being Crandall and Gregorius (1977) and Jeffreys (1979), who used the size and number of the anterior protrusions as a guide to the choice of an anterior or posterior procedure achieving improvement in approximately 80% by using either technique as indicated. It seems likely that this latter approach of improving the methods of selecting which technique to use in different clinical pictures will provide the best results.

## Rheumatoid Arthritis

Although not a degenerative process, it is convenient to consider the involvement of the cervical spine by rheumatoid arthritis at this point. In 1890, Garrod first described rheumatic cervical spine disease and it has been increasingly recognized as a common occurence especially in the more severe and longstanding cases of rheumatoid arthritis. The cervical spine is affected in two ways: namely at the atlanto-axial joint and in the midcervical spine. Atlanto-axial involvement with subluxation (Fig. 22.4) occurs in 25% of patients though not all of these are symptomatic (Mathews 1969). Mathews also described the apparent upward migration of the odontoid which occurs by the process known as 'cranial setting' leading to herniation of the odontoid into the foramen magnum with resulting brain stem compression (Fig. 22.5). He found this process occurring at least to some degree in 8% of his series; over a period of 5 years, 33% of

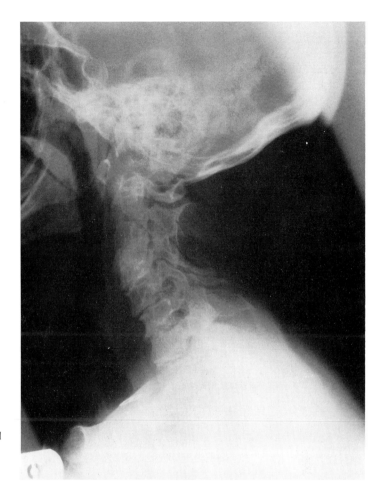

**Fig. 22.4** Obvious atlanto-axial subluxation in a patient with moderate midcervical rheumatoid disease.

the patients with simple atlanto-axial subluxation developed cranial setting.

The development of atlanto-axial subluxation is due to a combination of the destructive effects of the rheumatoid process on the soft tissue and ligamentous constituents of this joint, the dependence of this joint on such tissues for much of its stability and to erosive changes in the bones themselves. The subluxation may be: asymptomatic; cause severe upper cervical pain often with occipital neuralgia; or a high cervical myelopathy due to cord compression. This latter problem is particularly likely in the presence of cranial setting.

Asymptomatic cases pose a considerable dilemma. As many of these cases do not develop

clinical problems the case for prophylactic fusion of all cases cannot be sustained. However, they are undoubtedly at increased risk of cord damage following a fall and many physicians will prescribe a collar. Such a collar to be effective must include the chin and occiput and is not very comfortable to wear. Serial radiography is essential as progressive subluxation should be considered as a strong indicant for stabilization.

Patients presenting with intractable pain or myelopathy have to be considered for stabilization. Neurological examination in these patients is very difficult as the associated joint deformities make assessment of power and reflexes difficult. Much greater dependence must be placed on the clinical history as this often will

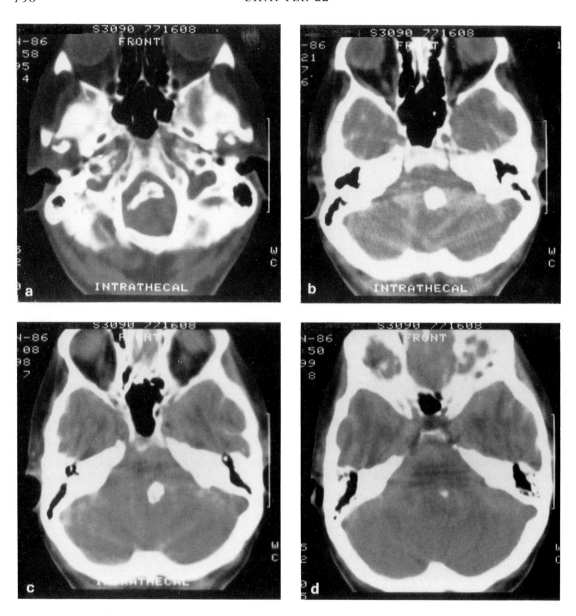

**Fig. 22.5** CT scan showing dramatic 'cranial settling' with the tip of the odontoid reaching a level parallel to the posterior clinoids. At transoral surgery it was found that the odontoid had penetrated the dura and was imbedded in the brain stem. The patient made a full recovery from a pre-operative severe quadriparesis.

give evidence of myelopathy. As the deformity or the degree of myelopathy becomes more severe, the surgical difficulties and risks increase dramatically. In addition the surgeon is often presented with these patients as a last resort when all conservative attempts at control have failed, by which time not only is there severe neurological handicap but the general medical condition of these patients is also very poor. There is therefore a strong case for surgical intervention at an earlier stage of the disease when it is clear that the deformity is progressive.

Assessing these patients for surgery demands careful consideration of the general medical condition as the patients are often undernourished with considerable cardiovascular instability and often suffering from the longer term complications of the disease such as amyloid or the steroid therapy. Full radiological investigation of the atlanto-axial area is essential to determine the degree of instability by stress films and the degree of anterior compression of the cord. The latter is best seen by CT scanning with some inthrathecal contrast as this graphically displays whether the compressing agent is anteriorly placed or caused by the posterior arch of the atlas. In the majority of patients with myelopathy it will be found that compression is anterior due to either the odontoid itself or the associated soft tissue changes occurring around the odontoid particularly posteriorly and compressing the cord.

The standard surgical approach to patients with atlanto-axial subluxation has been to fuse either C1 to C2 or, more occasionally, the occiput to C2 by a posterior approach. Several different fusion techniques have been described for posterior fusion and it has to be said that they do achieve a high degree of stabilization. However, especially in the presence of anterior cord compression as discussed above, there is a reprted risk of producing quadriplegia or a peroperative death with this approach ranging from 15% to 50% (Cregan 1966, Crellin et al. 1970, Boyle 1971). There is now increasing evidence that the transoral approach established by Fang and Ong for C1 tubercular lesions followed at the same stage with posterior fusion allows not only a safer decompression and stabilization but results in improved neurological recovery (Bonney & Williams 1985, Crockard et al. 1986). An alternative approach where a wide posterior fossa decompression with excision of the arch of the atlas is combined with posterior fusion with spinal instumentation has been described (Flint et al. 1986). However, it is likely that the great advantage of the actual excision of the compressing odontoid by trans oral surgery will give the best results.

Midcervical rheumatoid disease produces problems similar to sever sponylotic myelopathy but there is a much greater incidence of instability. Multiple level subluxations may be present without myelopathy but increasing degrees of instability can produce severe myelopathy. In such a situation surgery is mandatory but often requires preoperative reduction with skull traction. The major operative problem is not so much achieving decompression but rather in achieving stabilization. There is considerable debate as to whether an anterior or posterior approach is best but there does seem to be a trend towards fusion techniques such as Cloward's. Whichever route is chosen, achieving good bony fusion is difficult in view of the very osteoporotic bones at both the operative and donor sites. All such patients require postoperative external support while fusion is occurring, although the addition of a simple posterior wiring procedure at the time of anterior cervical fusion does seem to reduce the need for this.

## References

ABOULKER J., METZGER, DAVID M et al. (1965). Neurochirurgie, 11, 87.
ADAMS C. B., & LOGUE V. (1971a) Brain, 94, 557.
ADAMS, C. B. & LOGUE V. (1971b) Brain, 94, 569.
ALEXANDER G. L. (1946) Proc. roy. Soc. Med., 39.
ALLEN K. L. (1952) J. Neurol. Neurosurg. Psychiat., 15, 20.
ALSHARIF H., EZZAT S. L., HAY A. et al. (1979) Acta Neurochir., 48, 83.
ARMSTRONG J. R. (1965) Lumbar Disc Lesions, 3rd Edn. Livingstone, Edinburgh.
BARNES M. P. & SAUNDERS M. (1984) J. Neurol. Neurosurg. Psychiat., 47, 17.
BEADLE O. A. (1931) The Intervertebral Discs. MRC Special Report Series 161. HMSO, London.
BISHARA S. N. (1971) J. Neurol. Neurosurg. Psychiat., 34, 393.
BOBECHKO W. T. & HIRSCH C. (1965) J. Bone Jt Surg., 47B, 574.
BONNEY G. & WILLIAMS J. P. R. (1985) J. Bone Jt. Surg., 67B, 691.
BOWDEN R. E., ABDULLAH S. & GOODING M. R. (1967) In Cervical Spondylosis and Other Diseases of the Cervical Spine (Eds. Lord Brain & Wilkinson M.) p. 10. Heinemann, London.
BOYLE A. C. (1971) Proc. roy. Soc. Med. 64, 1161.
BOYLE R., THOMAS M. & ADAMS J. H. (1980) Postgrad. med. J., 56, 149.
BRADFORD D. S., COOPER K. M. & OEGEMA T. R. (1983) J. Bone Jt. Surg., 65A, 1220.
BRADLEY W. G. & BANNA M. (1968) Brit. J. Radiol., 41, 608.

BRAIN W. R. (1948) *Proc. roy. Soc. Med.*, **41**, 509.

BRAIN W. R. (1977) In *Brain's Diseases of the Nervous System*, p. 550. (Ed. Walton J. N.) Oxford University Press.

BRAIN W. R. & WILKINSON M. (1967) *Cervical Spondylosis and Other Diseases of the Cervical Spine*. Heinemann, London.

BRAIN W. R., NORTHFIELD D. W. & WILKINSON M. (1952) *Brain*, **75**, 187.

BREIG A. (1960) *Biomechanics of the Central Nervous System*. Almqvist, Stockholm.

BRENDLER S. J. (1968) *J. Neurosurg.*, **28**, 105.

BRIGGS H. (1948) *J. med. Soc. New Jersey*, **45**, 404.

BROWN M. (1982) In *The Spine* (2nd Edn.) p. 510. (Eds. Rothman R. H. & Simeone F. A.) Saunders, Philadelphia.

BULL J. W. (1948) *Proc. roy. Soc. Med.*, **41**, 513.

BURROWS E. H. (1963) *Clin. Radiol.*, **14**, 77.

CASOTTO A. & BUONCRISTIANI P. (1981) *Acta Neurochir.*, **57**, 275.

CLARKE E. & ROBINSON P. K. (1956) 79, 483.

CLOWARD R. B. (1958) *J. Neurosurg.*, **15**, 602.

COLLIE J. (1913) In *Malingering and Feigned Sickness*. Boeber P. B. (Edin), New York.

COLONNA P. C. & FRIEDENBERG Z. (1949) *J. Bone Jt. Surg.*, **31A**, 614.

CONLON P. W., ISDALE I. C. & ROSE B. S. (1966) *Ann. Rheum. Dis.*, **25**, 120.

CONNOLLY E. S., SEYMOUR R. J. & ADAMS J. E. (1965) *J. Neurosurg.*, **23**, 431.

CRAAFORD C., HIERTONN T., LINDBLOM K. *et al.* (1958) *Acta. Orthrop. Scand.*, **28**, 103.

CRANDALL P. H. & GREGORIUS F. K. (1977) *Spine*, **2**, 139.

CRAWSHAW C., FRAZER A. M., MERRIAN W. F., *et al.* (1984) In press.

CREGAN J. C. (1966) *Ann. Rheum. Dis.*, **25**, 242.

CRELLIN R. Q., MacCABE J. J. & HAMILTON E. B. D. (1970) *J. Bone. Jt. Surg.*,**52B**, 244.

CROCKARD H. A., POZO J. L., RANSFORD A. Q. *et al.* (1986) *J. Bone. Jt. Surg.*, **68B**, 351.

DAVIDSON R. I., DUNN E. J. & METZMAKER J. N. (1981) *Spine*, **6**, 441.

DePALMA A. & ROTHMAN R. (1946) *Clin. Orthop.*, **63**, 162.

DePALMA A. & ROTHMAN R. (1970) *The Intervertebral Disc.* W. B. Saunders & Co, Philadelphia.

DePALMA A., ROTHMANN R., LEWINNECK G. *et al.* (1972). *Surg. Gynecol. Obstet.*, **134**, 755.

DHSS (1979) *Cochrane Report: Working Group on Back Pain*. HMSO, London.

DOPPMANN J. L. (1975) *Invest. Radiol.*, **10**, 543.

DYCK P. (1979) *Spine*, **4**, 89.

EDGAR M. A. & PARK W. M. (1974) *J. Bone Jt. Surg.*, **56B**, 658.

ELSBERG C. A. (1928) *Surg. Gynec. Obstet.*, **46**, 1.

EL NEGAMY E. & SEDGWICK E. M. (1979) *J. Neurol. Neurosurg. Psychiat.*, **42**, 238.

EJESKAR A., NACHEMSON A., HERBERTS P. *et al.* (1983) *Clin. Orthop.*, **174**, 236.

EPSTEIN J. A., JANIN Y., CARRAS R. *et al.* (1982) *Acta. Neurochir.*, **61**, 89.

FAGER C. A. (1977) *Clin. Neurosurg.*, **24**, 488.

FAHRNI W. H. (1966) *Can. J. Surg.*, **9**, 44.

FANG H. S. Y. & ONG G. B. (1962) *J. Bone Jt. Surg.*, 44A, 1588.

FORFAR H. F. (1977) *Orthop. Clin. N. Amer.*, **8**, 9.

FEINSOD M., DAN BLAU P. E., FINDLER G. *et al.* (1982) *Neurosurgery*, **11**, 506.

FINDLAY G. F. G. (1986) *J. Neurol. Neurosurg. Psychiat.*, **49**, 470.

FLINT G. A., HOCKLEY A. D. & McMILLAN J. J. (1968) *J. Neurol. Neurosurg. Psychiat.*, **49**, 1329.

FRIEDENBERG Z. & MILLER W. (1963) *J. Bone Jt. Surg.*, **45A**, 1171.

FRYKHOLM R. (1951) *Acta. Chirg. Scand.*, Suppt. 160.

GALASKO C. S. B. & DOYLE F. H. (1972) *Clin. Radiol.*, **23**, 295.

GARROD A. E. (1980) *A Treatise on Rheumatism and Rhuematoid Arthritis*, pp. 1–342. Griffin, London.

GETTY C. J. (1980) *J. Bone Jt. Surg.*, **62B**, 481.

GETTY C. J., JOHNSON J. R., KIRWAN E. O. *et al.* (1981) *J. Bone Jt. Surg.*, **63B**, 491.

GLEDHILL R. F., HARRISON B. M. & McDONALD N. I. (1973) *Exp. Neurol.*, **38**, 472.

GOODING M. R., WILSON C. B. & HOFF J. T. (1975) *J. Neurosurg.*, **43**, 9.

GORTER K. (1976) *Acta. Neurochir.*, **33**, 265.

GRAINGER R. G., KENDALL B. E. & WYLIE I. G. (1976) *Brit. J. Radiol.*, **49**, 996.

GREENFIELD J. G. (1953) *Rev. méd. Suisse rom.*,**73**, 227.

HAMPTON A. O. & ROBINSON J. M. (1936) *Amer. J. Roentgenol.*, **36**, 782.

HAUGHTON Y. M., ELDVIK O. P., MAGNES B. *et al.* (1982) *Radiology*, **142**, 103.

HENDRY N. (1968) *J. Bone Jt. Surg.*, **40B**, 132.

HIRSCH C. L. (1948) *Acta. Othop. Scand.*, **17**, 240.

HIRSCH C. L. (1960) *Acta. Orthop. Scand.*, **30**, 172.

HIRSCH C. L. & NACHEMSON A. (1963) *Clin. Orthop.*, **29**, 189.

HIRSCH C. L., ROSENCRANTZ M. & WICKBOM I. (1969) *Acta. Radiol.*, **8**, 54.

HITSELBERGER W. E. & WITTEN R. M. (1968) *J. Neurosurg.*, **28**, 204.

HODGSON A. R. & STOCK F. E. (1956) *Brit. J. Surg.*, **44**, 266.

HUDGINS W. R. (1970) *J. Neurosurg.*, **32**, 152.

HUGHES J. T. (1966) *Pathology of the Spinal Cord*. Lloyd-Luke, London.

HUGHES J. T. & BROWNELL B (1964) *Neurology*, **14**, 1073.

HULME A. (1960) *J. Neurol. Neurosurg. Psychiat.*, **23**, 133.

JACOBS B., KREUGER E. G. & LEIVY D. M. (1970) *J. Amer. med. Ass.*, **211**, 2135.

JEFFREYS R. V. (1979) *Acta Neurochir.*, **47**, 293.

JENNETT W. B. (1956) *J. Neurol. Neurosurg. Psychiat.*, **19**, 109.

JOHNSON R. M., OWEN J. R., HART D. L. *et al.* (1981) *Clin. Orthop.*, **154**, 34.

JONES A. B. & LLEWELLYN L. J. (1917) *Malingering or the Simulation of Disease*. Heinemann, London.

JUNGHANNS H. (1929) *Dtsch. Z. Chir.*, **213**, 332.

KAHN E. A. (1947) *J. Neurosurg.*, **4**, 191.

KANE W. J. (1980) Personal communication.

KIKUCHI S., MACNAB I. & MOREAU P (1981) *J. Bone Jt. Surg.*, **63B**, 272.

KIRKALDY-WILLIS W. H., WEDGE J. H., YONG-HING K. *et al.* (1978) *Spine*, **3**, 319.

KNIGHT G. C. (1964) *Proc. roy. Soc. Med.*, **57**, 165.

LANE W. A. (1885) *Guy's Hosp. Reps.*, **43**, 321.

LARSON S. J., HOLST R. A., HEMMY D. C. *et al.* (1976) *J. Neurosurg.*, **45**, 628.

LAWRENCE J. S., BREMNER J. M. & BIER F. (1966) *Ann. Rheum. Dis.*, **25**, 1.

LEES F. & TURNER J. W. (1963) *Brit. med. J.*, **1**, 1607.

LEYSHON A., KIRWAN E. O. & WYN PARRY C. B. (1981) *J. Bone Jt. Surg.*, **63B**, 71.

LINDBLOM K. & HULTQVIST G. (1950) *J. Bone Jt. Surg.*, **32A**, 557.

LOGUE V. (1952) *J. Neurol. Neurosurg. Psychiat.*, **15**, 227.

LOGUE V. (1957) In *Modern Trends in Neurology* (2nd series) p. 259. (Ed. Williams D. J.) Butterworths, London.

LOMBARDI G. & PASSERINI A. (1964) *Spinal Cord Diseases*. Williams & Wilkins, Baltimore.

LOVE J. G. & KIEFER E. J. (1950) *J. Neurosurg.*, **7**, 62.

LUNSFORD L. D., BISSONETTE D. J., JANNETTA P. J. *et al.* (1980) *J. Neurosurg.*, **53**, 1.

MACNAB I. (1971) *J. Bone Jt. Surg.*, **53A**, 891.

MACNAB I. (1977) *Backache*. Williams & Wilkins, Baltimore.

MACNAB I., ST LOUIS E. L., GRABIAS S. L. *et al.* (1976) *J. Bone Jt. Surg.*, **58A**, 1093.

MACRAE I. F. & WRIGHT V. (1969) *Ann. Rheum. Dis.*, **28**, 584.

McCULLOCH J. A. (1977) *J. Bone Jt. Surg.*, **59B**, 45.

McCULLOCH J. A. & WADDELL G. (1978) *Brit. J. Radiol.*, **51**, 498.

McMURRAY G. N. (1982) *J. Bone Jt. Surg.*, **64B** 101.

McPHERSON P. & McPHERSON E. L. (1981) *Hlth Bull.*, **39**, 89.

MAIR W. G. & DRUCKMAN R. (1953) *Brain*, **76**, 70.

MARTIN A. N. (1976) *J. Neurosurg.*, **44**, 290.

MARTIN G. (1981) *Ann. roy. Coll. Surg. Eng.*, **63**, 244.

MATHEWS J. A. (1969) *Am. Rheum. Dis.*, **28**, 260.

MIDDLETON G. S. & TEACHER J. H. (1911) *Glas. med. J.*, **76**, 1.

MIXTER W. J. & BARR J. S. (1934) *N. Engl. J. Med.*, **211**, 210.

MODIC M. T. PARLICEK W. & WEINSTEIN M. A. (1984) *Radiology*, **152**, 103.

MOONEY V. & ROBERTSON J. (1976) *Clin. Orthop.*, **115**, 149.

NACHEMSON A. (1959) *Acta. Orthop. Scand.*, **28**, 269.

NACHEMSON A. (1965) *Acta. Orthop. Scand.*, **36**, 418.

NACHEMSON A. (1966) *Clin. Orthop.*, **45**, 107.

NACHEMSON A. (1981) *Spine*, **6**, 93.

NACHEMSON A. & MORRIS J. (1964) *J. Bone Jt. Surg.*, **46A**, 1077.

NACHLAS I. W. (1952) *J. Bone Jt. Surg.*, **34A**, 981.

NASHOLD B. & HRUBEC A. (1971) *Lumbar Disc Disease: A Twenty-Year Clinical Follow-Up Study*. Mosby, St Louis.

NORDBY E. J. & BROWN M. D. (1977) *Clin. Orthop.*, **129**, 79.

NORTHFIELD D. W. & OSMOND-CLARK H. (1967) In *Cervical Spondylosis and Other Diseases of the Cervical Spine*, p. 207, (Eds. Brain W. R. & Wilkinson M.) Heinemann, London.

NURICK S. (1972) *Brain*, **95**, 101.

NURICK S. (1975) *Brit. J. Hosp. Med.*, **15**, 668.

O'CONNELL J. E. (1943) *Brit. J. Surg.*, **30**, 315.

O'CONNELL J. E. (1946) *Brain*, **69**, 9.

O'CONNELL J. E. (1951) *J. Bone Jt. Surg.*, **33B**, 8.

O'LAOIRE, S. A., CROCKARD H. A. & THOMAS D. G. (1981) *Brit. med. J.*, **282**, 1852.

OTANI K., MANZOKU S., SHIBASAKI K. *et al.* (1977) *Spine*, **2**, 266.

OTANI K., NAKAI S., FUJIMARA Y. *et al* (1982) *J. Bone Jt. Surg.*, **64B** 340.

PATTERSON R. H. & ARBIT E. (1978) *J. Neurosurg.*, **48**, 768.

PAYNE E. E. & SPILLANE J. D. (1957) *Brain*, **80**, 571.

PENNING L. & VAN DER ZWAGG P. (1966) *Acta. Radiol.*, **5**, 1090.

PEROT P. L. & MUNRO D. D. (1969) *J. Neurosurg.*, **31**, 452.

PHILLIPS D. G. (1973) *J. Neurol. Neurosurg. Psychiat.*, **36**, 879.

PORTER R. W., HIBBERT C. & WELLMAN P. (1980) *Spine*, **5**, 99.

RANSOHOFF J., SPENCER F., SIEW F. *et al.* (1969) *J. Neurosurg.*, **31**, 459.

ROBERTSON J. T. (1973) *Clin. Neurosurg.*, **20**, 259.

ROBERTSON J. T. & JOHNSON S. D. (1980) *Clin. Neurosurg.*, **27**, 440.

ROBINSON R. A., WALKER A. E., FERLIE D. C. *et al.* (1962) *J. Bone Jt. Surg.*, **44A**, 1569.

ROBINSON R. A. & SMITH G. W. (1955) *Bull. Johns Hopkins Hosp.*, **96**, 223.

ROGERS L. (1961) *J. Neurosurg.*, **18**, 490.

ROSENØRN J., HANSEN E. B. & ROSENØRN M. (1983) *J. Neurosurg.*, **59**, 252.

ROSS J. C. & JAMESON R. M. (1971) *Brit. med. J.*, **3**, 752.

ROWE M. L. (1969) *J. occup. Med.*, **11**, 161.

SAUNDERS J. B. & INMAN V. T. (1940) *Arch. Surg.*, **40**, 389.

SCHLESINGER P. (1955) *J. Bone Jt. Surg.*, **37A**, 115.

SCHMORL G. & JUNGHANNS H. (1932) *Die gesunde und kranke Wirbelsäule im Roentgenbild*. Thieme, Leipzig.

SCHMORL G. & JUNGHANNS H. (1959) *The Human Spine in Health and Disease*. Grune & Stratton, New York.

SCOVILLE W. B. (1961) *J. Neurosurg.*, **18**, 423.

SEKHAR L. N. & JANNETTA P. J. (1983) *Neurosurgery*, **12**, 303.

SHANNON N. & PAUL E. A. (1979) *J. Neurol. Neurosurg. Psychiat.*, **42**, 804.

SHEPHARD R. H. (1959) *Brit. med. J.*, **2**, 1434.

SIIVOLA J., SULG I. & HEISKARI M. (1981) *Electroenceph. clin. Neurophysiol.*, **52**, 276.

SMITH L. (1964) *J. Amer. med. Ass.*, **187**, 137.

SMITH L., GARVIN P. J., GESLER R. M. *et al.* (1963) *Nature* 198:1311.

SPURLING R. G. (1956) *Lesions of the Cervical Intervertebral Disc*. Thomas, Springfield, Illinois.

SPURLING R. G. & SCOVILL W. B. (1944) *Surg. Gynaecol. Obstet.*, **78**, 350.

STOLTMAN H. F. & BLACKWOOD W. (1964) *Brain*, **87**, 45.

STOOKEY B. (1928) *Arch. Neurol. Psychiat.*, **20**, 275.

STOOKEY B. (1940) *Arch. Surg.*, **40**, 416.

SYMONDS C. P. (1939) *Proc. roy. Soc. Med.*, **32**, 1712.

TAYLOR A. R. (1953) *Lancet*, **1**, 717.

TAYLOR A. R. (1964) *Neurology*, **14**, 62.

TONDURY G. (1961) *Acta. Chirurg. Belg.*, **60**, 567.

TSAIRIS P., DYCH P. J. & MULDER D. W. (1972) *Arch. Neurol.*, **27**, 109.

VENNER R. M. & CROCK H. (1981) *J. Bone Jt. Surg.*, **63B**, 491.

VERBIEST H. (1954) *J. Bone Jt. Surg.*, **36B**, 230.

VERBIEST H. (1968) *J. Neurosurg.*, **28**, 191.

VERBIEST H. & PAZ Y GEUSE H. D. (1966) *J. Neurosurg.*, **25**, 611.

VIRGIN W. J. (1951) *J. Bone Jt. Surg.*, **33B**, 607.

VON LUSCHKA H. (1858) *Die Halbgelenke des menschlichen Körpers*. Karpress, Berlin.

WADDELL G. (1982) *Brit. J. Hosp. Med.*, **22**, 187.

WADDELL G., KUMMEL E. G., LOTTO W. N. *et al.* (1979) *J. Bone Jt. Surg.*, **61A**, 201.

WADDELL G., McCULLOCH J. A., KUMMELL E. G. *et al.* (1980) *Spine*, **5**, 117.

WADDELL G., MAIN, C. J., MORRIS E. W. *et al* (1982) *Brit. med. J.*, **284**, 1519.

WALTON G. L. & PAUL W. E. (1905) *Boston med. Surg. J.*, **153**, 114.

WALTZ T. A. (1967) *Brain*, **90**, 395.

WEBER H. (1978) *J. Oslo City Hosp.*, **28**, 36, 89

WHITE A. A., SOUTHWICK W. O., DePONTE R. J. *et al.* (1973) *J. Bone Jt. Surg.*, **55A**, 525.

WHITE J. G., STRAIT T. A., BINKLEY J. R. *et al.* (1982) *J. Neurosurg.*, **56**, 114.

WILBERGER J. E. & PANG D. (1983) *J. Neurosurg.*, **59**, 137.

WILKINSON M. (1960) *Brain*, **83**, 589.

WILKINSON M. (1967) In *Cervical Spondylosis and Other Diseases of the Cervical Spine* (Eds. Brain W. R. & Wilkinson M.) Heinemann, London.

WILLIAMS R. W. (1978) *Spine*, **3**, 175.

WILSON C. B. (1969) *J. Neurosurg.*, **31**, 499.

WILSON D. H. & CAMPBELL D. D. (1977) *J. Neurosurg.*, **47**, 551.

WILSON D. H. & HARBAOUGH R. (1981) *Neurosurgery*, **8**, 422.

WOLFE B. S., KILMANI M. & MALIS L. (1965) *J. Mt Sinai Hosp.*, **23**, 283.

# Chapter 23
# Head injury

J. D. MILLER

## Introduction

The high prevalence of head injury among civilian populations and the provision of adequate hospital services have become matters of worldwide concern. Both the Third and the Eighth International Congress of Neurological Surgery in 1965 and 1985 devoted a large part of the programme to the subject of head injury and during this interval a number of epidemiological and management studies have drawn attention to the dreadful toll that head injuries exact on society in terms of mortality and morbidity (Field 1976, Becker et al. 1977, Jennett et al. 1977, 1979, Bowers & Marshall 1980, Klauber et al. 1981, Turazzi et al. 1984).

Each year, between 200 and 300 per 100,000 of the population are admitted to hospital because of a head injury (Anderson & McLaurin 1980, Jennett & McMillan 1981). Four to five times that number of patients are seen in UK Accident and Emergency Departments because of head injury (Jennett & Teasdale 1981). Of the patients who are admitted to hospital the vast majority (70–80%) are males, and most injuries (85%) are minor cases in which the patient has been rendered unconscious only briefly but by the time of admission is talking and obeying commands (Miller & Jones 1985). A relatively small proportion (5%) of head injury admissions are for severe injuries in which the patient has become comatose; in approximately half of these severe cases the development of an intracranial haematoma or severe brain swelling will necessitate decompressive measures (Miller et al. 1981). This limited number of severely head injured patients commands much of the neurosurgeon's attention, as well as an even smaller number of

patients, less severely injured, who have depressed skull fractures, persistent CSF leaks or who develop an extradural or chronic subdural haematoma after a seemingly minor head injury. The neurosurgeon should be aware that his perspective of the major problems of head injured patients may be rather restricted.

The most common causes of head injury in the UK are road traffic accidents, falls at work or in the home and physical assault. With increasing severity of injury, road traffic accidents account for a higher proportion of the causes. Thus road traffic accidents account for 27% of minor head injuries but for 70% of severe head injuries.

Head injury is frequently associated with injuries to other parts of the body (Miller et al. 1978). This is particularly true of head injuries sustained in road traffic accidents in which a large amount of force is involved in the causation of the injury. Of patients with severe head injury, half can be expected to suffer from major systemic injuries, requiring the services of another group of surgeons. Of 551 persons admitted in one year to the Emergency Unit of the Birmingham Accident Hospital 42% had sustained more than one injury and the total number of injuries was 890. The most frequent sites of injury were head (53%), lower limb (45%), upper limb (23%), chest (17%), (London 1963). When the cases were divided into groups of mild, moderate and severe head injuries the distribution of systemic injuries was 9, 25 and 48% respectively.

In a series of 1919 head injured patients admitted to the Department of Surgical Neurology in Edinburgh in 1981, other injuries were present in half of the 93 severely injured cases and in a smaller proportion of the moderate and

Table 23.1 Combination of head and other injuries.

| Injury | Severe | Moderate | Minor | Total |
|--------|--------|----------|-------|-------|
| Head | 93 (100%) | 210 (100%) | 1616 (100%) | 1919 (100%) |
| Face | 18 (19%) | 29 (14%) | 173 (11%) | 220 (11%) |
| Limbs | 30 (32%) | 23 (11%) | 108 (7%) | 161 (8%) |
| Thorax | 26 (28%) | 16 (8%) | 90 (6%) | 132 (5%) |
| Abdomen | | | | |
| Spine | 6 (6%) | 3 (1%) | 83 (5%) | 92 (5%) |

minor head injuries (Table 23.1) (Miller & Jones 1985).

For many years, comparisons of the results of management of head injury were difficult because of a lack of clearly defined criteria of severity of injury. For example, the quotation of a 30% mortality rate for a series of patients with acute subdural haematoma is meaningless unless the reader knows whether the patients were conscious or comatose before surgical decompression was carried out. In the last 10 years the Glasgow Coma Scale has been widely adopted as the International standard by which the level of consciousness in head injured patients is assessed (Teasdale & Jennett 1974).

Table 23.2 The Glasgow Coma Scale.

| Eye Opening | Best Motor Response | Verbal Response |
|-------------|---------------------|-----------------|
| 4 Spontaneous | 6 Obeys commands | 5 Oriented speech |
| A ————————————————————————— A | | |
| 3 To command | | 4 Confused speech |
| 2 To pain | | 3 Words only |
| B ————————————————————————— B | | |
| | 5 Localizes pain | 2 Sounds only |
| | 4 Flexor withdrawal | |
| | 3 Abnormal flexion | |
| | 2 Extension | |
| 1 Nil | 1 Nil | 1 Nil |

Above line A = minor head injury (GC Sumscore 13–15)
Between lines
 A & B    = moderate head injury (GC Sumscore 9–12)
Below line B = severe head injury (GC Sumscore 3–8)

Allocation of head injured patients into the categories of severe, moderate and minor is now made on the basis of the patient's level of response after resuscitation has been carried out as measured on the Glasgow Coma Scale (Table 23.2).

Severe head injuries can be classified as being in coma when examined. This state is characterized, in terms of the coma scale, by failure to open the eyes even to painful stimuli, failure to obey simple commands and inability to utter any formed verbal response. Patients with moderate head injuries may open the eyes to painful or verbal stimuli, may obey commands but are not oriented to time or place. Patients with minor head injuries either score at the top level of the coma scale, that is open eyes spontaneously, obey commands and give an oriented verbal response or they may be drowsy and disorientated. In numerical terms, severe head injuries score 8 or less on the Glasgow Coma Score (but must have no eye opening), moderate head injuries score between 9 and 12 on the coma scale and minor head injuries score from 13 to 15 points (Rimel et al. 1981, 1982).

The mortality rate from head injury varies according to the severity of injury. Of severely head injured cases admitted alive to hospital, between 40 and 50% die, most within the first 24 hours. In patients with moderate head injury, between 2 and 5% mortality is to be expected, while less than 1% of minor head injury cases should die as a result of injury (Miller et al. 1981, Miller & Jones 1985). The overall mortality rate of any given series of head injured patients depends, therefore, upon the relative numbers of severe, moderate and minor head injuries included in the series.

The causes of death from head injury fall broadly into three groups, the primary effects of injury on the brain and its vascular network, secondary intracranial factors such as haematoma, brain swelling, intracranial hypertension or intracranial complications such as infection or epilepsy; the third group of causes are systemic, related in the early stages to injuries to other parts of the body producing haemorrhage or hypoxia, or later systemic complications such as infection, embolism or other medical complications of trauma and prolonged coma (Miller 1982).

The same schema can be used to explain the morbidity from head injury. The primary injury produces contusions on the brain surface, particularly at the frontal and temporal poles, and diffuse axonal injury due to shear stresses in the brain subjected to sudden acceleration and/or deceleration (Adams 1975, 1984). The widespread nature of these injuries helps to explain the diversity of neurological dysfunction that may follow a head injury but it appears to be the case that the more severe the acceleration force applied to the brain the more likely it is that the diffuse injury will extend centrally to involve the brain stem. In patients who die at the time of or within the first few minutes after impact, extremely severe brain stem injuries are frequently found including complete transection of the midbrain at the pontine level. In the minutes and hours that follow the injury, arterial hypotension, hypoxaemia and anaemia all play a part in impairing the function of the already damaged brain (Price & Murray 1972, Kohi et al. 1984). Such secondary insults are strongly associated with the presence of multiple injuries (Miller et al. 1978).

Disability following head injury is an enormous problem. Of severely head injured patients 40–50% die, 10% remain severely disabled or vegetative, dependent on the help of others for some or all of their activities of daily living, while the remaining 50% recover to the point of being independent in terms of such functions. Only about a third of severely head injured patients are able to return to their previous level of employment and detailed testing will almost always reveal persisting physical, mental or behavioural deficits.

Even among those who suffer only a minor head injury, there is a significant degree of disability following the injury. Rimel et al. (1981) noted at 3 months from the time of a minor head injury, one third of a series of 424 patients had still not been able to return to their former level of activity and in a sample of those patients subjected to psychometric testing there was clear evidence of cognitive and memory deficits.

The problems of caring for the survivors of severe head injury, and the need to render as many patients as possible self-sufficient and employable, has invoked a renewed interest in rehabilitation and a slowly improving understanding that the needs of head injured patients are different from both physically and mentally handicapped patients (Lewin et al. 1979, Rosenthal et al. 1983, Brooks 1984).

Recognition of the importance of protecting the head from injury developed in the first World War. The high incidence of fatal head injury in motor cyclists led to the compulsory use of crash helmets by British Army motor cyclists in 1941 and the subsequent adoption of this policy by civilian riders. The value of a satisfactorily designed helmet in minimizing the affects of head injury is now well established. It protects the skull from local injury by spreading the blow over a larger area and by reducing the speed of impact diminishes the intensity and extent of brain damage (Cairns & Holbourn 1943, Lewin & Kennedy 1956). For the occupants of motor vehicles protection has been developed along three lines.

1 Restraining seat belts which prevent the occupant from being flung forwards against the dashboard or through the windscreen, the wearing of which by drivers and front seat passengers became compulsory in the UK in February 1983. This preventive measure has reduced the incidence of head injury in drivers and front seat passengers but has particularly reduced the numbers of severe combined craniofacial injuries (Rutherford et al. 1985). Similar legislation will probably be enacted to make the wearing of seatbelts by rear seat passengers compulsory.

2 The provision of support for the back of the head and neck to prevent violent extension and flexion movements, the so-called whiplash injury, when the car is struck from the rear. Not only does this mechanism damage the muscular and ligamentous structures of the neck, but it

plays a part in producing loss of consciousness (Ommaya & Gennarelli 1974).

3   Improvements in the design of motor vehicle bodies so that the occupants are shielded at the front and rear by parts of the car that will crumple on impact and absorb much of the force.

Other examples of preventive measures against head injury are the compulsory wearing of hard hats on construction sites, better design of headgear for horse riders, cyclists and mountaineers and increasing awareness of the cumulative effects of relatively minor head injury leading to stricter regulations affecting hard contact sports, such as rugby and association football, boxing and the other martial arts.

## Nature of the injuries

### Injury to the scalp

Scalp wounds are clinically important because they draw attention to, and indicate the site of, an injury to the head. They may be the source of bleeding sufficient to cause shock, particularly in the very young, and even when insignificant in size can indicate a penetrating injury from which infection may spread to bone and intracranial structures. The tough structure of the scalp and its tight application to the underlying smooth skull influence the patterns of injury. These may comprise abrasions or denudation of skin, simple linear splits as though cut with a knife, ragged multilimbed lacerations with crushing and devitalization of edges or elevation of large flaps approximating to scalping in severe cases. The rich blood supply of the scalp frequently results in significant blood loss but also promotes ready healing, providing surgical treatment has been adequate.

The capacity of the scalp to slide on the skull means that a scalp laceration can be located at some distance from an underlying skull fracture, yet the fracture is still a compound injury.

Haematomas of the scalp may be subgaleal, the common variety, or subperiosteal, more frequent in infants. Subgaleal haematomas can reach large dimensions because of the looseness of the subgaleal tissue plane and in a young child may contain considerable blood loss. Subperiosteal haematomas remain restricted by suture lines, but new bone may form during their resolution.

### Skull fractures

There is clinical justification for the grouping of fractures of the skull into those of the vault and those of the base, although both may separately be present in the same patient and both parts of the skull may be involved in one fracture. Fractures through the skull base have certain common features in presentation and complications. In general they are associated with more severe degrees of brain injury. As with fractures elsewhere there is an important distinction between simple (closed) and compound (open) fractures and the risk of infection. Vault fractures are assumed to be open if there is any nearby breach of the skin. Fractures of the base of the skull which involve the cribriform plate, the sphenoid sinus, the paranasal sinuses and the petrous temporal bone are compound if the adjacent mucosa is torn. This is usually the case with ethmoidal air sinus injuries. Violence which causes pharyngeal mucosa to tear at the time of fracture of the basisphenoid usually causes fatal brain damage.

Fractures of the vault may be linear and with so little separation when they are short that they are difficult to discern radiologically. When extensive, so that they traverse a considerable area of convexity, separation may be marked. Such fractures may extend circumferentially around the skull, or be vertically disposed with continuation into the base. This is frequent in the frontal, temporal and occipital regions. Several linear fractures may radiate from a point of impact to form a stellate pattern. Comminuted fractures may be restricted to a relatively small area or may be widespread with large fragments. The former pattern is commonly due to violence from a small round blunt object such as a hammer; the latter pattern occurs when the impact is with a flat heavy object or when the head has been thrown violently against a hard immobile surface. This causes deformation of the entire skull and fracturing occurs along lines of bending of the skull; this is sometimes referred to as a bursting fracture. Fractures of the vault may be depressed. In adults there is usually comminution; in infants the thin and elastic bone may be indented with little or no fracture, the 'pond' depression. The former are usually compound, the latter usually simple. The degree of depression and of comminution depends upon the momentum of the object striking the skull and the duration of the impact. Small high velocity missiles perforate the skull relatively cleanly but project within its cavity small fragments of bone that may be widely dispersed. Fracture fragments may be occasionally displaced outwards relative to the cranial contour. This may be seen in severe bursting injuries and is usually associated with an adjacent diffuse deformation. An unusual remote phenomenon is downward depression and comminution of the roof of the orbit from severe injury to the forehead or vertex. The converse of this injury is encountered in the upwards bursting fracture of the roof of the orbit with intracranial displacement following a severe blow to the eyeball or orbit. In both cases the thin orbital roof gives way downwards or upwards under the piston like effect of the blow.

In adults, suture lines have little influence over the pattern of vault fractures. In children, diastasis (separation) of sutures may replace a fracture or a fracture may extend into a suture and thence be continued as diastasis.

Fractures of the base of the skull tend to be grouped in well defined patterns, splitting the relatively weak panels of bone and passing around intervening thick buttresses. Much was made of these patterns in older writings but they are significant only in their clinical connotations, such as the liability of those in the anterior fossa to be compound via paranasal sinuses, the part they play in producing cranial nerve palsy and the evidence they provide that the violence of

impact has been severe. Although there is much individual variation in the precise situation of these fractures, there are really two basic patterns, those fractures disposed about the anteroposterior axis and those which run in a transverse axis across the middle fossa. The line of the fracture is a continuation of the axis of the striking force and separation is greatest at the point of impact. The fracture runs parallel to or obliquely around a buttress whose length lies approximately in the same axis but passes transversely across the buttress where this directly opposes its path. The line of the fracture may be deflected at this point. Frontal blows split the floor of the anterior cranial fossa often with much splintering of thin bone, usually to one side of the midline and may pass through into the ipsilateral middle fossa or cross the sphenoid bone at the weak area of the pituitary fossa to enter the contralateral middle fossa. Occipital blows often give rise to a clean linear fracture to one side or other of the thickened midline and pass obliquely towards the foramen magnum. The fracture may deviate round the margin of the foramen or break through the rim. These fractures cross the groove of the transverse sinus and may extend towards the vertex. A blow on the side of the head may fracture the floor of the middle cranial fossa (great wing of sphenoid) in the transverse cranial axis. It may extend in this general direction across the sphenoid to the opposite side. The fracture may take an oblique direction to encounter the petrous bone which it crosses transversely at the area weakened by the middle and inner ear. Russell and Schiller (1949) studied the injuries produced in the cadaver skull when it was compressed from side to side or from before backwards. The particular feature of importance was the effect of these forces on the petrous temporal bone, which was liable to be avulsed from the greater wing of the sphenoid, and from the squamous temporal bone to be rotated back on an axis so that the petrous apex was displaced backwards, opening up the foramen lacerum. This explains the high incidence of traction injury to the abducens, the opthalmic division of the trigeminal nerve and

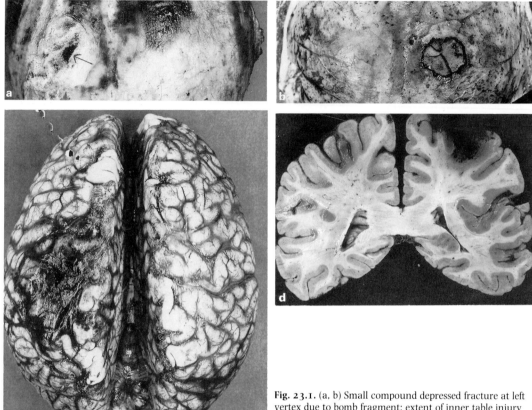

**Fig. 23.1.** (a, b) Small compound depressed fracture at left vertex due to bomb fragment; extent of inner table injury greater than outer (arrow). (c, d) Widespread haemorrhagic contusion and laceration of subjacent brain.

the auditory nerves which characterize such crushing injuries in life.

The mechanics of skull fractures were extensively studied by Gurdjian (Gurdjian & Lissner 1944, Gurdjian *et al.* 1950). They showed that the calvarium is momentarily bent inwards at the site of impact causing an abrupt rise of intracranial pressure, while at distant, often opposing points, there is a corresponding outward bending of the skull. With indentation of bone at the site of impact there is also a concentric outbending. These deformations rapidly subside and the entire cycle of events lasts about 5 milliseconds. Increasing force of a blow increases the degree of indentation but does not alter the time course.

Gurdjian's studies explain the common experience that in small depressed fractures the inner table gives way more than the outer table (Fig. 23.1). Sharp edges of inner table may penetrate the dura mater and brain to an unexpected degree. In some cases there may be no obvious fracture of the external table although the inner can be splintered and depressed. Such lesions of the skull are usually worse than they appear radiologically and can cause marked damage to the brain surface. These types of injury account for the observation that scalp wounds without fractures produced by tangential missile tracks can be associated with neurological signs because of contusion of the underlying brain.

## Brain injury

Although the macroscopic lesions of the brain found at necropsy following head injury and the lethal effects of brain compression by intracranial haematoma have long been familiar to pathologists and surgeons, knowledge of the finer changes and of the mechanisms of their production are more recent acquisitions. Interest in this subject was stimulated during the second World War. Indeed, the first notable contribution (Denny-Brown and Russell 1941) resulted from work started during the early months of 1940 when the medical services in Britain were being reorganized at the outbreak of hostilities. To a considerable extent, methods of experimental study had to wait the evolution of recording techniques which could discern physical events of the duration of fractions of a second, and present several simultaneous events on one record. Pathological observations have been enriched by illuminating studies of the brains of patients who have sustained severe injuries but who survived many months in a state of prolonged coma. Historical reviews of the development of understanding of brain damage include those of Mettler and Mettler (1945), Pudenz and Shelden (1946), Denny-Brown (1945), Adams (1975, 1984). Ambroise Paré is thought to have introduced the term *commotio cerebri* or concussion. It has been to the elucidation of this phenomenon that much experimental investigation has been directed. Definition of the word 'concussion' has varied from time to time, but common to all is loss of consciousness which is instantaneously brought about by a blow on the head of adequate degree. Opinions have varied as to the degree to which macroscopic lesions of the brain such as petechial contusions and oedema play a role in causing unconsciousness and whether they should be included in the term concussion. A few authenticated cases have been recorded in which concussion has been rapidly fatal but no naked eye abnormality could be found in the brain and yet there was no other cause of death than the blow. It is a banal observation that a person struck on

the head may lose consciousness only briefly and may fully recover from all effects shortly afterwards save for failure to remember the blow. Traumatic unconsciousness leaves its mark on cerebral functions in the form of traumatic amnesia. Trotter's classical definition emphasizes the minimum end of the scale of cerebral disturbances consequent upon trauma: 'an essentially transient state due to head injury which is of instantaneous onset, manifests widespread symptoms of a purely paralytic kind, does not as such comprise any evidence of structural cerebral injury, and is always followed by amnesia for the actual moment of the accident' Trotter (1924). The emphasis upon the minimal requirements to qualify concussion which is essentially a clinical state has been valuable in the experimental elucidation of the mechanisms involved. Macroscopic brain lesions may be caused by similar mechanisms but they are not themselves an essential part of the picture of concussion. The definition therefore, seeks to invoke a purely functional disorder, but histological studies have shown that even in minimal degrees of experimental concussion it is possible to demonstrate abnormal and damaged neurons in the brain stem both in the acute stage and months later (Windle *et al.* 1944, Jane *et al.* 1982). Clinical and experimental observations have also shown that repeated concussion produces additive effects. The most notable example is the traumatic encephalopathy seen in some professional boxers (Roberts 1969). Some believe that concussion is never a totally reversible disorder but that structural damage always occurs even if it is of minimal degree. Riddoch proposed this in 1931. Trotter's definition has however led to much confusion because of its emphasis on transience. Has the patient who suffers a severe injury and remains for many months in coma not suffered concussion? Autopsy on such patients may reveal no macroscopic evidence of brain lesions, though widespread microscopic lesions may be found in the brain (Strich 1961). Symonds (1928) chose to label as concussion traumatic unconsciousness from which full clinical recovery had occurred in 24 hours. He believed that such speedy recovery was incompatible with structural damage to the brain. Patients who suffered longer lasting effects, whether or not they were unconscious, were deemed to have sustained both concussion and a more severe damage which was loosely identified with contusion. This was an arbitrary convention which persisted for many years because post-mortem study offered no better explanation. The distinction was, however, purely artificial and Jefferson (1931) perceived the difficulty in using the two terms concussion and contusion in describing the effects of head injury because of 'our inability to set a period to the duration of concussion and to know with exactitude when it merges into contusion. The author's own inclination is to dispense with concussion altogether, not that it is meaningless but that it suggests too many unproven possibilities'. Jefferson preferred to regard traumatic unconsciousness and its sequelae as the result of a general contusion of the brain but recognized that the term contusion implied haemorrhages. The view of the neuropathologist (Greenfield 1928) was 'contusion suggests, if it does not actually postulate, haemorrhagic bruising of some part of the brain, a condition which can easily be seen at the time in fatal cases'. Because these focal lesions seemed to have no close relationship with the primary disorder, Greenfield put forward the view that concussion and contusion were 'purely clinical terms indicating varying degrees of severity of symptoms that should be replaced by terms which do not suggest a difference in pathological effects'. Twenty years later, Greenfield retained the term concussion, summarized the experimental work undertaken to elucidate its mechanism and described the macroscopic and microscopic changes which characterize 'diffuse injuries of the brain' (Greenfield 1958). The current view is that concussion comprises the state of traumatic unconsciousness, for however long this lasts, which occurs as an immediate and direct consequence of injury. Clinical severity is a reflection of the degree of underlying pathological disturbance, not of a qualitative variation. It excludes the role played by focal contusions,

by intracranial haemorrhage, by brain oedema or swelling and by systemic disorders. Any or all of these may aggravate, prolong or modify the clinical state.

*Concussion*

The important experiments of Denny-Brown and Russell (1941) showed that the phenomena of concussion were most readily produced by a blow on the cranium when it was free to move. When the cranium was rigidly supported a much greater force was required to produce the same effects. A blow to the mobile head was delivered by a weighted pendulum and with a mass equal to or greater than that of the head a minimum impact speed of 28 ft/s was necessary. They regarded this speed as a threshold value in the animals used in these experiments, cats, dogs and monkeys. When struck by the mass the stationary head is abruptly accelerated to take up the speed of the striker. The mass of the striker, and therefore its momentum at the moment of impact, is significant in so far as it is sufficient to provide the critical degree of acceleration to the head. Too small a mass at 28 feet per second will not shift the heavier heads sufficiently rapidly; a larger mass at the same speed will not only concuss but will cause additional brain damage. A large mass moving more slowly will displace the head without harm. A small mass such as a missile travelling at great speed will perforate the skull without necessarily producing loss of consciousness. The physics of the rate of change of velocity are identical whether the change is positive (acceleration) or negative (deceleration). Consequently the mechanisms of concussion due to the moving head suddenly striking a hard immobile object, abrupt deceleration, will be identical to that produced by acceleration. Denny-Brown and Russell estimated that the velocity of the moving head required to produce concussion at the time of impact was approximately 25 ft/s. Gurdjian *et al.* (1953) carried out experiments using apparatus which could measure and record the degree of acceleration imparted to the mobile head and concluded that between 250 and 500 g over a period of 5–10 milliseconds was necessary to produce a concussive effect. More recently, Gennarelli and his colleagues have used a much more sophisticated experimental model to produce graded angular acceleration to the head of the experimental primate without the requirement to produce any impact. The brain can therefore, be accelerated and decelerated over a period of 8–12 milliseconds and controlled variations can be made in the radius, angle and plane of movement (Gennarelli *et al.* 1982). Using this device, these workers have been able to reproduce the entire clinical spectrum of head injury from transient loss of consciousness to prolonged coma (Adams & Gennarelli 1982). In even the most briefly concussed animals, however, evidence of brain damage is demonstrable. Thus in monkeys awake 2 minutes following the injury, and appearing normal thereafter, application of the Fink–Heimer technique for axonal degeneration revealed clear cut abnormalities in the brain stem reticular formation (Jane *et al.* 1985).

Injury to the head by simultaneously opposed forces in which the head does not move significantly are uncommon. These crushing injuries of the head result from purely compressive forces; they may produce severe fractures of the skull base and extensive cranial nerve damage, yet loss of consciousness or concussion is rare. Russell and Schiller (1949) reported 15 cases in which consciousness was unimpaired throughout the accident in 12.

The physiological accompaniments of concussive acceleration/deceleration injuries have been characterized by Denny-Brown and Russell (1941) and many other subsequent investigators. At the time of impact there is an abrupt rise and fall of intracranial pressure of between 1000 and 4000 mmHg. Denny-Brown and Russell showed that experimental concussion could be produced by this mechanism alone by transmitting a pulse of increased pressure from a syringe to the intracranial cavity. This model for producing experimental concussion was subsequently refined by Lindgren and Rinder

(1969), by Stalhammar (1975) and by Sullivan *et al.* (1976). This extremely rapid rise of intracranial pressure must be differentiated from the lower increase of intracranial pressure which will bring about the phenomena described by Cushing. Denny-Brown and Russell found a wide range of other physiological effects of concussive injury, confirmed by later investigators. These included loss of corneal and pinna reflexes, brief abolition of respiration, and a steep rise of blood pressure with a gradual fall to normal. The reduction of arterial pressure from the postinjury peak appears to be related to release of endogenous opioids, since it is reversed by administration of naloxone experimentally (Hayes *et al.* 1983).

The rise of blood pressure, a constant feature, was associated with an increase in cerebral blood flow and peripheral vasoconstriction. Slowing of the heart rate often accompanied the elevated blood pressure and could be prevented by previous section of vagal nerves, although this did not affect the respiratory disturbance. Further criteria of experimental concussion were absence of haemorrhagic lesions in the brain and cervical spinal cord and of fracture of the skull. More severe blows caused progressive failure of blood pressure and death; from a variety of observations they considered that this circulatory failure was due to primary surgical shock. Their general conclusions were that the signs of experimental concussion were due to paralysis of various brain stem mechanisms. Similar results were obtained in decerebrate animal preparations and showed that the cerebral cortex played no part in the physiological response to concussional injury. The cardiac sequelae of experimental head injury have been studied in detail by Crockard *et al.* (1977) and Lewelt *et al.* (1980). Cholinergic blockade with atropine appeared to ameliorate these effects, whereas alpha or beta adrenergic blockade accelerated the deterioration in cardiac function after head injury. Parallel changes in cardiac function in patients with head injury have been noted by McLeod *et al.* 1982.

Electroencephalographic recordings during experimental concussion have provided helpful information on concurrent events at different levels of brain activity. Williams and Denny-Brown (1941) found an instantaneous generalized diminution in the surface EEG persisting after reflex activity had returned then succeeded by abnormally slow waves. Similar findings were reported by Sullivan *et al.* in 1976. Local trauma to the brain produces similar but localized, EEG changes.

The critical part played by acceleration in the aetiology of concussion which Denny-Brown and Russell established in their experiments led Holbourn (1943, 1944, 1945) to a theoretical analysis of the physics of the event.

He considered that only skull bending and rotation of the head are important. Abrupt movement of the head in space, without rotation and without deformity, purely linear acceleration, develops strains of compression within the brain; because of its extreme incompressibility Holbourn thought that such strains were unimportant in the production of concussion. He quoted the ability of nerves to maintain electrical conduction, despite being subjected to a compression strain of many thousand pounds per square inch provided that this was equally distributed. Brain tissue however, offers little resistance to change in shape because it has a very small modulus of rigidity and can readily suffer damage, when movement takes place between one point and another within its substance. This will occur in the immediate vicinity of the impact if the skull bends inwards or fractures as a result of the shearing stress and is the cause of the subjacent contusion or laceration. Rotational acceleration of the head gives rise to widespread shearing strains throughout the brain which vary in their intensity at different points. The position of the axis about which rotation takes place influences the incidence of strains and their consequent effects. Holbourn constructed a simple model representing the brain in its skull case and recorded the intensity and distribution of the shear strains set up by blows at various points. The correspondence between his experimental model and the distribution of contusions on post-mortem specimens is striking. The

importance of this analysis however, lay not in explaining the location of contusions but in postulating rotational acceleration as the cause of shearing forces, capable of affecting the entire brain with varying degrees of intensity. Deformation of the brain as a result of movement had been graphically demonstrated by Pudenz and Shelden (1946) who replaced the skull cap of primates by transparent perspex so that the cortex of the brain could be photographed during experimental concussion. Swirling movements of the cortex were seen which followed, after a brief interval and at a slower pace, the movement of the skull produced by the blow. The falx and the tentorium played an important part in controlling the direction of, and in dampening the movements of the brain, but in doing so they were responsible for localized brain damage. Similar lesions are seen on the dorsolateral aspect of the midbrain and corpus callosum in human material.

The relationship between shear strain and disturbance of the brain stem in experimental concussion was studied by Gurdjian and Lissner (1961) using a model similar to that of Holbourn. They demonstrated the presence and pattern of shear strains of the foramen magnum evoked by blows to the head. Loss of consciousness has been reported in 'whiplash' injury of the neck, and Friede (1961) produced 'concussion' in cats by sudden axial traction to the neck. The effects of boxing injury on head movement and loss of consciousness have been dramatically examined by Unterharnscheidt and Sellier (1971).

Observations on the changes in the cerebral circulation which immediately follow experimental concussion are relatively few. Denny-Brown and Russell (1941) showed that impact was followed by increased cerebral blood flow, considered to be due to the rise in arterial pressure. This has recently been confirmed by De Witt *et al.* (1981) using radioactive microspheres to measure blood flow in several regions of the brain. Pial window studies of brain surface vessels after concussion injury, reported by Walker (1966) showed that after the preliminary dilatation and increased flow there was segmental vasoconstriction and slowing of blood flow. This accords with the observations of Ommaya (1966) who found angiographic evidence of circulatory slowing in the brain 90 minutes after experimental concussion in primates.

Studies of intraparenchymal vascular dysfunction following experimental concussive brain injury have been carried out (Povlishock et al. 1978, 1979, Povlishock & Kontos 1982). In the arteriolar and capillary vasculature of the midline raphe and reticular core of the cat brain transient alterations in vascular permeability to horseradish peroxidase have been found. This permeability was produced by an increase in transendothelial vesicular transport. This protein passage could occur without evidence of intraparenchymal haemorrhage, but with injuries of increasing intensity microscopic petechial haemorrhages could be observed. Detailed examination by transmission and scanning electron microscopy of intraparenchymal vessels was carried out. These studies revealed maintenance of the tight interendothelial junctions but widespread evidence of damage to the endothelial surface with appearance of numerous plasmalemmal pits and endothelial craters. Parallel physiological studies in the same experimental preparation have demonstrated loss of vascular responsiveness to changes in perfusion pressure and arterial blood concentrations of carbon dioxide and oxygen as well as a depression of metabolic activity within the cerebral blood vessel wall (Wei et al. 1980, Lewelt et al. 1980, 1982). It appears, therefore, as if even minor concussional head injuries produce a temporary suspension of many normal cerebrovascular responses, rendering the concussed subject vulnerable to the superimposition of any systemic insult such as arterial hypotension of hypoxia (Miller & Becker 1982).

### Morbid anatomy of brain injury

The literature contains many excellent descriptions of the diverse appearances of the injured brain (Adams 1984). These are valuable in drawing attention to certain general patterns, but cannot replace assiduous attendance at post-mortem examinations and at demonstrations of sectioned fixed brains. The correlation of clinical record and autopsy finding is as important educationally (in the broadest sense) in these cases as in obscure cases of tumour; the course of events should, so far as possible, be explained by the terminal findings.

The macroscopic primary lesions of the brain may be loosely placed in three categories; haemorrhage, single or multiple, petechial or larger, some with well defined boundaries free from surrounding laceration; contusion, a localized area of softened swollen brain, often haemorrhagic; laceration, implying a breach of the pia and underlying brain, generally associated with intracerebral and surface haemorrhage. Secondary changes include oedema, displacement of brain and internal herniations due to the space occupying effects of swollen injured tissue, or of surface clot. It is important to distinguish the secondary haemorrhagic infarctions consequent upon these changes from primary haemorrhages (Fig. 23.2). The pathology of extra cerebral haemorrhage is considered separately. The analysis of Freytag (1963) of the post-mortem findings in a large series, is of interest. In 6% death was 'instantaneous' and no gross lesions were found; primary lesions were present in about 90%, and constituted the only findings in 24%; secondary lesions were present in 71%. In about one third the primary macroscopic lesions were in the basal ganglia and corpus callosum and in about one quarter in the brain stem. The cervical cord may be damaged in severe head injury (Davis et al. 1971).

Discrete punctate haemorrhages may occur in apparently random distribution or may be grouped in certain areas, in the walls of the ventricle subjacent to the ependyma and around the aqueduct, in the midbrain, pons and medulla, the last of which may be associated with bruising of the lower parts of the cerebellar lobes and tonsils suggesting a sudden piston-like displacement of the hind brain into the foramen

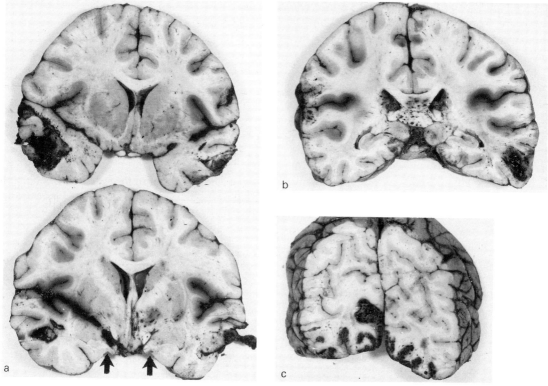

**Fig. 23.2.** The brain of a female aged 50 years, who died 4 days after being knocked down by a car. Shortly after the accident she was unresponsive to speech but reactive to painful stimulation; spontaneous movements of right arm, a left hemiparesis, spasms of extensor rigidity, pupils equal and reactive to light. Right parieto-occipital scalp bruising, limb injuries. Condition deteriorated; pupils became nonreactive to light, right larger than left; Breathing rapid and shallow, later irregular with periods of apnoea; angiography performed 2 days after injury showed alight shift of midline structures to right, and exploratory burr holes revealed only thin film of subdural blood over left convexity. Deep coma, rapid pulse and falling blood pressure which did not respond to pressor drugs. Post-mortem examination revealed numerous areas of cortical laceration and bruising, subarachnoid bleeding, areas of intracerebral haemorrhage more marked on left side, and petechiae. Flattened convulutions, bilateral hippocampal herniation.
(a) Haemorrhage in right temporal lobe (a similar one was present in right frontal lobe) and slight subfalcine herniation. Blood in sulci, other lacerations of cortex. Punctate haemorrhages in left hypothalamus and wall of third ventricle. lateral ventricles narrow, wharpened upper and outer angles. Hippocampal herniation (arrows).
(b) Petechial haemorrhages in splenium of corpus callosum and hippocampal gyri.
(c) Bilateral haemorrhagic infarction of occipital cortex. There was no macroscopic abnormality of brain stem and cerebellum.

magnum (Lindenberg & Freytag 1960). Haemorrhages in the grey matter of a group of contiguous gyri may occur at a site opposite to the blow to the head and, in the opinion of Unterharnscheidt, are due to the negative pressure created at this pole. Such injuries are common in the frontal temporal and occipital poles, the uncus and hippocampal gyri.

Distinction between primary and secondary brain stem haemorrhages is often difficult. The former are usually small, round and irregularly scattered. The latter are irregular in size and shape but often one or more are quite large, and there may be adjacent softening or necrosis of brain suggestive of an infarctive origin. Isolated haemorrhages, at times several centimetres across, may be found in the basal ganglia and internal capsule.

Contusions and lacerations vary in size from a few centimetres to the bulk of a lobe. Depending upon the duration of survival, the affected brain may be much swollen by haemorrhage and oedema, producing secondary pressure effects. In some cases of contusion there is little to see on the surface of the brain save swollen gyri and narrowed sulci with a few subpial petechiae. Within, however, the brain substance is swollen, soft, even diffluent, with varying degrees of haemorrhage. A large intracerebral haemorrhage surrounded by ragged necrotic tissue may lie hidden beneath almost normal cortex. Blood may break through into the ventricles. Contusions and lacerations are most frequent at frontal and temporal poles particularly on their inferior surfaces and between the lips of the Sylvian fissure. This distribution is determined by the irregular bone pattern of the floor of the anterior and middle cranial fossae and the buttress-like prominence of the sphenoidal ridge. The relative lack of cerebrospinal fluid in the subarachnoid space on the under surface of the brain probably aggravates the effect of the disruptive forces. Occipital pole contusions are less common, one reason being the smooth contour of the tentorium and inner aspect of the occipital bone. The severest degrees of contusion and laceration in blunt injuries occur at the side of the head opposite the blow as a result of deceleration.

Some less common sites of brain injury deserve comment. The corpus callosum was damaged in 16–25% of head injury specimens examined by Lindenberg et al. (1955) and Nevin (1967). The lesion may consist of only a small a haemorrhagic area or may involve the majority of its length. In severe cases, the lesion consists of haemorrhagic linear tear situated off the midline and often sparing the dorsal surface. It has been attributed to violent contact with the sharp edge of the falx but this seems improbable. Lindenberg considered that shear strains between one hemisphere and the other were the most likely cause. The lesion is not lethal in itself but is an important pathological finding as it is a frequent con-

comitant of extensive diffuse axonal injury (Adams et al. 1977, 1982).

Bruising may be found in the deep parts of the temporal lobes involving the hippocampus and hippocampal gyrus. Such lesions are to be distinguished from ischaemic lesions in the distribution of the posterior cerebral artery of the type linked to temporal lobe herniation. This primary lesion is attributable to shear strains inflicted by the tentorium. Haemorrhagic lesions of the dorsolateral aspect of the midbrain have also been attributed to forcible contact with the tentorial edge at the time of impact.

Daniel and Treip (1961) detected traumatic infarction of the pituitary gland in 5% of autopsies on head injured patients, associated most commonly with complete or partial section of the pituitary stock. In all such cases the skull had been fractured. Hypothalamic lesions have been described by Crompton (1971a) and visual field disturbances and blindness are well recognized. Observations on damage to this part of the brain provide an immediate explanation for diabetes insipidus following head injury but impairment of functions of the anterior pituitary lobe is a rare sequel of head injury.

Brain oedema is well marked in areas of contusion and laceration. It adds to local bulk and thereby aggravates brain displacement and its consequences. In this situation there is an increase in brain tissue water content and increased permeability of blood vessels in and around the damaged area. The oedema is therefore of the vasogenic type (Klatzo 1972, Fishman 1975), but of more acute origin than the vasogenic oedema which is associated with brain tumour or abscess. What is much more controversial is whether there is such an entity as generalized brain oedema following, and attributable to, concussional head injury. Greenfield (1938, 1958) was sceptical. Diffuse brain swelling due to vascular engorgement of the traumatized brain seems to be a much more likely explanation for the collapse of ventricles and disappearance of the subarachnoid space seen on computerized tomography soon after injury in severe cases. If this swelling is persistent and

associated with severe intracranial hypertension, generalized brain ischaemia may ensue,
with the development of cyototoxic oedema due
to perfusion failure. This phenomenon is more
common in children than in adults (Bruce *et al.*
1981). The major difficulty is to know whether
the cause of the problem lies in an episode of
severe arterial hypotension or hypoxia which
caused the injured brain to swell. At the present
time any link between concussional brain injury
and generalized brain oedema seems tenuous
(Corales *et al.* 1980, Miller *et al.* 1980).

The late macroscopic changes which occur in
survivors from head injury can be assessed by
radiological investigations, during operations or
from autopsy when such patients die from other
causes. The sites of contusion and laceration
become represented by loss of brain tissue leaving
smooth irregular depressions on the surface of
the brain, occupied by lakes of cerebrospinal fluid
with a variable degree of adherent arachnoid
membrane. The cavities are usually stained
faintly yellow and there may be trough-like excavation of the summits of gyri with sparing of the
sulci. Cysts may be found within white matter,
discoloured yellow, the sites of absorbed intracerebral haemorrhage. The tissue around old
injuries becomes firm from scarring and gliosis
over time. Spillane (1962) has noted rupture of
the septum lucidum as a characteristic of old
boxing injuries.

Previous temporal lobe herniation maybe
adduced by persistent grooving of the uncus and
hippocampal gyrus and toughening of the neighbouring brain. Irregular shrinkage, cavitation
and firmness may indicate the healed areas of
infarction in the medial temporal structures.
Similar changes in the cingulate gyrus may
provide evidence of previous mid-line sub-falcine
herniation. These tell-tale signs of previous brain
shift correlate closely with prior occurrence of
raised intracranial pressure (Adams & Graham
1976).

The ventricles often become dilated after a
serious head injury (Fig. 23.3). This may be
generalized and symmetrical, may affect one
lateral ventricle much more than its fellow, or

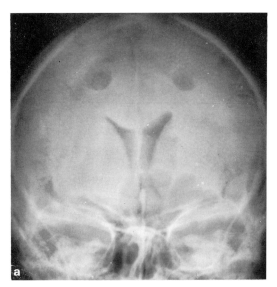

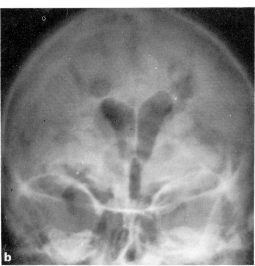

**Fig. 23.3** Ventriculogram in a case of head injury, female
aged 28: shortly after accident response only to pain, right
pupil dilated and nonreactive to light, left small and reacted
sluggishly, complete right and partial left ptosis, limbs rigid
in extension. Left parietal scalp bruise. (a) One day after
injury: no midline shift, upper and outer angle of right lateral
ventricle pointed, body of ventricle narrow.
(b) Seven weeks after injury: large ventricles, left more than
right, sulci dilated (poor definition). Her recovery was slow
but ultimately she was able to fulfil all family duties: residual
dysarthia and ataxic spastic gait.

comprise a local bulging which in some cases
has the appearance of a diverticulum (Northfield
1944). In all cases it is likely that loss of white

matter from nerve fibre destruction plays the major role in determining enlargement of the CSF space. Recognition of ventricular dilatation on CT one to three months after severe head injury is an ominous sign, suggesting survival in a severely disabled state. Generalized shrinkage of the cerebral cortex may be seen in some patients who have sustained severe head injury but cortical atrophy was absent in the severely injured brains of younger patients studied by Strich (1961). In a small number of cases of ventricular dilatation, obstruction of CSF pathways by blood and debris in the acute stage and later by leptomeningial fibrosis may contribute to hydrocephalus. This is rare however. While ventricular dilatation was observed in more than 20% of a consecutive series of survivors from severe head injury by Roberson *et al.* (1979), in only 4 cases was it considered likely that true hydrocephalus due to CSF pathway obstruction was present. In the remaining cases the dilatation of the ventricular system was considered to be occurring *ex vacuo* due to white matter tissue loss (Meyers *et al.* 1983). Focal bulging of the ventricle or porencephaly is determined by damage and shrinkage of the white matter at the site of severe contusion and/or haemorrhage. Ventricular pulsion against the localized area of softening is thought to be an important factor. This mechanism becomes much more pronounced when a bony decompression of the skull has been carried out overlying the area of damaged brain. Atrophy of the cerebellum and brain stem in the posterior cranial fossa has been observed on CT in patients suffering from dysarthria and ataxia after severe head injury (Van Dongen & Braakman 1980).

*Microscopic lesions*

The effects of brain damage are apparent in nerve cells within a few hours of injury. Two types of response can be distinguished, firstly, due to ischaemia, the other attributable to physical forces. In 1956, Strich made a notable contribution to the pathology of head injury by describing widespread degeneration of the white matter in the brains of persons who had died many months after severe injury. In 1961, she reported the results of histopathological examination in 20 cases, mostly young patients and all uncomplicated by brain compression from intracranial haematoma. The survival of these patients had varied from several weeks to two years, all patients had been deeply unconscious from the time of injury, some recovered sufficiently to swallow and utter a few words but only one had been able to leave the hospital, and was severely handicapped both mentally and physically. In spite of the severity of the brain injuries the skull had been fractured in only two of the 20 cases. Naked eye changes in the brain were few and inconspicuous. There was no cortical atrophy and the white matter looked normal. The ventricles were dilated and in some also the aqueduct. Small areas of old haemorrhage and softening could be detected. In all 20 cases the corpus callosum was damaged and in 12 cases the superior cerebellar peduncles. Two important findings were seen on microscopical examination. When survival had been only weeks, many nerve fibre retraction balls were found in the white matter; these were considered to represent flow of axoplasm from the free end of ruptured axions. In longer surviving cases there were widespread areas of myelin degeneration. These foci of degeneration were found in the white matter, converging in the fibre tracts in the brain stem and spinal cord. No abnormality could be detected in the cerebral cortex but Strich pointed out that cortical cell loss can not be assessed unless it reaches at least 33%. Secondary shrinkage of the thalami was present and Strich emphasized the widespread distribution of the lesions and their asymmetry. Assuming that they are the result of shear strains, tearing or rupturing axons, Strich pointed out that the asymmetry was in accord with the predictions made by Holbourn (1943). Rotational acceleration will affect the mirror image structures of the hemispheres to a different degree on each side, depending upon the relationship between the axis of rotation and that of the structure. That the axonal damage is immediate, is shown by the prompt development of abnormal neurological signs from the time of impact. Strich related a case in which the accident had been witnessed by a trained nurse. The patient 'took up her characteristic posture with both legs and the right arm rigidly extended and the left arm flexed as soon as she struck the ground'. Evidence of this sort concerning the immediate effects of head injury derived from an expert witness must be rare but is of great value. (A similar observation of prolonged apnoea immediately following head injury has been recorded by Levine and Becker 1979.) Spasticity, involuntary movements and abnormal posturing may be seen in patients admitted to hospital soon after a severe head injury but by then secondary events within the brain may well have modified the initial event. Oppenheimer (1968) also studied these micro-scopic lesions. By the use of appropriate stains he demonstrated multiple minute foci of microglial reaction in the white matter within 24 hours of injury. These microglial stars were visible also in the brains of patients who had survived many months and appeared to relate closely to the lesions described by Strich. The great importance of Oppenheimer's paper was that in 5 of the cases in which microglial clusters had been found, the concussion had been trivial and death due to other causes. This supports the contention that in even minor degrees of concussion there is structural damage to the brain. Oppenheimer also puts forward evidence that tearing of nerve fibres by stress may be determined by the direc-tional relationship between the axis of a small blood vessel and the axis of the nerve fibres between which it is situated.

Crompton (1971b) reported on the post-mortem findings in a consecutive series of 106 patients dying soon after head injuries. In only 14 specimens was there no macroscopic or microscopic lesion in the brain stem. In 32 there were primary and in 63 secondary brain stem lesions and in 3 both were present. In the case of primary lesions of the brain stem there was a preponderance of occipital impacts, survival was shorter than in the cases of secondary lesion

and a lucid interval was recorded in only 6% of primary as compared with 38% of secondary brain stem lesions. In an earlier study Crompton et al. (1966), found in cases in which death had followed prolonged coma with no lucid interval and there had been no epiphenomena to cause secondary brain stem lesions, all of the brains showed primary damage to the brain stem. Jel-linger and Seitelberger (1970) also carried out detailed necropsy studies in head injured patients. In their series, cases of haematoma were included, which probably accounts for the 83% incidence of secondary brain stem lesions. They found that all of the brain stem lesions were primary in cases where death had occurred within one hour of the accident, mixed primary and secondary lesions were found when death occurred between one and 48 hours after the accident, and all brain stem lesions were con-sidered to be secondary in cases dying after a longer interval.

An extensive study of the pathology of diffuse brain damage of immediate impact type was reported by Adams et al. (1977, 1982). From a series of 151 fatal head injuries, 19 patients were identified and 26 subsequent cases added, all of whom had been continuously in coma from the time of impact without any lucid interval. In the early stages after injury the patients had shown abnormal motor posturing, usually extensor rigidity, and frequently autonomic dysfunction. In this group of patients skull fracture was rela-tively uncommon. The features of raised intra-cranial pressure or brain compression were entirely absent and a rather stereotyped neur-opathological picture was recognized. Few surface contusions of the brain were present but there was always a small lesion in the corpus callosum and commonly one in the superior cer-ebellar peduncle. In cases studied within the first two weeks after injury, numerous axonal retrac-tion balls were found. Microglial stars appeared within a few days and by two weeks were extremely prominent. In patients who survived more than six weeks Wallerian degeneration of white matter could be shown affecting the ascending and decending tracts in the brain stem and the white matter of the cerebral hemispheres. Although such lesions were commonly present in the brain stem, in not a single case of Adam's series were brain stem lesions found in isolation. They were always accompanied by extensive diffuse white matter damage in the hemispheres. Adams proposed that these pathological findings corresponded to the hypothesis of Ommaya and Gennarelli (1974) that in acceleration injury the brain is damaged centripetally from the subcortex, so that with increasing severity of injury there is an increasing tendency for the diffuse axonal injury to extend to the brain stem.

Microscopic evidence of brain damage of a different type is also seen. In Adams' total series of 151 fatal head injuries, 91% had evidence of ischaemic brain damage and 83% had pathological evidence that raised intracranial pressure had previously been present (Adams & Graham 1976, Graham et al. 1978). More than three quarters exhibited both of these forms of secondary brain damage. The most common areas of the brain to exhibit ischaemic brain damage were the hippocampus and basal ganglia. Ischaemic damage in the medial occipital cortex was seen in 30% of cases and could be directly related to tentorial herniation during life, with compression of the posterior cerebral artery. Ischaemic brain damage in other areas of the cortex is even more common however, and instances of both boundary zone ischaemia between the territories of distribution of the anterior and middle and middle and posterior cerebral arteries was seen, as well as ischaemic damage located squarely in the territories of distribution of the main cerebral vessels. Boundary zone ischaemia could be related to the occurrence during life of reductions in cerebral perfusion pressure caused either by arterial hypotension or intracranial hypertension. Arterial hypoxaemia was also considered to be an important contributor to the development of damage in the cortex and in the hippocampus.

*Meninges*

Subarachnoid haemorrhage is found in most cases of fatal brain injury. It may spread from torn cortical vessels at the site of contusions and lacerations or from intraventricular haemorrhage. Its pathological consequences are described in Chapter 11 on aneurysms. It should be understood however, that the most frequent cause of blood in the subarachnoid space is trauma, rather than aneurysmal rupture, and in cases where the haemorrhage is extensive, the patient is exposed to all of the sequelae associated with spontaneous subarachnoid haemorrhage. Cerebral vasospasm undoubtedly occurs in patients with head injury. Unfortunately, there are no reliable data on the prevalence of this problem in head injured cases of a given degree of severity. Nowadays, angiography is performed so seldom on head injured patients that this information will never be available. MacPherson and Graham (1978), noted that 35% of a series of fatal head injuries had shown significant cerebral vasospasm on angiography during life. The distribution of ischaemic brain damage at autopsy was in part related to the location of the regions affected most severely by vasospasm. The combination of cerebral vasospasm and raised intracranial pressure is likely to be particularly important in the genesis of ischaemic brain damage in head injured patients (Miller & Gudeman 1980).

Subdural haemorrhage was found in approximately two thirds of a series of fatal head injuries of Freytag (1963). Fracture of the skull was present in about half of these cases and in most specimens there was naked eye evidence of cerebral contusion. In approximately 20% of subdural haematomas there was however, no contusion and in such cases a fracture was uncommon. This is in keeping with clinical experience, that in a proportion of subdural haematomas there is little or no evidence of primary traumatic damage to the brain. The origin of bleeding in such cases may be a tear in a dural cortical or sinus vein or, more rarely, a cortical artery (Drake 1961). The subdural course of the superior cortical veins as they pass to the superior sagittal sinus renders them easily torn by swirling movements of the cortex during rotational acceleration. The vein of Labbé may also be torn where it leaves the posterior temporal lobe for the sigmoid sinus by the same movements of the brain. The high incidence of subdural haematoma after minor head impact in elderly patients can be attributed to the shrinkage of the brain consequent upon age which allows a greater degree of movement and therefore an increased liability to extend a vein beyond its limits. Chronic subdural haematoma in middle aged patients is rare, but when it occurs is often in patients with brain atrophy, due usually to excessive alcohol consumption

In cases of severe brain injury, blood may seep from cortical lacerations into the subdural space, this process may be bilateral with diffuse extension of a thin layer of subdural clot over the hemisphere. In cases of severe contusion and laceration of the temporal pole a large subdural collection may form, producing upward displacement of the Sylvian fissure and contralateral shift of the midline structures.

If the amount of bleeding or associated brain injury is insufficient to prove fatal, the blood may slowly clot and a reactionary membrane forms around it. In some cases this may develop into a firm fibrous capsule, the thickest part of which is applied to the dura. The wall of the encysted haematoma consists of fibrous tissue merging with vascular granulation tissue which lines the cavity. The contents of the haematoma vary with duration. In the early stages they consist of thick opaque brownish or tarry fluid with loose fragments of liquefying clot. Later the contents become less viscous, paler, more recognizably red or orange turning later to even thinner yellow fluid. These changes represent the evolution of a chronic subdural haematoma, the size of which is frequently such as to make it unlikely that the original haemorrhage could have been of similar volume. The eventual contents of the sac are not equivalent to simple liquefaction of blood but are more dilute. It has been suggested that the capsule of the haematoma begins to act as a

semipermeable membrane and the highly proteinaceous fluid contents attract water through the membrane by osmosis (Gardner 1932). Weir (1971) measured the osmolality of subdural haematoma fluid and showed that this mechanism was most unlikely. Greenfield (1958) considered that the increase in the volume of the contents was due to episodes of recurrent haemorrhage into cavity. Fresh red blood cells can usually be identified in the fluid content. In infants the wall of a chronic subdural haematoma may become so thick and rigid that it is feared that expansion of the brain will be prevented. In the past, excision of the subdural membrane has been advocated but this procedure is fraught with risks of damage to the cerebral cortex and the procedure is seldom carried out today (Fig. 23.4). In cases where there is persistent collection of subdural

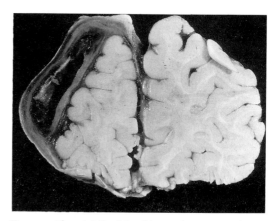

Fig. 23.4. Chronic left subdural haematoma in an infant aged 18 months: symptoms commenced at age of 8 months with attacks of screaming and stiffening of limbs, big head and papilloedema. Repeated subdural aspiration failed to cure the condition and death followed craniotomy for excision of membranes.

fluid despite repeated tapping of the cavity, the insertion of a subdural to peritoneal drain provides a satisfactory solution.

The term hygroma is sometimes applied to the collections of clear or yellow stained fluid of the consistency of CSF found in the subdural space following head injury.

While it has been considered that subdural hygroma may represent a further stage of evolution of chronic subdural haematoma, the usual lack of any membrane and the watery nature of the fluid make it more likely that these fluid collections are caused by small tears in the arachnoid, functioning as a one way valve permitting gradual expansion of the subdural space with CSF, from which some fluid content is subsequently absorbed so as to increase the protein content. These collections of fluid seldom, if ever, function as space occupying lesions. Effusions of yellow, usually sterile fluid in the subdural space may arise in the course of acute meningitis in children. In a series of 116 cases of subdural haematoma and effusion in infancy Till (1968) found that 40% were due to trauma and 5% to meningitis. No definite cause could be identified in the remaining 55% of the cases.

Extradural haemorrhage was evident in 15% of the cases of Freytag and this was accompanied by a skull fracture in 98%. The haemorrhage usually arises from vessels of the dura mater, the middle meningeal artery and vein being particularly liable to injury owing to the thinness of the squamous temporal bone, rendering it particularly susceptible to fracture, and to the course of these vessels in a deep groove or even tunnel in the inner table of the bone. Bleeding may also arise from damage to the superior sagittal sinus and transverse sinus or unnamed venous channels. It may also arise from diploic vessels of small depressed skull fractures in which the outer table is firmly impacted preventing egress of blood while the edges of the fractured inner table are separated exposing the diploe to the dura. In large depressed fractures the dura mater is often split and blood enters the lacerated brain. The absence of fracture in a small proportion of cases of extra dural haemorrhage, mainly in children, suggest that the distortion of the skull at the time of impact, the in-bending and out-bending, separates the dura mater from the bone and at the same time ruptures the vessels. A potential space is thus provided into which the vessels can bleed and gradually the dura mater is stripped from the bone over a wider area. Unlike the subdural haematoma, extradural haemorrhage remains localized although it may attain a large size both in thickness and extent. Extradural haematomas do not become encapsulated like subdural haematomas. They threaten life by cerebral compression within hours, days or occasionally weeks. Powers of absorption from the extradural space are slight and slow.

Surface collections of blood add to the dangers of head injury because they occupy space in the craniospinal cavity. In some cases of acute subdural haemorrhage the brain has already sustained intrinsic lesions and if these are overwhelmingly lethal the removal of the clot only delays the inevitable end. In many other cases however, the primary brain damage is not of lethal degree and in such cases evacuation of haematoma is a vital matter. Surface haematomas give rise to progressive displacement of the brain, beginning with progressive flattening of the subjacent gyri and the distant effects of dislocation in the form of brain herniation, brain stem displacement, infarctions and secondary haemorrhages. Infarction may occur in the territory of a major vessel supplying the brain immediately subjacent to the haematoma. This may be produced by a combination of local pressure effects and an episode of systemic arterial hypotension. Haematomas in the posterior cranial fossa cause direct pressure upon the medullary centres but, if prolonged, may displace the cerebellum upwards, crowding into the tentorial hiatus compressing the aqueduct and producing an obstructive hydrocephalus.

The practice of obtaining computerized tomographic scans in severely head injured patients as soon as possible after arrival at the hospital has shed important new light on the frequency and course of subdural and extradural haemorrhage. Sizeable intracranial haematomas are present in 40–50% of comatose patients, regardless of the clinical evolution of the case (Becker et al. 1977). Acute subdural haematoma, mainly in the frontotemporal location, may be observed within two hours of an injury in which the patient has been comatose from the moment of impact. Excepting the case of acute subdural hematomas related to a cortical arterial haemorrhage, there does not appear to be a marked tendency of acute subdural haematoma to increase in size. Progressive brain compression is more likely to be due to swelling of the subjacent brain than expansion of the haematoma.

The situation is entirely different with extra-dural haematoma in which computerized tomography carried out too soon after the injury may fail to demonstrate what subsequently develops into a sizeable extradural haematoma. Acute subdural haematoma is approximately 3 times as common as extradural.

Penetrating injuries of the brain may arise as a complication of depressed skull fracture, from relatively low velocity impacts with perforation of the skull by an object of small calibre or from high velocity missiles. With the first two forms of injury, the damage may range from a small dural tear and superficial brain laceration to extensive brain destruction. In the case of missile injury the damage depends on the velocity, size and shape of the missile. Injuries produced by irregular fragments or bullets from hand guns punch out an opening in the bone and dura mater and much of the brain damage is due, not to the missile fragment itself, but to the shower of small bone fragments driven in from the entrance wound. The missile fragment may traverse the brain and leave the skull, creating a much larger and irregular opening. Spent bullets may fail to leave the skull being reflected by the inner table back into the brain to create haemorrhage at the site of reflection and possibly a further trail of brain destruction. Initial examination of the missile track soon after injury may give an impression of a relatively restricted area of tissue damage. The walls of the track however are de-vitalized over a considerable radius and the track soon becomes surrounded by an extensive area of oedema while the damaged ischaemic tissues in the track become diffluent (Raimondi & Samuelson 1970). High velocity missiles such as rifle bullets produce even more widespread disruption of tissue when they traverse the brain as a consequence of the explosive force exerted by the passage of the high speed missile. Cant-ation and gas bubble formation in the brain is produced and if the missile begins to tumble as

it traverses the brain the degree of damage is increased even more.

In depressed skull fractures much of the energy of impact has been dissipated in fracturing the skull and the brain may suffer much less con-cussional injury. Fifty per cent of a large series of patients with depressed skull fracture reported by Miller and Jennett (1968) had either never been unconscious or were only rendered briefly so. In large depressed fractures produced by violent blunt impact, severe acceleration forces may be transmitted to the brain as a whole and coma will be produced.

One of the most important factors in pen-etrating injuries is the breach of the dura mater. This is normally a reliable barrier against intra-cranial infection; when it has been breached and contaminated tissue and foreign bodies driven into the brain the risks of intracranial infection rise hour by hour. In cases of depressed skull fracture the most common source of infection is indriven hair, while in cases of low velocity missile injury it is the indriven fragments of bone that seem to contribute most to the later occur-rence of infection (Carey et al. 1971). The met-allic fragments themselves seem less important and are surgically removed only if accessible; all indriven bone fragments must however be removed if intracranial infection is to be avoided. Loss of continuity of the dura mater allows fibroblasts from the extradural part of the injury to proliferate into the area of injured cortex uniting the scar in the brain with that of its coverings. This results in formation of a men-ingocerebral cicatrix continuous with bone and scalp. This may relate in some cases to the development of post traumatic epilepsy.

## Clinical manifestations of closed head injury and its sequelae

It is a banal observation, but it bears repetition, that the importance of a head injury depends first upon the degree of primary brain damage and secondly upon the nature and intensity of complications which may develop. Jefferson

(1933) emphasized the importance of distinguishing between these two sets of events for a clear understanding of the diagnosis and treatment of head injury and introduced for them the terms 'basic state' and 'epiphenomena'. The basic state comprises levels of consciousness and subsequent mental disorders, vital signs, general and focal abnormal neurological signs and accompanying symptoms. The epiphenomena included the manifestations of increased intracranial pressure and progressive neurological deficit due to oedema, haemorrhage or infection which were added to the clinical picture of the basic state.

At the outset, loss of consciousness is usually profound and at this early phase, its duration, rather than its depth, is the measure of the severity of injury. Thereafter, and by the time the patient reaches hospital, the level of consciousness is the most important and reliable single sign of progress. Anxiety persists while the level is low and steadily diminishes as it rises. A fall in the level of consciousness may herald the onset of brain compression, infection, metabolic disorder or other complications such as fat embolism. A regular and frequent record of the state of unconsciousness is as essential in management as that of the vital signs. The use of the descriptive terms coma, semicoma and stupor is deprecated because they convey different meanings to different observers. The level should be assessed in terms of the response elicited in the patient by a particular stimulus. In 1974 Teasdale and Jennett advocated the Glasgow Coma Scale, in which 3 features were independently observed (eye opening, motor response and verbal performance) so as to assess arousal and the capacity to respond to change in the environment, which are the two features of consciousness (Table 23.2). Eye opening was taken to be an indication of arousal. The eyes may open spontaneously, only when the patient is spoken to, when the patient is given a painful stimulus or not even to painful stimuli. The motor response in the limbs was tested by first of all determining whether the patient could obey commands. If not, two standardized stimuli were

used, pressure on the nail bed of the finger or toe using a hard object and supra-orbital pressure. If the hand moves towards the source of the pain the response is recorded as localizing. If localization is not present, the next level of response is normal flexor withdrawal of the upper limb in which the arm is pulled away from the nail bed stimulus. At the next level of response the flexor movement is said to be abnormal because of its association with pronation of the upper limb, wrist flexion and, in some cases, tucking of the thumb across the palm of the hand. The next level of response below abnormal flexor is extensor, referring to extension at the elbow upon applying painful stimulation. While the arm is usually pronated with the wrist flexed, as in the characteristic decerebrate posture, this is not always the case and is one reason why the term extensor response is preferred. The final level on the motor scale is when no response whatsoever occurs in response to painful stimuli. This seldom occurs for long in the lower limbs because of the development of spinal reflex withdrawal but it is frequent in the upper limbs and it is crucial in such cases to ensure that supra-orbital painful stimuli are included in the examination. Patients with coexistent head and spinal injury may show no limb responses because of quadriplegia yet examination above the neck reveals them to be scoring at a much higher level on the coma scale. A similar problem can arise in the neurological evaluation of patients who have been resuscitated following cardiac arrest, when patients who are recovering may show a functional transection of the upper cervical cord. On the verbal performance scale, speech is classified as normal orientated conversation, confused verbal response with disorientation, inappropriate words, sounds only or no vocalization whatsoever.

Coma is defined as a state in which there is no eye opening even to painful stimuli, failure to obey commands or to utter recognizable words. Under certain circumstances it may not be possible to elicit responses on this scale. Eye opening may be prevented by peri-orbital swelling, speech may be impossible to test because of the presence of endotracheal tube. When this is the case this part of the assessment is simply omitted, the reason noted and the conscious level score made on the basis of the remaining part of the examination. This objective scaling system is extremely repeatable and robust whether used by doctors or nurses, specialist or generalized. It has been widely adopted throughout the world and since 1976 has formed the basis for comparison of head injury results in many different centres and the development of management programmes and prognostic algorithms relating the clinical state of the head injured patient to his eventual outcome (Langfitt 1978, Jennett *et al.* 1979, Miller *et al.* 1981).

Evolution through the levels on the coma scale is recognizable in all cases of concussional head injury although in mild cases it may be compressed into minutes while in severe cases it extends into weeks. With the return of responsiveness, spontaneous mental activity may be expressed in restlessness, incoherent speech, confusion, delirium, excitement and negativistic attitudes amounting at times to violent resistance to attention. The development of more fluent speech reveals evidence of the patient's awareness of his surroundings and is often accompanied by offensive remarks and antisocial activities due to continuing inhibition or interruption of the controlling habits of normal social life. The feelings of thirst, hunger, headache, a full bladder or the desire to evacuate the bowel may trigger off extreme restlessness. After this, islands of normal behaviour and speech emerge, current happenings are recorded and can subsequently be recalled. These episodes enlarge and ultimately fuse in a continuity of normality. The patient may be considered fully conscious by now but after severe head injuries disturbances of behaviour, of spatial and temporal orientation, of cognition, memory and attention persist from varying periods of time. For the duration of disturbed consciousness memory recording is in abeyance resulting in post-traumatic amnesia (PTA), and memory of events leading up to the accident may also be erased, retrograde amnesia. Retrograde amnesia is usually fairly brief, often

only a matter of seconds or minutes prior to the injury. In some patients with recovery of consciousness may come a realization of a prolonged period of retrograde amnesia extending sometimes to months or years prior to the injury. With the passage of time and further recovery however, the duration of retrograde amnesia virtually always shrinks considerably. The post-traumatic amnesia is usually of longer duration; it nearly always includes the moment of impact and extends for 3 or 4 times the duration of the observed loss of consciousness. In patients with minor head injuries, inability to recall the actual impact is acceptable evidence of concussion, even if only momentary. If the duration of post-traumatic amnesia is to be a measure of severity of concussion, its end point must be determined. Russell, who was the first to appreciate this yard stick, regarded as most reliable the patient's statements as to return of continuous memory taken when sufficiently recovered (Russell 1931). This form of measurement will include periods of clouded consciousness during which the patient may confabulate. The arbitrary divisions of concussion as suggested by Russell (1959) are shown in Table 23.3.

Table 23.3 Severity of injury and post-traumatic amnesia (PTA)

| Severity | Duration of PTA |
|---|---|
| Slight | less than 1 hour |
| Moderate | 1 to 24 hours |
| Severe | 1 to 7 days |
| Very severe | over 7 days |

*Vital signs*

Immediately after the impact the vital activities are reduced to a minimum, a state of acute surgical shock during which death may occasionally occur. The pulse is slow, irregular and feeble. There is a profound fall in blood pressure; respirations are shallow, irregular and reduced in rate, indeed prolonged apnoea may occur, just as in the physiological response to experimental concussion. If the person lies unattended for any length of time body temperature falls. These effects have usually disappeared by the time the patient is admitted to hospital and by then no such abnormality may be detected. It is common in slight to moderate degrees of concussion for the pulse rate to rise slightly for a day or so then fall below normal to 50–60 beats per minute for some days before once again returning to normal. This delayed bradycardia has been attributed by Denny-Brown (1961) to a medullary effect. He noted an acceleration of the pulse during restlessness and concluded that both abnormalities provided evidence of vasomotor instability. In severe injuries a progressive rise in the pulse rate occurs during the first 24 hours with little or no change in the blood pressure. A rapid and steep rise in pulse rate is a bad omen.

The blood pressure, having returned to a normal level usually remains steady in uncomplicated cases, though when brain damage is severe and overwhelming the blood pressure will fall as a preterminal event. Arterial hypotension is seen in 15% of severely head injured patients on admission to hospital (Miller *et al.* 1981). At this stage the cause of the fall in blood pressure is virtually always related to external or internal haemorrhage associated with multiple injuries. Nonhaemorrhagic arterial hypotension may result from severe damage to the spinal cord at a high cervical level.

The respiration rate rises and ventilation increases in depth in severe head injury, so that when first seen most severely head injured patients are hyperventilating (Froman 1968). Abnormalities of respiratory rhythm may develop. Several different forms of respiratory arrhythmia may be observed, including Cheyne–Stokes respiration, ataxic respiration, hyperventilation; more than one form of arrhythmia may be observed in a single patient. The correlation between brain damage in a particular locus and a specific type of respiratory abnormality is poor, but the more damage that occurs in the brain stem the more likely it is that some form of abnormal respiratory rhythm will result (North & Jennett 1974). Rhythmic deepening and acceleration of respiration often occurs in the patient with extensor rigidity, coincident with periodic episodes of increased spasticity. Respiratory abnormalities are also produced by mounting intracranial pressure. Obstruction of the airway is frequent in severe head injury and may arise in three ways. The first is a consequence of incorrect position of the unconscious patient. The paralysed tongue may fall back and block the oral pharynx if the patient is left lying on his back. The second cause of obstruction is an outpouring of excess mucus in the respiratory passages or inhalation of gastric contents after vomiting. The third, less common, is spasm of the glottis which causes a crowing noise during inspiration.

Most severely head injured patients hyperventilate, that is have an abnormally increased minute volume. Blood gases on the other hand often show a combination of hypocapnia but a relatively low arterial oxygen tension. This suggests that the alveolar–arterial oxygen tension gradient is increased indicative of pulmonary dysfunction resulting from the brain injury.

Temperature rises after the immediate tendency to fall and reaches approximately 38°C in the first 24 hours. Pyrexia for longer than 3 days is usually due to subarachnoid haemorrhage or an infective complication. A rapidly rising temperature during the first few hours after injury, like severe tachycardia, denotes a severe head injury and poor prognosis. The same applies to marked hypothermia.

Vomiting, though not a vital sign, may be conveniently mentioned here because it may have vital consequences. It is common in the early stages of recovery from concussion although it is not usually persistent. It is potentially dangerous because vomitus may be aspirated into the airways causing unexplained sudden death in unattended patients, unexplained that is, until autopsy reveals the presence of vomitus in trachea and bronchi. Evacuation of stomach contents by naso-gastric tube suction is an essential early step in the treatment of the drowsy or comatose head injured patient.

Neurological abnormalities immediately consequent upon impact indicate widespread paralysis. There is no voluntary movement, the muscles are flaccid, the pupils are dilated and do not react to light, all reflexes are absent. The brief, jerk-like, extensor spasms evoked in animal experiments at the time or within a few seconds of impact do not occur in humans. The duration of total neuronal paralysis is usually brief. By the time medical examination is performed flaccidity has usually passed, the pupils have returned to normal size and reflexes can be obtained. In minor concussive head injury the pupils become equal and reactive, corneal reflexes brisk, and tendon and abdominal reflexes are active. The plantar responses may be extensor at first but they become flexor within a short time, often one before the other.

In severe head injury, evidence of widespread neurological dysfunction is impressive and may persist for days or weeks in accord with the prolonged disturbance of consciousness. The pupils may be dilated or contracted, equal or irregular in shape and do not react to light. The ocular axis may be misaligned with skew deviation or there may be persistent conjugate deviation to one or other side, rarely upwards or downwards. At this stage, paralysis of an ocular muscle cannot really be identified. Corneal reflexes are absent, the limbs may be spastic on one or both sides and may adopt abnormal attitudes. Common postures are with the upper limbs adducted flexed and internally rotated across the trunk or extended at the elbow and flexed at the wrist and fingers, the lower limbs adducted extended at both hip and knee with the feet plantar flexed. The picture of extensor rigidity may be bilaterally symetrical, may affect one side more than the other or may be unilateral. The head may be maintained in extension by spasm of the neck muscles, a state of opisthotonus. It may be persistently rotated to one side in which event the eyes may be deviated towards that side. Passive head turning may alter the attitude and motor response in the arms and legs. The hyper-

tonus of the limbs, though loosely described as spasticity, is so intense that it has the nature of spastic dystonia as described by Denny-Brown (1966). Dystonic attitudes persist for hours or days before gradually subsiding, though at this stage of resolution they may still be readily evoked by a painful stimulus. Frequently they are intermittent from the beginning, the patient passing spontaneously within seconds from a condition of relaxed immobility to intense extensor rigidity, accompanied by changes in respiration, flushing of the face and outpouring of sweat. The episode lasts for about a minute or so and the patient returns to the former state. The cycle may be repeated at intervals, sometimes as a result of an obvious stimulus such as nursing attention, sometimes apparently spontaneously. Involuntary movements, usually of an upper limb, may occasionally be seen, though they may easily be mistaken for simple restlessness. Coarse, waving, ballistic movements may occur and generalized tremor may accompany dystonic states.

The two abnormal postures seen in severe closed head injury, the one with extended and the other with flexed, upper limbs must originate from diffuse lesions which differ in the localization of intensity. The former is probably determined by a preponderance of damage to the afferent fibres to the upper brain stem, the latter by a preponderance in the subcortical cerebral white matter and perhaps basal grey matter. The flexed posture corresponds to the picture of decortication. The observation recorded by Strich (1961), that abnormal postures of these types were seen in patients immediately after impact is unusual. In most cases of severe head injury these abnormal postures do not develop until an hour or so after impact. The delay in their appearance may be due to prolongation of the period of diffuse neuronal inactivity (the cerebral equivalent of spinal shock, perhaps) or may be due to the delayed effects of petechial haemorrhages which require time to attain a critical size and to influence the surrounding brain.

It is remarkable the extent to which dystonic

and spastic states may resolve in survivors. In some cases there may be complete recovery, in others posturing and rigidity subside, leaving a quadri- or hemiparesis. Other permanent neurological residua include abnormalities of the pupils and of the occular movements, nystagmus, dysarthria, ataxia, tremor and rarely sensory impairment, all suggestive of brain stem dysfunction. Kremer et al. (1947) have described in detail several examples and demonstrated dilatation of the aqueduct of Sylvius in some of their cases. More recently, Van Dongen and Braakman (1980) have made similar observations. In their study CT scan showed shrinkage of brain stem and cerebellar tissue in patients with persistent ataxia following severe head injury.

Focal neurological signs, indicating a localized area of brain injury, such as contusion are not usually apparent until the patient has recovered sufficiently to cooperate in a physical examination. Prior to this point observations are limited to detecting asymmetry of reflex eye movements and pupil responses and differences between the motor response on one side and the other. At a later stage, when the patient is able to collaborate more in the examination, detectable focal abnormalities include dysphasia, dyslexia and dyscalculia, hemianopia, sensory disorders of cortical type and hemiparesis. It may be difficult to decide whether hemiparesis is of cortical origin or due to shearing of corticospinal fibres sustained as part of diffuse axonal injuries. Hemiparesis of cortical origin related to brain contusions is usually more limited and less severe. If it is extensive one may anticipate involvement of adjacent areas of cortex as shown by the presence of dysphasia or by impairment of cortical sensory function as revealed in tests of joint sense, stereognosis, tactile localization and two point discrimination.

## Symptoms

Headache is common and often severe when the patient is sufficiently rational to voice a response. The headache may be generalized, frontal or occipital and nuchal, unilateral or concentrated in an area coincident with scalp bruising or skull fracture. Posture may influence the severity of head injury, physical and mental activity may aggravate it. Slight fever and neck stiffness will suggest that subarachnoid haemorrhage is the explanation. It is common experience that the more severe the head injury the less is the severity of the headache. At an early stage of recovery, a neurotic origin of headache should not be assumed in patients who have sustained mild injuries. The conclusion to be drawn is that in severe injuries the early causes of headache have subsided by the time the patient is sufficiently recovered to complain. It is important to note that in the natural course of events in uncomplicated concussive head injury, headache usually diminishes steadily. A reversal of this normal progress requires an explanation. While some cases may be explained by increasing intracranial pressure, or a developing extradural haematoma, often the explanation is obscure. Nausea and giddiness may be troublesome symptoms which will subside with rest although giddiness and headache may recur at a later stage and are then reconsidered below.

## Sequelae of head injury

Symonds (1962) defined head injury sequelae as those symptoms which continued after the end of the period of post-traumatic amnesia. They represent patterns of disordered cerebral function which emerge as the brain injury resolves. Resolution in some places means resumption of normal physiological processes, in others scavenging to clear away irreplaceably damaged nerve cells and axons. Lesions may be of microscopic size or may involve appreciable areas of grey and of white matter that are diffuse in distribution. Russell (1931b) thought it likely that all brain systems are damaged and the rate of recovery depends more on the complexity of the system than on a concentration of trauma to any one site in the brain. It seems necessary therefore to stress the relative vulnerability of different levels of cerebral activity.

## Memory

Impairment of memory for current events is probably the commonest sequel to head injury (Brooks 1972, 1983). Its mildest manifestation may be failure to recall names and unimportant passing of events and a need to keep an *aide-mémoire*. This may constitute no more than a minor embarrassment and give rise to no difficulty in performing routine work based on skills that have been acquired in the past. More severe impairment of memory, the inability to recall associations or the fruits of experience merges into impairment of intelligence. The higher the degree of previous educational attainments the more obvious will be the disorder and the more important its effect. To what extent failure to remember depends exclusively on diffuse neuronal damage or upon damage concentrated in certain areas remain conjectural. Its general coincidence with the severity of concussion and the primacy of amnesia among the manifestations of concussion makes diffuse brain damage the likeliest cause. However, the results of bitemporal ablations for epilepsy showed the important part played by these areas of the brain and in particular the hippocampus in the processes of memory. Post mortem studies have demonstrated that localized damage in deep parts of the temporal lobe is not uncommon in head injured patients. Bilaterality of damage is crucial for impairment of recording current events and bilaterality is a frequent finding in the microscopic lesions of head injury whether produced primarily, by contusion or by secondary infarction.

## Intelligence

Impairment of intellectual processes, or in children the capacity to develop them, probably occurs to some extent as a result of all but minor degrees of concussion and even these if they are frequently repeated as in professional boxers (Roberts 1969). Slight blunting of intelligence may be difficult to identify particularly in those already less well endowed. The effect is frequently obvious to the critical judgement of close relatives yet not revealed by direct examination. In this effect head injury is more serious in the elderly for they possess a smaller reserve of neurons. The subtle change which follows injury is commonly likened to sudden ageing. This was observed long ago, for Symonds (1962) quotes Astley Cooper (1836) 'the change that takes place in the intellect from injuries of the brain is very similar to the effects of old age. The patient becomes, as it were, suddenly old'. The less obvious defects of intelligence are in the highest levels of activities, abstract thought, organization, planning for future action, for which there may be little call in many forms of employment but the lack immediately renders a person unfit for administrative duties. More severe intellectual loss merits the term mild dementia and coupled with poor memory downgrades the patient's capacity at all levels of employment. Some 30 years or so ago opinion differed as to the validity of traumatic dementia, probably because of the high mortality of severe head injury at that time. But modern methods of rescue have provided indubitable evidence in survivors. All grades of dissolution of mental activity occur after head injury and in the worst examples there is little or no evidence of intelligent reaction.

While it is true to say that following head injury many patients perform less well on intelligence testing than they did or would have done when tested prior to injury, the concept that head injury impairs intelligence does require further examination. Performance in I.Q. tests reflects many factors including the intellectual habits of a lifetime, the cultural background and motivation of the individual as well as ability to remember and respond quickly to intellectual challenge. There are also differences in the way that verbal and nonverbal parts of the intelligence quotient test are affected by head injury.

The effect of the head injury on test results depends to a large extent on the location extent and severity of focal and diffuse brain injury. Focal brain injury associated with disorders of language or mathematical calculation will clearly be associated with specific deficits in the testing of those functions that depend upon on verbal or numerical concepts. Occipital and parietal lobe damage may specifically impair those nonverbal parts of the test that depend upon visuospatial orientation and response.

In general however, the two factors that impair overall performance appear to be disorders of short-term memory and a slow-down in the rate of processing information (Brooks 1983, Gronwall & Wrightson 1981). These can be found even after minor head injury (Barth *et al.* 1983, Macflynn *et al.* 1984).

*Behaviour*

Although the deleterious effect of head injury on performance may in some cases be difficult to identify, the change in behaviour is more apparent and disturbing to the family of the injured patient. It shows in shortness of temper, inability to accept adverse events or opposition, lack of ambition and drive, lack of self control and reduction in attention span and power of concentration. The more severe disturbances may render the patient antisocial and unable to fit into the community (McKinlay *et al.* 1981). These changes concern the affective emotional aspects of life. It will be apparent that the changes in attitude and behaviour which follow head injury are similar to some of those which were noted to follow the now discarded surgical procedure of bifrontal leucotomy. It was the need to avoid such responses which prompted the modified forms of this procedure. The similarity of effects raises the question of whether focal damage of the undersurface and white matter of the frontal lobes may not be the determining factor of personality change after head injury. Even in the acute stage, the observation on computerized tomography of bifrontal contusion should

prompt the neurosurgeon to alert the nursing staff to the possibility that the patient may develop an acute behaviour disturbance in the recovery phase.

The effects of head injury in children require special comment. Presumably as a result of the buffering effect of the more yielding and elastic skull, children seem to withstand the immediate effects of head injury better than adults. They have a lower mortality and a shorter duration of coma than adults similarly injured (Becker *et al.* 1977, 1981, Bruce *et al.* 1978, Berger *et al.* 1985). On the other hand, children show a greater capacity than adults to survive for indefinite periods in a comatose or vegetative state and in the survivors of very severe head injury the incidence of post-traumatic intellectual and behaviour disturbance may be extremely high. Rowbotham *et al.* (1954) analysed 1,000 head injuries in adults and 400 in children and noted the incidence of post-traumatic personality change as 21% of the adult survivors but in 33% of the children. Hjern and Nylander (1962) reported on the sequelae of severe head injuries in children who had been in a coma for 24 hours or longer and noted 82% of survivors to be suffering from mild to severe psychiatric symptoms.

In the child, the damage sustained by head injury has important consequences for learning. In the adult, the level of intelligence already developed and acquired by experience and by formal education may be lowered by damage but enough of the previous learned pattern may remain for practical purposes. In the child the formative years are yet to come and brain damage may be sufficient to impede the normal acquisition of experience, the limitless recording of memories and associations. Progress at school may be slowed or ended and the same disturbances may impair the development of normal emotional life. Thus head injured children may show considerable behaviour disturbances arising from a combination of impaired learning and impaired emotional control. These problems may render them unsuitable for education at a normal school and make them a considerable burden to family life because of hyperactivity and unreasoning, uncontrollable tantrums (Russell 1959, Pond 1967).

*Postconcussional syndrome*

This term has been in use for many years to cover a group of symptoms, the incidence of which has been shown to bear no statistical relationship to the severity of the injury (Russell & Smith 1961). Each symptom by itself is of little consequence but the combination often proves troublesome to the patient to a degree which may render re-employment difficult or impossible. The terminology also indicates the lack of agreement as to the cause of the symptoms, whether they are organic or psychological. The syndrome includes headache, dizziness, blackouts, undue fatigue, lack of concentration, anxiety, irritability and insomnia. It is characteristic that these symptoms develop when the patients leave hospital for home, or when work is restarted, having in some cases been free from symptoms since the subsidence of the immediate post-traumatic symptoms. The headache has no particular characteristics save that it is often aggravated by activity, noise and anxiety. Dizziness is used to convey a sense of insecurity of position, a fear of falling and in some patients a blurring or transient loss of vision or sense of imminent faintness. It is often aggravated by sudden changes in posture but does not usually amount to true vertigo. In some cases the sensation of dizziness progresses suddenly to a brief loss of consciousness usually described as a 'blackout'. In such episodes patients rarely hurt themselves; nor are there any convulsive movements or urinary incontinence. Such symptoms need to be clearly distinguished from epilepsy. The dizziness also needs to be distinguished from vertigo in which there is a hallucination of rotational movement of the environment. Vertigo is a consequence of injury to the vestibular pathways in the inner ear or in the brain stem. Tests of auditory and vestibular function, including elec-trohystagmography, can help to distinguish whether the end organ or its central connections are at fault when this problem occurs after head injury.

Opinions concerning the cause of the post-concussional syndrome have varied from time to time and have been influenced by the types of patient examined. When a large number of patients suffering from postconcussional symptoms are referred in the course of litigation, the examining neurosurgeon is likely to be impressed by the lack of signs of organic brain damage and by the prominence of the syndrome associated with the most minor degrees of concussive head injury. It was such selected experience that led Henry Miller (1966) to conclude that 'these cases are much closer to malingering than any form of mental illness genuinely outside the patients control'. Neurosurgeons who have observed large consecutive series of patients who have sustained minor concussional injuries are less impressed by these aspects and more concerned with the difficulty that such patients experience in enduring the symptoms and in returning to work. Rimel *et al.* (1981) observed that 3 months after a minor concussive head injury one third of a series of 434 patients were still unable to return to work, college or school as a result of disabling postconcussional symptoms. The differentiation into organic and psychogenic causes for postconcussional symptoms may be more apparent than real, for Cartlidge (1978), in examining a series of patients with post-concussional syndrome, noted minor disturbances of vestibular function, detected by oculonystagmography, in nearly half of his patients. In other patients there was found to be a pre-injury history of frequent visits to the doctor, and in such cases it was concluded that the head injury had been a nonspecific insult to a patient with a fairly precarious personality and who already depended heavily on the services of a doctor to cope with the stresses of daily life. Taylor and Bell (1966) noted slowing of the cerebral circulation in a number of patients who were symptomatic after a concussional head injury.

# Compression of the brain

This old-fashioned term is apt to be frowned upon, but is correct in denoting the effect of extradural and subdural haemorrhage and valuable in underlying the urgency of the situation. Compression causes displacement of the brain, distortion and internal herniations, embarrasses cerebral circulation and gives rise to mounting intracranial pressure. These effects have already been described and will not be repeated here save to emphasize certain points. Increased intracranial pressure after head injury may also be caused by brain oedema, by the immediate and late effects of subarachnoid bleeding, by meningitis and by obstruction of dural venous sinuses. The incidence of post-traumatic intracranial haematoma is somewhat difficult to determine because of variations in hospital admission policies and need to be revised since the introduction of CT. If only comatose patients are considered, the incidence of haematoma detected by CT, and requiring surgical decompression, ranges between 30 and 50% (Becker *et al.* 1977, Jennett *et al.* 1979, Miller *et al.* 1981, Bowers & Marshall 1980). Lewin (1966) found intracranial haematomas in 5.8% of a series of 1750 cases of head injury of all degrees of severity. Of these, 46 were extradural, 41 were acute and 6 chronic subdural and 9 intracerebral. In a more recent series, verified by computerized tomography, Miller and Jones (1985) analysed the incidence of intracranial haematoma in 1919 consecutive admissions for head injury over a period of one year in a unit that admitted head injuries of all degrees of severity. The overall incidence of intracranial haematoma was 4.3%, comprising 17 patients with extradural haematoma, 27 with acute subdural haematoma, 5 with chronic subdural haematoma and 34 with intracerebral haematoma. The relatively greater incidence of detection of intracerebral haematoma is an undoubted effect of CT scanning. The incidence of haematoma varied considerably according to the level of consciousness of patients on admission. Of 93 comatose patients, 43% had intracranial haematomas as compared with 9%

of 210 moderately injured patients (Glasgow Coma Score 9–12). In the remaining 1616 patients scoring 13 or above on the Coma Scale the incidence of detected intracranial haematoma was only 0.7%.

### Extradural haematoma

By far the commonest site is temporal (70%) and the next is frontal (10%); posterior and vertical parasaggital locations are relatively uncommon. The actual proportions in Hooper's (1960) series were 65, 18, 11 and 10% respectively. The interval between injury and onset of symptoms can vary between several hours and weeks but is usually between 6 and 12 hours. Hooper identified the origin of the bleeding in a number of cases and found evidence of a shorter interval associated with arterial sources of haemorrhage than after venous. Once started, the cycle of events in acute brain compression moves with increasing speed so that the final deterioration is often precipitous. This lesion constitutes a surgical emergency and hesitation in diagnosis or delay in treatment is likely to have fatal consequences. Extradural haemorrhage may result from relatively minor head injury; the triviality of the injury, and absence of loss of consciousness may lead to delay in diagnosis. Extradural haemorrhage may also complicate severe brain injury, and in such cases the persisting effects of the primary brain damage may mask the picture of brain compression (Gallagher & Browder 1968, Jamieson & Yelland 1968) (Fig. 23.5). Tomlinson (1964) estimated that one quarter of cases of extradural haemorrhage occurred without loss of consciousness at the time of impact. Headache is the outstanding symptom in those patients who have not been unconscious or who regain their senses after a brief concussion. The headache is distinguishable from post-traumatic headache by increasing severity, its paroxysmal throbbing character, unrelieved by variations in posture. It may be accompanied by vomiting, often violent and profuse, often called projectile.

Deterioration of consciousness is the most

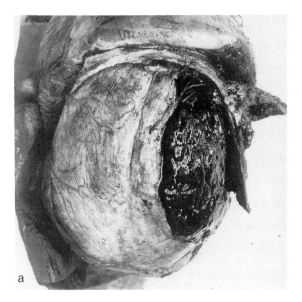
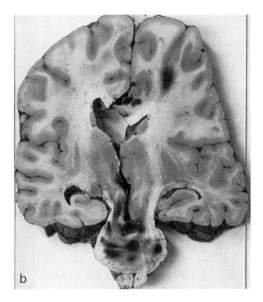

**Fig. 23.5.** Male aged 55 years, fell down lift shaft, admitted to hospital 1 hour later deeply unconscious, breathing stertorously, bleeding from both nostrils, fixed dilated pupils, all reflexes absent: died 8 hours after injury.
(a) Extensive extradural haematoma, comminuted fracture of skull (clot measured 13 × 9 × 3.5 cm).
(b) Flattening of right hemisphere, displacement of midline structures: haemorrhages in crura, pons, right cingulate gyrus (subfalcine) (corpus callosum, left globus pallidus and internal capsule in other sections); pronounced left hippocampal herniation.

important sign. It is obvious in patients who are conscious when first seen, but only one half of Hooper's patients followed the classical pattern of deterioration of consciousness after a lucid interval. Lethargy and drowsiness lead to compelling sleep and at this stage there is a real danger that the depression of conscious level may be mistaken for normal sleep and the error becomes apparent only when the patient cannot be roused much later. Drowsiness associated with headache, confusion, restlessness and incontinence is highly suspect. A high index of clinical suspicion, coupled with modern management can reduce the mortality from extradural haematoma well into single figures (Bricolo & Pasut 1984).

Slowing of the heart rate is common in the early stages of brain compression; later the pulse rate rises and the increase may be abrupt. This is an ominous sign. In the classical experiments of Cushing on the responses to rising intracranial pressure, bradycardia was accompanied by an increase of the blood pressure. This combined effect may also be seen in compression by intracranial haematoma; when it is observed it is well nigh pathognomonic but it may also be absent on many occasions and its absence should not reassure the neurosurgeon that brain compression is unlikely. Disturbances of respiratory rhythm and depth are also important signs of compression but their presence will not be detected unless the observer spends a few minutes looking and listening or employs some form of monitoring device. Several different disorders of respiratory pattern may be observed from the regular waxing and waning pattern of Cheyne–Stokes respiration to the complete irregularity of ataxic respiration.

These cardiorespiratory changes in brain compression result from embarrassment of the brain stem consequent on downward axial displacement, side to side compression and ischaema due to stretching of the perforating branches from the basilar and other main distributive cerebral

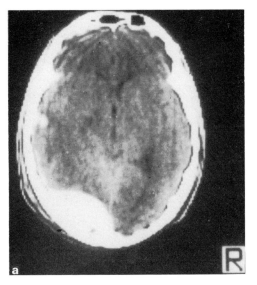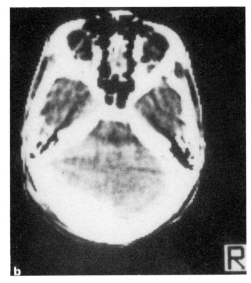

**Fig. 23.6.** Extradural haematoma shown on CT in a 27-year-old man who fell on the back of his head and had depression of consciousness to score 10 on Glasgow Coma Scale and no localizing neurological signs. a) typical lens shaped extracerebral opacity in left occipital area b) extending below tentorium (displacing transverse sinus) into posterior fossa.

arteries. Similar cardiorespiratory changes may of course follow immediately after severe primary injury and in such cases represent primary brain stem damage. The distinguishing feature from the two circumstances is the temporal sequence of events.

Extradural haematomas at sites other than the temporal area usually show modifications of the clinical picture outlined above. In general the clinical evolution is slower and the march of events through unilateral to bilateral is less clear cut. Patients with frontal extradural haematomas may show little or no evidence of lateralization; lowering of the level of consciousness may be followed shortly by bilateral pupillary abnormalities and increased tone of the limbs on both sides without any intervening hemiparesis. In extradural haematomas of the vertex, in which the sagittal sinus had been stripped from the bone, pyramidal signs may appear early and there may be marked engorgement of the retinal veins (Columella *et al.* 1968). In the posterior fossa the haemorrhage frequently lies both above and below the transverse sinus which is separated from the bone (Fig. 23.6a and b). Con-

sciousness is disturbed relatively late and there may be no abnormality of pupillary or limb function. Vital functions tend to be affected early, on the other hand, with tachycardia and slowing of the rate of respiration (Strang 1971). The particular danger of haematomas in this situation is the liability to sudden and unanticipated respiratory failure.

### Subdural haematoma

It was common practice to classify subdural collections of blood into the acute, subacute and chronic haematomas on an arbitrary basis accordingly to the interval between injury and emergency of symptoms. McKissock *et al.*(1960b) included under acute haematomas those with an interval of 3 days or less, under subacute those whose symptoms arose 4 to 21 days after injury, and under chronic those with a longer interval. This grouping, though convenient for retrospective data analysis, creates divisions where none exist, and the widespread use of CT scanning has led to the belief that the distinction between acute and subacute haematomas is particularly misleading. All of these collections of clotted blood are present soon after the injury. The later emergence of clinical symptomatology in the subacute cases is related to the degree and extent of brain oedema and swelling around the haematoma rather than to any change in the haematoma itself. It is worthwhile mentioning that whereas early computerized tomography will detect reliably virtually all acute subdural haematomas it is possible for scanning to be carried out so early that an extradural haematoma in evolution may be missed and the neurosurgical team falsely reassured. Repeat CT scanning is always warranted by the subsequent observation of neurological deterioration.

There is an undoubted distinction between the acute subdural haematomas, consisting of clotted blood, and the chronic subdural, consisting of a liquid collection, often of considerable size, and which presents so late after the head injury that there is a frequent diagnostic dilemma as to whether the patient is suffering from a post-traumatic lesion or from a brain tumour or stroke. For that reason chronic subdural haematomas require separate consideration.

Acute subdural haematoma gives rise to symptoms and signs (epiphenomena) similar to those of extradural haematoma but rarely shows the clear cut development of events often seen in extradural collections. There are several reasons for this. In the first place subdural bleeding causing symptoms shortly after injury commonly arises from cortical lacerations or from violent movements of the brain within the skull that are themselves associated with severe primary brain damage of the diffuse axonal type. This association between subdural haematoma and brain injury is reflected in a mortality which is much higher in acute subdural haematoma (30–80%) than in extradural haematoma (5–20%). Where the onset of symptoms of brain compression is delayed for several days the mortality is lower. In McKissock's series (1960b) mortality of acute haematomas was 54% and in subacute, 20%.

In acute subdural haematoma blood spreads more widely over the cerebral hemisphere

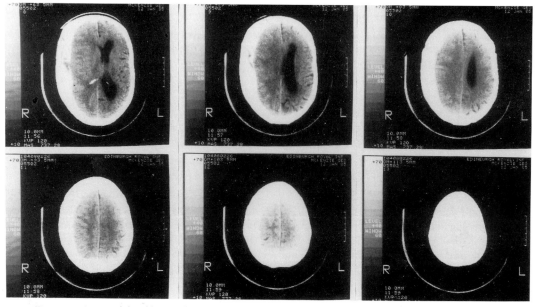

**Fig. 23.7.** Acute subdural haematoma on right side in 34-year-old man. Note the extent of the extracerebral opacity representing clotted blood and the small area of radiolucency at the centre of the haematoma which represented an area of liquid blood at the site of active haemorrhage, in this case a small cortical artery.

forming an appearance on CT of a concave–convex lesion of greater extent but of lesser thickness than the typically biconvex, lens-shaped appearance of the extradural haematoma (Fig. 23.7). The lesions are usually of increased density on CT but may conceal a pronounced isodense component, a feature that is much less common in extradural haematoma where virtually all lesions are of uniform increased density. Acute subdural haematomas are more likely to be bilateral than extradural haematomas. In one third of McKissock's cases subdural haematomas were bilateral compared to 2.4% of a series of extradural haematomas reported by the same authors (McKissock et al. 1960a).

Chronic subdural haematoma is most likely to develop in infancy and after the age of 60 years. A high incidence in the former is probably related to birth injury and a tendency to haemorrhage. In the older patients brain atrophy renders the cortical veins more susceptible to injuries as they traverse the subdural space. In addition, minor injuries to the head are more frequent in infants and in the elderly; in the former because righting reflexes have not yet been acquired or perfected in the latter because of their deterioration. When a chronic subdural haematoma is encountered in a younger adult patient the suspicion should be that the patient is also suffering from a degree of brain atrophy, often as a result of excessive intake of alcohol.

Although it is generally believed that injury to the head is the cause of subdural bleeding in most cases there are other well authenticated causes. These include rupture of a saccular or mycotic aneurysm or a vascular malformation, cortical venous thrombosis and brain tumour. Russell and Cairns (1934) described cases in which subdural bleeding had arisen from metastatic neoplastic infiltration of the dura mater. Early pathologists ascribed an inflammatory origin to the insisted subdural blood hence the term pachymeningitis interna haemorrhagica given by Virchow (Verbiest 1958). Trotter (1914) was the first to establish the traumatic origin of chronic subdural haematoma.

Infantile subdural haematoma is most common within the first six months of life and its recognition as an important illness of childhood was in the United States by Peet and Kahn (1932) who described 9 cases encountered in 3 years. Ingraham and Matson (1944) reported 98 cases seen over a 7 year period. The symptoms are those of rising intracranial pressure: drowsiness, fretfulness, vomiting, difficulty with feeding and weight loss. Convulsions are frequent and may be the first symptom. These infants commonly show enlargement of the head with bossing of the frontal bone, separation of sutures, malnutrition and pyrexia. Hemiparesis, papilloedema and retinal haemorrhages are occasional features. The clinical picture mimics that of hydrocephalus.

In adults chronic subdural haematoma may present in one of three ways: by raised intracranial pressure with no localizing signs; by fluctuating drowsiness, deteriorating to coma; and by progressive dementia with an akinetic state.

When raised intracranial pressure is present, headache, vomiting, drowsiness and papilloedema may all lead to the supposition that a neoplasm is present and the absence of localizing signs still does not permit a firm clinical diagnosis which must await computerized tomography or other neuroradiological study. When the predominant feature is a decline in the level of consciousness, this may take place during the course of days or even several weeks, beginning at first as a lack of alertness with a readiness to drop off to sleep which later becomes a true drowsiness with difficulty in arousal. Fluctuation of symptoms is often a conspicuous feature but during the drowsy periods ptosis, impairment of upward movement of the eyes and enlargement of the pupils with a sluggish light response may be present. These signs indicate tectal plate compression and represent posterior tentorial herniation, common when brain compression is bilateral or frontal in origin. When the presentation is associated with failing mental acuity this may wrongly be attributed in the elderly patient to senility or cerebral atherosclerosis. The course of the illness is however usually more rapid and progressive and a more likely diagnostic confusion is with an infiltrating frontal or corpus callosum glioma. The dulling of mental facilities is shown by apathy, lack of interest, failing memory, inability to carry out prior commitments and confusion. Incontinence of urine may be an early symptom.

In patients with chronic subdural haematoma abnormal neurological signs may be present but it is often difficult to interpret their significance. Of all circumstances in which false localizing signs may be found, subdural haematoma is perhaps the commonest. Sixth nerve palsy may occur and an extensor plantar or hemiparesis, when found, is often ipsilateral to the site of the haematoma. This feature was present in 29% of all subdural haematomas reported by McKissock et al. (1960b) and the feature is due to the so-called Kernohan's notch caused by lateral displacement of the brain stem. The contralateral cerebral peduncle impinges upon the edge of the tentorium on the opposite side, and caudal decussation of the motor pathway means that the weakness so produced is on the same side as the haematoma.

Intracerebral haemorrhage complicating head injury may be derived from surface contusions and lacerations or it may lie deep within the basal ganglia, but both forms can be linked to violent movements of the brain within the skull at the time of impact. As in acute subdural haematoma, there is an association between the presence of intracerebral haemorrhage and the occurrence of acute primary brain damage of diffuse type that relates to a common cause, but these may not be a cause and effect relationship between these two phenomena. It is the systematic computerized tomography of large series of head injured cases that has revealed intracerebral haemorrhage, or an appearance resembling densely haemorrhagic contusions, deep in the brain within hours of injury. The data of Miller et al. (1981) and of Miller and Jones (1985) show that acute subdural and intracerebral haemorrhage is relatively more common in the severely injured, comatose patient confirming the association between severity of primary brain damage and occurrence of bleeding in these sites.

By contrast, extradural haematoma is related more to the occurrence of skull fracture and shows less of an asociation with severity of brain injury.

In some cases of intracerebral haematoma, the term haemorrhagic necrosis would be a truer description. This process often occupies the temporal lobe and in some cases radical removal of the devitalized swollen tissue may be required because of brain compression (Becker et al. 1981). In other cases the haemorrhage is localized and forms a cavity within the brain. Courville and Blomquist (1940) distinguished between two varieties of traumatic intracerebral haematoma, 'adjacent' and 'central', observed at autopsy. The former type were situated immediately below an area of cortical damage, the latter were remote from any cortical lesion and lay deep within the white matter. Recent CT studies, therefore, confirm these earlier pathological observations.

## Cranial nerve injury

### Olfactory nerves

Testing the sense of smell requires cooperation from the patient. Consequently, disturbances of olfactory function are often not identified until the patient is convalescent. The test is often omitted from the examination at the time of discharge and the defect may be appreciated by the patient only by chance. The olfactory nerve or bulb may be involved in a local injury to the anterior cranial fossa but more commonly anosmia follows a diffuse type of closed head injury as a result of movements of the brain within the skull. Sumner (1964), who has made the most comprehensive study of the problem, noted that in many cases the impact had been occipital, and that the sense of smell was usually defective in both nostrils but could be partially or completely lost. He found an incidence of anosmia of 7% of all head injuries, but 30% in those cases with post-traumatic amnesia exceeding 24 hours. Recovery of function occurred in only one third of Sumner's cases; this took place within a month in half of these. Occasionally olfactory function is distorted as well as impaired so that when an odour is appreciated it is abnormal and usually unpleasant. If epileptic disturbances of an olfactory nature arise after head injury they tend to do so as a consequence of a seizure arising from deep temporal rather from frontal structures.

Patients with anosmia seldom complain spontaneously about this. They are much more likely to mention loss of the sense of taste, although when the primary taste function is tested this is usually found to be normal. The disorder is however one of the quality of taste or flavour in which olfactory stimulation plays such an important part. While it is not usually considered to be a great handicap, anosmia is potentially dangerous because the subject cannot detect a leak of gas or other possibly noxious fumes.

*The optic nerves and chiasma*

The optic nerve and more rarely the chiasma, may suffer damage as a result of local injury involving the orbit and neighbouring structures, even if this does not directly involve the optic foramen. Hooper (1951) described 58 examples of orbital injury in a series of 500 patients with head trauma and in approximately one half vision was impaired. A visual defect may follow head injury without evidence of extensive local damage although the impact is usually frontal (Turner 1943, Venables *et al.* 1978).

Goulden (1929) described various disturbances of the visual fields following injury including central scotoma, sector defects and vertical or altitudinal hemianopia. He pointed out that visual disturbance could range from slight to total, was usually restricted to one eye, and that optic atrophy took 2–6 weeks to develop. Hughes (1962) reviewed 90 cases and found that in two thirds the injury was thought to be in the canalicular portion of the optic nerve. In other cases there was funduscopic evidence of injury at the anterior end of the nerve and in

12% the field defects suggested involvement of the chiasmal end of the nerve or of the optic chiasma itself. The appearance at operation have been described by all of these authors and include haemorrhages and tears but the most common observation is of no external abnormality. It is thought that injury only occasionally tears the optic nerve or chiasma and that the damage is most commonly of ischaemic origin. Frontal impact may cause shearing stress at the junction of the fixed (canalicular) and free (intracranial) portions of the optic nerve; this may either affect the nerve directly or its nutritional vessels, or by compression from a haematoma (Skarf *et al.* 1984).

When trauma effects the optic chiasma hypothalamic damage may be anticipated. Of 30 cases of chiasmal injury collected from the literature by Traquair *et al.* (1935) polyuria occurred in 7 and progressive adiposity in 2. Traquair (1945) made the important point that chiasmal damage only occurs in severe head injury whereas optic nerve damage may occur as a result of minor injury.

In the early stages of recovery from coma, optic nerve damage may provide misleading clinical signs. The loss of afferent conduction in the optic nerve renders the pupil on that side moderately dilated and nonreactive to direct stimulation with light. The same pupil will of course contract promptly in response to light shone in the opposite eye, provided that the optic nerve is intact on that side (bilateral optic nerve damage is exceedingly rare) and the ipsilateral third nerve is undamaged by injury. Injury of both the second and third cranial nerves is nearly always due to severe orbital damage and is accompanied by local swelling, haematoma and involvement of the ocular muscles.

The full extent of visual field and acuity defects cannot be determined until the patient is sufficiently recovered to allow these to be plotted and measured. In the comatose patient the gradual development of optic atrophy will however confirm the diagnosis and allow the neurosurgeon to warn the family. Visual evoked potentials can be measured in the comatose patient by attaching light emitting diodes to the closed eyelids. Failure of transmission along the optic nerves can be detected, but only when this is complete. These tests are of limited value in the early detection of visual field disturbances.

Operative decompression of the affected optic nerve generally confers no benefit. This may be the consequence of leptomeningeal fibrosis or scarring within the optic canal and for this reason detailed examination of visual function should be accomplished as soon as possible. When vision has been lost the prognosis is poor. Hughes found that of his patients with canalicular optic nerve injury practically one half remained blind, 20% improved but none attained an acuity better than 6/12. Hooper (1969) reported that in 14 patients with complete unilateral blindness following head injury, vision returned in only 3 cases.

*Oculomotor, trochlear and abducens nerves*

These nerves may be injured within the orbit and the injury may select the branch to one muscle only (Cross 1945) or at the superior orbital fissure when basal skull fractures involve the sphenoid wing. The sixth nerve may be affected by a fracture across the apex of the petrous bone; Russell and Schiller (1949) found the sixth nerve to be frequently damaged in crushing injuries of the skull. The three nerves may all be subject to injury in cases of optic nerve trauma but the prognosis for recovery is generally better.

An important cause of diplopia following injury is fracture of the walls of the orbit with displacement of the eyeball producing misalignment of the ocular axis. These fractures may cause so much local swelling that displacement is not at first apparent, although it may be visible on computerized tomography. The patient may be unable to complain of diplopia because he is unconscious or because of eyelid closure. Early correction of the deformity is best and the neurosurgeon should take the earliest opportunity of consulting with his ophthalmological colleagues, who must be informed if the patient is to receive

an anaesthetic, so that examination under the anaesthesia can be performed.

Attention has been drawn to the signs of midbrain damage which may be seen in some comatose patients. These include abnormalities of pupil size and reaction and complex disturbances of conjugate ocular movements. Jefferson (1961) described some illustrative cases pointing out that consciousness is not necessarily lost in such patients at the moment of injury and that in some the appearance of ocular signs may be delayed.

*Trigeminal nerve*

Jefferson and Schorstein (1955) presented 66 cases and reviewed the literature on injuries to the fifth cranial nerve. In 14 cases the injury was penetrating and in these the ganglion and its divisions were equally liable to be affected. In the remaining 52 cases the injury was blunt and damaged the intracranial course of the nerve in 13 (9 ganglionic and 4 divisional) and its extracranial course in 39, the maxillary nerve or its branches being affected in 32 cases. Thus in half the total cases the sensory loss was in the distribution of the second division of the trigeminal nerve. Injury of the ganglion did not always affect the motor root; the resulting analgesia was usually dense and permanent. Pain was often troublesome in the early stages of peripheral injuries but *tic douloureux* was not a sequel of trigeminal injury. Injuries of the ganglion usually arise from a fracture of the base of the skull and the root may rarely be torn completely from the ganglion. Other cranial nerves are sometimes affected; in one of their patients there was an optic nerve lesion with total internal and external ophthalmoplegia. More recent papers (Summers & Wirtschafter 1979, Norman *et al.* 1982) have confirmed the observations of Jefferson and Schorstein (1955).

## Facial nerve

The facial nerve may be injured in its extra-cranial course as a result of a blow on the side of the head which may also fracture the ascending ramus or neck of the mandible. The injury may affect only part of the nerve as shown by the selective nature of the paralysis and in such cases recovery is usually complete. The nerve is however, more commonly injured in its course through the petrous bone as a result of a fracture; in these cases the palsy is usually complete and may be immediate or its onset may be delayed for some days. When facial nerve palsy is immediate it is usually assumed that conduction has ceased as a result of traction, torsion or tearing at the time of impact. Delayed facial palsy is usually considered to be the result of slow compression by haemorrhage or oedema within the facial canal or possibly due to ischaemia by damage to the arterial supply of the nerve.

The figures of Turner (1943) and Gurdjian and Webster (1958) suggest an incidence of trau-matic facial palsy of 3% of head injury cases admitted to hospital. Associated nerve deafness indicates that the injury is in the proximal part of the course of the nerve where the seventh and eighth nerve are travelling together. In these cases the fracture often traverses the petrous bone through the internal auditory meatus. The sense of taste on the anterior two thirds of the tongue will be impaired if the nerve has been injured proximal to the point of departure of the chorda tympani. The prognosis of traumatic facial paralysis is usually good, particularly when palsy is of the delayed type. Turner reported 27 complete and 6 incomplete recov-eries of 36 immediate facial palsies and 32 recov-eries of 34 delayed palsies. These excellent results form a strong case against the practice of surgical decompression of the facial nerve.

## Eighth nerve

Injuries of the middle and inner ears and of the eighth cranial nerve produce a wide variety of symptoms ranging from minor degrees of gid-diness and unsteadiness to severe vertigo, tin-nitus and deafness which may be conductive in type, or receptive, due to damage to the cochlear or to the auditory nerve. Some of these symptoms have been discussed under the sequelae of minor head injury. Giddiness may be due to laby-rinthine damage, to lesions in the vestibular pathways, or it may be a symptom of vasomotor instability or neurosis. Hughes (1964) gave an incidence of middle ear disorder of 7%, and of internal ear disorder of 1% in a series of head injuries. Of the patients with internal ear dis-orders deafness occurred in 63% and was accompanied by facial palsy in 33%.

An important item in the investigation of these cases is the radiological examination of the petrous bone. Proctor et al. (1956) studied these fractures in cadaver skulls and found that they occurred as an indirect result of impact in the vault which had a bursting effect. Two varieties of fracture are usually described: the common longitudinal form which runs the length of the petrous bone, determined by the eustachian and carotid canals, and the transverse fracture, at right angles to the long axis, which may traverse the internal auditory meatus and the jugular foramen or the internal meatus and the laby-rinth. With a longitudinal fracture of the petrous bone the facial and auditory nerves are likely to escape injury whereas with a transverse fracture the internal ear and both nerves are usually involved. Cawthorne (1945) considered that the vestibular end organs must also be damaged by the violent movement of the head at impact. In concussed patients referred for otological inves-tigation, he found a high incidence of abnormal caloric responses while hearing tests gave normal results in over half of these cases. Phillips (1945) made an otological study of 449 cases of head injury of which 30% complained of giddi-ness. Abnormal responses to vestibular tests were found in some patients without symptoms but a much greater degree of abnormality was detected in those patients who complained of giddiness. Of patients who had acoustic symp-toms, giddiness was present in approximately two-thirds often accompanied by nystagmus and blurred vision or diplopia. Deafness due to damage in the middle ear, may be expected to improve, whereas deafness due to internal ear damage is likely to be permanent.

Injuries of the petrous bone are commonly associated with rupture of the tympanum and cerebrospinal otorrhoea. Treatment in the early stages is aimed at avoidance of infection by keeping the ear clean and covered with a sterile pad. Such patients must be considered at risk from meningitis or mastoiditis and must be observed carefully. This risk is, of course, much higher if the ear has been previously involved in a chronic infective process. The use of prophylactic antibiotics in patients not primarily infected is considered controversial at the present time and routine practice varies from centre to centre. Post-traumatic CSF otorrhoea seldom persists more than a few days.

*Ninth, tenth, eleventh and twelfth nerves*

Injury of the last four cranial nerves is usually associated with a fracture of the basisphenoid and basiocciput and may be detected only *post mortem*. Most of the few recorded cases of traumatic injury to the lower cranial nerves have resulted from penetrating injuries rather than closed head trauma. Where persisting disorders of swallowing or vocal cord function occur after closed head injury these are usually in association with marked ataxia and are more probably due to the residua of primary brain stem damage than to injury of specific cranial nerves (Britt *et al.* 1980).

*Thrombosis of the carotid or vertebral artery*

A rare complication of head injury is vascular occlusion by thrombosis of a carotid or vertebral artery in the neck. Thrombosis of the internal carotid artery as a result of direct local neck injury is well recognized and an obvious example is that which follows a missile wound, the missile

passing close to and contusing the artery without lacerating it. Hughes and Brownell (1968) described three cases and reviewed the literature. They also pointed out the artery could suffer indirect injury leading to thrombosis if violent movements of the head and neck exerted longitudinal traction on the artery. Cairns (1942) and Sedzimir (1955) reported 7 cases in each of which there was a head injury with frontal impact. In two patients in whom autopsy was carried out there was a fracture across the body of the sphenoid bone and Sedzimir considered that the thrombosis might have arisen as a result of injury to the wall of the carotid artery at the point of its emergence from the cavernous sinus into the intracranial cavity. Thrombosis usually extends proximally and angiography does not reveal whether clotting started in the neck or in the cavernous portion of the artery.

Vertebral artery thrombosis may similarly complicate head injury. It is more likely to occur if there is damage to cervical vertebrae such as a fracture dislocation (Gurdjian *et al.* 1963).

# Treatment of head injury

The management of a case of head injury will be considered under the following six headings:

1 assessment of neurological dysfunction and risk of complications;
2 sequential observation of response;
3 care of the unconscious patient;
4 complications;
5 scalp wounds and fractures;
6 rehabilitation and prognosis.

**Assessment of neurological dysfunction and risk of complications**

A rapid preliminary general examination must be carried out to determine the degree of head injury, the presence of injuries elsewhere in the body, the state of the vital functions and evidence of shock (Table 23.4). If the patient is unconscious the airway must claim first attention. This

**Table 23.4** Initial assessment of the head injured patient.

Airway, respiration, oxygenation
blood pressure, heart rate, peripheral circulation

Conscious level (Glasgow Coma Scale)
Comparison of left with right side responses (focal signs)
Pupil sizes and direct vs consensual light response
Reflex eye movements (OCR or OVR)

Total injury inventory: skin, soft tissue, bone, viscera
Urine for blood
Abdomen for bleeding
X-rays: skull, lateral cervical spine, others as indicated

is true, whatever may prove to be the cause of loss of consciousness. The mouth should be cleared of mucus, blood, dentures, loose teeth, foreign bodies, and the pharynx and trachea cleared by aspiration of blood and secretions. An airway should be inserted or the body turned on the side or semi-prone, and the stomach emptied by nasogastric tube. Profuse bleeding from the scalp or a wound elsewhere should be temporarily controlled by a pressure pad, haemostat or temporary suture. The arterial pressure, heart rate and state of the peripheral circulation should be recorded. The general examination can now be carried out, with particular attention to evidence of local trauma to the head, discharge of blood or cerebrospinal fluid from nose and ears, sign of injury to the limbs, palpation of the spinal column for deformity or tenderness, injury to the thorax (surgical emphysema, pneumothorax or haemothorax) and to the abdomen.

The level of consciousness should be carefully assessed and recorded in terms of the best response on the Glasgow Coma Scale to standard stimuli of eye opening, motor response and verbal response. The corneal and pupillary light reflexes should be tested and the size of the pupils noted. The limbs should be observed for spontaneous or involuntary movement then tested for the motor response to command or pain. The findings should be recorded on a neurostatus chart together with the blood pressure and heart rate (Fig. 23.8) and repeated every 15 or 30 minutes. The facts concerning the accident and information concerning the past medical history

of the patient should be sought from the attendant or should be obtained by telephone from the relatives and/or a previous medical observer. It is the practice in many accident departments that, upon this assessment which is preliminary, X-rays are taken of the relevant areas before the patient arrives in the admission ward. The head and cervical spine should be included in the investigation provided the patient is not restless. No anaesthetic is permissible at this immediate stage, whether for radiological or other purposes. The indications for a skull X-ray after a recent head injury are as follows:

1 loss of consciousness or amnesia at any time;
2 neurological symptoms or signs;
3 discharge of cerebrospinal fluid or blood from the nose or ear;
4 suspected penetrating injury, scalp bruising, swelling or laceration;
5 alcohol intoxication making neurological evaluation difficult;
6 other difficulties in assessing the patient, for example children and patients with seizures.

It is at this stage of preliminary assessment in an accident and emergency department that a decision must be taken whether or not the patient should be admitted to hospital. The decision can be difficult when the injury has apparently been slight and the patient has fully recovered his senses by the time he is seen. The following criteria for admission to hospital after a recent head injury may be helpful:

1 confusion or any other depression of the level of consciousness at the time of examination;
2 skull fracture, clinical or radiological evidence;
3 signs of neurological dysfunction;
4 severe headache or vomiting;
5 difficulty in assessing the nervous system of the patient because of alcohol, being young, or epilepsy;
6 presence of serious coexisting medical conditions such as haemophilia, anticoagulant therapy, diabetes mellitus;

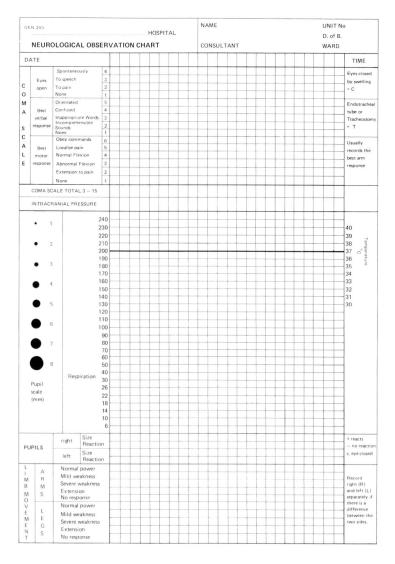

**Fig. 23.8.** Neurological observation chart for sequential evaluation of head injured patients, incorporating Glasgow Coma Scale, pupillary reactions and vital signs.

7   poor social conditions at the patient's home or a lack of a responsible adult or relative to carry out observations after discharge from hospital.

Patients with one or more of these factors should be admitted to hospital (Mendelow *et al.* 1982). It should be noted that a short period of post-traumatic amnesia with full recovery of mental function is not an indication for admission on its own (Weston 1981). If the patient is not admitted to hospital, he should return home provided he will not be alone there, and there is written information for his family and his doctor, to whom he should report any untoward symptoms and whom he should visit the next day. A patient who has been concussed should not be allowed to spend that night alone. If no companion can be arranged he should be admitted.

Since the advent of routine CT scanning, in most cases of moderate and severe head injury there is considerable information available concerning the combinations of clinical factors that are associated with the development of intracranial haematomas complicating head injury. The crucial observations at this early stage in observation and management of the patient are whether the patient is fully alert or drowsy and whether or not there is a skull fracture (Mendelow *et al.* 1983). In adult patients the combination of drowsiness or abnormal neurological signs with a skull fracture, increases the risk that that patient may be harbouring a traumatic intracranial haematoma several hundred times over the risk of haematoma developing in a patient who is alert with no skull fracture. The risk of an intracranial haematoma in a patient who is drowsy with a skull fracture can be as high as 25%. In a patient who is comatose when evaluated the risk is twice as high again (Becker *et al.* 1977). Based on these risk factors and other data, criteria can be evolved for those injured patients who are admited initially to general surgical units to decide which patients should be referred on to a neurosurgical unit. Criteria for neurosurgical consultation include one or more of the following:

1   coma that continues after resuscitation;
2   neurological deterioration since admission;
3   skull fracture in combination with:
    a)   confusion or other depression of the level of consciousness
    b)   focal neurological signs
    c)   epilepsy
4   suspected open injury of skull vault or base;
5   depressed fracture of the skull;
6   confusion or other neurological disturbance that persists for more than 12 hours if there is no skull fracture.

Great emphasis has been placed upon the presence of a skull fracture as increasing the risk of development of intracranial haematoma. This applies only to adult patients. Children may develop extra or subdural haematoma in the absence of any skull fracture, due presumably to the greater ease of in and out bending of the skull that can take place in the infant without fracture. The criteria shown above for admission for skull X-ray and for referral to a neurosurgical unit refer to adult patients. For children additional

vigilance is required. Depression of consciousness and motor dysfunction may be difficult to detect. In children there may be an abrupt transition from a flexor motor response with restlessness to flaccidity with no motor response at all. For this reason it is always safer in case of any doubt at all, to admit the head injured child to hospital for detailed and repeated observation.

### Sequential observation of response

Observation of the head injured patient at frequent regular intervals is an essential part of care, ensuring early detection of complications. The nursing staff of the neurosurgical unit make these observations and record them promptly and legibly on an observation chart that in most UK centres incorporates the features of the Glasgow Coma Scale, the pupillary light response, the relative strength of movements of the limbs on right and left sides and the

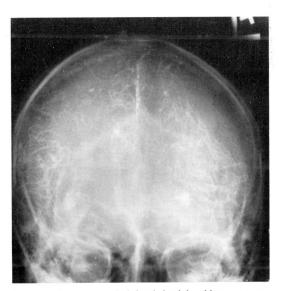

**Fig. 23.9** Angiogram of a left-sided subdural haematoma: avascular area beneath left parietal calvarium, subjacent vessels compressed, marked subfalcine displacement of midline vessels, 'crossed circulation' elicited by digital compression of right carotid artery. Both choroid plexuses calcified, the left is slightly displaced medially. Male aged 58 years, 2 weeks history of headache and weakness of right leg, no known head injury.

traditional chart of temperature, blood pressure, pulse rate and respiration rate (Fig. 23.9). The level of intracranial pressure may in some instances be included in this chart as well. The interval at which observations are recorded must vary with the severity of the injury; quarter or half hourly recording is advisable for the first 2 or 3 hours in all but minor cases, progressing to hourly then two hourly, four hourly and 12 hourly observations as the patient improves.

### Care of the unconscious patient

*Posture*

On theoretical grounds, elevation of the head and shoulders is regarded as the best position to promote venous drainage from the head and to facilitate diaphragmatic ventilation. In the comatose patient maintenance of an unobstructed air way must take precedence; in the absence of an endotracheal tube this can be assured only by nursing the patient in the horizontal position on the side or semiprone. If this position is adopted the under leg should be flexed at the hip and knee to provide a broad base for support, the upper leg should lie extended with thin pillows between the two limbs to protect pressure points. The underarm may be flexed under the trunk or placed in front or behind, the overarm should be supported on pillows; pillows placed behind the trunk prevent the patient from turning into the supine position and keep the weight of the over arm off the thorax where it can hinder respiratory movements. The head also lies on its side supported in such a way that the head lies with its midline axis in continuity with that of the trunk. Angulation or rotation may obstruct the great veins of the neck. The head should be turned slightly towards the pillow so that saliva or vomitus can trickle out of the lower corner of the mouth. If the patient is put in this position he should be turned from one side to the other at regular intervals, two hourly at first.

Patients who are treated by intubation and artificial ventilation are usually nursed more on their backs but they should also be turned partially to the side and particular attention must be paid to the pressure points; if possible the head of the bed should be elevated.

*Shock*

The preliminary assessment in the accident and emergency department may reveal the presence of systemic arterial hypotension (systolic blood pressure $< 95$ mmHg) and other signs of surgical shock. This complication is present in 15% of patients with severe head injury (Miller *et al.* 1981); when it is found it should immediately prompt a close search for evidence of a causative injury elsewhere, because surgical shock is almost never due to primary brain injury (Illingworth & Jennett 1965). Once an adequate airway has been established, the reversal of surgical shock must take precedence over all other treatment for the head injury; neurological evaluation of the patient is of no value until blood pressure has been restored to normal levels. Persistent arterial hypotension due to intracranial damage is unusual and usually indicates a lethal premorbid state. The exception to this is children, who may lose a significant part of their blood volume through simple scalp lacerations or even subgaleal haematoma.

The search for a source of haemorrhage in a shocked comatose patient must be urgent and thorough. It should include peritoneal lavage or mini laparotomy in all cases in whom intra-abdominal injury cannot be excluded. In a study of 60 severely head injured patients, in whom peritoneal lavage was carried out when intra-abdominal bleeding could not be excluded firmly, Butterworth *et al.* (1980) located 10 instances of intra-abdominal bleeding. All of these cases were submitted for laparotomy and in every case a significant intra-abdominal haemorrhagic lesion was found. It is of some interest that 4 of these 10 patients had entirely normal blood pressure at the time of the investigation and treatment. A rare, nonhaemorrhagic, source for arterial hypotension following head injury that should be kept in mind is a concomitant high spinal injury. In the elderly patient, head injury may precipitate cardiac arrythmias or myocardial infarction (Lewin 1966).

Whatever the cause, surgical shock requires immediate treatment with intravenous infusion of crystalloid solutions followed by blood or blood substitute. The foot of the bed should be elevated or inflatable trousers used if there is any difficulty in regaining a normal level of arterial pressure.

*Pulmonary ventilation*

A most important factor in saving life and reducing morbidity is the care given to respiratory efficiency, the avoidance of anoxic anoxia. This insult inflicts fresh widespread damage to the brain largely of an irreversible nature; it causes cerebral oedema and brain swelling which causes further damage. Hypoxia aggravates the neuronal damage already sustained by the traumatic brain injury and delays recovery. Emphasis has been placed on the need for simple methods of measuring ventilation and blood gases because clinical judgement may err. Hugh-Jones (1959) pointed out that cyanosis is a most insensitive test of hypoventilation and anoxaemia and that considerable retention of carbon dioxide can occur before there is any visible colour change in the skin or lips. Arterial oxygen tension is commonly reduced below 8 kPa before cyanosis is detectable.

Attention to the airway should be started at scene of the accident by the ambulance officer and should continue until the patient is sufficiently conscious for his reflexes to provide adequate protection against respiratory obstruction. Tracheobronchial suction and toilet when the patient is admitted to hospital often greatly improves respiration, when it has been embarrassed by inhaled vomitus. Correct positioning can enable gravity to promote the flow of mucus and foreign material from the upper lung into the trachae, pharynx and mouth which the attending nurse can clear. If the tongue or lips are swollen or if there is any faciomaxillary frac-

ture an airway should be inserted. Any fluid accumulating in the pharynx and nose should be removed by regular aspiration. Turning the patient from side to side on a two hourly basis ensures that each lung gets the benefit of gravity drainage and free expansion. If drainage from the lungs is unsatisfactory it can be aided by elevating the foot of the bed for short intervals of time. The physiotherapist can help considerably in improving ventilation and reducing pulmonary collapse. Every patient who has been unconscious for more than a few hours is very likely to acquire respiratory infection. Opinions vary as to the value of prophylactic antibiotics. They are certainly no substitute for regular physiotherapy and airway suction.

If efficient ventilation cannot be achieved and maintained by these methods endotracheal intubation should be considered, either through the mouth or nose. Typical indications for endotracheal intubation followed by artificial ventilation in a head injured patient are:

1  presence of an intracranial haematoma in a comatose patient;
2  deep coma with abnormal motor responses (abnormal flexor or extensor and indications of brain stem dysfunction);
3  respiratory indications (pulmonary contusion or collapse, fat embolism, concomitant head and chest injury).

An endotracheal tube can nowadays be maintained *in situ* for at least two weeks and sometimes longer. For that reason, tracheostomy is seldom performed in head injured patients today. Endotracheal intubation permits the patient to be nursed supine or in a semisitting position but frequent positional changes are still advisable for the proper aereation and emptying of the lungs and for care of the skin. The air breathed by the patient should be humidified and continuous vigilance is necessary to ensure that blockage of the tube by viscous mucus does not take place and that the tube does not migrate down into one main bronchus.

In virtually all cases where an endotracheal tube has been placed intermittent positive pressure ventilation is started and the patient treated with a combination of a sedative drug and a muscle relaxant.

Oxygenation of the head injured patient may become inadequate despite the presence of a satisfactory airway for any one of several reasons (Frost 1977, Baigelman & O'Brien 1981). Patients who have sustained a moderate or severe head injury have impairment of the cough reflex; aspiration of gastric contents is a constant hazard in the head injured patient. Even when a cuffed endotracheal tube is *in situ*, with the tube inflated, the patient is still not immune from the possibility of aspiration. Artificially ventilated patients who develop spontaneous respiration and make violent inspiratory efforts can suffer aspiration of gastric contents under these special circumstances. An increase in the perfusion by blood of poorly ventilated lung units results in shunting of blood and the development of an increased alveolar–arterial oxygen gradient. In comatose head injured patients a sizable alveolar arterial gradient for oxygen has been demonstrated in more than 80% of cases. Another cause of impaired oxygenation is the development of neurogenic pulmonary oedema. This phenomenon, seen in its most florid state in young patients, is associated with systemic vasoconstriction and pulmonary vasodilation, resulting in flooding of the pulmonary capillary bed with blood under increased pressure. This produces a considerable net outflow of water into the lung tissue, resulting in stiffening of the lung and impairment of oxygen exchange across the alveolar wall. Pulmonary oedema is also a feature of the adult respiratory distress syndrome, seen in multiply injured patients. A similar picture can result also from lung infection. Many severely head injured patients develop tachypnoea and hyperventilation and when this becomes excessive, oxygenation can be affected adversely. When pulmonary collapse is major and a large bronchus is affected then emergency bronchoscopy and direct toilet of the affected bronchi is indicated.

Head injuries do not always occur in isolation and many patients with head injury, particularly those who have sustained them in road traffic accidents, may have sustained concomitant injuries to the chest wall, lungs or diaphragm. The neurosurgeon should always be alert for the possibility of multiple rib fractures, producing an unsupported segment of chest wall, pneumothorax, haemothorax, lung contusion and traumatic rupture of the diaphragm. This last condition is frequently missed in the initial evaluation and about half of the recorded cases have presented late because of the effects of delayed herniation of an abdominal viscus into the thoracic cavity (Miller & Howie 1968).

Finally, it should be remembered that treatments applied to head injured patients may secondarily effect lung function or immunocompetence and the liability to pulmonary infection. High dose glucocorticoids fall into this category and so, probably, do barbiturates.

It is important that the adequacy of the patient's respiratory efforts be assessed frequently and a check made on blood gas levels and pH in arterial blood. In the patient who has a reduced level of consciousness, particularly the patient who is already in coma, any doubts about the adequacy of respiration should result in artificial ventilation being applied. In patients who are at the lower end of the coma scale, scoring 3, 4, or 5, it is probably wise to institute artificial ventilation regardless of the blood gas figures, as soon as it is clear that the patient is not going to make a rapid recovery. In most centres a large tidal volume and a relatively slow rate, for example 12/minute, is preferred. If hypoxaemia persists, the inspired oxygen fraction can be increased and/or positive end-expiratory pressure applied.

As indicated in Chapter 2, most processes which produce intracranial pressure, brain distortion and downward axial shift of the brain stem are likely to result in respiratory arrest. When this occurs suddenly as an unexpected event it is an emergency which should be treated vigorously, for it may have a remediable cause. If an airway is not already in place this must be established immediately and artificial respiration commenced, using an Ambu bag to start with and then the artificial ventilator. A decision must be made whether the respiratory arrest was due to raised intracranial pressure and whether relief of that increase in pressure can be provided quickly. Speed of decision and action are absolute requirements if spontaneous respiration is to be re-established. Every neurosurgeon will have experienced the gratifying relief of seeing the patient breathe once more, after an operative manœuvre to reduce raised intracranial pressure; many will also have had disappointments when such efforts have failed. The question often arose in the past concerning the length of time for which a patient should be maintained on artificial ventilation following an episode of several raised intracranial pressure. Once artificial respiration had been started there was a reluctance to discontinue it. The patient then remained in an unresponsive state somewhere between life and death, and could remain in that state for many days, a harrowing experience for relatives and for nurses. When death finally supervened, autopsy commonly disclosed advanced autolysis of the brain, indicating massive infarction of several days duration, the so-called ventilator brain.

### The definition of brain death

The introduction and widespread adoption of standardized criteria for the diagnosis of brain death were not easy to achieve, but have greatly clarified the procedure in the UK for deciding when to turn off the ventilator. This decision must be made by two doctors, one of whom should be the consultant in charge of the case and the other at least 5 years registered. These two doctors should see the patient on two occasions and should be able to verify that the patient is not hypothermic or under the influence of any relaxant, sedative or other drugs that depress brain function. The cause of the neurological deterioration should be known and declared; on examination, the patient should not exhibit any response to pain applied to the face and neck, and there should be no signs of brain stem reflex activity. Testing should include the pupil light response, the corneal reflex and the oculo vestibular response to irrigation of both ears with ice-cold saline. Patients who fail to give any response during this neurological examination may still exhibit withdrawal reflexes of the legs when painful stimuli are applied to the feet. Finally, a test to see whether spontaneous respiration is possible must be carried out. To do this, the patient is disconnected from the ventilator while the airway is flooded with oxygen from a tracheal catheter through which a gas flow of 6 litres/minute is suffused. Under these conditions the apnoeic patient does not become hypoxic over a period of several minutes, provided that lung function is satisfactory. During this period of testing, therefore, it is wise to monitor the heart rate, and blood pressure; at the end of the period of apnoeic oxygenation of 5 or more minutes an arterial blood sample should be drawn for measurement of gases and pH, immediately prior to the reconnection of the patient with the ventilator. If there has been no attempt at spontaneous respiration despite an increase in the arterial $PCO_2$ of more than 1 kPa from normal values, then the relatives are informed that the patient has shown no signs of sentient brain activity but that he has been reconnected to the ventilator, and the second and final test will be carried out at a specific time, usually about 6 hours later. The relatives are informed that if the patient fails to show any sign of brain function at the end of the second period of testing, the patient will be declared dead and the ventilator will then be switched off.

It is noteworthy that at no point in the test procedures for establishment of criteria of brain death in the UK is there a legal requirement to employ recording of the electroencephalogram, evoked potentials, or to use intravenous injections of radioisotopes. The decisions concerning brain death are made at the bedside.

*Nourishment of the head injured patient*

After head injury there is no need to give fluid
or food for the first 12 hours in a moderately or
mildly injured adult and in the first 6 hours in a
moderately or mildly injured child. In the
severely injured patient a nasogastric tube
should be passed but this should at first be used
to aspirate the stomach during the first 48 hours
after injury, to reduce the risk of aspiration of
gastric contents. Fluids should be provided by
the intravenous route. Once bowel sounds
return, then feeding by nasogastric tube can
commence starting with half strength milk and
gradually working up to a liquid feed of high
calorific content. The calorific requirements of
head injured patients are considerable particularly when the patient is experiencing spontaneous abnormal movements; 3,000 calories a
day may be required just to keep the patient in
balance (Clifton *et al.* 1985).

The total quantity of fluid given in each 24
hours should be governed by hourly measurements of the urinary output with sufficient
additional fluid to cover the insensible loss, as
well as other fluid losses, such as CSF drainage.
It is crucial to keep up with the urinary output
and not to adopt a regimen of a fixed volume of
fluid. This is particularly important in the patient
who has been given intravenous mannitol and
who may experience extensive diuresis or who
develops diabetes insipidus. The adages about
keeping the patient dry practiced in former years
probably erred on the conservative side, and in
some cases produced an undesirable element of
hypovolaemia. This may not produce any problem under normal conditions; but in patients
who are given any form of anaesthetic drug,
including agents to reduce intracranial pressure,
an underlying hypovolaemia is likely to result in
the development of arterial hypotension; this is
a severe insult to the brain of the head injured
patient that should be avoided at all costs
(Miller 1985).

When it becomes clear that the patient may
be able to swallow this should be started gently,
with clear fluids at first, semi solids and then the
full diet under careful and constant supervision.
If attempts to introduce food into the mouth
result in coughing or choking these should
immediately be discontinued. There is a very real
danger of aspiration of swallowed material into
the bronchial tree at this crucial stage in the
recovery of the head injured patient, and constant vigilance must be the rule.

*Temperature*

Patients with head injury may present with a
wide range of body temperatures ranging from
hypothermic to pyrexial. Low body temperature
may be the result of exposure associated with the
circumstances of the injury or, at a late stage in
an overwhelming brain injury when brain death
has occurred or impending, the patient may
become poikilothermic. It is not infrequently
necessary to warm up a patient in order to satisfy
the criteria for brain death testing. Hypothermia
due to exposure in the operating theatre or in
the ward is an especial hazard in young children.
Elevations of body temperature may be central
in origin or due to subarachnoid haemorrhage,
or intracranial or systemic infections. Whatever
the cause efforts should be made to reduce the
body temperature to normal because elevated
body temperature has definite ill effects on the
brain; cerebral blood vessels tend to dilate,
intracranial pressure rises and the rate of formation of vasogenic brain oedema is increased
(Clasen *et al.* 1974).

Cooling a pyrexial patient can be achieved by
the use of a bedside fan, by tepid sponging or
application of wet sheets and helped by aspirin
suppositories. Shivering may commence and this
will tend to elevate the body temperature. It may
be counteracted by the administration of chlorpromazine; this will induce vasodilatation of the
skin and reduce spontaneous shivering. Chlorpromazine does, however, have sedative effects
and the blood pressure, respiration and level of
consciousness should all be closely monitored if
this drug is used in a spontaneously breathing
patient. The goal of this treatment is to reduce

body temperature to normal. It is not to induce hypothermia. This therapeutic modality which was advocated some years ago by Rosomoff *et al.* (1961), is no longer in general use. Where it is necessary to warm up a hypothermic patient this is most easily achieved by the use of an insulating blanket.

### Bladder care

In severely head injured patients the use of an indwelling catheter is important, not to prevent wetting of the bed, but in order to ensure that an accurate measurement may be made of urine output. When fluid balance becomes less critical, wet beds can still be avoided by the use of a condom strapped to the penis and connected to drainage tubing. In the patient who is emerging from coma the desire to micturate may produce considerable restlessness and even quite violent behaviour. Well trained nursing staff will recognize this and arrange for the patient to be taken to the toilet at the appropriate time.

### Bowel care

Enemas are seldom required. Laxative suppositories may be used if needed. In some cases when the patient is on prolonged nasogastric tube feeding some adjustment of the composition of the feed may be necessary to avoid diarrhoea.

### Physiotherapy

It is never too early for the physiotherapist to begin working with the head injured patient (Rosenthal *et al.* 1983). In the initial phase the principal role of the physiotherapist will be to help with the care of the airway and to ensure that there is proper clearance of bronchial secretion. At this stage, attention to the limbs will be to ensure that a full range of passive movements continues to be available. These passive movements may be of great importance in 'imprinting' information about motor function during the early recovery phase. The physiotherapist will help in minimizing abnormal postures in the severely head injured patient by advising as to the best position in which the patient should be nursed making use of the relationship between the tonic neck reflexes and limb muscle tone. As the patient proceeds in his recovery, the help of the physiotherapist is invaluable in aiding the patient's ability to balance and coordinate, to restore muscle power and to ensure that gait and stance are as normal as possible.

### Sedative and analgesic drugs

The neurosurgeon is always extremely wary about the use of sedative and analgesic drugs in head injured patients. Requirement of these agents in the early stages after injury may be an indication for the institution of artificial ventilation. Moderate degrees of restlessness do not require drug therapy; spontaneous movement of the patient helps ventilation and limb circulation. Again it should be remembered that the urge to defaecate or the sensation of a distended bladder may be a powerful source of restless behaviour. In some patients however, who are recovering from the head injury, the degree of spontaneous activity is clearly excessive and there is a danger of the patient hurting himself or doing damage to other patients or staff. In these cases it may be necessary to prescribe a drug with a tranquillizing influence. Chlorpromazine, 25 mg repeated as required, is beneficial; its use should be attended by the appropriate caution. Chlormethiazole (Heminevrin) up to 10 mg/kg as an 0.8% intravenous solution may also be useful.

Headache and pain from other injuries may also cause restlessness and distress in a patient unable yet to express his symptoms clearly in words. In the early stages of recovery from head injury it is undesirable to give an analgesic which is so powerful that it may blur the clinical picture and obscure evidence of raised intracranial pressure. This may in fact be the source of the headache. Strong analgesic drugs should not be given until the possibility of cerebral compression has been excluded. Aspirin 600 mg or codeine phosphate 60 mg are often sufficient. Where there is a larger amount of pain from fractured ribs or another localized injury, control of the pain can sometimes be safely achieved by the use of local anaesthetic block or immobilizing the part. If a systemic agent has to be used, 10 mg of morphine, diluted to 10 ml and injected intravenously in aliquots of 1–3 ml will provide satisfactory pain relief. Once again however, great care should be taken to observe the patient for respiratory depression following administration of this drug. Where the patient is intubated and receiving artificial ventilation much greater freedom can be exercised in the administration of analgesic drugs. These may include phenoperidine up to 0.5 mg/kg, omnopan up to 0.2 mg/kg and fentanyl up to 3 $\mu$g/kg.

### Monitoring of intracranial pressure

Raised intracranial pressure is common in patients with severe head injury (Miller *et al.* 1977 & 1981, Narayan *et al.* 1982) and it is now recognized that there are particular indications for monitoring the intracranial pressure in head injured patients. In general, these would include all artificially ventilated patients, since the muscle relaxants and sedatives administered to these patients rob the neurosurgeon of the opportunity for neurological assessment. Thus monitoring would be carried out in comatose patients who have had a craniotomy for removal of a haematoma (risk of raised ICP 70%), patients without a haematoma, but whose best motor score is abnormal flexion or worse, and those in whom CT strongly suggests raised ICP. The most reliable sign on CT is effacement of the third ventricle and the perimesencephalic cisterns (Teasdale *et al.* 1984). When ICP rises over 25 mmHg treatment should be instituted.

### Therapy for raised intracranial pressure

Despite the advocacy of a wide number of anaesthetic drugs for control of raised intracranial pressure, the mainstays of treatment continue to be hyperventilation, CSF drainage, where this is possible and osmotherapy. Hyperventilation is simple to arrange when the patient is being artificially ventilated. Becker *et al.* (1977) emphasized the use of a large tidal volume and relatively slow rate. Arterial $PCO_2$ levels of 3 KPa should be aimed at; if the cerebral vessels are still responsive, a degree of cerebral vasoconstriction should result, with a consequent fall in cerebral blood volume and intracranial pressure. The dangers of production of cerebral ischaemia by hyperventilation have probably been overemphasized in the past; there is no evidence that structural damage to the brain can be produced by hyperventilation, although it is undeniable that temporary and reversible cerebral dysfunction can be produced in normal subjects induced to hyperventilate to extreme levels.

CSF drainage may be possible in some patients provided that the fluid is drained off continuously against a considerable positive pressure (usually 20 cm of water). This form of treatment however will not alleviate brain shift, indeed it may worsen it; it can be used only when there is a degree of brain swelling yet with preservation of some ventricular capacity. It is neither feasible nor advisable to attempt to drain CSF from the subarachnoid space. The abrupt evacuation of cerebrospinal fluid from an acute post-traumatic hygroma does not usually result in lasting benefit. When the hygroma fluid is under high pressure, this is likely to be because of swelling of the underlying brain, rather than a space-occupying effect of the hygroma fluid.

Osmotherapy continues to be widely used in patients with severe head injury. The most popular agent in mannitol, delivered intravenously as a rapid infusion. When the situation is extremely acute, as for example, just after the detection of an intracranial haematoma in a comatose patient, a large dose of 1 g/kg body weight should be administered over a period of ten minutes. Where the situation is less acute, and the patient is in the intensive care unit with intracranial pressure monitoring in progress, then an initial dose of 0.5 g/kg should be given and subsequent doses adjusted upwards or downwards, according to the effect observed. If mannitol is going to be effective, this should be apparent within a few minutes of the end of the infusion. The duration of effect is variable; in some patients with intracranial hypertension, no more than one or two doses of mannitol may be required to bring intracranial pressure down to a satisfactory level and thereafter it remains at those levels. In more severely injured patients with well developed brain swelling, repeated doses of mannitol must be given every few hours; in such cases the limiting factors are the effectiveness of the dose and the level of plasma osmolality just before the next dose is due. When this rises to more than 320 mmol/l further mannitol administration is inadvisable because of the danger of development of renal failure and metabolic acidosis.

The mechanism of effect of osmotic agents remains a controversial matter. The early assertions that osmotherapy withdrew fluid from areas of oedematous brain have been challenged. It has also been suggested that the maximum effect is an undamaged brain, where the blood–brain barrier is intact, and that water is withdrawn from this tissue to produce an overall reduction in the volume of water in the whole brain. Other postulates are that intravenous mannitol causes osmotic withdrawal of water from the CSF spaces across the ependyma and that mannitol acts on cerebral blood vessels both directly and via changes in viscosity. Finally, when mannitol is administered intravenously, the cardiac output increases considerably, and there is a marked increase in circulating blood volume; autoregulatory vasoconstriction may occur in response to this stimulus (Muizelaar et al. 1983, 1984).

Mannitol is not the only osmotic agent to be used; other substances include urea, no longer used extensively, and glycerol, which some claim has certain metabolic benefits over mannitol when administered intravenously. Glycerol has more usually been administered as a large oral dose but not in the context of severe head injury, for obvious reasons.

The use of barbiturates to lower intracranial pressure in head injured patients was advocated by Shapiro et al. (1974) (Marshall et al. 1979). The basis for this recommendation was that barbiturates reduce cerebral metabolism, reduce cerebral blood flow and blood volume and thereby result in lowering of intracranial pressure. In addition, barbiturates damp down cardiovascular responses and result in a more stable blood pressure and intracranial pressure, reducing the frequency of spontaneous waves of increased pressure, possibly due to a central mechanism first described by Ishii (1966).

Despite the claims made for the effectives of barbiturates in head injury, no solid evidence had yet emerged to demonstrate that outcome is improved, mortality lowered or the incidence of raised intracranial pressure lessened (Miller 1979a). Ward et al. (1985) have recently reported on a randomized trial of barbiturate therapy in patients with severe head injury. In this study 53 patients were randomized to a group in which any intracranial hypertension which occurred was treated by hyperventilation, CSF drainage and osmotherapy, and a barbiturate treated group where continuous administration of pentobarbitone was commenced as soon as the patients were admitted to the intensive care unit. The goals of the study were to determine whether barbiturate treated patients had a lower mortality and a lessened incidence of raised intracranial pressure. In the group of patients selected for study the anticipated mortality rate was 60% and the rate of intracranial hypertension expected was 75%. At the termination of the study there was no difference in the mortality rates which were however somewhat lower than expected (50%) in both groups but the incidence of intracranial hypertension was 75% in both control and treatment groups. Furthermore, the same number of patients in each group died as a result of fulminating intracranial hypertension. The only significant difference between the groups was the incidence of arterial hypotension. More than half of the barbiturate treated patients suffered significant reductions in arterial blood pressure despite elaborate precautions being taken to ensure that such problems were detected immediately and treated. A similar study with the same results was reported by Schwartz *et al.* (1984). In summary, therefore, in barbiturate therapy for intracranial hypertension in head injured patients, the hazards of the treatment appear to at least balance any possible benefits that may accrue from its administration. Particular mention should be made of the danger of administering barbiturates, or any anaesthetic agent, to patients with a reduced circulating blood volume, Such patients include the multiply injured, in whom fluid replacement had been inadequate, and patients who have had osmotic agents with a large diuresis which has been inadequately replaced.

The dangers of arterial hypotension following administration of barbiturates have prompted those responsible for the intensive therapy of head injured patients to look for alternative agents which might have similar effects on the brain but lesser effects on arterial blood pressure.

As part of the management of the severely head injured patient neurosurgeons have long sought to reduce the motor and vegetative accompaniments of severe head injury, consisting of spontaneous decerebrate extention of the limbs, sweating, flushing associated with increases in body temperature and marked changes in arterial pressure and heart rate. Chlorpromazine was widely used in the management of these vegetative disturbances and it is being used again, as studies of ECG and blood levels of catecholamines confirm that in association with severe head injury, there is a sympathetic over-activity (Clifton *et al.* 1981), ECG change reminiscent of myocardial ischaemia (Clifton *et al.* 1983) subendocardial haemorrhage and focal cardiac myocytolysis (Connor 1968). At various times, cholinergic, alpha and beta adrenergic receptor blocking drugs have been used, although it is still unclear whether

they are associated with an improvement in outcome from injury.

## Complications of head injury

*Intracranial haematoma*

The clinical manifestations of intracranial haematoma have already been described in detail but some points require emphasis:

1 In the conscious patient, increasing headache, vomiting and drowsiness provide important evidence for action, particularly if a skull fracture is known or suspected.

2 In the patient who is unconscious on arrival at the hospital, a history of earlier consciousness should be accepted as evidence of subsequent deterioration ('lucid interval').

3 If the patient is in coma when examined, with no eye opening to pain, not obeying commands and unable to give a formed verbal response, the likelihood that intracranial haematoma is present is at least 40%. If there is deepening of the level of consciousness or increasing restlessness the risk is even higher.

4 The progressive development of pupillary dilatation and paralysis, hemiparesis, spasticity, extensor rigidity, tachycardia or bradycardia, increasing blood pressure or respiratory disturbances are all phenomena which demand an explanation. Until proved otherwise these should be attributed to rising intracranial pressure with brain stem compression. They are all late manifestations because they result from internal herniations and it is quite improper to await their evolution before making a decision to take action. Even though a haematoma may be satisfactorily evacuated the mortality rate in patients exhibiting such 'paralytic signs' is high.

5 In patients without an intracranial haematoma on admission prolonged depression of the level of consciousness may indicate the delayeddevelopment of an intracranial haematoma; evaluation by computerized tomography

may need to be repeated after an interval of 24, 48 or 72 hours.

6 Patients in whom cerebrospinal fluid is leaking freely from the nose or ear may harbour an intracranial haematoma without manifestations of raised intracranial pressure. Connolly (1956) and Becker et al. (1977) drew attention to this small group of patients in whom the loss of fluid prevented a rise of intracranial pressure.

The success of operative evacuation of intracranial haematomas is proportionate to early diagnosis and action, with the proviso that the coexisting primary brain damage will determine the limits of outcome if the operation is performed before secondary ischaemic brain damage has been sustained. In the case of extradural haematoma, primary brain damage is often slight and in such patients early operation should carry a low mortality. This experience is exemplified by the series reported by Jamieson and Yelland (1968), Mendelow et al. (1979), and most graphically by Bricolo and Pasut (1984). In these series the lowest level of mortality, below 10%, was associated with patients in whom treatment was provided early, the level of consciousness had not been too greatly depressed and in whom there was no associated intradural haematoma. In the series of McKissock et al. (1960a) operative mortality varied from nil in patients who were alert to 50% in patients who were comatose prior to surgery. The interpretation is not that unconsciousness makes operations dangerous, but that coma denotes central brain damage, due either to the primary effect of trauma in patients comatose from the outset, or to secondary (ischaemic) effects of brain compression, or both. A similar relationship between increasing mortality and depth of coma and delay before decompression is seen in cases of acute subdural haematoma (Seelig et al. 1981).

Reilly et al. (1975) reviewed the autopsy findings in a series of 66 patients who had talked at some time after their head injury and noted that intracranial haematoma was the most important contributor to the subsequent death of the patients. This experience led Rose et al. (1977) to introduce the term 'avoidable factors' to those conditions or complications of head injury that can lead to death but which, if detected, can be treated or prevented. They reviewed 116 patients who had talked and subsequently died from their head injury, and identified one or more avoidable factors in 74%. By far the most common and important was delay in the detection and treatment of an intracranial haematoma. This experience led the neurosurgeons in this centre to modify and expand the criteria for transfer to the neurosurgical unit of patients suspected of harbouring an intracranial haematoma. This change in admission policy doubled the number of head injury referrals, doubled the number of intracranial haematomas detected and reduced the overall head injury mortality in their area (Teasdale et al. 1982). Meanwhile, Jeffreys and Jones (1981) were reporting that of 160 head injury deaths occurring in general hospitals in patients who had not been referred to the regional neurosurgical centre 33% were due to intracranial haematoma. The case for the use of guidelines for neurosurgical referral and for CT in head injured patients is now overwhelming.

The surgical significance of intracerebral haematoma is more difficult to determine. Only since the widespread adoption of computerized tomography in the investigation of the acutely head injured patient has the true incidence of intracerebral haematoma and haemorrhagic contusion has been evident. Intracerebral haematoma may be related to acute subdural haematoma, associated with laceration and haemorrhage at the temporal pole or in the subfrontal area; the proportion of haematoma that is subdural or intracerebral is variable and the decision in favour of surgical evacuation can often be made only during craniotomy for removal of the subdural component. In other instances, however, the intracerebral haemorrhage appears isolated, lies more deeply, and may represent bleeding into an area of previous infarction or be associated with diffuse axonal injury and shearing stress in the brain. There is considerable controversy as to the indications for surgical decompression in such cases, where the haematoma is almost entirely within the brain substance. Surgical decompression should be contemplated only when there is a significant shift of surrounding brain structures with shift of the midline in addition. Operative decompression of some intracerebral haematomas, quite unlike the decompression of extracerebral haematomas, may in certain cases be, with advantage, delayed for 24 or 48 hours. In the interim the intracranial pressure is continuously monitored and controlled.

Following the evacuation of intracranial haematomas, whether extradural, subdural or intracerebral, the incidence of postoperative intracranial hypertension remains high. This problem is least evident in patients with extradural haematoma, due presumably to the lower incidence of associated brain damage, but is most severe in patients who have required operative decompression of intracerebral haematomas. In these cases Miller and his colleagues (1981) found an 88% incidence of intracranial hypertension and in nearly half of these cases the elevation of intracranial pressure was of such severity to out-strip measures aimed at its control.

*Investigations for haematoma*

Without any doubt the premier investigation of the severely head injured patient is computerized tomography. This noninvasive investigation will not only reveal the existence of space-occupying mass lesions but will distinguish between areas of haemorrhage, oedema or infarction in the production of the mass effect. The indications and urgency for referral for CT are as follows:

1  Comatose patients (Glasgow Coma Score 8 or less) have a 40% risk of harbouring a significant haematoma and should be referred for immediate CT scan as soon as it is safe for the patient to leave the Accident and Emergency Department, i.e. the airway and circulatory status is secure.
2  Adult patients who have a skull fracture coupled with depression of the conscious level (GCS 9–14), development of abnormal neurological signs or recurrent seizures should be referred for CT within hours of admission.
3  Children without skull fracture but with severe headache and vomiting, persisting drowsiness or development of abnormal neurological signs should also be referred for CT.
4  Patients with drowsiness or confusion persisting for more than 24 hours, worsening of conscious level or development of abnormal neurological signs after admission to hospital should be referred for CT even if there is no skull fracture.
5  Patients with elevated intracranial pressure which can neither be easily controlled nor explained should be referred for CT or repeat CT.

Skull X-rays in head injured patients have been a source of controversy. While it has been asserted that too many skull X-rays are carried out in A & E Departments, the presence of a skull fracture in an adult patient greatly increases the probability that the patient will be harbouring an intracranial haematoma (Mendelow *et al.* 1983, Fowkes *et al.* 1984). If the clinical circumstances are such that CT scan is going to be carried out in any case it may be less important to carry out skull X-ray. The principal value of plain X-rays of the skull is in that group of patients who are seen in the Accident & Emergency Department following a head injury where consciousness has not been lost or only briefly lost. These patients should not be dismissed from the hospital until it has been established that no linear or depressed skull fracture is present; this should include plain X-rays of the skull, which must also be searched for intracranial air as evidence of a basal skull fracture.

*Other investigations*

If CT is unavailable, cerebral angiography is the most reliable means of locating a supratentorial intracranial haematoma (Fig. 23.9). Anterior fossa, middle fossa and extradural haematomas of the vertex are clearly depicted, as are subdural haematomas over the convexity of the hemisphere. It is less easy to distinguish swollen haemorrhagic contusion of the temporal lobe from subdural or extradural haematomas at this site. While displacement of cortical vessels away from the inner surface of the skull is pathognomonic of an extracerebral collection (extra or subdural) this may be difficult to distinguish on the anteroposterior views. Only rarely can contrast medium be seen leaking from the torn middle meningeal vessels in cases of extradural haematoma.

The displacement of angiography by CT as the investigation of choice in head injury has posed certain problems in neurosurgery. Diagnostic problems may arise in head injured patients which can be resolved only by angiography. One example is the patient who collapses during sport after only minimal head injury, another is the patient who falls over in the street without warning, striking the head as he falls. In such cases the original problem may have been a spontaneous subarachnoid haemorrhage or stroke; in addition, certain patients with injuries about the head and neck may proceed to develop signs of progressive cerebral hemispheric deficit, drowsiness, depression of consciousness into coma with dense hemiplegia. In all cases cerebral angiography is required; the first two instances may reveal an intracranial aneurysm or intracranial vascular occlusion, often of the middle cerebral artery; in the third example, traumatic occlusion of the carotid artery in the neck may be the cause of the progressive neurological syndrome.

During the course of management of patients with head injury, thrombosis, partial or complete, of the sagittal or transverse sinuses may be encountered. While it is a rare complication (Martin 1955), it should be remembered as a cause of diffuse persistent brain swelling on CT or angiography and associated severe intracranial hypertension. Another, and more frequently encountered, potential source of cerebral ischaemia is cerebral vasospasm, which can only be detected by angiography (Miller &

Gudeman, 1980). Wilkins and Odom (1970) and Suwanela and Suwanela (1972) have shown clearly that it is not uncommon after injury; Macpherson and Graham (1978) have demonstrated the link between cerebral vasospasm during life and ischaemic brain damage in fatal head injuries.

Ventriculography is rarely necessary because angiography is more generally informative and, if there is markedly raised intracranial pressure, is less dangerous. Ventriculography can however, be used extremely rapidly and is particularly helpful if a posterior fossa haematoma is suspected. Becker et al. (1977) used twist drill ventriculography with injection of only sufficient air to outline the position of the frontal horns of the ventricle in a series of 160 patients with severe head injury, detecting brain shift associated with intracranial haematoma formation in 40% of cases. In a subsequent series of 225 identically defined patients (Miller et al. 1981) 41% of cases were found by CT to be harbouring surgically significant intracranial haematomas. It seems therefore as if ventriculography is indeed reliable but practice is required to ensure reliable location of the usually small lateral ventricles of the head injured patient.

If ventriculography is to be carried out, a small quantity of air or positive contrast medium should be used, with as little disturbance to intracranial pressure as possible. If a sizeable posterior fossa haematoma is present the withdrawal or leakage of a substantial volume of CSF may reduce the supratentorial pressure too abruptly and precipitate lower brain stem ischaemia by upward herniation of the cerebellum through the tentorial hiatus propelled by the mass effect of the posterior fossa haematoma.

Air encephalography has never been indicated during the acute stage of head injury. In the past it was used at a later stage to evaluate the extent of post-traumatic brain atrophy of CSF pathway obstructions. Computerized tomography has entirely supplanted this investigation.

Electroencephalography has not proved in the past to be helpful in the diagnosis and management of acute complications of head injury, and in the UK the EEG is not required to make the diagnosis of brain death. Serial records have proved to have certain scientific and research value, and in a small number of patients the detection of electrical spiking has predicted successfully the development of post-traumatic epilepsy (Bricolo *et al.* 1979). In many more cases however, post-traumatic epilepsy has developed without any such changes (Jennett & Van de Sande 1975). At the present time it is not yet clear whether various forms of EEG data processing and compression such as the compressed spectral array or the cerebral function analyser will be of practical value in the management of the acutely head injured patient (Bricolo *et al.* 1978, Prior 1971). Multimodality evoked electrical potentials have a considerable research interest; abnormal recordings in head injured patients are of prognostic value, but the investigations are time consuming and elaborate and cannot at this stage be said to form part of the routine care of the severely head injured patient (Greenberg *et al.* 1977, Lindsay *et al.* 1981, Chiappa & Ropper 1982). It does appear however, that it will be technically feasible to have some form of continuous monitoring of electrical function in the brain that may play a role in the early detection of events such as hypoxia or arterial hypotension which produce secondary brain insults. This form of cerebral function monitoring may therefore come to play an important role in the management of the paralysed, ventilated head injured patient permitting early detection and treatment of such insults.

Lumbar puncture should not be undertaken if there is a suspicion of intracranial haematoma or any space occupying lesion in the craniospinal axis because of the grave risks of aggravating internal herniation, not only at the time of the lumbar puncture, but in the subsequent period of 24 hours, during which CSF leaks slowly from the small rent in the arachnoid made by the needle. The most important and urgent indication for lumbar puncture in the head injured patient and, in the opinion of some neurosurgeons, the only indication, is the detection of meningitis. Ideally, in cases of doubt, lumbar puncture should be preceded by CT. When neurological deterioration in a head injured patient cannot be explained by the formation of an intracranial haematoma or systemic factors such as hypoxia or hypotension then meningitis must always be considered as a possible diagnosis. Far too often the diagnosis is considered when it is too late and treatment is then to no avail. The characteristic signs of meningitis (headache, vomiting, irritability, photophobia, nuchal rigidity and elevation of temperature) may all be present already in the head injured patient who has traumatic subarachnoid haemorrhage. In such cases the only new finding is the generalized depression of conscious level and motor function (Miller 1976).

*Operative treatment of intracranial haematoma*

General anaesthesia should always be the rule in present day operations to relieve acute traumatic cerebral compression. A gastric tube should be passed and the stomach emptied prior to attempts to intubate the trachea. The nasal route should be avoided in the presence of basal skull fractures. When an intracranial haematoma has been detected or suspected it is a wise precaution to administer intravenous osmotic agents prior to the induction of anaesthesia in order to reduce as much as possible the elevations in intracranial pressure which may accompany these manœuvres. The use of local anaesthetics in the operative management of head injured patients should be restricted to patients in whom the operation will be limited to burr hole evacuation of chronic subdural haematoma or insertion of a ventricular catheter.

When CT has been performed beforehand, the location of the haematoma will be known and an appropriate bone flap can be planned. When the haematoma is subdural in location the flap should be large extending from the midline over the vertex down into the temporal fossa. The flap should be fashioned so as to make it possible for the surgeon to arrest bleeding from veins linking the cortex with the sagittal sinus, and at the same time to inspect the undersurface of the frontal and temporal lobes, where contusion and laceration are most likely to be located. Because time is of the essence in beginning surgical decompression of the haematoma, the first burr hole should be made over the clot and some of it removed before the full skin and bone flap is turned.

If the circumstances are such that no CT scan or angiography could be performed and the location of the intracranial haematoma is unknown then the surgeon may be faced with the need to do preliminary burr hole exploration, uncertain whether he is going to encounter an extradural, subdural or intracerebral haematoma. Two factors should guide the surgeon as to the location and order in which the burr holes are to be fashioned. The first is the pattern of clinical signs, in particular the location of unilateral pupillary dilatation. This indicates reliably the side on which the mass effect is present. Hemiparesis is somewhat less reliable as a guide to lateralization, because in a certain number of patients with subdural haematoma the motor dysfunction may be ipsilateral to the mass due to compression of the opposite cerebral peduncle against the free edge of the tentorium (Kernohan's notch). The other helpful factor is the location of a skull fracture. If the pupil dilates on the same side as a skull fracture it is most likely that the cause of the mass effect is an extradural haematoma and this will be located under or close to the site of the skull fracture. In such cases this is where the first burr hole should be made. When the pupillary dilatation and the skull fracture are on opposite sides the likelihood is that an acute subdural haematoma is present and this will be located on the side of the dilating pupil, contralateral to the skull fracture. In this event the first burr hole should be made in the temporal region just above the zygomatic arch on the side ipsilateral to the dilated pupil.

If the haematoma is not located in the site of the first burr hole the surgeon should proceed to make burr holes in the lateral frontal region close to the coronal suture and posteriorly over the parietal boss. This should be done on both sides. The skull must be completely shaved in all cases of head injury who require any form of surgical exploration. This is most important. Only when the scalp has been shaved is it possible to see lacerations or areas of bruising which may provide valuable evidence of the site of an underlying fracture and save considerable time in the location of an extradural haematoma.

If the burr hole is successful in locating extradural haematoma the findings are unmistakable. A dark, crumbling, liver-like mass of clotted blood extrudes through the opening. If none presents immediately some investigation of the surrounding area is possible by sweeping a periosteal elevator around the margins of the burr hole in the extradural space. If the dura mater is bulging or bluish in appearance it should be incised and a search made for subdural blood and evidence of cortical contusion. Acute subdural haematoma is also formed of clotted blood, so fresh bleeding may follow the evacuation of some clot. If the brain looks normal and there is no subdural haematoma it should not be explored with a brain cannula. If the exploration is negative at all burr holes then CT or angiography are strongly indicated. If these are not available an attempt can be made to tap the lateral ventricles through the frontal burr holes and to insert a ventricular catheter. It may then be possible to inject some contrast medium into the ventricle to assess whether there is ventricular enlargement suggestive of a posterior fossa lesion or midline ventricular shift. Location of the compressed lateral ventricle is extremely difficult from a lateral frontal burr hole. To reach the lateral ventricle the coronal burr hole should be made in line with the inner canthus of the eye and the cannula aimed for the bridge of the nose. This is more medial than the usual frontal route for ventricular cannulation.

If it is not possible to locate the lateral ventricles then an intracranial pressure monitoring device should be inserted with the subdural space through the right frontal burr hole.

The use of exploratory burr holes has been scathingly referred to as 'woodpecker surgery'.

When employed with critical judgement however, and with as accurate a clinical diagnosis as the available information will allow, it has proved successful in the past and continues to be the only method available to a general surgeon confronted with the grave emergency of a rapidly deteriorating patient who is harbouring an extradural haematoma. In certain geographical areas time cannot permit the transfer of such a seriously ill patient to a regional neurosurgical unit. A reasonable guideline in the UK is that if more than one hour is to be required to transfer the patient to the nearest neurosurgical unit and the patient has already deteriorated to the stage of coma, then the surgeon on the spot would be better to initiate the exploratory surgery himself. The education of a general or traumatic surgeon is incomplete if he has not received training in the surgical relief of extra- and subdural haematoma. By being prepared and able to deal with these emergencies he can save lives. Having found a clot by burr hole exploration the burr hole need only be enlarged sufficiently to enable the primary surgeon to remove some of the haematoma and allow it to extrude itself. If the surgeon then wishes, the skin can then be loosely closed and, during the period of immediate improvement, the patient can be transferred to the nearest neurosurgical centre for completion of the procedure (Potter 1965).

Detection and surgical management of the source of an intracranial haematoma may not be without its problems. The source of an extradural haematoma may lie in the floor of the middle cranial fossa and be associated with fractures running across the base of the skull. The use of wax, or cotton impregnated with wax, may be necessary to arrest the haemorrhage in such cases. In patients with acute subdural haematoma the source of the bleeding may be the ragged edge of a cerebral laceration, a torn bridging vein linking the brain to the superior sagittal sinus, the petrosal sinus or the lateral sinus. In some instances it may be a small cortical artery which can be seen spurting on the surface when the haemaoma is removed. In patient with acute

subdural haematoma the use of a large osteoplastic flap is essential if satisfactory location and control over the bleeding point is to be attained.

Controversy still exists as to the need for removal of brain tissue after evacuation of an extra cerebral haematoma. Where brain is considerably pulped and disorganized it will be removed by most surgeons, but some have advocated the need for excising contusions that extend to the cortical surface, asserting that such lesions act as a focus for the later development of brain oedema. Miller et al. (1981) pointed out, however, that in cases where this had been done the incidence of postoperative intracranial hypertension remained extremely high. In cases where the brain remains extremely tight after a haematoma has been evacuated it may be necessary to amputate the temporal pole or some of the tip of the frontal lobe. In many severe cases, however, brain soon swells to fill any decompression thus created.

Some surgeons also advocate leaving the bone flap out and performing a dural plastic procedure to provide a large temporal decompression. While this may be of benefit in a small number of cases, in many others leaving a temporal decompression merely encourages the development of further swelling and a possible cortical venous infarction of extensive areas of brain due to compression of vessels in the herniated brain around the margin of the bony decompression. While the patient may be saved from the life threatening occurrence of intracranial hypertension, this may be at the expense of developing a severe and permanent neurological deficit. The most usual surgical practice is to replace the bone flap wherever this is possible, leaving it out only when the swelling is so severe as to preclude this manoeuvre.

When brain swelling occurs in the operating theatre after the removal of an extracerebral haematoma, and the cause is not immediately apparent in the form of poor positioning of the patient's head and neck, or obstruction of the airway, then the neurosurgeon should consider the possibility that there is a contralateral extracerebral haematoma.

In the past some surgeons proposed that in patients who showed signs of brain stem compression the attempt should be made to lift the temporal lobe out of the tentorial hiatus and a few surgeons even advocated dividing the tentorium. While it may be beneficial to disimpact the medial part of the temporal lobe to allow CSF to emerge from the tentorial hiatus, the practice of sectioning the tentorium is mentioned only to be condemned. In experimental studies this has been shown to prevent the development of the clinical signs of tentorial herniation but to encourage the earlier development of medullary coning with arrest of respiration (Jennett & Stern 1960).

Sometimes the brain which has been compressed by a surface haematoma fails to reexpand or does so only very slowly after the blood has been removed. This phenomenon is most common in chronic subdural haematomas removed from elderly patients. In such cases a period of subdural drainage may be helpful and the patient should be kept flat for several days assuming the upright position only gradually after removal of the drain.

A cavity persisting after the removal of an intracranial haematoma provides a dead space in which a recurrent haematoma may readily collect. Haemostasis must therefore be as perfect as possible, and tenting suture to hold the dura close to the inner table of the skull should be used liberally. A postoperative haematoma is a disaster and patients who have managed to tolerate a first episode of brain compression with only moderate depression of consciousness, tolerate a second insult of brain compression much less well. Neurological deterioration on this occasion is usually rapid and severe and non-reversible.

Chronic subdural haematoma is always liquid, the consistency ranging from thin watery orange-stained fluid to thick tarry material. Within the same haematoma there may be a considerable variation in the consistency of the fluid and when the patient is lying supine on the operating table the thickest blood is found in the most inferior part of the cavity. Two burr holes should be made in the lateral frontal and parietal regions in patients with chronic subdural haematoma on one side and a soft rubber catheter should always be passed posteriorly from the posterior burr hole in order to permit drainage of the thickest part of the haematoma in this location. The cavity should be washed out with normal saline at body temperature and the decision as to whether or not a subdural drain is left in is a personal one. The author usually drains the subdural space only if the brain fails to re-expand after evacuation of the haematoma. In only a few instances is it necessary to make a third burr hole in the anterior temporal region. The possibility of bilateral chronic subdural haematoma should always be borne in mind and especially when CT shows a somewhat smaller midline brain shift than can be accounted for by a large, apparently unilateral, haematoma. At a certain stage in their evolution chronic subdural haematomas may on CT examination be completely isodense with the underlying brain. If there is any serious doubt, a burr hole on the opposite side will quickly settle the matter.

Infantile subdural haematomas and effusions provide different problems in treatment. If the condition remains undiagnosed for several months subdural capsular membranes may become extremely thick and even if fluid is evacuated there is concern that the membrane may prevent expansion of the compressed brain. Ingraham and Matson (1944) believed that excision of this membrane was necessary after preliminary aspiration of fluid, the aim being to release the underlying brain. Unfortunately this operation carried a considerable morbidity and membrane excision is no longer carried out. Another problem in treatment results from the capacity for enlargement of the skull that can occur in young children. When the haematoma fluid has been evacuated the subdural space may not readily be obliterated because the skull has already enlarged and the subdural effusion may persist despite repeated tapping of the subdural space. Since repeated insertion of a needle into the space carries an increasing risk of fresh haemorrhage or infection, Ransohoff (1957) advocated the use of a subdural peritoneal shunt, a suggestion which was taken up by many other surgeons including Collins (1968) and Till (1968). Late results have shown that intelligence in children with subdural effusions and haematomas develop normally in 86% of infants treated by subdural peritoneal shunting compared with 66% of those treated with craniotomy for removal of subdural membrane.

*Post-traumatic brain oedema*

The general topic of cerebral oedema has been discussed in an earlier chapter but it is appropriate to reintroduce the topic in the context of head injury. While the term 'post-traumatic brain oedema' is widely used it appears that in most instances true oedema, an increase in volume due to an increase in brain tissue water content, is not present and the phenomenon is more likely to be due to congestive brain swelling in which the volumetric increase lies mainly within the vascular system (Miller 1979b, Miller *et al.* 1980). The only exception to this is in the case of perifocal oedema around cerebral contusions, whether these lie near the frontal or temporal poles or deeper within the brain substance. Sampling of brain tissue from the vicinity of these haemorrhagic lesions has confirmed an increase in tissue water content and it is felt that these areas are an example of vasogenic oedema (Bullock *et al.* 1985, Galbraith, personal communication). In terms of the symptomatology of brain swelling and oedema such arguments about definition are of little importance. The symptomatology is due to a combination of raised intracranial pressure, brain shift and focal neurological dysfunction. The arguments about brain swelling versus oedema are important however when the question of treatment is considered. The diffuse swelling of the brain which may follow concussive head injury is not affected in any way by therapy with corticosteroids, agents which produce excellent effects in patients with brain tumour associated with perifocal oedema. It is possible

that steroid therapy is of benefit in patients with oedema surrounding cerebral contusions but at the present time no definitive trial has been carried out. All the current evidence concerns the use of steroid therapy in 'normal' or high dose regimens applied to patients with severe, coma producing, head injuries. In most studies steroids have been found to influence neither the mortality nor the incidence of raised intracranial pressure (Braakman *et al.* 1983, Cooper *et al.* 1979, Gudeman *et al.* 1979). Earlier studies (Faupel *et al.* 1976, Gobiet *et al.* 1976) had suggested that high dose steroid therapy might be of value but later studies have failed to confirm this. Recent studies of methylprednisolone therapy suggests a small advantage for high dose therapy (Giannotta *et al.* 1984, Saul *et al.* 1981). Management of acute traumatic brain swelling therefore, depends upon control of the intracranial pressure using the methods and agents already dealt with.

*Metabolic disorders in head injury*

The severely head injured patient is placed in a particularly vulnerable position for the following reasons:

1   the patient becomes entirely dependent upon others for provision of all fluids and nutrition;
2   damage to the brain and to other parts of the body may induce alterations in the normal mechanisms for regulation of the balance of fluids, electrolytes and other blood constituents;
3   treatment may be necessary, such as osmotherapy, that has a profound effect upon fluid balance, inducing massive diuresis that must be replaced.
4   following injury to the brain the caloric requirements of the body are increased just as in the phase following systemic injury or surgical procedures.

The role of the neurosurgeon caring for the severely head injured patient must be to try to preserve a normal balance of fluids, electrolytes and an adequate calorie intake. This means the rigorous measurement of all aspects of fluid intake and output including urinary catheterization to ensure that all urinary output is measured on an hourly basis. To this must be added the volume of fluid removed by nasogastric aspiration, by CSF drainage and by insensible loss, bearing in mind that the insensible loss through sweating may be considerably increased in the head injured patient.

Care must be taken to ensure that fluid losses that are coupled to losses of sodium and chloride are not replaced by water in the form of 5% dextrose solutions. The surgeon should also be on the lookout for development of the syndrome of inappropriate ADH secretion associated with decreased serum sodium concentration and osmolality, increased total body water and passage of urine with high osmolality. Post-traumatic diabetes insipidus is another possible problem in which there will be a polyuria, with passage of urine of low specific gravity.

Hyponatraemia is the most important electrolyte disturbance for the head injured patient. If serum sodium falls to 120 mEq/L brain swelling is extremely likely and measures should be undertaken urgently to restore the fluid and electrolyte balance to normal. In the case of the syndrome of inappropriate ADH secretion, fluid restriction may be all that is necessary but if this is severe infusion of hypertonic saline may

be required. In diabetes insipidus, administration of DDAVP will be required.

A caloric intake of 3,000 calories/day may be required in a fit young adult. This is best given by nasogastric tube but clearly this cannot commence until bowel sounds and other indications of normal gastrointestinal function return following the initial paralytic phase immediately following the head injury. In some patients a prolonged period of intolerance of nasogastric feeding may occur and in these cases intravenous nutrition may be required for a time. Intravenous infusion of fat, amino acid and glucose solutions requires the use of a long intravenous line terminating centrally and this carries with it the danger of septicaemia. Nasogastric feeding always carries the risk of aspiration of material into the airway and the appropriate nursing supervision must be provided.

*Cerebral fat embolism*

This is an occasional complication of head injury, particularly when other injuries have occurred which involve the marrow-containing bones (Sevitt 1962). The fall in conscious level that occurs in the absence of focal abnormality is usually accompanied by, and may be caused by arterial hypoxaemia due to the associated

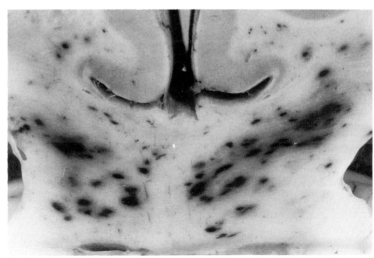

**Fig. 23.10.** Coronal section of brain showing petechial haemorrhages due to fat embolism, particularly numerous around the corpus callosum.

pulmonary fat embolism (Bergentz 1968). The petechial haemorrhages that are said to be pathognomonic are rarely seen and the clinical picture is dominated by tachycardia, respiratory distress and a fall in the level of consciousness (Fig. 23.10). Therapy is directed towards returning oxygenation to normal levels and the management of any episodes of intracranial hypertension by the means already described.

*Gastrointestinal complications of head injury*

A rare complication of severe brain injury is rupture of the oesophagus. Necropsy reveals a narrow slit-like tear in the lower end of the oesophagus with blackening due to digestive changes in adjacent tissues. This terminal complication may also be seen in patients with brain tumours or other serious diseases of the central nervous system. Maciver *et al.* (1956) found rupture of the oesophagus in 19 of 1590 necropsies. Fifteen of these cases were associated with an intracranial lesion of which 9 were traumatic in origin. In 77 of the 19 cases lesions were also found in the stomach and duodenum.

Erosion, ulceration and haemorrhage in the stomach and duodenum are much more common occurrences following head injury than rupture of the oesophagus. Cushing (1932) drew attention to the association between cerebral lesions and gastric and duodenal erosions and ulcers. Sheehan (1940) reviewed the association between gastric activity and pathological change with stimulation or injury of the hypothalamus. Measurements of gastric acidity in comatose head injured patients have been carried out by Watts and Clark (1969) and Gudeman *et al.* (1983). Acidity is increased to levels comparable to those seen in patients with active duodenal peptic ulceration, but not to the excessive levels seen in patients with Zollinger-Ellison Syndrome. The degree of gastric acidity is not related to the presence of decerebrate rigidity, evidence of brain stem dysfunction or the height of the intracranial pressure. There is however, an association between increased gastric acidity, gastric haemorrhage and the presence of gastric and duodenal erosions seen on endoscopy. Halloran *et al.* (1980) showed that the administration of a histamine-2 receptor antagonist drug to severely head injured patients reduced the volume and degree of gastric acidity, and reduced the amount of haemorrhage from the gastrointestinal tract, but did not influence the prevalence of endoscopically observed erosions in the stomach and duodenum.

These findings suggest that while the degree of gastric acidity may be related to the tendency of the eroded gastric mucosa to bleed, the cause of the erosions themselves is not related to gastric acidity. Mucosal ischaemia related to sympathetic discharges from the damaged brain have been postulated as a cause of breakdown of the protective mechanisms in the mucosa and development of erosion.

In a very small number of cases, oval punched-out ulcers in the stomach, duodenum or proximal jejunum may be associated with severe head injury. In parallel with peptic ulcers, those situated in the posterior wall of the viscus tend to cause severe haemorrhage due to erosion into a major vessel, while those on the anterior wall of the stomach or duodenum or jejunum are more likely to be associated with perforation. In either event there is a dramatic deterioration in the state of the patient and the diagnosis may be difficult to make unless the alert neurosurgeon keeps the possibility in mind. The management of these patients is the same as for the acute complications of peptic ulceration although the mortality is extremely high.

**Scalp wounds and fractures**

All wounds of the scalp should be regarded as potentially serious for three reasons:

1 Improperly treated, they may become infected and from this infection may arise osteomyelitis, purulent meningitis, dural sinus thrombosis, extradural or even intracerebral abscess.

Even if no intracranial complication occurs a septic scalp wound causes considerable inconvenience and may take many weeks to heal (Botterell & Jefferson 1942). In rare occasions the infection may spread widely in the subgaleal space producing a considerable collection of thin liquid pus. In cases where the infection becomes established in the subperiosteal space it is limited by the attachment to the suture lines and results in the rare but characteristic appearance of Pott's Puffy Tumour.

2 A scalp laceration may overlie a fracture which enhances the chance of intracranial infection. Particularly important is the small, apparently insignificant, wound caused by a sharp object which penetrates both the scalp and the skull. Because of the mobility of the scalp over the skull the scalp wound may not directly overlie the fracture but be located at a distance of up to one inch from the bone lesion.

3 The location of a scalp injury indicates the site of impact and thereby provides important information for the localization of a suspected intracranial haematoma. The possibility of more than one impact must not be overlooked, the head may have been struck by a moving object and struck again at a different site when the body hit the ground. The location of a scalp injury may also provide an explanation for abnormal neurological signs due to a local cerebral contusion. This may occur without fracture of the overlying skull, particularly in children (Jefferson 1919).

In all cases of scalp wounds the skull should be X-rayed in order to detect a fracture. In addition foreign bodies such as glass and road grit may be demonstrated in the wound. All wounds of the scalp should be clearly defined by shaving at least one inch of the scalp around the margins of the lacerations, they should be thoroughly cleaned, the edges debrided and sutured. Longer more ragged or irregular lacerations with contused edges require careful excision of any non-viable skin edges, retraction for inspection, meticulous cleansing of sub galeal pockets with removal of foreign bodies and dirt which may be forced deeply under the galea. These wounds should be closed by interrupted sutures.

Fractures of the skull require surgical treatment if they are depressed and compound. Miller and Jennett (1968) reported that 90% of their series of 400 consecutive depressed skull fractures were compound. Closed linear fractures and multiple or burst fractures without depression do not require specific surgical treatment although associated complications of intracranial haemorrhage may of course demand urgent operative relief.

The indications for elevation of closed depressed skull fractures are more complex. In a certain number of cases the indications for operative elevation are entirely cosmetic, particularly when the fracture is located in the middle of the forehead in an area not covered by hair. In a limited number of cases the appearances of the fracture with deep depression of fragments may suggest that there is associated dural tearing or in an even small number of cases the fracture may be associated with an extra or subdural haematoma. There is no evidence that elevation of closed depressed fractures decreases the severity of cerebral contusion or the risk of post-traumatic epilepsy. It should be appreciated that the appearances of depression of bone fragments on X-ray indicate only the final lodging place of the indriven bone. At the time of impact it is likely that the fragments were momentarily driven more deeply into the cranial cavity.

In young children, a subgaleal collection of cerebral spinal fluid may form over a closed linear fracture because of an associated tear of the dura mater. A false meningocele can develop, and over a period of time the edges of the fracture may be resorbed, producing the classical appearance of growing fracture of the skull. While a firm padded bandage may prevent the expansion of the subgaleal collection, once such sac has become established it requires excision, obliteration of the neck and repair of the dural defect (Pia & Tönnis 1953).

Fractures involving the base of the skull become compound if they extend into the paranasal sinuses, the roof of the masopharynx or the middle ear. They may provide a pathway for the escape of cerebrospinal fluid or the ingress of air to the cranial cavity. In the days immediately following the injury attention is directed to the possibility of development of meningitis. There is considerable controversy concerning the role of antibiotics at this stage in the prevention of infection. One view is that penicillin and a sulphonamide drug should be given to all patients with CSF rhinorrhoea, aimed at the prevention of the most common form of meningitis complicating such injuries, pneumococcal meningitis (Leech & Paterson 1973, Wehrle *et al.* 1967). The opposing view is that the administration of penicillin merely encourages colonization of the nasopharynx by other organisms which may produce an even more virulent form of meningitis (MacGee *et al.* 1970). Cessation of the CSF leak is not necessarily evidence of closure of the fistula as the flow of CSF may be obstructed by prolapse of brain tissue into the dural defect. This also has the effect of preventing spontaneous dural repair. Subsequent head injury or violent head movement may dislodge the prolapsing tongue of brain and reopen the cranionasal fistula. The indications for closure of a persistent cerebrospinal fistula are considered later.

*Treatment of compound depressed skull fractures*

The sometimes difficult issues relating to the elevation of closed depressed skull fractures have been mentioned but the treatment of compound fractures is not subject to question. This comprises excision of the wound, location and removal of indriven fragments of bone and foreign bodies and hair, evacuation of pulped brain and haematoma, repair of the dura mater and, in most cases, replacement of the larger bone fragments (Rowbotham 1964). These measures are taken in order to avoid the risk of infection spreading into the brain if the dura mater is penetrated, to diminish brain damage due to haematoma and oedema and to facilitate resolution of the contusional brain injury that underlies the depressed fracture. Miller and Jennett (1968) analysed 400 cases of depressed skull fracture and emphasized some of the important complications that may attend these injuries. In 25% of their series Miller and Jennett encountered intracranial haemorrhage, infection, or actual and potential difficulties relating to the location of the depressed fractures over or close to a major dural venous sinus. The infection rate for the entire series was 10% due in most cases to failure to recognize the injury, under estimation of its severity or inadequate surgical treatment (Fig. 23.11). Intracranial haematomas were encountered in 7% of the series and were most commonly intracerebral in location. This is in contrast to head injuries associated with linear skull fractures, where most intracranial haematomas are extracerebral. Dural venous sinuses were involved by the fractures in 11% of the series and in half of these cases the sagittal or transverse sinus had been torn by the fracture. Such cases can prove extremely difficult to treat and transfusions of large volumes of blood may be required. Before embarking on the surgical repair of such cases it is wise to ensure the secure placement of at least two widebore intravenous lines. The occurrence of such actual or potential complications of depressed skull fracture was associated with a significant increase in the mortality, morbidity and incidence of post-traumatic epilepsy in Miller and Jennett's cases.

Because detection and delineation of the depressed fracture is so important it is essential that good quality X-ray films are available, employing such projections as will best demonstrate the details of the fracture. These will usually include tangential views. The possibility of the scalp laceration being located at a distance from the depressed skull fracture has been mentioned. It is also important to realize that in depressed skull fractures the area of the inner table fracture is greater than that of the outer table. For this reason a burr hole should always be made with great care at the margin of the visible fracture and the bone nibblers employed so as to lift fragments from the brain without the possibility of tilting a sharp edged fragment so

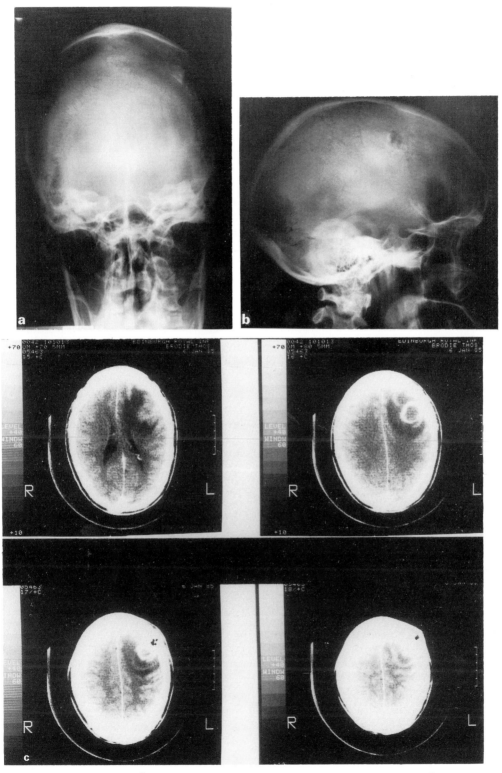

**Fig. 23.11.** Compound depressed skull fracture caused by a blow from a sickle in left frontoparietal area. No loss of consciousness, skull not X-rayed at initial hospital visit. Patient presented 6 days later with focal epilepsy. Skull X-rays shows small fracture on a) antero-posterior and b) lateral skull X-rays. c) CT showed brain abscess underlying fracture.

that its deep portion can penetrate or lacerate the brain tissue further.

A small but important group of compound skull fractures deserves special mention. These comprise penetrating or perforating wounds via the roof of the orbit. The paper thin bone is easily entered at this site and subsequent swelling of the periorbital tissues may completely obscure the entry wound. That a serious injury has been sustained is often not appreciated until intracranial complications, notably haemorrhage, meningitis or abscess, occur. In children there is often no satisfactory history of the accident and the diagnosis will only be made by a neurosurgeon who has considered the possibility beforehand. Guthkelch (1960) described an instructive series of such cases.

*High velocity penetrating injuries*

Major advances in the treatment of war wounds of the head occurred during successive wars. In the First World War the application of meticulous care in excision of the wound and primary suture saved the lives of rather more than half of those in whom there had been dural penetration. Infection of the brain remained the most important cause of death inspite of the use of antiseptics and disinfectants (Cushing 1918, Jefferson 1919). In the Second World War and the Korean conflict further improvements were made in the treatment of penetrating head wounds due to policies of early definitive operative treatment provided by trained neurosurgeons located in advanced posts. The definitive operation consisted of meticulous excision of wounds, removal of indriven bone fragments, foreign material and missile fragments where accessible, watertight closure of the dura mater, employing a graft if necessary, and accurate scalp closure. Sulphonamide, then antibiotic, therapy was introduced at this stage but it was considered that the lowering of the infection rate in the Korean conflict was due in greater part to the provision of early definitive surgery than to the employment of antibiotics. The importance of detecting

and evacuating intracranial haematomas was emphasized and attention drawn to tangential wounds of the head in which large extra or subdural haematomas could form under a glancing injury of the skull in which no fracture had been sustained (Schorstein 1947).

Established cerebritis continues to carry a high mortality. Meirowsky and Harsh (1953) described a method of treatment by which the wound was widely opened, the affected portion of brain tissue excised, and the dura mater and wound left open, covered by a bulky nonadherent dressing. Antibiotics were used and increased intracranial pressure was treated. Secondary closure was then performed after some days when the infection and brain swelling had subsided.

In more recent conflicts such as the Vietnam war the same surgical principles were adhered to, but the availability of rapid helicopter transport enabled the definitive neurosurgical team to be more safely placed at some greater distance from the actual theatre of conflict; patients were able to be delivered from the site of injury to the operating theatre typically in 30–60 minutes. While this rapid transport ensured that early definitive treatment of brain wounds could be rendered, it also meant that a number of patients with overwhelmingly severe multiple injuries were delivered to the medical care team; cases where death would formerly have supervened long before medical attention could be rendered. Because of the addition of such cases in the Vietnam war the average blood transfusion requirements rose to enormous levels.

*Cerebrospinal fluid rhinorrhoea*

Leakage of cerebrospinal fluid from the nose after a fracture of the base of the skull and the associated danger of meningitis have long been recognized. Dandy (1926) described the use of a graft of fascia lata to repair the site of such a leak from the anterior cranial fossa. Cairns (1937) described a series of such cases treated by grafting and was responsible for the development of an aggressive policy of operating in such patients in order to prevent meningitis. He and his colleagues outlined the anatomical problems and assessed the relative risks of conservative and of surgical treatment (Calvert & Cairns 1942, Lewin and Cairns 1951, Lewin 1966). Lewin pointed out that pyogenic meningitis could be of dramatic onset and fatal within hours and Wehrle *et al.* (1967) reported a mortality of 21% in cases of pneumococcal meningitis, the commonest form to complicate CSF rhinorrhoea. After repair of CSF leaks, recurrent meningitis

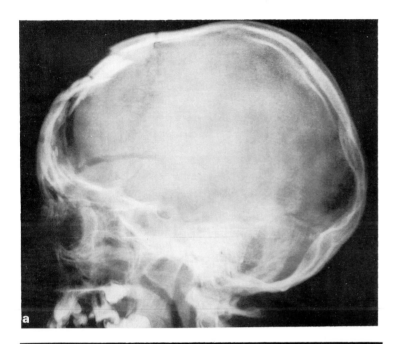

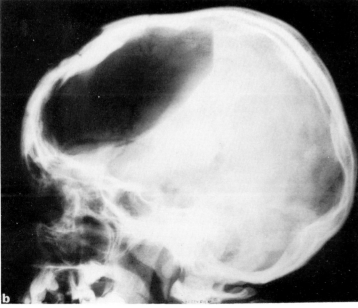

Fig. 23.12. This 23-year-old woman sustained frontal craniofacial injuries in a head-on collision in which she was a front seat passenger. a) Lateral skull X-ray on admission showed multiple linear fractures. b) Skull X-rays 5 days later when she was complaining of severe frontal headache shows an extensive aerocele.

was exceptional while in the absence of repair repeated attacks of meningitis were possible.

Basal fractures likely to cause cerebrospinal fluid rhinorrhoea are those involving the anterior cranial fossa. Rarely a middle fossa fracture passing through the tegmen tympani produces leakage of cerebrospinal fluid into the middle ear, draining into the nasopharynx through the Eustachian tube. Leakage of fluid and subsequent invasion of the intracranial cavity by microorganisms depends upon the presence of a tear in the dura mater and arachnoid. Operative and post-mortem findings indicate that such tears in the dura mater rarely heal by firm fibrous scar, because the margins of the tear are separated by a prolapsing plug of brain tissue or arachnoid. A fluid leak may be deferred until the plug of tissue shrinks or there is a sudden rise of intracranial pressure or a sudden movement of the head that may dislodge the plug. In a series of cases reviewed by Lewin (1966) two thirds of the patients leaked CSF within 48 hours of the accident and in one third the CSF leak was within 3 months; in a small number of patients the leakage of CSF was delayed for more than one year from the time of injury.

Cerebrospinal fluid rhinorrhoea may also complicate fractures of the anterior cranial fossa that are mainly associated with facial fracture Jefferson and Reilly (1972) have pointed out that in such cases cerebrospinal fluid leak virtually always ceases when the facial fracture is reduced; in such cases exploration of the anterior cranial fossa is not rewarding.

In cases in which the fluid leak is a complication of a predominantly cranial injury neurosurgeons vary in their readiness to recommend anterior cranial fossa exploration and repair. Most frequently however, the indications for anterior cranial fossa repair are leakage of cerebrospinal fluid which persists for more than one week after the injury, the development of a large aerocele and any occurrence of meningitis following a head injury associated with aerocele or cerebrospinal fluid leakage (Fig. 23.12). When, as in most cases, the cerebrospinal fluid

leak ceases within a few days of the injury most neurosurgeons will opt to take a conservative line. This policy has the additional benefit of avoiding anterior cranial fossa exploration in the first few days after injury when the frontal lobes are swollen and haemorrhagic and where retraction of the brain may cause lasting neurological deficit.

When anterior cranial fossa exploration is required, this should be conducted intradurally with location of the dural defect usually by the protruding tongue of fibrotic brain tissue. The defect, once defined, can be closed with a periosteal graft from the skull, fascia lata or dura mater substitute. Where there is extensive bone destruction and a defect in the paranasal sinuses underlying the dural fistula, this can be packed with fat after stripping of the mucosa from the wall of the sinus. In a small number of cases a more extensive reconstruction of the bony floor of the anterior fossa may be required using squamous temporal bone or rib graft.

It is fortunate that persistent cerebrospinal fluid otorrhoea following head injury is a much less frequent problem. Most cases of CSF leakage from the ear cease spontaneously within a few days of injury and do not recur. In the rare case in which the leakage is persistent, location and obliteration of the fistula may be extremely difficult and persistence of the CSF leak after operative exploration and attempted repair is a well recognized problem among neurosurgeons.

*Spontaneous cerebrospinal fluid rhinorrhoea*

Although these cases are not traumatic in origin it is convenient to consider this matter here. Three main groups of cases can be distinguished. In the first, the fistula is created by erosion of bone due to a local lesion that can be identified by radiological investigation. This group will therefore include intrasellar and parasellar tumours, invasive osteomas or malignancies of the orbital ethmoidal area and cancers of the paranasal sinuses. Treatment of a pituitary adenoma by bromocriptine, surgery or radiation may so reduce the lesion that cerebrospinal fluid leaks through the floor of the sella previously eroded by the adenoma. This is a variety of the so-called empty sella syndrome.

In the second group of cases of spontaneous CSF rhinorrhoea, raised intracranial pressure due to a lesion remote from the floor of the anterior cranial fossa may cause bone erosion and development of a CSF fistula. In the majority of cases, the lesion also produces obstructive hydrocephalus. The leak of fluid may be through an erosion in the posterior wall of the frontal sinus or in the cribriform plate.

The third group of cases most precisely warrants the description 'spontaneous' because, although the site of the leak may be successfully identified, its aetiology remains obscure. The fistulous opening is usually through the cribriform plate but careful examination may be necessary to detect the small opening. In other cases the leak may occur through the floor of the sella turcica and when hydrocephalus is present the enlarged third ventricle may extend into the sella enlarging it and thinning its floor. These problems have been extensively reviewed by Ommaya *et al.* (1968) and Rovit *et al.* (1969).

Investigations in such cases of CSF rhinorrhoea have two aims. To identify the fluid as cerebrospinal fluid and to ascertain the anatomical location of the leak. The presence of glucose in the fluid has long been accepted as a means of distinguishing CSF from the results of severe allergic rhinitis. Injection of radioisotopes into the CSF and retrieval of that isotope from packs placed in the nose, so as to differentiate leakage via the sphenoid, ethmoid and frontal sinuses has been employed but is in practice often inconclusive in supplying evidence other than that one nostril is more involved than the other. If the leakage of cerebrospinal fluid is profuse it may be visualized by cisternal injection of metrizamide and computerized tomography.

## Rehabilitation and prognosis

The process of rehabilitation after head injury can be seen as the planned, phased, withdrawal of intensive nursing care and the supervised resumption of normal physical activities, with skilled help being provided for the assessment and treatment of specific neuropsychological deficits. The goal of the rehabilitation process should be the restoration of full independence of the patient and resumption of most of his or her former activities. Where this is not possible, the aim should be to provide the patient with greatest degree of independence possible. Effective rehabilitation after head injury must be based on a sound understanding of the constellation of behavioural, psychological, neurological, physical and social problems that may confront the head injured patient during the recovery process (Rosenthal *et al.* 1983).

The activities of a modern rehabilitation service must therefore cover an extremely wide field using a multidisciplinary team approach. The team should include a neurosurgeon or neurologist, clinical psychologist, physiotherapist, speech and occupational therapists, nursing staff skilled in rehabilitation and a social worker, providing core support for the patient. The services of many other individuals may be required, including orthopaedic or urological surgeons, disablement resettlement officers, psychiatrists and many others. The particular problems requiring consideration in the recovering head injured patient, may be grouped as follows:

1 *The general symptoms and disabilities following concussive head injury* These include headache, dizziness, difficulty in concentration with a short attention span and poor memory. Cairns (1942) was largely responsible for introducing a regime of graduated increasing activity for patients after they had fully recovered consciousness following head injury. It was felt that such graduated increases in activity hastened the recovery of patients and reduced the incidence of post-traumatic headache and dizziness. The general aim of rehabilitation therefore, is directed towards a

steady progressive increase of physical activity at first amounting to no more than freedom from restraint with bedrest terminating within a few days of recovery of consciousness, leading on to remedial exercises designed to promote adjustments in posture and improve protective reflexes. These can lead in due course to simple games and group exercises.

2 *Emotional and behavioural disturbances* Along with physical education, attention must be paid to this important aspect of the head injured patient. A cheerful and optimistic attitude on the part of the therapeutic team is of great importance, because the lassitude, lack of concentration and initiative and poor memory may cause the patient to believe that his mind has failed as a result of the injury and will never recover. It is of great importance that members of the nursing and therapy team realize that apparent indifference, forgetfulness and inability to stick to a task are common sequels of head injury; they will improve and they certainly do not indicate that the patient does not desire or require rehabilitative treatment.

3 *Neurological deficits* Special attention will be required for focal neurological deficits, in particular disturbances of speech and motor function. Speech therapy is of great help, not only in facilitating relearning of tongue and lip movement, breath control and formation but in graduated increase in the vocabulary, memory and fluency of expression. Hillblom (1961) has pointed out that recovery from post-traumatic dysphasia is often better than that due to stroke. Other neurological deficits may require special measures. Strabismus for example, may require orthoptic exercises.

4 *Return to home and return to work* Decisions on these two important milestones are of outstanding importance in the eyes of the patient and his family. The return to home should however, be viewed within the context of a progressive rehabilitation programme and is often best achieved in phases, with the patient returning home at weekends only, and returning to the rehabilitation unit to continue inpatient therapy during the week. This not only boosts the

patient's morale but provides a real insight on the part of the family into the problems that are likely to be encountered in coping with the disabled patient at home. Home visits by the occupational therapist are of considerable importance in planning the extent of physical aid and modifications to the house that may be required before the patient returns home full-time.

The clinical psychologist has a vital role to play in determining the timing and mode of the patient's return to school, college or to the place of work. Before the patient is exposed to the risk of humiliating failure, his capacity for concentrating, decision making as well as his physical abilities should be carefully explored. Judgements must also be made concerning the nature of the work which may be unsuitable on grounds of noise, excess of surrounding activity or responsibility. Resumption of work in stages can sometimes be arranged with sympathetic employers provided that the rehabilitation team take the initiative.

As soon as it is clear that the patient is going to be permanently unfit for his previous occupation, this should be made clear to the patient and his family. Such a determination can almost always be made within one year of injury. To postpone this information, keeping the patient and his family vainly hoping for an improvement that does not come, is not only to postpone, but to ultimately make worse, the disappointment.

*Prognosis*

The art of predicting outcome from a head injury has always been considered of great importance. In the hours and days following a severe head injury the major concern of the family is the patient's chance of survival. Once survival is assured, concern focuses on whether there will be a satisfactory return of mental and physical function. During the succeeding weeks and months, as recovery proceeds, increasing concern will be expressed as to the extent of recovery and whether the patient will be able to resume his former occupational and recreational activities. In 1975 Jennett and Bond published details of a 5-point scale denoting the recovery status of patients who had sustained a severe head injury, the Glasgow Coma Scale. In this scale *Good Recovery* indicated ability to return to the pre-injury level of activity or occupation; *Moderate Disability* denoted patients who were independent for activities of daily living but unable to return to the former level of activity for physical or psychological reasons; *Severely disabled* patients were dependent upon the help of others for one or more of the activities of daily living; the remaining categories were the *Permanent Vegetative State* and *Death*.

Prediction of death versus survival in cases of severe head injury has been studied in great depth by Jennett *et al.* They have emphasized the importance of age, the level of consciousness in the hours following injury, the presence of intracranial haematoma and of signs of dysfunction or damage to the brain stem structures. Following from this, Narayan *et al.* (1981) evaluated the prognostic role of computerized tomography, measurement of intracranial pressure and of evoked potentials in predicting outcome as compared with the clinical factors of age and neurological status. While correct predictions as to whether death or survival will occur can be obtained in up to 90% of severely head injured patients such predictions can only be made with confidence (95% certainty) in about two thirds of cases. Addition of information from computerized tomography or other investigations does not increase the total number of cases correctly predicted but does improve the confidence of predictions made. In all of these exercises however, the predictions are limited to whether or not the patient survives. Predictions of the severity of disability have proved to be much more difficult (Bricolo *et al.* 1980). Miller *et al.* (1981) have suggested that observation of moderately increased intracranial pressure in severely head injured patients is predictive of a higher rate of severe disability in survivors. In contrast, observation of severe eleva-

tion of intracranial pressure is predictive of early death.

In the clinical examination, observation of clinical signs of brain stem dysfunction consisting of bilateral absence of the pupil light response and impairment or absence of the oculocephalic and oculovestibular responses, coupled with the observation of abnormal motor responses (abnormal flexion or extension) which persist more than a few days are predictive of persisting disorders of balance and gait during the recovery phase. Another indication of prolonged disability is the development on serial computerized tomography of progressive dilatation of the ventricles with enlargement of the subarachnoid spaces indicative of a progressive loss of brain substance (Narayan *et al.* 1981).

Information concerning the time course of recovery from severe head injury is of considerable importance in the provision of reasoned advice to the family and patient. Bond and Brooks (1976) followed a series of severely head injured patients for a two year period and found that in terms of overall outcome category as graded on the five point Glasgow Coma Outcome Scale (Jennett & Bond 1975) more than 90% of patients had reached their final outcome status by six months from the time of injury with virtually no change in outcome categorization between 1 and 2 years from the time of injury. A more detailed study of intellectual function and memory after head injury suggested that virtually all of the recovery that took place after a severe head injury was accomplished within the first 12 months. It is not to be denied that further improvements in those functions of which the patient is already capable do take place in the second and third year after a head injury, but the improvements are virtually never of sufficient magnitude to alter the outcome status from the categories of severe and moderate disability.

With current methods of management, typical figures for the six months outcome of patients who are in coma following head injury (no eye opening, not obeying commands and not uttering recognizable words) are 30% good recovery,

20% moderately disabled, 10% severely disabled or vegetative and 40% mortality. These would be classed as severely head injured patients. In moderately head injured patients scoring between 8 and 12 on the Glasgow Coma Scale, the anticipated mortality is 5% or less and in patients with minor head injuries, that is the group of patients that may have been unconscious but who on arrival at the hospital are alert and orientated or awake but disorientated, the anticipated mortality rate is well below 1% (Miller & Jones 1985).

In the less severely injured patient, the duration of post traumatic amnesia is of considerable prognostic value. When PTA lasts longer than 24 hours difficulties with return to school, work or social activities can be anticipated. It is recognized that there is an interaction between severity of injury, age, state of the brain prior to injury and the duration of PTA. Thus an elderly patient may have a longer PTA after a less severe injury than a younger patient. Regardless, in both cases, the quality of outcome is likely to be related to the duration of PTA.


### Post-traumatic epilepsy

Much has been written about epilepsy following head injury. Jennett (1975) consulted some 500 publications but listed less than 100 because of 'serious deficiency in the information' given in the remainder. Relatively few contributions have been based on sufficiently large numbers of unselected cases to provide an accurate and useful enquiry. Observation over a sufficiently long period of time is essential, for in at least one fifth of patients with epilepsy the first fit is delayed for more than one year after the injury. Large numbers of cases are also necessary in order to give significance to subgroups, to the incidence of epilepsy following different degrees of severity, and different varieties, locations and complications of the injury. A bald statement that the incidence of post-traumatic epilepsy is 5% is of little practical value, for according to the factors operating in subsets of cases, the inci-

dence may vary from no more than that observed in the general population up to 80%. The information required when considering a particular patient is the incidence in that subgroup which most closely matches the circumstances of the case under consideration. Even that item of information provides only an estimated probability, for as yet there is no method of accurately predicting whether the patient will or will not develop epilepsy. Statistical studies have their most practical application in litigation and it is in the best interests of all concerned that probability data should rest on accurate information. From the strictly medical angle the information may also be valuable in deciding whether prophylactic anticonvulsant drugs should be given, though whether these drugs are of value in preventing seizures has not yet been conclusively proven.

If a fit is thought to have been due to a precedent head injury, it is necessary to lay down criteria. The duration of post-traumatic amnesia is now widely accepted as a measure of the severity of a given head injury. The status of the patient on the Glasgow Coma Scale on admission and after resuscitation is an accepted measure in those whose conscious level is still depressed at the time of arrival in hospital. Local brain injury can however, occur without loss or depression of consciousness, particularly in cases of low velocity penetrating or perforating injuries and a number of depressed skull fractures. For this reason fractures of the skull and major scalp lacerations are also acceptable criteria of the occurrence of significant head injury. The definition of what constitutes an epileptic fit following a head injury may not always be straightforward. Transient loss of consciousness preceded by giddiness or faintness or mistiness of vision is a frequent sequel of head injury but does not necessarily constitute an epileptic fit. The association of many such episodes with sudden changes of posture, abnormalities of vestibular function, previous signs of brain stem injury, vasomotor instability and subsequent resistance to anticonvulsant therapy all speak against an epileptic nature of such phenomena. On the other hand, attacks of more than transient duration which are associated with some confusion of thought, speech or action suggest temporal lobe epilepsy. It is widely agreed that petit-mal in the true sense of the term is never of traumatic origin. Some investigators excluded cases with a solitary post-traumatic seizure from the definition of post-traumatic epilepsy on the grounds that a single seizure does not provide evidence of a persistent susceptibility to fits. A solitary fit is uncommon however. Walker and Jablon (1961) found that only 13% of their series of cases of post-traumatic epilepsy had a single seizure during the 9 year period of follow up. The difficulties of making a decision as to when to label a patient as suffering from post-traumatic epilepsy is not an easy one and should be considered by the neurosurgeon on an individual basis.

### Missile wounds of the brain

Wounds of the brain produced by missiles which penetrate the skull and dura mater provide a well defined and homogenous group of patients in whom a consistently high level of post-traumatic epilepsy has been observed in a series of studies extending from and before the first World War through the Second World War to the Korean and Vietnam conflicts. The observed incidence of post-traumatic epilepsy in patients suffering from missile wounds of the brain has ranged from 19 to 50% and it is likely that a realistic figure is at least 30% (Wagstaffe 1928, Credner 1930, Ascroft 1941, Russell & Whitty 1952, Walker & Jablon 1959, Caveness & Liss 1961, Jennett 1962).

Although it has been suggested that wounds in one particular area of the brain carry a greater risk of post-traumatic epilepsy than wounds in another, there is no general agreement about this, nor is it agreed whether the persistence of indwelling metal fragments in the brain increases the risk of subsequent epilepsy. There is no doubt however, about the influence of infection. Ascroft (1941) found that in healed wounds

the epilepsy incidence was 36%. When brain wounds remained unhealed after 60 days the incidence of epilepsy was 57% and after abscess formation the incidence increased to 73%. Epilepsy is an almost invariable sequel of an infective herniation of the brain ('brain fungus') occurring in 86 and 92% of the cases of Walker and Jablon (1961) and Caveness et al. (1962) respectively.

Although missile wounds of the brain produce a localized lesion, the pattern of epilepsy does not correspond. Only a minority of patients suffer exclusively from focal epilepsy (13–31%). The majority of patients have generalized seizures.

### Blunt injury to the head

The overall incidence of epilepsy in such cases is much lower than with missile wounds ranging in report series between less than 1% and 20% (Penfield & Shaver 1945, Phillips 1954, Jennett 1975, Walker 1964).

There is general agreement that the majority of patients with post-traumatic epilepsy have their first fit within a year of injury, the figures ranging from 71% to 83%. There has long been an opinion among British clinicians however, that fits arising within the first few days of an injury do not carry the same prognostic significance as do those of later onset. These early fits are related to the acute damage sustained by the brain and do not bespeak persistent epilepsy. In 1943, Denny-Brown was apprehensive that such patients having had a single early seizure might be labelled epileptic when the likelihood of further fits was remote. Lewin arbitrarily divided his cases into early epilepsy, those with fits in the first week, and late epilepsy, those who had seizures after that first week. In support of this Jennett and Lewin pointed out that in the period from the second to the tenth week after injury, the only patients in a very large series who developed seizures had all subdural haematomas. Furthermore, Jennett and Lewin (1960) pointed out significant differences in the type and pattern of seizure occurring early and late. Early seizures were more common in children, focal motor fits were frequent while temporal lobe seizures did not occur at all at this early stage. In contrast temporal lobe seizures are a common form of late post-traumatic epilepsy and when seizures occur late they are much more likely to recur and present the persisting problem of post-traumatic epilepsy. The studies of Jennett revealed that although early seizures by themselves did not amount to a diagnosis of post-traumatic epilepsy, the presence of such fits increased the likelihood that late post-traumatic epilepsy would follow.

Late epilepsy was calculated by Jennett (1975) to occur in about 5% of surviving head injuries. Phillips calculated the incidence at 6% overall. In addition to the presence of early fits in determining the incidence of late post-traumatic epilepsy, other factors noted as important by Jennett included the presence of an intracranial haematoma, whether extradural, subdural or intracerebral, intracranial infection, depressed skull fracture, particularly when dural tearing was present, and prolonged post-traumatic amnesia.

*Anticonvulsant drugs*

Convincing statistical evidence concerning the effects of the prophylactic administration of anticonvulsant drugs has not yet been presented. Walker (1957) in a series of 246 cases of battle injury found that 15% of the patients did not take drugs and this group was equally distributed amongst those whose fits had remitted and those whose fits had persisted. Walker also noted that the nature of the drug taken was not important, clearly in such early studies the problems of patient compliance could not be assessed but in more recent studies supported by the use of measurements of drug level in the blood the controversy remains. Randomized trials of anticonvulsant therapy carried out by Young *et al.* (1983) and McQueen *et al.* (1983) have failed to demonstrate any effect of phenytoin in the prevention of either early or late post-traumatic seizures.

In the light of this recent information what should the neurosurgeon do when confronted by the individual head injured patient? It seems that there are two choices, either to await the development of post-traumatic epilepsy before applying treatment or to identify those individual patients in whom the risk of epilepsy seems sufficiently high (more than 30%) to warrant the administration of anticonvulsant drugs, bearing in mind that this must also entail regular withdrawal of blood samples to check satisfactory levels of the anticonvulsant. At the present time most neurosurgeons probably follow the latter approach (Deutschman & Haines 1985). It should be recognized however, that it is equally important to identify those head injured patients in whom the risk of post-traumatic epilepsy is low, so as to avoid the use of anticonvulsant drugs in such cases. These would include patients with a short period of post-traumatic amnesia, those who do not have intracranial haematomas or infection and in whom the dura mater has not been torn.

If anticonvulsant therapy has been started for how long should it be continued? Since epilepsy has declared itself by the end of the second year in about 80% of cases, that would be a responsible minimum period if no fits have occurred following the injury. If fits have occurred, however, what minimum length of time should be considered as a remission after which drugs might be stopped? This is still a matter of opinion. Northfield felt that if fits had previously been frequent, 12 or more per annum, a minimum of five years of freedom from seizures was advisable before ceasing drugs.

# References

ADAMS J. H. (1975) In *Injuries of the Brain and Skull, Handbook of Clinical Neurology*, Vol. 23 (Eds Vinken P. J. & Bruyn G. W.) pp. 35–65. North Holland, Amsterdam.

ADAMS J. H. (1984) In *Greenfield's Neuropathology*, 4th edition (Eds. Adams J. H., Corsellis J. A. N. & Duchen L. W.) pp. 85–124. Arnold, London.

ADAMS J. H. & GENNARELLI T. A. (1984) In *Recent Advances in Neuropathology* (Eds. Smith W. T. & Cavanagh J. B.) pp. 165–190. Churchill Livingstone, Edinburgh.

ADAMS J. H. & GRAHAM D. I. (1976) *Neuropath. Appl. Neurobiol.*, **2**, 323.

ADAMS J. H., GRAHAM D. I., MURRAY L. S. & SCOTT G. (1982) *Ann. Neurol.*, **12**, 557.

ADAMS J. H., MITCHELL D. E., GRAHAM D. I. & DOYLE D. (1977) *Brain*, **100**, 489.

ANDERSON D. W. & McLAURIN R. L. (1980) *J. Neurosurg.*, Suppl., S1.

ASCROFT P. B. (1941) *Brit. med. J.*, **1**, 739.

BAIGELMAN W. & O'BRIEN J. C. (1981) *Neurosurgery*, **9**, 729.

BARTH J. T., MACCIOCHI S. N., GIORDANI B., RIMEL R., JANE J. A. & BOLL T. J. (1983) *Neurosurgery*, **13**, 529.

BECKER D. P., GUDEMAN S. K. & MILLER J. D. (1981) in *Goldsmith's Practice of Surgery*, pp. 1–42. Harper & Row, Philadelphia.

BECKER, D. P., MILLER J. D., WARD J. D., GREENBERG R. P., YOUNG H. F. & SAKALAS R. (1977) *J. Neurosurg.*, **47**, 491.

BERGENTZ S. E. (1968) *Progr. Surg.*, **6**, 85.

BERGER M. S., PITTS L. H., LOVELY M., EDWARDS M. S. B. & BARTKOWSKI H. M. (1985) *J. Neurosurg.*, **62**, 194.

BOND M. R. & BROOKS D. N. (1976) *Scand. J. rehab. Med.*, **8**, 127.

BOTTERELL E. H. & JEFFERSON G. (1942) *Brit. med. J*, **1**, 781.

BOWERS S. A. & MARSHALL L. F. (1980) *Neurosurgery*, **6**, 237.

BRAAKMAN R., SCHOUTEN H. J. A., BLAAUW-VAN DISHOECK M. & MINDERHOUD J. M. (1983) *J. Neurosurg.*, **58**, 326.

BRICOLO A. & PASUT I. M. (1984) *Neurosurgery*, **14**, 8.

BRICOLO A., TURAZZI S. & FACCIOLI F. (1979) *Acta Neurochir.*, **Suppl 28**, 35.

BRICOLO A., TURAZZI S., FACCIOLI F., ODORIZZI F., SCIARETTA G. & ERCULIANI P. (1978) *Electroencephogr. clin. Neurophysiol.*, **45**, 211.

BRICOLO A., TURAZZI S. & FEFIOTTO G. (1980) *J. Neurosurg.*, **52**, 625.

BRITT R. H., HERRICK M. K., MASON R. T. & DORFMAN L. J. (1980) *Neurosurgery*, **6**, 623.

BROOKS D. N. (1972) *J. nerv. ment. Dis.*, **155**, 350.

BROOKS D. N. (1975) *Cortex*, **11**, 329.

BROOKS D. N. (1983) in *Rehabilitation of the Head Injured Adult* (Eds Rosenthal M., Griffith E. R., Bond M. R. & Miller J. D.) pp. 185–96. Davis, Philadelphia.

BROOKS D. N. (1984) *Closed head Injury: Psychological, Social and Family Consequences.* Oxford University Press.

BRUCE D. A., ALAVI A., BILANUIK L., DOLINSKAS C., OBRIST W. & UZZELL B.(1981) *J. Neurosurg.* **54**, 170.

BRUCE D. A., SCHUT L., BRUNOL A., WOOD J. H. & SUTTON L. N. (1978) *J. Neurosurg.*, **48**, 679.

BULLOCK R., SMITH R., FAVIER J., DUTREVOU M. & BLAKE G. (1985) *J. Neurosurg.*, **63**, 64.

BUTTERWORTH J. F., MAULL K. I., MILLER J. D. & BECKER D. P. (1980) *Lancet*, **ii**, 759.

CAIRNS H. (1937) *J. Laryng.* **52**, 589.

CAIRNS H. (1942a) *Proc. roy. Soc. Med.*, **35**, 299.

CAIRNS H. (1942b)) *Proc. roy. Soc. Med.*, **35**, 809.

CAIRNS H. (1947) *Brit. J. Surg.* (War Surgery Suppl 1), 9.

CAIRNS H. & HOLBOURN H. (1943) *Brit. med. J.*, **1**, 591.

CALVERT C. A. & CAIRNS H. (1942) *Proc. roy. Soc. Med.*, **35**, 805.

CAREY M. E., YOUNG H., MATHIS J. L. & FORSYTH J. (1971) *J. Neurosurg.*, **34**, 145.

CARTLIDGE N. E. F. (1978) *Scott. med. J.*, **23**, 103.

CAVENESS W. F. & LISS H. R. (1961) *Epilepsia*, **2**, 123.

CAVENESS W. F., WALKER A. E. & ASCROFT P. B. (1962) *J. Neurosurg.*, **19**, 122.

CAWTHORNE T. (1946) *Proc. roy. Soc. Med.*, **36**, 270.

CHIAPPA K. H. & ROPPER A. H. (1982) *New Engl. J. Med.*, **306**, 1140.

CLASEN R. A., PANDOLFI S., LAING I. & CASEY D. (1974) *J. Neurosurg.*, **41**, 576.

CLIFTON G. L., ROBERTSON C. S. & COUTANT C. F. (1985) *J. Neurosurg.*, **62**, 186.

CLIFTON G. L., ROBERTSON C. S., KYPER K., TAYLOR A., DHEKNE R. & GROSSMAN R. G. (1983) *J. Neurosurg.*, **59**, 447.

CLIFTON G. L., ZIEGLER M. G. & GROSSMAN R. G. (1981) *Neurosurgery*, **8**, 10.

COLLINS W. F. (1968) *Clin. Neurosurg.*, **15**, 394.

COLUMELLA F., GAIST G., PIAZZA G. & CARAFFA T. (1968) *J. Neurol. Neurosurg. Psychiat.*, **331**, 315.

CONNOLLY C. (1965) *Brit. med. J.*, **2**, 1154.

CONNOR R . C. R. (1968) *Brit. med. J.*, **3**, 29.

COOPER A. (1836) *The Principles and Practice of Surgery*, p. 151. Cox, London.

COOPER P. R., MOODY S., CLARK W. K., KIRKPATRICK J., MARAVILLA K., GOULD A. L. & DRANE W. (1979) *J. Neurosurg.*, **51**, 307.

CORALES R. L., MILLER J. D. & BECKER D. P. (1980) In *Intracranial Pressure IV* (Eds Shulman K., Marmarou A. & Miller J. D.) pp. 280–3. Springer Verlag, Berlin.

COURVILLE C. B. & BLOMQUIST O. A. (1940) *Arch. Surg.*, **41**, 1.

CREDNER L. (1930) *Z. ges. Neurol. Psychiat.*, **26**, 721.

CROCKARD H. A., BROWN F. D., CALICA A. B., JOHNS L. M. & MULLAN S. (1977) *J. Neurosurg.*, **46**, 784.

CROMPTON M. R. (1971a) *Brain*, **94**, 165.

CROMPTON M. R. (1971b) *Lancet*, **1**, 669.

CROMPTON M. R., TEARE R. D. & BOWEN D. A. L. (1966) *Lancet*, **2**, 938.

CROSS A. G. (1945) *Trans. Lymph. Soc. UK*, **65**, 20.

CUSHING H. (1918) *Brit. J. Surg.*, **5**, 558.

CUSHING H. (1932) *Surg. Gynec. Obstet.*, **55**, 1.

DANDY W. (1926) *Arch. Surg.*, **12**, 949.

DANIEL P. M. & TREIP C. S. (1961) In *Modern Trends in Endocrinology 2* (Ed. Gardiner-Hill H.) p. 55. Butterworth, London.

DAVIS D., BOHLMAN H., WALKER S. A., FISHER R. & ROBINSON R. (1971) *J. Neurosurg.*, **24**, 603.

DENNY-BROWN D. (1943) *Amer. J. Psychiat.*, **100**, 585.

DENNY-BROWN D. (1945) *Physiol. Rev.*, **25**, 296.

DENNY-BROWN D. (1961) *Arch. Neurol.*, **5**, 13.

DENNY-BROWN D. (1966) *The Cerebral Control of Movement.* Liverpool University Press.

DENNY-BROWN D. & RUSSELL W. R. (1941) *Brain*, **64**, 93.

DEUTSCHMAN C. S. & HAINES S. J. (1985) *Neurosurgery*, **17**, 510.

DE WITT D. S., JENKINS L. W., LUTZ H., WEI E. P., KONTOS H. A., MILLER J. D. & BECKER D. P. (1981) *J. Cereb. Blood Flow Metabol.*, **1**, (Suppl 1) S579.

DRAKE C. G. (1961) *J. Neurosurg.*, **18**, 597.

FAUPEL G., REULEN H. J., MULLER D. & SCHURMANN K. (1976) In *Dynamics of Brain Edema* (Eds Pappius H. M. & Feindel W.) pp. 337–43. Springer Verlag, Berlin.

FIELD J. H. (1976) *Epidemiology of Head Injuries in England and Wales.* HMSO, London.

FISHMAN R. A. (1975) *New Engl. J. Med.*, **293**, 706.

FOWKES F. G. R., EVANS R. C., WILLIAMS L. A., GEHLBACH S. H., COOKE B. R. B. & ROBERTS C. J. (1984) *Lancet*, **2**, 795.

FREYTAG E. (1963) *Arch. Path.*, **75**, 402.

FRIEDE R. L. (1961) *Arch. Neurol.*, **4**, 449.

FROMAN C. (1977) *Neurosurgery*, **1**, 300.

GALLACHER J. P. & BROWDER E. J. (1968) *J. Neurosurg.*, **29**, 1.

GARDNER W. J. (1932) *Arch. Neurol. Psychiat.*, **27**, 847.

GENNARELLI T. A., SEGAWA H., WALD U., CZERNICKI Z., MARSH K. & THOMPSON C. (1982) In *Head Injury: Basic and Clinical Aspects* (Eds Grossman R. G. & Gildenberg P. L.) pp. 129–140. Raven Press, New York.

GIANNOTTA S., WEISS M. H., APUZZO M. L. J. & MARTIN E. (1984) *Neurosurgery*, **15**, 497.

GOBIET W., BOCK W. J., LIESEGANG J. & GROTE W. (1976) In *Intracracranial Pressure III* (Eds Beks J. W. F., Bosch D. A. & Brock M.) pp. 231–235. Springer Verlag, Berlin.

GOULDEN C. (1929) *Trans. ophthal. Soc. UK.*, **49**, 333.

GRAHAM D. I., ADAMS J. H. & DOYLE D. (1977) *J. Neurol. Sci.*, **39**, 213.

GREENBERG R. P., MAYER D. J., BECKER D. P. & MILLER J. D. (1977) *J. Neurosurg.*, **47**, 150.

GREENFIELD J. G. (1938) *Proc. roy. Soc. Med.*, **32**, 43.

GREENFIELD J. G. (1958) *Neuropathology*, p. 408. Arnold, London.

GRONWALL S. K. & WRIGHTSON P. (1981) *J. Neurol. Neurosurg. Psychiat.*, **44**, 889.

GUDEMAN S. K., MILLER J. D. & BECKER D. P. (1979) *J. neurosurg.*, **51**, 301.

GUDEMAN S. K., WHEELER C. B., MILLER J. D., HALLORAN L. G. & BECKER D. P. (1983) *Neurosurgery*, **12**, 175.

GURDJIAN E. S., HARDY W. G., LINDNER D. W. & THOMAS L. M. (1963) *J. Neurosurg.*, **20**, 418.

GURDJIAN E. S. & LISSNER H. R. (1944) *J. Neurosurg.*, **1**, 393.

GURDJIAN E. S. & LISSNER H. R. (1961) *J. Neurosurg.*, **18**, 59.

GURDJIAN E. S., LISSNER H. R., LATIMER F. R., HADDAD B. F. & WEBSTER J. E. (1953) *Neurology*, **3**, 417.

GURDJIAN E. S. & WEBSTER J. E. (1958) *Head Injuries*. Little Brown, Boston.

GURDJIAN E. S., WEBSTER J. E. & LISSNER H. R. (1950) *J. Neurosurg.*, **7**, 106.

GUTHKELCH A. N. (1960) *Brit. med. J.*, **2**, 842.

HALLORAN L. G., ZFASS A. M., GAYLE W. E., WHEELER C. B. & MILLER J. D. (1980) *Amer. J. Surg.*, **139**, 44.

HAYES R. L., GALINAT B. J., KULKARNE P. & BECKER D. P. (1983) *J. Neurosurg.*, **58**, 720.

HILLBLOM E. (1961) *Acta Psychiat. Scand.*, (Suppl.), **15**, 265.

HJERN B. & NYLANDER I. (1951) *Arch. dis. Childh.*, **37**, 113.

HOLBOURN A. H. S. (1943) *Lancet*, **2**, 438.

HOLBOURN A. H. S. (1944) *J. Neurosurg.*, **1**, 190.

HOLBOURN A. H. S. (1945) *Brit. med. Bull.*, **3**, 147.

HOOPER R. S. (1951) *Brit. J. Surg.* **39**, 126.

HOOPER R. S. (1960) *Brit. j. Surg.*, **47**, 71.

HOOPER R.S. (1969) *Patterns of Acute Head Injury*. Arnold, London.

HUGHES B. (1962) *Bull. John Hopk. Hosp.*, **111**, 98.

HUGHES B. In *Acute Injuries of the Head* (Ed. Rowbotham G. F.) Fourth edition, p. 408. Livingstone, Edinburgh.

HUGH-JONES P. (1959) *Proc. roy. Soc. Med.*, **52**, 412.

ILLINGWORTH G. & JENNETT W. B. (1965) *Lancet*, **2**, 511.

INGRAHAM F. D. & MATSON D. D. (1944) *J. Pediat.*, **24**, 1.

ISHII S. In *Head Injury: Conference Proceedings* (Eds Caveness W. F. & Walker A. E.) pp. 276–299. J. B. Lippincott, Philadelphia.

JAMIESON K. G. & YELLAND J. D. N. (1968) *J. Neurosurg.*, **29**, 13.

JANE J. A., RIMEL R. W., POBERESKIN L. H., TYSON G. W., STEWARD O. & GENNARELLI T. A. (1982) In *Head Injury: Basic and Clinical Aspects* (Eds Grossman R. G. & Gildenberg P. L.) pp. 229–237. Raven Press, New York.

JANE J. A., STEWARD O. & GENNARELLI T. (1985) *J. Neurosurg.*, **62**, 96.

JEFFERSON A. (1961) *Trans. ophthal. Soc. UK.*, **81**, 595.

JEFFERSON A. & REILLY G. (1972) *Brit. J. Surg.*, **59**, 585.

JEFFERSON G. J. (1919) *Brain*, **43**, 93.

JEFFERSON G. J. (1931) *Proc. roy. Soc. Med.*, **24**, 742.

JEFFERSON G. (1933) *Brit. med. J.*, **2**, 807.

JEFFERSON G. & SCHORSTEIN J. (1955) *Brit. J. Surg.*, **42**, 561.

JEFFREYS R. V. & JONES J. J. (1981) *Lancet*, **2**, 459.

JELLINGER K. & SEITELBERGER F. (1970) *J. neurol. Sci.*, **10**, 33.

JENNETT B. (1962) *Epilepsy After Blunt Head Injuries*. Heinemann, London.

JENNETT B. (1975) *Epilepsy After Non-Missile Head Injuries*, 2nd edition, pp. 1–179. Heinemann, London.

JENNETT B. & BOND M. R. (1975) *Lancet*, **1**, 480.

JENNETT B. & LEWIN W. (1960) *J. Neurol. Neurosurg. Psychiat.*, **23**, 295.

JENNETT B. & MCMILLAN R. (1981) *Brit. med. J.*, **282**, 101.

JENNETT B., MURRAY A., CARLIN J., MCKEAN M., MCMILLAN R. & STRANG I. (1979) *Brit. med. J.*, **2**, 955.

JENNETT W. B. & STERN W. E. (1960) *J. Neurosurg.*, **17**, 598.

JENNETT B. & TEASDALE G. (1981) *Management of Head Injuries*, pp. 1–361. Davies, Philadelphia.

JENNETT B., TEASDALE G., GALBRAITH S., PICKARD J., GRANT H., BRAAKMAN R., AVEZAAT C., MAAS A., MINDERHOUD J., VECHT C. J., HEIDEN J., SMALL R., CATON W. & KURZE T. (1977) *J. Neurol. Neurosurg. Psychiat.*, **40**, 291.

JENNETT B. & VAN DE SANDE J. (1975) *Epilepsia*, **16**, 251.

JENNETT B., TEASDALE G., BRAAKMAN R., MINDERHOUD J., HEIDEN J. & KURZE T. (1979) *Neurosurgery*, **4**, 283.

JENNETT B., TEASDALE G., FRY J., BRAAKMAN R., MINDERHOUD J., HEIDEN J. & KURZE T. (1980) *J. Neurol. Neurosurg. Psychiät.*, **43**, 289.

KLATZO I. (1972) In *Steroids and Brain Edema* (Eds Reulen H. J. & Schurmann K.) pp. 1–8.

KLAUBER M. R., MARSHALL L. F., BARNETT-CONNOR E. & BOWERS S. A. *Neurosurgery*, **9**, 236.

KOHI Y. M., MENDELOW A. D. & TEASDALE G. M. (1984) *Injury*, **16**, 25.

KREMER M., RUSSELL W. R. & SMYTH G. E. (1947) *J. Neurol. neurosurg. Psychiat.*, **10**, 49.

LANGFITT T. W. (1978) *J. Neurosurg.*, **48**, 673.

LEECH P. J. & PATERSON A. (1973) *Lancet*, **1**, 1013.

LEVETT J. M., JOHN L. M., REPLOGLE R. L. & MULLAN S. (1980) *Surg. Neurol.*, **13**, 59.

LEVINE J. E. & BECKER D. P. (1979) *New Engl. J. Med.*, **301(2)**, 109.

LEWELT W., JENKINS L. W. & MILLER J. D. (1980) *J. Neurosurg.*, **53**, 500.

LEWELT W., JENKINS L. W. & MILLER J. D. (1982) *J. Neurosurg.*, **56**, 332.

LEWIN W. (1966a) *The Management of Head Injuries*. Ballière Tindall Cassell, London.

LEWIN W. (1966b) *Clin Neurosurg.*, **12**, 237.

LEWIN W. & CAIRNS H. (1951) *Brit. med. J.*, **1**, 1.

LEWIN W. & KENNEDY W. F. C. (1956) *Brit. med. J.*, **1**, 1253.

LEWIN W., MARSHALL T. F. D. & ROBERTS A. H. (1979) *Brit. med. J.*, **2**, 1533.

LINDENBERG R., FISHER R. S., DURLACHER S. H., LOVITT W. V. & FREYTAG E. (1955) *Amer. J. Path.*, **31**, 297.

LINDENBERG G. & FREYTAG E. (1960) *Arch. Path.*, **69**, 440.

LINDGREN S. & RINDER L. (1966) *Acta Physiol. Scand.*, **76**, 340.

LINDSAY K. E. W., CARLIN J., KENNEDY I., FRY J., McINNES A. & TEASDALE G. M. (1981) *J. Neurol. Neurosurg. Psychiat.*, **44**, 796.

LONDON P. S. (1963) *Proc. roy. Soc. Med.*, **56**, 821.

MACFLYNN G., MONTGOMERY E. E., FENTON G. W. & RUTHERFORD W. (1984) *J. Neurol. Neurosurg. Psychiat.*, **47**, 1326.

MACIVER I. N., SMITH J. B., TOMLINSON B. E. & WHITBY J. D. (1956) *Brit. J. Surg.*, **43**, 505.

McGHEE E. E., CAUTHEN J. C. & BRACKETT C. E. (1970) *J. Neurosurg.*, **33**, 312.

McKINLAY W. W., BROOKS D. N., BOND M. R., MARTINAGE D. P. & MARSHALL M. M. (1981) *J. Neurosurg. Psychiat.*, **44**, 527.

McKISSOCK W., RICHARDSON & BLOOM W. H. (1960a) *Lancet*, **2**, 167.

McKISSOCK W., RICHARDSON A. & BLOOM W. H. (1960b) *Lancet*, **7**, 1365.

McLEOD A. A. M., NEIL-DWYER G., MEYER C. H. A., RICHARDSON P. L., CRUICKSHANK J. & BARTLETT J. (1982) *Brit. Heart J.*, **47**, 221.

MACPHERSON P. & GRAHAM D. I. (1978) *J. Neurol. Neurosurg. Psychiat.*, **41**, 122.

McQUEEN J. K., BLACKWOOD D. H. R., HARRIS P., KALBAG R. M. & JOHNSON A. L., (1983) *J. Neurol. Neurosurg. Psychiat.*, **46**, 899.

MARSHALL L. F., SMITH R. W. & SHAPIRO H. M. (1979) *J. Neurosurg.*, **50**, 26.

MARTIN J. P. (1955) *Brit. med. J.*, **2**, 467.

MEIROWSKY A. M. & HARSH G. R. (1953) *J. Neurosurg.*, **10**, 373.

MENDEKOW A. D., CAMPBELL D. A., JEFFREY R. R., MILLER J. D., HESSETT C., BRYDEN J. & JENNETT B. (1982) *Brit. med. J.*, **285**, 1530.

MENDELOW A. A., KARMI M. Z., PAUL K. S., FULLAR C. A. G. & GILLINGHAM F. J. (1979) *Brit. med. J.*, **1**, 1240.

MENDELOW A. D., TEASDALE G., JENNETT B., BRYDEN J., HESKETT C. & MURRAY G. (1983) *Brit. med. J.*, **287**, 1173.

METTLER F. A. & METTLER C. C. (1945) *Res. Publ. Ass. nerv. ment. Dis.*, **24**, 1.

MEYERS C. A., LEVIN H. S., EISENBERG H. M. & GUINTO F. C. (1983) *J. Neurol. Neurosurg. Psychiat.*, **46**, 1092.

MILLER H. (1966) *Proc. roy. Soc. Med.*, **59**, 257.

MILLER J. D. (1976) In *Handbook of Neurology* (Ed. Braakman R.) Vol 24, pp. 215–230. North Holland, Amsterdam.

MILLER J. D. (1979a) *Ann. Neurol.*, **6**, 189.

MILLER J. D. (1979b) *Brit. J. hosp. Med.*, **20**, 152.

MILLER J. D. (1982) *Clin. Neurosurg.*, **29**, 103.

MILLER J. D. (1985) *Brit. J. Anaesth.*, **57**, 120.

MILLER J. D. & BECKER D. P. (1982) *J. roy. Coll. Surg. Edin.*, **27**, 292.

MILLER J. D., BECKER D. P., WARD J. D., SULLIVAN H. G., ADAMS W. E. & ROSNER M. (1977) *J. Neurosurg.*, **47**, 503.

MILLER J. D., BUTTERWORTH J. F., GUDEMAN S. K., FAULKNER J. E., CHOI S. C., SELHORST J. B., HARBISON J. W., LUTZ H., YOUNG H. F. & BECKER D. P. (1981) *J. Neurosurg.*, **54**, 289.

MILLER J. D. & GUDEMAN S. K. (1980) In *Cerebral Arterial Spasm* (Ed Wilkins R. H.) pp. 476–79. Williams and Wilkins, Baltimore.

MILLER J. D., GUDEMAN S. K., KISHORE P. R. S. & BECKER D. P. (1980) In *Brain Edema* Eds Cervos-Navarro J. & Ferzt R.) Vol. 28, pp. 413–422. Raven Press, New York.

MILLER J. D. & HOWIE P. W. (1968) *Brit. J. Surg.*, **55**, 423.

MILLER J. D. & JENNETT W. B. (1968) *Lancet*, **2**, 91.

MILLER J. D. & JONES P. A. (1985) *Lancet*, **1**, 1141.

MILLER J. D., SWEET R. C., NARAYAN R. & BECKER D. P. (1978) *J. Amer. med. Ass.*, **240**, 439.

MUIZELAAR J. P., LUTZ H. A. & BECKER D. P. (1984) *J. Neurosurg.*, **61**, 700.

MUIZELAAR J. P., WEI E. P., KONTOS H. A. & BECKER D. P. (1983) *J. Neurosurg.*, **59**, 822.

NARAYAN R., GREENBERG R. P., MILLER J. D., ENAS G. G., CHOI S. C., KISHORE P. R. S., SELHORST J. B., LUTZ H. A. & BECKER D. P. (1981) *J. Neurosurg.*, **54**, 751.

NARAYAN R., KISHORE P. R. S., BECKER D. P. & WARD J. D. (1982) *J. Neurosurg.*, **56**, 650.

NEVIN N. C. (1967) *J. Neuropath. exp. Neurol.*, **26**, 77.

NORMAN J. E., DAN N. G. & ROGERS P. A. (1982) *Orbit*, **1**, 259.

NORTH J. B. & JENNETT S. (1974) *Arch. Neurol.*, **31**, 338.

NORTHFIELD D. W. C. (1944) *J. Neurol. Neurosurg. Psychiat.*, **7**, 1.

OMMAYA A. K. (1966) *Ann. roy. Coll. Surg. Eng.*, **39**, 317.

OMMAYA A. K., DICHIRO G., BALDWIN M. & PENNYBACKER J. B. (1968) *J. Neurol. Neurosurg. Psychiat.*, **31**, 214.

OMMAYA A. K. & GENNARELLI T. A. (1974) *Brain*, **97**, 633.

OPPENHEIMER D. R. (1968) *J. Neurol. Neurosurg. Psychiat.*, **31**, 214.

PEET M. & KAHN E. A. (1932) *J. Amer. med. Ass.*, **98**, 1851.

PENFIELD W. & SHAVER M. (1945) *Res. Publ. Ass. nerv. ment. dis.*, **24**, 620.

PHILLIPS D. G. (1945) *J. Neurol. Neurosurg. Psychiat.*, **8**, 79.

PHILLIPS G. (1954) *J. Neurol. Neurosurg. Psychiat.*, **17**, 1.

PIA H. W. & TÖNNIS W. (1953) *Zbl. Neurochirurg.*, **13**, 1.

PLUM F. & POSNER J. B. (1980) *The Diagnosis of Stupor and Coma*, third edition. F. A. Davis Company, Philadelphia.

POND D. A. (1967) In *Modern Trends in Neurology*, fourth edition (Ed Williams D.) p. 125. Butterworth, London.

POTTER J. M. (1965) *Brit. med. J.*, **2**, 1477.

POVLISHOCK J. T. BECKER D. P., MILLER J. D., JENKINS L. W. & DIETRICH W. D. (1979) *Acta Neuropath.*, **47**, 1.

POVLISHOCK J. T., BECKER D. P., SULLIVAN H. G. & MILLER J. D. (1978) *Brain Res.*, **153**, 223.

POVLISHOCK J. T. & KONTOS H. A. (1982) In *Head Injury: Basic and Clinical Aspects* (Eds Grossman R. G. & Gildenberg P. L.) pp. 15–30. Raven Press, New York.

PRICE D. J. E. & MURRAY A. (1972) *Injury*, **3**, 218.

PRIOR P. F., MAYNARD D. E., SHEAFF P. C., SIMPSON B. R., STRUNIN L., WEAVER E. J. M. & SCOTT D. G. (1971) *Brit. med. J.*, **2**, 737.

PROCTOR B., GURDJIAN E. S. & WEBSTER J. E. (1956) *Laryngoscope*, **66**, 16.

PUDENZ R. H. & SHELDEN C. H. (1946) *J. Neurosurg.*, **3**, 487.

RAIMONDI A. & SAMUELSON G. H. (1970) *J. Neurosurg.*, **32**, 647.

RANSOHOFF J. (1957) *Pediatrics*, **20**, 561.

REILLY P. L., GRAHAM D.I., ADAMS J. H. & JENNETT B. (1975) *Lancet*, **2**, 375.

RIDDOCH G. (1931) *Proc. roy. Soc. Med.*, **24**, 735.

RIMEL R. W., GIORDANI B., BARTH J. T., BOLL J. T. & JANE J. A. (1981) *Neurosurgery*, **9**, 221.

RIMEL R. W., GIORDANI B., BARTH J. T. & JANE J. A. (1982) *Neurosurgery*, **1**, 344.

ROBERSON F. C., KISHORE P. R. S., MILLER J. D., LEIPER M. H. & BECKER D. P. (1979) *Surg. Neurol.*, **12**, 161.

ROBERTS A. H. (1969) *Brain Damage in Boxers*, Pitman, London.

ROSE J., VALTONEN S. & JENNETT B. (1977) *Brit. med. J.*, **2**, 615.

ROSENTHAL M., GRIFFITH E. R., BOND M. R. & MILLER J. D. (1983) *Rehabilitation of the Head Injured Adult* pp. 1–454. Davis, Philadelphia.

ROSOMOFF H. L. (1961) *J. Neurosurg.*, **18**, 753.

ROVIT R. L., SCHECHTER M. M. & NELSON K. (1969) *J. Neurosurg.*, **30**, 406.

ROWBOTHAM G. F. (1964) *Acute Injuries of the Head*, fourth edition. Livingstone, Edinburgh.

ROWBOTHAM G. F., MACIVER I. N., DICKSON J. & BOUSFIELD M. E. (1954) *Brit. med. J.*, **1**, 726.

RUSSELL D. S. & CAIRNS H. (1934) *Brain*, **57**, 32.

RUSSELL W. R. (1931a) *Trans. med. chir. Soc. Edinb.*, **46**, 25.

RUSSELL W. R. (1931b) *Proc. roy. Soc. Med.*, **24**, 751.

RUSSELL W. R. (1959) *Brain Memory and Learning*. Calendar Press, Oxford.

RUSSELL W. R. & SCHILLER F. (1949) *J. Neurol. Neurosurg. Psychiat.*, **12**, 93.

RUSSELL W. R. & SMITH A. (1961) *Arch Neurol.*, **5**, 4.

RUSSELL W. R. & WHITTY C. W. M. (1952) *J. Neurol. Neurosurg. Psychiat.*, **15**, 93.

RUTHERFORD W. H., GREENFIELD T., HAYES H. R. M. & NELSON J. K. (1985) *The Medical Effects of Seatbelt Legislation in the United Kingdom*, pp. 1–175. HMSO, London.

SAUL T. G., DUCKER T. B., SALCMAN M. & CARRO E. (1981) *J. Neurosurg.*, **54**, 596.

SCHORSTEIN J. (1947) *Brit. J. Surg.* War Surgery Suppl., **1**, 96.

SCHWARTZ M. L., TATOR C. H., ROWED D. W., REID S. R., MEGURA K. & ANDREWS D. F. (1984) *Canad. J. Neurol. Sci.*, **11**, 434.

SEDZIMIR C. B. (1955) *J. Neurol. Neurosurg. Psychiat.*, **18**, 293.

SEELIG J. M., BECKER D. P., MILLER J. D., GREENBERG R. P., WARD J. D. & CHOI S. C. (1981) *New Engl. J. Med.*, **304**, 1511.

SELHORST J. B., GUDEMAN S. K., BUTTERWORTH J. F., HARBISON J. W., MILLER J. D. & BECKER D. P. (1985) *Neurosurgery*, **16**, 357.

SEVITT S. (1962) *Fat Embolism*. Butterworth, London.

SHAPIRO H. M., WYTE S. R. & LOESER J. (1974) *J. Neurosurg.*, **40**, 90.

SHEEHAN D. (1940) *Res. Publ. Ass. nerv. ment. Dis.*, **20**, 589.

SKARF B., DAVIS R. L., BIRSNER H. A. & HOYT W. F. (1984) *Arch. Neurol.*, **41**, 58.

SPILLANE J. D. (1962) *Brit. med. J.*, **2**, 1205.

STALHAMMAR D. (1975) *Acta Neurol. Scand.*, **52**, 27.

STRANG F. A. (1971) *Proc. roy. Soc. Med.*, **64**, 14.

STRICH S. J. (1956) *J. Neurol. Neurosurg. Psychiat.*, **19**, 163.

STRICH S. J. (1961) *Lancet*, **2**, 443.

SULLIVAN H. G., MARTINEZ J., BECKER D. P., MILLER J. D., GRIFFITH R. & WIST A. O. (1976) *J. Neurosurg.*, **45**, 520.

SUMMERS C. G. & WIRTSCHAFTER J. D. (1979) *J. Neurosurg.*, **50**, 508.

SUMNER D. (1964) *Brain*, **87**, 107.

SUWANELA C. & SUWANELA N. (1972) *J. neurosurg.*, **36**, 314.

SYMONDS C. P. (1962) *Lancet*, **1**, 1.

SYMONDS C. P. (1982) *Brit. med. J.*, **2**, 829.

TAYLOR A. R. & BELL T. K. (1966) *Lancet*, **2**, 178.

TEASDALE E., CARDOSO E., GALBRAITH S. & TEASDALE G. (1984) *J. Neurol. Neurosurg. Psychiat.*, **47**, 600.

TEASDALE G., GALBRAITH S., MURRAY L., WARD P., GENTLEMAN D. & MCKEAN M. (1982) *Brit. med. J.*, **285**, 1695.

TEASDALE G. & JENNETT B. (1974) *Lancet*, **2**, 81.

TILL K. (1968) *Brit. med. J.*, **3**, 400.

TOMLINSON B. E. (1970) *J. clin. Path.* (23 Suppl) **4**, 178.

TRAQUAIR H. M. (1946) *Trans. ophthal. Soc. UK.*, **65**, 64.

TRAQUAIR H. M., DOTT N. M. & RUSSELL W. R. (1935) *Brain*, **58**, 398.

TROTTER W. (1914) *Brit. J. Surg.*, **2**, 271.

TROTTER W. (1924) *Lancet*, **1**, 935.

TURAZZI S., BRICOLO A. & PASUT M. L. (1984) *Acta Neurochir.*, **2**, 167.

TURNER J. W. A. (1943) *Brain*, **66**, 140.

UNTERHARNSCHEIDT F. & SELLIER K. (1971) *Fortschr. Neurol. Psychiat.*, **39**, 109.

VAN DONGEN K. J. & BRAAKMAN R. (1980) *Neurosurgery*, **7**, 14.

VENABLES H. B., WILSON S., ALLAN W. C. & PRENSKY A. L. (1978) *Neurology*, **28**, 1066.

VERBIEST H. (1958) *Folia Psychiat. nederl.*, **61**, 652.

WAGSTAFFE W. D. (1928) *Lancet*, **2**, 561.

WALKER A. E. (1957) *J. Amer. med. Ass.*, **164**, 1636.

WALKER A. E. (1964) In *Acute Injuries of the Head*, fourth edition. (Rowbottom G. F. Ed.) p. 486. Livingstone, Edinburgh.

WALKER A. E. & JABLON S. (1959) *J. Neurosurg.*, **16**, 600.

WALKER A. E. & JABLON S. (1961) *A Follow-up Study of Head Wounds in World War II*. US Government Printing Office, Washington DC.

WARD J. D., BECKER D. P., MILLER J. D., CHOI S. C., MARMAROU A., WOOD C., NEWLON P. & KEENAN R. (1985) *J. Neurosurg.*, **62**, 383.

WATTS C. W. & CLARK K. (1969) *J. Neurosurg.*, **30**, 107.

WEHRLE P. F., MATHIES A. W. & LEEDOM J. M. (1967) *Clin. Neurosurg.*, **14**, 72.

WEI E. P., DIETRICH W. D., POVLISHOCK J. T. & KONTOS H. A. (1980) *Circ. res.*, **14**, 72.

WEIR B. (1971) *J. Neurosurg.*, **34**, 528.

WESTON P. P. A. M. (1981) *Brit. J. Surg.*, **68**, 633.

WILKINS R. H. & ODOM G. L. (1970) *J. Neurosurg.*, **32**, 626.

WILLIAMS D. & DENNY-BROWN D. (1941) *Brain*, **64**, 223.

WINDLE W. F., GROAT R. A. & FOX C. A. (1944) *Surg. Gynec. obstet.*, **79**, 561.

YOUNG B., RAPP R. P., NORTON J. A., HAACK D., TIBBS P. A. & BEAN J. R. (1983) *J. Neurosurg.*, **58**, 231.

# Chapter 24
# Spinal injury

P. M. FOY, G. F. G. FINDLAY

## Introduction

In civilian practice the great majority of cases of spinal cord injury occur as the indirect effect of violence applied to the spinal column. Flexion or vertical compression causes vertebral fracture, dislocation or both; the cord is crushed or bruised by occlusion of the spinal canal and by fragments of bone or of ruptured intervertebral disc. The cord may sustain injury, usually transient, if the spine is violently struck without causing fracture or dislocation. In the cervical region sudden hyperextension can narrow the spinal canal sufficiently to squeeze the cord, particularly in patients with spondylosis. Direct injury of the cord requires penetration by a foreign object, usually a bullet or other high velocity missile, rarely by stabbing with a sharp weapon. Missiles may also injure the cord indirectly, from bone splinters or from the impact of missile on bone when it is deflected and fails to enter the spinal canal. These glancing injuries on the vertebral column produce widespread bruising of the cord similar to that in the brain beneath a tangential cranial injury. This type of injury has been described by earlier writers as concussion of the spinal cord (Holmes 1915, Claude & Lhermitte 1919) but this term should perhaps be restricted to a different clinical syndrome, that of transient traumatic paraplegia, considered later; Thorburn (1887) mentioned the phenomenon but had never encountered an example. Except for an unusual form of assault by stabbing to be described, direct and therefore compound injuries of the spinal cord are rare in civil practice but they cause the majority of traumatic paraplegias in military warfare. Wannamaker (1954)

reported on 300 spinal injuries sustained in the Korean campaigns: 85% were penetrating.

Stabbing is an unusual mode of injury. The protection given by the laminae means that the sharp weapon must be driven home to one side of the middle line and in an oblique direction. The majority of the lesions are partial but total division of the cord can be achieved. Lipschitz and Block (1962) have reported 130 examples: they formed the remarkably high proportion of 60% of all their cases of traumatic paraplegia.

The regional incidence of injury and the proportion with a complete lesion is given in the following table. This is derived from information given by Guttmann (1959) concerning 1047 cases of injury treated at Stoke Mandeville Hospital.

|  | (per cent) | Complete lesion in (per cent) |
|---|---|---|
| Cervical | 10 | 30 |
| Upper thoracic (1–5) | 10 | 77 |
| Lower thoracic (6–12) | 50 | 79 |
| Cauda equina | 30 | — |

Lucas and Ducker (1979) reported a series of over 500 cases of acute spinal injury in which complete lesions occurred in 60% of the cervical injuries and over 70% of the thoracic and upper lumbar injuries.

It will be noted that injuries are more common in the lower half of the spinal cord and that the thoracic cord is more likely to sustain complete functional transection than the cervical. This is probably related to the greater violence and more severe vertebral damage involved in thoracic injuries than to the relatively small size and tight fit of the spinal cord in the thoracic spinal canal. The mobility of the cervical spine provides a measure of protection; fracture or fracture dislocation usually occurs at the apex of its normal curve rather than at the transitional zone between mobility and immobility. Road traffic accidents account for 30–50% of spinal cord injuries and industrial accidents for a further 30%. The remainder comprise a mixed group of which sports and domestic injuries are the most prominent. The great majority of cases are young males, for example Sutton (1973) reported a series of 232 tetraplegics of whom 72% were under 40 years of age and 87% were male.

Early mortality from spinal injury has declined steadily from up to 80% before 1944 to between 5 and 15% in recent years.

## Morbid anatomy of spinal cord injury

*Concussion* is a term applied loosely to transient states of loss of function which may follow violent blows on the spinal column (without causing fracture dislocation): whiplash injuries, sudden flexion of the head in patients with abnormalities around the foramen magnum and so forth. Paralysis is immediate and flaccid and the subject falls to the ground; recovery takes place in minutes or hours and is complete. Whether all functions of the spinal cord can be temporarily interrupted in this way is an open question, for the opportunity of making a meticulous neurological examination immediately after an injury rarely occurs. Benes (1966) diagnosed concussion in 5% of 202 injuries and in none was complete loss of function recorded. The term is adopted from head injury parlance, for the clinical similarity with cerebral concussion is close, in the immediate dramatic result of trauma, the sudden paralysis of nervous function which quickly recovers. But like cerebral injury, there is no line of demarcation between 'concussion' and more severe injury in which recovery is slow and incomplete. There are at least two fairly convincing animal models of cerebral concussional injury: the fluid percussion model and

the nonimpact head acceleration device, as described in the previous chapter. There has been no convincing experimental model of the phenomenon in the spine and the anatomy of the cranial contents is so different from the spinal that it is likely that the physical processes are also entirely different. The most widely used experimental model of spinal cord injury involves a weight dropping from a measured height onto the exposed spinal cord or the dura to produce a range of levels of dysfunction in the spinal cord, including complete interruption of function with an area of haemorrhagic necrosis in the central cord (Dohrmann *et al.* 1978). It seems improbable that rotation which is so important in the aetiology of cerebral concussion plays any part in spinal cord injury but violent pressure waves propagated through the deep tissues may exert a direct effect upon fibre tracts. Sudden extreme neck movement in cases of unstable atlanto-axial articulation presumably pinches the cord momentarily though insufficiently to cause structural damage. Hughes (1966) states that there is 'no acceptable histopathological counterpart'. The use of the phrase 'concussion of the spinal cord' can only be justified on clinical grounds, to denote retrospectively a closed injury of minimal degree, with complete neurological recovery.

*Contusion* of the spinal cord implies structural damage; in its most severe form the cord is destroyed by pulping or is torn asunder. Hughes recognizes three stages, early, intermediate and late.

*Early* pathological changes are found within the first few weeks after injury. The affected portion of cord is swollen and may fit the theca tightly, discoloured from petechial haemorrhages and from venous stasis. It is soft, to a degree that liquefied cord may exude if the pia is pricked. On section there may be central necrosis and haemorrhage more conspicuous in the grey matter but a localized haematomyelia is unusual. Myelin sheaths are swollen and broken up, axones ruptured and neurons degenerate. There are oedema and infiltration with red cells and leucocytes. Subarachnoid bleeding is insignificant in closed injuries but may be considerable in penetrating injuries. Extradural haemorrhage occurs to a variable extent, usually on the ventral aspect in conjunction with tearing of the posterior longitudinal ligament; those seen by Wolman (1965) at autopsy were not sufficiently large to cause compression of the cord. Morbid changes are not confined to the crushed portion of cord but extend through adjacent segments above and below. The more obvious are irregular cavities containing necrotic material which Holmes noted were larger at their distal extremities and communicated by narrow tracks with the main lesion. They tend to occur in the ventral part of the dorsal columns, in the peripheral field of the anterior spinal artery, and consequently an area most likely to suffer ischaemic softening. Holmes (1915) noted that fibre tracts bordering these cavities appeared compressed and concluded that the cavities were due to the seepage under pressure of necrotic material and exudate from the main lesion. With haemorrhage and softening they were regarded by Holmes as the cause of the delayed deterioration in neurological status often encountered within the first few days of injury. The spread of oedema (in rostral and caudal directions) from the site of damage is similar to that which occurs in the brain. In experimental studies it shows the features of vasogenic oedema.

*Intermediate* changes may persist for several years. Swelling subsides, oedema resolves and the infiltration with red cells and polymorphs is replaced by lymphocytes and compound granular cells active in cleaning up the products of tissue destruction. Gliosis occurs unless traumatic necrosis has destroyed the glial cells as well as nerve cells and processes.

*Late* and final changes are seen after many years. Severely damaged cord is entirely replaced by a connective tissue scar which blends with the dura mater. In lesser degrees of injury there is a dense gliosis.

*Delayed myelopathy and syringomyelia*

A rare sequel to thoracic and lumbar injuries is the extension in a rostral direction of manifestations of cord dysfunction. It occurs after a varying latent interval of several or many years. The cervical enlargement is most affected and the clinical picture resembles syringomyelia. Myelography usually reveals evidence of expansion of the cord, more marked at the cervical extremity. Surgical exploration in a few cases has confirmed the presence of a distended cavity within the spinal cord. The aetiology is obscure but it is generally accepted that such a cavity corresponds with those described by Holmes. No satisfactory explanation has been offered for the long latent period before cystic distension gives rise to clinical signs. Barnett *et al.* (1966) described 8 cases in detail, encountered in an experience of 591 cases of traumatic paraplegia. In 2 cases reported by Rossier *et al.* (1968) drainage of the cyst into the subarachnoid space was followed by improvement and reference is made to other cases in which operation was beneficial. With the advent of magnetic resonance imaging of the spinal cord, it is becoming apparent that post-traumatic syringomyelia is by no means as rare as previously thought.

## Injury to blood vessels

It is probable that interruption of the circulation plays an important role in cord damage. Wolman noted thrombotic occlusion of small pial and intramedullary arteries in about one-third of specimens with necrosis of the cord, but stated that occlusion of a major spinal artery was rare. Venous thrombosis may be responsible for remote changes in the cord (Jellinger 1964). The vertebral artery may be damaged at the site of dislocation of the neck with consequent infarction of the spinal cord. Autopsy specimens have been described by Hughes (1964) and by Wolman (1965); the latter quotes a case in which coma and respiratory failure due to cerebellar infarction occurred 18 days after injury; artificial respiration and operative removal of swollen cerebellum was followed by recovery. Schneider and Crosby (1959) record a case in which an injury at C4–5 with necrosis of the cord at that level was accompanied by infarction six segments lower attributable to the precarious circulation in upper thoracic segments. They point out that the vertebral artery may also be damaged in atlanto-axial dislocations and brain stem signs may develop. Collier (1916) described cases in which the whole spinal cord distal to the injury necrosed, in the adult and in the infant following birth injury. It probably depends on damage to major spinal arteries, perhaps aggravated by the severe systemic hypotension which may accompany spinal injury.

## Injury to the spine

Only a brief and simplified account of the spinal injury will be given; text books of orthopaedic surgery should be consulted.

*Cervical.* Violence causes damage by flexion, rotation, compression or hyperextension. Flexion–rotation ruptures the posterior intervertebral ligaments, causes an oblique shearing fracture through the body or ruptures the intervertebral disc, or a combination of both; the upper segment of spine is driven forwards on the lower as a result of dislocation or of fracture of the zygapophyseal processes on one or both sides. Schneider and Kahn (1956) have drawn attention to a particular pattern of compression fracture of the vertebral body in some cases; the postero-inferior margin may be split off and displaced backwards into the spinal canal.

The neurosurgeon must recognize certain patterns of bone injury at the upper end of the cervical spine. Fracture of the ring of the atlas was described by Jefferson (1920) and bears his name today. It is not usually associated with neurological damage, and is generally considered a stable injury. The fracture is most easily recognized on the anteroposterior view by widening of the ring of the atlas with lateral displacement of the C1 facets.

The two recognizable injuries of the axis are a fracture of the odontoid process, a dangerous and unstable injury (Fig. 24.1), and the 'hangman's' fracture (Fig. 24.2). This latter injury is a fracture across both sides of the neural arch of C2 resulting in separation of the body from the arch. The hangman's and Jefferson's fractures can be satisfactorily managed by wearing a cervical collar. In contrast, odontoid process fractures require reduction and more rigid fixation, either externally by a halo apparatus, or internally, by wiring and/or fusion.

The mechanism by which the cord is injured probably varies. It has been generally assumed that the cord is crushed between the postero-superior margin of the lower vertebral body and the inferior edge of the neural arch above and that spinal nerves are squeezed or stretched in their course to and through the intervertebral foramina; this is probably the common mechanism. Fragments of bone displaced backwards into the spinal canal will injure the cord and increase the shearing effect of dislocation. Jefferson (1936) expressed the view that extruded pulped disc material played a major role and later (1948) pointed out that Thorburn in 1909 had observed this at necropsy. In the experience of Munro (1965) displacement of disc cartilage occurred in 5.6% of cervical injuries, and Harris (1966) reported a somewhat similar incidence of 7%. Schneider (1955) reported 12 cases selected for operation because the clinical picture suggested that the anterior aspect of the cervical cord had received the brunt of the injury: extruded disc material was found in only 3. Flexion injuries of the cervical spine are classified by orthopaedic surgeons as 'unstable', because of the rupture of the posterior ligaments (Fig. 24.3). Instability implies a tendency for the displacement to recur after reduction, avoided by prolonged immobilization or by operative fusion (Holdsworth 1966).

In flexion injuries of the cervical spine, with disruption of the ligaments around the posterior facet joints, restitution of normal vertebral

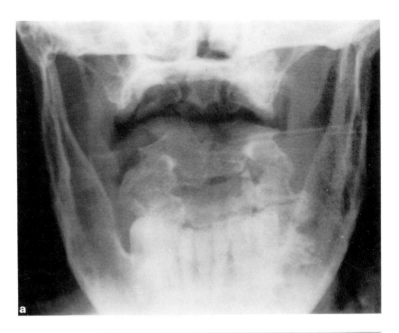

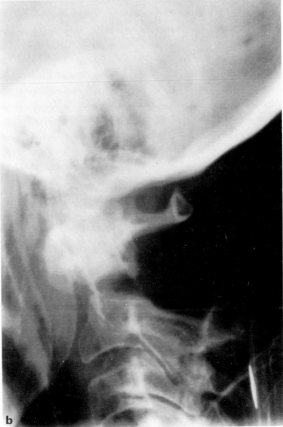

**Fig. 24.1** Displaced fracture of odontoid process a) anteroposterior, b) lateral projection.

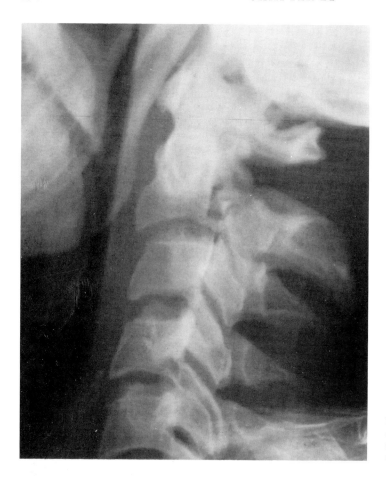

**Fig. 24.2** Fracture through the arch of C2 with anterior displacement of the body of C2 on C3: 'hangman's fracture'.

alignment may be prevented by 'jumping' of the facets so that locking occurs and the upper vertebral body remains displaced and angulated forward upon the lower. The displacement and angulation is easy to recognize on lateral X-rays of the cervical spine when both facet joints are affected (Fig. 24.4). When unilateral locking of a facet joint occurs the condition is much less easy to recognize because the upper vertebra is rotated upon the lower and there may be little of this displacement or angulation viewed from the lateral aspect. Loss of alignment of the shadows of the vertebral spines on the anteroposterior view should be a clue to this problem but irregularities in spinal alignment are sufficiently common to make this unreliable (Fig. 24.5). In practice, oblique views targeted on the facet

joints, or tomography may be required to define the problem. In keeping with the degree of displacement of the vertebral bodies and the extent to which the spinal canal is occluded, spinal cord damage and dysfunction is much more likely with bilateral than with unilateral facet dislocation. On the other hand, bilateral facet dislocation is more easily reduced with closed spinal traction than unilateral dislocation which more often requires operative reduction.

Hyperextension of the cervical spine may result in dislocation, or there may be no radiological evidence of trauma. Barnes (1948) and Taylor and Blackwood (1948) showed that the anterior longitudinal ligament ruptures, an intervertebral disc may be torn asunder and the hyperextension which this allows leads to

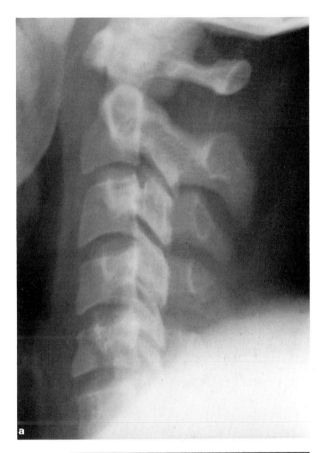

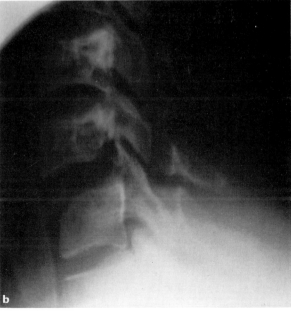

Fig. 24.3 Fracture through body of cervical vertebra a) C5 fracture without displacement: note that only the top of C6 is shown: this is not an adequate X-ray examination. b) Fracture through upper anterior rim of the body of C6 with some displacement. Due to associated ligamentous tearing produced by flexion injury this is an unstable and dangerous injury.

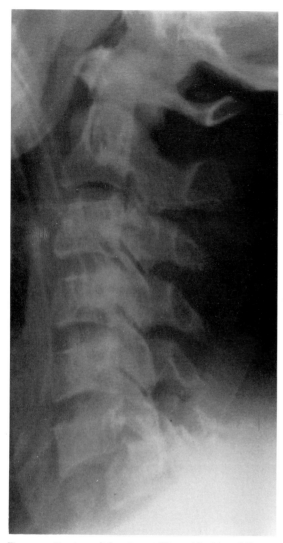

**Fig. 24.4.** Fracture: dislocation at C6–7 with almost full diameter displacement of the vertebral body and bilateral facet locking.

coming to post-mortem had relatively minor pathological changes when severe neurological deficit had been present in life. If dislocation occurs as a result of rupture of posterior spinal ligaments the posterior longitudinal ligament is torn from the vertebral bodies and the cord is crushed between the postero-inferior border of the upper vertebra and the neural arch below. Violent hyperextension is a frequent and serious cause of spinal cord contusion in patients with cervical spondylosis, causing severe neurological disturbance when none was previously present, or severely aggravating a pre-existing myelopathy. Barnes (1948) noted that among 7 hyperextension injuries, 6 occurred in elderly persons with spondylosis and little radiological evidence of recent injury. A common story is of a fall forwards or downstairs striking the face and forcing the head backwards, although Symonds (1953) described cases in which injury resulted from little more than normal movement. Among their 45 cases of spondylosis, Brain *et al.* (1952) found that in 8 trauma was immediately followed by symptoms, there having been none previously. Illustrations of the acute necrosis of the cord which may follow these accidents will be found in that paper and in that of Wilkinson (1960). The cord is squeezed between the spondylotic excrescences jutting into the spinal canal and the infolded ligamenta flava. In the post-mortem specimens examined by Hughes and Brownell (1963) the indentation and contusion of the cord corresponded 'exactly to the largest spondylotic bulge'. If the spinal canal is narrow by development, the cord will be damaged by a lesser degree of extension. The mechanism is discussed in greater detail in the section on cervical myelopathy. Wilkinson (1960) suggests that the adherence of the dura mater to the floor of the spinal canal and of the spinal root sleeves to the intervertebral foramina anchors the spinal cord and renders it more liable to injury. Schneider and Schemm (1961) have suggested that the cord damage in hyperextension injuries of the neck may not be due to contusion, but to temporary impairment of vertebral circulation. The evidence of this is slender, though indubitably

lengthening of the spinal canal and distraction of the spinal cord: the cord lesion may be rostral to the vertebral. When the head and neck revert to the neutral position, if dislocation has not taken place there is no radiological abnormality and even post-mortem examination may not reveal the spinal damage unless a careful search is made. Bohlman (1979) showed in his review of 300 cervical spine injuries that some of those

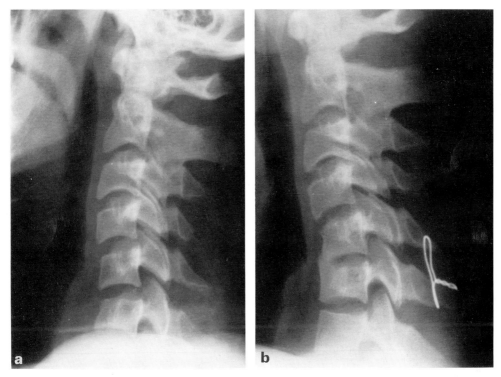

**Fig. 24.5.** Partial dislocation and loss of alignment at C5–6 that should raise suspicion of unilateral facet displacement. Lateral view a) before, and b) after open reduction and posterior wiring followed by anterior interbody fusion.

the vertebral arteries may be damaged in dislocation.

*Thoracolumbar* spinal injuries are commonly due to violent hyperflexion combined with torsion, or to vertical compression. The former occurs when heavy masses of rock or masonry fall on the shoulders: the latter when the subject falls from a height and lands on the feet. The compressive injury is often combined with fractures of the calcaneum. If the posterior ligaments successfully resist, the vertebral body is crushed but no dislocation occurs and the cord frequently escapes injury. As with cervical injuries, tearing of the ligaments permits shearing movement; articular processes fracture, the vertebral body is fractured obliquely in a plane governed by the force applied, with or without rupture of the disc. Remarkable degrees of displacement in the sagittal or coronal axes may be encountered, to an extent that the adjacent vertebrae may be entirely disengaged; there may be marked angu-

lation. Instability may be such that gross displacement has become largely corrected by the time the spine is X-rayed, having occurred during the movements of placing the patient on a stretcher or other flat surface. The presence of instability must then be inferred from the pattern of bony injury, or neurological damage.

### Neurology of spinal cord injury

The Goulstonian Lectures by Holmes (1915) were a massive contribution to the knowledge of the effects of spinal injury in man and provide an essential introduction to the subject. Other important early papers were those of Collier (1916), Riddoch (1917, 1918) and Head and Riddoch (1917). Although the cases upon which these studies were made comprised mainly penetrating war injuries, the observations are of equal application to closed civilian injuries.

If the injury is sufficiently severe, there is immediate total interruption of function at the level of the lesion and in the distal portion of the cord. Paralysis is complete and flaccid, reflexes are abolished (with certain provisos to be mentioned later) and all forms of sensibility are lost. Interruption of function may be structural or physiological in origin and at an early stage it is not possible to differentiate. Only the passage of time will reveal whether and to what relative extents total interruption of cord function is anatomical or physiological. Restitution of conduction physiologically blocked occurs within hours or a day or so, and its detection depends on repeated and thorough physical examination. It should be noted that signs of conduction may be few and meagre (therefore easily overlooked) for the great majority of axons may have suffered more than physiological interference. As a result of clinical experience it is now generally agreed that if there are no signs of recovery of function within 48 hours of an injury causing initial total motor and sensory paralysis, then none will occur subsequently: anatomical 'transection' has been inflicted. Kahn (1959) goes further than this for he states that 'if the paralysis is immediate, complete and lasts for a period of 24 hours function of the spinal cord will not return' and that he had never seen recovery from complete paralysis following thoracic spinal injury. Guttmann (1959) has seen exceptions to this general rule. Michaelis (1976a) estimated that a wrong prognosis of a permanently complete lesion may be made in 1–5% of cases, basing this estimate on the analysis of 3,500 cases of spinal cord trauma including about 1,000 tetraplegics. He cited two factors which may be overlooked: the history given by the patient may indicate that the lesion was not complete immediately after trauma, and the time from the injury to the initial neurological examination may allow oedema and haemorrhage to draw a veil over sacral sparing which reappears on later examination.

The diagnosis of anatomical transection of the cord has a commanding influence over treatment for it follows that operation upon the vertebral injury can have no beneficial effect upon neurological function. It may be thought necessary for other reasons, but not for the treatment of the spinal cord lesion. On the other hand, operation may be advisable for the relief of compression or traction on spinal nerves for they are more resistant to trauma than the cord and their function may ultimately return. A particular example is in injury involving the conus and the cauda equina; the former may be permanent but relief of pressure upon the latter may provide recovery of activity in muscles supplied by nerves derived from the cord above the level of destruction.

In lesions partial from the outset, motor function is generally affected much more severely than sensory. This greater susceptibility of the corticospinal tract to the effects of trauma appears in some respects to be similar to its susceptibility to the effects of compression from, say, a tumour, as was considered in the section on compression paraplegia. The greater disturbance of motor function is also related to the phenomenon of 'spinal shock', considered later, which magnifies temporarily the effect of trauma upon the descending spinal pathways. Extensive sensory loss particularly if all forms are affected is an ominous sign, indicating denser structural damage than would be the case with severe motor loss. Partial lesions present diverse neurological pictures. Sensory pathways may be entirely preserved, may show a suspended type of dissociated loss like syringomyelia, may conform to a Brown-Sequard distribution, or may be irregular and asymmetrical suggesting a lesion of patchy density. Paralysis may be unilateral or worse on one side than the other; it may predominate in the upper limbs in cervical lesions, indicating that destruction has affected the anterior horns more than the lateral columns, a pattern particularly associated with extension injuries of the neck and to which further attention will be given.

*Special features*

1. *Spinal shock* denotes certain characteristics of the paralysis which follows sudden interruption of the descending spinal pathways. The muscles are flaccid and waste rapidly and superficial and deep reflexes are abolished, except for the plantar reflex which may show varied responses. Holmes observed that in complete lesions the response was entirely absent for several weeks; in severe partial lesions a normal but reduced flexor response was noted for several days and then became extensor. Collier emphasized that if an early flexor response is encountered it is reduced in degree; he frequently saw in succession no response, reduced flexor and then extensor responses and in patients whose condition was deteriorating this succession was exhibited in reverse. In unilateral lesions, the flaccidity and areflexia are also unilateral; in unequal bilateral lesions Collier stated that there may be on one side a reduced flexor plantar response and on the other side an extensor response. Spinal shock subsides after a varying period of time; the muscles innervated by distal segments become spastic, the tendon reflexes return to an exaggerated degree and the plantar reflexes become extensor: voluntary movement may be detected as the muscles recover tone. In the early stages of returning movement it may be difficult to determine whether these are volitional, or reflex in response to touching the limb or to a movement of the bed. Recovery from spinal shock is influenced by the general state of the patient's health. It is prolonged by anaemia, low plasma proteins, metabolic disorder and infection (urinary, cutaneous and respiratory being the commonest); spinal shock may recur if these complications arise. It is a traditional view that while muscles are flaccid there is hope for the return of voluntary power but with increasing spasticity the likelihood of this diminishes. It is true that this is a useful guide, but the argument is faulty. Persistent flaccidity (in an upper motor neuron lesion) denotes spinal shock, and until this wears off voluntary movement cannot be initiated: spasticity will then develop in those

muscles whose descending fibre tracts have been too severely injured to conduct the impulses necessary for voluntary movement. There is no clear-cut separation, for a group of muscles may recover some power and also show spasticity.

The cause of spinal shock is obscure. It is usually ascribed to a reduction of synaptic activity of the motor neurons in the isolated segments of cord, consequent upon the cessation of descending impulses which maintain an adequate excitatory state in the motor neuron pool: 'the loss of some subsidy of excitatory process derived from higher levels of the nervous system' (Denny-Brown 1966). Illis (1967) suggests that the spinal network of neurons has a plastic rather than an anatomically determined organization, and that when its normal functions are upset, as by the loss of particular inputs, the network is reorganized. This requires time, the period of 'shock' and the reorganization is evident later in the recovery of and change in the nature of the reflexes. Illis has investigated the changes which take place on the surface of a motor neuron distal to section of the cord and after posterior root section. Within 24 hours there are marked alterations in the *boutons terminaux* many thousands of which stud the cell surface and proximal parts of its dendrites. After some days areas of cell surface become bare as a result of the degeneration and absorption of boutons; later boutons reform and their numbers become nearly normal. Illis concludes that this represents a reorganization of input contacts due to the re-innervation of bare areas from intact fibres.

2. *Vegetative disturbances.* During the period of spinal shock there is paralysis of the bladder and of the intestinal tract. The bladder passively distends until overflow incontinence occurs. Abdominal distension may lead to vomiting; absorption from the gut is defective; defecation ceases. Dependent upon the level of the lesion the blood pressure falls as a result of loss of vasomotor tone and with this there may be marked hypothermia (or hyperthermia) according to the extent to which after the accident the

body is protected from the ambient temperature: its reactions are poikilothermic. Shivering of muscles above the level of the lesion has been observed (Collier 1916). The pulse rate slows and Holmes noted a lethargic state of the mind; he recognized the similarity of this state to hibernation.

3. *Posture of limbs.* As spasticity develops the paraplegic limbs tend to adopt a position of flexion or of extension.

*Paraplegia-in-flexion* corresponds to the position taken up in the flexor withdrawal reflex: flexion of hip and knee and dorsiflexion of ankle and toes. (Although dorsiflexion of the distal joints of the extremity is performed by muscles nominated as extensors, their action is to shorten the limb and thus to act physiologically as flexors. The 'extensor plantar response' is the minimal degree of the flexor withdrawal reflex). Head and Riddoch (1917) described the mass-reflex which is an exaggerated flexor withdrawal reflex and evoked by stimuli applied anywhere below the lesion. The trunk responds with the lower limbs by violent flexion, the bladder and rectum evacuate and profuse sweating occurs which involves the whole body if the lesion lies above the cervical sympathetic outflow. Riddoch (1918) drew attention to the exhausting nature of the mass reflex and the need to adopt nursing techniques least likely to evoke it. Holmes observed in severe or total lesions automatic movements of the lower limbs, which alternately slowly flexed and extended, representing rudimentary stepping. He also described reflex arm movements in high cervical lesions, comparable to withdrawal: a stimulus applied to the inner aspect of the arm caused the limb to rotate inwards and to adduct.

*Paraplegia-in-extension* occurs if there is a preponderance of hypertonus in the extensors, the antigravity muscles, and represents a reflex maintenance of the standing posture; it can be compared with decerebrate rigidity.

On the basis of his experience Riddoch (1917) came to the conclusion that paraplegia-in-flexion developed in those patients with total severance

of the cord: operation revealed a gap between two ends of cord, created by a missile. Paraplegia-in-extension he believed to occur when the cord was severely but not totally destroyed, but he quoted no detailed pathological description of such an example in support of his belief. Riddoch noted differences in the reflexes of flexed and of extended paraplegics and on these based the assumption that one could distinguish partial from complete lesions, although there might be no other neurological evidence of conduction through the damaged segments of the cord. Walshe (1915) argued that for extensor hypertonus to arise there must be preservation of pontospinal connections. The tacit correlation of paraplegia-in-flexion and in-extension with total and with subtotal isolation of the caudal portion of the cord respectively, dates from these papers by Walshe (1915) and Riddoch (1917). It is open to criticism. It is difficult to visualize a traumatic lesion which spares pontospinal connections but interrupts all others. Guttmann (1966a, 1970) has categorically expressed disbelief in the concept. His experience has taught him that the final posture greatly depends on the position of the limbs in the initial stages of the paraplegia. If the legs are from the beginning maintained in extension and abduction, little flexion occurs and in many cases of complete transection the final result is spasticity-in-extension; conversely in patients with partial lesions, severe spasticity in flexion may develop if the position of the legs is neglected, i.e. if they are allowed to lie flexed. The studies on spasticity in paraplegics by Dimitrijevic and Nathan (1967) give considerable support to Guttmann's contention. They emphasize that there is considerable idiosyncrasy among patients as to which muscle groups are susceptible to low threshold stimulation, so that one particular group may always contract powerfully. They also found that 'a posture of flexion generally favours further flexion and one of extension further extension'. For recent reviews on this subject and spasticity in general see Simpson (1965), Rushworth (1966), Whitteridge (1966), Brodal (1969), Michaelis (1976b).

4. *Cervical cord injuries* carry the highest mortality, 20% in the series of Holdsworth (1966) and over 50% in those of Taylor and Gleave (1962) and Durbin (1961). Complete transection at a high level accounted for the majority of the deaths. Wolman (1965) reported on the post-mortem findings in 73 fatal cases of cord damage secondary to spinal injury: in 60% the injury was cervical, whereas the general incidence of injury in this region is only about 10%. Two-thirds of the patients dying after cervical injury survived for less than 11 days; acute respiratory failure and pulmonary oedema were the commonest causes of death. In low cervical lesions pulmonary ventilation is seriously impaired by the intercostal paralysis; if the lesion involves C3 and C4 segments, by direct contusion or by secondary upward extension, diaphragmatic paralysis is added and death rapidly ensues unless artificial ventilation or phrenic nerve stimulation is employed. Cheshire and Coates (1966) examined the various factors which lead to impaired ventilation: in addition to obvious paralysis, they emphasize pulmonary collapse due to inhalation of vomitus and retention of respiratory secretions due to the ineffective cough. Injury of the cervical enlargement produces a picture of mixed upper and lower motor neuron damage. This is of course true in any region of the cord but the effects in the cervical and thoracolumbar region are more easily recognized because of the limb dysfunction, and are of greater significance. The distinction between the two forms of lesion has been described elsewhere but until spinal shock has subsided they cannot be differentiated, for all paralysed muscles will be flaccid and without reflex response. Holmes considered that localization of the upper limit of damage was more reliably determined by the examination of the motor system than of the sensory, particularly in partial lesions. The lower motor neuron paralysis may be due to grey matter damage or to spinal root damage; the latter may recover, the former will be permanent.

Hyperextension injuries often produce a similar clinical picture. When spinal shock has passed it is found that the upper limbs are more severely affected than the lower and the weakness is predominantly of the lower motor neuron type while the lower limbs show a banal spastic weakness; sphincter disturbance is frequent, proprioceptive sensory loss is usually more marked than impairment of pain and temperature sensibility. Very considerable recovery of power in the lower limbs and of sphincter control is usual, but in the upper limbs is delayed and usually imperfect, particularly in the long flexors and extensors of digits and in the intrinsic muscles. The final state of the upper limbs shows a mixture of upper and lower motor neuron lesions. The neurological pattern indicates damage of the cervical enlargement, with a particular incidence upon anterior horns, upon the posterior rather than the anterior columns, and more upon corticospinal fibres to the cervical segments than to the distal segments; that is to say the lateral (more peripheral) corticospinal fibres tend to be spared or injured less severely. The residual neurological signs are very similar to the signs found in severe spondylotic myelopathy. The anatomical interpretation would be a lesion of central areas of the cord extending into the posterior columns. Schneider and his colleagues (Schneider *et al.* 1954, 1958) have given an identity to the syndrome by calling it 'acute central cervical cord injury' and have provided pathological evidence (1958) that the major changes are within the grey matter and extending into the posterior columns. Central necrosis has of course long been recognized as a frequent finding in the traumatized spinal cord, and Holmes noted that paresis affecting the arms more than the legs characterized injury to the cervical enlargement. In their earlier paper Schneider *et al.* (1954) give diagrams of a model used to study the stresses induced by compression. Factors which may influence the determination of this pattern of injury are the relative 'slowness' of hyperextension compared with fracture dislocation, the forces are compressive and not shearing as in dislocation and the relatively large amount of grey matter in the cervical enlargement.

Injury in the cervical region may interrupt descending fibres which ultimately provide the cervical sympathetic outflow causing dryness of the face and upper limbs (paroxysmal reflex sweating envelopes the whole body in total lesions) and Horner syndrome. This may not be readily recognized if both sides are involved. Nystagmus may occasionally be seen; it was recorded in 3 of 63 cervical injuries observed by Holmes, who found that it rapidly disappeared.

Thorburn (1887) described an unusual position which the upper limbs may adopt in cervical injuries and eponymously named after him. They are abducted and externally rotated at the shoulder and flexed at the elbows so that they lie against the bed above the patient's head. The lesion was considered to extend as high as C7, and the posture was attributed to unopposed activity of the muscles supplied by the intact fifth and sixth segments. It is unlikely that the explanation is quite so simple since traumatic lesions do not end so abruptly that the muscles supplies by one segment would have an overpowering effect on those supplied by the next lower and injured segment. Of importance are certain reported cases in which tonic spasm of muscles were observed in nontraumatic lesions. Penry et al. (1960) described two cases with postmortem findings of necrotic lesions in the cervical cord and attribute the posture imposed by tonic spasm to the result of damage to interneurons. Rushworth et al. (1961) reported a case of intense muscle spasm in the arms arising in the course of an intramedullary glioma: they attributed the spasm to 'isolation' of anterior horn cells.

5. *Lumbar cord and cauda equina injuries.* Injuries of the lower part of the spinal column involve a greater number of cord segments than those higher in the spine owing to the greater height of the vertebral bodies and the closer approximation of the spinal cord segments. Thus all the lumbar segments lie opposite vertebrae T10 and T11: a bony injury damaging L1 segment may also damage roots as high as T10. An injury of L2 vertebra should theoretically spare the conus

and inflict damage only on the roots of the cauda equina: the neurological consequences may include motor and sensory loss as high as L2. Thus a greater number of roots may be directly injured or compressed the further caudal that the trauma occurs. The importance is twofold. First, pain in spinal injuries is largely dependent on damage to roots and consequently persistent extensive pain is more often a feature of cauda equina injury than cervical injury, once the initial skeletal pain of trauma has subsided. Secondly, although the cord has virtually no resistance to the forces imposed on it by injury, nerve roots are tough structures by comparison. The cord may be irretrievably crushed and no recovery can follow correction of bony deformity; but, if carried out promptly, correction of deformity and therefore of persistent compression and traction on nerve roots may allow them to recover, at any rate partially.

The effects upon the function of the bladder and the rectum in lesions of the sacral segments and cauda equina have been described in the section on compression paraplegia.

## Management

The vital importance of the necessity to prevent further increase in, or the production of, neurological deficit results in a pronounced emphasis on the early treatment of spinal injury. Indeed, the need for treatment to start immediately indicates that therapeutic and preventive measures should ideally have commenced prior to any radiographic investigations, on suspicion of spinal injury. It is appropriate, therefore, to discuss investigation and treatment as conjoint disciplines under the heading of management.

To emphasize that management is concerned with the whole patient and not merely with his lesion is banal but is the guiding principle in spinal injury. Whilst in some patients it may be obvious that a spinal injury has occurred and is the major factor, in others the evidence of injury may be concealed by associated coma due to head injury. Indeed, in certain instances the spinal injury may adopt a lower priority in the face of, for example, airway obstruction or major haemorrhage. Nevertheless, it is the early recognition and subsequent treatment of a spinal injury which can not only prevent the development of neurological deficit but also in certain circumstances promote its recovery. The effective management of such cases in the longer term further exemplifies the need to look at all aspects of the problem. The needs of the spinal cord lesion and those of the damage to the vertebral column may require differing consideration, as in the situation of certain total cord lesions where, on occasions, it may be better to allow early mobilization accepting a less than perfect spinal reduction. In all patients, whether with or without a cord lesion, it is essential also to place great effort on producing a healthy urinary tract, intact skin, adequate respiration and good psychological state. While experience in the latter part of this century has shown that these factors are most likely to be achieved by specially organized management teams in spinal rehabilitation centres, the early management of spinal injury does not always occur in such centres. Many neurosurgical and orthopaedic units are called upon to participate in early management and, in particular, the highly dangerous and (in road traffic accidents) common combination of head and spinal injury necessitates initial management in neurosurgical centres.

### Immediate treatment

The extrication and conveyance of the patient from the scene of the accident to hospital requires special care in order to avoid any movement which might exaggerate displacement of an unstable fracture or dislocation and thereby increase the extent of the cord injury. It has been estimated that in at least 3% of cases, the cord suffers damage or the damage worsens at an interval after the accident; in part of this fraction, aggravation was due to incautious handling of the patient (Geisler *et al.* 1966). To ambulance attendants and first-aid personnel the presence

of paralysed limbs in a conscious patient may be obvious and a spinal injury should be assumed. It should also be assumed if there is pain, tenderness, bruising or deformity at some point along the spine. The following precautions are taken:

1　Traction is applied gently to head and to feet, the limbs are straightened and the patient is gradually rolled on to his back; maintaining the position of the head relative to the body.
2　With preferably four attendants, two exerting traction on head and feet and two supporting the trunk the patient is lifted on to a firm stretcher. All movements should be performed in unison so that the subject is moved 'in one piece'.
3　All hard objects in pockets etc., which may be under the patient, and footwear are removed.
4　The small of the back and the legs (not the heels) are supported on soft pillows or folded blankets.
5　If the injury appears to be in the neck, the head should be in the neutral or slightly extended position and slight traction should be maintained. Blankets should be applied to prevent loss of heat.
6　At all times the necessity to provide an adequate airway overrules the above precautions.

On arrival at hospital, and assuming an adequate airway and blood pressure, the first step should be to perform a brief but adequate neurological examination. This should be carefully recorded and forms a baseline from which improvement or deterioration may be assessed as this profoundly affects management. Any evidence of movement or preserved sensation is of major significance. Priapism is an ominous sign of severe cord damage. Evidence of either a neurological level or the pain, tenderness and deformity associated with the vertebral lesion may indicate the level of injury. Deformity plays a major role in indicating an otherwise unsuspected injury to the cervical spine in a comatose patient.

Once the patient's general condition has been stabilized, radiological examination of the spine

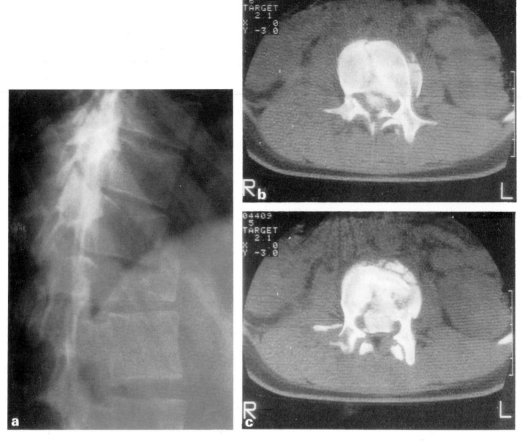

**Fig. 24.6.** Crush fracture of lumbar spine. a) lateral view. Computerized tomography shows much more clearly the extent of bone damage and displacement, including b) fracture across right pedicle and body, and c) posterior displacement of fragment into the spinal canal. (By courtesy of Dr Robin Sellar.)

may be performed. Ideally, the whole spine should be examined. This is initially performed by anteroposterior and lateral films taking great care in the placement of cassettes for anteroposterior views and for chest X-ray. Certain areas in the cervical spine may call for special views to show difficult regions such as the odontoid process and in particular the cervicothoracic area where fractures or dislocations can be easily missed. The lateral cervical spine X-ray must show the vertebral column clearly to the body of C7. If it does not, the film should be repeated with downward traction applied to the arms, so as to lower the shoulders, or one arm should be derated as in the 'swimmer's view'. When

dislocation is obvious, no great diagnostic difficulty exists but many patients may show only relatively minor radiographic evidence of damage on a static film, such as minor body avulsions, paravertebral soft tissue swelling or a retropharyngeal haematoma, even in the presence of an unstable lesion. Some authorities advocate myelography as an aid to evaluating the injury. However, not only is this difficult and may be dangerous to perform adequately in this early phase but with cord swelling it is difficult to interpret. There is sometimes a place for myelography however at a later stage in showing the occasional case when the neurological injury is due to disc rupture.

For many years, elucidation of radiodiagnostic problems related to injury, such as nondisplaced linear fractures, unilateral facet locking or bursting fractures of the vertebral body with extension into the spinal canal, depended upon tomography. Now, computerized tomography is supplanting this and can rapidly provide complete information about the extent of bony spinal injury, as soon as the level has been established by clinical examination and plain radiology. (Keene *et al.* 1982, Fig. 24.6).

By this stage, ideally, a diagnosis of spinal injury will have been made. The most important decision consequent to this diagnosis is to distinguish between injuries with and those without neurological deficit by means of clinical examination. It is also important to attempt to deduce the mechanism of the injury from both clinical (for example evidence of site of impact) and radiological evidence. Injury to the spine is usually the result of indirect force transmitted through the body causing abnormal stresses on the spine. Such stresses are primarily those of flexion, extension, rotation and compression. They may act singly or in unison and the effects of their various combinations have been defined by Holdsworth (1970), and Braakman and Penning (1976). Interpretation of the mechanism of injury may be very difficult and indeed the final radiological effects of hyperflexion and hyperextension can be very similar. However, it is vital to make some assessment of whether flexion or extension has occurred, and often the site of bruising, such as on the forehead in a hyperextension cervical injury, is a strong indicant. For example, if a flexion injury is treated or transported in a flexed position then further neurological damage is likely. The other factor of importance is to ascertain whether rotation has occurred in addition to a flexion injury. This is often indicated by a small chipped shear fracture from the anterosuperior border of the vertebral body and the presence of such a finding strongly suggests an unstable fracture. Having decided whether or not there is neurological deficit and attempted to define the mechanism of injury, it is then important to decide whether any fracture

is stable or unstable as this obviously alters management. This decision, although often simple as in a stable wedge fracture, may be very difficult. For further details of the early assessment of injury and radiographic interpretation, the reader is referred to more specific texts. Indeed, the reader will also find detailed assessments of the various types of fractures which occur at differing spinal levels in these texts as such detailed discussion is beyond the scope of this general chapter.

Having transferred the patient with appropriate care to the area where formal treatment is to be undertaken, a decision then has to be taken as to how to manage the vertebral injury. The guiding principle is that if a dislocation or gross displacement is present it should be reduced as quickly as possible in order to return the cross-sectional area of the spinal canal to normal in an attempt to either facilitate recovery or prevent deterioration. There are in essence two ways of achieving this: nonoperative and operative. In the thoracolumbar spine, reduction may be achieved by postural means by the careful positioning of the patient using lumbar rolls or pillows as described in detail by Guttmann (1959). Nonoperative reduction in the cervical spine may be achieved in two ways. The most commonly used is that of inserting calipers for skull traction (such as Gardner's tongs) and to then exert traction in an appropriate direction (either flexion or extension) to achieve reduction. In the presence of a fracture dislocation where the facets are locked traction is exerted and the load is gradually increased over a few hours with frequent check X-rays until the edges of the facet joints are linearly opposed. This may involve temporary application of traction weights of up to 40 or 45 lbs in a large patient. When reduction has reached this point, the load is dramatically reduced and placed in slight extension to hopefully allow the joints to slip back into their normal position. A word of caution regarding traction weights used in the stabilization of fractures of C1, C2 and C3 is necessary as there is only limited muscular counteraction in this area and any weight greater than 3–4 pounds normally carries a considerable risk of over-distracting the fracture. A simple guide to maintenance traction weights for cervical spine injuries is that the weight in pounds should not greatly exceed the sum of the two vertebrae involved, for example C5/6 and 11 pounds. Acute reduction of a cervical fracture should only be attempted by very experienced practitioners (Holdsworth 1966). This requires either full general anaesthesia or deep neuroleptanalgesia to reduce muscle tone. Having inserted skull traction, the neck is then carefully and gradually moved in a direction appropriate to the individual fracture under image intensification control until reduction can be achieved by reversing and reducing the traction pull. If there is only a unilateral locked facet (and this may require tomography for identification) then a rotatory element is required in the reduction. Most neurosurgeons, however, prefer in such cases to proceed directly to operative, open reduction of this type of subluxation.

Acute operative intervention is usually used in the cervical spine when the above methods have failed to achieve reduction. Facets can be unlocked by various manoeuvres performed during the course of an anterior cervical fusion procedure (Cloward 1961) but usually they are best reduced via a posterior approach which is then combined with a stabilization procedure using bone and/or wire, though other fusion techniques are available (Fig. 24.5). Operative reduction of thoracolumbar fractures may involve various techniques. Harrington distraction instrumentation is popular in many centres (Dickson et al. 1978), especially for the reduction of burst fractures. The technique depends on an intact posterior longitudinal ligament which, when stretched during distraction should reduce fragments of the vertebral body which had been displaced posteriorly into the spinal canal. However, Gertzbein et al. (1982) found a high rate of loss of correction using this technique. Other authorities prefer a direct anterior approach to the spine via a thoraco-abdominal incision so that the dura may be decompressed under direct vision but, if these

patients are to be mobilized early, they also require some form of posterior instrumentation. The previously common method of posterior placement of plates on the spine to achieve stability (for example, Williams 1963) is now widely accepted as being ineffective unless accompanied by prolonged recumbency (McKibbon 1982). The only effective posterior instrumentation for early mobilization is some type of segmental spinal fixation as developed for scoliosis surgery (for example, Luque & Cardoso 1977, Allan & Ferguson 1982). On some occasions patients with fracture dislocation and locked facets are not recognized at the time of injury. If the delay is such that the situation is not recognized until 7 or 10 days after the injury, then reduction by any means is hazardous and should not ordinarily be attempted.

Further management of the vertebral injury may either be by maintaining the position in traction or by operative stabilization. There is no clear indication which method is best. The use of traction requires a lengthy period of skilled nursing during which the patient is kept recumbent on a special turning frame or electric bed to prevent pressure sores and this obviously has its own hazards. On the other hand, operative stabilization carries not only the risk of increasing the neurological deficit but also has a significant mortality especially if the anterior cervical route is used in the first few days after injury. If operative stabilization is chosen then it is probably best deferred until towards the end of the second week. It does have the advantage that the patient may be mobilized at that stage. At the moment the choice of treatment seems best to be left to decisions based on individual cases, though opinions differ widely. Some advocate operative intervention in cases only with an established complete cord lesion to allow the early start of a rehabilitative programme; others suggest the same only in cases with no deficit and use conservative methods in patients with a cord injury. The development of halothoracic and halopelvic traction offers a middle course in cervical spine injury as such apparatus will maintain the reduced fracture whilst allowing mobilization. The proper application of such equipment, however, requires considerable expertise.

With regard to patients with an established cord lesion, either partial or complete, there is great debate as to whether conservative or operative treatment gives better neurological results. Guttmann (1959) and Bedbrook (1981) amongst others have strongly advocated conservative therapy. There are many reports of early surgical intervention (for example, Bradford *et al.* 1977), but few attempts at any controlled consideration of such techniques. It seems on balance that the final neurological result is similar in groups of patients treated either conservatively or operatively. There is however one absolute indication for operative intervention and that is a patient with a deteriorating neurological status. Such patients are uncommon but this stresses the importance of early and then repeated neurological examination to identify such cases as well as to assess prognosis (*see* below). No one operative technique is applicable to all spinal fractures and operative management is best decided on an individual basis by a surgeon skilled in all types of approaches to the spine. Further discussion of individual procedures and the differing management of the various types of fracture which occur throughout the spine is beyond the scope of this text. One fact is clear, however, and that is that laminectomy alone is dangerous, having not only a high mortality but also a considerable risk of worsening the neurological deficit (Bohlman 1979) and increasing spinal instability.

## General care

The aims of the care devoted to management of patients who cannot be immediately mobilized are: to maintain spinal alignment; to protect the skin; to maintain nutrition; to keep the respiratory and urinary tracts free of infection; to preserve comfort and morale; and to maintain free joint movement. It is best to transfer patients with irreversible severe neurological deficit as

soon as is feasible to a specialized spinal unit, should such a facility be available.

*Skin care*

Great attention has to be paid to preserving an intact and healthy skin in the pressure areas, especially in those patients with sensory loss. This is achieved only by skilled nursing using regular turning of the patient either by logrolling, a Stryker bed or some type of electrically moved bed. In the case of cervical injuries the method used must allow for continuous traction in the same position and axis. The skin must be kept scrupulously clean and free from urinary or faecal soiling.

*Nutrition*

In the early stages following the injury the patient will enter into a negative catabolic phase and will require appropriately increased caloric, nitrogenous and fluid requirements. This may be difficult to achieve via the gastrointestinal tract as often there is a period of ileus and parenteral nutrition may be required. Loss of autonomic control in complete injuries may cause difficulties in the maintenance of blood pressure and body temperature. The development of respiratory or urinary infection or of pressure sores considerably increases nutritional requirements.

*Respiratory care*

All patients with spinal injury require expert frequent chest physiotherapy to help maintain good respiratory function. The situation is especially critical in cervical injury where there may be intercostal and, if the lesion is above $C_4$, diaphragmatic paralysis. Such patients may require ventilation and sometimes in long term cases of diaphragmatic paralysis, phrenic nerve stimulation may be useful.

*Urinary tract care*

Guttmann advocated intermittent catheterization as the ideal way of managing urinary retention. He found that with this technique two-thirds of patients discharged from his unit had sterile urine. The technique and results have been described in detail and analysed by Guttmann and Frankel (1966). In the first few days after the injury renal secretion is reduced; as judged by its palpable size, the bladder may not need to be emptied in the first 24 hours and only twice a day in the next day or so. Thereafter it is emptied three times in the 24 hours, or more if the post-traumatic diuresis renders it necessary. Various antibiotics and chemotherapeutic agents have been used prophylactically but now reliance is largely placed on maintaining an acid urine. An indwelling catheter and bladder irrigation is employed temporarily if severe infection develops. The main disadvantage of this technique lies in the demands which it makes upon staff.

An indwelling catheter is preferred in some centres. Irrigation is necessary and, although the bladder can be kept empty, the catheter is likely to induce urethritis and indeed can produce ulceration unless properly managed.

Whatever method of drainage is used, the aim is to prevent infection and to encourage the development of reflex micturition. When the bladder can be emptied by either abdominal compression or by eliciting reflex contraction and a residual volume of less than 100 mls regularly obtained, then catheterization may be omitted. It is now possible in some cases to stimulate micturition electrically via implanted electrodes.

### Preservation of morale

This is of course of vital importance. It is necessary to maintain a positive attitude of hope and encouragement, tempered by realism and honesty. False hopes should not be raised. Once the diagnosis of complete cord injury is certain, the patient should be appraised of the situation and likely future. The formation of spinal rehabilitation centres has allowed expertise to develop in managing this difficult problem. In such centres this can be combined with a con-structive rehabilitation programme, tailored to the individual, to teach the patients to accept their disability and yet maximize their remaining potential.

### Care of joints

The role of the physiotherapist in early respiratory care has been stressed. There is a further role of vital importance in the maintenance of free movements of joints by passive movements. The prevention of contractures is vital as not only can they impair recovery but their development in a patient with even a total lesion can lead to major problems in positioning, especially sitting.

### Other therapeutic measures

Much experimental and some clinical effort has been employed on attempting to limit or prevent the effects of injury on the cord. It is fair to state that none of these have found universal application. Many of the factors which improve or limit the cord injury experimentally exert their effect only if given prior to or very soon after the injury and thus are impossible to apply clinically. Most attention has been given to the use of glucocorticoids, such as dexamethasone. Some feel that their use especially in high dosage does confer benefit (for example, Young & Flamm 1982) but there are a similar number of reports which deny this and even suggest that they increase mortality (for example, Faden et al. 1984). Other agents and techniques which have been applied include: hyperbaric oxygen (Yeo et al. 1978); hypothermia localized to the cord (Albin et al. 1967); hypothermia combined with methysergide (Howitt & Turnbull 1972); barbiturates (Oldfield et al. 1982); opiate-receptor antagonists such as naloxone (Young et al. 1981; Faden et al. 1981) and thyrotropin releasing hormone (Faden et al. 1982). To date there is no firm evidence that any of these agents confer significant benefit.

## Prognosis

There are basically two elements to prognosis following spinal injury: mortality risk and the outlook for neurological recovery. Spinal injury without associated neurological deficit or other injury carries a good prognosis for full recovery provided the diagnosis of vertebral column injury is made promptly and appropriate care given. With regard to prognosis of neurological recovery in a patient with a deficit, this is highly variable but depends largely on the extent of neurological damage. Patients with incomplete lesions fare better than those whose lesion is complete. The degree of recovery from an incomplete lesion, however, is highly variable and this factor has caused major problems in the assessment of the efficacy of many differing types of treatment. Reports of surgical intervention claiming good results and neurological improvement have to be balanced with the knowledge that conservative measures also may allow major neurological recovery. Attempts at controlled series are infrequent, primarily as it is so difficult to ensure comparable groups of patients. The term 'complete cord lesion' refers only to the situation of total absence of motor, sensory and sphincteric function below the level of the lesion. Many patients present such a picture in the first few hours following injury and there is debate as to the time from which persistence of such a state indicates that there is no hope of recovery. Most authorities align with Schneider (1962) who felt that persistence of a complete cord lesion beyond 24 hours signified that there was no hope of recovery. Holdsworth (1963) agreed with this but observed that it was only true with regard to lower limb recovery, pointing out that in a cervical injury there could be some root recovery. However, others (for example, Michaelis 1976c) believed that the interval should be as long as six weeks. Certain factors which may be present on initial examination make the likelihood of recovery even more remote. These include: priapism; malignant Strumpell reflex (a slow, sustained flexor response by the great toe to plantar stimulation); and the development after their initial absence of spinal reflexes such as the anal and cremasteric reflex. 'Spinal shock' is a condition of temporary cessation of all cord function including reflex activity below the lesion. During this phase no assessment of prognosis may be made but the appearance of the cord-mediated reflexes mentioned above indicates the end of 'spinal shock'. The appearance of these reflexes without any return of voluntary motor or sensory function indicates that there is indeed a complete cord lesion which is likely to be irrecoverable.

The diagnosis of a complete and irrecoverable lesion indicates only that no useful cord function will return. The prognosis of the patient as a whole should not be seen to be as gloomy. With the expertise available in rehabilitative spinal injury units it is possible to preserve and promote a very satisfactory quality of life despite the cord handicap. It is obvious that the level of the lesion is a major determinant in the quality of life with higher lesions producing greater handicap. With regard to mortality the level of the lesion is again of vital importance with high cervical lesions carrying the greatest risk. Upper cervical cord damage with respiratory paralysis will result in immediate death unless resuscitation is performed. Early mortality following spinal injury is usually due to: associated injury (especially to the head); pulmonary infection or embolus; and gastrointestinal haemorrhage. Late mortality is usually related to either the debilitating effect of decubitus ulceration or to renal failure secondary to either infection, calculus or amyloid (Tribe & Silver 1969); although unfortunately suicide also plays a role. The dramatic efficacy of spinal units is shown in two ways: firstly, by achieving such a high quality of survival for their injured patients; and secondly, by the low mortality rate in patients who have survived long enough to reach such a unit. As long ago as 1959, Guttmann could report a mortality rate of only 8.2%.

# References

ALBIN M.S., WHITE R.J., LOCKE G.S. *et al.* (1967) *Anesth. Analg.*, **48**, 8.

ALLEN B.L. & FERGUSON R.L. (1982) *Spine*, 7, 276.

BARNES R. (1948) *J. Bone Jt. Surg.*, 30B, 234.

BARNETT H.M., BOTTERELL E.H., JOUSSE A.T. & WYNN-JONES M. (1966) *Brain*, **89**, 159.

BEDBROOK G.M. (1981) *The Care and Management of Spinal Cord Injuries*, Springer-Verlag, New York.

BENES V. (1966) Proc. Third Int. Cong. Neurol. Surg. Int. Cong. Series No. 110, p. 343. Exc. Med. Foundation, Amsterdam.

BOHLMAN H.H. (1979) *J. Bone Jt. Surg.*, **61A**, 1119.

BRAAKMAN R & PENNING L. (1976) In Vinken P.J. & Bruyn G.W. (eds) *Handbook of Clinical Neurology*, Vol. **25**, pp. 227–380. Elsevier-North Holland, Amsterdam.

BRADFORD D.S., AKBARNIA B.A., WINTER R.B. & SELGESKOG E.L. (1977) *Spine*, **2**, 185.

BRAIN W.R., NORTHFIELD D.W.C. & WILKINSON M. (1952) *Brain*, **75**, 187.

BRODAL A. (1969) *Neurological Anatomy in relation to Clinical Medicine.* Oxford University Press, London.

CHESHIRE D.J.E. & COATS D.A. (1966) *Paraplegia*, **4**, 1.

CLAUDE H. & LHERMITTE J. (1919) *Lancet*, 1, 67.

CLOWARD R.B. (1961) *J. Neurosurg.*, 18, 201.

COLLIER J. (1916) *Lancet*, 1, 711.

DENNY-BROWN D. (1966) *The Cerebral Control of Movement.* The Eighth Sherrington Lecture. Liverpool University Press, Liverpool.

DICKSON J.H., HARRINGTON P.R. & ERWIN W.D. (1978) *J. Bone Jt. Surg*, 60A, 799.

DIMITRIJEVIC M.R. & NATHAN P.W. (1967) *Brain*, **90**, 1.

DOHRMANN G.J.,PANJABI M.M., BANKS D. (1978) *J. Neurosurg*, **48**, 993.

DURBINN F.R. (1961) *Proc. roy. Soc. Med*, **54**, 367.

FADEN A.I., HALLENBECK J.M., BROWN C.Q. (1982) *Neurology*, **32**, 1083.

FADEN A.I., JACOBS T.P., MOUGEY E., HOLADAY J.W. (1981) *Ann. Neurol.*, **10**, 326.

FADEN A.I., JACOBS T.P., PATRICK D.H. & SMITH M.T. (1984) *J. Neurosurg*, **60**, 712–717.

GEISLER W.O., WYNNE-JONES M. & JOUSSE A.T. (1966) Proc. Third Int. Cong. Neurol. Surg. Int. Cong. Series No. 110, p. 331. Exc. Med. Foundation, Amsterdam.

GERTZBEIN S.D., MacMICHAEL . & TILE M. (1982) *J. Bone Jt. Surg.*, **64B**, 526–9.

GUTTMANN L. (1959) In *Modern Trends in Diseases of the Vertebral Column* (ed. Nassim R. & Burrows H.J.) p. 245. Butterworth, London.

GUTTMANN L. (1966a) *Paraplegia*, **4**, 148.

GUTTMANN L. (1970) *Paraplegia*, **8**, 100.

GUTTMANN L. & FRANKEL H. (1966) *Paraplegia*, **4**, 63.

HARRIS P. (1966) Proc. Third Int. Cong. Neurol. Surg. Int. Cong. Series No. 110, p. 347. Exc. Med. Foundation, Amsterdam.

HEAD H. & RIDDOCH G (1917) *Brain*, **40**, 188.

HOLDSWORTH F.W. (1963) *J. Bone Jt. Surg*, **45B**, 6.

HOLDSWORTH F.W. (1966) Proc. Third Int. Cong. Neurol. Surg. Int. Cong. Series No. 110, p. 323 Exc. Med. Foundation, Amsterdam.

HOLDSWORTH M.B. (1970) *J. Bone Jt. Surg.*, **52A**, 1534.

HOLMES G. (1915) *Brit. med. J.*, **2**, 769.

HOWITT W.M; & TURNBULL I.M. (1972) *Canad. J. Surg.*, **15**, 179.

HUGHES J.T. (1964) *Paraplegia*, **2**, 2.

HUGHES J.T. (1966) *The Pathology of the Spinal Cord*, Lloyd-Luke, London.

HUGHES J.T. & BROWNELL B. (1963) *Lancet*, **1**, 687.

ILLIS L.S. (1967) In *Modern Trends in Neurology*, (ed. Williams D.) No. 4 p. 53. Butterworth, London.

JEFFERSON G. (1920) *Brit. J. Surg.*, **7**, 407.

JEFFERSON G. (1936) *Lancet*, **2**, 430.

JEFFERSON G. (1948) *J. Bone Jt. Surg.*, 30B, 232.

JELLINGER K. (1964) *Acta Neuropath.*, **3**, 451.

KAHN E.A. (1959) *J. Bone Jt. Surg.*, **41A**, 6.

KEENE J.S., GOLETZ T.H., LILLEAS F., ALTER A.J., SACKETT J.F. (1982) *J. Bone Jt. Surg.*, **64A**, 586.

LIPSCHITZ R. & BLOCK J. (1962) *Lancet*, **2**, 169.

LUCAS J.T. & DUCKER T.B. (1979) *Amer. Surg.*, **945**, 151–8.

LUQUE E.R. & CARDOSO A. (1977) *Orthop. Trans.*, **1**, 136.

McKIBBON B (1982) *J. Bone Jt. Surg.*, **64B**, 517–8.

MICHAELIS L.S. (1976a) In Vinken P.J. & Bruyn G.W. (eds), *Handbook of Clinical Neurology*, Vol **26** pp., 307–12. North-Holland Publishing Company, Amsterdam.

MICHAELIS L.S. (1976b) In Vinken P.J, & Bruyn, G.W. (eds.) *Handbook of Clinical Neurology*, Vol **26**, pp. 477–8. North-Holland Publishing Company, Amsterdam.

MICHAELIS L.S. (1976c) In Vinken P.J. & Bruyn G.W. (eds) *Handbook of Clinical Neurology*, Vol , pp. **25**, pp. 141–3. North-Holland Publishing Company, Amsterdam.

MUNRO D. (1965) *Paraplegia*, **3**, 97.

OLDFIELD E.H., PLUNKETT R.J., NYLANDER W.A. & MEACHAM, W.F. (1982) *J. Neurosurg.*, **56**, 511.

PENRY J.K., HOEFNAGEL D., DEN NOORT S. & DENNY-BROWN D. (1960) *Arch. Neurol.*, **3**, 500.

RIDDOCH G. (1917) *Brain*, **40**, 264.

RIDDOCH G (1918) *Lancet*, **2**, 839.

ROSSIER A.B., WERNER A., WILDI E. & BERNEY J. (1968) *J. Neurol. Neurosurg. Psychiat.*, **31**, 99.

RUSHWORTH G. (1966) *Paraplegia*, **4**, 130.

RUSHWORTH G., LISHMAN W.A., HUGHES J.T. & OPPENHEIMER D.R. (1961) *J. Neurol. Neurosurg. Psychiat.*, **24**, 132.

SCHNEIDER R.C. (1955) *J. Neurosurg.*, **12**, 95.

SCHNEIDER R.C. (1962) *Clin. Neurosurg*, **8**, 157.

SCHNEIDER R.C. & CROSBY E.C. (1959) *Neurology*, **9**, 643.

SCHNEIDER R.C. & KAHN E.A. (1956) *J. Bone Jt. Surg.*, **38A**, 985.

SCHNEIDER R.C. & SCHEMM G.W. (1961) *J. Neurosurg.*, **18**, 348.

SCHNEIDER R.C., CHERRY G. & PANTEK H. (1954) *J. Neurosurg.*, **11**, 546.

SCHNEIDER R.C., THOMPSON J.C. & BEBIN J. (1958) *J. Neurol. Neurosurg. Psychiat.*, **21**, 216.

SIMPSON J.A. (1965) In *Symposium on Spinal Injuries.* Royal College of Surgeons of Edinburgh, (ed. Harris P.) p. 10. Morrison & Gibb, Edinburgh.

SUTTON N.G. (1973) *Spinal Cord Injuries* London, Butterworth.

SYMONDS C. (1953) *Lancet*, **1**, 451.

TAYLOR A.R. & BLACKWOOD W. (1948) *J. Bone Jt. Surg.*, 30B, 245.

TAYLOR G.R. & GLEAVE J.R.W. (1962) *Proc. roy. Soc. Med.*, **55**, 1053.

THORBURN W. (1887) *Brain*, **9**, 510.

TRIBE C. R. & SILVER J. R. (1969) *Renal Failure in Paraplegia*. Pitman Medical Pub., London.

WALSHE F. M. R. (1915) *Brain*, **37**, 269.

WANNAMAKER G. T. (1954) *J. Neurosurg.*, **11**, 517.

WHITTERIDGE D. (1966) *Paraplegia*, **4**, 127.

WILKINSON M. (1960) *Brain*, **83**, 589.

WILLIAMS E. W. (1963) in Matthews D. N. (ed) *Recent Advances in the Surgery of Trauma*, pp. 171–86. Churchill, London.

WOLMAN L. (1965) *Paraplegia*, **2**, 213.

YEO J. D., LOWRY C. & MCKENZIE B. (1978) *Med. J. Aust.*, **2**, 572.

YOUNG W., FLAMM E. S., DEMOPOULOS H. B., TOMASULA J. J. & DECRESCITO V. (1981) *J. Neurosurg.*, **55**, 209.

YOUNG W. & FLAMM E. S. (1982) *J. Neurosurg.*, **57**, 667.

# Index